International Neurology

Dedication

To my many teachers and mentors over the years, most especially Lewis Rowland, Robert Fishman, Sidney Carter, Donald Silberberg, Donald Schotland, and Arthur Asbury in neurology, Burton Zweiman in immunology and clinical immunology, Marian Kies in neuroscience, neurochemistry and glial biology, and Elvin Kabat in immunology. To my collaborators, colleagues, students, residents, fellows, and patients over the years. And finally and most importantly to my family, including my late parents Irving and Sylvia Lisak, my sister Nancy Lisak Sager, my wife Deena, my children Ilene and Michael, and my grandchildren Samuel, Isabella, Vivienne, and Sophie.

RPL

To my mother Cam Tran, my wife Diane Truong, and my friend Marcia Manker for whose support I am indebted, to my associates Thong Nguyen, Mayank Pathak, Karen Frei, Anumantha Kanthasamy, Rae Matsumoto, KK Tai, Phuong Pham, Steven Jenkins, Dave Brown and Christina Nguyen whose loyalty I cherish, and to Emily Gelskey, Suzanne Mellor, Gianni Pezzoli, Khalid Sheikh, Erik Wolters and Rick Warren from whose wisdom I learn.

DDT

To my wife Kathryn and our daughters Gemma, Bonita, and Laura, I thank you for your support, encouragement, and forbearance, and I thank all who have contributed so unstintingly to make this textbook truly unique.

WMC

To my beloved grandmother Pranom Chivakiat, my parents Mitr and Nisaratana Bhidayasiri, my family, Nucharee Yoovidhya and Bhiradej Yoovidhya Bhidayasiri, for their continuing support, love, and understanding, all my teachers of neurology, and lastly my patients who have taught me much about neurology.

RB

International Neurology
Second edition

Edited by

Robert P. Lisak
MD FAAN FRCP(E) FANA

Parker Webber Chair in Neurology
Professor of Neurology
Professor of Immunology and Microbiology
Wayne State University School of Medicine
Attending Neurologist, Detroit Medical Center
Detroit, MI, USA

Daniel D. Truong
MD FAAN

Clinical Professor, University of California, Riverside
Riverside, CA, USA
The Truong Neuroscience Institute
Orange Coast Memorial Medical Center
Fountain Valley, CA, USA

William M. Carroll
MBBS MD FRACP FRCP(E)

Clinical Professor of Neurology,
Western Australian Neuromuscular Research Institute
University of Western Australia,
Sir Charles Gairdner Hospital,
Perth, Western Australia
Australia

Roongroj Bhidayasiri
MD FRCP FRCPI

Professor of Neurology and Director
Chulalongkorn Center of Excellence for Parkinson's Disease & Related Disorders, Faculty of Medicine,
Chulalongkorn University Hospital
Bangkok, Thailand

Department of Rehabilitation Medicine, Juntendo University,
Tokyo, Japan

Foreword by John Walton (Lord Walton of Detchant)

WILEY Blackwell

Library of Congress Cataloging-in-Publication Data

Names: Lisak, Robert P., editor. | Truong, Daniel, editor. |
    Carroll, William M., editor. |
    Bhidayasiri, Roongroj, editor.
Title: International neurology / edited by Robert P. Lisak, Daniel D. Truong,
    William M. Carroll, Roongroj Bhidayasiri ; foreword by John Walton (Lord
    Walton Of Detchant).
Description: Second edition. | Chichester, West Sussex ; Hoboken, NJ : John
    Wiley & Sons, Inc., 2016. | Includes bibliographical references and index.
Identifiers: LCCN 2015046045 (print) | LCCN 2015048295 (ebook) | ISBN
    9781118777367 (cloth) | ISBN 9781118777350 (pdf) | ISBN 9781118777343
    (epub)
Subjects: | MESH: Nervous System Diseases | Neurology—methods
Classification: LCC RC346 (print) | LCC RC346 (ebook) | NLM WL 140 | DDC
    616.8—dc23
LC record available at http://lccn.loc.gov/2015046045

A catalogue record for this book is available from the British Library.

Contents

Editors

Robert P. Lisak MD, FAAN, FRCP(E), FANA
Parker Webber Chair in Neurology
Professor of Neurology
Professor of Immunology and Microbiology
Wayne State University School of Medicine
Attending Neurologist, Detroit Medical Center
Detroit, MI, USA

Daniel D. Truong MD, FAAN
Clinical Professor, University of California, Riverside
Riverside, CA, USA
The Truong Neuroscience Institute
Orange Coast Memorial Medical Center
Fountain Valley, CA, USA

William M. Carroll MBBS, MD, FRACP, FRCP(E)
Clinical Professor of Neurology,
Western Australian Neuromuscular Research Institute
University of Western Australia,
Sir Charles Gairdner Hospital,
Perth, Western Australia
Australia

Roongroj Bhidayasiri MD, FRCP, FRCPI
Professor of Neurology and Director
Chulalongkorn Center of Excellence for Parkinson's
Disease & Related Disorders, Faculty of Medicine,
Chulalongkorn University Hospital
Bangkok, Thailand

Section Editors

Zohar Argov MD
Kanrich Professor of Neuromuscular Diseases
Hadassah-Hebrew University Medical Center
Jerusalem, Israel

Roongroj Bhidayasiri MD, FRCP, FRCPI
Professor of Neurology and Director
Chulalongkorn Center of Excellence for Parkinson's
Disease & Related Disorders, Faculty of Medicine,
Chulalongkorn University Hospital
Bangkok, Thailand

Francisco Javier Carod-Artal MD, PhD
Visiting Professor of Neurology
Universitat Internacional de Catalunya (UIC)
Barcelona, Spain
Consultant Neurologist and Neurology Service Lead,
Neurology Department, Raigmore Hospital
Inverness, UK

William M Carroll MBBS, MD, FRACP, FRCP(E)
Clinical Professor of Neurology,
Western Australian Neuromuscular Research Institute
University of Western Australia,
Sir Charles Gairdner Hospital,
Perth, Western Australia
Australia

Marc C. Chamberlain MD
Department of Neurology and Neurological Surgery
University of Washington
Fred Hutchinson Cancer Research Institute
Seattle Cancer Care Alliance
Seattle, Washington, USA

Oscar H. Del Brutto MD
Professor of Neurology, School of Medicine,
Universidad Espíritu Santo – Ecuador
Department of Neurological Sciences
Hospital-Clínica Kennedy
Guayaquil, Ecuador

Marianne de Visser MD
Professor of Neurology
Department of Neurology, Academic Medical Centre,
University of Amsterdam
Amsterdam, Netherlands

Don Gilden MD
Louise Baum Endowed Chair and Professor
Departments of Neurology and Microbiology and
Immunology, University of Colorado School of
Medicine
Aurora, CO, USA

Christopher C. Giza MD
Professor of Neurosurgery and Pediatric Neurology
Director, UCLA Steve Tisch BrainSPORT Program
UCLA Brain Injury Research Center
David Geffen School of Medicine & Mattel Children's
Hospital
University of California, Los Angeles
Los Angeles, CA, USA

Murray Grossman MDCM, PhD
Departments of Neurology and Psychiatry
Penn FTD Center
Neuroscience Graduate Group, Bioengineering
Graduate Group
University of Pennsylvania
Philadelphia, PA, USA

Chung Y. Hsu MD, PhD
Chair Professor, China Medical University, Taichung,
Taiwan
Principal Investigator, Ministry of Health Clinical Trial
Center of Excellence, Taichung, Taiwan
Executive Trustee, Board of Trustees, National Health
Research Institute, Chunan, Taiwan

Robert P. Lisak MD, FAAN, FRCP(E), FANA
Parker Webber Chair in Neurology
Professor of Neurology
Professor of Immunology and Microbiology
Wayne State University School of Medicine
Attending Neurologist, Detroit Medical Center
Detroit, MI, USA

Friedhelm Sandbrink MD
Director, EMG Laboratory
Director, Pain Management Program
Department of Neurology
Veterans Affairs Medical Center Georgetown University
Washington, DC, USA

Raman Sankar MD, PhD
Professor and Chief of Pediatric Neurology
Rubin Brown Distinguished Chair
David Geffen School of Medicine Pediatric Neurology
UCLA and Mattel Children's Hospital UCLA
Los Angeles, CA, USA

Marylou V. Solbrig MD
Professor, Departments of Internal Medicine
(Neurology) and Medical Microbiology
University of Manitoba
Winnipeg, MB, Canada

Barbara E. Swartz MD, PhD
Director, Epilepsy Center and Neurophysiology
Laboratory
Professor, Renown Neuroscience Institute
University of Nevada
Reno, NV, USA

Ann Tilton MD
Professor of Neurology and Pediatrics
Department of Neurology
Louisiana State University Health Sciences Center
Children's Hospital
New Orleans, LA, USA

Daniel D. Truong MD, FAAN
Clinical Professor, University of California, Riverside
Riverside, CA, USA
The Truong Neuroscience Institute
Orange Coast Memorial Medical Center
Fountain Valley, CA, USA

Aleksandar Videnovic MD, MSc
Director, Program on Sleep, Circadian Biology and
Neurodegeneration
Department of Neurology, Massachusetts General
Hospital
Assistant Professor of Neurology, Harvard Medical
School
Boston, MA, USA

David B. Vodušek MD, DSc
Professor of Neurology
Medical Faculty, University of Ljubljana
Medical Director, Division of Neurology
University Medical Centre Ljubljana
Ljubljana, Slovenia

Melanie Walker MD
Clinical Associate Professor
Departments of Neurology and Neurological Surgery
University of Washington School of Medicine
Seattle, WA, USA

List of contributors

Angela Abicht PD Dr. med.
Fachärztin für Humangenetik
Medizinish Genetisches Zentrum
München, Germany

Hussam Abou Al-Shaar MD
Division of Neurology, Department of Neurosciences
King Faisal Specialist Hospital and Research Centre
College of Medicine, Alfaisal University
Riyadh, Saudi Arabia

Oded Abramsky MD, PhD
Professor of Neurology
Hadassah Hebrew University Medical Center
Jerusalem, Israel

Assiya Akanova MD
Asfendiyarov Kazakh National Medical University
Department of Neurology Almaty Kazakhstan.

Farida Balkhi Alam MD
Consultant Clinical Oncologist
Clatterbridge Cancer Centre NHS Foundation Trust
Wirral, Merseyside, UK

Yuri Alekseenko MD, PhD
Associate Professor
Chairman of the Department of Neurology
and Neurosurgery
Vitebsk State Medical University
Vitebsk, Republic of Belarus

Jasem Yousef Al-Hashel MD, FRCPC, FAHS
Department of Neurology
Ibn Sina Hospital
Safat, Kuwait

Zarina S. Ali MD
Department of Neurosurgery
University of Pennsylvania
Philadelphia, PA, USA

Yves Allenbach
Département de Médecine Interne et Immunologie
Clinique,
Centre de Référence Maladies Neuro-Musculaires Paris Est
Assistance Public – Hôpitaux de Paris Hôpital
Pitié-Salpêtrière
UMRS 974, INSERM, Université Pierre et Marie
Curie (UPMC)
Paris, France

Monica L. Andersen PhD
Associate Professor
Department of Psychobiology
Universidade Federal de São Paulo
São Paulo, Brazil

Abelardo Q. C. Araujo MD, MSc, PhD
Head, Laboratory for Clinical Research in
Neuroinfections
National Institute of Infectology (INI),
Oswaldo Cruz Foundation (FIOCRUZ),
Brazilian Ministry of Health
Associate Professor of Neurology, Institute of Neurology,
Federal University of Rio de Janeiro (INDC-UFRJ)
Rio de Janeiro, Brazil

Zohar Argov MD
Kanrich Professor of Neuromuscular Diseases
Hadassah-Hebrew University Medical Center
Jerusalem, Israel

Kimiyoshi Arimura MD, PhD
Okatsu Neurology and Rehabilitation Hospital
Kagoshima University
Kagoshima, Japan

Ovidiu-Alexandru Bajenaru MD, PhD
Faculty of Medicine, University of Medicine and
Pharmacy "Carol Davila" Bucharest
Director of the Department of Neurosurgery and
Psychiatry with Clinical Neurosciences
Chairman of the Department of Neurology
University Emergency Hospital Bucharest
Bucharest, Romania

Marek Baláž MD, PhD
Associate Professor
First Department of Neurology, Faculty of Medicine,
Masaryk University,
St. Anne's Teaching Hospital
Brno, Czech Republic

Kelly J. Baldwin MD
Clinical Assistant Professor
Department of Neurology, Neuro-Infectious Disease
Geisinger Medical Center
Danville, PA, USA

Brenda L. Banwell MD
Professor of Neurology at the Children's
Hospital of Philadelphia
Division of Neurology
Philadelphia, PA, USA

Delwyn J. Bartlett PhD
Clinical Associate Professor
University of Sydney Central Clinical School
Medical Psychology/Sleep & Circadian Group
Woolcock Institute of Medical Research
Sydney, Australia

Idan Ben-Horin MD
Neuro-Oncology Service, Division of Oncology
Tel-Aviv Sourasky Medical Center
Tel-Aviv, Israel

Olivier Benveniste MD
Département de Médecine Interne et Immunologie
Clinique, Centre de Référence Maladies
Neuro-Musculaires Paris Est
Assistance Public – Hôpitaux de Paris Hôpital
Pitié-Salpêtrière
UMRS 974, INSERM, Université Pierre et Marie
Curie (UPMC)
Paris, France

Joseph R. Berger MD, FACP, FAAN, FANA
Professor of Neurology and Chief of the MS Division
Perelman School of Medicine, University of
Pennsylvania
Philadelphia, PA, USA

Ute Berweiler MD, MA
Kliniken Sindelfingen, Klinikverbund Südwest
Sindelfingen, Germany

Pratik Bhattacharya MD, MPH
Vascular Neurologist, Michigan Stroke Network
Director of Stroke Quality,
Saint Joseph Mercy Oakland, MI, USA

Roongroj Bhidayasiri MD, FRCP, FRCPI
Professor of Neurology and Director
Chulalongkorn Center of Excellence for Parkinson's
Disease & Related Disorders, Faculty of Medicine,
Chulalongkorn University Hospital
Bangkok, Thailand

Rohini Bhole MD
Vascular Neurology Fellow
University of Tennessee Health Science Center
Memphis, TN, USA

Lia R. A. Bittencourt MD, PhD
Associate Professor
Department of Psychobiology
Universidade Federal de Sao Paulo
Sao Paulo, Brazil

David J. Blacker MBBS, FRACP
Clinical Professor of Neurology
University of Western Australia
Department of Neurology
Sir Charles Gairdner Hospital
Western Australian Neuroscience Research Institute
Nedlands, Western Australia

Deborah T. Blumenthal MD
Co-Director of Neuro-oncology Service
Division of Oncology
Tel-Aviv Sourasky Medical Center
Tel-Aviv, Israel

Enver I. Bogdanov MD
Professor and Head
Department of Neurology and Rehabilitation
Kazan State Medical University
Kazan, Russia

Saeed Bohlega MD, FRCPC, FAAN
Professor and Senior Consultant
Division of Neurology, Department of Neurosciences
King Faisal Specialist Hospital and Research Centre
Riyadh, Saudi Arabia

Michael Brada MD
Professor of Radiation Oncology
Department of Molecular and Clinical Cancer
Medicine, University of Liverpool
Department of Radiation Oncology, Clatterbridge
Cancer Centre NHS Foundation Trust
Wirral, Merseyside, UK

Stefen Brady MBBCh, BAO, DPhil
Consultant Neurologist
Department of Neurology
Southmead Hospital
Bristol, UK

Alba A. Brandes MD
Department of Medical Oncology
Azienda USL – IRCCS Institute of Neurological
Science
Bologna, Italy

Bruce J. Brew MBBS, MD, FRACP
Professor of Neurology
University of New South Wales
Department of Neurology
St Vincent's Hospital
Sydney NSW, Australia

Herbert Budka MD, MScDhc
Professor of Neuropathology
Neuropathology Consultant,
University Hospital Zurich; and
Professor and Institute Director, ret., Medical
University Vienna.

Sergio Cabrera MD
Fellow in Neuro-Oncology
Department of Neurology, division of Neuro-Oncology
at the University of Toronto
Pencer Brain Tumor Centre
Toronto, ON, Canada

Bernardo Cacho-Díaz MD
Neuro-oncologist, Neuroloscience Unit
Chief, Instituto Nacional de Cancerología
Mexico City, Mexico

Louis R. Caplan MD
Neurologist, Beth Israel Deaconess Medical Center,
Department of Neurology
Professor of Neurology, Harvard Medical School
Boston, MA, USA

Rosanna Cardani MD
Laboratory of Muscle Histopathology and Molecular
Biology, IRCCS Policlinico San Donato
Milan, Italy

Patrick W. Carney PhD, FRACP
Florey Institute of Neuroscience and Mental Health
Heidelberg, VIC, Australia

**Francisco Javier Carod-Artal
MD, PhD**
Visiting Professor of Neurology
Universitat Internacional de Catalunya (UIC)
Barcelona, Spain
Consultant Neurologist and Neurology Service Lead,
Neurology Department,
Raigmore Hospital Inverness, UK

Jonathan Carr MBChB, PhD
Head, Division of Neurology
University of Stellenbosch
Stellenbosch, South Africa

**William M. Carroll MBBS, MD,
FRACP, FRCP(E)**
Clinical Professor of Neurology,
Western Australian Neuromuscular Research Institute
University of Western Australia,
Sir Charles Gairdner Hospital,
Perth, Western Australia
Australia

John Caviness MD
Professor of Neurology
Chair, Mayo Clinic Movement Disorders Division
Department of Neurology, Mayo Clinic
Scottsdale, AZ, USA

Stephen Cederbaum MD
Professor Emeritus of Psychiatry,
Pediatrics and Human Genetics
University of California, Los Angeles
Los Angeles, CA, USA

Thomas C. Cesario MD
Professor and Dean Emeritus
University of California Irvine School of Medicine
Orange County, CA, USA

Jong-Hee Chae MD, PhD
Associate Professor
Department of Pediatrics,
Seoul National University College of Medicine
Division of Pediatric Neurology, Seoul National
University Children's Hospital
Seoul, Korea

Salim Chahin MD, MSCE
Instructor
Division of Multiple Sclerosis
Department of Neurology
University of Pennsylvania
Philadelphia, PA, USA

Marc C. Chamberlain MD
 Professor, Department of Neurology and Neurological
Surgery
University of Washington
Fred Hutchinson Cancer Research Center
Seattle Cancer Care Alliance
Seattle, WA, USA

Bernard P. L. Chan MRCP
Senior Consultant, Director of Stroke Neurology
Department of Medicine
National University Health System
Singapore

**Christopher Li-Hsian Chen
MD, PhD**
Associate Professor
Department of Pharmacology
National University of Singapore
Singapore

Shih-Pin Chen MD, PhD
Attending Physician, Department of Neurology
Neurological Institute, Taipei Veterans General Hospital
Assistant Professor, Faculty of Medicine,
National Yang-Ming University School of Medicine
Taipei, Taiwan

Olivier L. Chinot MD
Professor and Chief of Neuro-Oncology
Neuro-Oncology Department
Aix-Marseille University AP-HM
Marseille, France

Anna Cho MD
Assistant Professor
Department of Pediatrics,
Ewha Womans University School of Medicine
Seoul, Korea

Young-Chul Choi MD, PhD
Professor
Department of Neurology
Yonsei University College of Medicine
Gangnam Severance Hospital
Seoul, Korea

Heng Thay Chong MD
University of Melbourne
Department of Neurology
Western Hospital, Melbourne, VIC, Australia
University of Malaya, Malaysia

Nai-Shin Chu MD, PhD
Professor
Department of Neurology,
Chang Gung Memorial Hospital
Chang Gung University, College of Medicine
Taipei, Taiwan

Morad Chughtai MD
Orthopedic Research Fellow
Rubin Institute for Advanced Orthopedics
Center for Joint Preservation and Replacement
Sinai Hospital of Baltimore, Baltimore, MD

Luis A. Chui MD
Clinical Professor, Department of Neurology
University of California, Irvine
Orange, CA, USA

Aurauma Chutinet MD
Instructor in Neurology
Division of Neurology
Department of Medicine
Chulalongkorn University
Bangkok, Thailand

Anthony Ciabarra MD
Neurology Center of North Orange County
Fullerton, CA, USA

Cynthia L. Comella MD, FAAN
Professor of Neurology
Rush University Medical Center
Department of Neurological Sciences
Chicago, Illinois, USA

Patricia K. Coyle MD, FAAN, FANA
Professor of Neurology
Vice Chair (Clinical Affairs)
Department of Neurology
Stony Brook University Medical Center
Stony Brook, NY, USA

Liying Cui MD
Professor
Department of Neurology
Peking Union Medical College Hospital
Beijing, China

Anna Czlonkowska MD, PhD
Professor of Neurology
Institute of Psychiatry and Neurology,
and Warsaw Medical University
Warsaw, Poland

Marie Dagonnier MD
Florey Institute of Neurosciences and Mental Health
University of Melbourne
Melbourne Brain Center
Heidelberg, VIC, Australia

Marinos C. Dalakas MD
Professor of Neurology
Thomas Jefferson University
Philadelphia, PA, USA

Josep Dalmau MD, PhD
Professor of Neurology
Institució Catalana de Recerca i Estudis Avançats (ICREA)
Institut d'Investigació Biomèdica August Pi i Sunyer
(IDIBAPS)
ICREA Research Professor
Department of Neurology, Hospital Clínic
University of Barcelona
Barcelona, Spain

Larry E. Davis MD
Chief, Neurology Service
New Mexico VA Health Care System
Distinguished Professor of Neurology and Molecular
Genetics and Microbiology
University of New Mexico School of Medicine
Albuquerque, NM, USA

Stephen M. Davis AM, MD, FRCP, Edin, FRACP
Director, Melbourne Brain Centre
Royal Melbourne Hospital
Professor of Translational Neuroscience
University of Melbourne
Parkville, VIC, Australia

Marianne de Visser MD, PhD
Department of Neurology
Academic Medical Centre, University of Amsterdam
Amsterdam, Netherlands

Oscar H. Del Brutto MD
Professor of Neurology
School of Medicine, Universidad Espíritu
Santo – Ecuador
Department of Neurological Sciences
Hospital-Clínica Kennedy
Guayaquil, Ecuador

Antonio V. Delgado-Escueta MD, FAAN
Professor of Neurology
University of California, Los Angeles
Los Angeles, CA, USA

Stephen R. Deputy MD, FAAP
Associate Professor of Neurology, Louisiana State
University School of Medicine
Louisiana State University Health Sciences Center
New Orleans, LA, USA

Anneke J. van der Kooi MD, PhD
Department of Neurology, Academic Medical Centre
University of Amsterdam
Amsterdam, The Netherlands

Günther Deuschl MD, PhD
Professor
Department of Neurology
Christian-Albrechts-University
University-Hospital-Schleswig-Holstein, Campus Kiel
Kiel, Germany

Salvatore DiMauro MD
Lucy G. Moses Professor of Neurology
Columbia University Medical Center
College of Physicians and Surgeons
New York, NY, USA

Geoffrey A. Donnan MD, FRCP, FRACP
Director, Florey Institute of Neurosciences and
Mental Health
University of Melbourne
Department of Neurology, Austin Health
Melbourne Brain Center
Heidelberg, VIC, Australia

Ira J. Dunkel MD
Professor
Department of Pediatrics
Weill Cornell Medical College
New York, USA

Jennifer Durphy MD
Indiana University School of Medicine
Indianapolis, IN, USA

Jeffrey J. Ekstrand MD, PhD
Assistant Professor
Department of Pediatrics, Division of Neurology
University of Utah School of Medicine
Primary Children's Hospital
Salt Lake City, UT, USA

Colin A. Espie BSc, MAppSci, PhD, DSc, FBPsS, CPsychol, CSci
Professor of Sleep Medicine
Senior Research Fellow, Somerville College
Sleep & Circadian Neuroscience Institute (SCNi)
Nuffield Department of Clinical Neurosciences
University of Oxford
Sir William Dunn School of Pathology
Oxford, UK

Bruno Estañol-Vidal MD
Neurophysiologist
Neurology and Neurophysiology Department
Instituto Nacional de Ciencias Médicas y Nutrición
Salvador Zubiran
Mexico City, Mexico

Stanley Fahn MD
H. Houston Merritt Professor of Neurology
Department of Neurology
Columbia University Medical Center
New York, NY, USA

Aisylu T. Faizutdinova MD, PhD
Docent
Department of Neurology and Rehabilitation
Kazan State Medical University
Kazan, Russia

Anna Katharina Flügel MD
Department of Neurology
Klinikum Frankfurt Höchst GmbH
Frankfurt, Germany

Enrico Franceschi MD
Department of Medical Oncology
Bellaria-Maggiore Hospital
Azienda USL of Bologna - IRCCS Institute of
Neurological Sciences
Bologna, Italy

Birgit Frauscher MD
Associate Professor,
Department of Neurology
Innsbruck Medical University
Innsbruck, Austria

Karen P. Frei MD
Associate Professor
Loma Linda University Medical Center
Loma Linda, CA, USA

Jared Fridley MD
Department of Neurosurgery
Baylor College of Medicine
Houston, TX, USA

Janice Fuentes MD
Associate Professor of Neurology
Department of Neurology,
Loma Linda University Medical Center
Loma Linda, CA, USA

Steven Galetta MD
Professor and Chair
Department of Neurology
NYU Langone Medical Center
Ambulatory Care Center
New York, USA

Guillermo García-Ramos MD
Neurologist
Neurology and Neurophysiology Department
Instituto Nacional de Ciencias Médicas y Nutrición
Salvador Zubiran
Mexico City, Mexico

Caterina Garone MD, PhD
Investigator Scientist
Medical Research Council
MRC Mitochondrial Biology Unit
Cambridge, UK

Ellen Gelpi MD, EFN
Neurological Tissue Bank of the Biobank-Hospital
Clinic-Institut d'Investigacions Biomediques August Pi
i Sunyer (IDIBAPS), Barcelona, Spain.

Don Gilden MD
Louise Baum Endowed Chair and Professor
Departments of Neurology and Microbiology
and Immunology
University of Colorado School of Medicine
Aurora, CO, USA

Nils Erik Gilhus MD
Professor, Department of Clinical Medicine
University of Bergen
Department of Neurology
Haukeland University Hospital
Bergen, Norway

Christopher C. Giza MD
Professor of Neurosurgery and Pediatric Neurology
Director, UCLA Steve Tisch BrainSPORT Program
UCLA Brain Injury Research Center
David Geffen School of Medicine & Mattel Children's
Hospital
Los Angeles, CA, USA

David Gloss MD, MPH&TM
Geisinger Health System
Danville, PA, USA

Hans-Hilmar Goebel MD
Department of Neuropathology
Charité – Universitätsmedizin Berlin, Berlin
Department of Neuropathology
University Medicine
Johannes Gutenberg University, Mainz
Germany

Volodymyr Golyk MD, PhD
Chair, Neurology and Border States Department
Ukrainian State Institute of Medical and Social
Problems of Disability
Ministry of Public Health of Ukraine
Dnipropetrovs`k, Ukraine

Marc Gotkine MD
Department of Neurology
Agnes Ginges Center for Human Neurogenetics
Hadassah University Hospital
Hebrew University Hadassah Medical School
Jerusalem, Israel

Namita Goyal MD
Associate Clinical Professor, Department of Neurology,
Associate Director, UC Irvine-MDA ALS and
Neuromuscular Center
University of California, Irvine, CA, USA

Murray Grossman MDCM, PhD
Departments of Neurology and Psychiatry and Penn
FTD Center
Neuroscience Graduate Group, Bioengineering
Graduate Group
University of Pennsylvania
Philadelphia, PA, USA

Vesselina T. Grozeva MD, PhD
Assistant Professor
Neurology Department
Medical University – Sofia
Multiprofile Hospital for Active Treatment in
Neurology and Psychiatry "St. Naum", Sofia, Bulgaria

Alla Guekht MD
Professor of Neurology
Russian National Research Medical University
and Director
Moscow Research and Clinical Center for
Neuropsychiatry
Moscow, Russia

Christian Guilleminault MD
Professor, Stanford University Sleep Medicine Division
Stanford Outpatient Medical Center
Redwood City, CA, USA

James Ha MD
Assistant Clinical Professor
Department of Neurology,
University of California, Davis
Sacramento, CA, USA

Yael Hacohen MBBS, DPhil
Nuffield Department of Clinical Neurosciences
John Radcliffe Hospital, University of Oxford
Oxford, UK

Michael G. Hanna PhD
Professor in Clinical Neurology
MRC Centre for Neuromuscular Diseases
UCL Institute of Neurology
London, UK

Kapila Hari MD
Lecturer, University of the Witwatersrand
Johannesburg, South Africa

Gregory G. Heuer MD, PhD
Assistant Professor
Department of Neurosurgery
University of Pennsylvania
Children's Hospital of Philadelphia
Philadelphia, PA, USA

David Hilton-Jones
Honorary Senior Lecturer, Nuffield Department of
Clinical Neurosciences (Clinical Neurology), University
of Oxford, John Radcliffe Hospital,
Oxford, UK

Silvia Hofer MD
Consultant Medical Oncologist
Division of Oncology, Luzerner Kantonsspital
Luzern, Switzerland

Birgit Högl MD
Associate Professor of Neurology, Head of the Sleep
Disorders Clinic, Department of Neurology, Medical
University of Innsbruck, Austria

Sarah E. Hopkins MD, MSPH
Assistant Professor of Clinical Neurology
The University of Pennsylvania Perelman School of
Medicine/The Children's Hospital of Philadelphia,
Philadelphia, PA, USA

Chung Y. Hsu MD, PhD
Chair Professor, China Medical University
Taichung, Taiwan
Principal Investigator, Ministry of Health Clinical Trial
Center of Excellence, Taichung, Taiwan
Executive Trustee, Board of Trustees, National Health
Research Institute, Chunan, Taiwan

Chin-Chang Huang MD
Professor of Department of Neurology
Chang Gung Memorial Hospital
Chang Gung University, College of Medicine
Taipei, Taiwan

Marcel Hungs MD, PhD
Adjunct Associate Clinical Professor of Neurology
Department of Neurology, University of Minnesota
Minneapolis, MN, USA

Jae-Won Hyun MD
Department of Neurology
Research Institute and Hospital of National
Cancer Center
Goyang, Korea

**Sergey N. Illarioshkin MD,
PhD, DSc**
Vice-Director
Research Center of Neurology, Russian Academy of
Medical Sciences
Moscow, Russia

David J. Irwin MD
Instructor of Neurology
Department of Neurology, Frontotemporal
Degeneration Center (FTDC)
University of Pennsylvania Perelman School of
Medicine
Hospital of the University of Pennsylvania
Philadelphia, PA, USA

Takeshi Iwanaga MD
Florey Institute of Neurosciences and Mental Health,
University of Melbourne
Melbourne Brain Center
Heidelberg, VIC, Australia

Nauman Jahangir MD
Zeenat Qureshi Stroke Institute
St. Cloud, MN, USA

Regina I. Jakacki MD
Children's Hospital of Pittsburgh
Pittsburgh, PA, USA

**Altynshash Jaxybayeva
MD, PhD**
Chief Science Officer
National Research Center for Maternal and Child
Health
Astana, Kazakhstan

Miran Jeromel MD, PhD
Assistant Professor of Radiology
Department for Neuroradiology,
University Medical Centre Ljubljana,
Ljubljana, Slovenia.
General Hospital Slovenj Gradec,
Slovenj Gradec, Slovenia

Onanong Jitkritsadakul MD, MSc
Instructor in Neurology
Chulalongkorn Centre of Excellence for Parkinson's
Disease & Related Disorders
Faculty of Medicine, Chulalongkorn University,
Bangkok, Thailand

Nanette C. Joyce DO
Assistant Clinical Professor
Department of Physical Medicine and Rehabilitation
University of California, Davis
Sacramento, CA, USA

Babita Jyoti MD
University of Florida Health Proton Therapy Institute
Jacksonville, FL, USA

Saltanat Kamenova MD
Professor, Head of Department of Neurology in
Asfendiyarov Kazakh National Medical University
Almaty, Kazakhstan

Andres M. Kanner MD, FANA
Professor of Clinical Neurology
Director, Comprehensive Epilepsy Center and Head,
Epilepsy Section
Department of Neurology, University of Miami,
Miller School of Medicine
Miami, FL, USA

Kevin A. Kerber MD, MS
Associate Professor
Department of Neurology, University of Michigan
Ann Arbor, MI, USA

Emilia Kerty MD, PhD
Professor of Neurology
Neurology Department
Oslo University Hospital/Rikshospitalet
University of Oslo
Oslo, Norway

Ismail A. Khatri MD
Associate Professor, King Saud bin Abdulaziz
University for Health Sciences
Consultant Neurologist, King Abdulaziz Medical City
National Guard Health Affairs
Riyadh, Kingdom of Saudi Arabia

Ho Jin Kim MD, PhD
Head of MS Clinic and Department of Neurology
Research Institute and Hospital of National Cancer
Center
Goyang, Korea

Jun-Ichi Kira MD
Professor and Chairman, Department of Neurology
Neurological Institute, Graduate School of Medical
Sciences
Kyushu University, Japan

Yasuhisa Kitagawa MD, PhD
Professor of Neurology
Tokai University School of Medicine
Tokai University Hachioji Hospital
Tokyo, Japan

Andreas Koch MD, Capt (MC)
Professor of the Section for Maritime Medicine
German Naval Medical Institute
Christian-Albrechts-University
Vice-President, German Society of Diving and
Hyperbaric Medicine
Kiel, Germany

Aida Kondybayeva MD
Department of Neurology
Asfendiyarov Kazakh National Medical University
Department of Neurology
Almaty Kazakhstan

Vladimir Kostić MD, PhD
Profesor of Neurology
Faculty of Medicine, University of Belgrade
Institute of Neurology, CCS
Belgrade, Serbia

Srivicha Krudsood MD
Professor
Departments of Tropical Hygiene
Faculty of Tropical Medicine
Mahidol University
Bangkok, Thailand

Aoife Laffan MBBCh, BAO, MD, MRCPI
Departments of Neurology and HIV Medicine
Peter Duncan Neuroscience Unit
St Vincent's Centre for Applied Medical Research
St Vincent's Hospital
Sydney, NSW, Australia

Nigel G. Laing MD, PhD
Professor
Centre for Medical Research
University of Western Australia
Harry Perkins Institute of Medical Research and
Neurogenetics Unit
Department of Diagnostic Genomics, Path West,
Department of Health, Western Australia
Nedlands, WA, Australia

Sandi Lam MD, MBA
Assistant Professor
Department of Neurosurgery/Division of Pediatric
Neurosurgery
Baylor College of Medicine/Texas Children's Hospital
Houston, TX, USA

Dronacharya Lamichhane MD
Department of Neurology
University of Maryland Medical Center
Baltimore, MD, USA

Phillipa J. Lamont MBBS, FRACP
Professor of Neurology
University of Western Australia
Department of Neurology
Royal Perth Hospital
Perth, Western Australia

Nicola Latronico MD
Professor of Anesthesia and Critical Care Medicine.
Department of Anesthesia, Critical Care and
Emergency, Spedali Civili University Hospital,
Brescia, Italy
Department of Medical and Surgical Specialties,
Radiological Sciences and Public Health, University of
Brescia, Italy

Minh Le MD
Senior Lecturer on Neurology
Head, Department of Neurology, University
Medical Center
Ho Chi Minh City, Vietnam

Emilie Le Rhun MD
Breast Unit, Department of Medical Oncology
Centre Oscar Lambret, Lille
Department of Neurooncology, Hopital Roger Salengro
Hospital, Lille University Hospital
PRISM Laboratory, INSERM U1192, Villeneuve d'Ascq
France

Jason T. Lerner MD
Associate Professor
Director, Pediatric Neurophysiology Lab
Director of Training, Pediatric Neurology
Division of Pediatric Neurology, David Geffen School
of Medicine at UCLA
Los Angeles, CA, USA

Thomas W. Leung MD, MRCP, FAHA
Lee Quo Wei Associate Professor of Neurology
Department of Medicine and Therapeutics
The Chinese University of Hong Kong
Shatin, Hong Kong

Steven R. Levine MD, FAHA, FAAN, FANA
Professor of Neurology & Emergency Medicine
Executive Vice Chair, Neurology
Chief of Neurology, University Hospital of Brooklyn
Associate Dean for Clinical Research & Faculty
Development
Department of Neurology/Stroke Center, SUNY
Downstate Health Science Center
Brooklyn, NY, USA

Arnold I. Levinson MD
Emeritus Professor of Medicine and Neurology
Perelman School of Medicine
University of Pennsylvania
Philadelphia, PA, USA

Richard A. Lewis MD
Professor of Neurology,
Department of Neurology
Cedars-Sinai Medical Center
Los Angeles, CA, USA

Marco A. Lima MD, MSc, PhD
Senior Researcher
Laboratory for Clinical Research in Neuroinfections
National Institute of Infectology (INI)
Oswaldo Cruz Foundation (FIOCRUZ), Brazilian
Ministry of Health
Adjunct Professor of Neurology, Department of
Internal Medicine, the Federal University of Rio de
Janeiro
Rio de Janeiro, Brazil

Yu-Wei Lin MD
Attending Physician
Department of Neurology, Taiwan Adventist Hospital
Taipei City, Taiwan

Alfred Lindner MD
Professor and Head Department of Neurology
Marienhospital Stuttgart
Stuttgart, Germany

**Li Ling Lim MBBS, MRCP (UK),
MPH (USA), Dip. ABPN, ABSM,
ABEM, ABCN (USA)**
Medical Director & Consultant Neurologist
Singapore Neurology & Sleep Centre
Visiting Consultant Neurologist
National Neuroscience Institute
Visiting Consultant Neurologist
Department of Medicine, Khoo Teck Puat Hospital
Singapore

**Robert P. Lisak MD, FAAN,
FRCP(E), FANA**
Parker Webber Chair in Neurology
Professor of Neurology
Professor of Immunology and Microbiology
Wayne State University School of Medicine
Attending Neurologist, Detroit Medical Center
Detroit, MI, USA

Tomasz Litwin MD, PhD
Assistant Professor
Institute of Psychiatry and Neurology, Sobieskiego
Warsaw, Poland

Mingsheng Liu MD
Professor
Peking Union Medical College Hospital
Department of Neurology
Beijing, China

Albert C. Ludolph MD
Professor of Neurology
Universitäts- und Rehabilitationskliniken Ulm
Ärztlicher Direktor
Abteilung für Neurologie
Ulm, Germany

Adrian Marchidann MD
Assistant Professor of Neurology
Department of Neurology/Stroke Center
SUNY Downstate Health Science Center
Brooklyn, NY, USA

Warren P. Mason MD, FRCPC
Professor of Medicine, Department of Neurology,
Division of Neuro-Oncology, University of Toronto,
Pencer Brain Tumor Centre
Toronto, ON, Canada

**Frank L. Mastaglia MBBS, MD,
FRACP, FRCP**
Professor of Neurology
Institute for Immunological and Infectious diseases,
Murdoch University,
Perth, Australia

Diana Matallana PhD
Department of Psychiatry and Institute on Aging
Pontificia Universidad Javeriana
Bogota, Colombia

Radoslav Matěj MD, PhD
Associate Professor
Department of Pathology and Molecular Medicine
National Laboratory for Diagnostics of Prion Diseases
Thomayer Teaching Hospital
Prague, Czech Republic

Catherine Maurice MD, FRCPC
Department of Neurology, division of Neuro-Oncology
at the University of Toronto
Pencer Brain Tumor Centre
Toronto, ON, Canada

Marco T. Medina MD, FAAN
Professor of Neurology and Dean
Faculty of Medical Sciences,
National Autonomous University of Honduras
Tegucigalpa, Honduras

Marco Medina-Montoya MD
Faculty of Medical Sciences
National Autonomous University of Honduras
Tegucigalpa, Honduras

**Giovanni Meola MD, PhD, FAAN,
FANA**
Professor and Chair of Neurology
Department of Biomedical Sciences for Health
University of Milan
Laboratory of Muscle Histopathology and Molecular
Biology, IRCCS Policlinico San Donato
Milan, Italy

Ivan G. Milanov MD, PhD, DSc
Academic Professor
Neurology Department, Medical University – Sofia
University Hospital for Active Treatment in Neurology
and Psychiatry, St. Naum
Movement Disorders Clinic
Sofia, Bulgaria

Andre Mochan MD
Lecturer, University of the Witwatersrand
Johannesburg, South Africa

**Girish Modi MBBCh (Wits), MSc
(Lond), PhD (Lond), FCP (SA),
FRCP (Lond)**
Professor, Chief Specialist, Chair of Neurology
University of the Witwatersrand
Johannesburg, South Africa

Eric Momin MD
Resident Neurosurgeon
Department of Neurosurgery
Baylor College of Medicine
Houston, TX, USA

Philip K. Moskowitz MD
Department of Internal Medicine
NYU Langone Medical Center
New York, USA

Tahseen Mozaffar MD
Professor
Departments of Neurology and Orthopedic Surgery
University of California, Irvine
Orange, CA, USA

Maria A. Nagel MD
Department of Neurology
University of Colorado School of Medicine
Aurora, CO, USA

Sona Narula MD
Division of Neurology
Children's Hospital of Philadelphia
Perelman School of Medicine at the University of
Pennsylvania
Philadelphia, PA, USA

**Merrilee Needham MBBS, PhD,
FRACP**
Associate Professor of Neurology
Department of Neurology, Fiona Stanley Hospital and
Institute for Immunological and Infectious diseases,
Murdoch University,
Perth, Australia

Yoram Nevo MD
Professor of Neurology
Director, Neurology Institute
Schneider Children's Medical Center of Israel
Petah Tikva, Israel

Adam L. Numis MD
Mattel Children's Hospital UCLA
Los Angeles, CA, USA

Hirokazu Oguni MD, PhD
Professor of Pediatrics, Department of Pediatrics
Tokyo Women's Medical University
Tokyo, Japan

Humphrey Okechi MD
Attending Neurosurgeon
Department of Neurosurgery
Kijabe Hospital
Kijabe, Kenya

Björn Oskarsson MD
Associate Professor, Department of Neurology
University of California, Davis,
Sacramento, CA, USA

Bruce Ovbiagele MD, MSc, MAS
Admiral Pihl Professor and Chairman
Department of Neurology and Neurosurgery
Medical University of South Carolina
Charleston, SC, USA

Shelly Ozark MD
Assistant Professor of Neurology,
Department of Neurology and Neurosurgery
Medical University of South Carolina
Charleston, SC, USA

George W. Padberg MD, PhD
Professor Emeritus of Neurology
Department of Neurology
Radboud University Medical Center
Nijmegen, The Netherlands

**Chrysostomos P.
Panayiotopoulos MD**
Consultant Emeritus, Department of Clinical
Neurophysiology and Epilepsies
St. Thomas' Hospital
London, UK

Margaret Park, MD, DABSM, DABPN/Sleep Medicine
Chicago Sleep Health
Chicago, IL, USA

Janesh Patel MD
Stanford University Sleep Medicine Division
Stanford Outpatient Medical Center
Redwood City, CA, USA

Mary Payne MD
Department of Neuroscience
Marshall University
Huntington, WV, USA

Kammant Phanthumchinda MD
Professor of Medicine
Department of Medicine, Faculty of Medicine
Chulalongkorn University
Bangkok, Thailand

Claudio Podesta MD
Head of Sleep Medicine Unit
FLENI Foundation
Buenos Aires
Argentina

Simon Podnar MD, PhD
Associate Professor of Neurology
Institute of Clinical Neurophysiology
Division of Neurology
University Medical Centre Ljubljana
Ljubljana, Slovenia

Anuchit Poonyathalang MD
Associate Professor of Ophthalmology
Department of Ophthalmology
Ramathibodi Hospital, Mahidol University
Bangkok, Thailand

Sudesh Prabhakar MD (Medicine), DM (Neurology), FAMS
Director Neurology
Fortis Hospital
Chandigarh, India

Paul B. Pritchard III MD
Professor of Neurology
Medical University of South Carolina
Charleston, SC, USA

Leon D. Prockop MD
Founding Chairman, Emeritus Professor of
Department of Neurology
University of South Florida
Chair, Environmental Neurology Research Group
(ENRG)/World Federation of Neurology (WFN)
Tampa, FL, USA

Adnan I. Qureshi MD
Professor of Neurology, Neurosurgery, and
Radiology
Zeenat Qureshi Stroke Research Center,
University of Minnesota, Minneapolis. MN

Mushtaq H. Qureshi MD
Zeenat Qureshi Stroke Institute
St. Cloud, MN, USA

Malcolm Rabie MBBCh (Wits), FCP (SA) (Neurol.)
Physician
Neurology Institute, Schneider Children's Medical
Center of Israel
Petah Tikva, Israel

Jan Raethjen MD, PhD
Neurology Clinic, Kiel
Adjunct Professor
University of Kiel,
Kiel, Germany

Jeffrey Raizer MD
Professor of Neurology
Director, Medical Neuro-Oncology
Northwestern University, Chicago, IL, USA

Kumar Rajamani MD, DM
Associate Professor of Neurology
Wayne State University School of Medicine
Detroit, MI, USA

Nathan J. Ranalli MD
Assistant Professor of Neurosurgery and Pediatrics
University of Florida Health Science Center –
Jacksonville
Division of Pediatric Neurological Surgery at Lucy
Gooding Pediatric Neurosurgery Center
Wolfson Children's Hospital
Jacksonville, FL, USA

Katya Rascovsky PhD
Department of Neurology and Penn Frontotemporal
Degeneration Center
University of Pennsylvania Perelman School of
Medicine
Philadelphia, PA, USA

Frank A. Rasulo MD
Department of Medical and Surgical Specialties
Radiological Sciences and Public Health
University of Brescia
Brescia, Italy

Narendra Rathi MD, DNB, FIAP
Consultant Pediatrician
Pediatric Infectious Disease Consultant
Rathi Children Hospital
Akola, India

Ivan Rektor MD, CSc
Professor, Masaryk University; Brno Epilepsy
Centre, St. Anne's Hospital; Central European
Institute of Technology, Neuroscience Centre,
Brno, Czech Republic

Irena Rektorová MD, PhD
First Department of Neurology
Faculty of Medicine, Masaryk University
St. Anne's Teaching Hospital
Brno, Czech Republic

Steven P. Ringel MD
Department of Neurology
University of Colorado School of Medicine
Aurora, CO, USA

John M. Ringman MD, MS
Helene and Lou Galen Endowed Professor of
Clinical Neurology
Department of Neurology
Keck School of Medicine of USC
Center for the Health Professionals
Los Angeles, CA, USA

Luis C. Rodríguez Salinas MD
Honduras Medical Center, Tepeyac
Tegucigalpa, Honduras

Ildefonso Rodríguez-Leyva MD
Professor Medicine Faculty, San Luis Potosi State
University of San Luis Potosi, Mexico

Yvonne D. Rollins MD, PhD
Regional West Physicians Clinic – Neurology,
Scottsbluff, NE, USA

Karen L. Roos MD
Professor of Neurology
Indiana University School of Medicine
Indiana University Neuroscience Center
Indianapolis, IN, USA

Raymond L. Rosales MD, PhD
Professor of Neurology, Neurosciences and Psychiatry
The Royal and Pontifical University of Santo Tomas,
Manila
Head of Center for Neurodiagnostic and Therapeutic
Services (CNS)
Metropolitan Medical Center, Manila Philippines

Myrna R. Rosenfeld MD, PhD
Professor of Neurology
Hospital Clínic/IDIBAPS, Department of Neurology
Barcelona, Spain

Roberta Rudà MD
Assistant Professor of Neuro-Oncology
Department of Neuro-Oncology
University of Turin
Turin, Italy

Sabine Rudnik-Schöneborn MD
Professor
Sektion Humangenetik
Medizinische Universität Innsbruck
Innsbruck, Austria

Robert Rusina MD, PhD
Associate Professor
Department of Neurology, First Faculty of Medicine,
Charles University,
Thomayer Teaching Hospital
Prague, Czech Republic

Gérard Said MD, FRCP
Professor
Centre Médical Bastille, Paris, France

Sabahattin Saip MD
Professor of Neurology
Department of Neurology, Istanbul University
Cerrahpaşa School of Medicine
Istanbul, Turkey

Friedhelm Sandbrink MD
Director EMG Laboratory and
Director Pain Management Program
Department of Neurology, Veterans Affairs Medical
Center and Georgetown University
Washington, DC, USA

Raman Sankar MD, PhD
Professor and Chief
Pediatric Neurology - UCLA
Rubin Brown Distinguished Chair
David Geffen School of Medicine UCLA and Mattel
Children's Hospital UCLA
Los Angeles, CA, USA

Ulrike Schara MD
Neuropädiatrie, Entwicklungsneurologie und
Sozialpädiatrie
Klinik für Kinderheilkunde I, Universitätsklinikum
Essen, Germany

Josef Schill MD
Geschäftsführender Oberarzt
Klinik für Neurologie und Neurogeriatrie
Klinikum Darmstadt
Darmstadt, Germany

Jacques Serratrice MD
Assistant Professor
Internal Medicine Department
Hôpitaux Universitaires de Genève
Geneva, Switzerland

Lisa M. Shulman MD
Professor of Neurology
Eugenia Brin Professor in Parkinson's Disease and
Movement Disorders
Rosalyn Newman Distinguished Scholar in Parkinson's
Disease
Director, University of Maryland PD & Movement
Disorders Center
University of Maryland School of Medicine
Baltimore, MD, USA

Donald Silberberg MD
Professor Emeritus
Department of Neurology
University of Pennsylvania Medical Center
Philadelphia, PA, USA

Stephen D. Silberstein MD
Professor of Neurology
Jefferson Medical College, Thomas Jefferson University
Director, Jefferson Headache Center, Thomas Jefferson
University Hospital
Philadelphia, PA, USA

David M. Simpson MD, FAAN
Professor of Neurology
Director, Clinical Neurophysiology Laboratories
Director, Neuromuscular Division
Director, Neuro-AIDS Program
Icahn School of Medicine at Mount Sinai Dept of
Neurology, New York, NY

Simran Singh DO
Medical Neuro-Oncology
Northwestern University, Chicago, IL. USA

**Kay Sin Tan MBBS (Melb), FRCP
(Edin), FAMM**
Professor and Senior Consultant Neurologist
Department of Medicine, Faculty of Medicine
University of Malaya
Kuala Lumpur, Malaysia

Marcus Tulius Silva MD, MSc, PhD
Senior Researcher and Consultant Neurologist
The Laboratory for Clinical Research in
Neuroinfections, National Institute of Infectious
Diseases (INI), Oswaldo Cruz Foundation (FIOCRUZ),
Brazilian Ministry of Health
Rio de Janeiro, Brazil

Gagandeep Singh MD, DM
Professor & Head, Department of Neurology
Dayanand Medical College & Hospital
Punjab, India

Simran Singh DO
Department of Neurology
Northwestern University
Chicago, IL, USA

Aksel Siva MD
Professor of Neurology
Department of Neurology, Istanbul University
Cerrahpaşa School of Medicine
Istanbul, Turkey

Riccardo Soffietti MD
Professor of Neurology/Neuro-Oncology
Department of Neuro-Oncology
University of Turin
Turin, Italy

Marylou V. Solbrig MD
Professor
Departments of Internal Medicine (Neurology) and
Medical Microbiology, University of Manitoba
Winnipeg, MB, Canada

Sopio Sopromadze MD
Department of Neurology
N. Kipshidze Central University Clinic
Tbilisi, Georgia

Mark M. Souweidane MD
Memorial Sloan Kettering Cancer Center
Department of Neurosurgery
New York Presbyterian Hospital Weill Cornell Medical
College, Department of Neurological Surgery
New York, USA

Jirada Sringean MD
Chulalongkorn Centre of Excellence for Parkinson's
Disease & Related Disorders
Faculty of Medicine
Chulalongkorn University
Bangkok, Thailand

Mark Stacy MD
Professor of Neurology and Vice Dean
Duke Institute for Brain Sciences
Duke University
Durham, NC, USA

Kara Stavros MD
Assistant Professor of Neurology
The Warren Alpert Medical School of Brown
University
Rhode Island Hospital
Providence, RI, USA

Elka Stefanova MD, PhD
Professor of Neurology
Faculty of Medicine, University of Belgrade
Institute of Neurology, CCS
Belgrade, Serbia

Thorsten Steiner MD
Department of Neurology
Klinikum Frankfurt Höchst GmbH
Frankfurt, Germany
Department of Neurology
Heidelberg University Hospital, Heidelberg,
Germany

Rick Stell MBBS, FRACP
Director of Movement Disorders Unit, Western
Australian Neuromuscular Research Institute
Sir Charles Gairdner Hospital, Nedlands
Perth, WA, Australia

Werner Stenzel MD
Professor of Neuropathology & Neuroimmunology
Department of Neuropathology
Charité – Universitätsmedizin Berlin
Berlin, Germany

Barney J. Stern MD
Interim Chair
Stewart J. Greenebaum Endowed Professor in Stroke
Neurology
Department of Neurology
University of Maryland School of Medicine
Baltimore, MA, USA

Chiara S. M. Straathof MD, PhD
Department of Neurology
Leiden University Medical Center
Leiden, The Netherlands

Karen Suetterlin MD
MRC Centre for Neuromuscular Diseases
UCL Institute of Neurology
London, UK

Valerie Suski DO
Assistant Professor
Department of Neurology
University of Pittsburgh Medical Center
Pittsburgh, PA, USA

Nijasri C. Suwanwela MD
Professor of Neurology
Division of Neurology
Department of Medicine
Chulalongkorn University
Bangkok, Thailand

Barbara E. Swartz MD, PhD
Director, Epilepsy Center and Neurophysiology
Laboratory
Professor, Renown Neuroscience Institute
University of Nevada
Reno, NV, USA

Takeshi Tabira MD, PhD
Department of Diagnosis
Prevention and Treatment of Dementia
Graduate School of Medicine, Juntendo University
Tokyo, Japan

Sophie Taillibert MD
Department of Neurology Mazarin and Department
of Radiation Oncology
Pitié-Salpétrière Hospital University Pierre et
Marie Curie
Paris, France

Chong Tin Tan MD
Professor
University of Malaya, Malaysia

Noppadon Tangpukdee MD
Assistant professor
Department of Clinical Tropical Medicine
Faculty of Tropical Medicine, Mahidol University
Bangkok, Thailand

Stacey K. H. Tay MD
Associate Professor
Department of Paediatrics
Yong Loo Lin School of Medicine
National University of Singapore
Singapore

Hock L. Teoh MD, MRCP
Florey Institute of Neurosciences and Mental Health
University of Melbourne
Melbourne Brain Center
Heidelberg, VIC, Australia

Ann Tilton MD
Professor of Neurology and Pediatrics
Louisiana State University Health Sciences Center
Department of Neurology
Children's Hospital
New Orleans, LA, USA

Manjari Tripathi MD, DM
Professor of Neurology
Department of Neurology, Neurosciences Centre
All India Institute of Medical Sciences
New Delhi, India

Daniel D. Truong MD, FAAN
Clinical Professor, University of California, Riverside
Riverside, CA, USA
The Truong Neuroscience Institute
Orange Coast Memorial Medical Center
Fountain Valley, CA, USA

Alex Tselis MD, PhD
Professor of Neurology
Wayne State University School of Medicine
Detroit, MI, USA

**Alexander Tsiskaridze MD, PhD,
DSc, FESO**
Professor of Neurology
Department of Neurology, Tbilisi State University
Tbilisi, Georgia

Sergio Tufik MD, PhD
Professor
Department of Psychobiology, Universidade Federal
de São Paulo
São Paulo, Brazil

Ugur Uygunoglu MD
Associate Professor of Neurology
Department of Neurology, Istanbul University
Cerrahpaşa School of Medicine
Istanbul, Turkey

Sanjeev N. Vaishnavi MD, PhD
Instructor
Department of Neurology, Perelman School of
Medicine, University of Pennsylvania
Philadelphia, PA, USA

Frank J. E. Vajda MD, FRCP, FRACP
Professor
Department of Medicine and Neuroscience
Royal Melbourne Hospital
Parkville, VIC, Australia

Minh Hoang Van MD
Senior Lecturer on Dermatology
Department of Dermatology
University of Medicine and Pharmacy
Ho Chi Minh City, Vietnam

Martin J. van den Bent MD
Brain Tumor Center at Erasmus MC Cancer Institute
Rotterdam, The Netherlands

Gregory P. van Stavern MD
Associate Professor
Departments of Ophthalmology and Visual Sciences
and Neurology, St. Louis School of Medicine,
Washington University
St. Louis, MO, USA

Arousiak Varpetian MD
Department of Neurology, Keck School of Medicine
University of Southern California
Downey, CA, USA

**Narayanaswamy
Venketasubramanian FRCP**
Consultant Neurologist
Raffles Neuroscience Centre, Raffles Hospital
Singapore

Rachel Ventura MD, PhD
Multiple Sclerosis Fellow,
New York University Langone Medical Center
Department of Neurology
New York, NY, USA

John Vissing MD, PhD
Professor, Copenhagen Neuromuscular Center
Department of Neurology
University of Copenhagen
Copenhagen, Denmark

David B. Vodušek MD, PhD
Professor of Neurology, Medical Faculty
University of Ljubljana
Medical Director, Division of Neurology
University Medical Centre Ljubljana
Ljubljana, Slovenia

Melanie Walker MD
Clinical Associate Professor
Departments of Neurology and Neurological
Surgery
University of Washington School of Medicine
Seattle, WA, USA

Shuu-Jiun Wang MD
Vice Director, Neurological Institute
Taipei Veterans General Hospital
Professor and Chairman, Faculty of Medicine
National Yang-Ming University School of Medicine
Taipei, Taiwan

Mohamad Wasay MD, FRCP, FAAN
Professor of Neurology
The Aga Khan University
Karachi, Pakistan

Thomas Weber MD
Department of Neurology, Marienkrankenhaus
Hamburg, University Clinic Hamburg-Eppendorf
Hamburg, Germany

Thomas Wieser MD
Department of Neurology and Pain Medicine
Fachkrankenhaus Jerichow
Jerichow, Germany

Polrat Wilairatana, MD
Professor
Department of Clinical Tropical Medicine,
Faculty of Tropical Medicine, Mahidol University,
Bangkok, Thailand

**Einar P. Wilder-Smith MD
(Heidelberg), DTM&H (London),
FAMS (Neurology)**
Professor and Senior Consultant
National University of Singapore
Singapore

**Ernest Willoughby MB
ChB, FRACP**
Neurologist
Department of Neurology
Auckland City Hospital
Auckland, New Zealand

David A. Wolk MD
Associate Professor
Co-Director, Penn Memory Center
Department of Neurology, Perelman School
of Medicine
University of Pennsylvania
Philadelphia, PA, USA

Lidia Yamada MD
Department of Neurology and Neurosurgery
Medical University of South Carolina
Charleston, SC, USA

Eric L. Zager MD
Professor of Neurosurgery
Department of Neurosurgery
University of Pennsylvania
Philadelphia, PA, USA

Afawi Zaid MD, MPH, PhD
Coordinator, Genetics of Epilepsy Research
Tel-Aviv Sourasky Medical Center,
Tel-Aviv, Israel

Jorge A. Zavala MD
Florey Institute of Neurosciences and Mental Health
University of Melbourne
Melbourne Brain Center
Heidelberg, VIC, Australia

Klaus Zerres MD
Professor and Chairman
Institut für Humangenetikder RWTH Aachen
Aachen, Germany

Foreword

I was delighted and honoured a few years ago when Robert Lisak, a neurologist of outstanding ability and merit and former editor of the *Journal of Neurological Sciences*, invited me to write a foreword to the first edition of this book. I then said that, whereas many notable textbooks on clinical neurology exist, I was not aware that there were any which dealt as comprehensively with international neurology as did that volume, which has proved, as I anticipated, to be outstandingly successful. It is therefore a great pleasure, in my 93rd year, to welcome this second edition, substantially expanded with much new material added, but deploying the same kind of comprehensive and inclusive approach which characterised the first edition. Dr Lisak's co-editors have recruited an outstanding group of internationally notable colleagues, who have succeeded in bringing this volume and all of its contents well up to date. This new edition represents in my opinion a remarkable achievement, and its contents will be invaluable, not only to neurologists in tropical and developing countries whose interests are fully covered, but also to many of those in the Western world who are interested in international developments in their respective fields of study and practice. All those who will study this work in depth, and also all those who dip into individual chapters in which they have particular expertise or interest, will find it an outstanding teaching tool, a remarkable guide to clinical practice in different countries, and a veritable powerhouse of knowledge which will be widely read and consulted to the profit of its readers. I congratulate Bob Lisak and his co-editors on planning such a remarkable volume and bringing it to fruition.

John Walton (Lord Walton of Detchant) Kt TD MA MD DSc
FRCP FmedSci
Former Professor of Neurology and Dean of Medicine, University
of Newcastle upon Tyne, UK
Former President, World Federation of Neurology

Endorsement from the World Federation of Neurology

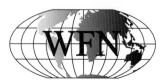

The world of neurology has changed. The spectrum and depth of all the conditions affecting the nervous system are now galloping ahead. Clinicians need to keep abreast of the new world. This book is an excellent effort to gather 200 authors from across the globe to distil their knowledge in well-laid-out sections. The true international nature of the authorship is most impressive and gives the reader the ability to see how neurology has changed firstly in its breadth, and secondly in the ability to encompass experts with differing backgrounds yet able to produce a cohesive narrative and message. The shrinking globe in the age of the internet has led to an explosion of knowledge in a manner which is exemplified by the authorship of this book. Moreover, this second edition in six years means that this is a continuous live project both for editors and authors.

The editors are to be congratulated in bringing together all this in one volume and allowing readers access to the most up-to-date information. The World Federation of Neurology is proud to see the wide collaboration, which really represents the ethos of true internationalism.

Raad Shakir MD FRCP
President World Federation of Neurology
June 2015

Preface

The first edition of this text, *International Neurology: A Clinical Approach*, grew out of the involvement of the editors in international meetings held in Vietnam and was published in 2009. The "shrinking of the globe," with people traveling for pleasure and business, has made it likely that physicians may see individuals as patients who have diseases they have not personally encountered or patients with different manifestations of diseases they have seen. This is true of visitors from developing countries who may become ill in North America, Europe, and other 'Westernized' nations as well as the converse. In most texts, some chapters are by authors writing about diseases or groups of diseases they themselves only know from their reading. Other texts deal with disorders seen worldwide, but only emphasize the clinical features encountered in a limited geographic region. We chose authors and section editors who were familiar with and expert in neurological diseases and asked them to cover these diseases as they present in different populations and areas of the world. The section editors and authors were from all regions of the world. They took into account differences in genetic, environmental, and demographic factors as well as therapeutic approaches. In the latter area treatments not based on evidence, or for which clinical evidence was lacking, were not included. Although all of the chapters included sections on etiology and pathogenesis, the emphasis was on clinical neurology, not basic science. To take into account the expense of medical texts, we tried to limit the length of chapters and bibliographies and framed those as suggested further reading. We also limited colored figures.

We were pleased with the acceptance of our efforts and that of the authors and section editors and when approached to consider a second edition, we decided to go forward with the project. We have made some changes in organization, section editors, and authors, and asked authors to update their chapters to capture the exciting changes that are occurring in neurology. We have once again asked them to emphasize, where present, differences in diseases and their manifestations in different populations and locales.

We once again would like to thank the authors and section editors for their efforts and contributions as well as Sally Osborne, Angela Cohen and our Editors at Wiley Blackwell, Devender Gupta of Aptara India and Lisa Bauer for their assistance and support in the project

Robert P. Lisak MD FAAN FRCP(E) FANA
Daniel D. Truong MD FAAN
William M. Carroll MBBS MD FRACP FRCP(E)
Roongroj Bhidayasiri MD FRCP FRCPI

PART 1 Vascular Disorders

1 Overview of stroke

Christopher Li-Hsian Chen[1] and Chung Y. Hsu[2]
[1] Department of Pharmacology, National University of Singapore, Singapore
[2] China Medical University, Taichung, Taiwan

Stroke, encompassing both ischemic and hemorrhagic types, is a major health burden globally, affecting 15 million people each year. It is the second leading cause of death for people above the age of 60 years and the fifth leading cause for those aged 15 to 59 years. Stroke is the most common cause of adult disability and the second most important cause of dementia worldwide. According to World Health Organization (WHO) figures, global stroke deaths were 5.8 million in 2005 and are projected to increase to 6.5 million in 2015 and 7.8 million in 2030. Stroke is the most common disease that practicing neurologists manage. Stroke patients constitute approximately two-thirds of the inpatient neurology ward in virtually every hospital, with comprehensive neurology services in most countries around the world. With advances in evidence-based medicine, consensus on the diagnosis and treatment of selected types of strokes has gradually emerged across national boundaries.

Stroke mortality and incidence declined in developed countries during the 1980s and early 1990s, but this trend appears to have slowed recently. Despite the lack of reliable data on stroke statistics from several developing regions of the world, there are indications that the age-standardized mortality rate of stroke in developing nations may be substantially higher than in developed countries. The burden of stroke is accordingly greater due to relatively larger populations in developing countries. Furthermore, as a result of demographic transition, rapid urbanization, and industrialization, many developing regions show a trend of increased life expectancy, as well as a changing profile of risk factors for developing cardiovascular diseases, including stroke. This may contribute to a looming epidemic of stroke in medium- to low-income nations, as a greater population in these countries is at increased risk of stroke.

Stroke is a preventable disease. Implementation of effective primary and secondary prevention strategies is likely to have an enormous impact in reducing its burden. However, reducing stroke risk factors remains a challenging task, particularly in developing countries. It is appropriate that the WHO has set a priority on stroke prevention with the implementation of practical, accessible, cost-effective, and socially acceptable strategies.

Between the first and second editions of *International Neurology*, several important therapeutic advances have been made in the treatment of acute stroke and in stroke prevention: (1) endovascular intervention to remove blood clots in the proximal intracranial artery has been found to be safe and efficacious in patients with acute ischemic stroke beyond the approved therapeutic window of tPA (tissue plasminogen activator; 4.5 hours after stroke onset) and in particular in patients who failed intravenous tPA; (2) stroke prevention in patients with atrial fibrillation has been expanded from warfarin and/or heparin to novel oral anticoagulants that can spare patients frequent and inconvenient laboratory monitoring and show a favorable trend in reducing the risk of intracerebral hemorrhage, which is a serious side effect associated with traditional anticoagulants; (3) dual antiplatelets (aspirin plus clopidogrel) have been shown to be more effective than aspirin alone in preventing stroke in a critical period (within three weeks) after minor stroke and TIA.

Therapeutic attempts at applying neuroprotective agents, however, have failed in a series of large clinical trials and have highlighted the obstacles that remain to be overcome in translating promising therapeutic effects in animals in preclinical studies to clinical care for stroke patients based on evidence from clinical trials. Much soul searching has led to recommendations for improvements in the standards for preclinical studies including randomization, blinding, and sample-size calculations for interventional studies in animals, so as to improve the rigor of preclinical data and guide more appropriate selection of novel agents for trials in humans. The use of surrogate efficacy end points in early-phase studies has also been advocated so as to determine a possible efficacy signal before large, costly trials using clinical end points are undertaken. Neuroimaging has also been investigated as a means of selecting patients who would benefit most from treatment while minimizing the risk of serious side effects. Despite the slow rate of progress, it is essential that more clinical studies be undertaken to understand the pathophysiology of stroke, in order to develop appropriate clinical trial protocols to validate promising therapeutic strategies coming out of preclinical investigations.

In developing international standards for stroke prevention and therapy, the differences in stroke etiology and pathology among various ethnic groups cannot be overemphasized. Obvious examples are the higher incidence of intracerebral hemorrhage and higher prevalence of intracranial atherosclerosis in non-white

International Neurology, Second edition. Edited by Robert P. Lisak, Daniel D. Truong, William M. Carroll and Roongroj Bhidayasiri

populations, including people of Hispanic, Asian, and African origin. It is encouraging that recent major stroke trials have been expanded to cover non-Western countries. A notable example is the multinational stroke trial to explore the effect of rapid blood pressure lowering in reducing the risk of hematoma expansion following acute intracerebral hemorrhage.

Although modest progress has been made in improving functional recovery after stroke, more research effort is urgently required, including clinical trials to validate innovative rehabilitation measures. Cognitive impairment and consequent dementia after stroke remain a substantial burden in chronic care and there is a great need for developing evidence-based preventive and treatment strategies.

It is essential that integrated stroke care covers not only treatment of patients in the acute setting, but also post-stroke care, including the prevention of stroke recurrence and complications as well as adequate rehabilitative measures to maximize functional recovery. The guidelines developed by the American Heart Association/American Stroke Association and recommendations from the World Stroke Organization encourage stroke prevention and the implementation of timely and adequate standards of care, especially in the acute setting and post-stroke. These are addressed in the relevant chapters to follow, each of which aims to provide an important source of reference to maintain high-quality stroke prevention and care.

2 Ischemic stroke and transient events, TIA

Lidia Yamada, Shelly Ozark, and Bruce Ovbiagele
Department of Neurology and Neurosurgery, Medical University of South Carolina, Charleston, SC, USA

The relevance of timely and appropriate management of a transient ischemic attack (TIA) lies in its frequent role as a forerunner of an impending stroke, which is a leading cause of death, disability, and dementia. We will outline in this chapter the historical context, epidemiology, clinical features, evaluation, and management of TIA patients.

History

Since the seventeenth century, the term "stroke" has represented acute non-traumatic lingering neurological deficits of vascular origin, but it was only in the 1950s that Charles Miller Fisher described the concept of symptomatic yet transient cerebral ischemia received attention. Indeed, it was in 1965 that a consensus term "transient ischemic attack" was introduced to better characterize the occurrence of acute focal, neurological symptoms due to vascular causes that would last "for a shorter period of time." A key controversy over the ensuing 40 years involved agreeing on the actual length of this period of time. Although an arbitrary 24-hour window was originally chosen, several clinicians observed that most of these transient spells would actually last for just a few minutes, at the most no more than a few hours. Another aspect of contention that has arisen relatively more recently following the advent of multimodal neuroimaging has been whether a tissue-based definition of TIA is more precise and prognostic of stroke risk than a time-based definition. Several studies have revealed that a considerable number of TIA patients actually had initial radiographic evidence of ischemic brain injury, a finding that persisted on follow-up brain imaging in many cases. Thus, in 2009, a committee of experts proposed a new pathological definition of TIA, which emphasized a lack of sustained vascular brain injury: "a transient episode of neurological dysfunction caused by focal brain, spinal cord, or retinal ischemia *without acute infarction*." With the introduction of this new tissue-based definition, the old time-based definition for TIA has increasingly fallen into disuse in clinical studies and clinical practice.

Epidemiology

Although the identification of a TIA is considered of major importance to prevent subsequent stroke, estimating its incidence and prevalence can be a challenge. Not infrequently, TIA patients fail to seek medical attention given the transitory nature of symptoms and insufficient knowledge. For other patients, historical details become blurred with time or the symptoms experienced were neurologically non-specific. Therefore, current statistics likely underestimate the real occurrence of TIA around the world. In spite of these limitations, several studies have examined the incidence and prevalence of classically defined TIAs. Johnston *et al.* showed that among 10,112 Americans with TIA symptoms, only 64% sought care within 24 hours of the event. In the United Kingdom, a study by Chandratheva and colleagues observed that only about 67% of patients with TIAs contacted a healthcare provider after symptoms. In Switzerland, a survey of 422 habitants of Bern showed that just 64% of the population interviewed had "good knowledge" of stroke warning signs. In all three studies, lower income and fewer years of education were associated with lesser knowledge of stroke risk factors and the need to seek immediate medical attention in the event of stroke-like symptoms.

A study in Rochester, Minnesota, noted a crude age- and sex-adjusted incidence rate of 68 per 100,000 persons per year for the years 1985–89. TIA incidence rose with age, increasing to 584 per 100,000 persons for those aged 75–84 years. There was no clear sex predilection, but rates were slightly higher among men. In this study, 75% of the TIAs were due to carotid circulation insufficiency, and the rest due to problems in the vertebrobasilar circulation. Approximately 18% of the TIAs were transient monocular blindness (amaurosis fugax). Lower age- and sex-adjusted incidence rates for TIA have been reported from other populations, from a low of 18 per 100,000 persons per year from 1987–88 in Novosibirsk, Russia, to a high of 37 per 100,000 persons per year from 1970–73 in Estonia. Data from England, France, Japan, and Sweden showed similar incidence rates. According to Kokubo, the overall incidence rates of TIA in the European population aged 55–64 years were 0.52–2.37 in men and 0.05–1.14 in women. For the age range 65–74 years, men and women had rates of 0.94–3.39 and 0.71–1.47, respectively. Finally, among those aged 75–84 years, women's TIA incidence ranged from 3.04–7.20, while men's was 2.18–6.06. Overall, time-based TIA incidence rates appear to have remained stable over time. It has been estimated that adopting a tissue-based definition of TIA in the United States would lower estimates of the annual incidence of TIA by 33%, from approximately 180,000 to about 120,000. Studies on TIA prevalence vary widely, but generally run at between 1% and 6% and not surprisingly increase with age.

Risk factors for TIA are congruent to those for stroke. Conventional yet modifiable risk factors include hypertension, smoking,

International Neurology, Second edition. Edited by Robert P. Lisak, Daniel D. Truong, William M. Carroll and Roongroj Bhidayasiri
© 2016 John Wiley & Sons, Ltd. Published 2016 by John Wiley & Sons, Ltd.

diabetes, atrial fibrillation, aortocervicocephalic atherosclerosis, and recent large myocardial infarction.

Comparisons across distinct studies suggest that the 90-day stroke risk is 10–20% after TIA, with the highest risk occurring in the first 48 hours following the TIA, and that when these strokes happen they are disabling or fatal in up to 85% of patients. Some studies suggest that patients with transient monocular blindness have half the risk of stroke compared to patients with a hemispheric TIA, and those with purely sensory symptoms tend to have a lower risk of stroke than patients with motor symptoms or aphasia. Taking into consideration differences between study designs, reviews of prospective emergency department investigations have pointed to the fact that about 1 in 20 patients with a TIA will have a stroke in the next 48 hours, with a 15% chance of the stroke being a fatal event and a 60% risk of sustaining long-term disability. Unfortunately, mounting data indicate that an unacceptably high proportion of TIA patients (vs. stroke patients) are underinvestigated and undertreated during the period of the highest risk of stroke.

Pathophysiology

Although there have been several modifications since, the criteria for subdividing stroke events by their underlying mechanism developed in the original TOAST (Trial of ORG 10172 in acute stroke treatment) study are widely used to classify cerebrovascular events into three major types.

Atherosclerosis of great vessels

Atherosclerosis of great vessels is defined by obstruction of blood flow due to a localized occlusive disease within large arteries. Atherosclerosis resulting from years of gradual plaque formation is considered to be the main cause of luminal obstruction. These stenotic lesions are most commonly seen in the internal carotid arteries and middle cerebral arteries, as well as in the posterior circulation, affecting the vertebrobasilar system.

Occlusion of small vessels

In small artery disease, especially small perforator arterioles, lipohyalinosis is considered to be the main pathological obstructive process, mostly secondary to poorly controlled hypertension.

Cardioembolism

In cardioembolism, a thrombus formed in the heart is dislodged and occludes one of the arteries in the cervicocephalic arterial tree.

The TOAST criteria include two other categories: acute stroke of other determined etiology, which includes patients with rare causes of stroke, such as non-atherosclerotic vasculopathies, hypercoagulable states, or hematologic disorders; and stroke of undetermined etiology, which is estimated to account for approximately 25% of all cerebrovascular events.

The occurrence of non-focal transient cerebral ischemia also deserves mention. TIAs can happen due to reduced blood flow to brain tissue as a result of lower systemic perfusion pressure. Most commonly, this is related to decompensated heart failure, myocardial infarction, cardiac arrhythmias, or hypovolemia. Border zones between major vascular territories, also referred to inaccurately as "watershed territories," are usually more susceptible to these insults. Therefore, many of these events can occur bilaterally, but it is important to keep in mind that a territory supplied by an already stenosed vessel can be more susceptible to ischemia in the face of systemic hypoperfusion.

Clinical features

In most cases, by the time a TIA patient is evaluated by a healthcare provider, his or her neurological deficits have resolved. Therefore, identifying the symptoms as having a vascular origin can be a challenge. A high level of suspicion is fundamental in preventing these "warning signs" from being missed. Some symptoms, such as hemiparesis or dysarthria, are non-specific regarding the location of the vascular injury, since this can be seen in both anterior and posterior circulation ischemia. Other deficits can suggest more specific areas of insult. Aphasia and amaurosis fugax are commonly seen in anterior circulation; that is, carotid territory ischemia. On the other hand, homonymous hemianopia, ataxia, vertigo, diplopia, bilateral weakness, and numbness are mostly ascribed to vertebrobasilar circulation. One should be aware of the so-called stroke and TIA mimics (Table 2.1), especially due to the fact that other neurological processes, such as seizures or demyelinating diseases, also require attention and treatment.

Investigations

Major discussions exist throughout the world regarding the extent of investigation that transient focal neurological signs deserve. To assess the risk of short-term stroke after a TIA, risk factor prediction scores have been created. One of the most commonly used is the ABCD2 score (Table 2.2), where a score of 0–3 is considered "low risk," with a 2-day stroke risk of 1.0%; a score of 4 or 5 is considered "moderate risk," with a 2-day stroke risk of 4.1%; and a score of 6 or 7 is considered "high risk," with a 2-day stroke risk of 8.1%.

Table 2.1. Comparison of typical features of a transient ischemic attack (TIA) to mimics.

Features to suggest TIA	Features more suggestive of TIA mimics	Can be seen in TIAs or TIA mimics (non-specific)
Decreased strength in one limb or in two ipsilateral limbs	Generalized tonic or clonic motor activity	Unilateral involuntary movements in one limb or two limbs (could be due to seizures or "limb-shaking TIA"
	Light-headedness, decreased consciousness, confusion, or amnesia in the absence of other symptoms	
	Positive sensory symptoms, such as tingling	
Complete visual loss in one eye or visual field cut in both eyes (quadrantanopia or homonymous hemianopia)	Scintillating scotomas	
	Bowel or bladder incontinence	
	Headache during or after the event	

Table 2.2. Components and scoring of the ABCD 2 score.

Risk factor	Value	Number of points
Age	>60 years	1 point
Blood pressure	Systolic >140 mmHg or diastolic >90 mmHg	1 point
Clinical symptoms	Unilateral weakness Speech impairment without weakness	2 points 1 point
Duration of symptoms	>60 minutes 10–59 minutes	2 points 1 point
Diabetes	Present	1 point

Despite being considered "low-risk" patients, studies have shown that those with ABCD2 scores of 3 or less should not be ignored and deserve to be carefully investigated. Regarding the decision of whether patients with transient focal neurological symptoms should be hospitalized or not, recent investigations have shown hospitalization to be cost-effective for patients with a 2-day risk of stroke of 4% or higher. Observation of the patient in an inpatient setting allows rapid administration of tissue plasminogen activator in the case of recurrent stroke symptoms and facilitates prompt evaluation and initiation of secondary prevention therapies.

By utilizing the ABCD2 scores, most recent guidelines consider it reasonable to hospitalize patients with TIA symptoms if they present within 72 hours of the event with any of the following criteria: ABCD2 score of 3 or more; ABCD2 score of 0–2 and uncertainty that diagnostic workup can be completed within 2 days as an outpatient; or ABCD2 score of 0–2 and other evidence that indicates the patient's event was caused by focal ischemia.

TIA patients should be evaluated as soon as possible after the occurrence of symptoms. The initial assessment should include a full blood count, serum electrolytes and creatinine, fasting blood glucose and lipids, as well as electrocardiogram. Other laboratory studies may be undertaken based on the history and other clinical features, such as concern for hypercoagulable states.

Regarding imaging, most recent TIA guidelines suggest that patients with suspected ischemic events should have neuroimaging performed within 24 hours of symptom onset. Brain MRI (magnetic resonance imaging) with DWI (diffusion-weighted imaging) sequence is the preferred imaging modality, especially when small vessel lesions are suspected, since these can be easily missed on CT (computer tomography) scans in the acute setting.

Non-invasive evaluation of extracranial vasculature should be performed in all patients with suspected ischemic events. In this case, use of either Doppler ultrasonography of the neck, CT, or MRI angiograms is adequate to assess extracranial internal carotid disease. Intracranial vasculature evaluation is considered to be reasonable in cases when the finding of intracranial stenosis can change management. For these, transcranial Doppler ultrasonography, as well as CT and MRI angiograms, can also be used. In specific cases, catheter angiography might be necessary to detect the presence or degree of intracranial arterial disease.

Finally, regarding cardiac evaluation, an electrocardiogram should be performed by the time of the initial assessment, as already mentioned. Preferably, these patients should be kept under telemetry cardiac monitoring for evaluation of possible paroxysmal arrhythmias, such as atrial fibrillation. In cases where an embolic origin is suspected, the use of continuous prolonged cardiac monitoring for 30 days after hospital discharge is suggested. It is reasonable for all TIA patients to have a transthoracic echocardiogram performed as part of the etiological investigation. A transesophageal echocardiogram can be considered for those who had no identifiable etiology of their symptoms despite the aforementioned evaluation.

Treatment

Understanding the ischemic event's pathophysiologic mechanism is crucial to defining what secondary stroke prevention path must be taken. Those with non-cardioembolic etiology of TIA should be started immediately on an antiplatelet agent. Aspirin (50–325 mg/day) is the first-line antiplatelet agent for stroke prevention after a diagnosis of TIA has been made. Clopidogrel (75 mg/day) is an alternative antiplatelet agent for those patients who cannot tolerate aspirin.

Major studies have been published in the last few years regarding whether there is ever a benefit to the use of dual antiplatelet therapy versus aspirin or clopidogrel alone. In 2011, the Stenting vs. Aggressive Medical Management for Preventing Recurrent Stroke in Intracranial Stenosis (SAMMPRIS) trial was published, showing benefit of dual antiplatelet therapy with aspirin plus clopidogrel for three months for patients with recently symptomatic intracranial large vessel atherosclerosis. After this 90-day period, patients should be continued on monotherapy antiplatelet regimen. More recently, the Chinese Clopidogrel in High-risk Patients with Acute Non-disabling Cerebrovascular Events (CHANCE) trial evaluated 5170 patients within 24 hours of TIA or minor ischemic stroke symptoms. They were randomized to either dual therapy with clopidogrel and aspirin (clopidogrel 300 mg loading dose followed by 75 mg/day for 90 days, added to aspirin 75 mg/day) or to placebo and aspirin 75 mg/day. This study showed a significant efficacy in secondary stroke prevention in the dual antiplatelet therapy arm compared to the aspirin-only group. It is important to mention that it included patients with high-risk TIA only and excluded patients with isolated dizziness, isolated visual changes, and isolated sensory symptoms with no evidence of acute infarction on neuroimaging. It should also be taken into consideration that the Chinese population appears to have a higher rate of intracranial large vessel atherosclerosis as compared to Caucasians.

In patients with known embolic etiology of a cerebral ischemic event, anticoagulation with warfarin or one of the new oral anticoagulant agents, such as dabigatran, rivaroxaban, apixaban, or edoxaban, is recommended. The therapy of choice will depend on multiple factors, such as cost, patient preference, renal function, and drug interaction. Of note is that there is still no strong evidence that the new agents are appropriate for treating patients with thrombus formed by valvular heart disease. For this population, warfarin remains the therapy of choice. If a cardioembolic source is suspected but not confirmed, it is reasonable to continue to evaluate the patient for arrhythmias after hospital discharge with prolonged cardiac monitoring (for approximately 30 days).

Recognized as an important stroke and TIA risk factor, hypertension should be carefully identified and treated. Blood pressure–lowering agents are indicated for those with a known history of hypertension or newly diagnosed patients who after a TIA have an established systolic blood pressure greater than 140 mmHg or diastolic greater than 90 mmHg. It is considered reasonable to set a goal of systolic blood pressure lower than 140 mmHg and a diastolic lower than 90 mmHg for secondary ischemic event prevention.

Identifying those with diabetes mellitus by ordering HbA1c levels is of major importance and should be part of the evaluation of all patients presenting with focal neurological symptoms. Patients should also be screened for obesity. Although there is no clear evidence regarding the usefulness of weight loss among patients with a recent TIA and obesity, the known beneficial effects of weight loss on cardiovascular risk factor control should be taken into consideration. It is the healthcare provider's role to counsel these patients regarding physical activity and balanced nutrition. Tobacco use has been clearly associated with overall increased risk of vascular disease and patients should be strongly advised regarding smoke cessation, as well as avoiding passive tobacco exposure.

Given the results of the Stroke Prevention by Aggressive Reduction in Cholesterol Levels (SPARCL) trial, aggressive lipid lowering is recommended for the prevention of secondary cerebral ischemic events. Currently, a low-density lipoprotein (LDL) goal of <100 mg/dL is strongly advised, some suggesting an even lower level (<70) for those with a concomitant diagnosis of diabetes. For patients in whom atherosclerotic disease is thought to be the etiology of their event, current guidelines recommend high-dose statin therapy regardless of baseline LDL.

Recent recommendations have been made for those patients with suspected or established diagnosis of obstructive sleep apnea. Treatment of sleep apnea improves outcome in patients with a stroke or TIA. Therefore, it is reasonable to consider formal sleep studies for this population, especially when there is a high level of suspicion for sleep apnea.

In the matter of carotid disease, based on multiple studies in the past decade regarding symptomatic carotid atherosclerosis, current recommendations are the following for patients with a TIA within the past six months:

- Ipsilateral 70–99% (severe) carotid artery stenosis: open procedure carotid endarterectomy (CEA) is the treatment of choice if the perioperative morbidity and mortality risk is estimated to be <6%.
- Ipsilateral 50–69% (moderate) carotid stenosis: CEA is recommended depending on the patient's age, sex, and comorbidities, also if the perioperative morbidity and mortality risk is <6%.
- Ipsilateral <50% stenosis: CEA or carotid stenting is not recommended.

It is reasonable to perform the surgery in the first two weeks after the ischemic event rather than delaying it. Carotid stenting can be considered in those with symptomatic carotid disease, severe carotid stenosis, and average or low risk of complications associated with endovascular intervention. Also, for younger patients, carotid stenting is currently being considered equivalent to CEA regarding risk for periprocedural complications and long-term risk for ipsilateral stroke.

Conclusions

Over 60 years after Miller Fisher's initial description of transient ischemic attacks, it is extremely important for patients with these events to be promptly identified and appropriately managed. Better identification will involve intensified efforts at routine and regular education of the lay public and the medical enterprise, as well ongoing dissemination of new knowledge and reminders to clinicians caring for people with, or at risk for, stroke. A TIA should be treated as a warning sign, a narrow window of opportunity to target patients at imminent risk of experiencing the devastating consequences of permanent brain ischemia, with proven interventions for preventing stroke.

Further reading

Adams HP, Bendixen BH, Kappelle LJ, et al. Classification of subtype of acute ischemic stroke: Definitions for use in a multicenter clinical trial. TOAST. Trial of Org 10172 in Acute Stroke Treatment. *Stroke* 1993;24(1):35–41.

Chandratheva A, Lasserson DS, Geraghty OC, Rothwell PM; Oxford Vascular Study. Population-based study of behavior immediately after transient ischemic attack and minor stroke in 1000 consecutive patients: Lessons for public education. *Stroke* 2010;41(6):1108–1114.

Chimowitz MI, Lynn MJ, Derdeyn CP, et al. Stenting versus aggressive medical therapy for intracranial arterial stenosis. *N Engl J Med* 2011;365(11):993–1003. doi:10.1056/NEJMoa1105335

Easton JD, Saver JL, Albers GW, et al. Definition and evaluation of transient ischemic attack: A scientific statement for healthcare professionals from the American Heart Association/American Stroke Association Stroke Council; Council on Cardiovascular Surgery and Anesthesia; Council on Cardiovascular Radiology and Intervention; Council on Cardiovascular Nursing; and the Interdisciplinary Council on Peripheral Vascular Disease. *Stroke* 2009;40(6):2276–2293.

Johnston SC. Short-term prognosis after a TIA: A simple score predicts risk. *Cleveland Clin J Med* 2007;74(10):729–736.

Johnston SC, Fayad PB, Gorelick PB, et al. Prevalence and knowledge of transient ischemic attack among US adults. *Neurology* 2003;60(9):1429–1434.

Kernan WN, Ovbiagele B, Black HR, et al. Guidelines for the prevention of stroke in patients with stroke and transient ischemic attack: A guideline for healthcare professionals from the American Heart Association/American Stroke Association. *Stroke* 2007;45(7):2160–2236.

Kokubo Y. Epidemiology of transient ischemic attack. *Front Neurol Neurosci* 2014;33:69–81. doi:10.1159/000351892

Nedeltchev K, Fischer U, Arnold M, Kappeler L, Mattle H. Low awareness of transient ischemic attacks and risk factors of stroke in a Swiss urban community. *J Neurol* 2007;254(2):179–184.

Ovbiagele B, Kidwell CS, Saver JL. Epidemiological impact in the United States of a tissue-based definition of transient ischemic attack. *Stroke* 2003;34:919–992.

Wang Y, Wang Y, Zhao X, et al. Clopidogrel with aspirin in acute minor stroke or transient ischemic attack. *N Engl J Med* 2013;369(1):11–19.

3 Atherothrombotic disease

Nijasri C. Suwanwela
Department of Medicine, Chulalongkorn University, Bangkok, Thailand

Atherosclerosis is one of the major causes of ischemic stroke worldwide. Among patients presenting with acute ischemic stroke, atherosclerosis of the large arteries accounts for 20–45% of cases. Classic risk factors for atherosclerosis are classified as modifiable risks such as hypertension, diabetes, dyslipidemia, smoking, and high C-reactive protein, and non-modifiable risks that include advanced age and male sex.

Site of atheroslerosis

Although atherosclerosis is a generalized condition involving various vascular beds, atherosclerotic plaque formation tends to be a strategically focal process at the arterial branch points and bifurcations. For arteries supplying the brain, common sites of atherosclerosis include the carotid bifurcation in the neck, the carotid siphon, the proximal portion of intracranial arteries around the circle of Willis, the proximal and distal portions of the vertebral artery, the basilar artery, and the ascending aorta.

Atherosclerosis of extracranial arteries in the neck

Disease of the carotid arteries in the neck, especially at the carotid bifurcation and origin of the internal carotid artery, has long been known to be common among Caucasians. The risk of stroke depends on the degree of stenosis as well as atherosclerotic plaque characteristics. More severe stenosis (>70%) and plaque with evidence of lipid core, intraplaque hemorrhage, irregular surface, or ulceration carry a greater risk of ischemic stroke in the ipsilateral cerebral hemisphere. The proximal part of the vertebral artery is another site of atherosclerosis, and is generally underdiagnosed.

Atherosclerosis of the intracranial arteries

Atherosclerosis of the intracranial arteries is more prevalent in Asians, black people, and Hispanics. Studies from Asia demonstrate that intracranial atherosclerosis accounts for at least one-fourth of all ischemic strokes. The explanation for this ethnic difference is still unclear. Some genetic and environmental factors have been proposed. Common sites of intracranial atherosclerosis are the proximal middle cerebral artery, carotid siphon, midbasilar artery, distal vertebral artery, and proximal anterior and posterior cerebral arteries.

Ascending aorta

Atherosclerosis of the ascending aorta, especially when plaque thickness is greater than 4 mm, has been shown to be associated with embolic stroke.

Mechanisms of stroke and clinical manifestations

The mechanism of stroke in patients with atherosclerosis can be classified into three main categories.

Arterial to arterial embolism

Arterial to arterial embolism is the major mechanism of stroke among patients with atherosclerosis in the extracranial cervical artery and ascending aorta. It is the cause of stroke in some patients with intracranial disease. Embolic stroke occurs when a portion of thrombus or atherosclerotic plaque that originates in stenotic arteries, especially those with an irregular surface, dislodges and travels into the distal arteries.

Clinically, patients with extracranial carotid stenosis with arterial to arterial embolism present with ischemic stroke in the cortical and subcortical areas of the anterior circulation, particularly in the middle cerebral artery territory. Preceding non-stereotyped repeated transient ischemic attack (TIA) involving the same hemisphere and transient monocular blindness are common. In patients with intracranial atherosclerosis with distal embolism, ischemic stroke with fluctuation, stepwise, or progressive symptoms can be found. Emboli from atherosclerosis in the posterior circulation can occlude the branches of the vertebral and basilar arteries. The embolism may travel to the distal end or top of the basilar artery, causing thalamic, midbrain, occipital lobe, and sometimes cerebellar infarction. Frequently, multiple small emboli that travel to distal arteries are asymptomatic. They can only be demonstrated by diffusion imaging as multiple small infarcts or by transcranial Doppler ultrasound monitoring for microembolic signals.

Low-flow state secondary to severe arterial stenosis or occlusion

This mechanism of stroke and TIA is usually found in patients with severe arterial stenosis or occlusion with inadequate distal perfusion and insufficient collateral circulation. Stroke or TIA usually occurs in the distal territories or border-zone areas between the major cerebral arteries. The TIAs are generally stereotyped and may be aggravated by systemic hypoperfusion. Although uncommon, very severe extracranial carotid stenosis can cause low-flow TIA with stereotypic focal limb weakness and sometimes limb-shaking episodes resembling focal seizures, which is called limb-shaking TIA. Low-flow stroke in patients with intracranial atherosclerosis may present with progressive or fluctuating symptoms in the affected vascular territory. Special precautions have

International Neurology, Second edition. Edited by Robert P. Lisak, Daniel D. Truong, William M. Carroll and Roongroj Bhidayasiri
© 2016 John Wiley & Sons, Ltd. Published 2016 by John Wiley & Sons, Ltd.

to be taken in the posterior circulation, especially basilar artery disease, since the progression of symptoms may extend over 7–10 days and basilar occlusion has a very high fatality rate.

Occlusion of the perforating arteries due to atherosclerotic plaque

In patients with atherosclerosis of the intracranial arteries, atherosclerotic plaque may occlude the orifice of the perforating arteries, causing infarction in the deep areas of the brain such as the basal ganglia in middle cerebral artery disease, and the pons and midbrain in basilar atherosclerosis. The clinical syndrome of these patients may resemble lacunar infarction, but the areas of infarction on brain imaging are usually larger.

Investigations

The diagnosis of atherosclerosis is based on two important findings: direct evidence of atherosclerotic plaque in the arterial wall and indirect evidence of luminal stenosis.

Atherosclerotic plaque can be visualized by imaging the arterial wall. Ultrasonography is the most widely available non-invasive method to visualize the vascular wall of the extracranial arteries. Using B-mode and duplex ultrasound, plaque components and surface as well as the degree of stenosis can be determined. Carotid duplex ultrasound is the most useful tool for the diagnosis of extracranial internal carotid stenosis, which may require surgical management.

Transesophageal echocardiogram is another ultrasound technique used for evaluation of the ascending aorta as a source of embolic stroke.

In some patients, especially those with atherosclerosis of intracranial arteries, the details of the arterial wall cannot be visualized using ultrasonography. The diagnosis of atherosclerosis is generally made by the presence of arterial stenosis at the common site, together with the established atherosclerotic risk factors. Significant intracranial artery stenosis can be diagnosed by the changes in flow velocity and pattern on transcranial ultrasound, and arterial lumen narrowing can be visualized on magnetic resonance (MRI) angiography and computed tomography (CT) angiography. These vascular imaging techniques can evaluate localization, degree of stenosis, and collateral circulation. Recently, high-resolution MRI and CT scanning has also been used to visualize the arterial wall of the intracranial arteries. Cerebral angiography is only recommended in cases with inconclusive results from non-invasive studies and for which intravascular procedures are indicated.

Management of large vessel atherosclerosis

The management of acute ischemic stroke due to large vessel atherothrombosis consists of rapidly establishing the pathophysiology of the arterial lesion responsible for the ischemia, as well as the location and extent of infarct. In the acute phase of stroke, intravenous thrombolytics should be considered in eligible patients. Endovascular intervention for acute ischemic stroke due to occlusion of the internal carotid artery or proximal middle cerebral artery, with retrievable stent following intravenous recombinant tissue plasminogen activator (rtPA) within six hours of symptom onset, has been shown to be effective. The treatment has been added as a new evidence-based therapy (Class I and Level of evidence A) in the American Heart Association/American Stroke Association

guidelines of June 2015. Antiplatelets should be given as early as possible. Anticoagulants may be used in patients with large vessel atherosclerosis who have progressive or unstable neurological symptoms, but this recommendation is not based on evidence from randomized controlled trials. In the case of progressive or fluctuating stroke, blood pressure should be monitored closely to avoid hypotension and extreme hypertension, since patients with severe stenosis of the large artery may sometimes be blood pressure sensitive. Adequate hydration and keeping the patient's head flat on the bed are also recommended.

In patients with transient ischemic attack or minor stroke who presented within 24 hours of the event, loading of clopidogrel 300 mg followed by 75 mg/day plus aspirin for three weeks was proven to be effective in preventing early recurrence without increasing risk of bleeding. In patients who received statin treatment prior to stroke, the medication should not be discontinued.

Special consideration has to be paid to the prevention of recurrent events, since it has been shown that patients with large vessel atherosclerosis have a poorer prognosis than those with other types of ischemic stroke. Moreover, these patients tend to have a greater risk of major coronary events and vascular death.

For symptomatic extracranial internal carotid atherosclerosis with more than 70% stenosis, a revascularization procedure is recommended. Among such procedures, carotid endarterectomy and carotid artery stenting have been shown to have similar short- and long-term outcomes. However, perioperative stroke was significantly higher in the stenting group, with the benefits of endarterectomy more pronounced in elderly patients. The surgery should be performed as soon as the symptomatic stroke is stable, preferably within two weeks after stroke. In patients with significant stenosis of the extracranial internal carotid artery with evidence of microemboli on transcranial ultrasound monitoring, the combination of aspirin and clopidogrel has been shown to temporarily reduce the number of emboli as well as recurrent TIA and stroke. However, if there are no contraindications, carotid endarterectomy should be performed without delay.

For patients with intracranial atherosclerosis, long-term secondary prevention by dual antiplatelets with aggressive risk factor modification was shown to be superior to endovascular treatment. A combination of aspirin and clopidogrel or aspirin and cilostazol for 3–6 months followed by a long-term single antiplatelet is reasonable for secondary prevention.

Lifestyle modification and risk factor management, as well as medical treatment including long-term antiplatelet therapy, can reduce the risk of recurrent stroke. Reduction of blood pressure to less than 140/90 mmHg and low-density lipoprotein to less than 100 mg/dL with statins is generally recommended. Moreover, prevention of further atherosclerotic plaque progression and possibly regression has been observed in patients treated with angiotensin-converting enzyme inhibitors, angiotensin receptor blockers, and statins.

Further reading

Caplan LR, Wong KS, Gao S, Hennerici MG. Is hypoperfusion an important cause of strokes? If so, how? *Cerebrovasc Dis* 2006;21(3):145–153.

Derdeyn CP, Chimowitz MI, Lynn MJ, *et al.*; Stenting and Aggressive Medical Management for Preventing Recurrent Stroke in Intracranial Stenosis Trial Investigators. Aggressive medical treatment with or without stenting in high-risk patients with intracranial artery stenosis (SAMMPRIS): The final results of a randomised trial. *Lancet* 2014;383(9914):333–341.

Kwon SU, Hong KS, Kang DW, *et al*. Efficacy and safety of combination antiplatelet therapies in patients with symptomatic intracranial atherosclerotic stenosis. *Stroke* 2011;42(10):2883–2890.

Lee DK, Kim JS, Kwon SU, Yoo SH, Kang DW. Lesion patterns and stroke mechanism in atherosclerotic middle cerebral artery disease: Early diffusion-weighted imaging study. *Stroke* 2005;36(12):2583–2588.

Mantese VA, Timaran CH, Chiu D, *et al*.; CREST Investigators. The Carotid Revascularization Endarterectomy versus Stenting Trial (CREST): Stenting versus carotid endarterectomy for carotid disease. *Stroke* 2010;41(10 Suppl):S31–S34.

Suwanwela N, Koroshetz WJ. Acute ischemic stroke: Overview of recent therapeutic developments. *Annu Rev Med* 2007;58:89–106.

Wang Y, Wang Y, Zhao X, *et al*.; CHANCE Investigators. Clopidogrel with aspirin in acute minor stroke or transient ischemic attack. *N Engl J Med* 2013;369(1):11–19.

Wong KS, Chen C, Fu J, et al.; CLAIR Study Investigators. Clopidogrel plus aspirin versus aspirin alone for reducing embolisation in patients with acute symptomatic cerebral or carotid artery stenosis (CLAIR Study): A randomised, open-label, blinded-endpoint trial. *Lancet Neurol* 2010;9(5):489–497.

4 Occlusive disease of small penetrating arteries

Marie Dagonnier, Takeshi Iwanaga, Hock L. Teoh, Jorge A. Zavala, and Geoffrey A. Donnan
The Florey Institute of Neurosciences and Mental Health, University of Melbourne, Heidelberg, VIC, Australia

Durand-Fardel first introduced the terms "lacunes" as small cavities seen in the core of cerebral infarcts and "état criblé" as perivascular space dilatation in 1843. From 1965, Fisher studied small, deep infarcts and described the classical lacunar syndromes as the result of penetrating artery occlusion. It is now known that most lacunar infarcts occur within the lenticulostriate, thalamoperforators, and pontine paramedian arterial territories. Lacunar infarcts are usually due to occlusion of a single penetrating artery.

Epidemiology

In hospital-based series, the proportion of lacunar syndrome ranges from 14–28% of all ischemic strokes. In community-based incidence studies, lacunar strokes represent a similar proportion of all strokes except in some Asian countries, such as China and Japan, where they are reported to account for 38–54% of ischemic strokes (Table 4.1).

Hypertension is the most important modifiable risk factor for ischemic stroke, and is present in more than half of patients. The risk of lacunar infarction is increased five- to ninefold in hypertensives, which is not unexpected since microatheroma and lipohyalinosis are linked to hypertension (see later discussion).

There is about a two- to threefold increased risk of lacunar stroke in individuals with diabetes mellitus. Smoking is a significant risk factor for lacunar strokes, with some suggestion that it may play a more important role as a risk factor in this type of stroke than for other forms of ischemic stroke. Heart disease, including ischemic heart disease (IHD), is a risk factor for ischemic stroke, but may be less so for lacunar syndromes.

Pathophysiology

Lacunar infarcts occur in the territory of penetrating arteries. Table 4.2 shows their branches and territories. Fisher demonstrated in autopsy studies that lacunar infarcts are caused by two forms of arteriopathy: lipohyalinosis and microatheroma. Lipohyalinosis is a destructive small lesion in penetrating arteries (40–200 μm in diameter) characterized by fibrinoid necrosis, loss of normal wall structure, and collagenous sclerosis. It probably accounts for many of the asymptomatic smaller lacunes. Microatheroma (200–800 μm in diameter) can lead to occlusive thrombus and infarcts that tend to be larger than those associated with lipohyalinosis (5 mm or more in diameter) and are usually symptomatic (Figure 4.1).

Although the mechanism of lacunar infarction is traditionally held to be *in situ* small vessel disease, there is some evidence for an embolic cause in a small proportion of cases. Indeed, aortic arch atheroma has been demonstrated to be a risk factor for lacunar infarction. Whether this is a reflection of diffuse cardiovascular atheromatous load rather than an embolic source is uncertain.

Table 4.1. Lacunar strokes in community-based studies.

Study	Total number of ischemic strokes	Lacunar ischemic strokes
Mayo Clinic, United States (1991)	1382	159 (11.5%)
Oxfordshire Project, Europe (1993)	2740	660 (26.7%)
Takashima, Japan (2004)	M 781 F 608	427 (54.7%) 324 (53.3%)
China (2007)	3905	1650 (42%)
Canada (2008)	11503	2196 (19.1%)
Barcelona, Spain (2009)	M 2274 F 2318	375 (16.2%) 488 (21.5%)
Bergen, Norway (2013)	1886	317 (16.8%)
Lombardia, Italy (2012)	8564	1983 (23%)

Table 4.2. Penetrating arteries, their branches, and regions supplied.

Penetrating arteries	Branch	Regions supplied
Lenticulostriate	Medial lenticulostriate artery Lateral lenticulostriate artery	Lateral globus pallidus, medial putamen Lateral putamen, external capsule, upper internal capsule, corona radiata
Thalamoperforating	Tuberothalamic artery Paramedian artery Thalamogeniculate artery Posterior choroidal artery	Anteromedial and anterolateral thalamus Posteromedial thalamus Ventrolateral thalamus Pulvinar and posterior thalamus
Paramedian	–	Basis pons, ventral part of tegmentum

International Neurology, Second edition. Edited by Robert P. Lisak, Daniel D. Truong, William M. Carroll and Roongroj Bhidayasiri
© 2016 John Wiley & Sons, Ltd. Published 2016 by John Wiley & Sons, Ltd.

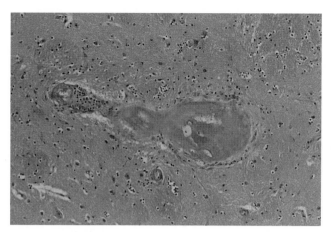

Figure 4.1 Lipohyalin mural change in a caudate nucleus arteriole, with possible microaneurysm formation. (Hematoxylin and eosin stain x200.) For color details, please refer to the color plates section.

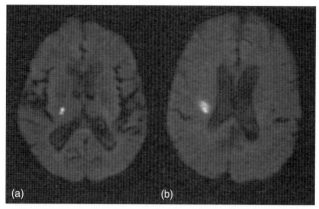

Figure 4.2 Diffusion-weighted images (DWI) showing lacunar infarcts (a) in the posterior limb of the right internal capsule; (b) in the right corona radiata.

Clinical features

Traditionally, lacunar infarction has been associated with five clinical syndromes. Pure motor hemiparesis is the most common syndrome (about 50% of all cases) and involves complete or incomplete facial, arm, and leg paresis. The most common site of infarction is the posterior limb of the internal capsule. Other sites are the corona radiata, pons, and medial medulla.

Sensorimotor stroke is the second most common lacunar syndrome (about 20%). The combination of ipsilateral hemiparesis and hemihypesthesia is the main distinguishing feature. The most common site is the posterior limb of the internal capsule.

Pure sensory stroke is characterized by face, arm, and leg numbness on one side, with absence of weakness and higher cortical dysfunction. In 10% of cases the symptoms may be transient. The most common site of infarction is the thalamus.

Ataxic hemiparesis encompasses hemiparesis combined with an ipsilateral cerebellar-like ataxia. Common infarct sites are the pons and internal capsule. Facial weakness, severe dysarthria, and dysphagia combined with mild weakness and hand clumsiness are the features of the dysarthria clumsy hand syndrome. The site of infarction is frequently the internal capsule. Subcortical transient ischemic attacks (TIA) comprised of transient lacunar syndromes occur in brief clusters (the 'capsular warning syndrome'), and may evolve into capsular infarction.

In general, lacunar infarction carries an overall good prognosis. In contrast with other strokes, functional disability is relatively mild. The five-year survival rate is over 80%, and five-year stroke-free survival rates are over 60%. Predictors of recurrent stroke are age, degree of neurological dysfunction, functional disability, diabetes mellitus, and leukoaraiosis.

Contrary to the historical belief that the classic lacunar syndromes did not include cognitive impairment, there is now undoubtedly a body of evidence to suggest that the development of cognitive impairment and dementia may be features of cerebral small vessel infarction. Cognitive function is often intact in the acute phase, but may progressively decline over the long term. Cognitive impairment as measured by performance on the Mini Mental State Examination (MMSE) one year after stroke is present in 5%, and rises to 11% after three years. There is an overall estimated 11–23% risk of developing dementia following a lacunar stroke, and this risk increases with recurrent lacunar events and the presence of concurrent white matter disease.

Investigations

Computed tomography (CT) is the most widely used neuroimaging diagnostic method in the acute setting. However, CT often fails to reveal lesions in the first 48 hours or those that are smaller than 10 mm. Magnetic resonance imaging (MRI) has been shown to be more sensitive than CT in the diagnosis of strokes, particularly for small, deep infarcts. Diffusion-weighted MRI (DWI) is especially useful in showing lacunar infarcts soon after symptoms begin, and in separating recent infarcts from old infarcts. Hence, MRI is the preferred method, either in the acute subset or for patient follow-up (Figure 4.2).

Treatment

Previously, lacunar strokes were not studied on their own but as a subgroup in large stroke trials. Recently, however, there has been increasing interest in the specific treatment of lacunar stroke.

Acute stroke therapy

In a meta-analysis of large trials (International Stroke Trial and Chinese Acute Stroke Trial), early aspirin significantly reduced the risk of recurrent ischemic stroke (including lacunar stroke), accompanied by a minor increase in the risk of hemorrhagic stroke or hemorrhagic transformation. Aspirin also reduces the overall risk of death or dependency. Thrombolysis with intravenous recombinant tissue plasminogen activator (rtPA) within 4.5 hours improves the overall clinical outcome of ischemic stroke, and there is currently no evidence that lacunar strokes should not benefit from thrombolysis as do other stroke subtypes.

Secondary prevention

Lacunar stroke patients are often included in secondary prevention trials because their level of impairment is usually low. Indeed, they are often overrepresented in these trials ('lacunarization' of secondary prevention trials). Hence, secondary prevention of stroke with antiplatelet agents (aspirin, clopidogrel, aspirin plus dipyridamole), blood pressure lowering with perindopril and indapamide or ramipril, and cholesterol lowering with atorvastatin are most likely effective for lacunar strokes as well as for ischemic stroke overall. Recently, in the Study of Prevention of Small Subcortical Strokes (SPS3) trial in which secondary prevention in lacunar strokes was studied, it was shown that careful blood pressure management (systolic below 130 mmHg, with any medication) was associated with a reduction of symptomatic intracerebral hemorrhage, but not ischemic stroke recurrence. In the same trial it was shown that the addition of clopidogrel to aspirin did not significantly reduce the risk of recurrent stroke, but did significantly increase the risk of bleeding and death.

Further reading

Donnan G, Norrving B. Lacunes and lacunar syndromes. *Handb Clin Neurol* 2009;93:559–575.

Donnan G, Norrving B, Bamford J, Bogousslavsky J. *Subcortical Stroke* (2nd edn). Oxford: Oxford University Press; 2002.

Fisher CM. Lacun ar strokes and infarcts: A review. *Neurology* 1982;32:871–876.

IST-3 Collaborative Group. The benefits and harms of intravenous thrombolysis with recombinant tissue plasminogen activator within 6 h of acute ischaemic stroke (the Third International Stroke Trial [IST-3]): A randomised controlled trial. *Lancet* 2012;379:2352–2363.

Pantoni L, Gorelick P. *Cerebral Small Vessel Disease.* Cambridge: Cambridge University Press; 2014.

SPS3 Study Group. Blood-pressure targets in patients with recent lacunar stroke: The SPS3 randomised trial. *Lancet* 2013;382:507–515.

5 Ischemic white matter disease (Binswanger's disease)

Saltanat Kamenova, Aida Kondybayeva, and Assiya Akanova
Asfendiyarov Kazakh National Medical University, Department of Internship and Residency by Neurology, Almaty Kazakhstan.

Binswanger's disease, also known as subcortical arteriosclerotic encephalopathy or subcortical leukoencephalopathy, is a type of vascular dementia characterized pathologically by cerebral hemispheric white matter lesions and clinically by progressive dementia or other neurological disorders related to white matter damage, as well as episodes of acute focal symptoms. First described by Dr. Otto Binswanger in 1894, it was Dr. Alois Alzheimer who, in 1902, suggested the name "Binswanger's disease" in recognition of the fact that this condition was a distinct nosological entity.

Epidemiology

Historically, diagnosis of Binswanger's disease was made only post-mortem. Binswanger's disease is listed as a "rare disease" by the Office of Rare Diseases (ORD) of the US National Institutes of Health (NIH). This means that Binswanger's disease, or a subtype of it, affects fewer than 200,000 people in the US population. With the introduction of neuroimaging techniques into clinical practice, Binswanger's disease has been noted more frequently and it is now recognized to represent approximately one-third of all cases of vascular dementia. More than 80% of patients with Binswanger's disease have onset between the ages of 50 and 70 years. The disease evolves gradually.

The main risk factor for developing Binswanger's disease is resistant arterial hypertension, which is present in 75–90% of patients. In the elderly, another risk factor may be arterial hypotension.

Pathophysiology

Binswanger's disease is frequently characterized by recurrent transient ischemic attacks and "small strokes," with reversible hemiparesis and pure motor weakness, uneven reflexes, akinesia, and other mild neurological deficits. Microangiopathy can be a pathological feature of amyloid angiopathy, as in the hereditary types such as cerebral autosomal dominant arteriopathy with subcortical infarcts and leukoencephalopathy (CADASIL). Compared to most cases of subcortical progressive encephalopathy, CADASIL occurs at a relatively younger age. The pathological feature that may underlie clinical manifestations of dementia in Binswanger's disease is the presence of diffuse lesions in subcortical white matter as a consequence of arterial hypertension, with accompanying severe cerebral arteriosclerosis involving deep penetrating arteries and arterioles in both hemispheres, leading to chronic cerebral hypoperfusion and white matter ischemia. Increase in blood–brain barrier permeability caused by arterial hypertension is compounded by expansion of the perivascular space in the brain parenchyma. White matter–impregnated edematous fluid contains plasma proteins. Persistent edema, along with progressive loss of fibers in white matter, is the most important factor in the development of spongiosis, which results in the destruction of oligodendroglia and disintegration of myelin. Consequently, diffuse lesions develop in subcortical white matter, primarily periventricular, with foci of incomplete necrosis, loss of myelin, partial disintegration of axons, and diffuse proliferation of astrocytes. Pathophysiologically, dementia in Binswanger's disease is a disconnection syndrome; that is, it is characterized by the separation of cortical–subcortical connections as a result of subcortical white matter lesions. Disconnections may extend to the basal ganglia and thalamus.

Clinical features

In general, Binswanger's disease begins with mild confusion, apathy, personality changes, and memory loss. It is characterized by a steady progression of dementia, usually over a 5–10-year period. However, intervals of stabilization may be noted between deteriorating phases. In late-stage disease, cognitive impairment may be punctuated by misjudgment, disorientation, inability to synthesize and process information, difficulty in decision making, and lack of self-care. Pyramidal or cerebellar dysfunction with gait disturbance may also develop. As the disease progresses further, incontinence and pseudobulbar palsy may set in. Seizures and myoclonia have also been noted in some patients.

Investigations

As proposed by Bennett *et al.*, the diagnostic criteria for Binswanger's disease include: (1) dementia; (2) two of the following three features: vascular risk factors or signs of systemic vascular disease, evidence of focal cerebrovascular disease, or evidence of subcortical cerebral dysfunction (e.g., Parkinsonian rigidity, incontinence); and (3) bilateral leukoaraiosis on computed tomography (CT) or bilateral multiple or diffuse lesions in the white matter of the cerebral hemispheres larger than 2 cm on magnetic resonance imaging (MRI). These criteria may not be valid if the patient has multiple or bilateral cortical lesions on CT or MRI, or severe dementia.

International Neurology, Second edition. Edited by Robert P. Lisak, Daniel D. Truong, William M. Carroll and Roongroj Bhidayasiri
© 2016 John Wiley & Sons, Ltd. Published 2016 by John Wiley & Sons, Ltd.

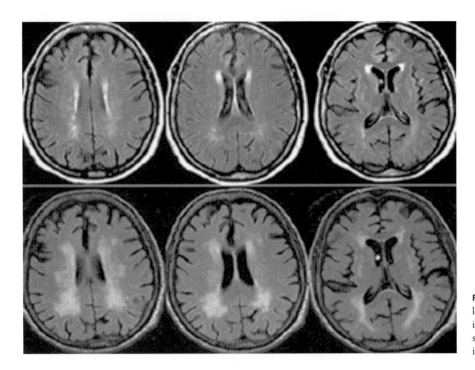

Figure 5.1 On the horizontal section at the level of the lateral ventricles (MRI T2-weighted image) in the periventricular white matter are seen multiple areas of increased signal intensity in the form of leukoaraiosis.

The diagnosis of Binswanger's disease is confirmed by MRI (T2 and FLAIR) or CT based on the following findings: (1) diffuse bilateral density reduction in the white matter, especially around the frontal horns of the lateral ventricles (leukoaraiosis); (2) multiple small cysts in the white matter; and (3) expansion of the ventricle volume (Figure 5.1).

The severity of leukoaraiosis varies from patient to patient and may be related to the degree and duration of underlying hypertension. The most severe and widespread changes are likely to be seen in patients with malignant hypertension presenting with frequent vascular crises. Patients with early dementia may not present leukoaraiosis on neuroimaging.

The most widely criteria for dementia in clinical practice are those proposed by the American Psychiatric Association (DSM IV). The diagnosis of dementia syndrome is based on the clinical evaluation of cognitive, emotional, and social spheres of activity history and the dynamics of the disease. This is a clinical diagnosis that does not include visual methods.

Treatment

Treatment of Binswanger's disease should be directed at the underlying causes, primarily arterial hypertension. However, overtreatment of hypertension may cause clinical deterioration. Currently, there is no FDA- or EMA-approved drug for treating Binswanger's disease.

For primary prevention, if the patient has arterial hypertension a series of measures should be carried out to normalize the pressure. In terms of secondary prevention, there are reports that excessive reduction of blood pressure, especially before the advent of postural hypotension, can cause a condition similar to leukoaraiosis. From this it follows that for vascular dementia blood pressure should not be reduced to normal levels, and in postural hypotension treatment should strive to stabilize blood pressure. Patients are encouraged to adhere to a lifestyle that contributes to the prevention of cerebrovascular accident; that is, to pay attention to their diet, to control their blood pressure, to stop smoking, and not to abuse alcohol, which will avoid injury, hypoxia, and ischemia of the brain.

Further reading

Bennett DA, Wilson RS, Gilley DW, Fox JH. Clinical diagnosis of Binswanger's disease. *J Neurol Neurosurg Psychiatr* 1990;53:961–965.

Caplan L. Binswanger's disease – revisited. *Neurology* 1995;45:626–633.

Gold G. Vascular dementia: A diagnostic challenger. *Int Psychogeriatr* 2003;15: 111–114.

Hachinski V. Binswanger's disease: Neither Binswanger's nor a disease. *J Neur Sci* 1991;103:1.

Right Diagnosis. Prevalence and incidence of Binswanger's disease. http://www. rightdiagnosis.com/b/binswangers_disease/prevalence.htm#prevalence_intro (accessed November 2015).

Roman G, Erkinjuntti T, Wallin A, Pantoni L, Chui HC. Subcortical ischaemic vascular dementia. *Lancet Neurol* 2002;1:426–436.

6 Brain embolism

Bernard P. L. Chan[1], N. Venketasubramanian[2], and Chung Y. Hsu[3]

[1] Department of Medicine, National University Health System, Singapore

[2] Raffles Neuroscience Centre, Raffles Hospital, Singapore

[3] China Medical University, Taichung, Taiwan

Although the heart has traditionally been regarded as the major source of brain embolism, large artery disease (in the aortic arch, neck, and intracranial regions) frequently results in artery-to-artery embolism. Brain embolism can also occur during endovascular procedures for treating cerebrovascular diseases. This chapter focuses on the management of brain embolism of cardiac origin, hereafter referred to as cardiac embolism.

Epidemiology

Cardiac embolism constitutes approximately one-quarter of all ischemic strokes, with a higher incidence among young stroke patients. For individuals aged 45 years and younger, up to half of all strokes can be attributed to cardiac embolism.

Pathophysiology

Established causes of cardiac embolism are listed in Table 6.1. Atrial fibrillation (AF) is the most common cause of cardiac embolism

Table 6.1. Causes of cardiac embolism.

Atrial
Atrial fibrillation
Atrial flutter
Sick-sinus syndrome
Patent foramen ovale ± atrial septal aneurysm
Valvular
Prosthetic valve
Rheumatic mitral valve stenosis
Infective endocarditis
Non-bacterial thrombotic endocarditis
Ventricular
Recent myocardial infarction
Dilated cardiomyopathy/congestive heart failure
Akinetic/dyskinetic segment
Chagas' disease
Endomyocardial fibrosis/hypereosinophilic syndrome
Stress/Takotsubo cardiomyopathy
Left ventricular non-compaction
Cardiac tumors
Atrial myxoma
Papillary fibroelastoma
Iatrogenic
Cardiac surgery
Diagnostic/interventional cardiac catheterization
Intra-aortic balloon counter-pulsation
Left ventricular assist device
Inadvertent left heart pacing

and the leading cause of ischemic stroke in the elderly population, with increasing prevalence as age advances. In developing countries, rheumatic mitral stenosis remains an important cause of cardiac embolism. Cardiomyopathy resulting from Chagas' disease is prevalent in Latin America, whereas endomyocardial fibrosis related to hypereosinophilia with underlying helminthic infections is common in tropical regions of Africa. In developed countries, coronary artery disease and related cardiac surgeries are significant causes of cardiac embolism. Among young stroke patients without an established etiology (cryptogenic stroke), paradoxical embolization through the patent foramen ovale (PFO) is a possible cause in up to 40–56% of this subgroup of patients.

Clinical features

Presentation of cardiac embolism is frequently abrupt, with the worst deficit at onset followed by improvement thereafter. "Spectacular shrinking deficit" occasionally occurs, whereby occlusion of a large cerebral artery (e.g., the proximal middle cerebral artery) undergoes spontaneous early recanalization, resulting in dramatic clinical improvement. However, the clinical course of cardiac embolism does not always follow this pattern, and patient characteristics may be more suggestive of the underlying etiology of brain embolism. For example, patients with large cervicocerebral artery atherosclerosis tend to be older, harbor multiple vascular risk factors, or have preceding transient ischemic attacks (TIAs) in the absence of overt heart disease. Elderly patients with cardioembolic strokes are also likely to have clinically evident cardiac ailments, including AF or coronary artery disease. However, the coexistence of risk factors for both thrombotic and embolic strokes is not uncommon in the elderly. Young stroke patients without apparent risk factors should raise a high index of suspicion of cardiac embolism.

Particular neurological symptoms and signs have been used to predict the likelihood of cardiac embolism. For example, emboli from the heart are believed to be larger than emboli from carotid plaques. Consequently, cardiac emboli tend to occlude the proximal middle cerebral artery (MCA), intracranial internal carotid artery (ICA), or even the carotid bifurcation in the neck, causing more severe strokes; whereas carotid artery emboli tend to cause superficial cortical infarcts associated with milder neurological deficits. Unfortunately, the opposite scenarios also occur frequently. Even in case series of lacunar infarcts mainly caused by penetrating artery disease, about 10% of these strokes are likely cardioembolic in nature. In general, the MCA and its branches carry a substantially

International Neurology, Second edition. Edited by Robert P. Lisak, Daniel D. Truong, William M. Carroll and Roongroj Bhidayasiri
© 2016 John Wiley & Sons, Ltd. Published 2016 by John Wiley & Sons, Ltd.

larger load of emboli than the anterior cerebral artery or the posterior circulation in proportion to the volumes of blood flowing into the respective vascular beds. Nevertheless, cardiac embolism to the vertebrobasilar territory is not uncommon.

Investigations

Computed tomography (CT) and magnetic resonance imaging (MRI) are widely used to localize the infarcts. Like the clinical presentation, neuroimaging may not always be reliable for differentiating embolic from thrombotic stroke. Unilateral infarcts in the watershed territories or border zones are usually associated with hypoperfusion with ipsilateral ICA occlusion. Diffusion-weighted MRI (DWI) can better depict the acute infarcts and may implicate the heart or the aortic arch as the embolic source by revealing multiple infarcts in different vascular territories (Figure 6.1).

As clinical and radiological features are not specific, and multiple potential stroke etiologies or embolic sources may coexist in individual patients, study of the neck and intracranial arteries is recommended in all ischemic stroke patients, using duplex ultrasonography and transcranial Doppler (TCD), CT angiography, or MR angiography.

Routine performance of transthoracic echocardiography (TTE) is associated with a low yield and may be omitted in selected stroke patients with normal cardiac examination, electrocardiogram (ECG), and cardiac enzyme levels, and without a history of heart disease. Transesophageal echocardiography (TEE) is better than TTE in detecting PFO, aortic plaques, and left atrial appendage thrombus, and is recommended in patients with cryptogenic stroke under age 55. Non-invasive screening of right-to-left shunt and plaques in the ascending aorta can be undertaken with TCD after intravenous (IV) injection of bubble-contrast and duplex ultrasonography respectively, before confirmation by TEE.

ECG monitoring to detect paroxysmal AF (PAF) has become more important in the prevention of embolic events, with evidence-based data showing effective stroke prevention by long-term anticoagulant therapy using warfarin or novel oral anticoagulants (NOACs). Traditional 24-hour ECG monitoring by telemetry or Holter device is associated with a low detection rate of PAF of about 2% and is cumbersome to use for more prolonged periods. Longer durations of monitoring up to 4 weeks can be performed with a small "patch" device that transmits real-time ECG recordings through a mobile phone to a central monitor. Recently, a small implantable loop recorder inserted subcutaneously into the precordium has become available, which enables very long durations of continuous ECG monitoring, up to 3 years. Ambulatory ECG monitoring for an additional 1–4 weeks may be considered in patients with cryptogenic stroke or a clinical profile suggestive of cardiac embolism and negative Holter results. However, the cost-effectiveness of more prolonged monitoring with the implantable device has not been established at present.

Treatment

Thrombolysis and mechanical clot retrieval

Fresh emboli from the heart are susceptible to thrombolysis, and IV tissue plasminogen activator (tPA) should be considered in all cardioembolic stroke patients who present within 4.5 hours of onset. The optimal dose of IV tPA for Asian stroke patients is a hotly debated issue, with the regular dose (0.9 mg/kg up to 90 mg) theoretically associated with better recanalization in cardiac embolism, and the lower dose (0.6 mg/kg up to 60 mg) being used in Japan possibly associated with a lower risk of intracerebral hemorrhage (ICH).

Endovascular therapy using new-generation stent retrievers has resulted in improved recanalization rates and significantly better outcomes in a number of recently published clinical trials, and should be considered when such expertise is available. Patients with proximal MCA occlusion (with or without tandem ICA occlusion), minimal early ischemic change on non-contrast CT brain scan, and preservation of collateral circulation to the ischemic territory on CT angiography are the best candidates to receive such therapy if the

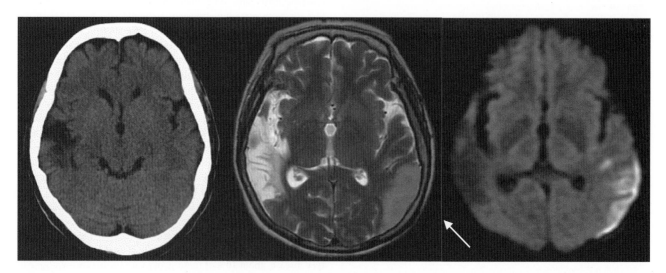

Figure 6.1 A 64-year-old woman in AF presented with acute cortical deafness but recovered over 2 months. CT of the brain (left) on admission showed an old right temporal infarct. T2 MRI (middle) 24 hours after admission revealed an additional recent left temporal infarct, confirmed by DWI (right). Bilateral cortical infarcts are typical of a cardiac source of embolism. Infarct in the territory of the posterior division of the MCA is also suggestive of embolism from a proximal source due to its more direct course from the proximal MCA. As long-term cortical deafness usually requires bilateral damages to the primary auditory cortices, sparing of the left primary auditory cortex likely accounted for the clinical recovery in this patient.

procedure can be initiated within 6 hours of stroke onset, including patients who have received IV tPA therapy within 4.5 hours according to current guidelines. Nevertheless, such aggressive treatment should be individualized and offered after careful consideration of potential risks and benefits among stroke neurologist, neurointerventionalist, patients, and their caregivers.

Although endovascular therapy is currently approved up to 8 hours after stroke onset, every effort should be made to expedite acute stroke evaluation and treatment. Whether it is IV thrombolysis and/or endovascular intervention, the time from stroke onset to possible arterial recanalization should be as short as possible to optimize clinical outcome and reduce the risk of ICH. Currently, a "door-to-needle" time of within 30 minutes for IV thrombolysis can be achieved in experienced stroke centers, whereas CT angiography to procedure and reperfusion times of 60 minutes and 90 minutes respectively were specifically aimed for in some of the successful endovascular treatment trials.

Prevention of recurrent cardiac embolism

Anticoagulation starting with heparin followed by warfarin is evidence-based therapy to prevent recurrent cardiac embolism once it has been established as the cause of stroke. There are small case series showing the safety and benefit of early anticoagulation immediately after stroke onset that outweighed the risk of ICH. However, timing of anticoagulation after acute brain embolism should be individualized. Early anticoagulation may be considered in selected patients with a high risk of recurrent brain embolism (e.g., early stroke recurrence, presence of intracardiac thrombus, increasing number of DWI lesions on repeat brain MRI, or frequent microembolic signals on TCD) and a low risk of cerebral hemorrhage (e.g., absence of large cerebral infarct, hemorrhagic transformation on neuroimaging, concomitant antiplatelet therapy, and uncontrolled hypertension). Prevention of recurrent cardiac embolism in selected conditions is further elaborated later in this chapter.

Infective endocarditis

Thrombolytic and antithrombotic therapies are contraindicated in stroke secondary to infective endocarditis because of the hemorrhagic risk associated with mycotic aneurysms. High-dose IV antibiotic therapy is the mainstay of treatment. Urgent surgery may be indicated in patients with infective endocarditis or cardiac tumors (e.g., atrial myxoma, papillary fibroelastoma) who present with recurrent brain embolism or cardiac failure.

Atrial fibrillation

AF patients with a history of cerebral ischemia or peripheral embolism should be treated with long-term warfarin with dosage adjusted to the target international normalized ratio (INR) of 2.5 (range 2.0–3.0), unless contraindicated. Those without a prior history of embolism should be risk stratified using the $CHADS_2$ score. Recently, the CHA^2DS_2-VASc score has been proposed to improve risk stratification in AF patients with a $CHADS_2$ score of 0–1. Patients with a CHA_2DS_2-VASc score ≥ 2 should take warfarin. Aspirin may suffice in patients with a score of 1. No antithrombotic therapy may be necessary for those with a score of 0 (Table 6.2). Patients with PAF or atrial flutter are treated with the same guidelines as described for AF, as their stroke risks are nearly comparable. Patients with sick-sinus syndrome or carrying a pacemaker require special attention. The former condition is frequently associated with PAF, whereas detection of AF on routine ECG in patients implanted with

a pacemaker may require reprogramming of the pacemaker to lower ventricular rates.

Asian stroke patients with AF on long-term warfarin therapy are recognized to have a higher risk of ICH compared to patients of other ethnic groups. Use of the HAS-BLED score (Table 6.2) can help to assess this risk, with scores ≥ 3 predictive of higher risks of major bleeding and intracranial hemorrhage. Patients with high HAS-BLED scores should be closely monitored while on warfarin, with special efforts to control risk factors associated with bleeding (e.g., elevated blood pressure, labile INR, concomitant aspirin or NSAID [non-steroidal anti-inflammatory drug] therapy).

The recent introduction of NOACs represents a major advance in stroke prevention in patients with AF. One direct thrombin inhibitor (dabigatran) and three direct Factor Xa inhibitors (rivaroxaban, apixaban, and edoxaban) are at least as effective as warfarin in stroke prevention and are associated with half the risk of ICH among AF patients without valvular disease (non-valvular AF, NVAF). In addition, these NOACs are prescribed as fixed doses with drug levels usually not affected by food or concomitant medications. Furthermore, frequent blood draws to check INR for dose adjustment are not needed. Besides higher costs, NOACs have several limitations, however. NOACs are excreted by the kidney. Patients with renal dysfunction may have a higher risk of developing bleeding complications on NOACs and need to have the doses more carefully adjusted based on renal function. With the exception of apixaban, the risk of gastrointestinal bleeding is higher with NOACs than with warfarin. Due to their quick onset of action, NOACs should not be commenced in acute stroke patients with a large infarct or uncontrolled hypertension who are at higher risk of ICH. Compliance

Table 6.2 Stroke and bleeding risk scores for atrial fibrillation patients.

CHADS₂	Score
Congestive heart failure	1
Hypertension	1
Age ≥ 75 years	1
Diabetes mellitus	1
Stroke/TIA/embolism	2
≥ 2: Long-term anticoagulant	
0-1: Aspirin	

CHA₂DS₂-VASc	Score
Congestive heart failure	1
Hypertension	1
Age ≥ 75 years	2
Diabetes mellitus	1
Stroke/TIA/embolism	2
Vascular disease (CAD, PVD) 1	
Age 65–74 years	1
Sex category (Female)	1
≥ 2: Long-term anticoagulant	
1: Aspirin	
0: No antithrombotic	

HAS-BLED	Score
Hypertension (uncontrolled BP)	1
Abnormal renal/liver function	1 or 2
Stroke	1
Bleeding tendency	1
Labile INR while on warfarin	1
agE >65 years or frail condition 1	
Drugs (aspirin, NSAID) or alcohol abuse	1 or 2
≥ 3: High risk of major/intracranial bleeding	

with NOAC medication should be emphasized, as missing even one or two doses may raise stroke risk due to the short plasma half-lives of these agents. Caution should be exercised in prescribing NOACs to the elderly, pregnant women, and children because of limited experience in these patient populations. In contrast to warfarin, there is no antidote for NOACs to restore normal coagulation in the event of a major bleeding complication or emergency surgery. NOAC-induced ICH is addressed in Chapter 10.

If long-term anticoagulation is a contraindication, percutaneous closure of the left atrial appendage (LAA) using one of the available devices (e.g., Watchman, ACP, or Lariat) is an option, since the majority of cardiac emboli in NVAF patients originate from the LAA. However, device closure of the LAA is associated with periprocedural complications that include death, bleeding, device leakage, pericardial effusion/tamponade, cardiac perforation, and air or device embolization. Moreover, initial anticoagulation followed by combined aspirin–clopidogrel therapy is usually required for a few months after LAA closure. The Watchman device is the only one to date shown to be non-inferior to warfarin therapy in a trial of 707 patients. Large-scale randomized trials comparing LAA closure with anticoagulation using NOACs are needed to establish the safety and efficacy of LAA closure with mechanical devices, and to identify subgroups of NVAF patients who may benefit more from device closure than from long-term anticoagulation.

Catheter ablation of AF to restore normal sinus rhythms is an option as a first-line therapy. Catheter ablation of AF demands procedural expertise and can be successfully executed only in a limited number of centers around the world. Catheter ablation of AF, like LAA closure, is associated with a number of periprocedural complications and is compounded by a relatively high probability of AF recurrence, therefore it may not be able to obviate the need for long-term anticoagulant therapy in AF patients. The effect of catheter ablation of AF in stroke prevention remains to be established.

Valvular diseases

Patients with mechanical heart valves should be treated with long-term warfarin. Those with bioprosthetic valves should take warfarin for three months after valve replacement, followed by aspirin. For patients with rheumatic mitral valve stenosis in sinus rhythm, primary stroke prevention with warfarin may be considered in those with an enlarged left atrium, or when TTE or TEE reveals thrombus or spontaneous echo contrast in the left atrium. Although one trial demonstrated that dabigatran was inferior to warfarin in patients after mechanical heart valve replacement, whether NOACs offer advantages over warfarin for patients with other valvular conditions remains to be determined.

Acute myocardial infarction/left ventricular dysfunction

Patients with acute myocardial infarction (MI) have increased stroke risks when AF, ST elevation, anterior wall involvement, significant left ventricular (LV) dysfunction, or LV thrombus is present. In addition to global severe LV dysfunction, focal LV dyskinesia or aneurysm may also be a source of cardioembolism, especially when the apical region is involved. In patients with stroke secondary to acute MI, or global or focal ventricular dysfunction, warfarin for 3–6 months together with appropriate medical treatments for MI and heart failure is recommended, with TTE repeated to monitor the LV status. Warfarin therapy may be continued if high-risk features such as severe LV dysfunction or LV thrombus persist on TTE.

Patent foramen ovale

PFO is present in up to 35% of the general population. Features that increase the chance of a PFO being responsible for paradoxical embolism include cryptogenic stroke at age 55 or younger, concomitant venous thrombosis with or without pulmonary embolism, large right-to-left shunt demonstrated on TCD or TEE, coexisting atrial septal aneurysm, hypercoagulable condition, and history of cough or Valsalva maneuver before stroke onset. In these patients warfarin may not be more effective than aspirin for stroke prevention. In selected patients, percutaneous device closure of PFOs may be considered.

Further reading

Camm AJ, Lip GY, De Caterina R, *et al*. 2012 focused update of the ESC Guidelines for the management of atrial fibrillation: An update of the 2010 ESC Guidelines for the management of atrial fibrillation. *Eur Heart J* 2012;33:2719–2747.

Goyal M, Demchuk AM, Menon BK, *et al*. Randomized assessment of rapid endovascular treatment of ischemic stroke. *N Engl J Med* 2015;372:1019–1030.

Heidbuchel H, Verhamme P, Alings M, *et al*. European Heart Rhythm Association practical guide on the use of new oral anticoagulants in patients with non-valvular atrial fibrillation. *Europace* 2013;15:625–651.

Holmes DR, Reddy VY, Turi ZG, *et al*. Percutaneous closure of the left atrial appendage versus warfarin therapy for prevention of stroke in patients with atrial fibrillation: A randomised non-inferiority trial. *Lancet* 2009;374:534–542.

January CT, Wann LS, Alpert JS, *et al*. 2014 AHA/ACC/HRS Guideline for the management of patients with atrial fibrillation: A report of the American College of Cardiology/American Heart Association Task Force on Practice Guidelines and the Heart Rhythm Society. *J Am Coll Cardiol* 2014;64:e1–e76.

Jauch EC, Saver JL, Adams HP, *et al*. Guidelines for the early management of patients with acute ischemic stroke: A guideline for healthcare professionals from the American Heart Association/American Stroke Association. *Stroke* 2013;44:870–947.

Kernan WN, Ovbiagele B, Black HR, *et al*. Guidelines for the prevention of stroke in patients with stroke and transient ischemic attack: A guideline for healthcare professionals from the American Heart Association/American Stroke Association. *Stroke* 2014;45:2160–2236.

Sanna T, Diener HC, Passman RS, *et al*. Cryptogenic stroke and underlying atrial fibrillation. *N Engl J Med* 2014;370:2478–2486.

7 Systemic hypotensive injury (border-zone infarction)

Thomas W. Leung
Department of Medicine and Therapeutics, Chinese University of Hong Kong, Hong Kong

The border zone (or watershed) is the junction between adjacent non-anastomosing arterial perfusion beds where the perfusion pressure is the lowest. Two distinct supratentorial border zones have been described: (1) the cortical (or external) border zone, which refers to the strips of brain lying between the territories of blood supply from the anterior cerebral artery (ACA), middle cerebral artery (MCA), and posterior cerebral artery (PCA); and (2) the internal border zone, which refers to the white matter alongside and above the body of the lateral ventricles between the territories of ascending branches of lenticulostriate arteries and inward medullary branches of the pial-arachnoidal circulation.

Epidemiology

Border-zone infarction (BI) represents approximately 10% of all brain infarcts in autopsy series, which might be an underestimate as unilateral BI is less likely to be fatal. In a European study that included ischemic stroke patients of all subtypes, more than two-thirds of BI identified by computed tomography were related to large artery disease. BI is the most common type of infarction distal to an occluded internal carotid artery. In head-and-neck cancer survivors with strokes attributed to radiotherapy-induced vasculopathy, BI is frequent and associated with diffuse bilateral carotid and vertebral artery steno-occlusions. BI also constitutes up to one-fourth of ischemic strokes after cardiac surgery owing to perioperative hypotensive episodes.

Pathophysiology

Acute bilateral BI is classically associated with profound systemic hypotension, although a mild transitory hypotension may precipitate BI in patients with critical large artery disease accompanied by an exhausted perfusion reserve. Hemodynamic factors that may cause BI include hypotension as a side effect of antihypertensive therapy, reduced cardiac output induced by paroxysmal arrhythmias or cardiomyopathies, massive acute bleeding, hypovolemia, and hypotensive complications during cardiopulmonary bypass surgery.

BI is frequently observed in the ipsilateral cerebral hemisphere of severe carotid artery or MCA steno-occlusive disease without a preceding hypotensive event. In these patients, microembolization and chronic cerebral hypoperfusion interact inextricably in the pathogenesis of BI. Autopsy studies have revealed occlusion of terminal branches of leptomeningeal and pial arteries at the border zone by small cholesterol emboli of 50–300 μm in diameter. High-intensity transient signals compatible with microemboli have been consistently captured by transcranial Doppler ultrasound in patients with critical carotid stenosis and BI. It has been postulated that microemboli that might originate from unstable atherosclerotic plaques are prone to lodge at the hypoperfused border zone where the low-flow circulation fails to wash out the emboli. The absence of effective collaterals further impedes clearance of the microemboli.

Clinical features

The clinical presentation of BI is diverse. Small, discrete BI may be clinically silent or manifest as transient ischemic attacks or lacunar syndromes. Dependent on the extent of permanent ischemic injury, BI can be described as partial or confluent based on neuroimaging (see the next section). Most patients with confluent BI develop dizziness or syncope as a prodromal symptom, followed by a fluctuating but progressive neurological deficit consisting of hemiparesis, hemisensory loss, cortical signs, or, rarely, focal limb shaking.

Investigation

BI is usually identified by computed tomography (CT) or magnetic resonance imaging (MRI). Cortical border-zone infarction (CBI) between the ACA and MCA produces a thin fronto-parasagittal wedged infarct extending from the anterior horn of the lateral ventricle to the cortex, which is termed the "anterior border zone." CBI between the MCA and PCA causes a temporo-parieto-occipital wedged infarct extending from the occipital horn of the lateral ventricle to the cortex, referred to as the "posterior border zone." At the level of the upper centrum semiovale, CBI involving the three cerebral arteries results in a continuous strip extending from the frontal pole along the convexity of the cerebral hemisphere in a parasagittal line to the occipital pole, which is also called the "superior border zone." Internal border-zone infarction (IBI) affects the corona radiata, between the territories of the deep and medullary (or superficial) MCA perforators or the centrum semiovale between the superficial perforators of ACA and MCA. Considerable individual variation of cortical and internal border zones may result from developmental anomalies (e.g., non-competent Circle of Willis or hypoplasia of intracranial arteries) or high-grade steno-occlusion of cranial arteries (e.g., critical carotid or MCA stenosis).

Compared with CT, MRI is more sensitive and reliable in the detection of BI (Figure 7.1). Diffusion-weighted MRI is useful to

International Neurology, Second edition. Edited by Robert P. Lisak, Daniel D. Truong, William M. Carroll and Roongroj Bhidayasiri
© 2016 John Wiley & Sons, Ltd. Published 2016 by John Wiley & Sons, Ltd.

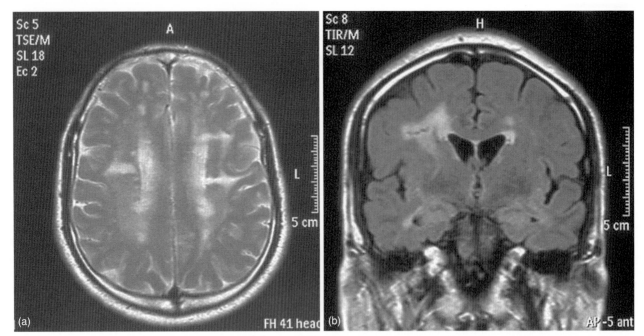

Figure 7.1 A classic "C-shaped" bilateral total cortical border-zone infarct, in which a linear chain of subcortical hyperintensity extends from the frontal pole and back along the convexity of the cerebral hemisphere in a parasagittal line to the occipital pole (a, MRI T2 axial view) and then forward again to involve the temporal lobe (b, MRI FLAIR coronal view).

differentiate acute infarcts from those associated with chronic white matter hypoperfusion. Based on the extent of involvement on imaging, BI can be categorized as partial or confluent. Partial BI represents smaller, single or multiple, discrete infarcts in the corresponding border zones. Multiple partial BI form a linear, rosary-like chain of lesions. In its confluent form, CBI appears as a wedged infarct and IBI as a cigar-shaped infarct extending the length of the lateral ventricle at the level of the centrum semiovale.

Treatment

While the majority of patients with small, partial BI make an excellent recovery with minor or no residual disability, many patients with confluent BI are left with major motor disability. Bilateral watershed infarcts after cardiac surgery are associated with poor short-term outcome. Long-term prognosis and successful prophylaxis of BI depend on identification and treatment of the underlying pathological mechanism. Patients with large artery disease are prone to recurrence, particularly in the first year after the index stroke. Imaging studies for carotid and intracranial stenosis should be conducted routinely and early for secondary stroke prevention. Carotid Doppler ultrasound is a convenient bedside tool to screen for proximal carotid artery disease. Contrast CT or MR angiography can readily detect intracranial and/or extracranial large artery disease of both anterior and posterior circulation in a single examination with sensitivity and specificity >90%. For patients with a diagnosis of atherosclerotic large artery disease risk factors such as hyperlipidemia, diabetes and hypertension should be rigorously controlled. Aggressive medical therapy with dual antiplatelets for 90 days, statins, and antihypertensives, coupled with lifestyle modifications regarding diet, regular exercise, and abstinence from smoking, is the mainstay for treating

symptomatic intracranial atherosclerotic disease. The usefulness of angioplasty with and without stenting is unknown and is still considered investigational for treating intracranial atherosclerosis.

Patients with symptomatic proximal internal carotid artery high-grade (>60%) stenosis may benefit from carotid endarterectomy (CEA) at centers where the rate of perisurgical stroke or death is <6%. The benefit of CEA in reducing stroke risk may be greater if surgery is performed sooner after the stroke. Carotid angioplasty and stenting (CAS) may be effective at centers where the rate of periprocedural stroke or death is <6%. CAS may be an alternative to CEA, especially in younger patients with arterial anatomy more favorable for endovascular intervention, or when carotid stenosis is present bilaterally or is radiotherapy induced. For patients with carotid occlusion, revascularization including extracranial/intracranial bypass is not indicated despite an annual ipsilateral stroke rate of 6%. Readers are referred to American Heart Association/American Stroke Association guidelines for more detailed evidence-based ratings of medical, surgical, or endovascular interventions for secondary prevention of stroke in patients with intracranial or/and extracranial arterial stenosis or occlusion.

Apart from large artery disease, evidence of hypotensive episodes should be sought. Holter monitoring may record occult cardiac arrhythmia. Charting of erect and supine blood pressure identifies orthostatic hypotension and may suggest autonomic failure. Calcium channel blockers and vasodilators are most commonly implicated in drug-induced hypotension. For patients with chronic cerebral ischemia and systemic hypertension, angiotensin-converting enzyme inhibitors or angiotensin receptor blockers can be an appropriate alternative given their lower propensity to cause orthostatic hypotension.

In summary, secondary prevention of BI clings to the use of antiplatelet agent, aggressive cardiovascular risk factor control, revascularization for extracranial high-grade stenosis, and avoidance of systemic hypotension.

Further reading

Bogousslavsky J, Regli F. Borderzone infarctions distal to internal carotid artery occlusion: Prognostic implications. *Ann Neurol* 1986;20(3):346–350.

Caplan LR, Wong KS, Gao S, Hennerici MG. Is hypoperfusion an important cause of strokes? If so, how? *Cerebrovasc Dis* 2006;21:145–153.

Del Sette M, Eliasziw M, Streifler JY, *et al.*; for the North American Symptomatic Carotid Endarterectomy (NASCET) Group. Internal borderzone infarction: A marker for severe stenosis in patients with symptomatic internal carotid artery disease. *Stroke* 2000;31(3):631–636.

Gottesman RF, Sherman PM, Grega MA, *et al.* Watershed strokes after cardiac surgery: Diagnosis, etiology, and outcome. *Stroke* 2006;37(9):2306–2311.

Kernan WN, Ovbiagele B, Black HR, *et al.* Guidelines for the prevention of stroke in patients with stroke and transient ischemic attack: A guideline for healthcare professionals from the American Heart Association/American Stroke Association. *Stroke* 2014;45:2160–2236.

Leung WT, Wang L, Soo YOY, *et al.* Evolution of intracranial atherosclerotic disease under modern medical therapy. *Ann Neurol* 2015;77:478–486.

Momjian-Mayor I, Baron J-C. The pathophysiology of watershed infarction in internal carotid artery disease: Review of cerebral perfusion studies. *Stroke* 2005;36;567–577.

Salazar JD, Wityk RJ, Grega MA, *et al.* Stroke after cardiac surgery: Short- and long-term outcomes. *Ann Thorac Surg* 2001;72(4):1195–1201.

Zou XY, Leung WT, Yu S, *et al.* Angiographic features, collaterals, and infarct topography of symptomatic occlusive radiation vasculopathy: A case-referent study. *Stroke* 2013;44:401–406.

8 Dissection of the cervicocerebral arteries

Nijasri C. Suwanwela[1], Aurauma Chutinet[1], and Chung Y. Hsu[2]

[1] Division of Neurology, Department of Medicine, Chulalongkorn University, Bangkok, Thailand
[2] China Medical University, Ministry of Health Clinical Trial Center of Excellence, Taichung, Taiwan

Introduction and epidemiology

Dissection of the cervicocerebral arteries is cause of stroke that is relatively more common in young and middle-aged adults. Dissection is more likely to occur in the cervical section of the carotid or vertebral arteries, because this is the segment of both arteries that is highly movable and is susceptible to external impact to cause dissection. In this chapter, the term cervicocerebral arteries covers the cervical segment of both carotid and vertebral arteries. Less commonly, dissection may involve intracranial arteries.

In a population-based study, the annual incidence rate of cervicocerebral artery dissection was 2.6 per 100,000 population, with the internal carotid arteries affected more frequently than vertebral arteries in an approximately 2:1 ratio. The mean age of onset is 44 years, slightly older in men than in women. Recurrence of dissection is rare and probably does not exceed 1%. In the younger population, cervicocerebral artery dissection is a common cause of stroke, constituting up to 25% of stroke in patients under 45 years.

Dissection of the internal carotid generally occurs just distal to the carotid bulb or between the level of the second cervical vertebra and the base of the skull. The dissection frequently extends to the intracranial part of the internal carotid artery. Vertebral artery dissection generally occurs at the V3 segment, where it travels along the lateral aspect of C1 and C2 and is susceptible to injury caused by rotation of the head. Another site of vertebral artery dissection is the V2 segment within the transverse foramen, which is susceptible to stretching, in addition to rotation, injury.

Etiology and pathophysiology

Cervicocerebral artery dissection typically starts with a tear between the intima and media of the arterial wall. However, in some cases with spontaneous dissection, intramural hematoma without an intimal tear may be observed. Less commonly, the tear is between the media and adventitia and is called a subadventitial dissection, which may result in aneurysm formation. Aneurysmal dilatations are more commonly noted in the carotid than the vertebral arteries.

Trauma is a well-established cause of cervicocerebral artery dissection. Carotid and vertebral artery dissection has been reported in 0.86% and 0.53% respectively of patients with blunt trauma. It is likely that dissection is underrecognized in patients with trauma. The movable cervicocerebral arteries may be susceptible to mild injury caused by hyperextension, rotation, or lateroversion of the neck. Chiropractic neck manipulation has been implicated as a cause of cervical artery dissection, primarily in adults younger than 45 years and affecting mostly vertebral arteries. Other than blunt injury and chiropractic neck manipulation, it is not uncommon that patients with cervical artery dissection are without a clear-cut cause. Trivial injury is frequently cited in case reports. Trivial incidents including vomiting, coughing, prolonged head tilting, painting a ceiling, riding on a roller coaster, and practicing yoga have been reported to be the precipitating events in 12–34% of patients with cervicocerebral artery dissection. These patients without obvious injury are categorized as spontaneous dissection. Among them, a small population (probably less than 5%) may have hereditary disorders affecting connective tissue. Weakening of the media and elastic tissue of the arterial wall, as seen in patients with fibromuscular dysplasia, Marfan syndrome, Ehlers–Danlos syndrome (type IV), osteogenesis imperfecta, autosomal dominant polycystic kidney disease, hyperhomocysteinemia, and other genetic conditions, has been associated with spontaneous dissection of cervicocerebral arteries. Infection, particularly respiratory tract infection, may trigger dissection. The greater frequency of upper respiratory tract infection among patients with dissection than among controls and the peak incidence of dissection in the fall season support the possible association.

Accumulation of intramural blood in the subintimal region results in reduced blood flow in the distal territory. Moreover, exposure of the blood to the subintimal arterial structure may activate the coagulation cascade, leading to intraluminal thrombus formation. Clot formation in the lumen may embolize distal intracranial arteries, causing transient ischemic attack or stroke. Subadventitial dissection may expand the vessel size to result in aneurysm formation and compress the surrounding structures such as the nearby cranial nerves.

Clinical features

The dilated arteries may exert pressure effects on surrounding structures including the adjacent nerves to cause characteristic symptoms and signs, including head, neck, and facial pain, sympathetic nerve dysfunction resulting in Horner's syndrome, and lower cranial nerve palsies. The onset of these symptoms and signs related to local arterial injury frequently precedes those caused by cerebral ischemia secondary to artery occlusion or distal emboli by hours or days. The sequence of pain, ophthalmological and lower cranial

International Neurology, Second edition. Edited by Robert P. Lisak, Daniel D. Truong, William M. Carroll and Roongroj Bhidayasiri
© 2016 John Wiley & Sons, Ltd. Published 2016 by John Wiley & Sons, Ltd.

nerve findings followed by cerebral ischemia is a helpful clinical feature for directing clinicians to reach the correct diagnosis.

Less commonly, dissection may involve intracranial arteries. The clinical presentation depends on the site of dissection and the vascular territory supplied by the affected artery.

Dissection of the extracranial internal carotid artery

The presenting symptoms and signs of carotid dissection are generally based on two major mechanisms: (1) the pressure effect of the dissected arterial wall on surrounding structures; and (2) blood accumulation/hematoma formation/luminal stenosis/distal emboli leading to cerebral ischemia in the internal carotid artery territory.

Extracranial carotid dissections usually begin 2 cm distal to the carotid bifurcations. The classic triad of extracranial carotid artery dissection is pain, Horner's syndrome, and ischemia. However, the combination of the classic triad is found in only 30% of patients. Headache, neck pain, and facial pain are generally confined to the side of the dissection. Unilateral pain may be noted in the upper anterolateral neck, face, teeth, or orbit. Headache in the frontotemporal area is noted in more than two-thirds of cases and is the initial symptom in up to 60% of patients. Ipsilateral headache with a constant steady aching or throbbing character resembling migraine and/or sharp pain in the face, neck, and jaw may be the presenting symptoms. The sympathetic nerve and lower cranial nerves, especially cranial nerves IX–XII, are commonly affected, with Horner's syndrome reported in 50% and dysgeusia involving chorda tympani or glossopharyngeal nerve in 10% of patients. Isolated Horner's syndrome may make the diagnosis of carotid or vertebral artery dissection more difficult. Pulsatile tinnitus is reported by 25% of patients. About three-quarters of patients with carotid dissection show symptoms and signs of ischemic events, including amaurosis fugax (ischemic optic neuropathy), transient ischemic attack, or ischemic stroke in the carotid territory. A small number of patients may remain asymptomatic.

Dissection of the vertebral artery

Vertebral artery dissection tends to involve the distal (V3) portion near the C1 and C2 vertebrae, which is highly movable and therefore the most vulnerable segment. Bilateral dissection of the vertebral arteries is not uncommon. Ipsilateral neck or occipital pain usually precedes neurological deficits by hours or days. The median interval is 2 weeks. Stroke is caused by embolization distal to the posterior circulation, resulting in brainstem, cerebellar, or occipital infarction. Transient ischemic attacks are less common in vertebral artery than carotid artery dissection. Intracranial dissection involving the V4 segment, either primary intracranial or as an extension of extracranial dissection, may present with lateral medullary syndrome. Dissection of the intracranial vertebral artery may extend to the basilar artery, leading to ischemic insult in pons, midbrain, or other territories in the posterior circulation. Formation of pseudoaneurysm may cause subarachnoid hemorrhage.

Investigations

Advances in neuroimaging allow diagnosis of cervicocerebral artery dissection with non-invasive approaches. New imaging techniques now offer visualization of the vascular wall in detail superior to conventional angiographic findings.

For extracranial carotid dissection, B-mode ultrasound may demonstrate tapering of the arterial lumen above the carotid bifurcation, with possible differentiation between true and false lumens. Abnormal flow patterns can also be detected by Doppler study. Color duplex sonography has been reported to be of high sensitivity and specificity in spontaneous dissection of the internal carotid artery with severe stenosis or occlusion. However, in patients with isolated Horner's syndrome, ultrasound may not be a reliable method. For conventional arteriography, the most distinctive feature is the string sign, which is a long, irregular filling defect due to lumen compression by blood in the vessel wall. Other rare but pathognomonic features are double-barrel lumen and mural flap. Occasionally, pseudoaneurysm can be found.

Magnetic resonance imaging (MRI) and computed tomography (CT) can demonstrate enlargement of arterial diameter and, more importantly, blood or blood products in the arterial wall. High-resolution MRI may be capable of differentiating the crescent sign changes of a mural hematoma from the adjacent perivertebral venous plexus. Together with information derived from MRI or CT angiographic findings, full delineation of the cervicocerebral artery dissection with accompanying vascular changes is possible to reach a firm clinical diagnosis.

Treatment

There have been no randomized controlled trials to guide the management of dissection. Patients with cervicocerebral artery dissection have been placed on intravenous or intra-arterial thrombolysis. While the efficacy of thrombolysis remains to be established, no adverse effect has been noted in recent studies. Within the 4.5-hour therapeutic window, thrombolysis is an option for managing patients with ischemic stroke secondary to cervicocerebral artery dissection. For the prevention of recurrent stroke, the American Heart Association/American Stroke Association guidelines recommend that antiplatelet or anticoagulant therapy for 3–6 months is "reasonable" and that endovascular therapy (stenting) "may be considered" if medical therapy fails. The Cervical Artery Dissection in Stroke Study (CADISS) showed no difference in efficacy between antiplatelet and anticoagulant therapies in the prevention of stroke and death in patients with symptomatic carotid and vertebral artery dissection. Surgery has a limited role, but "may be considered" if medical therapy and endovascular interventions fail, according to the American Heart Association/American Stroke Association guidelines.

For intracranial artery dissection, especially if it involves the vertebral artery, there is a concern of arterial rupture resulting in subarachnoid hemorrhage. Therefore, anticoagulant therapy is usually not recommended.

The prognosis of patients with dissection largely depends on the location and extent of the initial ischemic insult. In general, outcomes based on functional assessment have been excellent, with a modified Rankin scale (mRS) score of 2 or less in the majority of patients. More than 70% of the lesions resolve within a few months. Recanalization of occluded vessels occurs less frequently. Smoking and older age are associated with poor recanalization. The results of a population-based survey suggest that recurrence of dissection is rare.

In conclusion, dissection of the cervicocerebral artery is a common cause of stroke in the young. History of neck injury can be found in some cases, but spontaneous dissection after or without history of trivial trauma is more common. Clinical features include TIA or ischemic stroke in the same arterial territory, together with the symptoms and signs of pressure effect to the surrounding structures of the dissecting artery. Head and neck pain is another common presentation that warrants the diagnosis. To date, MRI with wall imaging and MRA are useful for diagnosis. Antiplatelet or anticoagulant therapy is generally recommended for the prevention of recurrent stroke.

Further reading

Biller J, Sacco RL, Albuquerque FC, *et al.* Cervical arterial dissections and association with cervical manipulative therapy: A statement for healthcare professionals from the American Heart Association/American Stroke Association. *Stroke* 2014;45:3155–3174.

Dziewas R, Konrad C, Dräger B, *et al.* Cervical artery dissection: Clinical features, risk factors, therapy and outcome in 126 patients. *J Neurol* 2003;250:1179–1184.

Fisher CM. The headache and pain of spontaneous carotid dissection. *Headache* 1982;22:60–65.

Kernan WN, Ovbiagele B, Black HR, *et al.* Guidelines for the prevention of stroke in patients with stroke and transient ischemic attack: A guideline for healthcare professionals from the American Heart Association/American Stroke Association. *Stroke* 2014;45:2160–2236.

Zinkstok SM, Vergouwen MD, Engelter ST, *et al.* Safety and functional outcome of thrombolysis in dissection-related ischemic stroke: A meta-analysis of individual patient data. *Stroke* 2011;42:2515–2520.

9 Coagulation and Hematological Disorders in Stroke

Kay Sin Tan
Department of Medicine, University of Malaya, Kuala Lumpur, Malaysia

Coagulation and numerous hematological disorders increase the risk of thrombosis in the cerebral vasculature. "Hypercoagulable state" is a term frequently applied to any underlying coagulopathy that increases the risk of stroke, including cerebral venous or sinus thrombosis or ischemic stroke of arterial origin. "Thrombophilia" is another term used in reference to increased thrombotic tendency. Hypercoagulable states may be caused by inherited hemostatic abnormalities such as activated protein C resistance due to factor V Leiden or prothrombin gene mutation, protein C, protein S, or antithrombin (AT) III deficiency. Antiphospholipid antibody syndrome is a common acquired disorder. Hypercoagulable states may occur during pregnancy or puerperium, in patients on oral hormonal contraception, and in patients with malignancy. Coagulation disorders predispose to strokes involving cerebral veins and sinuses more frequently than cerebral arteries. Hemorrhagic stroke is rare and more commonly noted in patients with coagulation disorders secondary to autoimmune diseases.

In practice, most patients with ischemic stroke do not have well-defined coagulation disorders. As such, coagulation disorders are uncommon causes of stroke, contributing to less than 10% of strokes in young patients and less than 1% of all patients with ischemic stroke. The epidemiology of coagulopathies and stroke varies between different regions and ethnic groups. For example, factor V Leiden is a common mutation in the West and results in the resistance of factor Va to activated protein C (APC). The prevalence of this condition is highest in Europe, but extremely rare in Asia, Africa, and indigenous populations in Australia. Therefore, it is important to be cognizant of the relevant local literature and the ethnic composition of the various regions. Commonly encountered pathophysiological conditions leading to hypercoagulable states and increased stroke risk are described in this chapter.

Hyperviscosity disorders

Sickle cell anemia

Hemoglobin is the oxygen-carrying protein–iron complex in erythrocytes. The incidence of stroke in patients with sickle cell anemia is related to the composition of this protein–iron complex. The incidence of stroke in hemoglobin SS (homozygous) and hemoglobin SC (heterozygous) is 10% and 2–5%, respectively. Hyperviscosity induced by sickle cell anemia affects blood flow, with long-term detrimental effects on vascular integrity. The resultant vascular damage leads to a progressive, segmental narrowing of the distal internal carotid artery and proximal branches of major intracranial arteries. In turn, these changes contribute to large arterial or watershed infarcts. Briefly, large arterial strokes can be diagnosed clinically according to classic cortical localization. Presentations of border-zone infarctions vary depending on the implicated locations: precentral, postcentral, corticosubcortical, exclusively subcortical, or a combination of these infarcted regions. Sickle cell plugging of microcirculation and cerebral veins has also been observed. Intracerebral hemorrhage is not an uncommon event.

Intracerebral arteriopathy can be monitored with non-invasive imaging such as transcranial Doppler ultrasound and magnetic resonance imaging (MRI). Regular blood transfusion has been shown in randomized clinical trials to reduce stroke risk. The risk of stroke recurrence in children increases if blood transfusion is stopped. Hydroxyurea, antiplatelet therapy, and bone marrow transplantation are possible treatment options, but remain to be tested in valid clinical trials to confirm their efficacy in stroke prevention. Outside of Africa, sickle cell anemia is most prevalent in North America, with 8.5% of African Americans carrying the sickle trait and 0.16% manifesting the disease. Sickle cell anemia is increasingly reported in Europe as a result of immigration from countries where it is more common. It is uncommon in Asia, except in the Middle East Asian region.

Polycythemia rubra vera and thrombocytosis

Myeloproliferative disorders such as polycythemia rubra vera and essential thrombocytosis are recognized risk factors for stroke. The pathophysiological mechanisms of neurovascular symptoms in these conditions occur through a hyperviscosity-related reduction in cerebral blood flow. Coexisting atherosclerosis and dysfunctional platelets also contribute to cerebral thrombotic events. Clinical features of these events differ according to the degree of blood flow reduction, manifesting as headaches, lethargy, drowsiness, and strokes. Aspirin has been proven to be effective in reducing stroke risk in patients with polycythemia rubra vera and has been validated in randomized clinical trials. Measures to reduce platelet counts include platelet pheresis, hydroxyurea, and recombinant interferon-α.

Prothrombotic disorders

Prothrombotic coagulation abnormalities are complex. Knowledge of these conditions is expanding. Inherited thrombophilias, including deficiency in AT III, protein C, and protein S, predispose carriers to cerebral venous thrombosis, peripheral venous thrombosis, and, rarely, arterial thrombosis. Cerebral venous thrombosis has a wide spectrum of symptoms and signs that are most frequently progressive over several days. Headache, seizures, nausea, vomiting, focal neurological deficits, altered consciousness, and papilledema are recognized clinical features. Overall, the prevalence of these mutations is higher in Western populations.

International Neurology, Second edition. Edited by Robert P. Lisak, Daniel D. Truong, William M. Carroll and Roongroj Bhidayasiri
© 2016 John Wiley & Sons, Ltd. Published 2016 by John Wiley & Sons, Ltd.

AT III deficiency

AT is an inhibitor of thrombin and other activated clotting factors. Deficiency in AT has a prevalence of 1 in 250–500 and is not restricted to any particular ethnic group. It is inherited in an autosomal dominant pattern. The prevalence of hereditary AT deficiency is 0.5–1% among patients after a first thrombotic event. Clinical events are usually precipitated by pregnancy, surgery, infection, or oral contraceptive use. For treatment of symptomatic inherited AT deficiency, anticoagulant therapy is recommended. AT deficiency is resistant to anticoagulation with heparin. Alternatively, replacement AT is available for short-term therapy or during episodes of high risk.

Protein C and protein S deficiencies

Protein C is an important inhibitor of plasma coagulation. It is activated when clotting is initiated on the endothelial surface. Protein S acts as a non-enzymatic cofactor for activated protein C (APC). APC and protein S collectively confer anticoagulant actions and also activate fibrinolysis. Most affected adult patients are heterozygous for protein C deficiency, with a prevalence of 1 in 200–500 worldwide. The prevalence of protein S deficiency is estimated at 1 in 700–3000.

Both conditions are inherited in an autosomal dominant pattern with partial expression. Premature stroke may also affect children and young adults heterozygous for protein C deficiency, especially when conventional stroke risk factors are also present. Acquired protein C deficiency may occur with liver disease, vitamin K malabsorption, infection, sepsis, disseminated intravascular coagulation, or malignancy. Homocystinuria in association with protein C deficiency has been recognized to cause thrombotic episodes. Acquired protein S deficiencies can also occur in patients with nephrotic syndrome, HIV infection, and L-asparaginase chemotherapy, in addition to being associated with oral contraceptive use and liver dysfunction.

Activated protein C resistance may be due to genetic mutations such as factor V Leiden G1691A. This and other point mutations such as prothrombin G20210A offer genetic insights into the pathogenesis of hypercoagulable states.

Homocysteinemia

Case-control studies and meta-analyses have demonstrated that an increase in plasma homocysteine is a significant independent risk factor for ischemic stroke. Genetic errors in the metabolism of sulfur-containing amino acids result in plasma hyperhomocysteinemia and homocystinuria. Hyperhomocysteinemia may activate coagulation via endothelial injury, creating an occlusive vasculopathy. Acquired conditions such as vitamin B_{12} and folate deficiency, renal failure, hypothyroidism, and drugs such as anticonvulsants predispose to hyperhomocysteinemia. Previous large randomized controlled trials using folate and vitamin B supplements to lower homocysteinemia failed to reduce the risk of ischemic stroke. However, a recent Chinese trial using combined use of enalapril and folic acid among adults with hypertension and low baseline folate levels significantly reduced the risk of first stroke.

Antiphospholipid syndrome

Antiphospholipid syndrome (APLS) is one of the most common acquired thrombophilias and is associated with an increased risk of stroke. Clinical features of primary APLS include recurrent migraine-like headaches, fetal loss, mild thrombocytopenia, and false-positive Venereal Disease Research Laboratory (VDRL) tests. Furthermore, arterial or venous cerebrovascular events may present with encephalopathy and seizures.

Secondary APLS occurs with lupus erythematosus, immune complex diseases, cancer, and in association with some drug reactions. The majority of these patients have significant titers of either lupus anticoagulant or anticardiolipin antibody. Low-titer APLS is found in 1–2% of the normal population. APLS also occurs transiently after infection, tissue injury such as myocardial infarction, or as a reaction to drugs, and is usually not associated with thrombotic events. In addition, the presence of both anticardiolipin (aCL) and lupus anticoagulant (LA) confers the highest risk of recurrent thrombotic events.

Aspirin or warfarin is routinely used in the prevention of recurrent stroke in patients with primary or secondary APLS. However, these strategies have been based on relatively small randomized controlled studies showing clinical outcomes with wide confidence intervals. As such, the optimal length and intensity of anticoagulation therapy are uncertain. A moderate-intensity anticoagulation range of international normalized ratio (INR) 2.0–3.0 may be sufficient. There is evidence that a higher INR range of 3.0–4.5 is not superior to moderate anticoagulation and may be associated with a higher risk of major bleeding events. Immunosuppression and the addition of aspirin to anticoagulation for individuals with recurrent cerebral ischemia are possible therapeutic alternatives.

Platelet dysfunction disorders

Thrombotic thrombocytopenic purpura (TTP) is a consumptive coagulopathy characterized by microangiopathic hemolytic anemia, thrombocytopenia, and central nervous system disorders, including ischemic stroke. Most of the microvascular occlusions in TTP are secondary to multiple microvascular platelet-fibrin thrombi that involve subintimal deposits in small arteries and capillaries. These changes contribute to multiple organ damage in the brain and kidney. Clinically, TTP may present with fluctuating encephalopathic signs and seizures. Computed tomography (CT) or MRI findings may show ischemic changes, cerebral edema, or intracerebral hemorrhage. Therapeutic measures including the use of high-dose corticosteroids, repeat plasma exchanges, antiplatelet agents, and splenectomy have shown varying degrees of success. Heparin-induced thrombocytopenia is a disorder in which patients develop antibodies against heparin. These antibodies are directed toward platelets, causing activation.

Other coagulopathies

Rare genetic disorders may predispose carriers to hypercoagulable states with defective heparin cofactor II and fibrinolysis factors such as plasminogen, tissue plasminogen activator, and excessive formation of plasminogen activator inhibitor-1. The role of these rare hereditary conditions in venous thrombosis and stroke remains incompletely defined. An acquired hypercoagulable state is not uncommonly noted in patients with advanced malignancy. These patients are at increased risk of stroke as well.

Investigations

Routine hematological tests should be conducted in the evaluation of patients with stroke. These tests include clotting profile (prothrombin time [PT] and activated partial thromboplastin time [aPTT]) and a complete blood count. Blood dyscrasias or hypercoagulability should be suspected in patients with ischemic stroke exhibiting selected clinical profiles such as younger age (<50), absence of stroke risk factors, history of recurrent strokes of undetermined etiology, history of peripheral or cerebral venous thrombosis, family history of thrombosis, and abnormalities of coagulation profile on routine tests.

PT is used for diagnosis of deficiencies of factors I, II, V, VII, and X or for detection of inhibitors of these coagulation factors. It is also used to monitor warfarin therapy and to screen for vitamin K deficiency. aPTT is used for diagnosis of deficiencies in factors VIII, IX, XI, and XII or von Willebrand factor, and for detection of inhibitors of these coagulation factors. It is also used to monitor heparin therapy and serves as a screening test for lupus anticoagulant (LA).

Additional tests may be needed for selective hypercoagulable states. Thrombin time is used for the diagnosis of fibrinogen deficiencies, assessment of possible heparin resistance, and monitoring fibrinolytic therapy. Antiphospholipid antibodies of the immunoglobulin (Ig) G class and LA may be indicated in selected patients with or without clinical systemic lupus.

Fasting homocysteine level is measured by high-performance liquid chromatography (HPLC) or immunofluorescence techniques. Hyperhomocystinemia is associated with arterial and venous thrombosis and is to be distinguished from autosomal recessive homocystinuria. Elevated homocysteine levels are also encountered in numerous acquired conditions, described earlier.

Hemoglobin electrophoresis enables the detection of hemoglobin SS and SC. This test should be considered in ethnic groups at high risk for sickle cell disease.

Proteins C and S and AT III activity may also be measured to screen for prothrombotic states. The respective protein antigens are required as confirmatory tests. Resistance to APC is the most common inherited risk factor for thrombosis in Western populations. An Activated Protein C Resistance V (APCRV) ratio <2.2 indicates a high likelihood of APC resistance. Genetic studies including factor V Leiden and prothrombin 20210A gene mutations could be considered if a hereditary hypercoagulable state is suspected. These defects are rare in Asian populations, and routine screening is not recommended.

Treatment

Anticoagulant therapy with heparin is the mainstay for treating cerebral venous or sinus thrombosis. Anticoagulant therapy is also needed for the prevention of stroke or other thrombotic events in patients with stroke caused by hypercoagulable states. The duration of anticoagulant therapy may be dictated by the risk of recurrent thrombotic events. In most patients with hypercoagulable states, anticoagulant therapy for at least three months may be needed.

Underlying causes such as sickle cell anemia, polycythemia rubra vera, thrombocytosis, malignancy, autoimmune disorders, and others should also be specifically treated as already described under selected hematological disorders.

Further reading

Derksen RHWM, de Groot PG. Towards evidence-based treatment of thrombotic antiphospholipid syndrome. *Lupus* 2010;19:470–474.

Gruppo Italiano Studio Policitemia. Polycythemia vera: The natural history of 1213 patients followed for 20 years. *Ann Intern Med* 1995;123:656–664.

Levine SR, Brey RL, Tilley BC, *et al.* Antiphospholipid antibodies and subsequent thrombo-occlusive events in patients with ischemic stroke. *JAMA* 2004;291(5):576–584.

Toole JF, Malinow MR, Chambless LE, *et al.* Lowering homocysteine in patients with ischemic stroke to prevent recurrent stroke, myocardial infarction and death: The Vitamin Intervention for Stroke Prevention (VISP) randomized controlled trial. *JAMA* 2004;291:565–575.

VITATOPS Trial Study Group. B vitamins in patients with recent transient ischaemic attack or stroke in the Vitamins to Prevent Stroke (VITATOPS) trial: A randomized, double blind, parallel, placebo controlled trial. *Lancet Neurol* 2010;9(9):855–865.

Yong Huo, Jianping Li, Xianhui Qin, et. al. Efficacy of Folic Acid Therapy in Primary Prevention of Stroke Among Adults with Hypertension in China. The CSPPT Randomized Clinical Trial. JAMA. 2015;313(13):1325–1335.

10 Hemorrhagic strokes

Anna Katharina Flügel[1], Thorsten Steiner[1,2], Josef Schill[3], Nauman Jahangir[4], Morad Chughtai[5], Mushtaq H. Qureshi[4], and Adnan I. Qureshi[6]

[1] Department of Neurology, Klinikum Frankfurt Höchst GmbH, Frankfurt, Germany

[2] Department of Neurology, Heidelberg University Hospital, Heidelberg, Germany

[3] Klinikum Darmstadt, Darmstadt, Germany

[4] Zeenat Qureshi Stroke Institute, St. Cloud, MN, USA

[5] Rubin Institute for Advanced Orthopedics, Center for Joint Preservation and Replacement, Sinai Hospital of Baltimore, Baltimore, MD, USA

[6] Zeenat Qureshi Stroke Research Center, University of Minnesota, Minneapolis. MN, USA

Hemorrhagic strokes are acute bleeding events in the intracranial cavity that are more serious than ischemic strokes and have a higher mortality. In this chapter, hemorrhagic strokes will be covered in four categories based on causes and pathological features: (1) primary or spontaneous intracerebral haemorrhage (ICH); (2) subarachnoid hemorrhage (SAH); (3) arteriovenous malformations (AVM); and (4) cerebral amyloid angiopathy (CAA).

Primary intracerebral hemorrhage

Primary or spontaneous intracerebral hemorrhage refers to bleeding into the parenchyma of the brain as a result of spontaneous blood vessel rupture and in the absence of trauma or surgery. Primary ICH accounts for two-thirds of hemorrhagic strokes. Every year approximately 37,000–52,000 people suffer ICH in the United States and the number of patients with ICH is expected to increase due to the accelerated aging of the population.

Epidemiology

Primary ICH constitutes 10–25% of all strokes. Ethnic differences in ICH incidence have been noted. In Western countries, ICH accounts for 10–17% of all strokes and in Asian countries up to 25%. In the United States, ICH incidence in the African American (32 per 100,000) or Asian American (61 per 100,000) populations is higher than among white Americans (7–12 per 100,000). Environmental (e.g., diets, salt intake) and genetic factors could account in part for the ethnic/racial differences in ICH prevalence. Among patients with atrial fibrillation who are on anticoagulant treatment, the same trend for higher incidence of ICH in the non-white population also holds. Each year, more than 20,000 patients in the United States die of ICH. The 30-day mortality rate of ICH is 44%. Brainstem hemorrhage has a mortality rate of 75% at 24 hours.

Risk factors

The most important ICH risk factor is hypertension. The crude odds ratio (OR) for hypertension is 3.68 and the frequency of hypertension in ICH is 70–80%. Another major risk factor is age, with an OR of 1.97 for increase in age by every 10 years. For current smokers the crude OR is 1.31 and for those with diabetes 1.30. With regard to alcohol consumption, the quantity is a significant variable. High intake (>56 g/day, OR 4.00) results in greater risk than moderate consumption (<56 g/day, OR 2.05). Drug abuse (e.g., cocaine,

amphetamines) is also associated with increased ICH risk, as well as low cholesterol (<150 mg/dl). ICH incidence is lower among those with higher cholesterol levels. Modifying these risk factors plays an important role in lowering ICH risk. Iatrogenic causes of ICH are not uncommon. Oral anticoagulants, especially those prescribed for elderly patients with atrial fibrillation, have drawn increasing attention to ICH as a serious adverse side effect. A meta-analysis shows that the risk of ICH is approximately half with the novel oral anticoagulants (NOACs) in comparison to warfarin treatment. Traumatic head injury may cause acute or delayed ICH, especially in victims on oral anticoagulants. Traumatic ICH is beyond the scope of coverage in this chapter. Thrombolytic therapy of ischemic stroke with tissue plasminogen activator (tPA) increases the risk of symptomatic ICH 10-fold. Approximately 0.5% of patients who underwent carotid endarterectomy experienced ICH after surgery. Other procedures such as intracerebral electrode placement or angioplasty and stenting of the internal carotid artery or its branches may also cause ICH.

Pathophysiology

Primary ICH constitutes 80–85% of all hemorrhagic strokes, with secondary ICH that can be ascribed to discrete vascular lesions, including AVM, and aneurysm comprising the remaining 15–20%. Secondary ICH will be reviewed in the subsequent sections on AVM and aneurysm, respectively.

Over 50% of primary ICH cases are attributed to hypertension, with location in the basal ganglia, the most common site of bleeding, accounting for approximately 40%. Other frequent locations of hypertensive ICH include the thalamus (30%), cerebral cortex (20%), and cerebellum and brain stem (10%). The remaining cases of primary ICH are mainly those associated with CAA, which has been found to increase with age and is described in a later section. ICH is often caused by rupture of a small artery with subsequent hematoma formation and expansion. Miliary aneurysms (Charcot–Buchard's aneurysms) and lipohyalinosis, both associated with hypertension, are the key pathological features in autopsy series of ICH. Following arterial rupture in ICH, the subsequent pathophysiological processes can be divided into three phases: (1) accumulation of extravascular blood leading to hematoma formation; (2) continuation or resumption of bleeding resulting in hematoma expansion; and (3) development of perihematomal edema.

International Neurology, Second edition. Edited by Robert P. Lisak, Daniel D. Truong, William M. Carroll and Roongroj Bhidayasiri
© 2016 John Wiley & Sons, Ltd. Published 2016 by John Wiley & Sons, Ltd.

Hematoma expansion or enlargement secondary to continuous bleeding or rebleeding has gained attention in recent years because of the possibility of therapeutic interventions applying hemostatic agents or more rigorous control of extremely high blood pressure (>180 mmHg systolic) at a very early stage of ICH. In view of the clinical and therapeutic implications, hematoma enlargement and perihematomal edema formation are reviewed in more detail.

Progressive enlargement of a hematoma is the most serious complication in patients with ICH. It is not clear whether rebleeding or continuous bleeding is the cause of hematoma growth. Hematoma increases by about 33% in size in approximately one-third of patients within the first 4 hours of onset. In another 12% of patients the hematoma expands within the next 20 hours. Neurological deterioration follows hematoma enlargement. The following predictors of hematoma expansion have been identified: large initial blood volume, irregular bleeding contours, liver dysfunction, hypertension, hyperglycemia, and history of high alcohol consumption. An ominous pathophysiological process following ICH is bleeding into intraventricular space, which is associated with higher mortality and morbidity. Intraventricular hemorrhage (IVH) is a dynamic process and is present in 38% of ICH patients at onset and in 45% 24 hours after onset.

Brain edema can be observed in the acute and subacute stages of ICH. Perihematomal edema volume increases by approximately 75% during the first 24 hours after ICH. Edema usually progresses for up to 14 days after ICH onset. Based on magnetic resonance imaging (MRI) and positron emission tomography (PET) studies, edema plays a minor role in the development of perihematomal ischemia, in contrast to a more significant pathophysiological role of brain edema in ischemic stroke. Brain edema following ICH is thought to involve activation of the coagulation mechanism and release of osmotic substances from the clot, rather than impairment of the blood–brain barrier. In the presence of very high intracranial pressure and low cerebral perfusion pressure, the risk of global ischemia is high. A variable reperfusion phase lasts from 2–14 days, and a normalization phase develops after 14 days, with re-establishment of normal cerebral blood flow in all viable regions.

ICH in patients on anticoagulant therapy with iatrogenic coagulopathy is accompanied by a lesser magnitude of perihematomal edema.

Clinical features

It may be difficult to distinguish hemorrhagic from ischemic stroke based on bedside clinical evaluation. The presence of one or more of the following features suggests ICH: sudden onset of focal neurological deficit along with symptoms caused by a sudden increase in intracranial pressure (headache, nausea and vomiting, altered level of consciousness, and acute hypertensive response with systolic blood pressure greater than 180 mmHg and diastolic blood pressure greater than 110 mmHg) and a patient on anticoagulation therapy. Patients with supratentorial hemorrhage often present with contralateral hemiplegia, hemisensory loss, aphasia, neglect, gaze abnormalities, and hemianopia. Infratentorial hemorrhages manifest with signs of brainstem dysfunction, cranial nerve abnormalities, ataxia, nystagmus, and cerebellar signs. In patients with supratentorial ICH, conjugate eye deviation is frequently observed secondary to a relatively smaller thalamic hematoma. Approximately 10% of patients with ICH in the lobar areas also experience seizures at onset or in the first 24 hours after symptom onset. One study demonstrated that the mean ICH volume was independently associated

with seizures. An increase of 1 mm^3 in hematoma volume increased the seizure rate by 2.7%. Blood may leak into the ventricles and the subarachnoid space. A large hematoma may also compress structures like the brainstem and thalamus and may cause herniation clinically manifesting as coma, bilateral plantar extensor reflexes, pupillary abnormalities, or Cheyne–Strokes breathing. In a case of worsening hemorrhage, death may occur as a result of the compromise of vital centers secondary to brainstem compression. Predictors of early death include age, initial score on the Glasgow coma scale (GCS), volume of the hematoma, presence and quantity of ventricular blood volume, and increase in the size of the hematoma.

Investigations
Patients with clinical features suggestive of ICH require immediate neuroimaging for prompt diagnosis. Non-contrast computed tomography (CT) is a sensitive procedure for detecting or excluding acute ICH. Acute bleeding presents as a hyperdense area on CT. However, in patients with low hematocrits, even an acute hematoma may appear isodense. The area of the hematoma becomes iso- and hypodense during the course of hematoma breakdown and absorption. With the implementation of susceptibility-weighted T2* sequences, MRI has become a useful diagnostic tool to supplement CT in detecting hyperacute and acute ICH. In hyperacute hemorrhage these sequences reveal characteristic hyperintense signals. In the chronic stage, hemosiderin causes a hypointense signal on T2- and T2*-weighted sequences. Follow-up imaging may not be necessary unless hematoma enlargement in patients with deteriorating clinical course or unusual causes of ICH (e.g., bleeding caused by a brain tumor) is suspected. In younger patients without known risk factors such as hypertension or in patients with suspected secondary bleeding (e.g., lobar bleedings or so-called atypical ICH), further diagnostic workup is required to define the etiology of the hemorrhage. CT angiography (CTA), MR angiography (MRA), and digital subtraction angiography (DSA) are useful in these patients. CTA is recommended as a rapid method of identifying the underlying vascular pathology when emergency surgical evacuation of the hematoma is required. Aneurysms larger than 3 mm and AVM can be detected effectively by using this technique, as larger ICH can cause hemodynamic changes in AVM that may then not be detected by MRA or CTA. Under this circumstance, DSA should be performed. MRI is the best technique to reveal underlying vascular malformation of the low-pressure system or the venous system (cavernoma, hemorrhagic tumors). Using contrast-enhanced magnetic resonance venography or CTA, sinus/venous thrombosis can be clearly diagnosed.

Medical management
Initial management
According to guidelines from the American Heart Association/American Stroke Association, management of patients with ICH should take place in an intensive care unit setting. Initial management is commonly started in the emergency department and is focused on airway support, blood pressure control, intracranial pressure treatment, and anticoagulation reversal. A number of observational studies have shown that about 30% of patients with supratentorial hemorrhage and almost all patients with brainstem or cerebellar hemorrhage present with either a decrease in or loss of consciousness or with bulbar muscle dysfunction mandating the need for intubation. Clinical features including rapid deterioration of consciousness, evidence of mass effect, obstructive hydrocephalus on imaging, and signs of transtentorial herniation may demand

emergent neurosurgical consultation for intraventricular catheter placement or surgical evacuation, along with the use of hyperventilation and intravenous mannitol treatment. It is very important to assess patients frequently in the first 24 hours after symptom onset due to the increased risk of neurological deterioration and cardiovascular instability.

Whether the administration of hemostatic agents can prevent hematoma enlargement to improve outcomes is still the subject of clinical research. Prevention of deep vein thrombosis and pulmonary embolism in immobilized ICH patients remains a therapeutic dilemma. Surgical evacuation of hematoma is not generally recommended, but may be an exception in some patients who may benefit from neurosurgical interventions.

Management of increased intracranial pressure

Increased intracranial pressure secondary to mass effects caused by hematoma, perihematoma edema, and obstructive hydrocephalous should be aggressively treated. It is a major cause of death in ICH patients. Intubation for hyperventilation is frequently the best option for lowering intracranial pressure in a timely manner. Mannitol is also used commonly to lower intracranial pressure. In cases of ventricular obstruction, drainage of cerebrospinal fluid with intracranial monitoring is indicated. Mannitol may cause renal failure. It is very important to monitor fluid and electrolyte balance during mannitol therapy. Routine use of mannitol is not recommended as it may diffuse into the hematoma, consequently aggravating edema and mass effect. Intensive care leading to controlled cerebral perfusion pressure of 50–70 mmHg may improve outcome.

Acute hemostatic therapy

With ICH, it is very important to prevent the growth of the hematoma using an early hemostatic therapy. Factor VII in its activated form (fVIIa) reduces hematoma enlargement after ICH and is limited to the area of injury without systemic activation of the coagulation cascade. A Phase III fVIIa for Acute Hemorrhagic Stroke Treatment (FAST) trial assessed patients who presented within 3 hours of symptom onset for the safety and efficacy of fVIIa. Of the total of 821 patients enrolled, 263 received placebo, 265 received 20 µg/kg, and 293 received 80 µg/kg of fVIIa. At 3 months, 26% and 29% of patients who were given 20 µg/kg and 80 µg/kg of fVIIa had died or experienced disability compared to 24% of the patients who were given placebo, and the rate of arterial thrombosis was also higher in patients treated with 80 µg/kg of fVIIa (10%) than in those treated with placebo (5%) or 20 µg/kg of fVIIa (6%). The results suggest that while fVIIa was effective in reducing haematoma expansion, it did not improve functional outcome or reduce mortality.

Management of acute hypertensive response

Generally, treatment recommendations for elevated blood pressure in patients with ICH are more aggressive compared to those with acute ischemic stroke. Management of elevated blood pressure should be based on individual factors, including age, past history of hypertension, elevated intracranial pressure, cause of hemorrhage, and time interval since onset of hemorrhage. American Stroke Association guidelines recommend that "until ongoing clinical trials of blood pressure intervention for ICH are completed, physicians must manage blood pressure on the basis of the present incomplete evidence," by maintaining systolic blood pressure at less than 180 mmHg in the acute setting with short half-life intravenous antihypertensive drugs if (1) systolic BP (SBP) is >200 mmHg (or mean arterial pressure [MAP] is >150 mmHg); or (2) SBP is >180 mmHg (or MAP >130 mm Hg) and there is suspicion of increased intracranial pressure (ICP).

Importantly, these guidelines recommend careful and near-continuous monitoring (every 5–15 minutes) of patients with acute ICH on antihypertensive therapy to assess for worsening of neurological status or drop in cerebral perfusion pressure. Each of these recommendations is graded C, indicating a low level of evidence.

New evidence-based recommendations for managing patients with ICH were published in August 2014 by the European Stroke Organization (ESO). In acute ICH within 6 hours of onset, intensive blood pressure reduction (systolic target <140 mmHg in <1 h) is safe and may be superior to a systolic target of <180 mmHg. The ESO does not recommend a specific agent.

The Intensive Blood Pressure Reduction in Acute Cerebral Hemorrhage Trial II (INTERACT II) aimed to assess the safety and efficacy of early and intensive lowering of systolic BP to below 140 mmHg, as compared to below 180 mmHg within 6 hours, in patients who presented with acute ICH. INTERACT II enrolled 2839 ICH patients from 21 countries, with 2793 eligible for assessment of death or major disability as the primary outcome. The results show that more aggressive management of systolic BP below 140 mmHg did not improve the primary outcome. An ancillary ordinal analysis of modified Rankin scores suggests better functional outcomes in the group with intensive systolic BP lowering to below 140 mmHg.

The lack of clear-cut therapeutic effects of aggressive BP lowering prompted another multinational clinical trial, Antihypertensive Treatment of Acute Cerebral Hemorrhage (ATACH-II). This is a five-year, multicenter, randomized controlled, Phase III trial with blinded outcome ascertainment to determine the efficacy of early, intensive antihypertensive treatment using intravenous nicardipine for acute hypertension in subjects with primary supratentorial ICH. The primary hypothesis of ATACH II is that intensive systolic blood pressure reduction to 110–140 mmHg using intravenous (IV) nicardipine with treatment initiated within 4.5 hours of ICH onset and continued for 24 hours reduces the risk of death or disability at 3 months after ICH by 10% or greater, compared with systolic blood pressure reduction to 140–180 mmHg. While avoiding extremes of systolic blood pressure (i.e., >180 mmHg or <110 mmHg) seems prudent, defining an optimal blood pressure range in all patients with ICH will likely be difficult, especially with the notion that blood pressure in ICH patients often fluctuates markedly over short periods of time due to impaired cerebral autoregulation. ATACH-II hopefully will provide a higher level of evidence on blood pressure management in the acute setting of primary ICH.

Intracerebral hemorrhage related to use of oral anticoagulants

In the past four years, NOACs including apixaban, rivaroxaban, edoxaban, factor Xa inhibitors, and dabigatran, a thrombin inhibitor, have been increasingly prescribed for stroke prevention in patients with atrial fibrillation. While differences in pharmacological actions and variable results are noted among large-scale Phase III trials, NOACs outperform warfarin on safety and efficacy in individual trials and in meta-analyses, such that they are favored for stroke prevention in patients with atrial fibrillation. NOACs are also favored in reducing ICH, a complication of anticoagulant therapy, by half as compared to warfarin. Furthermore, the need for frequent monitoring of prothrombin time and possible interference of food and concomitant medications during warfarin therapy can be obviated with NOACs. In ICH patients on warfarin, rapid correction of coagulopathy is needed to prevent continuous bleeding. Rapid reversal of systemic anticoagulation may be accomplished with a combination of intravenous vitamin K, prothrombin complex concentrates, or fresh frozen plasma and fVIIa, preferably within 2 hours of onset. If necessary, transfusion of fresh frozen plasma along with vitamin K may be given. Platelet concentrate may also be needed in patients receiving massive transfusion. Some physicians may be reluctant to prescribe NOACs because of a lack of antidotes, which are still under development.

Treatment of ICH related to fibrinolysis

Symptomatic ICH occurs in 3–9% of patients with acute ischemic stroke treated with intravenous recombinant tissue plasminogen activator (rtPA). "Symptomatic" should be differentiated from "any" hemorrhage found in stroke patients treated with rtPA. "Symptomatic" ICH is defined as clinical deterioration that is attributed to ICH, with the understanding that hemorrhage in the brain may occur in approximately 30% of patients with acute ischemic stroke who received rtPA thrombolysis. In cases of symptomatic hemorrhage, this tends to be serious, sometimes multifocal. The 30-day death rate can be 50% or higher. Recommended treatments include platelets and factor VIII substitution to correct the systemic fibrinolytic state rapidly. Cryoprecipitate has been recommended in order to increase the level of fibrinogen to at least 150 mg/dl.

Surgical treatment

Mass effect–resulting brain herniation is a common cause of early death in patients with ICH. Timely surgical management of ICH is directed toward impending brain herniation, which may be predicted by hematoma volume with related structural shift noted on neuroimaging, persistently intracranial hypertension, and deteriorating neurological condition or consciousness level. In prospective controlled randomized trials, surgical intervention has not been shown to offer advantages over conservative treatment. The largest group was examined in the Surgical Trial in Spontaneous Intracerebral Haemorrhage (STICH). In a pooled analysis of several surgical trials including the largest prospective trials (STICH and in STICH II), a selected group of patients might benefit from early surgery. Taking all available information together, early evacuation of hematoma might be considered in conscious patients showing a deteriorating consciousness level with a superficial hematoma (less than 1 cm from the cortical surface). It should be noted that in another series of studies, no patient with an ICH volume greater than 85 cc survived, regardless of treatment modality.

In ICH patients with elevated ICP, surgical intervention may be an option to lower ICP. However, the benefit of surgical reduction of ICP remains to be established. Another indication for surgical intervention is brainstem compression.

Infratentorial cerebellar ICH is considered for surgical evacuation in patients with a GCS ≤13 and a hematoma diameter ≥4 cm or greater. If the GCS score is ≥14 or the ICH is <4 cm, conservative treatment is recommended. Patients who present with absent brainstem reflexes and flaccid quadriplegia should not undergo intensive therapy in the notion that a loss of brainstem function due to direct compression may not be always irreversible. Caution should be exercised under such circumstances so that patients who may benefit from active interventions are not denied them.

The Minimally Invasive Surgery plus Tissue Plasminogen Activator for Intracerebral Hemorrhage Evacuation (MISTIE-III) trial is currently underway to assess the efficacy of removing hematoma by applying a minimally invasive surgical technique coupled with thrombolysis by rtPA. Clot Lysis, Evaluating Accelerated Resolution of Intraventricular Hemorrhage, a Phase III trial, is ongoing to investigate the efficacy of adding tPA to extaventricular drainage in patients with IVH.

Obstructive hydrocephalus may result from obstruction of the ventricular system, either indirectly from the mass effect of ICH in the cerebellum or directly by IVH extension. Both conditions result in a poor outcome. These events can be treated by external ventricular drainage catheters to reduce ICP. A thrombolytic agent administered through ventricular catheters leads to a faster resolution of IVH as compared to external ventricular drainage alone, and may result in mortality reduction, as reported in two systematic reviews of clinical studies.

Subarachnoid hemorrhage

A subarachnoid hemorrhage (SAH) is characterized by the leakage of blood into the subarachnoid space between the arachnoid and the pial membranes. It constitutes 5% of all strokes, but the mortality rate and the extent of disability are significant. The cause of SAH is rupture of a cerebral aneurysm in approximately 80% of patients, with the remaining 20% showing no aneurysm on neuroimaging and angiographic investigation. SAH is associated with high rates of mortality and severe complications. Other rare causes of SAH include AVM, bleeding diathesis, intracranial arterial dissection, amyloid angiopathy, vasculitides, and illicit drug use (e.g., cocaine, amphetamines).

Epidemiology

The incidence of SAH varies around the world, ranging from 4.2 (South and Central America) to 21.9 (Japan) cases per 100,000 person-years. Every year roughly 21,000–33,000 people suffer from SAH in the United States. In the European Union, 36,000 cases are registered per year. The mortality rate is about 60% within 6 months. An age-dependent increase in SAH incidence has been consistently noted, with a mean age of 55 years. A gender difference is also evident, with women having a risk 1.6 times higher than that of men. Higher prevalence is noted with a family history of aneurysms. African Americans are 2.1 times more likely to suffer from SAH than the white population. The prognosis is influenced by a number of non-modified factors and by the availability of therapeutic interventions and intensive care management.

Pathophysiology

Approximately 2.3% of the adult population without specific risk factors are estimated to have intracerebral aneurysms. This proportion increases with age. Important modifiable risk factors for SAH are hypertension, cigarette smoking, heavy alcohol use, and drug abuse (e.g., cocaine, amphetamines). These factors can double the risk of developing SAH. Between 5% and 20% of patients have a positive familial history. Increased risk of subarachnoid hemorrhage can persist even after the cessation of cigarette smoking. Connective tissue diseases, including Ehler–Danlos disease IV, neurofibromatosis type I, Marfan's syndrome, polycystic kidney disease, fibromuscular dysplasia, and pseudoxanthoma elasticum, are associated with a higher prevalence of intracerebral aneurysm and SAH. In contrast, hormone replacement therapy among women, hypercholesterolemia, and diabetes mellitus reduce the risk of aneurysm.

The risk of aneurysmal rupture increases as the tension in the wall of the aneurysm increases. According to the La Place theory, the radius of an aneurysm and the pressure gradient across its wall determine the tension in the wall of the aneurysm. The vast majority of intracranial aneurysms are round in shape and are called saccular or berry aneurysms. Saccular aneurysms are mostly located at the bifurcation of the circle of Willis or a nearby branching point. An international study has reported that the cumulative risk of rupture in 5 years is 0 for aneurysms smaller than 7 mm, 2.6% for dimensions between 7 and 12 mm, 14.5% for dimensions between 13 and 24 mm, and 40% for aneurysms greater than 25 mm. The risk increases by 2.5%, 14.5%, 18.4%, and 50%, respectively, for aneurisms located in the posterior circulation. Most intracerebral aneurysms never rupture, but small aneurysms are frequently seen in patients with SAH due to the fact that small aneurysms are much more prevalent than large ones.

Perimesencephalic non-aneurysmal SAH occurs due to blood leakage into the cisterns around the midbrain, pons, or at the level of the quadrigemina cistern. Generally, hemorrhage does not extend to the Sylvian fissure or interhemispheric fissure. A small amount of blood may leak into the ventricular system. Perimesencephalic SAH is usually not due to aneurysmal malformation and is associated with a better outcome. Gross hemorrhage in the ventricular system or brain parenchyma suggests other etiologies. Undiagnostic angiographic findings suggest that SAH may be of venous origin, featuring rupture of a prepontine or interpeduncular vein. In these patients the perimesencephalic veins frequently drain directly into the dural sinuses instead of the vein of Galen, predisposing them to venous congestion.

Clinical features
A hallmark of SAH is an acute (thunderclap) headache, which the patient may describe as "the worst headache of my life." Other symptoms include nausea, vomiting, and neck stiffness. Blood in the subarachnoid space irritates meninges, resulting in the appearance of meningeal signs with neck pain and stiffness. Other signs of meningeal irritation include positive Lasegue, Kernig, or Brudziski signs. Meningeal signs can take 3–12 hours to develop and can be completely absent in the case of coma or minimal blood extravasation. Thus, the absence of neck stiffness cannot exclude the diagnosis of subarachnoid hemorrhage. Reduced level of consciousness, confusional state, hemiparesis, and other focal neurological symptoms are common in severe SAH. Preretinal hemorrhage (Terson's syndrome) indicates a more abrupt increase in ICP and is associated with higher mortality. Linear streaks of blood or flame-shaped hemorrhage appear in the preretinal layer (subhyaloid), usually near the optic disc. Aneurysm can cause single or combined cranial nerve palsies, depending on the size and localization. Painful third nerve palsy is highly suspicious of aneurysm of the posterior communicating artery. Sixth nerve palsy is a non-localizing finding that is due to increased intracranial pressure. Seizures may present in 7% of all patients. Young age (<40 years), bleeding location, presence of acute hydrocephalus, and early rebleeding are the main risk factors for early seizures, while vasospasms with cortical ischemia, intraparenchymal bleeding, and neurosurgical, instead of endovascular, inteventions are risk factors for late-onset seizures.

In the absence of classic symptoms, SAH might be misdiagnosed. In these cases, patients tend to be less ill and the results of neurological examination are normal or showing only subtle signs. Sentinel or thunderclap headaches may be the only symptom of "warning leaks." It is essential to distinguish these sentinel headaches from benign headaches for early therapeutic intervention. As many as half of patients who present to physicians for the first time with SAH are misdiagnosed. This is due to failure either to obtain a proper imaging study, perform a lumber puncture, or interpret a cerebrospinal fluid analysis correctly. Most commonly these patients are labeled with a diagnosis of migraine and tension-type headache. In these cases, signs and symptoms are generally less severe and characteristic neurological features are not present at onset, resulting in delayed diagnosis or misdiagnosis.

Systemic features that can be associated with SAH in the acute phase are severe hypertension, hypoxemia, and electrocardiographic (ECG) changes, which may mimic acute myocardial infarction and lead to erroneous examinations and treatment. In about 3% of patients, cardiac arrest occurs at onset of SAH, requiring resuscitation. Mass effect caused by hematoma and vasoconstriction after hemorrhage may present with clinical features similar to stroke.

For rating SAH severity based on clinical findings, the World Federation of Neurological Surgeons (WFNS) and the classification by Hunt and Hess can be applied in therapeutic decision making.

Complications of SAH
In as many as 50% of cases, complications develop subsequent to the initial ictus and include rebleeding, vasospasm, hydrocephalus, and others.

Recurrence of SAH
Rebleeding of symptomatic aneurysms is a very severe complication and should therefore be prevented by early aneurysmal occlusion with surgical or endovascular measures. Rebleeding is a common event within 2 weeks, with 15% occurring within the first few hours after the initial haemorrhage. The mortality of patients who suffer rebleeding is about 50%.

Vasospasm and delayed ischemic deficit
Vasospasm of the cerebral arteries (mostly first- and second-order branches) occurs within the first 2 weeks after SAH. Vasospasm can cause delayed ischemic neurological deficit, leading to ischemic stroke and death in one-third of patients through a critical reduction of cerebral perfusion. Transcranial sonography is a common modality for detecting and monitoring vasospasm.

Hydrocephalus
Acute, subacute, or chronic hydrocephalus is a common complication of SAH. Hydrocephalus occlusus is caused by a blockage of cerebrospinal fluid (CSF) drainage from the fourth ventricle/aqueduct. Blood in the subarachnoid space may lead to ineffective reabsorption of cerebrospinal fluid because of malfunction of pacchionian granulation, resulting in non-obstructive or communicating hydrocephalus. Intermittent external ventricular catheter drainage (EVD) may be required for both obstructive and non-obstructive hydrocephalus to prevent elevated ICP (target value between 10–20 mmHg). In about a third of patients non-obstructive hydrocephalus is asymptomatic. However, other patients may need CSF drainage with a ventriculo-peritoneal, ventriculo-atrial, or ventriculo-pleural shunt.

Other complications
Seizures, pulmonary edema, cardiovascular dysfunction secondary to increased autonomic discharges, hyponatremia, inappropriate secretion of antidiuretic hormone, or cerebral salt wasting are known pathophysiological processes complicating the management of SAH.

Diagnostic investigations

CT scan

A CT scan is the first investigation if SAH is suspected. The ability to detect SAH is dependent on the amount of subarachnoid blood, the interval after symptom onset, the resolution of the scanner, and the skills of the radiologist. The sensitivity of CT performed within the first 12 hours after onset is 98%, but is down to 85% by the fifth day and to under 30% by 2 weeks after onset. Conventional catheter angiography is the gold standard for detecting aneurysms. It should be performed if the bleeding source was not found with CTA or if the patient has a typical perimesencephalic basal SAH pattern on CT. Because the incidence of multiple aneurysms is up to 15%, all cerebral vessels should be carefully evaluated. The examination should be repeated 7–14 days after initial presentation in patients suspected of having SAH and in whom initial imaging results were negative. On the first day, subarachnoid blood can be detected by CT in more than 95% of patients, but this proportion falls sharply with the passage of time as blood in the subarachnoid space is recirculated. Bleeding from an intracranial aneurysm may not be confined within the subarachnoid space or cisterns and can rupture into the brain tissue, the ventricular system, or on rare occasions the subdural space. The site of aneurysm can be more reliably identified with the location of hematoma than the cisternal blood alone. Diffuse brain swelling can sometimes result in a false positive diagnosis of SAH because a hyperdense image in the subarachnoid space may represent blood in congested subarachnoid blood vessels. Cerebral vasospasm and poor outcome may be predicted with CT findings. A diffuse thick blood clot in the subarachnoid space increases the risk of cerebral vasospasm and ischemia. The Fisher Grade classifies the appearance of blood on a CT scan. A higher grade is predictive of an increased risk of developing cerebral vasospasm.

Lumber puncture

If suspicion of SAH is high clinically but neuroimaging is negative, then CSF examination should be performed. The most informative CSF test is obtained 6–12 hours after symptom onset to look for the presence of bilirubin and hemoglobin catabolites in CSF that show characteristic xanthochromia. An elevated opening pressure is frequently noted during the procedure. Spectrophotometric examination of CSF provides more sensitive qualitative and quantitative assessment of blood products in CSF.

MRI

It is extremely important to assess the anatomy of cerebral circulation for the site of an aneurysm and also to identify whether multiple aneurysms are present. Approximately 25% of patients have multiple aneurysms. If the initial CT scan is negative, then a repeat CT scan should be performed after 1–2 weeks. If the second evaluation does not reveal any significant finding, the next step should be MRI to uncover an aneurysm or vascular malformation of the brain, brainstem, or spinal cord. The sensitivity of MRI with FLAIR sequences, performed on the first day, is equal to that of CT, but MRI has a higher sensitivity for subacute SAH.

Angiography

Angiographic studies not only help to identify one or multiple aneurysms, but also provide sufficient anatomical details of the aneurysm in relation to adjacent arteries for selection of therapeutic modalities, either surgical and/or endovascular interventions. Conventional angiography, which is 95% sensitive for detection of a ruptured aneurysm, is the gold standard. CTA and MRA have gained in popularity and are frequently used for the detection of aneurysms. CTA and MRA are also helpful for planning the treatment of large and complex aneurysms because of the possibility of three-dimensional visualization. A great advantage of CTA over MRA and catheter angiography is the speed with which it can be undertaken, preferably immediately after the CT scan of the brain by which the diagnosis of aneurysmal hemorrhage is made, and while the patient is still in the scanner. CTA and MRA resemble each other in terms of test characteristics and are well suited for screening people at high risk of intracranial aneurysms, but are less feasible for SAH patients who are restless or need mechanical ventilation.

Conventional catheter angiography should be performed if the bleeding source was not found with CTA or MRA and the patient has a typical perimesencephalic basal SAH pattern on CT. Because the incidence of multiple aneurysms is up to 15%, all cerebral vessels should be carefully evaluated. The examination should be repeated 7–14 days after initial presentation in patients suspected of having aneurysmal hemorrhage and in whom initial imaging results were negative. In a patient with a pattern of hemorrhage on CT scanning that is compatible with a posterior circulation aneurysm, an angiogram cannot be considered without both vertebral arteries fully visualized. Aneurysms arising from the posterior inferior cerebellar artery or other proximal branches of the vertebral artery will be missed with imaging of a single vertebral artery only. Also three-dimensional imaging of the region in which the aneurysm is suspected can identify an aneurysm not visible on routine projections. Catheter angiography has certain risk in patients with SAH: the rate of ischemic neurological complications (transient or permanent) is 1–8% and the overall risk of aneurysm re-rupture during the procedure is 1–2%.

Medical treatment

Patients with SAH must be evaluated and treated as an emergency in a neurocritical setting. First of all, the cardiovascular and respiratory functions should be checked and managed appropriately as needed, because of the risk of developing pulmonary edema, cardiac failure, cerebral edema, and electrolyte imbalances. Acute hypertensive response must be controlled promptly with appropriate use of IV antihypertensive drugs such as nicardipine, labetalol, or urapidil. Reduction and maintenance of systolic blood pressure (BP) to values below 140 mmHg are recommended. In the absence of the aneurysm blood pressure management can be less intensive. After the stabilization of vital functions including BP, further treatment should be carried out at centers where neurovascular expertise is available (neurosurgery and neuroradiology). The most important steps are to prevent rebleeding and other complications that can adversely affect the patient prognosis.

Hypomagnesemia is present in approximately 50% of SAH patients. Hypotension should be avoided to reduce the risk of hypoperfusion, even though a desirable BP range in the setting of SAH has not been established. Headache can be managed with medical treatment. Parenteral analgesics are recommended, including morphine derivatives to ensure adequate pain relief. Hyperpyrexia should be managed appropriately, with the recommended body temperature being 37.2 °C. Hyperglycemia should also be controlled, with blood glucose levels kept in the range of 80–120 mg/dl.

Stress peptic ulcers can be prevented by proton pump inhibitors. After appropriate management of the ruptured aneurysm with rebleeding risk removed, low molecular weight heparin may be used for the prevention of deep vein thrombosis. The risk of cerebral vasospasm leading to ischemia can be reduced by nimodipine 60 mg orally every 4 hours for 21 days. The benefit of nimodipine therapy in lowering the probability of poor outcome (death or dependency) is supported by Cochrane revision, with absolute risk reduction of 5.1% and relative risk reduction of 18% (95% CI 7–28%). Correction of hypomagnesemia with intravenous magnesium sulfate has been noted to be of no benefit in a Phase III study. Antifibrinolytic agents, which may increase the risk of cerebral ischemia and systemic thrombosis, are used to prevent rebleeding. Rebleeding can also be prevented by tranexamic acid from 11–2.4%. It should be noted, however, that the advantages of antifibrinolytic or thrombostatic agents may be offset by their adverse effects in inducing ischemic complications.

Surgical and endovascular management

For the prevention of rebleeding, surgical or endovascular intervention is frequently needed. Early occlusion of symptomatic aneurysms with microsurgical clipping or by endovascular procedure with a detachable platinum coil device is commonly implemented to reduce the risk of early and fatal recurrence of hemorrhage. The decision for surgical or endovascular intervention depends on a number of factors, including age, medical condition, and aneurysm characteristics, such as location, size, and morphology.

The International Subarachnoid Aneurysm Trial (ISAT) compared endovascular coiling and surgical clipping prospectively in patients who had aneurysms that were considered to be equally amenable to both treatment modalities. The ISAT investigators noted more favorable outcomes, defined as survival free of disability at one year, in patients receiving endovascular coiling. The risk of epilepsy was lower also in the endovascular group. However, the risk of rebleeding and incomplete occlusion of the aneurysm was higher in those who underwent endovascular coiling as compared to microsurgical clipping.

Factors that favor microsurgical clipping include aneurysms with a wide neck, arising from the dome or base, accompanied by a large intraparenchymal hematoma or local mass effect. Factors that favor endovascular coiling include neck to dome diameter ratio less than or equal to half, location deep in the skull base, aneurysms of the vertebrobasilar system, and patients who are elderly and cannot tolerate the stress of surgery. Hospital factors should also be considered, as it is recommended that treatment of aneurysms should be in a hospital setting with expertise in both surgical and endovascular treatment options.

Complications of SAH that may require surgical attention include vasospasm and hydrocephalus. Patients suffering from vasospasm refractory to medical treatment should undergo urgent cerebral angiography and receive either local vasodilator infusion or angioplasty to resolve severe regional vasospasm.

The rebleeding rate is approximately 7% after SAH. Patients with rebleeding have a higher risk of permanent neurological disability and a higher mortality rate, reaching 50%. Rebleeding is more likely to occur in the first two weeks after initial ictus, with the highest risk within the first 24–48 hours. In the ISAT trial, the risk of rebleeding from a ruptured aneurysm after one year was 2 per 1276 patient-years in the endovascular and 0 per 1081 patient-years in the microsurgical clipping group.

Cerebral arteriovenous malformation

Cerebral arteriovenous malformation (AVM) refers to a heterogeneous group of cerebrovascular anomalies that predispose approximately half of those who harbor one of these discrete vascular lesions to bleeding events at various stages of life. AVMs appear to derive from structural and functional vascular anomalies during development, with no risk factors firmly established, although occasional cases are associated with other abnormalities (see the later discussion). AVM is likely to form during fetal development, because the unusual angioarchitectures fall within congenital anomalies of RASopathies caused by mutations of genes that control signal transduction (e.g., the Ras subfamily and Mitogen-activated protein kinases).

Epidemiology

In population-based studies, the incidence of AVM is approximately 1 per 100,000 per year. The Cooperative Study of Intracranial Aneurysms and SAH and early autopsy series estimate that approximately 0.14–0.50% of the population bear AVM, which affects men and women equally. Autopsy studies have shown that only 12% of AVMs become symptomatic during life. AVM-related hemorrhage constitutes 2–3% of all hemorrhagic strokes. The risk for recurrent hemorrhage is higher after an AVM has bled. The risk of death associated with initial AVM rupture is approximately 10%, and the mortality rate increases with each subsequent hemorrhage. Bleeding caused by rupture of AVM tends to occur at an earlier age than primary ICH. The mean age of AVM hemorrhage is between 30 and 40 years. AVMs may be associated with other vascular anomalies. For instance, 10–23% of patients with AVM harbor cerebral aneurysms. Congenital disorders that have been associated with AVM include Osler–Weber–Rendu disease and the Sturge–Weber syndrome. AVMs are not regarded as familial, and the overwhelming majority of cases are sporadic. Because of the relatively low incidence of AVM and the lack of epidemiological studies across countries, racial or ethnic differences in AVM incidence have not been reported.

Pathophysiology

AVMs are vascular anomalies with heterogeneous vascular structures. A consistent morphological finding of AVM is the lack of a capillary bed between arteries and veins, resulting in the evolving changes on the venous side. Gross characteristics of AVMs include single or multiple vascular shunting systems that lead to increased blood flow and higher pressure inside the affected arterial and venous channels. Microscopically, arterial and venous blood vessels are hypertrophic. Smooth muscle cells in the tunica media of arteries and veins develop hyperplasia due to increased blood flow and elevated pressure. Generally, the arteries in AVM have an intact elastic lamina, but some deficiencies or degradation may be seen. Absence of capillaries and high-pressure blood flow due to arteriovenous (AV) shunting increase the risk of hemorrhage in veins that have incompetent elastic lamina and a thick fibromuscular layer. Parenchyma surrounding the AVM can develop gliosis with hemosiderin deposits if hemorrhage has occurred.

AV shunting and related destruction of the vascular wall increase bleeding tendency. Brain tissue receiving blood supplies from vessels containing AVM may not be able to maintain normal function, resulting in neurological deficits or a lower threshold for seizure attacks. Most AVMs (approximately 90%) are located in supratentorial regions, predisposing the patient to headaches and seizures. The Spetzler–Martin scale based on specific characteristics (size, location, drainage) is a grading system for characterizing morbidity and mortality and for selecting patients for surgical interventions.

Clinical features

Patients with cerebral AVM may present with intracranial hemorrhage, seizures, and headaches. About half of patients with AVMs present with ICH that may be difficult to distinguish from primary ICH. However, the age of onset of ICH secondary to AVM is likely to be younger and common stroke risk factors such as hypertension and a history of smoking may be absent. Bleeding of a ruptured AVM frequently leads to the detection of the lesion. With the increasing utility of new imaging tools including CT and MRI, patients with an unruptured AVM may present with headache, subtle neurological deficit, or seizure disorders, which lead to the neuroradiological workup and the diagnosis of AVM prior to catastrophic ICH. The technique of digital-substraction angiography is necessary for assessment of the angioarchitectural characteristics of an AVM, particularly if it is a small one. Functional MRI may be used to assess the risk of cerebral dysfunction with surgical intervention.

In general, ICH secondary to AVM rupture bears a lower mortality (5–10%) and morbidity than primary ICH. Patients with AVM hemorrhage also fare better in functional outcome (30–50% with permanent neurological deficit). Among patients with ICH caused by AVM, higher morbidity is noted in those with parenchymal than non-parenchymal location. Recurrence of bleeding is expected in 18% of patients in the 12 months following the first AVM hemorrhage.

Other potential risk factors for hemorrhage include (1) AVM with exclusively deep venous drainage (typically defined as drainage through the periventricular, galenic, or cerebellar pathways); (2) AVM associated with aneurysms; (3) AVMs deep in location; and (4) AVM in infratentorial location. The risk of hemorrhage can be as high as 34.4% with risk factors for deep AVM location or deep venous drainage. Another study has estimated 6.93% risk of hemorrhage in AVMs associated with aneurysms compared with a risk of 3.9% in AVMs with no associated aneurysms.

Approximately 18–40% of cerebral AVMs can present with seizure. Seizure does not appear to increase the risk of ICH. The type of seizure most commonly associated with AVMs is generalized seizures (30%). Headaches can occur in 5–14% of patients with AVMs. Headaches are non-specific and can be unilateral or bilateral. Patients can also present with migraine-like features with or without aura.

Focal neurological deficit can occur in 1–40% of patients with cerebral AVMs. Progressive deficits not related to hemorrhage are noted in 5–15% of patients. The vascular steel phenomenon may develop when an increased amount of cerebral blood is channeled toward the low-resistance arteriovenous shunting system, leading to decreased blood flow and pressure in the feeding arteries and surrounding brain tissue. Mass effect with pressure on brain tissue surrounding the dilated veins may also result in ischemic changes.

Diagnostic studies

Modern imaging modalities including CT and MRI are the mainstays in the diagnosis of AVM. Past bleeding events may be detected by hemosiderin deposition. Preoperative MRI is helpful in planning the surgical approach, which may affect the structures surrounding the AVM. Conventional cerebral angiogram remains the gold standard in the evaluation of AVM. An angiogram provides sufficient details on the feeding arteries, location of nidus, venous drainage, presence or absence of associated varices, aneurysms, or stenosis in the affected vessels. Feeding arteries and shunting are also better characterized with angiography for developing treatment strategies.

AVMs must be searched for among younger patients with ICH, particularly those with lobar or so-called atypical bleeding locations.

Treatment

The risk of bleeding is relatively lower with the diagnosis of AVM than with arterial aneurysm. Risk assessment is a crucial step in developing therapeutic strategies, which include conservative managment or using a single or multiple therapeutic modalities consisting of surgical resection, radiosurgery, and/or embolization. Conservative medical management is recommended for patients with a low risk of developing ICH. Annual or biannual surveillance can be performed with MRI. Seizures, headaches, and hypertension can be managed medically.

Endovascular embolization and radiotherapy are often used to reduce the lesion size in preparation for surgery or when the AVM is difficult to access surgically. The treatment is selected according to the size of the AVM, proximity to eloquent areas, venous drainage, and accessibility. The ARUBA study compared medical management alone with medical management plus interventional therapy for the prevention of death or stroke in patients with an unruptured AVM. The results show that the risk of death or stroke was significantly lower in the medical management alone group than in the interventional therapy group after a mean follow-up of 33 months.

Cerebral amyloid angiopathy

Cerebral amyloid angiopathy (CAA) is a disorder of the central nervous system in which amyloid protein, usually in beta-pleated sheet configuration, is deposited in the media of small arteries (arterioles), veins (venules), and the adventitial component of capillaries in leptomeninges and the cortex of the brain.

The hereditary form of CAA is rare, but may be more severe in clinical presentation at an earlier age. Sporadic CAA is more common and is a major cause of cognitive decline in the elderly with ICH.

Epidemiology

CAA is a frequent autopsy finding in the elderly. CAA is present in approximately 80% or more of the brains of patients with Alzheimer's disease and 10–40% in the elderly population. The Harvard Brain Tissue Resource Center's analysis concluded that the more severe form of CAA is present in 2.3% of 65–74-year-olds, 8.0% of 75–84-year-olds, and 12.1% of those over 85 years. Spontaneous ICH in the elderly that can be attributed to CAA ranges from 10–20% in autopsy series and 34% in clinical series. CAA-related ICH (CAA-ICH) accounts for 5–20% of all spontaneous (non-traumatic) ICH in elderly subjects.

Pathophysiology

The cascade of events that promotes cerebrovascular amyloid-β (Aβ) accumulation is still not fully understood, but an imbalance between Aβ production and clearance is likely to play a key role. Aβ precursor protein (APP) is cleaved to yield Aβ peptide. Aβ requires two enzymatic events to be generated from APP: cleavage at the carboxyl terminus by γ-secretase followed by a proteolytic cleavage at the amino terminus of the Aβ sequence by β-secretase, resulting in a β-sheet structure with conformational change in soluble Aβ forms via an unknown mechanism. This β-sheet structure is prone to fibrillization, oligomerization, and deposition, which trigger a cascade of events that include complement system activation, release of inflammatory mediators, and alteration of the blood–brain barrier. These events lead to disruption of the vascular architecture, microaneurysm formation, fibrinoid necrosis, hyaline degeneration, intimal changes, and perivascular leakage of blood products.

The apolipoprotein E (APOE) ε4 and ε2 alleles are genetic aberrants associated with a risk of developing sporadic CAA-related ICH. The ε2 allele predisposes to the rupture of diseased vessels by inducing the vasculopathic changes and hematoma expansion in lobar ICH, whereas the ε4 allele is related to the severity of amyloid deposition within the vessel wall. More recently, the CR1 gene has also been linked to a risk of CAA-related ICH.

In familial forms of CAA, the cause of Aβ buildup is likely due to increased production rather than poor clearance. Mutations in the amyloid precursor protein (APP), presenilin (PS) 1, and PS2 genes have been shown to accelerate cleavage of APP and increase Aβ deposition to cause early onset of CAA.

Clinical features

CAA can be completely asymptomatic because amyloid deposition is part of the normal aging processes. Diseased blood vessels due to amyloid deposition can lead to both asymptomatic microbleeds and lobar ICH. Amyloid deposits can also occlude the lumen of the diseased blood vessels, leading to ischemia and related clinical manifestations such as cerebral infarction and leukoaraiosis. These pathophysiological mechanisms may also lead to progressive cognitive decline, dementia, focal neurological deficits, disturbances of consciousness, and death. Increasing evidence is emerging that CAA may be a risk factor for thrombolysis-related ICH. CAA patients can be asymptomatic, whereas hemorrhagic stroke is the defining clinical characteristic, raising concern that CAA is a risk factor for symptomatic ICH following rtPA therapy for acute ischemic stroke. Headache, focal neurological deficits, seizures, and an altered level of consciousness occur in patients with ICH. Spontaneous bleeding due to CAA, as previously mentioned, can also be small and asymptomatic and is commonly referred to as microbleeds. Microbleeds are an important hint in the clinical diagnosis of CAA and also have been shown to correlate with a risk of lobar ICH, functional dependence, and cognitive decline.

Diagnostic studies

A definitive diagnosis of CAA requires histopathological examination with either Congo red staining for amyloid or immunohistochemistry with fluorescent antibodies specific for Aβ. In clinical practice, specimens obtained from surgery for ICH or post-mortem examination are the major mechanisms for confirming the diagnosis of CAA. MRI sequences such as gradient-recalled echo (GRE) and susceptibility-weighted imaging (SWI) can assist in identifying not only major bleeding in the brain but also microbleeds. Cerebral microbleeds project as hypointense signals in GRE due to the formation of hemosiderin. Hemosiderin is engulfed by macrophages, which stay in brain tissue for an extended duration. Therefore, MRI provides an estimate of hemorrhagic burden in CAA patients for the risk assessment of possible deterioration of neurological functions and future ICH.

Using a combination of clinical, neuroimaging, and pathological data, the Boston Criteria establish the levels of certainty for the diagnosis of CAA.

Positive emission tomography (PET) imaging with Pittsburgh Compound B (PiB) has also been applied to measure the burden and location of brain fibrillar Aβ deposits in animal models and in humans with Alzheimer's disease or CAA. At present, PiB-PET use is still considered investigational by the US Food and Drug Administration for the diagnosis of Alzheimer's disease or CAA. Other amyloid-binding compounds using the longer-lasting radionuclide fluorine-18 have more recently been tested to detect amyloid with potential diagnostic value in clinical practice in the future.

Cerebrospinal fluid (CSF) can aid in the diagnosis of cerebral amyloid angiopathy. Patients with Alzheimer's disease and non-demented CAA subjects have decreased cerebrospinal fluid concentrations of Aβ42 and Aβ40 and increased tau proteins.

Management

Currently, there is no specific preventive or therapeutic strategy available for CAA or ICH secondary to CAA. However, corticosteroid treatment has been shown to result in symptomatic improvement by inhibiting CAA-related inflammation and reducing vasogenic edema. In the Perindopril Protection Against Recurrent Stroke study (PROGRESS), blood pressure lowering using perindopril plus optional indapamide was noted to reduce the risk of both ischemic and haemorrhagic stroke. Anticoagulation with warfarin or NOACs for stroke prevention in patients with atrial fibrillation and rtPA thrombolysis in the setting of acute ischemic stroke may predispose patients with CAA to a higher risk of ICH. Greater caution should be exercised and more conservative approaches should probably be entertained when elderly patients with a possible diagnosis of CAA are considered for anticoagulation for stroke prevention or thrombolysis for acute ischemic stroke.

Further reading

Biffi A, Greenberg SM. Cerebral amyloid angiopathy: A systematic review. *J Clin Neurol* 2011;7(1):1–9.

Broderick J, Connolly S, Feldmann E, et al. Guidelines for the management of spontaneous intracerebral hemorrhage in adults: 2007 update: A guideline from the American Heart Association/American Stroke Association Stroke Council, High Blood Pressure Research Council, and the Quality of Care and Outcomes in Research Interdisciplinary Working Group. *Stroke* 2007;38(6):2001–2023.

Caldeira D, Barra M, Pinto FJ, et al., Intracranial hemorrhage risk with the new oral anticoagulants: A systematic review and meta-analysis. *J Neurol* 2015;262(3):516–522.

Qureshi AI, Mendelow AD, Hanley DF. Intracerebral haemorrhage. *Lancet* 2009; 373(9675):1632–1644.

Qureshi AI, Jahangir N, Qureshi MH, et al. A population-based study of the incidence and case fatality of non-aneurysmal subarachnoid hemorrhage. *Neurocrit care* 2015;22(3):409–413.

Mendelow AD, Gregson BA, Rowan EN, et al. Early surgery versus initial conservative treatment in patients with spontaneous supratentorial lobar intracerebral haematomas (STICH II): A randomised trial. *Lancet* 2013;382(9890):397–408.

Mohr JP, Parides MK, Stapf C, et al. Medical management with or without interventional therapy for unruptured brain arteriovenous malformations (ARUBA): A multicentre, non-blinded, randomised trail. *Lancet* 2014;383:614–621.

Steiner T, Juvela S, Unterberg A, et al. European Stroke Organization guidelines for the management of intracranial aneurysms and subarachnoid haemorrhage. *Cerebrovasc Dis* 2013;35:93–112.

Steiner T, Al-Shahi Salman R, Beer R, et al. European Stroke Organization (ESO) guidelines for the management of spontaneous intracerebral hemorrhage. *Int J Stroke* 2014;9:838–839.

van Gijn J, Rinkel GJ. Subarachnoid haemorrhage: Diagnosis, causes and management. *Brain* 2001;124:249–278.

11 Strokes in children and young adults

Alfred Lindner[1] and Ute Berweiler[2]

[1] Department of Neurology, Marienhospital Stuttgart, Stuttgart, Germany
[2] Kliniken Sindelfingen, Klinikverbund Südwest, Sindelfingen, Germany

Cerebrovascular diseases in children cause considerable morbidity and are among the top ten causes of death in children worldwide. The incidence of arterial ischemic stroke ranges from 2–13 per 100,000 children under the age of 18 years annually in Europe and North America. A variety of diseases and disorders are associated with stroke in children.

Etiology and epidemiology

Unlike in adults, non-atherosclerotic arteriopathies seem to be the most important risk factors for stroke in children. In many cases more than one risk factor can be identified.

Abnormalities of the intracranial vessels have been found in almost 80% of children with ischemic stroke in a case series from the United Kingdom. The most common abnormalities were narrowing or occlusion of proximal large arteries such as the distal internal carotid artery or proximal middle cerebral artery.

Arterial dissection is found in up to 20% of children with ischemic stroke. In children, unlike adults, intracranial dissection in the anterior circulation without a trauma is more common than extracranial dissection. If a diagnosis of stroke in the posterior circulation is made, vertebral artery dissection should always be considered, especially since posterior circulation stroke is rare in children. Pain is not a prominent presenting feature, with headache reported in only half of patients, and neck pain rarely noted. This contrasts to adults, in whom pain is often recorded as the most common presenting feature.

Cervicocerebral artery dissections are less frequent in children than in young adults.

Moyamoya arteriopathy typically involves the small, fragile, basal, collateral vessels (puff of smoke). The manifestation is usually bilateral, but may also be unilateral and in more severe cases may involve the posterior circulation as well. The pathogenesis of moyamoya syndrome is unknown. Children present with ischemic stroke during the first decade of life and young adults present with intraparenchymal, intraventricular, or subarachnoid hemorrhage, as well as ischemic stroke during the third decade of life. Seizures and involuntary movement disorders may also occur in the pediatric population.

In patients with transient cerebral arteriopathy, typical clinical and radiological features can be found. All were previously healthy children, with acute hemiplegia as the initial symptom. Imaging studies revealed small subcortical infarcts located in the internal capsule or the basal ganglia. Conventional arteriography in the acute stage showed multifocal abnormalities of the cerebral arterial wall, with focal stenosis or segmental narrowing in the distal internal carotid and the proximal anterior, middle, or posterior cerebral arteries. Over time most of the patients had complete regression, improvement, or stabilization. The underlying condition is probably a transient inflammation of the arterial wall (angiitis) due to prior viral infection such as varicella. There are also case reports of transient cerebral arteriopathy triggered by enteroviral or HIV infection.

Fibromuscular dysplasia is a segmental, non-inflammatory, non-atheromatous angiopathy affecting small and medium-sized arteries of unknown etiology. It most commonly affects the renal and internal carotid arteries, but has also been described in almost every arterial bed in the body.

Vasculitis (inflammatory changes in the cerebral vessels) can be primary or secondary. Primary vasculitides associated with stroke include primary angiitis of the central nervous system, giant cell arteritis, Kawasaki disease, polyarteritis nodosa, and Takayasu arteritis.

At least one-third of pediatric strokes are caused by infectious diseases such as meningitis, encephalitis, human immunodeficiency virus (HIV) infection, varicella zoster virus infection, or systemic sepsis.

Underlying pathogenetic mechanisms include direct inflammation of blood vessels of the brain, hypercoagulopathy due to infection, or cardiovascular causes related to endocarditis or hypotension. Typical findings in children with postvaricella angiopathy are stenosis of the distal internal carotid and proximal cerebral arteries as well as subcortical ischemic lesions.

Other hereditary arteriopathies such as CADASIL (cerebral autosomal dominant arteriopathy with subcortical infarcts and leukoencephalopathy) have to be considered when family history is present or a MRI scan shows typical signs.

Cardiac diseases, including congenital and acquired heart diseases, are also among the most common causes of stroke in children, accounting for up to 50% in case series. They are often associated with other risk factors for stroke, including anemia, arteriopathies, or coagulation factor abnormalities (see the later discussion).

Sickle cell disease (SCD) is the most common cause of stroke in black children. Stroke occurs by the age of 20 in about 11% of patients with SCD. Untreated, two-thirds of these children will have a recurrence.

Several acquired and genetic coagulation factor abnormalities have been associated with pediatric stroke. Small case series and case-control studies found various abnormalities such as the

International Neurology, Second edition. Edited by Robert P. Lisak, Daniel D. Truong, William M. Carroll and Roongroj Bhidayasiri
© 2016 John Wiley & Sons, Ltd. Published 2016 by John Wiley & Sons, Ltd.

prothrombin mutation G20210, the presence of the factor V Leiden G1691A mutation, antiphospholipid antibodies, deficiency of natural anticoagulants protein C, protein S, and antithrombin III, elevations in homocysteine, and lipoprotein A.

Overall, prothrombotic abnormalities have been identified in 20–50% of children presenting with acute ischemic stroke and 33–99% of children with cerebral sinus venous thrombosis. Iron-deficiency anemia is an important risk factor for stroke in children, since it is easy to treat. It is found in more than 25% of children with stroke and is probably due to thrombocytosis related to low iron stores.

Metabolic conditions, such as Fabry disease (X-linked lysosomal storage disorder due to deficiency of a-galactosidase), homocystinuria, Menkes' disease, or deficiency of adenosine deaminase 2 (DADA2) can be associated with ischemic stroke, generally through effects on the vessel wall.

MELAS (mitochondrial encephalomyopathy with lactic acidosis and stroke-like episodes) is characterized by stroke-like episodes resulting in hemiparesis, hemianopia, or cortical blindness, caused by mutations of mitochondrial DNA. Other common features include recurrent migraine-like headaches, hearing loss, muscle weakness, focal or generalized seizures, short stature, and nausea. The syndrome usually manifests in childhood after a normal early development. A relapsing–remitting course is often seen.

The mechanism of stroke-like episodes in MELAS differs from that of "classic strokes" and may be related to regional metabolic energy failure and/or an impairment of cerebral artery vasodilation causing or exacerbating these episodes.

Vascular malformations are the reason for about 50% of hemorrhagic strokes in children and adolescents. Among these, arteriovenous malformations (AVM) are the most common cause, followed by cavernous hemangioma and aneurysms.

The incidence of sinus venous thrombosis (SVT) in children is 0.6/100,000 children per year and is highest in the first year of life. More than 40% occur within the neonatal period. Most of the SVT are located within the superior sagittal sinus with or without thrombosis of the lateral sinus. Approximately 50% of children with SVT present with seizures or focal abnormalities, but clinical presentation can also be subtle. This may lead to underdiagnosis, as well as early recanalization of the sinus. Risk factors include neck and head infections, perinatal complications, dehydration, and coagulation disorders.

Clinical features

Clinical presentation varies from hemiparesis with or without hemisensory signs or visual field defects to unexplained altered consciousness. If headache is present, venous thrombosis or arterial dissection should be considered. Seizures, with or without focal neurological deficit, are a common presentation of cerebral venous thrombosis. If deterioration in the level of conciousness occurs, large middle cerebral territory infarcts, posterior fossa strokes, and intracranial hemorrhage should be considered, which require transfer to a pediatric neurological and neurosurgical intensive care unit.

Differential diagnosis in children presenting with an acute hemiparesis includes central nervous system infections (e.g., abscess, focal encephalitis), trauma (e.g., subdural or epidural hematoma, traumatic intracerebral hemorrhage, and brain contusion), tumor, and demyelinating diseases such as acute demyelinating encephalomyelitis (ADEM). Todd's paresis and hemiparesis due to migraine must be carefully excluded.

Stroke severity is similar in children and young adults. Outcome at 3–6 months does not differ between children and adolescents. It is considered to be better than in adults due to the plasticity of the brain. About 60% of children and young adults have a favorable outcome. Mortality is similar among children and young adults (4% vs. 6%) and in children is often predisposed by the underlying disease.

Investigations

Intracranial hemorrhage must be excluded by emergency computed tomography (CT) or magnetic resonance imaging (MRI), since urgent neurosurgical intervention may be neccessary. MRI and MR angiography can provide more important information about intra- and extracranial vessels, venous sinus, and other pathologies confirming vascular diseases. If arterial dissection is suspected, additional MRI of the neck with fat suppression is indicated. Standard digital substraction cerebral angiography (DSA) should be strongly considered in cases with equivocal or negative findings on MRI or where no other explanation can be identified. Transcranial color-coded duplex sonography (TCCS) enables the reliable assessment of intracranial stenoses, occlusions, and cross-flow through the anterior and posterior communicating arteries, as well as midline shift in hemispheric infarcts. TCCS is also useful for diagnosis and monitoring of vasospasm and detection of supratentorial hematomas and aneurysms, and may identify arteriovenous malformations.

Electroencephalography (EEG) should be urgently performed if postictal hemiparesis (Todd's paresis) is suspected. On EEG epileptic activity can be found. On the other hand, seizures may also be caused by stroke. Hemiplegic migraine usually shows unilateral slow background activity, and without MRI no clear destinction between migraine and stroke can be made.

Cardiac examinations should include transthoracic echocardiogram (TTE) with agitated saline for detection of patent foramen ovale (PFO). Transesophageal echocardiography (TEE) should be considered if TTE is non-diagnostic, or if there is a high index of suspicion for a cardioembolic source. TEE is the gold standard for detection of valve vegetations in endocarditis and structural cardiac abnormalities.

Laboratory evaluation includes blood cell and platelet count, hemoglobin, electrolytes, liver and renal functions, HIV, Venereal Disease Research Laboratory (VDLR), fasting lipid profile, C-reactive protein, antinuclear antibody, and erythrocyte sedimentation rate.

Lactate, plasma amino acids, urine amino, and organic acids should be quantified if homocystinuria or MELAS is suspected. Analysis of the cerebrospinal fluid is the diagnostic clue for stroke caused by vasculitis due to infections of the central nervous system.

Numerous prothrombotic disorders can be associated with ischemic strokes in children and young adults. Screening laboratory evaluation includes detection of possible underlying acquired and genetic coagulation factor abnormalities (see the earlier discussion).

Treatment

At present, acute management and treatment are based on extrapolation from the literature on adults and expert opinion, as no evidence-based guidelines exist regarding management of children and adolescents, except in sickle cell anemia. International, multicenter trials are ongoing and should provide some answers over the next few years.

Aspirin is considered the first-line antiplatelet agent in children and adolescents. The efficacy and optimal dose of aspirin in the treatment of children with acute arterial ischemic stroke are not known. It is commonly used at a dose of 3–5 mg/kg/day. Most experts recommend aspirin for secondary stroke prevention in children. Experience with other antiplatelet drugs such as clopidogrel hardly exists in children.

Alteplase (rtPA) is not approved for use in patients less than 18 years of age with ischemic stroke. Data from case reports and international registries of intravenous or intra-arterial thrombolysis use exist only in small numbers of children. Effectiveness, safety, and dose of rtPA for the treatment of children with arterial ischemic stroke have not been established. For children with acute ischemic stroke, current consensus guidelines recommend not using thrombolysis or mechanical thrombectomy outside of specific research protocols or clinical trials.

There is no consensus regarding the use of thrombolysis for older adolescents. However, recognizing that safety and efficacy data are lacking in patients younger than 18 years of age, it may be reasonable to consider thrombolytic treatment on an individual basis for older adolescents (age 15 and older) with acute arterial ischemic stroke. Strict adherence to the accepted time limits, care, and attention to contraindications criteria used in adults have to be ensured if thrombolytic therapy is employed for older adolescents.

As many pediatric stroke centers have experience with acute treatment of childhood stroke, they are likely capable of making acute care decisions about fibrinolysis in children on a case-by-case basis in conjunction with patient and parental consent.

The use of anticoagulation in children with cardiac embolism is controversial. It involves balancing the risk of precipitating hemorrhagic transformation of the infarct with the potential to prevent further embolic events. The decision may be influenced by several factors including time elapsed since stroke, neurological and imaging findings, and pathology of the cardiovascular system.

In SCD, chronic blood transfusion is effective for secondary and primary prevention.

Supportive care should ensure adequate hydration, ventilation, oxygenation, and blood pressure management. Infarct volume and outcome may be related to body temperature during the first days of the stroke. Blood glucose levels should be maintained in the normal range. Seizures in the acute stage should be treated rapidly.

A change in the level of arousal may be the first sign of expanding brain edema. Surgical decompression in children presenting with coma with large ischemic infarcts of the middle cerebral artery may be necessary, which are very often lethal if managed conservatively.

Data regarding endovascular interventional treatment in childhood stroke are limited to case reports. Outcome data are not available in all reports, so clinical relevance is unclear. An individualized approach to decisions regarding the appropriateness of endovascular therapy in children is recommended by most experts and should likely be limited to centers familiar with childhood stroke.

In patients with moyamoya-related strokes revascularization surgery using different techniques has been reported to be successful.

In summary, stroke in children and young adults is an important cause of morbidity and mortality. The clinical presentation varies, and adequate diagnosis requires rapid use of multidisciplinary approaches to reduce the probability of serious neurological consequences. Clinical trials are needed to confirm the efficacy in children of selected therapies now used in adults.

Further reading

Bernard TJ, Rivkin MJ, Scholz K, et al. Thrombolysis in Pediatric Stroke Study. Emergence of the primary pediatric stroke center: Impact of the thrombolysis in pediatric stroke trial. *Stroke* 2014;45(7):2018–2023.

Bigi S, Fischer U, Wehrli E, et al. Acute ischemic stroke in children versus young adults. *Ann Neurol* 2011;70(2):245–254.

Cnossen MH, Aarsen FK, Akker SLJ, et al. Pediatric arterial ischaemic stroke: Functional outcome and risk factors. *Dev Med Child Neurol* 2010;52(4):394–399.

Dlamini N, Billinghurst L, Kirkham FJ. Cerebral venous sinus (sinovenous) thrombosis in children. *Neurosurg Clin N Am* 2010;21(3):511–527.

Ellis MJ, Amlie-Lefond C, Orbach DB. Endovascular therapy in children with acute ischemic stroke: Review and recommendations. *Neurology* 2012;79(13 Suppl 1):S158–S164.

Ishekhlee A, Geller T, Mehta S, et al. Thrombolysis for children with acute ischemic stroke: A perspective from the kids' inpatient database. *Pediatr Neurol* 2013;49(5):313–318.

Jordan LC, Hillis AE. Hemorrhagic stroke in children. *Pediatr Neurol* 2007;**36**(2):73–88.

Monagle P, Chan AK, Goldenberg NA, et al. Antithrombotic therapy in neonates and children: Antithrombotic therapy and prevention of thrombosis, 9th ed: American College of Chest Physicians Evidence-Based Clinical Practice Guidelines. *Chest* 2012;141(2 Suppl): 737S–801S.

Poisson SN, Schardt TQ, Dingman A, Bernard TJ. Etiology and treatment of arterial ischemic stroke in children and young adults. *Curr Treat Options Neurol* 2014;16(10): 315.

12 Other cerebrovascular syndromes

David J. Blacker

University of Western Australia, Department of Neurology, Sir Charles Gairdner Hospital, and the Western Australian Neuroscience Research Institute, Nedlands, Western Australia

This chapter addresses a miscellaneous collection of cerebrovascular conditions not covered elsewhere in Part I. These include stroke associated with migraine, stroke associated with substance abuse, cerebral autosomal dominant arteriopathy with subcortical infarcts and leukoencephalopathy (CADASIL) and related conditions, hypertensive encephalopathy and posterior reversible encephalopathy syndrome (PRES), periprocedural, postoperative, and in-hospital stroke, and some rare stroke syndromes. These conditions might be encountered in a wide variety of medical settings around the world.

Stroke and migraine

The relationship between stroke and migraine is complex. Migraine is a risk factor for stroke. Patients suffering from migraine with aura have a higher risk of developing stroke than those with migraine without aura. Migraine as a stroke risk factor is more prominent among women on oral contraceptives and among smokers. Migraine may also be caused by stroke. Migraine and stroke are intertwined in a number of diseases, notably several hereditary disorders with patients presenting both migraine and stroke. Genetic vasculopathies are remarkable in that migraine and stroke together form a characteristic phenotype, providing genetic insight into the possible vascular mechanisms that are shared between migraine and stroke. Common vasculopathic mechanisms for both migraine and stroke include heightened susceptibility to cortical spreading depression and degenerative changes in the vascular wall affecting media and endothelial dysfunction. CADASIL is the most extensively studied genetic vasculopathy. CADASIL and other genetic vasculopathies are detailed in a later section of this chapter.

Headache mimicking migraine may present in patients with dissection of cervicocerebral vessels (see Chapter 8 for characteristic features of head pain). Patent foramen ovale (PFO) is a comorbidity for both migraine and stroke. Closure of the PFO may prevent paroxysmal embolism, which is a cause of stroke. However, reversal of right-to-left shunt with closure of PFO may not prevent migraine. Those who suffer from migraine also have a higher prevalence of cardiovascular risk factors. Previously, it was thought that migraine sufferers harbor antiphospholipid antibodies more frequently than controls to provide a link of migraine to stroke. However, recent studies failed to verify this speculation.

Migrainous infarction is rare. Estimates of the incidence of migrainous infarction vary among a number of studies, probably related to difference in adherence to the International Headache Society (IHS) diagnostic criteria. The range is from 0.5–1.5% of all ischemic strokes and up to 10–14% of stroke in young patients (<45 years).

The IHS criteria suggest that the infarction results from hypoperfusion during an aura, and thus the stroke symptoms are similar to that of the aura. However, exceptions are frequently noted. Stroke may develop following migraine without aura. Imaging modalities measuring cerebral blood flow have demonstrated oligemia associated with cortical spreading depression that may become critical when cerebral blood flow is compromised in the setting of transient ischemic attack or stroke. One third of migrainous infarcts are located in the occipital lobe, the usual site of origin of spreading depression.

Investigation of migrainous infarction is essentially a diagnosis of exclusion and is similar to that routinely done for ischemic stroke. Secondary preventive measures include the usual antithrombotic therapies and management of vascular risk factors. Specific concerns include cessation of smoking, discontinuation of oral contraceptives and other hormone therapies, and avoidance of vasoactive migraine treatments such as ergot derivatives and triptans, which may trigger vasoconstriction and cerebral hypoperfusion.

Stroke and substance abuse

A tragic and eminently avoidable stroke syndrome is stroke associated with substance abuse. Although "legal" drugs such as nicotine and alcohol probably contribute to a large majority of strokes, the focus of this section will be on illicit substances commonly used as recreational drugs that have been implicated in causing both ischemic and hemorrhagic stroke. The major recreational drugs associated with stroke are psychomotor stimulants, including amphetamine and its derivatives. It should be noted that other recreational drugs such as cannabis, opioids, and psychotomimetic drugs, gammahydroxybutyrate (GHB) and methylenedioxypyrovalerone (MDPV), have been reported to cause stroke. Weight-loss medications such as phenylpropanolamine are implicated in hemorrhagic stroke. A systemic approach to strokes caused by substance abuse is outlined in what follows.

Cardiac

Infective endocarditis caused by intravenous drug use, hypertension and arrhythmias induced by cocaine and methamphetamine, and cardiomyopathy in alcoholics are the major cardiovascular causes of stroke among people with substance abuse.

Extracranial large arteries

Methamphetamine and cocaine have been associated with dissection of cervicocerebral arteries resulting in stroke. It is likely that

---

International Neurology, Second edition. Edited by Robert P. Lisak, Daniel D. Truong, William M. Carroll and Roongroj Bhidayasiri
© 2016 John Wiley & Sons, Ltd. Published 2016 by John Wiley & Sons, Ltd.

these drugs may have a direct vasculopathic effect. However, it is also possible that trauma-induced dissection may occur as a consequence of aberrant behaviors following ingestion of psychoactive substances such as cocaine or methamphetamine.

Intracranial vessels

As already noted, methamphetamine and cocaine may have direct toxic effects on blood vessels as well as causing vasospasm, vasculitis, and hypertension, resulting in ischemic or hemorrhagic stroke.

Other

Metabolic disturbances such as hyponatremia associated with methamphetamine use may lead to stroke-like symptoms. Complications of intravenous drug use and long-term alcoholism include hepatic failure with development of coagulopathy to cause hemorrhagic stroke. Heroin-related nephropathy may lead to renal failure, hypertension, and other concomitant stroke risk factors. Cannabis use is known to cause stroke and other arterial diseases as well, primarily in younger patients.

Cerebral autosomal dominant arteriopathy with subcortical infarcts and leukoencephalopathy (CADASIL) and related conditions

CADASIL is an inherited microangiopathy characterized by migraine with aura, recurrent strokes, and cognitive impairment at an early age. Stroke caused by CADASIL is typically subcortical, often presenting with classic lacunar syndromes. Rarely, it may present as an acute encephalopathy or intracerebral hemorrhage. CADASIL is caused by mutations in the NOTCH3 gene on chromosome 19, a discovery that has been a major breakthrough in our understanding of genetic vasculopathies. Various mutations have been unraveled, including an autosomal recessive form in a Japanese population.

Magnetic resonance imaging (MRI) typically shows marked periventricular and subcortical white matter T2 signal hyperintensities, which may be differentiated from hypertensive leukoaraiosis by predilection for the external capsule and anterior temporal lobes. Differential diagnoses also include Binswanger's disease and multiple sclerosis.

No specific treatment for CADASIL is currently available.

Other genetic vasculopathies include mitochondrial encephalopathy lactic acidosis and stroke (MELAS), hereditary endotheliopathy with retinopathy, neuropathy, and stroke (HERNS), retinovasculopathy and cerebral leukodystrophy (RVCL), and hereditary infantile hemiparesis, retinal arteriolar tortuosity, and leukoencephalopathy (HIHRATL).

Hypertensive encephalopathy posterior reversible encephalopathy syndrome (PRES) and reversible cerebral vasoconstrictive syndrome (RCVS)

Stroke physicians may encounter patients with hypertensive encephalopathy PRES or RCVS that have some similarities to patients with ischemic or hemorrhagic stroke who may be hypertensive. Hypertensive encephalopathy occurs when cerebral autoregulation is overwhelmed by a sudden rise in blood pressure, usually to extreme levels in the vicinity of 250/150 mmHg. Vasodilatation of intracranial vessels, cerebral hyperperfusion, and exudation of fluid may lead to elevated intracranial pressure. Renal disease, pheochromocytoma, sympathomimetic drugs, systemic vasculitides, or pregnancy may be the predisposing condition. Previously normotensive patients may be more vulnerable than chronic hypertensives (particularly if the change is abrupt), since in the latter cerebral autoregulation is already "shifted to the right."

Clinical features include headache, nausea and vomiting, visual symptoms, such as blurring or cortical blindness, impaired consciousness, and seizures. Physical findings include retinal hemorrhages and hyperreflexia. Focal neurological deficits usually are compatible with those seen in patients with hemorrhagic or ischemic stroke. Imaging findings are described shortly. Parenteral antihypertensive agents (e.g., sodium nitroprusside) are the mainstay in treating hypertension in this setting, with caution to be exercised to avoid excessive reduction in blood pressure leading to cerebral hypoperfusion.

Since the first descriptions of PRES in the mid-1990s, it has become recognized that this syndrome may not necessarily be posterior in location and may not be reversible. The typical presentations of PRES are headache, seizures, and visual loss, with accelerated hypertension, often in patients taking immunosuppressant medications such as cyclosporin and tacrolimus. The pathogenesis is proposed to be vasogenic edema without infarction secondary to disruption of normal cerebral autoregulation. The white matter of the parieto-occipital region is most commonly involved, possibly related to the degree of sympathetic innervation in the arteries supplying this area. Diffusion-weighted MRI (DWI) and apparent diffusion coefficient (ADC) sequences may be helpful in studying the vasogenic and cytotoxic components of brain edema for predicting the regions that are destined for recovery or infarction. Treatment includes antihypertensive and anticonvulsant agents and adjustment of immunosuppressant medications (also see Chapter 16).

Reversible cerebral vasoconstrictive syndrome (RCVS) is thought to be a transient disturbance of cerebral arterial vascular tone, sometimes precipitated by sympathomimetic or seretonergic drugs, postpartum state, or surges in blood pressure related to exercise or sexual intercourse. It typically presents with thunderclap headache, nausea, and vomiting, and sometimes seizures or focal neurological signs, if complicated by subarachnoid hemorrhage, or stroke. Headaches may recur over 1–4 weeks before resolving. Precipitating causes (especially drugs) need to be identified and ceased, and primary angiitis of the central nervous system should be considered. Treatment with calcium channel blockers or magnesium may be helpful.

Periprocedural, postoperative, and in-hospital stroke

There is an expanding literature on stroke related to medical procedures, perhaps driven by medicolegal concerns, but also reflecting the reality that stroke does occur in patients who are hospitalized. In-hospital stroke offers opportunities for timely interventions. Cardiac and carotid surgeries and neurosurgical procedures carry stroke risk inherent to the nature of the surgeries, and due to the fact that patients undergoing these procedures frequently have stroke risk factors. Patients receiving other types of surgeries may also be predisposed to stroke because of interruption of antiplatelet or antithrombotic medications, and other factors such as thrombogenic milieu generated or hemodynamic alterations induced during and after surgery. One large series of general surgery cases noted a perioperative stroke risk of 0.2%. Prospective studies of coronary artery bypass grafting show a stroke risk of approximately 2% on average, but risk varies greatly depending on the age of the patient and the invasiveness of the procedure.

Patients on medical wards may also be at risk, particularly cardiac patients who share common stroke risk factors such as atrial fibrillation and are predisposed to stroke by undergoing angiographic studies or are on intense antithrombotic therapy. General medical patients with infection, dehydration, and renal impairment may also be at risk. Cancer patients with either hyperviscosity or coagulopathy, especially those with hematological malignancies, are at higher risk.

Acute therapeutic options may be limited by the risk of bleeding from the fresh surgical site, but intra-arterial techniques may provide a potential treatment option for ischemic stroke in this setting.

Rare stroke syndromes

There are a number of rare, non-inflammatory cerebral vasculopathies that may lead to stroke. These include Fabry's disease, postpartum vasculopathy, and those with predominantly ophthalmological features such as Eale's and Susac's diseases.

Conclusion

This chapter has outlined a heterogenous group of vascular-related conditions that are rare, but often need consideration and sometimes expert management in the setting of a stroke service.

Further reading

Blacker DJ. In-hospital stroke. *Lancet Neurol* 2003;2:741–746.

Caplan LR. Lacunar infarction and small vessel disease: Pathology and pathophysiology. *J Stroke* 2015;17(1):2–6.

Fonseca AC, Ferro JM. Drug abuse and stroke. *Curr Neurol Neurosci Rep* 2013;13(2):325.

Peezzini A, Del Zotto E, Giossi A, *et al.* The migraine-ischemic stroke relation in young adults. *Stroke Res Treat* 2011;Dec 9. doi:10.4061/2011/304921

Stott VL, Hurrell MA, Anderson TJ. Reversible posterior leukoencephalopathy syndrome: A misnomer reviewed. *Int Med J* 2005;35:83–90.

13 Cerebral venous disease

Patrick W. Carney[1] and Stephen M. Davis[2]

[1] Florey Institute of Neuroscience and Mental Health, Heidelberg, VIC, Australia
[2] Melbourne Brain Centre, Royal Melbourne Hospital, and University of Melbourne, Parkville, VIC, Australia

Diseases of the cerebral venous system lead to cerebral venous sinus thrombosis (CVST). CVST may present as a cause of stroke or chronically with symptoms of intracranial hypertension. The prevalence and cause of CVST are variable and to some extent relate to cultural and economic factors.

Epidemiology

The epidemiology of CVST is difficult to define. CVST used to be thought of as an uncommon serious condition, with the diagnosis predominantly made at autopsy. However, recent developments in neuroimaging have established that CVST is much more prevalent than previously thought. A Saudi Arabian study found that 7 cases per 100,000 hospitalized patients had CVST. In India CVST is believed to cause up to 30% of strokes in the young. A Canadian review of pediatric stroke presentations estimated a population incidence of 0.67 cases per 100,000 per year. Mortality from CVST is approximately 8%. In a substantial proportion of patients, the cause of death could be attributed to underlying diseases that led to the sinus thrombosis. Functional outcome for survivors, however, is generally excellent, with minimal disability. Furthermore, recurrence rates are very low.

CVST commonly affects young people. The mean age of onset in several series is approximately 37 years. Younger patients with CVST often have different underlying causes and a better outcome. The condition predominantly affects women, with a female-to-male ratio of 3:1, and is strongly related to hormonal factors, including pregnancy and oral contraceptive use (see later discussion).

Pathophysiology

A variety of risk factors for the development of CVST have been identified (Table 13.1). CVST may occur due to systemic or local intracranial factors. Both acquired and inherited thrombophilic risk factors can lead to spontaneous cerebral venous thrombosis. Local processes, such as infection or intracranial tumors, may also cause venous obstruction leading to venous stasis and thrombosis. As a consequence of this there may be local complications such as venous infarction, due to occlusion of cortical veins, or a generalized increase in intracranial pressure.

Spontaneous venous sinus thrombosis is particularly a disorder of women and occurs in frequent association with hormonal factors, including pregnancy and the oral contraceptive pill (OCP). Increasingly, it has been recognized that inherited hypercoagulability disorders may lead to the development of CVST in isolation, or

Table 13.1 Recognized causes of dural sinus thrombosis

1. Systemic diseases/factors
   a. Hormonal
      i. Pregnancy and the puerperium
      ii. Oral contraceptive pill
      iii. Other hormone supplements
   b. Coagulation disorders
      i. Inherited
         1. Factor V Leiden
         2. Prothrombin gene mutation
         3. Protein C and S deficiencies
      ii. Acquired
         1. Antiphospholipid antibodies/lupus anticoagulant
         2. Disseminated intravascular coagulation
   c. Other hematological disorders
      i. Polycythemia vera
      ii. Thrombocythemia
   d. Systemic inflammatory cisease
      i. Systemic lupus erythematosis
      ii. Behcet's disease
   e. Malignancy
   f. Other
      i. Systemic infections
      ii. Nephrotic syndrome
      iii. Any cause of dehydration
2. Local diseases/factors
   a. Infection
      i. Extradural
         1. Mastoiditis
         2. Sinusitis
      ii. Intradural
         1. Meningitis
         2. Abscess
         3. Empyema
   b. Neurosurgical procedures including lumbar puncture
   c. Head injury
   d. Tumor

more commonly in conjunction with risk factors such as pregnancy or OCP use. Commonly identified risk factors include activated protein C resistance associated with the factor V Leiden mutation, the prothrombin gene mutation, and isolated factor deficiencies such as protein C, S, and anti-thrombin III. The identification of one risk factor should not halt the search for other potential causes.

Although local infection leading to venous sinus thrombosis is becoming increasingly rare, sepsis remains an important potential cause of CVST in the developing world. Infections including otitis media, mastoiditis, and paranasal sinusitis may lead to local venous sinus thrombophlebitis. Systemic sepsis also increases the risk of thrombosis, including cerebral venous thrombosis. The largest prospective study of CVST, the International Study on Cerebral Vein

International Neurology, Second edition. Edited by Robert P. Lisak, Daniel D. Truong, William M. Carroll and Roongroj Bhidayasiri
© 2016 John Wiley & Sons, Ltd. Published 2016 by John Wiley & Sons, Ltd.

and Dural Sinus Thrombosis, found an increased rate of infections leading to CVST among African and Asian populations, although obstetric factors remain the most significant cause.

CVST may arise as a complication of traumatic brain injury and should be considered as a cause of further neurological deterioration.

Clinical features

The clinical presentation of venous sinus disease is highly variable and relates to the underlying cause and the effect of venous obstruction. Venous sinus obstruction leads to a generalized increase in intracranial pressure associated with reduced venous outflow and impaired cerebrospinal fluid (CSF) absorption. This leads to headaches, impairment of consciousness, cognitive deficits, and visual blurring due to papilledema. Persistently elevated intracranial pressures leading to visual loss are uncommon. Symptoms relating to increased intracranial pressure may be acute, subacute, or chronic in their presentation. Chronic presentations occurred in approximately 7% of cases in the largest prospective analysis of CVST, typically with idiopathic intracranial hypertension. These patients are frequently women and have an overall better outcome than those who experience venous infarction.

If sinus thrombosis is complicated by occlusion of cortical veins, venous infarction, often accompanied by hemorrhage, may occur. Such patients present acutely with focal neurological deficits such as hemiplegia, hemiparesis, sensory and visual inattention, and receptive and expressive speech deficits relating to the site of stroke damage.

Seizures are a common presenting symptom of venous infarction and are seen more commonly than in arterial stroke. Seizures may occur in patients with venous sinus disease without stroke, related to increased intracranial pressure or underlying causes such as infection or trauma.

The overall prognosis of those presenting with CVST is very good. The most common complication during the follow-up of patients after CVST is ongoing seizures (occurring in up to 10%), while recurrent thrombotic events may also occur. However, recurrent CVST is relatively uncommon, particularly when there is no clear precipitant or there are treatable risk factors. Importantly, CVST appears to occur rarely during subsequent pregnancies in women who had CVST in a previous pregnancy.

Investigations

The diagnosis of CVST has been transformed by cerebral imaging. Plain computed tomography (CT) scan is useful for identifying venous infarction. The empty delta sign of low-attenuation thrombus surrounded by a triangular area of enhancement may be seen on contrast CT scan. However, CT is not sufficiently accurate to rule out CVST. CT venography is a further advance in the assessment of cerebral venous anatomy, with a sensitivity of up to 95%.

Traditionally, cerebral angiography with venography was the diagnostic test of choice for cerebral sinus disease. However, magnetic resonance imaging (MRI), particularly with MR venography (MRV), has largely replaced angiography and is generally considered the definitive investigation in the diagnosis of CVST. This modality not only enables imaging of thrombosed venous sinuses that are hyperintense on T1- and T2-weighted sequences (Figure 13.1), but also shows an absence of flow within the venous sinus. Furthermore, venous infarction and hemorrhage can be clearly identified.

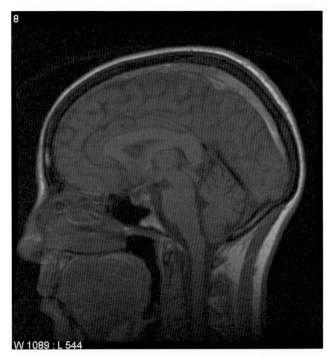

Figure 13.1 T1-weighted Sagittal image of a patient with Sagittal sinus thrombosis. The thrombosed sinus is hyperintense compared to the normal brain parenchymal signal. Courtesy of Dr. G. Fitt.

Cerebral angiography remains helpful for some difficult cases where MRI/MRV is not definitive. It is also used as the basis for the delivery of topical thrombolysis.

Treatment

The approach to managing CVST involves investigation and treatment of the underlying cause and specific therapy for the sinus thrombosis. The mainstay of therapy is systemic anticoagulation. A meta-analysis performed on three small studies of anticoagulation in CVST showed a trend toward benefit with anticoagulation, although it was not statistically significant. In contrast, expert opinion strongly supports acute anticoagulation, based on a dramatic reduction in case fatality rates in modern case series where heparin use has been routine. There is a paucity of evidence from randomized controlled trials to support treatment of CVST. However, a recent study in India randomized patients to either low molecular weight heparin (LMWH) or unfractionated heparin (UFH), and found a significantly higher mortality rate when therapy was instituted with UFH. Subtherapeutic anticoagulation occurred in over half of patients in the UFH group and was likely to have contributed to this result. Anticoagulation with heparin is followed by a variable period of warfarin therapy, even in the presence of parenchymal hemorrhage, due to clear research evidence in support of anticoagulation even in the presence of intracerebral hemorrhage.

The appropriate duration of oral anticoagulation therapy remains unclear. Commonly warfarin would be used for 6 months, but longer term if there is a demonstrated persisting coagulopathy. With these guidelines, recurrence is very rare. MRI can be used to follow the progress of sinus recanalization, but this may be incomplete and is not a reliable guide to the duration of therapy.

Both systemic and local thrombolysis have been employed to treat CVST. These approaches may lead to a more frequent and rapid restoration of venous flow, but there are no randomized controlled trials of thrombolysis versus anticoagulation. A systematic review of intravenous thrombolysis has demonstrated good outcomes, but has highlighted the risk of *de novo* intracranial hemorrhage. Local thrombolysis and other endovascular techniques have been used successfully in adult and pediatric populations, particularly with extensive thrombosis or poor prognostic signs, with good outcomes and favorable complication rates.

In the acute phase of the illness the main cause of death is brain herniation, resulting from either a hemorrhagic lesion or diffuse cerebral edema. It would appear that cerebrospinal fluid shunting is insufficient treatment in this circumstance, while decompressive craniectomy has been demonstrated to be safe and effective.

Further reading

Ferro JM, Canhao P, Stam J, Bousser MG, Baringagarrementeria F. Prognosis of cerebral vein and dural sinus thrombosis: Results of the International Study on Cerebral Vein and Dural Sinus Thrombosis. *Stroke* 2004;35:664–670.

Guo XB, Guan S, Fan Y, Song LJ. Local thrombolysis for severe cerebral venous sinus thrombosis. *Am J Neuroradiol* 2012;33:1187–1190.

Misra UK, Kalita J, Chandra S, Kumar B, Bansai V. Low molecular weight heparin versus unfractionated heparin in cerebral venous thrombosis: A randomized controlled trial. *Eur J Neurol* 2012;19:1030–1036.

Stram J. Thrombosis of the cerebral veins and sinuses. *N Engl J Med* 2005;352:1791–1798.

Viegas LD, Stolz E, Canhao P, Ferrro JM. Systemic thrombolysis for cerebral venous and dural sinus thrombosis: A systematic review. *Cerebrovasc Dis* 2014;37:43–50.

14 Spinal cord strokes

Rohini Bhole[1] and Louis R. Caplan[2]
[1] University of Tennessee Health Science Center, Memphis, TN, USA
[2] Beth Israel Deaconess Medical Center, Harvard Medical School, Boston, MA, USA

Spinal cord strokes represent a minute fraction of all central nervous system vascular diseases. As in the brain, spinal cord strokes can be divided into two large groups: ischemic and hemorrhagic. They account for about 1% of all strokes and about 5–8% of acute myelopathies. The rarity of spinal cord strokes and lack of accessibility to study the spinal cord vascular system in a timely manner have prevented a thorough understanding of spinal cord vascular diseases.

Spinal cord vascular supply

The arterial supply of the spinal cord is unique. A large single anterior spinal artery runs in the ventral midline rostrally from the spinomedullary junction at the foramen magnum to the filum terminale caudally. In contrast, paired smaller posterior spinal arteries are located on the dorsal surface, and often form a plexus of small vessels (Figure 14.1). The central portion of the cord between the two zones of blood supply has often been called the border-zone or watershed region of the spinal cord.

The anterior spinal artery originates from the two vertebral arteries at the base of the skull, feeds the medulla, and descends in the midline through the foramen magnum to supply the cervical spinal cord. The anterior spinal artery is fed by 5–10 radicular arteries. Blood supply is most marginal in the upper thoracic region (T4–T8) and has been referred to as the longitudinal watershed region of the spinal cord. The largest radicular artery, the artery of Adamkiewicz, arises from the aorta most often in the T9–T12 region.

In contrast to the ventral cord, there is a rich plexus of vessels that lie on the dorsal cord. Posteriorly, there are the paired posterior spinal arteries that supply the dorsal columns and posterior gray matter. The blood supply of the dorsal cord is much richer than that of the ventral cord, which is more vulnerable to ischemic insult. The blood supply to the ventral cord is vulnerable to becoming decompensated by the occlusion of a large radicular branch or lesions in the aorta.

Spinal cord ischemia and infarction

The evolution of the understanding of spinal cord infarction parallels the evolution of knowledge about the mechanism of brain infarction. Spinal cord infarctions can be subdivided into the following six types: (1) bilateral, predominantly anterior (Figure 14.2A) – clinical features are bilateral motor and spinothalamic sensory deficits and posterior column sensory functions (vibration and position sense) are spared; (2) unilateral, predominantly anterior

(Figure 14.2B) – the clinical findings are hemiparesis below the lesion and contralateral spinothalamic tract sensory loss, a partial Brown-Séquard syndrome; (3) bilateral, predominantly posterior (Figure 14.2C) – posterior column sensory loss below the lesion is the consistent finding associated with bilateral pyramidal tract signs of variable magnitude; (4) unilateral, mostly posterior (Figure 14.2D) – ipsilateral hemiparesis is accompanied by posterior column sensory loss; (5) central (Figure 14.2E) – bilateral pain and temperature loss sparing posterior column and motor functions are similar to the sensory deficit seen with a syrinx; and (6) transverse – loss of motor, sensory, and sphincter functions are noted below the level of the lesion and anterior patterns are more prominent than posterior, especially after aortic surgery.

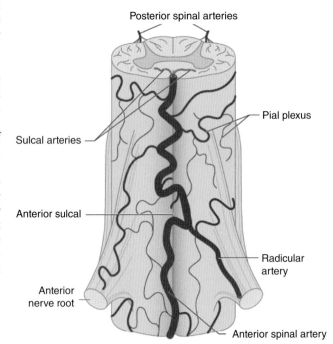

Figure 14.1 Cross-section of spinal cord showing arterial patterns of blood supply. The anterior spinal artery is a single midline artery that courses in the anterior fissure. The artery divides into left and right sulcal arteries, which supply the anterior horn and white matter. There are usually two posterior spinal arteries, one on each side, which anastomose and then branches emerge to supply the posterior gray horn and posterior columns. Source: Caplan 2009. Reproduced with permission of Elsevier.

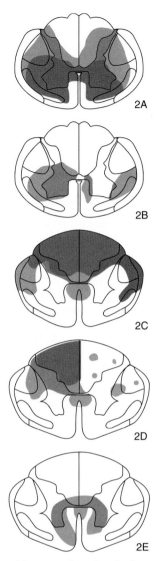

Table 14.1 Causes of spinal cord ischemia/infarction.

Arterial	Aortic disease	Aortic aneurysms	
Arterial		Aortic dissection	
		Traumatic rupture	
		Aortic surgery	Aortic aneurysm repair
	Embolic disease	Bacterial endocarditis	
		Atrial myxoma	
		Non-bacterial endocarditis	
		Fibrocartilaginous	Disc herniation, pregnancy, puerperium
	Dissections	Vertebral artery dissection	Cervical cord infarction
		Aortic dissection	Block orifices of spinal radicular arteries
	Infections and inflammations	Tuberculosis, syphilis	Spinal arteritis
		Fungal (cryptococcosis, coccidiomycosis)	
		Lyme's disease	
		Schistosomiasis	Parasite invading blood vessel or granulomatous inflammation
	Toxic	Heroin injection	Prolonged vasoconstriction
		Cocaine inhalation	
	Global ischemia	Severe hypotension Clinical shock Cardiac arrest	T4–T8 vulnerable segment (longitudinal watershed zone)
	Iatrogenic	Endovascular procedures involving aorta	Plaque dislodged that embolizes to spinal radicular arteries
Venous	Spinal arteriovenous malformations or dural fistulas		Venous thrombosis precipitating spinal cord infarction
	Spinal cavernous angiomas		

Figure 14.2 Cartoons of patterns of spinal cord infarction. Dark pink indicates the usual extent while light pink shows potentially large areas of ischemia. (A) Anterior bilateral infarction. (B) Anterior predominantly unilateral infarction. (C) Posterior bilateral infarction. (D) Posterior predominantly unilateral infarction. (E) Central spinal cord infarction. Source: Caplan 2009. Reproduced with permission of Elsevier.

Causes of spinal cord ischemia

The major causes of ischemia in the spinal cord are described in this section and in Table 14.1.

Disease of the aorta

This is undoubtedly the most commonly recognized cause of spinal cord infarction. Paraplegia is not an uncommon finding after repair of thoracic and abdominal aortic aneurysms. During surgical repair of the aorta, blood flow through radicular arteries to the anterior spinal artery is compromised. Similar findings are noted in unruptured aneurysms of the aorta, dissections of the aorta, traumatic rupture of the aorta, thromboembolic aortic occlusions, and ulcerative aortic plaque disease. Thrombi and plaques can obstruct the orifices of the radicular arteries. Dissections can tear or interrupt

the orifices of the feeding arteries to the spinal cord, occasionally spanning a long segment affecting a large number of arteries. Cholesterol crystals and other plaques may cause embolization in spinal arteries and branches. In some patients, the spinal ischemia may develop insidiously, giving the clinical impression of diabetic amyotrophy or even motor neuron disease because of selective involvement of anterior horn neurons or the pyramidal tract.

Embolism

Bacterial endocarditis is a recognized cause of embolic strokes in the brain and spinal cord. Atrial myxoma and non-bacterial thrombotic (marantic) endocarditis are other causes of embolic insults to the spinal cord. Fibrocartilaginous embolism presumably arises from disc herniations, predominantly affects young women, and nearly always involves the cervical spinal cord. This group of patients is characterized by the thromboembolic state specific for women during pregnancy or puerperium, or in those taking oral contraceptives. Minor trauma, sudden neck motion, or lifting have been identified as precipitating events.

Dissections

Vertebral artery dissection with cervical cord infarction has been reported. As already described, aortic dissections can block the orifices of the spinal radicular arteries leading to spinal cord infarction.

Infections and inflammation

Inflammation of the meningeal coverings of the spinal cord may spread to the spinal arteries, causing acute spinal cord stroke. This phenomenon is similar to Heubner's arteritis found in the brain in the presence of tuberculosis and syphilis. Chronic adhesive arachnoiditis from any cause may also lead to scarring and obliteration of the spinal penetrating arteries, resulting in ischemia of the central spinal cord.

Drug abuse

Spinal cord ischemia has been reported after heroin injection and cocaine inhalation. The most likely mechanism of spinal cord stroke after drug abuse is intense and prolonged vasoconstriction.

Global ischemia

Spinal cord ischemia may also develop during severe hypotension, shock, or cardiac arrest. In the literature, the spinal cord watershed region, which is most vulnerable to global ischemia caused by severe hypotension or cardiac arrest, is between segments T4 and T8. However, in a recent report on systematic examination of 145 patients who died of cardiac arrest or severe hypotension, ischemic myelopathy was noted in more than 95% at the lumbosacral level, sparing the mid-thoracic cord.

Iatrogenic

Endovascular procedures and arteriography involving the aorta may cause spinal cord infarction by dislodging plaques that result in embolization of the spinal radicular arteries.

Venous infarction

Venous spinal cord infarction is less common than venous brain infarction. Venous spinal cord infarction is most often caused by mechanical compression, infection, or inflammation that obliterates veins. Venous hypertension is an important contributor to spinal cord infarction in patients with spinal dural fistulas. Thrombosis of spinal veins or increased pressure in the venous system may also cause spinal cord infarction. Venous occlusions may occur in patients with spinal vascular malformations. In some patients, venous occlusion is caused by a hypercoagulable state, as seen in patients with visceral cancer or septic thrombophlebitis. Venous spinal cord infarction can also be caused by spinal tumors with venous compression.

Spinal vascular malformations

Spinal vascular malformations include telangiectasis, venous malformations (angiomas), varices, cavernous malformations, arteriovenous malformations (AVMs), and dural malformations. The most common two entities are described in this section.

Dural malformations

The more frequently encountered spinal dural malformations can be divided into two large groups; those with (type I) and without (type II) intradural venous drainage. Spinal dural fistulas oc-

cur predominantly in men (4:1 ratio with women) between 40–70 years of age, involving mostly the lower thoracic and lumbosacral segments, usually with one arterial feeder. Clinical presentation of spinal dural fistulas is characterized by progressive neurological worsening, punctuated by acute deteriorations. Less common is an acute apoplectic onset. Dural fistulas usually do not cause subarachnoid hemorrhage (SAH), except when the lesions are at the cervical level. The cervical fistulas that cause SAH are fed by the vertebral arteries and are often located near the cervicomedullary junction. Thoracic, lumbar, and sacral fistulas rarely present with epidural hemorrhage or SAH. Spinal transient ischemic attacks (TIAs) are more frequent in patients with spinal dural fistulas than with other spinal vascular lesions. These lesions cause symptoms because of venous hypertension and occasional thrombosis of the venous drainage system. Intradural malformations can be intra- or extramedullary or located outside the spinal cord. Usually there are multiple dilated veins with venous hypertension.

Arteriovenous malformations

Spinal AVMs, unlike AVMs in the brain, often present with ischemia rather than hemorrhage. Veins draining an arteriovenous malformation can become occluded and venous angiomas often undergo thrombosis, precipitating spinal infarction. About 10% of patients with spinal AVMs develop SAH.

Investigations and management

Spinal cord ischemia

Diffusion-weighted magnetic resonance imaging (MRI) scans often show acute spinal cord infarction. Recent ischemia causes edema with increased signal on T2-weighted scans. Older infarcts show abnormally increased T2 signals. A key finding that suggests the presence of a dural fistula is serpiginous dilated veins on the surface of the spinal cord. These are often seen on T2-weighted and gadolinium-enhanced images and on contrast-enhanced MR angiography (MRA). Using MRA techniques, phase display after contrast injection may show the direction of flow within the epidural veins to indicate the likely location of the arterial feeders. The coiled serpiginous veins are usually visible along the dorsal cord surface during myelography, which still has a place in diagnosis. Figure 14.3 is an intraoperative photo showing enlarged veins on the surface of the spinal cord. Myelographic films should be taken with the patient lying supine to show the abnormal veins.

Intradural AVMs are referred to as low-flow vascular abnormality, because angiography usually shows slow, low-volume filling of the lesions. Selective spinal arteriography in expert hands often shows the feeding arteries, but occasionally the feeding arteries do not get opacified. Advances in imaging allow better strategic planning for therapeutic interventions. Surgical exploration is recommended when clinical findings are characteristic and abnormal veins are clearly shown with myelography or MRA. The venous structures have to be removed as well. In most patients in whom dural fistulas are well delineated, effective therapies may improve muscle strength and gait, although sacral spinal cord dysfunction (urination, defecation, sexual function) often remains unchanged. Surgical treatment is not as successful for intradural AVMs as for the dural entities. If cavernous angiomas are identified, they can be surgically removed.

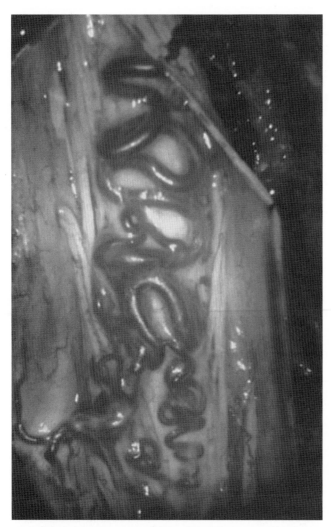

Figure 14.3 Intraoperative view of the surface of the spinal cord after the dura has been opened. Tortuous dilated veins can be seen along the surface of the spinal cord. Courtesy of Roberto Heros, MD, University of Miami. Source: Caplan 2009. Reproduced with permission of Elsevier.

Spinal hemorrhages

Hematomyelia refers to bleeding into the spinal cord parenchyma. The most common cause is trauma. Onset can be immediate or delayed. Usually the area around the central canal and gray matter is involved, most often in the cervical region. The usual signs are neck pain, weakness, and areflexia in the arms, associated with a cape-like distribution of pain and temperature loss. Other causes include AVMs, anticoagulation, hemophilia and other bleeding disorders, and hemorrhage into a spinal cord tumor (ependymoma, melanoma, angioblastoma) and less frequently syrinxes. The MRI shows a swollen blood-filled cord.

Spinal epidural hematoma is approximately four times more common than spinal subdural hematoma. Epidural or subdural hematoma may develop in patients who are on anticoagulants. Some patients may have severe liver disease with portal hypertension. Lumbar puncture has been known to precipitate epidural or subdural hematoma in patients on anticoagulants. The earliest symptom is pain in the dorsal region, more prominent in the neck than the back. This is followed by radicular pain, usually in one or both arms. The early symptoms may not be distinguished from those caused by disk herniation. Within hours, or rarely days, sensory and motor signs develop in the legs, bowel, and bladder, followed by sexual dysfunction. Usually, weakness and sensory loss are symmetric, but unilateral hemiplegia or paraplegia and dissociated hemisensory losses characteristic of Brown–Séquard syndrome may be noted. MRI is superior to computed tomography (CT) scanning in defining the location and extent of hematoma. Signs are almost invariably progressive unless the hematoma is evacuated. Anticoagulation should be reversed using vitamin K, fresh frozen plasma, or prothrombin complex concentrates, particularly those enriched with factor VII, factor X, and prothrombin. Decompression is urgent and should be pursued as soon as feasible with the international normalized ratio (INR) level under consideration. Outcome depends on the severity of the deficit before surgery, the duration of spinal cord compression, and the rapidity of onset of the paraplegia.

Further reading

Brust JCM. Stroke and substance abuse. In: Bogousslavsky J, Caplan LR (eds.). *Uncommon Causes of Stroke*. Cambridge: Cambridge University Press; 2001:132–138.

Caplan LR. *Spinal Cord Vascular Disease in Caplan's Stroke: A Clinical Approach*, 4th ed., Philadelphia, PA: Elsevier; 2009.

Cha YH, Chi JH, Barbaro NM. Spontaneous spinal subdural hematoma associated with low molecular-weight heparin: Case report. *Neurosurg Spine* 2005;2:612–613.

De Sèze J, Stojkovic T, Breteau G, et al. Acute myelopathies: Clinical, laboratory and outcome profiles in 79 cases. *Brain* 2001;124:1509–1521.

Duggal N, Lach B. Selective vulnerability of the lumbosacral spinal cord after cardiac arrest and hypotension. *Stroke* 2002;33:116–121.

Jacob A, Weinshenker BG. An approach to the diagnosis of acute transverse myelitis. *Semin Neurol* 2008;28:105–120.

Jellema K, Canta LR, Tijssen CC, et al. Spinal dural arteriovenous fistulas: Clinical features in 80 patients. *J Neurol Neurosurg Psychiatry* 2003;74:1438–1440.

Luetmer PH, Lane JI, Gilbertson JR, et al. Preangiographic evaluation of spinal dural arteriovenous fistulas with elliptic centric contrast-enhanced MR angiography and effect on radiation dose and volume of iodinated contrast material. *AJNR Am J Neuroradiol* 2005;26:711–718.

Morandi X, Riffaud L, Chabert E, Brassier G. Acute nontraumatic spinal subdural hematomas in three patients. *Spine* 2001;26:E547–E551.

Novy J, Carruzzo A, Maeder P, Bogousslavsky J. Spinal cord ischemia: Clinical and imaging patterns, pathogenesis, and outcomes in 27 patients. *Arch Neurol* 2006;63:1113–1120.

Saraf-Lavi E, Bowen BC, Quencer RM, et al. Detection of spinal dural arteriovenous fistulae with MR imaging and contrast-enhanced MR angiography: Sensitivity, specificity, and prediction of vertebral level. *AJNR Am J Neuroradiol* 2002;23:858–867.

Zampakis P, Santosh C, Taylor W, Teasdale E. The role of non-invasive computed tomography in patients with suspected dural fistulas with spinal drainage. *Neurosurgery* 2006;58:686–694.

PART 2   Disorders of Cerebrocascular Autonomic Control

15   Reversible cerebral vasoconstriction syndrome (RCVS)

Shih-Pin Chen and Shuu-Jiun Wang
Department of Neurology, Neurological Institute, Taipei Veterans General Hospital, and Faculty of Medicine, National Yang-Ming University School of Medicine, Taipei, Taiwan

Reversible cerebral vasoconstriction syndrome (RCVS) is a syndrome characterized by severe headaches with hyperacute onset and reversible segmental vasoconstrictions of cerebral arteries. RCVS was proposed as a unifying term in 2007 for varieties of historical nomenclature such as Call–Fleming syndrome, thunderclap headache (TCH) with reversible vasospasm, benign angiopathy of the central nervous system, postpartum angiopathy, drug-induced cerebral arteritis or angiopathy, or migraine angiitis. RCVS can be either primary or secondary to various factors, but regardless of etiological heterogeneity, the clinical and radiological characteristics are distinctively similar. With accumulating data, the clinical features, disease course, and neuroimaging findings of RCVS have been well characterized, and its pathophysiology is also being elucidated.

Epidemiology

The actual incidence and prevalence of RCVS are unknown, but it is not exceedingly rare. Large case series have been reported in Asia, Europe, and America, suggesting its worldwide distribution. In our hospital-based headache clinic in Taiwan, RCVS accounts for nearly 2% of headache patients (from a cohort of ~150,000). The peak age at onset is around 40–50 years in women and 30–40 years in men, but elderly and pediatric patients have been increasingly reported. Female predominance (F:M 2.6:1 to 10:1) has been found among different ethnic groups, despite variable clinical settings and inclusion criteria across studies.

Pathophysiology

Because RCVS has heterogeneous etiologies, the underlying mechanisms are likely multifactorial. Open brain biopsy and full autopsy have not demonstrated any evidence of arterial inflammation or infection, but only subendothelial thickening in the posterior cerebral artery in one case report. Dysregulation of cerebral vascular tone is probably the central element in the pathogenesis of RCVS. A sudden alteration of central vascular tone might lead to segmental cerebral vasoconstriction and compensatory vasodilatation in distal small arterioles, which could trigger the severe headaches by abruptly stretching the nociceptive fibers surrounding the vessel walls. Clinical observations such as blood pressure surge, triggers with elevated sympathetic tone, and the association with sympathomimetic agents, pheochromocytoma, and hypertensive crises indicate the role of sympathetic overactivity. A 24-hour heart rate variability study has revealed sympathetic overactivity and parasympathetic hypofunction in acute and remission stages in patients with RCVS. Furthermore, brain-derived neurotrophic factor (BDNF) is known to cause perivascular inflammation and vasoconstriction under circumstances of sympathetic overactivity, and the *BDNF Val66Met* polymorphism has been linked to the vasoconstriction in patients with RCVS. In addition, the level of 8-iso-prostaglandin F2α, an oxidative stress marker and potent vasoconstrictor, is higher in patients with RCVS and is correlated with the severity of vasoconstriction, supporting a detrimental role of oxidative stress to endothelial function and vascular reactivity. Patients with RCVS also have reduced circulating endothelial progenitor cells, suggesting an impaired capacity of the endothelial repairing system. Hence, it is plausible that the complex interaction of sympathetic overactivity, oxidative stress, and endothelial dysfunction contributes to dysregulated vascular tone in RCVS. This is further supported by the known pathogenesis of the overlapping syndrome or spectral disorder of RCVS, such as posterior reversible encephalopathy syndrome (PRES), pre-eclampsia, or eclampsia. Sex hormones might also contribute to the pathogenesis, but this speculation remains to be proved.

PRES is found in up to one-third of patients with RCVS, and nearly 90% of patients with PRES have been found to have vasoconstrictions or vasculopathies. In addition, acute severe headaches are commonly seen in patients with PRES. Immunosuppressive or cytotoxic agents that might cause RCVS are also common causes of PRES. Previous studies have indicated that the autoregulation in PRES is impaired, which leads to progressive increases of vascular resistance (phenomenologically presented as vasoconstriction) and permeability of the blood–brain barrier (which contributes to vasogenic edema). When vasoconstrictions become severe and involve more proximal vessels, irreversible ischemic change over the border zones develops.

International Neurology, Second edition. Edited by Robert P. Lisak, Daniel D. Truong, William M. Carroll and Roongroj Bhidayasiri
© 2016 John Wiley & Sons, Ltd. Published 2016 by John Wiley & Sons, Ltd.

Postpartum angiopathy, one of the secondary causes of RCVS, has been considered a spectral disorder of eclampsia and pre-eclampsia. Concentrations of placental growth factor (PlGF), soluble PlGF receptor (sFlt-1), and a soluble transforming growth factorβ1 receptor (soluble endoglin) correlate with the presence of eclampsia; the ratio of sFlt-1 to PIGF also predicts the occurrence of pre-eclampsia. The balance of these antiangiogenic and proangiogenic factors might also play a role in the pathogenesis of postpartum angiopathy.

Clinical features

The most important clinical hallmark of RCVS is thunderclap headache (TCH), which denotes an unanticipated, severe headache reaching maximum intensity within one minute. Repeated attacks of TCHs have been noted in more than 80% of patients with RCVS, and most of the TCHs have identifiable triggers such as Valsalva-like maneuvers (exertion, defecation, sexual activity, urination, or cough), bathing, or emotional disturbance. In atypical cases, the headaches might not reach maximal intensity within one minute, but these headaches are nonetheless acute and severe. Absence of headache is exceptional. When a patient experiences multiple TCHs within a short period, RCVS is the most probable diagnosis, but aneurysmal subarachnoid hemorrhage (SAH) should always be excluded first. TCHs tend to remit within 2–3 weeks, while vasoconstriction is usually at its worst point on headache remission and takes up to 3 months to recover. Blood pressure surges accompanying headache attacks have been reported in more than one-third of patients. Some patients might develop mild persistent headaches after remission of TCH. New diagnostic criteria for headaches attributed to RCVS have been proposed in the International Classification of Headache Disorders, 3rd edition beta version (ICHD-3 (beta), code 6.7.3; Table 15.1).

Primary RCVS (spontaneous or evoked by triggers) accounts for 39–94% of cases in large series, while secondary RCVS accounts for 6–61% of cases, depending on study setting, patient selection criteria, or ethnic differences. Vasoactive substances (such as cannabis, ecstasy, cocaine, amphetamine, serotonergic drugs, or sympathomimetics) and postpartum state are the most common secondary causes. Immunosuppressants or cytotoxic agents, exposure to blood products, catecholamine-secreting tumors, or extra- or intracranial arterial disorders or procedures are occasionally the culprits.

Table 15.1 Diagnostic criteria of headaches attributed to reversible cerebral vasoconstriction syndrome (RCVS) in the International Classification of Headache Disorders, 3rd edition beta version (ICHD-3 (beta), code 6.7.3). Source: International Classification of Headache Disorders. Reproduced with permission of Sage Publications.

Diagnostic criteria of RCVS in the ICHD-3 (beta)
A. Any new headache fulfilling criterion C
B. Reversible cerebral vasoconstriction syndrome (RCVS) has been diagnosed
C. Evidence of causation demonstrated by at least one of the following:
1. headache, with or without focal deficits and/or seizures, has led to angiography (with "strings and beads" appearance) and diagnosis of RCVS
2. headache has either or both of the following characteristics:
a. recurrent during ≤1 month, and with thunderclap onset
b. triggered by sexual activity, exertion, Valsalva maneuvers, emotion, bathing and/or showering
3. no new significant headache occurs >1 month after onset
D. Not better accounted for by another ICHD-3 diagnosis, and aneurysmal subarachnoid hemorrhage has been excluded by appropriate investigations.

Patients with RCVS are complicated by seizure (up to 21%), transient ischemic attacks (TIA, up to 16%), PRES or brain edema (9–38%), ischemic strokes over border zones (4–54%), convexity subarachnoid hemorrhage (SAH, up to 34%), intracerebral hemorrhage (ICH, up to 20%), or subdural hemorrhage (2%). Severity of vasoconstriction is associated with ischemic complications, while female sex and history of migraine are risk factors for hemorrhagic complications. Focal neurological deficits are reported in 9–63% of patients, while mortality has been noted in a few cases. In a prospective series, 12% of patients with RCVS had cervical artery dissection, and 7% of patients with cervical artery dissection were found to have RCVS. This strong association implicates a shared pathophysiology of both conditions and also underscores the need for prompt investigations for cervical artery dissections in RCVS patients with associated neck pain.

Investigations

Detailed history taking and neurological examinations are the keys to accurate diagnosis, but comprehensive neuroimaging studies are also indispensable to investigate the causes of TCH and to demonstrate reversible cerebral vasoconstrictions. For patients who present with the first episode of TCH, an emergent computed tomography (CT) scan of brain and/or cerebrospinal fluid (CSF) studies are mandatory to exclude aneurysmal SAH. If a patient has experienced multiple TCH without overt meningeal signs, brain magnetic resonance imaging (MRI) is the study of choice for differential diagnosis and evaluating complications. The MR sequences should include T1/T2 to exclude intracranial structural lesions that could lead to TCH, such as pituitary apoplexy, aneurysmal SAH, retroclival intracerebral hematoma, and so on; fluid-attenuated inversion recovery imaging (FLAIR) to evaluate convexity SAH, white matter hyperintense lesions, PRES, and distal hyperintense vessels; gradient-echo (T2*) or susceptibility-weighted imaging to evaluate subtle aneurysmal or convexity SAH; diffusion-weighted imaging (DWI) and apparent diffusion coefficient (ADC) mapping plus perfusion-weighted imaging or arterial spin labeling to evaluate PRES or ischemic stroke; magnetic resonance angiography (MRA) to exclude cerebral aneurysms or arterial dissections and to evaluate the severity of vasoconstrictions; and venography (MRV) to exclude venous sinus thrombosis. If the headache is orthostatic, T1 with contrast plus MR myelography is recommended to exclude spontaneous intracranial hypotension. If there is accompanying unilateral neck pain, cervical T1 fat saturation with contrast should be considered to exclude cervical artery dissection.

It is hypothesized that vasoconstrictions in RCVS evolve centripetally from distal arterioles or small arteries, so that an angiographic study performed in the initial days of headache onset might not be able to capture vasoconstriction. The presence of distal hyperintense vessels on FLAIR imaging might be an early imaging sign indicating a diagnosis of RCVS. Vasoconstrictions in RCVS are usually string and beads in appearance (Figure 15.1), pervasive, and outlast headache resolution. Regular follow-ups are required.

Morphologically, RCVS greatly resemble primary angiitis of the central nervous system (PACNS), but the headaches in PACNS are usually milder and less acute. CT angiography and CT perfusion scan are good alternative tools for diagnosis, but the concern about radiation exposure makes them less feasible choices for repetitive follow-ups. Transcranial color-coded sonography (TCCS) is a useful non-invasive tool to monitor hemodynamic changes and predict

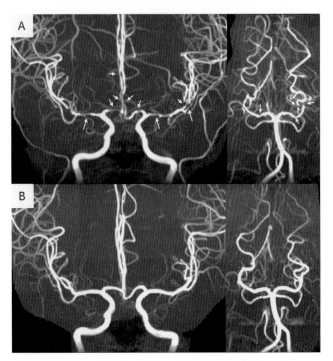

Figure 15.1 Typical imaging findings of reversible cerebral vasoconstriction syndrome. (A) Vasoconstriction during acute stage (indicated by arrows). (B) Reversal of vasoconstrictions.

risks of ischemic complications. Conventional angiography should be reserved for highly equivocal cases, because patients with RCVS are vulnerable to complications of angiography.

Laboratory tests should include thorough surveys of autoimmune profiles. In patients with abrupt blood pressure surges, 24-hour catecholamines should be checked. CSF study is mandatory to exclude aneurysmal SAH, infection, or inflammation of the central nervous system. Biopsy should generally be avoided.

Treatment

RCVS should be treated as an emergency. Patients using vasoactive drugs should be asked to discontinue them and to avoid triggers for TCH during the acute stage. There have not been any prospective randomized case-controlled trials, but calcium channel blockers, especially nimodipine (given 30–60mg every 4 hours orally or 0.5–2 mg/h via central venous catheter), was found to be effective in aborting TCH in 64–83% of patients in an open-label series. Blood pressure should be monitored closely when the patients are placed on calcium channel blockers, because hypotension might exacerbate cerebral hypoperfusion and worsen the condition in some patients. Magnesium sulfate has been shown to have acceptable outcomes

in a small subset of patients with postpartum angiography; nonetheless, large-scaled controlled trials are required. Glucocorticoids have been found to be independent predictors of poor outcome and should be avoided. Intra-arterial nimodipine, verapamil, or the phosphodiesterase inhibitor milrinone has been employed in some cases with refractory vasoconstrictions; however, this intra-arterial treatment should be limited to very experienced hands and risk of reperfusion injury should be considered.

Vasoconstrictions usually resolve within three months, but some patients have been found to have a more protracted course. Most patients recover from RCVS with excellent outcome, albeit permanent neurological deficits have been noted in 3–9% of patients in prospective studies, and 9–29% in retrospective series. Although RCVS generally runs a monophasic course, recurrence is possible. In a prospective long-term follow-up study, 10.7% of patients with RCVS experienced relapse of TCH, and half of these patients were found to have recurrent RCVS 6–87 months after the first episode. Having sexual activity as a trigger for thunderclap headaches (hazard ratio = 5.68) was an independent predictor of recurrent RCVS. Hence, long-term follow-up for patients with RCVS even after remission or appropriate education on the possibility of recurrent RCVS should be considered. Once patients develop new thunderclap-like headaches, clinicians should be aware that the recurrence of this potentially devastating disorder is highly probable.

Conclusion

RCVS is an important but underrecognized neurovascular disorder with potentially devastating ischemic or hemorrhagic complications. Diagnosis of RCVS should focus on excluding secondary causes of TCH, especially aneurysmal SAH, and demonstrating reversible cerebral vasoconstrictions with detailed craniocervical neurovascular imaging studies. A normal angiographic study during the initial days of disease onset does not exclude RCVS, and a follow-up study is mandatory. Sympathetic overactivity, endothelial dysfunction, and oxidative stress might play roles in the pathogenesis of RCVS. Calcium channel blockers, especially nimodipine, might be effective for TCHs in RCVS, but randomized placebo-controlled trials are still needed to optimize treatment strategies.

Further reading

Chen SP, Fuh JL, Lirng JF, Wang YF, Wang SJ. Recurrence of Reversible Cerebral Vasoconstriction Syndrome: a Long-Term Follow-up Study. Neurology 2015;84:1–7.

Chen SP, Fuh JL, Chang FC, et al. A transcranial color doppler study for reversible cerebral vasoconstriction syndromes. Ann Neurol 2008;63:751–757.

Chen SP, Fuh JL, Wang SJ, et al. Magnetic resonance angiography in reversible cerebral vasoconstriction syndromes. Ann Neurol 2010;67:648–656.

Ducros A. Reversible cerebral vasoconstriction syndrome. Lancet Neurol 2012;11:906–917.

Singhal AB, Hajj-Ali RA, Topcuoglu MA, et al. Reversible cerebral vasoconstriction syndromes: Analysis of 139 cases. Arch Neurol 2011;68:1005–1012.

16 Posterior reversible encephalopathy syndrome (PRES)

Pratik Bhattacharya
Michigan Stroke Network, Saint Joseph Mercy Oakland, Pontiac, MI, USA

Posterior reversible encephalopathy syndrome (PRES) was first described in 1996. It was initially called reversible posterior leukoencephalopathy syndrome (RPLS). However, magnetic resonance imaging (MRI) evaluations demonstrated gray and white matter involvement with edema, thereby giving it the present name. It is important for clinicians to consider PRES in the differential diagnosis for encephalopathy in the appropriate setting, as it is potentially reversible with prompt and aggressive treatment.

Epidemiology
PRES is not limited to any geographic location or race. Depending on the underlying etiology (Table 16.1), the disease can occur in both men and women, and in all age groups.

Table 16.1. Medications, diseases, and other conditions associated with PRES

Medications

Calcineurin inhibition: cyclosporin A, tacrolimus, sirolimus
Angiogenesis inhibition: bevacizumab, trastuzumab, bortezomib, carfilzomib, sorafenib, vemurafenib, regorafenib, sunitinib, axitinib, cediranib, pazopanib, thalidomide
Other chemotherapeutic agents: cisplatin, oxaliplatin, cytarabine, vincristine, gemcitabine, tiazofurin, cyclophosphamide, doxorubicin, etoposide, ipilimumab, alemtuzumab, methotrexate, vinorelbine
Immunosuppresive therapies: high-dose corticosteroids, intravenous immunoglobulin, mycophenolate mofetil, rituximab, azathioprine, fingolimod, infliximab, etanercept
Antibiotics: linezolid, ciprofloxacin
Hormonal therapies: anastrozole, enzalutamide
Others: erythropoietin, interleukin, interferon alpha, granulocyte stimulating factor, dihydroergotamine, nitroglycerine

Diseases

Eclampsia–pre-eclampsia
Accelerated hypertension
Sepsis
Kidney disease: nephrotic syndrome, glomerulonephritis, Goodpasture syndrome, microscopic polyangiitis, sickle glomerulopathy, hepatorenal syndromes, dialysis disequilibrium syndrome, granulomatous interstitial nephritis, exercise-induced acute renal failure
Inflammatory/autoimmune diseases: systemic lupus erythematosus, systemic sclerosis, granulomatosis with angiitis, polyarteritis nodosa, Behcet's disease, psoriasis, idiopathic thrombocytopenic purpura, Grave's disease, Guillain–Barré syndrome, Hashimoto thyroiditis, antiphospholipid antibodies, Takayasu arteritis, neuromyelitis optica, Crohn's disease, ulcerative colitis, primary sclerosing cholangitis, rheumatoid arthritis, autoimmune hepatitis, Sjögren syndrome, thromboangiitis obliterans
Other disease associations: myeloproliferative disease, subarachnoid hemorrhage with triple H therapy, cystinosis, thrombotic thrombocytopenic purpura, hemolytic uremic syndrome, autonomic dysreflexia in multiple system atrophy and spinal cord injury, acute intermittent porphyria, mitochondrial disease

Toxins

Substance abuse: cocaine, methamphetamine, marijuana, alcohol withdrawal and intoxication, lysergic acid diethylamide, licorice, mephedrone
Environmental toxins: snake bite (pit viper venom), scorpion, wasp and bee stings, organophosphate poisoning, starfruit intoxication
Infectious agents: influenza A, parainfluenza, plasmodium falciparum malaria, HHV 6, HIV-1 infection (in isolation and with opportunistic infections such as histoplasmosis, varicella zoster, blastomycosis, tuberculosis, mycobacterium avium intracellulare, indinavir-based antiretroviral regimens)

Miscellaneous
Perioperative blood pressure fluctuations
Contrast media
Large-volume blood transfusion
Dural puncture

Pathophysiology
The precise pathophysiology of edema in PRES is unknown. Three hypotheses have gained acceptance: (1) Rapid rise in blood pressure and the consequent increased blood flow overwhelm the autoregulatory systems in the small vessels and arterioles, which are normally maintained by endothelial cells and the blood–brain barrier. Failed autoregulation induces cerebral edema. Structures in the vertebrobasilar territory have relatively sparse sympathetic innervation, and therefore experience a preferential disruption of autoregulatory mechanisms. (2) Severe hypertension may lead to an overreaction of autoregulatory compensatory mechanisms, resulting in vasoconstriction and hypoperfusion. The consequent ischemia alters the integrity of the blood–brain barrier, leading to vasogenic edema. (3) Many clinical conditions associated with PRES result in immune system activation, suggesting an immunological basis for PRES. Inflammatory cytokines stemming from immune activation cause endothelial cell activation and damage, leading to fluid and protein leakage into the interstitium and subsequent vasogenic edema.

Etiology
The list of diseases and medications associated with PRES is long and continues to grow (Table 16.1). The association of certain diseases (e.g., eclampsia and hypertension) and medications (e.g., calcineurin inhibitors and angiogenesis inhibitors) with PRES are well established. Some other disease associations are supported by case reports. However, with all diseases and medications, the pathophysiological pathways already described mediate the development of PRES. For example, a patient with lupus nephritis may develop

International Neurology, Second edition. Edited by Robert P. Lisak, Daniel D. Truong, William M. Carroll and Roongroj Bhidayasiri
© 2016 John Wiley & Sons, Ltd. Published 2016 by John Wiley & Sons, Ltd.

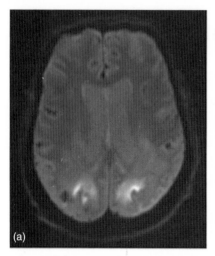 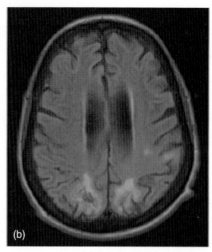 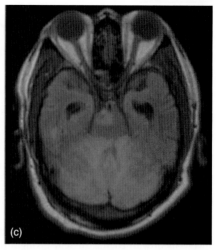

Figure DWI (Panel A) and FLAIR (Panel B) hyperintensities in the posterior parietal and occipital lobes on MRI in a patient with lupus nephritis. Panel C illustrates cerebellar and brainstem edema with obstructive hydrocephalus in a second patient with accelerated hypertension. Optic nerve head edema is also noted.

PRES due to accelerated hypertension from glomerulonephritis and due to immune mediated endothelial dysfunction.

Clinical features

PRES is a clinical neuroradiological syndrome occurring in children and adults that classically presents with headache, decline in cognition, seizures, and visual loss. Seizures may be focal or generalized, sometimes presenting with status epilepticus. The visual loss may present as unilateral or bilateral blurring, hemianopia, or cortical blindness. Rarely, PRES may also involve the retinal microcirculation, leading to macular edema. In severe cases, cerebral edema leads to increased intracranial pressure and rarely herniation and death.

Investigations

The classic MRI description is T2 hyperintensities involving the bilateral posterior parietal and occipital lobes (Fig). The areas show high signal on acquired diffusion coefficient (ADC) maps, suggestive of vasogenic edema. Other structures in the vertebrobasilar distribution such as the brainstem, thalamus, cerebellum, and rarely the splenium of the corpus callosum can also be involved. Cervical spinal cord, basal ganglia, and superior frontal gyrus edema have been described.

In atypical cases the MRI may show areas of decreased ADC signal, an indication of infarction. Gyriform gadolinium enhancement can occur rarely. PRES can result in foci of hemorrhages, generally within the area of edema. Subarachnoid bleeding has also been described. Hemorrhage is not associated with the severity of edema or the degree of blood pressure elevation, and does not seem to influence clinical outcome.

Vascular imaging in PRES sometimes demonstrates vasoconstriction in large and moderate-sized intracerebral arteries, reminiscent of another disease process, reversible cerebral vasoconstriction syndrome (RCVS). Loss of autoregulatory vascular tone is central to both processes. Involvement of the microcirculation versus the large and moderate-sized arteries will determine whether the patient will present with PRES, RCVS, or an overlap syndrome.

Treatment

Early identification and removal of the inciting factor are the hallmarks of treatment for PRES. Seizures may need antiepileptic therapy. Aggressive blood pressure lowering, treatment of underlying renal dysfunction, treatment of eclampsia with magnesium infusion, and discontinuing the offending medications are paramount to reversing PRES.

Prognosis

Most cases of PRES are reversible. Up to one-third of patients have irreversible injury, particularly if the diagnosis is delayed or the course of the underlying disease is protracted. Areas of infarction develop in the border zones between vascular territories. Temporal lobe epilepsy can ensue. Focal gyriform atrophy and laminar necrosis can occur. Bilateral parietal encephalomalacia can result in long-term perceptual impairments and problems with depth perception.

Conclusion

It is important for clinicians to consider PRES in the differential for encephalopathy in the appropriate setting or with the implicated medications, as the condition is potentially reversible. MR imaging will assist in the diagnosis. If the underlying disease runs a protracted course or if treatment is delayed, patients may be left with long-term and often disabling deficits.

Further reading

Hinchey J, Chaves C, Appignani B, *et al.* A reversible posterior leukoencephalopathy syndrome. *N Engl J Med* 1996;334:494–500.

Rykken J, McKinney A. Posterior reversible encephalopathy syndrome. *Semin Ultrasound CT MR* 2014;35:118–135.

Staykov D, Schwab S. Posterior reversible encephalopathy syndrome. *J Intensiv Care Med* 2012;27:11–24.

17   Extracranial and intracranial granulomatous arteritis (giant cell arteritis)

Gregory P. Van Stavern

Departments of Ophthalmology and Visual Sciences and Neurology, St. Louis School of Medicine, Washington University, St. Louis, MO, USA

Giant cell arteritis (GCA) is a relatively common systemic vasculitis with a predilection for large and medium-sized arteries, usually affecting patients older than 55 years. It is a necrotizing granulomatous arteritis involving the aorta and its major branches, especially the extracranial branches of the carotids.

Epidemiology

Giant cell arteritis is the most frequent systemic vasculitis in the elderly, predominantly affecting the Caucasian population, with the incidence being higher in Scandinavia, Northern Europe, and North America (17–18 cases/100,000 population aged >50 years). It rarely occurs in Asians, black people, and Hispanics. Women are affected twice as often as men, and the incidence increases with age (the mean presentation age is 71 years).

Pathogenesis

Converging lines of evidence suggest a genetic predisposition and emphasize the role of immune pathways in the pathogenesis of GCA. Studies have shown a higher prevalence of the major histocompatibility complex antigens HLA-DR 1, 3, 4, and 5, with expression of an HLA-DRB1*04 allele in the majority of patients. Both cellular and humoral immunity are involved in the pathogenesis of the disease. The pathogenesis represents a convergence of factors, including cumulative damage to the vascular endothelium from repetitive insults as well as age-related structural changes in the blood vessel wall, an aging immune system with weakening of adaptive immunity and inability to maintain tolerance, and intrinsic genetic factors. There is recent evidence that implicates varicella zoster virus (VZV) as a possible causative factor in at least some cases of GCA. It is unclear at this time whether the VZV antigens and DNA found in serial sectioning of temporal artery (TA) biopsies represent a primary stimulus triggering the immunological cascade in GCA, or whether this represents an epiphenomenon due to reactivation of the virus from surrounding inflammation.

Cellular immunity (vascular lesion)

The vessel wall infiltrates of GCA are a consequence of inappropriate activation of the CD4+ T-cells, macrophages, and multinucleated giant cells. T-cells enter the artery through the vasa vasorum, encounter stimulatory signals in the adventitia, and clonally expand to release interferon gamma. Interferon gamma recruits macrophages into the adventitia (to produce interleukins, IL-1 and 6) and the media (to produce metalloproteinases causing fragmentation of the elastic lamina). The multinucleated giant cells and macrophages lining the fragmented internal lamina produce growth factors that promote smooth-cell migration toward the lumen, causing intimal hyperplasia.

GCA commonly affects the superficial-temporal, occipital, vertebral, ophthalmic, and posterior-ciliary arteries (PCA), and sometimes the aorta, coronary arteries, and the carotid circulation (inflammatory involvement may be related to the amount of elastic tissue in the artery; consequently, the intracranial arteries are spared).

Histological criteria for diagnosis as defined by the American College of Rheumatology (ACR) include segmental cellular infiltrates of the vessel wall with T-helper and suppressor lymphocytes, plasma cells, and macrophages. The presence of giant cells is not essential for pathological diagnosis.

Humoral immunity

The systemic inflammatory response of GCA, best described as an acute-phase response, is a result of humoral immunity. Circulating monocytes produce IL-6, which stimulates production of acute-phase hepatic proteins, many of which are elevated in GCA.

Clinical manifestations

Systemic manifestations

Symptoms of systemic inflammation are present in most patients. New-onset temporal/occipital headache (sensory-fiber stimulation within inflamed extracranial arteries) and temporal scalp tenderness are common. Jaw claudication (pain/fatigue of masticatory muscles brought on by chewing and relieved by rest) is a classic and may be the most specific symptom of GCA. Low-grade fever and symmetric proximal myalgias around the shoulder girdle may be present in association with polymyalgia rheumatica (PMR). The temporal artery may feel normal, tender, nodular, or pulseless.

International Neurology, Second edition. Edited by Robert P. Lisak, Daniel D. Truong, William M. Carroll and Roongroj Bhidayasiri
© 2016 John Wiley & Sons, Ltd. Published 2016 by John Wiley & Sons, Ltd.

However, up to 8% of patients may have so-called occult GCA and present with visual loss and no systemic symptoms. These patients often have normal laboratory markers of inflammation. Therefore, although the systemic symptoms are helpful clues, their absence does not exclude the diagnosis of GCA, and the clinician must maintain a high index of suspicion in any elderly patient presenting with new-onset visual loss.

Neuro-ophthalmic manifestations
Patients with GCA may present with eye pain, diplopia, muscle paresis, or most commonly with irreversible visual loss (arteritic anterior ischemic optic neuropathy [A-AION], posterior ischemic optic neuropathy, or central retinal artery occlusion). Transient monocular visual loss (TMVL) with GCA (31% of patients) may be due to transient ischemia of the optic nerve head or retina (signifying impending blindness). The most common cause of visual loss (81.2%) in GCA is secondary to A-AION, resulting from occlusive inflammation in the PCA causing optic nerve-head infarction. Of affected eyes 50% have hand-movement vision or worse, with a relative afferent pupillary defect, and an inferior altitudinal visual field defect. In the acute stage, optic disk edema and pallor with peripapillary splinter hemorrhages may be seen. It is important to differentiate A-AION from non-arteritic anterior ischemic optic neuropathy (N-AION). Patients with N-AION have no systemic symptoms, less severe visual loss, and TMVL is extremely rare. Fundus fluorescein angiography shows delayed optic disc and choroidal filling in A-AION, whereas only optic disc filling is delayed in N-AION.

Neurological manifestations
Both the central and peripheral nervous systems can be involved. GCA may commonly manifest as neuropathies (14%) including mononeuropathies, peripheral polyneuropathies of the arms/legs, and rarely ischemic strokes (1%) or dementia. Patients with permanent visual loss or jaw claudication are more prone to ischemic strokes that affect the areas supplied by the carotid or vertebrobasilar arteries.

Large vessel arteritis
Large vessel arteritis affecting the aorta, subclavian, and axillary arteries is a recognized complication of GCA, with approximately 50% of these cases having negative temporal artery biopsy (TAB) results; the diagnosis in these cases is made by vascular imaging. Aortic involvement has been estimated in 4–7% of patients, although the actual incidence may be higher. At this time, routine screening with magnetic resonance angiography (MRA) or computed tomography angiography (CTA) in asymptomatic patients is not recommended.

Polymyalgia rheumatica
A variable portion of patients with GCA (about 50%) have PMR, a clinical syndrome characterized by pain and stiffness in neck, shoulder girdle, and pelvic girdle. Despite a suggestion that PMR and GCA belong to the same clinical continuum, they seem to be distinct conditions, as evidenced by differences in the HLA Class II associations. Patients with PMR aged <70 years without typical cranial features of GCA carry a low risk of vasculitis and visual loss.

Systemic inflammatory syndrome with arteritis
Arteritis can present in the absence of intimal hyperplasia, luminal stenosis, or tissue ischemia. In these cases, the systemic inflammatory syndrome (malaise, anorexia, weight loss, fever, night sweats, and depression) dominates clinical manifestations. The risk for visual loss may be less than that in cranial arteritis. A TAB is the procedure of choice and should be performed even in the absence of arterial tenderness/nodularity.

Diagnostic approaches to GCA

Laboratory findings
The erythrocyte sedimentation rate (ESR) is usually higher than 50 mm/hour, but a lower value has been reported in <5% of GCA patients. C-reactive protein (CRP), a dynamic acute-phase protein, is usually elevated. Since either ESR or CRP may be normal (more commonly ESR) in the presence of the elevation of the other, using both tests in combination provides greater sensitivity for diagnosis. Anemia of chronic disease, raised liver enzymes, and thrombocytosis are frequent. Thrombocytosis has a high specificity and positive predictive value (PPV) in diagnosis. There is evidence that IL-6 may be particularly sensitive in detecting the disease-associated acute-phase response. It is important to remember that all of these paraclinical tests must be interpreted in the context of the clinical setting, and the pretest probability of the disease being present. For example, an ESR of 60 in a 50-year-old African American man with vision loss and no systemic symptoms carries a different connotation than a similar ESR in a 75-year-old woman with profound visual loss and jaw claudication.

Diagnosis
A definite diagnosis of GCA requires histological examination of arterial tissue (TAB). This is important, given the low specificity of the clinical and laboratory markers, and implications of prolonged corticosteroid therapy. Because vascular inflammation is discontinuous, arterial specimens of sufficient size (≥2.5 cm) with analysis of closely spaced sections (0.25–0.5 mm) is recommended. If frozen sections from the first temporal artery do not reveal inflammatory infiltrates, the contralateral side is biopsied if clinical suspicion is high. However, the diagnostic yield for bilateral, simultaneous TAB is not appreciably higher than unilateral TAB. The facial and occipital arteries are often affected by GCA and might be appropriate targets for biopsy for cases in which the TAB is negative or equivocal and suspicion remains high. The sensitivity of TAB is not significantly affected if the biopsy is performed within two weeks of starting therapy. An experienced pathologist may see signs of a "healed arteritis" even after months of corticosteroid treatment. Therefore, therapy should not be postponed while awaiting the biopsy.

Imaging
Imaging may play a role in patients with large vessel arteritis with negative TAB results. Conventional X-ray angiography, digital subtraction angiography, computed tomography, and magnetic resonance imaging have emerged as reliable methods to assess vessel anatomy and luminal status. The distal subclavian, any portion of the axillary, and the proximal brachial artery are susceptible sites. The lesions are typically smoothly tapered. If there is clinical evidence for cerebral ischemia, evaluation of the carotid and vertebral arteries is important. However, the findings on angiography are not pathognomonic for vasculitis and should not substitute for a definitive tissue diagnosis.

Newer neuroimaging modalities have been reported, including the use of high-contrast, fat-saturated, T1 axial contrast-enhanced images, which can detect intraluminal changes in the superficial cranial arteries. This technique has recently been shown to have high specificity and sensitivity for GCA. Further studies are needed to determine the role for this imaging modality in the diagnostic workup for GCA.

Ultrasonography has been used both as a guide to locate the temporal artery for biopsy and also for diagnosis. The diagnostic accuracy of ultrasonography (using a variety of techniques) is mixed. The abnormalities found in the TA include stenosis, occlusion, and a hypoechoic "halo sign." However, in many studies, investigators were not blinded to the subject's clinical findings. A large meta-analysis of studies including a total of 2036 patients found relatively high sensitivity and specificity of ultrasonography compared with TAB, ranging from 69–88%. However, at this time, ultrasonography is neither sufficiently sensitive nor specific enough to replace TAB for definitive diagnosis.

The criteria proposed by the ACR for diagnosis of GCA included age at onset >50 years, new headache, temporal artery abnormalities, ESR >50 mm/hour, and a positive TAB. However, these criteria have been found to have limitations, including a PPV of only 29%. Since patients will need to remain on corticosteroid therapy for an extended period, with the attendant risk of complications, confirming the diagnosis with tissue biopsy is recommended in even the most clear-cut cases.

Treatment

Systemic corticosteroids are the treatment of choice for GCA, although the initial dose has varied in the literature. Patients with suspected GCA should usually be started on oral prednisolone of 1 mg/kg/day. For patients with ocular or cerebrovascular symptoms of GCA, a higher dose (80–100 mg/day) or intravenous methylprednisolone is advocated. Intravenous high-dose corticosteroids have especially been recommended in patients who present with a history of amaurosis fugax, marked visual loss, or early signs of involvement of the second eye. Follow-up protocol should include ophthalmic evaluation, ESR, and CRP at least once a week when they are on high-dose oral steroids.

Tapering of steroid therapy in GCA must be individualized, guided by ESR and CRP levels (systemic symptoms may be unreliable), to be commenced only when the ESR and CRP have reached consistently low levels and remain stable, which takes approximately two weeks on the initial high doses of oral steroids. Subsequently, the goal should be to maintain the lowest achieved levels of ESR and CRP with the lowest possible prednisolone dose. Patients must

be carefully monitored for any ocular/visual problems and systemic side effects of corticosteroids.

The total duration of steroid therapy is usually prolonged, and when patients with visual loss are being treated, a longer duration is anticipated (some requiring indefinite treatment). A slow taper with the goal of reaching 10 mg/day by 6 months is generally effective in preventing recurrence of disease as well as avoiding steroid-related complications. However, therapy must be individualized and many patients require a longer therapy and slower taper, based on recurrence of presenting symptoms and/or elevation of ESR and CRP. There is little evidence supporting the routine use of steroid-sparing agents in GCA, although agents such as methotrexate can be employed in patients who cannot tolerate high-dose steroids.

Given the possibility of VZV triggering inflammatory changes, some have argued for concurrent treatment with antiviral medications such as acyclovir. However, such medications are not completely risk free, particularly when given intravenously, and it is not clear at this time whether antiviral therapy confers an added benefit over and above treatment with corticosteroids. Future studies are needed to clarify this issue, and to help identify patients who might be candidates for antiviral medications.

Prognosis

The overall life expectancy of GCA patients and the general population have been reported to be similar, but there is morbidity due to side effects of prolonged steroid use. Permanent visual loss is more common in patients who present with amaurosis, transient diplopia, or jaw claudication. The goal of treatment in cases with visual loss is to arrest further visual deterioration in the affected eye and to prevent involvement of the other eye. The visual prognosis of GCA if untreated is devastating visual loss in both eyes. Early diagnosis and prompt initiation of treatment may result in favorable visual outcomes.

Further reading

Gilden G, White T, Khmelevea N, *et al.* Prevalence and distribution of VZV in temporal arteries of patients with giant cell arteritis. *Neurology* 2015;84:1943–1955.

Hayreh SS. Acute ischemic disorders of the optic nerve: Pathogenesis, clinical manifestations and management. *Ophthalmol Clin North Am* 1996;9:407–442.

Hayreh SS, Podhajsky PA, Raman R, Zimmerman B. Giant cell arteritis: Validity and reliability of various diagnostic criteria. *Am J Ophthalmol* 1997;123:285–296.

Weyand CM, Goronzy JJ. Medium- and large-vessel vasculitis. *N Engl J Med* 2003; 349:160–169.

Weyand CM, Liao JY, Goronzy JJ. The immunopathology of giant cell arteritis: Diagnostic and therapeutic implications. *J Neuro-Ophthalmol* 2012;32:259–265.

18 Intracranial granulomatous arteritis (primary angiitis of the CNS)/idiopathic CNS vasculitis

Donald Silberberg

Department of Neurology, University of Pennsylvania Medical Center, Philadelphia, PA, USA

Introduction and nomenclature

The terms "intracranial granulomatous arteritis" and "primary angiitis of the central nervous system" are synonyms for central nervous system (CNS) vasculitis of unknown etiology, perhaps better termed idiopathic CNS vasculitis (ICNSV). To confound the situation further, this category surely includes disorders with multiple, yet to be identified causes. As an example, it is now becoming clear that many patients with granulomatous giant cell arteritis, previously called temporal arteritis, have varicella zoster virus in the affected vessels, in the so-called skip areas (see Chapter 17). ICNSV also often includes peripheral nervous system, ocular, and sometimes systemic manifestations during the course of the illness.

ICNSV is uncommon, but treatable, so its identification is very important. ICNSV is being increasingly recognized, and may account for up to 5% of cerebrovascular disease occurring in individuals below the age of 50 years. No information regarding geographic distribution is available; all relevant publications are from North America. It is important to consider the possibility that the patient has reversible cerebral vasoconstrictive syndrome (RCVS), which can have overlapping symptoms and signs with ICNSV as well as similar findings on digital subtraction angiography, magnetic resonance angiography, and computed tomography (CT) angiography, particularly when larger or midsize vessels are involved (see Chapter 15).

One must keep in mind that CNS, ocular, cranial nerve, peripheral nervous system, and muscle signs and symptoms are often the first manifestation of what proves to be a systemic disorder. For example, acute disseminated lupus erythematosus frequently begins with seizures, sarcoidosis may present as cranial nerve or diffuse cerebral dysfunction, and a vasculitis syndrome has been associated with the beginning of Hodgkin's disease.

Clinical course and diagnosis

Signs and symptoms suggestive of vasculitis, in the absence of evidence for another diagnostic entity, most of which are themselves idiopathic (Table 18.1), lead to consideration of ICNSV. The occurrence of CNS infarcts or hemorrhages in unrelated vascular distributions should suggest the possibility of vasculitis. By definition, systemic signs such as fever, arthralgia, and myalgia, or an elevated peripheral blood leukocyte count or erythrocyte sedimentation rate, are not present, at least initially. However, an elevated erythrocyte sedimentation rate occurs in up to 50% of cases. Common features include those of diffuse cerebral dysfunction: headache, confusion, paresthesias, hemiplegia, seizures, ataxia, and visual disturbances.

Cranial nerves are often affected, and peripheral neuropathy is present in up to 10% of patients at the time of presentation. Less commonly, ICNSV presents as an isolated mass lesion. The signs and symptoms are frequently long-lasting and recurrent. ICNSV is most common in adults, but also occurs in children. If untreated, ICNSV usually leads to death within 1–2 years or less. However, ICNSV affecting primarily small vessels may have a better prognosis than that involving medium-sized vessels.

Diagnostic aids include examination of the cerebrospinal fluid (CSF), electroencephalogram (EEG), CT and magnetic resonance imaging (MRI), including MRI angiography, fluorescein angiography where ophthalmoscopy is abnormal, intracranial arteriography, and brain and meningeal biopsy. CSF abnormalities, primarily elevated protein and lymphocytic pleocytosis, are present in 80–90% of individuals with ICNSV. CSF is more often normal or shows just a modest increase in total protein in RCVS. Diffuse EEG abnormalities are very common in ICNSV, and may help to monitor the course of the disorder. Intracranial imaging often reveals one or more infarctions or hemorrhages, and may show evidence of perivascular inflammation or meningeal enhancement. Alternatively, imaging studies may be normal. Conventional angiography reveals occlusions, focal narrowing, beading, distal attenuation, or aneurysms in no more than 50% of those with ICNSV. MRI angiography may show the same abnormalities with no risk to the patient, but no studies are available that compare sensitivity or specificity with conventional angiography. It has recently been suggested that high-resolution (3T) MRI vessel wall imaging may help distinguish RCVS from ICNSV and other true vasculitic disorders. Uniform vessel wall thickening and negligible to mild enhancement is the usual finding in RCVS.

Brain and meningeal biopsy seeks to reveal the characteristic perivascular, primarily periarterial, inflammation that includes a variety of lymphocytes, plasma cells, and often multinuclear giant cells. However, it is important to realize that even biopsy fails to reveal an abnormality in about 20% of patients who otherwise appear to have ICNSV. One explanation for negative biopsies is undoubtedly the very focal nature of the disorder in many individuals, similar to what characterizes systemic giant cell arteritis (temporal arteritis).

Treatment

In the face of these uncertainties, the decision as to whether or not to treat for ICNSV often must be made despite a lack of laboratory evidence to support the diagnosis. Since ICNSV is almost uniformly fatal if not treated, and the risk of treatment is acceptable, it is usu-

International Neurology, Second edition. Edited by Robert P. Lisak, Daniel D. Truong, William M. Carroll and Roongroj Bhidayasiri
© 2016 John Wiley & Sons, Ltd. Published 2016 by John Wiley & Sons, Ltd.

Table 18.1. Central nervous system (CNS) vaculitis.

Infectious

Bacterial (e.g., tuberculosis)

Chagas' disease

Viral (e.g., Varicella soster)

HIV

Malaria

Syphilis

Presumably non-infectious

Arthritis associated

Juvenile rheumatoid arthritis

Rheumatoid arthritis

Relapsing polychondritis

Seronegative (HLA-B27-associated) spondyloarthropathies

Ocular

Acute posterior multifocal placoid pigment epitheliopathy

Eales disease

Idiopathic retinal vasculitis

Other

Antiphospholipid antibody-associated vasculopathy

Behçet's disease

Churg–Straus syndrome

Cogan's syndrome

Giant cell arteritis

Hodgkin's disease

Polyarteritis nodosa

Sarcoidosis

Henoch–Schonlein purpura

Hypersensitivity vasculitis

Mixed cryoglobulinemia

Dermatomyositis

Sarcoidosis

Scleroderma

Sjögren's syndrome

Systemic lupus erythematosus

Takayasu's arteritis

Thromboangiitis obliterans

Granulomatosis with angiitis

Idiopathic intracranial granulomatous arteritis (primary angiitis of the CNS)

ally prudent to proceed. That said, one must recognize that what informs the clinician is experience in treating vasculitis in other settings, and uncontrolled, mostly small, case series that describe the

treatment of ICNSV. The small number of cases at any one institution has so far precluded organization of a randomized controlled clinical trial.

What has been observed is that treatment with a combination of synthetic corticosteroids with a more potent immunosuppressant agent is often effective in reducing the severity and duration of the initial episode, and in preventing recurrences. Prednisone or prednisolone is most often used (1 mg/kg/day), in combination with cyclophosphamide (2 mg/kg, maximum 150 mg/day) for the initiation of treatment. Since treatment must be maintained for a least a year in most individuals, azathioprine (2 mg/kg/day) is often substituted for cyclophosphamide for maintenance, and one seeks to use the lowest dose of steroids that seems to be effective for the long term.

Varicela zoster virus (VZV) arteritis is a relatively common cause of cerebral vasculitis, and can be treated successfully with intravenous acyclovir (10–15 mg/kg 3 times a day for 14 days). It is reasonable to undertake treatment if the clinical and radiologic picture suggests this possibility, even in the absence of detection of either VZV DNA or anti-VZV IgG antibody in CSF, since the incidence of untoward side effects is very small.

Efficacy can be judged on the basis of clinical response, absence of recurrence, absence of new MRI abnormalities, and reduction in EEG abnormalities. However, one must recognize that, as is the case for many known causes of vasculitis, very long-term treatment (1–3 years, or indefinitely) may be needed to limit the disorder.

Future developments

The factors that lead to the development of vasculitis in any organ system are complex, and mostly poorly understood. As these are elucidated, more specific, effective, and less toxic treatments will follow. The factors that lead to the selection of a particular vascular tree or its component parts as the target for an inflammatory response are beginning to be unraveled, an important step along the way.

Further Reading

Calabrese LH, Dodick DW, Schwedt TJ, Singhal AB. Narrative review: Reversible cerebral vasoconstriction syndromes. *Ann Intern Med* 2007;146(1):34–44.

Gilden D. Varicella zoster virus infections. Continuum 21:1692–1703, 2015.

Hajj-Ali RA, Calabrese LH. Diagnosis and classification of central nervous system vasculitis. *J Autoimmun* 2014;48–49:149–152.

Hoffman GS. Determinants of vessel targeting in vasculitis. *Ann NY Acad Sci* 2005;1051:332–339.

MacLaren K, Gillespie J, Shrestha S, Neary D, Ballardie FW. Primary angiitis of the central nervous system: Emerging variants. *QJM* 2005;98:643–654.

Obusez EC, Hui F, Hajj-Ali RA, *et al.* High-resolution MRI vessel wall imaging: Spatial and temporal patterns of reversible cerebral vasoconstriction syndrome and central nervous system vasculitis. *Amer J Neuroradiol* 2014;35:1527–1532.

West SG. Central nervous system vasculitis. *Curr Rheumatol Rep* 2003;5(2):116–1127.

19 Takayasu's arteritis

Yasuhisa Kitagawa
Tokai University School of Medicine, Tokai University Hachioji Hospital, Tokyo, Japan

Takayasu's arteritis is a chronic, non-specific arteritis of unknown cause characterized by stenosis and/or occlusion of the aorta and its branches. Its major features were first described by Davy in 1839 and independently by Savort and by Kussmaul in 1856. In 1905, a Japanese ophthalmologist, Takayasu, reported a case with wreath-like arterial-venous anastomosis in the central retinal artery and, based on his description, the term Takayasu's arteritis is now most commonly used worldwide.

Epidemiology

The reported incidence of Takayasu's arteritis is 2.6 cases per million per year in North America. In Japan, newly developed cases amount to more than 100 annually, and the prevalence is 33 cases per million. It is 9 times more frequent in females than in males in Japan. The age at onset ranges from 20–40 years in females, although there is no clear age peak in males. In China, the female-to-male ratio is 2.9:1. Although Takayasu's arteritis appears mainly in Asians, it can occur in all racial groups. The age of onset of Takayasu's arteritis in North American and European countries is later than that in Asian countries. The reason for the later onset could relate to two factors: (1) the slow progression of occlusive arteritis; and (2) the rarity of the disease in "Western" countries, which results in a longer delay in diagnosis compared with Eastern countries.

Pathophysiology

Pathology

In Takayasu's arteritis, the aortic arch with its main arterial trunks and the descending aorta, as well as renal arteries, are the main sites of inflammation. The pathologic lesion is a granulomatous angiitis. The initial involvement is characterized by mononuclear cell infiltration in the adventitia, followed by prominent fibrous proliferation in the media and intima. Inflammatory cell infiltration foci are accompanied by perinecrotic foci and Langhans-type multinucleated giant cell infiltration. Long-standing cases show fibrosis and hyalinization of intima, stenosis of the vascular lumen, and finally complete occlusion.

Pathogenesis

Takayasu's arteritis is more common in Asians than in people of other racial origins. Its etiology is unknown, but local predominance in Asia and in Central and South America is consistent with some involvement of genetic factors, perhaps acting in concert with environmental factors. A study of Japanese human leucocyte antigen (HLA) patterns in 1998 reported a significant correlation of HLA-B52, HLA-B39, and HLA-DR2 with Takayasu's arteritis. Recently, HLA-B67 was reported to show a higher odds ratio compared to HLA-B52 in Japan. However, North American studies have failed to identify any association of HLA with the disease.

Clinical features

Clinical manifestations originate from both the systemic inflammation and from local vascular complications. The most frequent manifestations of acute systemic generalized inflammation were low- or high-grade fever, fatigue, general malaise, myalgia, and weight loss. In the chronic stage, further progression of the disease causes destruction of the arterial wall media leading to vascular lesion.

Four types of aortic arch involvement are known in Takayasu's arteritis. Involvement is limited to the ascending aorta and aortic arch in type 1, to the infradiaphragmatic aorta in type 2, to the supra- and infradiaphragma in type 3, and to the pulmonary arteries in type 4.

Physical findings in Takayasu's arteritis include weakness or right-to-left difference of radial pulsation, weakness of femoral arterial pulsation, asymmetry of blood pressure, hypertension, cardiac murmur, bruit especially in the neck, supraclavicular, and anterior chest, and abnormal ocular findings.

The vascular manifestations arising from stenosis and occlusion of vessels are varied, and the geographic variations of clinical features and prognosis as reported in Japan, North America, Europe, Asia, and South Africa are shown in Table 19.1. Characteristic findings of the upper limbs are pulses, and/or a difference in arterial blood pressure between the right and left radial arteries is found in about half of cases. Hypertension has been found in about half of cases. Hypertension is caused by stenosis of the renal artery and by decreased elasticity of the aorta, which induces systolic hypertension. Cardiac symptoms are shortness of breath, palpitations, and chest discomfort. Aortic valve insufficiency has been noted and the comcomitant rupture of aortic aneurysm has been associated with a poor outcome. Systemic features include fever, general malaise, arthralgia, and myalgia in the acute phase of the disease.

A survey of Takayasu's arteritis in Japan reported that the most common initial symptoms were associated with ischemia of the extremities, including paresthesias, cold sensation, pulselessness, and claudication (73.8%), followed by systemic symptoms including fever and fatigue (60.1%). Symptoms related to cerebral ischemia,

International Neurology, Second edition. Edited by Robert P. Lisak, Daniel D. Truong, William M. Carroll and Roongroj Bhidayasiri
© 2016 John Wiley & Sons, Ltd. Published 2016 by John Wiley & Sons, Ltd.

Table 19.1 Geographical variation of clinical manifestations and prognosis of Takayasu's arteritis.

	Japan	North America	Germany	Italy	China	Korea	Thailand	India	South Africa
No. of cases	1318	60	17	104	530	129	46	83	272 (8% Caucasian)
Age (mean)	31	25	23	29	25.8	29.5	7-40	5-53	25 (14-66)
Female/male ratio	9:1	29:1	3.2:1	7:1	2.9:1	6.6:1	1.9:1	1.6:1	3:1
Affected artery	Subclavian Common carotid Innominate	Subclavian Aorta Common carotid	Subclavian Common carotid	Subclavian Carotid Renal	Subclavian Abdominal Renal	Subclavian Renal Common carotid	Abdominal aorta Renal Subclavian	Renal Abdominal aorta Subclavian	Subclavian Abdominal aorta Renal
Clinical features									
Cerebral ischemic symptom	42.3%	57%	35.3%	50%	30.6%	46%	24%	8%	20%
Stroke	11.9%	9%	11.8%	4%	5.4%	3%	24%	7%	11%
Visual	23.6%	8%	35.3%	—	9.6%	20%	—	22%	—
Cardiac	41.4%	38%	—	—	23.2%	46%	28%	14%	45%
Carotid bruit	—	70%	23.5%	—	47.4%	37%	—	25%	—
Hypertension	55.7%	33%	58.8%	60%	60.0%	40%	80%	81%	77%
Ischemia of extremities	73.8%	—	—	—	—	—	—	—	—
Claudication	—	70%	88.2%	59%	24.7%	21%	—	—	30%
Dim. or no pulse	—	62%	82.4%	75%	37.2%	72%	50%	46%	—
Cause of death	Cardiac failure 23.7% Rupture of aneurysm 20.3% Cerebral hemorrhage 5.1%	—	—	—	Cerebral hemorrhage 23.6% Cardiac failure 5.5% Cerebral thrombosis 3.6% Rupture of aneurysm 1.8%	—	—	Cardiac failure 36% Renal failure 18% Cerebral hemorrhage 9%	Cardiac failure 46% Renal failure 11% Rupture of aneurysm 11% Stroke 9.5%

such as dizziness, headache, and syncope, sometimes orthostatic, were noted in 42.3% of 1302 cases. Cerebral infarction, transient ischemic attack (TIA), and cerebral hemorrhage were found in 5.5%, 5.7%, and 0.7% of cases, respectively.

There is geographic variation in the pattern of affected arteries. In Japan, the most frequently involved artery is the subclavian artery, followed by the common carotid artery and innominate artery. The vertebral artery tends to be spared until the final stage. Takayasu's arteritis presents with similar cerebrovascular signs in Europe and Japan. It may present as the subclavian steal syndrome. On the other hand, the renal artery is the most common vascular involvement seen in India.

Causes of death in a series of 59 Japanese patients included heart failure in 14 patients, rupture of aortic aneurysm in 12, cerebral hemorrhage in 2, and other cerebrovascular syndromes in 2. In a Chinese study, 23.6% of patients suffered from cerebral hemorrhage, although cerebral infarction was found in only 3.6%. The higher incidence of cerebral hemorrhage in China compared to Japan could be related to a higher rate of renovascular hypertension.

Investigations

Laboratory findings include elevated erythrocyte sedimentation rate (ESR), C-reactive protein (CRP), and increased serum gamma globulin in a polyclonal pattern. Although serological tests specific for Takayasu's arteritis are not available, pentraxin 3 and metalloproteinases are emerging as promising new biomarkers. Angiography remains the cornerstone of diagnosis, revealing narrowing of large arteries arising from the aorta. The presence of vascular lesions and their progression can be detected by duplex ultrasonography. Homogenous circumferential intima-media thickening of the common carotid arteries in ultrasonography is highly specific, particularly in young women. Microembolic signals (MES) can be detected by transcranial Doppler ultrasound and have been reported to be present in 22% of patients with Takayasu's arteritis during the acute and chronic stages. Cerebrovascular disease-induced changes can be detected using functional imaging, such as SPECT (single photon emission computed tomography) and PET (positron emission tomography).

Differential diagnosis for Takayasu's arteritis include arteriosclerosis, Buerger's disease, congenital vessel anomalies, coarctation of aorta, dissecting aneurysm, collagen disease, and Behcet's disease.

Treatment

Treatment of Takayasu's arteritis involves control of general inflammation and neurological complications. Since there is no completed, placebo-controlled, randomized clinical trial, the level of evidence for management of Takayasu's arteritis is low, generally reflecting the results of open studies, case series, and expert opinion. The most commonly used agents include corticosteroids and conventional immunosuppressive agents such as methotrexate, azathioprine, mycophenolate mofetil, and leflunomide.

In the acute stage, corticosteroids are initiated (0.5–1.5 mg/kg/day), and the dosage is adjusted depending on the clinical findings and the degree of inflammatory reaction as monitored by ESR and/or CRP. Given glucocorticoid alone, 60% of patients respond to varying degrees. If blindness seems imminent, intravenous high-dose corticosteroid should be given on an urgent basis (1 g intravenous methyprednisolone/day for 3–7 days). If corticosteroid therapy is insufficient, immmunosuppressive therapy such as methotrexate is indicated. However, immunosuppressive treatment failed to induce remission in 25% of cases, and about half of those who achieved remission later relapsed. In patients who remain resistant and/or intolerant to the agents suggested, biological agents including tumor necrosis factor (TNF) inhibitors, rituximab, and tocilizumab seem promising.

Antiplatelet therapy is indicated for patients with TIA and cerebral infarction. Strict control of hypertension is essential to reduce the incidence of cerebral infarction and cerebral hemorrhage. Indications for surgery in the chronic stage include severe aortic insuffiency, coarctation of the aorta, subclavian steal syndrome, and renovascular hypertension. Angioplasty may be indicated for certain patients with subclavian steal syndrome or stenosis of the carotid and renal arteries. In the presence of short-segment, critical arterial stenosis, balloon angioplasty or stent graft replacement may be useful. On the other hand, long-segment stenosis with extensive periarterial fibrosis or occlusion requires surgical bypass. Both endovascular intervention and surgical procedures should be avoided during the active phase of the disease.

Further reading

Deyu Z, Dijun E, Lisheng L. Takayasu arteritis in China: A report of 530 cases. *Heart Vessels* 1992;7(Suppl):32–36.

Johnson SL, Lock RJ, Gompels MM. Takayasu arteritis: A review. *J Clin Pathol* 2002;55:481–486.

Kerr GS, Hallahan CW, Gierdant J, *et al.* Takayasu's arteritis. *Ann Intern Med* 1994;120:919–929.

Keser G, Direskeneli H, Aksu K. Management of Takayasu arteritis: A systematic review. *Rheumatology* 2014;53:793–801.

Koide K. Takayasu's arteritis. *Heart Vessels* 1992;7(Suppl):48–54.

Ringleb PA, Strittmater EI, Loewer M, *et al.* Cerebrovascular manifestations of Takayasu arteritis in Europe. *Rheumatology* 2005;44:1012–1015.

20 | Polyarteritis nodosa, eosinophilic granulomatosis with polyangiitis, and overlap vasculitis syndrome

Arnold I. Levinson[1] and Robert P. Lisak[2]

[1] Perelman School of Medicine at the University of Pennsylvania, Philadephia, PA, USA

[2] Wayne State University School of Medicine and Detroit Medical Center, Detroit, MI, USA

The systemic vasculitides are a heterogeneous group of disorders that share the common feature of blood vessel inflammation. They may be primary – that is, with no identifiable cause – or secondary – namely, associated with an underlying disease process or a trigger like a microbe or drug. In either case, the nervous system may be involved in the systemic vasculitides and this involvement may manifest with diverse clinical presentations. Historically the primary vasculitic syndromes have been classified on the basis of distinct clinical and histopathological features. In particular, emphasis is placed on the size of the affected vessel. Thus, the vasculitides are viewed as encompassing a spectrum ranging from involvement of small to large vessels, with further distinction relying on the nature of the associated inflammatory process. The most recent classification scheme of these syndromes was provided at the 2012 Chapel Hill Consensus Conference. Of note is that microscopic polyangiitis (MPA) was not formally distinguished from polyarteritis nodosa (PAN) until 1994. Thus, early reports on PAN were clearly contaminated by cases of MPA. The discussion that follows focuses on PAN, eosinophilic granulomatosis with polyangiitis (EGPA; formerly called Churg–Strauss syndrome), and overlap vasculitic presentations that share features of several of the individually designated vasculitic disorders.

Polyarteritis nodosa (PAN)

This disorder is characterized by the involvement of predominantly medium-sized muscular arteries with occasional involvement of small muscular arteries and without glomerulonephritis or vasculitis in arterioles, capillaries, or venules (Table 20.1). There is a predilection for areas of bifurcation and branch points. Multiple organs are involved, including most commonly the peripheral nervous system, skin, gastrointestinal tract, joints, and kidneys.

Epidemiology

The incidence of PAN is estimated at 5–77 cases per million persons per year, although early reports included case series that were contaminated by cases of microscopic polyangiitis (MPA), one of the ANCA-positive vasculitides. Recent data from Eoropean countries puts its prevalence at about 31 cases per million. The peak incidence occurs in the 5th to 6th decades of life. Prior to the advent of hepatitis B (HBV) vaccination, more than 33% of adults with PAN were infected with this virus. Now, however, only 5% of patients with PAN in developed countries are infected with HBV.

Table 20.1 Distinguishing features of polyarteritis nodosa (PAN) and eosinophilic granulomatosis with polyangiitis (EGPA).

Organ involvement	PAN	EGPA
Nervous system		
Central nervous system	Uncommon	Uncommon
Peripheral nervous system	(38–75%)	(70–75%)
Respiratory tract		
Upper	No	50–60% (sinusitis)
Lungs	No	Asthma (90–100%)
	No	Pulmonary infiltrates/ nodules (40–70%)
Glomerulonephritis	No	10–40%
Cardiac	5–30%	10–40%
Gastrointestinal tract	14–53%	30–50%
Skin	28–60%	50–55%
Arthralgias/arthritis	50–75%	40–50%
Vascular pathology		
Vessel involvement	Medium +/- small muscular arteries	Medium and small muscular arteries
Inflammatory process	Segmental infiltration in/around vessel walls by neutrophils and monocytes	Vascular and extravascular granulomas + eosinophilic infiltrates in/around vessel walls
Serology		
ANCA		
PR3-cANCA	Rare	3–35%
MPO-pANCA	Rare	2–50%

Pathophysiology

Etiological factors in adult PAN patients are limited largely to microbes, including HBV, hepatitis C virus, HIV, and certain drugs. Among the infectious agents, HBV is the most common offender, with the ensuing vasculitis caused by an immune complex (hepatitis B surface antigen/IgG anti-Hepatitis B surface antigen antibody)

International Neurology, Second edition. Edited by Robert P. Lisak, Daniel D. Truong, William M. Carroll and Roongroj Bhidayasiri
© 2016 John Wiley & Sons, Ltd. Published 2016 by John Wiley & Sons, Ltd.

mediated inflammatory process that becomes clinically manifest by about four months after infection. However, it is not known why this process selectively targets medium and small muscular arteries and leaves arterioles, venules, and capillaries unscathed. The latter are the targets in other forms of both spontaneous human and experimental immune complex–mediated vasculitis. Less is known about the pathogenesis of primary PAN where convincing evidence for an immune complex–mediated process is absent. Unlike several immune complex–mediated diseases, primary PAN is not associated with evidence of complement pathway activation. On the other hand, some researchers have suggested that cell-mediated immune processes may contribute to the pathogenesis of PAN. This is based on the finding of abundant CD4+ T-cells and dendritic cells within the infiltrates of involved vessels.

Clinical features

The presenting clinical features of PAN may include fever, hypertension, renal insufficiency, weakness, fatigue, and musculoskeletal symptoms. Curiously, the lungs are characteristically not involved. The distinction between PAN (typically ANCA negative) and MPA was not recognized until 1994. MPA is now viewed as part of the vasculitis spectrum, which includes granulomatous vasculitides like polyangiitis with granulomatosis (formerly called Wegener's granulomatosis) and eosinophilic granulomatosis with polyangiitis.

Central nervous system involvement

The frequency of central nervous system (CNS) involvement varies across reports, but may be as low as 5–10% of patients. In a recently reported study of PAN patients, 11 of 225 patients (4.1%) with primary PAN and 5 of 123 (4%) patients with HBV-associated PAN were observed to have CNS involvement. The most commonly reported clinical manifestation is diffuse encephalopathy, followed in frequency by focal deficits and seizures and cerebrovascular accidents (CVAs). CVAs generally are caused by peripheral small infarcts in the cerebral cortex and subcortical white matter, and in the past were attributed to thrombosis occurring as a consequence of the vasculitic process. However, there is also evidence to suggest that CVAs may be caused by lacunar strokes related to small deep cerebellar or pontine-penetrating artery thrombotic microangiopathy rather than vasculitis. Moreover, the vasculopathy may be aggravated by the use of corticosteroids. An additional etiology for CVAs in PAN patients that should be kept in mind is cardiovascular thrombotic emboli.

Peripheral nervous system involvement

The peripheral nervous system (PNS) is involved in PAN in 50–75% of cases. Several types of peripheral neuropathy are seen, including mononeuritis multiplex (MM), extensive mononeuritis, distal sensorimotor polyneuropathy, and cutaneous neuropathy. Of these, MM is most frequently encountered. In the recent survey referred to earlier, peripheral neuropathy was seen in a total of 153 of 225 patients (68%) with primary PAN. Of the 153 patients, 94.7% had MM. By contrast, peripheral neuropathy was more common in HBV-associated PAN, occurring in 105 of 123 patients (85.4%). Of these, similar to the patients with primary PAN, 96% presented with MM. MM occurs during the acute stage of the illness. It typically presents with both motor and sensory components. Subsequently, it may progress to a symmetric distal polyneuropathy. The vasculitis causes occlusion of the vasa nervorum supplying peripheral nerves and leads to a characteristic central fascicular pattern of nerve-fiber damage. The earliest clinical signs of MM include transient pain or paresthesias. This is followed by weakness and sensory loss in the distribution of one or more peripheral nerves. Extensive mononeuritis produces a severe distal weakness and sensory loss caused by the simultaneous infarction of multiple individual peripheral nerves. Rarely, cranial MM is seen, with the oculomotor (III), trochlear (IV), abducens (VI), facial (VII), and vestibulocochlear (VIII) nerves most commonly affected. Also rarely, the arteritis affects the spinal arterial branches supplying the spinal cord at any level. Patients present with acute or subacute transverse myelopathy.

Investigations

The diagnosis of PAN is confirmed by finding characteristic changes on tissue biopsy or arteriography. The hallmark finding on biopsy is necrotizing inflammation of the medium or small muscular arteries. Histopathological changes include infiltration in and around the vessel walls by polymorphonuclear cells and mononuclear cells, fibrinoid necrosis, and disruption of the internal and external elastic membranes. The arterial lesions tend to show a segmental distribution and typically represent chronologically different stages of the disease process. The finding of granulomas should suggest an alternative diagnosis.

Abnormalities on arteriography are most commonly seen in the renal, mesenteric, and hepatic vasculature and may show aneurysmal dilatation, stenosis, and beading of the involved vessels. The vascular abnormalities result in narrowing and thrombosis, causing ischemia and/or infarction of the tissue supplied by the affected vessel.

The diagnostic evaluation of a patient presenting with peripheral neuropathy and suspected vasculitis includes electrophysiological studies and a nerve biopsy. In PAN, the latter yields a fairly high rate of results, which is increased by the addition of a muscle biopsy. A biopsy of an electrophysiologically abnormal nerve is considered by some researchers to enhance the likelihood of finding histological evidence of vasculitis.

Treatment

A 5-year survival rate of 13% has been reported in untreated patients with PAN. In patients with mild, non-life threatening disease – that is, without CNS, cardiac, or gastrointestinal involvement – treatment is commenced with an oral glucocorticoid in the equivalent dose of prednisone, 0.5–1.5 mg/kg/day with tapering over a period of months. The addition of a glucocorticoid improves the survival rate to 48%. Life-threatening disease should be managed with intravenous administration of methylprednisolone 1 gm/kg/day for three days, followed by transition to oral glucocorticoid therapy, and cyclophosphamide administered via the oral or parenteral route. Cyclophosphamide should be maintained for at least 6 months following onset of improvement, and may be replaced by a less toxic immunosuppressive agent like Imuran (azathioprine) or CellCept (mycophenolate mofetil) as maintenance therapy for at least another 6–12 months. The use of combination glucocorticoid/cyclophosphamide therapy improved the survival rate to 80–90%.

Eosinophilic granulomatosis with polyangiitis (EGPA)

EGPA (formerly called Churg–Strauss syndrome) is a multisystem disease caused by vasculitis that affects medium and small arteries (Table 20.1). The telltale features of this disease are asthma, rhinosinusitis, and peripheral blood eosinophilia.

Epidemiology

Assessment of the epidemiology of EGPA is hindered by the absence of clearcut diagnostic guidelines. Nevertheless, its incidence is estimated to range between 0.5 and 6.8 new cases per million patients per year, with its prevalence ranging from 10.7 to 13 per million adults. There is no clear sex or ethnic predominance. It accounts for roughly 10% of patients who are diagnosed with a major form of vasculitis. EGPA is the least common entity among the three major types of vasculitis associated with antineutrophil cytoplasmic antibody (ANCA).

Pathophysiology

The pathogenesis of EGPA is multifactorial with, not surprisingly, evidence for both environmental and genetic factors. The former include infectious agents such as actinomyces and drugs, including sulfonamides and carbamazepam. The development of EGPA has also been associated with drugs used in the treatment of asthma, including leukotriene inhibitors and the monoclonal anti-IgE antibody omalizumab. The latter associations are now understood to reflect the "unmasking" of underlying EGPA that had been suppressed by corticosteroid therapy. Among contributing genetic factors, HLA-DRB4 appears to carry the greatest risk.

Th2 immune mechanisms are generally considered to underlie the pathogenesis of EGPA. This is not surprising given the development of this type of vasculitis in patients suffering from asthma and allergic rhinitis. The Th2 phenotype drives the production of a number of cytokines, which promote the differentiation, activation, and survival of eosinophils. These include IL-3, IL-5, and IL-13. Furthermore, both endothelial and epithelial cells can secrete chemokines that attract infiltrations of eosinophils, thus amplifying the local inflammatory responses. Activated eosinophils release a number of soluble tissue-damaging factors including eosinophilic basic protein, eosinophilic neurotoxin, and eosinophilic cationic protein. ANCAs, particularly those directed against myeloperoxidase, are detected in approximately 40% of patients. These antibodies have the potential to amplify vascular damage via their activation of neutrophils.

Clinical features

EGPA may present in any one of three phases, although the phases are not always distinguishable. The first is a prodromal phase that manifests as asthma and allergic rhinitis. The second, or eosinophilic, phase features peripheral blood eosinophilia and tissue infiltrates, particularly in the lung and gastrointestinal tract. Vasculitis affecting the small and medium-sized arteries of multiple organs is found in the third phase, with involvement of the lungs (pulmonary infiltrates, nodules), peripheral nerves (see the next section), skin (purpura, subcutaneous nodules), gastrointestinal tract (eosinophilic gastroenteritis, colitis), heart (heart failure, pericarditis, arrhythmias), and kidneys (necrotizing glomerulonephritis). Patients often present with constitutional symptoms including fever, myalgias, arthralgias, weight loss, and malaise. There is typically a hiatus of some 8–10 years between the prodromal phase and the vasculitic phase, which is often signaled by worsening asthma that requires therapeutic step-up to systemic glucocorticoids. The histopathological features include vascular and extravascular granulomas with eosinophilic infiltrates. EGPA is now considered to be one of the ANCA+ vasculitic syndromes, since up to 75% of patients are ANCA positive, most with a perinuclear pattern.

Neurological involvement

As was true for PAN, peripheral neuropathies far outnumber CNS events. They are seen in up to 75% of EGPA patients with acute and subacute mononeuritis multiplex, with sensory and motor involvement seen most frequently. Unchecked, the mononeuritis multiplex may progress to an asymmetric polyneuropathy. Initial symptoms include acute painful dysesthesias and edema in the dysesthetic portion of the distal limbs. With immunosuppressive therapy, the initial symptoms of peripheral neuropathy usually recede, but sequelae of axonal damage persist. Less commonly, axonal polyneuropathy and cranial neuropathies are seen. CNS event are rare and include subarachnoid and intracerebral hemorrhage and cerebral infarcts.

Treatment

Treatment of EGPA entails a similar approach to that used in PAN, with the same dosing of glucocorticoid for non-life-threatening disease, the addition of cyclophosphamide for severe disease, and substitution of a less toxic immunosuppressive agent for cyclophosphamide as maintenance therapy. The prognosis of EGPA has improved dramatically with the use of glucocorticoid therapy with or without an immunosuppressive agent. Prior to implementation of what is now standard therapy, all patients died, with 50% deceased within three months of vasculitis onset. This contrasts sharply with the 5-year survival rate of 70–90% in patients in the modern treatment era.

Overlap vasculitis

Although vasculitis syndromes have traditionally been classified by distinguishing clinical, pathological, and immunological characteristics by groups like the American College of Rheumatology (ACR) and the Chapel Hill Consensus Conference (CHCC), the early schemes were not precise. Indeed, the ACR scheme did not recognize MPA. The 1994 CHCC scheme recognized MPA as a distinct nosological entity and the importance of ANCA in the diagnosis, but neither this nor other surrogate markers were included in the definition. Further confounding the issue is that histopathological information is not always available. Not surprisingly, it has become apparent that patients sometimes present with overlapping features that defy pigeonholing into one of the established entities. This is particularly true when large, medium, and/or small vessels are sometimes involved in some vasculitic presentations.

As noted previously, prior to the revision of the vasculitis nomenclature at the CHCC in 1994, much of the PAN literature was contaminated by cases of microscopic polyangiitis. The addition of testing for ANCA (generally positive in MPA and negative in most cases of PAN) and appreciation that PAN does not typically affect the lungs or cause necrotizing glomerulonephritis, while MPA does, have helped to distinguish these disorders. Nevertheless, there are occasional cases when even these entities, and for that matter others, make it difficult to distinguish between medium and small vessel vasculitides, as some patients with largely medium-sized vasculitis will present with clinical features of small vessel vasculitis like palpable purpura. Further confounding definitive diagnosis are the occasional patients with clinical features of PAN who lack pulmonary involvement and evidence of glomerulonephritis, but who are ANCA positive. Moreover, patients with polyangiitis with granulomatosis (formerly called Wegener's granulomatosis) who present with eosinophilia may be difficult to distinguish from patients with EGPA. Adult patients with Henoch–Schoenlein purpura may be difficult to distinguish from patients with so-called hypersensitivity vasculitis in the absence of histological results, including immunofluorescence for IgA deposition. In such patients with features of overlap vasculitis, the best diagnostic arbiter is prolonged follow-up and clinical outcomes.

Further reading

Jennette JC, Falk RJ, Bacon PA, *et al.* 2012 revised International Chapel Hill Consensus Conference Nomenclature of Vasculitides. *Arthritis Rheum* 2013;65:1–11.

Moore PM, Cupps TR. Neurological consequences of vasculitis. *Ann Neurol* 1983;14: 155–167.

Pagnoux C, Guillevein L. Churg–Strauss syndrome: Evidence for disease subtypes? *Curr Opin Rheum* 2010;22:21–28.

Pangoux C, Seror R, Henegar C, *et al.* Clinical features and outcomes in 348 patients with polyarteritis nodosa. *Arthritis Rheum* 2010;62:616–626.

Provenzale JM, Allen NB. Neuroradiologic findings in polyarteritis nodosa. *Am J Neuroradiol* 1996;17:1119–1126.

Watts R, Lane S, Hanslik T, *et al.* Development and validation of a consensus methodology for the classification of the ANCA-associated vasculitides and polyarteritis nodosa for epidemiological studies. *Ann Rheum Dis* 2007;66:222–227.

21 Granulomatosis with polyangiitis (GPA)

Gerard Said
Centre Médical Bastille, Paris, France

Primary vasculitides are often classified according to the size of the vessels predominantly affected, but overlaps are common and the nomenclature of the systemic vasculitides remains enigmatic. The antineutrophil cytoplasmic antibody (ANCA) associated forms of vasculitis have been separated as a group, as opposed to immune complex small vessel vasculitis. When consensus was achieved eponyms were replaced by systematic names, such as granulomatosis with polyangiitis (GPA). GPA is a rare disease, often associated with neurological manifestations, especially with ophthalmoplegia and multifocal neuropathy.

Epidemiology

The prevalence of GPA is about 3 in 100,000, with a slightly higher prevalence in men than in women (3:2). The peak incidence of the disease is at 50 to 60 years of age.

Clinical features

GPA typically affects the upper and lower airways and kidneys; however, other organ systems can be affected, including the joints, eyes, skin, central nervous system, and, less commonly, the gastrointestinal tract, parotid gland, heart, thyroid, liver, and breast. Common manifestations include persistent rhinorrhea purulent or bloody nasal discharge; oral or nasal ulcers; polyarthralgia or myalgias; sinus pain; earaches/hearing loss; hoarseness; hemoptysis, cough, and dyspnea; nodules and opacities seen on chest radiography; plus non-specific complaints: fevers, night sweats, anorexia, weight loss, malaise.

Peripheral neuropathy has been observed in 25% of patients with GPA. Peripheral neuropathy is seldom the first manifestation of the disease. In a review of 324 patients with GPA, 109 had neurological manifestations at some stage; 53 patients had peripheral neuropathy, which was multifocal in 42. Cranial nerves were involved in 21/109, and ophthalmoplegia was present in 16/21. The mean interval between the onset of GPA and neurological manifestations was 8.4 months. However, in a recent study peripheral neuropathy was inaugural in a higher proportion of patients with GPA than previously thought, a finding that was not accepted by all commentators.

Investigations

GPA is an antibody-mediated autoimmune granulomatous vasculitis, in which antibodies against proteinase 3 and myeloperoxidase are demonstrable in the serum of patients. Serological demonstration of these antineutrophil cytoplasmic antibodies (ANCAs) is a sensitive and specific means by which to diagnose GPA, provided that a positive result on a screening leukocyte indirect immunofluorescence microscopic ANCA study is followed up by an enzyme-linked immunoabsorbent assay demonstration of antiproteinase 3 and antimyeloperoxidase.

Of patients with active generalized disease, 90% are ANCA positive. However, in patients with milder, limited forms of the disease, the ANCA test may be negative up to 40% of the time. A positive perinuclear (P)-ANCA result is less specific. Other frequent but non-specific laboratory findings include leukocytosis, thrombocytosis, an elevated erythrocyte sedimentation rate, and a normocytic, normochromic anemia. A tissue biopsy is essential for the definitive diagnosis of GPA.

Treatment

Severe disease with organ- or life-threatening manifestations should be treated with cyclophosphamide or rituximab plus high-dose glucocorticoids, followed by lower-dose steroid plus azathioprine or methotrexate. Additional plasmapheresis is effective for very severe disease, reducing dialysis dependence from 60% to 40% in the first year, but with no effect on mortality or long-term renal function, probably due to established renal damage. In milder forms of ANCA-associated vasculitis, methotrexate, leflunomide, or mycophenolate mofetil is effective. Mortality depends on initial severity: 25% in patients with renal failure or severe lung hemorrhage and 6% for generalized non-life-threatening AASV, but rising to 30–40% at 5 years.

Further reading

De Groot K, Schmidt DK, Arlt AC, Gross WL, Reinhold-Keller E. Standardized neurologic evaluation of 128 patients with Wegener granulomatosis. *Arch Neurol* 2001;58:1215–1221.

Duna GF, Galperin C, Hoffman GS. Wegener's granulomatosis. *Rheum Dis Clin North Am* 1995;21:949–986.

Lugmani RA. State of the art in the treatment of systemic vasculitis. *Front Immunol* 2014;5:471.

Morgan MD, Harper L, Williams J, Savage C. Anti-neutrophil cytoplasm-associated glomerulonephritis. *J Am Soc Nephrol* 2006;17:1224–1234.

Nishino H, Rubino FA, DeRemee RA, Swanson JW, Parisi JE. Neurological involvement in Wegener's granulomatosis: An analysis of 324 consecutive patients at the Mayo Clinic. *Ann Neurol* 1993;33:4–9.

Stern GM, Hoffbrand AV, Urich H. The peripheral nerves and skeletal muscles in Wegener's granulomatosis: A clinicopathological study of four cases. *Brain* 1965;88:151–164.

White FS, Lynch JP. Pharmacological therapy for Wegener's granulomatosis. *Drugs* 2006;66:1209–1228.

International Neurology, Second edition. Edited by Robert P. Lisak, Daniel D. Truong, William M. Carroll and Roongroj Bhidayasiri

22 Cerebrovascular disease associated with antiphospholipid antibodies

Adrian Marchidann and Steven R. Levine

Department of Neurology/Stroke Center, SUNY Downstate Health Science Center, Brooklyn, NY, USA

The antiphospholipid antibody syndrome (APS) is the most common cause of acquired thrombophilia. It is characterized by arterial, venous, or small vessel thrombosis associated with persistently positive antiphospholipid antibodies (aPL). aPL is a family of autoantibodies directed against phospholipids and phospholipid-binding proteins. The most common aPLs are lupus anticoagulant (LA) antibodies, anticardiolipin antibodies (aCL), and anti-β 2-glycoprotein I antibodies (β2GPI). APS may occur as a primary disorder or in association with systemic lupus erythematosus (SLE). APS is an important cause of thrombotic disorders like deep venous thrombosis (DVT), pulmonary embolism (PE), myocardial ischemia, and stroke. In addition, it is associated with pregnancy morbidity and other neurological disorders with mechanisms other than thrombosis alone.

Epidemiology

In the general population, the prevalence of aPL is 1–5%, but only a minority will develop APS. The incidence of APS is 5/100,000/year and the prevalence is 40–50/100,000. The prevalence increases in the elderly and in those with chronic disease. In patients with SLE the prevalence of APS is higher, between 15% and 86%. This wide range may be due to various definitions of APS used by different authors with regard to the threshold for positive testing, the number of positive tests, and the interval between them needed for definitive diagnosis. The choice of aPL tested, aCL being the most commonly used, may also account for the variability of the results.

Approximately 40% of patients with SLE and aPL develop APS, but only 5% of those with APS will develop SLE. A transient and low level of aCL is often seen in normal individuals or in patients with various disorders and has unknown significance. Bacterial, viral, and parasitic infections (including Lyme, cytomegalovirus, mumps, and Epstein–Barr virus), neoplasms, chronic systemic illnesses (sickle cell disease, diabetes mellitus), and medications (procainamide) may be associated with positive aPL.

Genetic factors may play a role in APS. Approximately one-third of the relatives of patients with aCL tested positive for aCL. In addition, the presence of aPL is associated with certain HLA subtypes, including HLA-DR7 in Canadians, Germans, Italians, and Mexicans and HLA-DQ7 in Americans. The IgG aCL is dominant in the Hispanic and African American population, whereas the IgA aCL is present in all Afro-Caribbean patients. The clinical features of APS correlate better with the aCL isotopes in Hispanics and African Americans than in Afro-Caribbean patients.

Healthy individuals with positive aPL without previous thrombosis have a 0–3.8% annual risk of thrombosis, probably closer to 1% based on prospective data. aPL were found in 25% of patients under the age of 45 with a stroke of unclear etiology and in 5–21% of patients with venous thrombosis. However, one positive aPL does not predict the rate of stroke recurrence. In children with stroke, aPL were found in 16–76% of cases. Patients with APS and Sneddon syndrome compared to those without the syndrome have a risk of stroke of 28.5% vs. 7.5% and the risk of limb ischemia is 100% vs. 30%, respectively . Venous thromboembolism (VTE) recurs less often compared with arterial or recurrent venous events.

Pathophysiology

Anti-β2GPI plays a central role in activation of the endothelial cells, monocytes, and platelets. This results in the upregulation of intercellular adhesion molecule-1, tissue factor, and expression of thromboxane A2. Inhibition of protein C, its cofactors, antithrombin activity, prothrombin, factor X, protein Z pathway, and plasmin diminishes coagulation factor inactivation and fibrinolysis. Additionally, complement activation leads to a heightened procoagulant state.

Placental histology in patients with APS reveals complement deposition in throphoblasts, vasculitis of the spiral arteries, perivascular inflammation, deciduitis, thrombosis, infarction, and a large number of endometrial killer cells. Moreover, the IgG-β2GPI complexes displace annexin5, an anticoagulant protein found in placenta, endothelial cells, and platelets.

The catastrophic antiphospholipid syndrome (CAPS) occurs on a background of increased aPL, sometimes combined with another genetic thrombophilia-like depression of the anticoagulant system, hypofibrinolysis, prothrombin G20210A mutation, or MTHFR C677T mutation. A trigger factor, usually an infection but it can also be an autoimmune reaction, leads to the production of cross-reactive anti-β2GPI that binds to the surface of endothelial cells and activates them. The cascade of signal transduction is mediated by the TLR-4 receptor. This leads to a massive release of interleukin IL-1, IL-6, and TNF, referred to as the "cytokine storm," and cell adhesion molecules. Apoptosis of the endothelial cells and platelet aggregation result in intravascular thrombosis, thrombocytopenia, and microangiopathic anemia. A dramatic systemic inflammatory response syndrome follows, associated with disseminated intravascular coagulation and multiorgan failure. The infections that trigger

International Neurology, Second edition. Edited by Robert P. Lisak, Daniel D. Truong, William M. Carroll and Roongroj Bhidayasiri
© 2016 John Wiley & Sons, Ltd. Published 2016 by John Wiley & Sons, Ltd.

CAPS are dengue and typhoid fever, but also urinary tract and upper respiratory tract infections.

Clinical features

The most common presentations of APS are deep venous thrombosis (38.9%), thrombocytopenia (29.6%), stroke (19.8%), pulmonary embolism (14.1%), superficial thrombophlebitis (11.7%), transient ischemic attack (11.1%), hemolytic anemia (9.7%), epilepsy (7%), and obstetric morbidity. Venous thrombosis is more likely associated with LA and the arterial events with aCL. Each type of thrombotic event is more likely to be followed by subsequent events of the same type.

Stroke is the most severe complication of APS. Patients with positive aPL are younger and more likely to be female than those without aPL. Amaurosis fugax is one of the most common manifestations of APS. Strokes can be also associated with vascular dementia, epilepsy, and chorea.

Sneddon's syndrome is the association of cerebrovascular disease and livedo reticularis. More than 40% of these patients have aPL (not always persistent), and the clinical course is more severe than in patients without aPL. Leukoaraiosis and small vessel disease are more often seen in patients with Sneddon's syndrome than in patients with APS, who tend to present with large artery occlusions.

Transverse myelitis occurs in less than 1% of patients with APS, in particular in patients with SLE. A direct interaction between aPL and spinal phospholipids is thought to be more important than ischemia caused by thrombosis.

Antibodies against phospholipids and nuclear antigens may be associated with Guillain–Barré syndrome. Mononeuritis multiplex, rarely seen in patients with APS, may be caused by thrombosis of the vasa nervorum with or without autoantibodies and deposition of immune complexes. In one study, 35% of patients with APS had nerve conduction abnormalities like pure sensory, sensorimotor distal axonal, sensorimotor demyelinating, and carpal tunnel syndrome. Prospective studies have failed to find a relationship between APS and migraine or multiple sclerosis.

The catastrophic antiphospholipid syndrome (CAPS) is an accelerated form of APS causing multiple organ failure. Less than 1% of patients with APS develop CAPS, but mortality is approximately 50% despite treatment. Diagnosis of CAPS requires at least three organs, systems, and/or tissues involved within one week of the initial event, presence of aPL, and evidence of small vessel occlusion in at least one organ or tissue on pathological examination. If there is no history of definite APS, aPL should be measured twice or more at least six weeks apart. The most common precipitating factors include infections, trauma or surgery, obstetric complications, malignancy, lupus flare, anticoagulation withdrawal, and oral contraceptives. Approximately 35% of CAPS have no apparent trigger.

Investigations

APS should be suspected in young (<50 years) patients with ischemic stroke or unprovoked proximal or unusual sites of DVT, PE or recurrent thrombosis, SLE or autoimmune disease and thrombosis, recurrent pregnancy morbidity, unexplained thrombocytopenia, prolongation of PT/aPTT, or livedo reticularis.

The diagnosis of APS requires at least one episode of arterial, venous, or small vessel thrombosis or pregnancy morbidity, and positive testing for aCL, LA, or anti-β2GPI.

Thrombosis may be proved by biopsy or other appropriate diagnostic means in the absence of an alternative diagnosis or cause. Pregnancy morbidity is defined as at least three spontaneous abortions before the 10th week, at least one unexplained death at or after 10 weeks, or at least one premature birth before 34 weeks. Abortions occurring in the absence of chromosomal, anatomical, or endocrine abnormalities in the mother or chromosomal abnormalities in the father as well as prematurity occurring in a morphologically normal fetus or neonate should raise the suspicion of APS. Although there may be an association between aPL and pre-eclampsia and placental insufficiency, screening of infertile patients for aPL is not recommended.

To avoid a false negative result, the LA blood sample should be collected with minimal venous stasis and processed within 1 hour by a specialized laboratory. Some laboratories can process LA while the patient takes anticoagulant medication. Both aCL and anti-β2GPI are detected through standardized enzyme-linked immunoassays (ELISA). The aPL measurement should be performed on two or more occasions at least 12 weeks apart, preferably outside the acute phase of the event. The diagnosis should not be made if less than 12 weeks or more than 5 years separate the clinical event from the positive test.

Treatment

Asymptomatic individuals with persistently positive aPL do not benefit from aspirin, as they are unlikely to develop thrombosis in the absence of cardiovascular risk factors. Risk factor control and low molecular weight heparin (LMWH) in high-risk situations (surgery, immobilization, and puerperium) are recommended. Patients with SLE or pregnant and with aPL alone may benefit from low-dose aspirin (LDA).

Untreated patients with APS had a recurrence rate of 19–29% per year in retrospective, highly referral-biased studies that are likely to be overestimates. No prospective, randomized trials have demonstrated superiority of anticoagulant treatment over antiplatelet therapy. Only an international normalized ratio (INR) of 2–3 on warfarin has been shown to be as effective but safer than an INR of 3–4.

Patients with previous stroke or venous thrombosis and one positive aPL should have repeat aPL testing. Until the result is available, warfarin at an INR of 2–3 for venous thrombosis and aspirin for an ischemic stroke is recommended.

Based on the limited available data, the following recommendations for stroke patients with APS have been suggested:

- If the first venous event (cerebral venous thrombosis), use warfarin at INR of 2–3.
- If an arterial stroke, use aspirin.
- If a recurrent event, use warfarin at INR 2–3, consider LDA or LMWH.
- In patients who need surgery, use bridging therapy with LMWH or unfractionated heparin in place of warfarin.

The new oral anticoagulants (NOACs) have a predictable dose effect, do not require routine monitoring, are not influenced by diet, and have fewer drug interactions. They include direct thrombin inhibitors (dabigatran) and direct factor Xa inhibitors (rivaroxaban, apixaban, and endoxaban). NOACs can be considered in a patient with warfarin allergy, intolerance, or poor anticoagulant control, but are contraindicated during pregnancy.

Major bleeding occurs at a rate of 2–3% per year in patients receiving anticoagulation. However, mortality is mostly due to recurrent thrombotic events.

If APS is refractory to warfarin in spite of optimal INR, LMWH may be used due to its excellent bioavailability. Long-term use of LMWH is limited by the route of administration, risk of heparin-induced thrombocytopenia, and osteoporosis. Addition of a statin, independent of the lipid profile, may be useful due to its antithrombotic properties. Hydroxychloroquine may also be used in patients with SLE. Refractory APS may respond well to rituximab. If thrombotic events are present, LMWH or warfarin at INR 2–3 may be added.

The treatment of CAPS targets the ongoing thrombotic event and the suppression of cytokine cascade. Intravenous heparin followed by warfarin is the mainstay of treatment. Intravenous heparin and methylprednisolone 1000 mg/day for 3 days should be associated with plasma exchange, intravenous immunoglobulin, or both in order to lower mortality. Rituximab may be useful in selected cases.

Further reading

American Heart Association Stroke Council, Council on Cardiovascular and Stroke Nursing, Council on Clinical Cardiology, and Council on Peripheral Vascular Disease. Guidelines for the prevention of stroke in patients with stroke and transient ischemic attack: A guideline for healthcare professionals from the American Heart Association/American Stroke Association. *Stroke.* 2014;45:2160–2236.

Cervera R, Rodríguez-Pintó I, Colafrancesco S, *et al.* 14th International Congress on Antiphospholipid Antibodies Task Force report on catastrophic antiphospholipid syndrome. *Autoimmun Rev* 2014;13(7):699–707.

Gómez-Puerta JA, Cervera R. Diagnosis and classification of the antiphospholipid syndrome. *J Autoimmun* 2014;48–49:20-25.

Ortega-Hernandez OD, Agmon-Levin N, Blank M, Asherson RA, Shoenfeld Y. The physiopathology of the catastrophic antiphospholipid (Asherson's) syndrome: Compelling evidence. *J Autoimmun* 2009;32(1):1–6.

Rodrigues CEM, Carvalho JF, Shoenfeld Y. Neurological manifestations of antiphospholipid syndrome. *Eur J Clin Invest* 2010;40:350–359.

23 Thromboangiitis obliterans (Buerger's disease)

Kumar Rajamani
Wayne State University School of Medicine, Detroit, MI, USA

Thromboangiitis obliterans (TAO) is a non-atherosclerotic idiopathic inflammatory disease of the blood vessels of the upper and lower extremities, predominantly involving medium-sized and small arteries as well as veins. There is a resultant segmental obliteration of the affected vessels. Persistent tobacco smoking has long been associated with TAO, although alternative forms of tobacco consumption such as chewing and sniffing have also been implicated. Chronic and often heavy exposure to tobacco use is implicated in the onset as well as the progression of the disease. Tobacco smoke is a complex mixture of various chemicals and toxins. Quiescent disease can be reactivated if the patient starts to smoke again, underlining the causal link. Patients demonstrate hypersensitivity to intradermally injected tobacco extracts.

Epidemiology

TAO occurs throughout the world, but higher incidences have been described in Japan, Eastern Europe, India, Israel, and the Middle East compared to Western Europe and the United States. The reason for this geographic distribution is not entirely clear and has been variably attributed to local smoking habits as well as genetic predisposition. For example, heavy consumption of homemade cigarettes made from raw tobacco may contribute to the higher incidence of the disease in the Indian subcontinent. A recent decline in the incidence of TAO has been reported in the United States and is likely due to a general decline in smoking, but application of stricter diagnostic criteria could also be contributory.

Males are more affected than females (6:1) and symptoms typically start in the third and fourth decades.

Pathophysiology

Although the target is yet to be convincingly demonstrated, an autoimmune process is implicated in the vascular endothelial dysfunction and inflammatory thrombi that characterize the endarteritis. The precise triggers and the subsequent molecular pathways are not definitely known. The endothelial cells are located on the interface of the blood vessel wall and the circulating blood and may be the site of the initial damage. CD4- as well as CD8-positive T-cells are observed near the internal lamina. S-100-positive dendritic cells also localize to the intima. The cellular response is particularly robust in the acute stages. Deposition of immunoglobulins and complement factors has been shown along the internal elastic lamina. There is increased cell-mediated sensitivity to types I and III collagen (both of which are present in vessel walls) and elevated titers of anticollagen and antiendothelium antibodies. However, these are non-specific and could be an epiphenomenon rather than the cause. Increased incidences of HLA-A9 and HLA-B5 antigens and reduced HLA-B12 have been described, supporting the notion of a genetic influence over the immune response in TAO.

In the acute phase there is a highly cellular inflammatory thrombus. There is progressive organization of the thrombus and the late stage is characterized by an organized thrombus and fibrosis of the vessel wall. Differentiation from arteriosclerosis may be difficult, but intimal inflammation, characteristic preservation of the internal elastic lamina, adventitial fibrosis without affection of the media, onion-like recanalized vessels, and swelling of the endothelium of the vasa vasorum are more characteristic of TAO.

Clinical features

Claudication pain begins in the feet and may progress to the calf. More than one limb can be affected. Isolated involvement of large proximal arteries without involvement of small vessels is unusual. Pain in the legs even without exercise (rest pain), non-healing ulcers of toes and fingers, and gangrene are later features. Raynaud's phenomenon and superficial thrombophlebilitis are characteristic features that could help distinguish TAO from arteriosclerosis. Coronary, cerebral, mesenteric, and multiorgan involvement are described, but are decidedly rare.

Investigations

There are no definite laboratory tests for the diagnosis of TAO. Tests to rule out other vasculitides include those for acute phase reactants, antinuclear antibodies, rheumatoid factor, serological markers for the CREST syndrome (calcinosis, Raynaud's phenomenon, esophageal dysmotility, sclerodactyly, and telangiectasia), scleroderma, and hypercoagulability. Angiography demonstrates more distal vascular occlusions, and characteristic "corkscrew" collaterals (Martorell's sign) without proximal lesions, but is not pathognomonic.

International Neurology, Second edition. Edited by Robert P. Lisak, Daniel D. Truong, William M. Carroll and Roongroj Bhidayasiri
© 2016 John Wiley & Sons, Ltd. Published 2016 by John Wiley & Sons, Ltd.

Treatment

Early treatment is important, with complete avoidance of tobacco consumption being the most effective approach. Nicotine patches and gum, often used to help with smoking cessation, should *not* be used as the nicotine delivered through these routes can keep the disease active. In spite of the role of inflammation, steroids and other anti-inflammatory medications have not been shown to be useful. Intravenous iloprost (a prostaglandin analogue that stimulates blood flow by vasodilation and antiplatelet effects) and subcutaneous treprostinil (prostacyclin) have been shown to be useful in critical limb ischemia to heal ulcers and prevent the dreaded complication of limb amputations. A double blind placebo-controlled trial of oral iloprost has shown efficacy in reducing rest pain.

Supportive care is needed for maximizing blood supply to the limb, mainly by avoiding injuries and emphasizing properly fitting footwear. Judicious and timely use of sympathectomy may alleviate pain and promote healing while avoiding amputation. Bypass vascular surgery is not generally possible or useful because of the diffuse and distal nature of the disease and problems with graft thrombosis. Gene therapy, growth factors such as vascular endothelial growth factor (VEGF), and autologous bone marrow, all of which are aimed at therapeutic angiogenesis, hold future promise.

Further reading

De Haro J, Bleda S, Acin F. An open-label study on long-term outcomes of bosentan for treating ulcers in thromboangiitis obliterans (Buerger's disease). *Int J Cardiol* 2014;177:529–531.

Eichhorn J, Sima D, Lindschau C, *et al*. Antiendothelial antibodies in thromboangiitis obliterans. *Am J Med Sci* 1998;315(1):17–23.

European TAO Study Group. Oral iloprost in the treatment of thromboangiitis obliterans (Buerger's Disease): A double-blind, randomized, placebo-controlled trial. *Eur J Vasc Endovasc Surg* 1998;15:300–307.

Ketha SS, Cooper LT. The role of autoimmunity in thromboangiitis obliterans (Buerger's disease). *Ann NY Acad Sci* 2013;1285:15–25.

Kurata A, Franke F, Machinami R, Schulz A. Thromboangiitis obliterans: Classic and new morphological features. *Virchows Arch* 2000;436:59–67.

Olin JW. Thromboangiitis obliterans (Buerger's disease). *N Engl J Med* 2000;343(12): 864–869.

Olin JW, Shih A. Thromboangiitis obliterans (Buerger's disease). *Curr Opin Rheumatol* 2006;18:18–24.

Puechal X, Fiessinger JN. Thromboangiitis obliterans or Buerger's disease: Challenges for the rheumatologist. *Rheumatology* 2007;46(2):192–199.

24 Susac syndrome

Rachel E. Ventura and Steven L. Galetta

Department of Neurology, New York University Langone Medical Center, New York, USA

Susac syndrome is characterized by the triad of encephalopathy, visual deficits due to branch retinal artery occlusions (BRAOs), and hearing loss. It is thought to be due to autoimmune-mediated microvascular occlusions in the brain, retina, and inner ear. The syndrome was named after John O. Susac due to his report of a patient with a microangiopathy of the brain and retina. While rare, it is important to consider Susac syndrome in the differential diagnosis of other more common neurological disorders such as multiple sclerosis and CNS vasculitis, as well as conditions producing neurosensory hearing loss, since treatment with immunosuppressants seems effective in stabilizing its course.

Epidemiology

Because Susac syndrome is so rare, the literature only has case reports, so it is challenging to assess its demographic distribution accurately. Dorr and colleagues compiled all 304 cases published and all continents were represented, with a distribution of 152 reports from North America, 126 from Europe, 10 from Asia, 8 from South America, 7 from Australia, and 1 from Africa. Of those cases with ethnicity reported, 81% of the patients were white, 4% black, 8% Asian, 1% Hispanic, and 5% Turkish. The male:female ratio in all the reported cases was 1:3.5 and most individuals were between 21 and 35 years of age. Of female patients, 5% were diagnosed in the context of pregnancy, including in the postpartum period, which could reflect peripartum changes in autoimmunity.

Pathophysiology

Susac syndrome is thought to be an autoimmune microangiopathy with microvascular infarcts occurring in the brain, cochlea, and retina. The antigen is unknown, although immunoglobin G (IgG) antiendothelial cell antibodies with a titer >1:100 can be found in about 25% of patients with Susac syndrome versus 4.3% of controls. Consistent with a humoral etiology of Susac syndrome, brain biopsy has shown complement c4d staining in the microvasculature.

Clinical features

The clinical triad of encephalopathy, retinal involvement, and hearing abnormalities is present in 13% of cases at disease onset, but then over the ensuing months to years the triad is seen in 85% of cases. Thus, a failure to find the complete triad should not immediately exclude the diagnosis.

Headache can be seen in about 80% of patients at diagnosis, and often precedes the development of encephalopathy by several months. Patients can develop cognitive changes, confusion, memory loss leading to dementia, and psychiatric disturbances, including behavioral changes and paranoia. Other neurological manifestations include dysarthria, dysmetria, vertigo, cranial nerve involvement, and seizures.

Visual findings are characteristically due to branch retinal artery occlusions (BRAOs; see Figure 24.1), which are usually bilateral, multiple, and can develop over several months. The BRAOs can cause scotomas, photopsias, and blurred vision. Ophthalmic examination typically shows an area of retinal infarction, often with cotton-wool spots, retinal artery occlusions, and areas of arterio-arterial retinal collaterals. At times there is also neovascularization of the optic disc and macular edema. Some patients with significant arteriolar involvement develop optic atrophy and constriction of the visual field.

Hearing loss is typically in the low or middle frequencies, but can also occur in higher frequencies as well, and may be accompanied by vertigo and tinnitus. Hearing loss can at times occur overnight in both ears, which has been referred to as "bang bang hearing loss."

Rennebohm and colleagues classified Susac syndrome into three types of clinical courses: monocyclic for those with an active period of less than 2 years without recurrence; polycyclic for those with relapses over more than a 2-year period; and chronic-continuous for those with a single, potentially fluctuating, active period lasting over 2 years. To date, 54% of reported cases can be described as having monocyclic disease, 42% had polycyclic disease, and 4% had the chronic-continuous disease.

Investigations

Brain MRI characteristically shows multifocal T2 hyperintensities in the central part of the corpus callosum (see Figure 24.1), which are usually small but may have a larger "snowball" appearance. These lesions tend to spare the peripheral part of the corpus callosum and thus can be distinguished from demyelinating disease. There may also be small T2 hyperintense foci and contrast enhancement in the white and gray matter throughout the brain, with occasional leptomeningeal enhancement.

Fluorescein angiography can help delineate the BRAOs, and typically shows multifocal fluorescence and retinal arterial wall plaques, or Gass plaques. In addition, leakage can be seen that indicates loss of integrity of the vessel walls and marks active disease. Optical coherence tomography can also help characterize the retinal pathology.

International Neurology, Second edition. Edited by Robert P. Lisak, Daniel D. Truong, William M. Carroll and Roongroj Bhidayasiri
© 2016 John Wiley & Sons, Ltd. Published 2016 by John Wiley & Sons, Ltd.

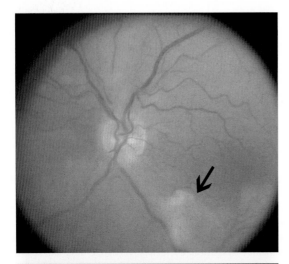

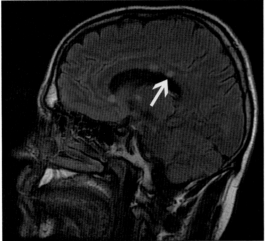

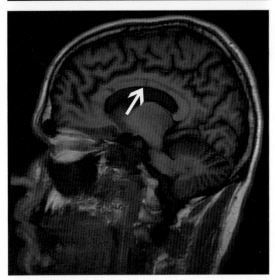

Pure tone audiometry reveals bilateral, asymmetric sensorineural hearing loss. Videonystagmography may show a deficit of the caloric response in the affected ear.

Laboratory tests may reveal elevated acute phase reactants. Cerebrospinal fluid (CSF) examination shows a lymphocytic pleocytosis and elevated protein levels. Typically, there are no oligoclonal bands or elevated IgG index.

Brain biopsy shows perivascular inflammation of the small vessels, microinfarcts, and complement staining.

Treatment

There are no randomized controlled trials to guide management. Nonetheless, it is generally thought that early, aggressive, and sustained immunotherapy improves outcomes. High-dose corticosteroids, such as oral prednisone with or without pulses of intravenous (IV) methylprednisolone, are the first-line therapy. Those who fail a trial of high-dose steroids such as prednisone 80 mg/day for 2 months can at times respond to other immunotherapies such as plasma exchange, IVIG, subcutaneous immunoglobulin, cyclophosphamide, mycophenolate mofetil, and rituximab. Combination therapy sometimes is necessary, such as prednisone with cyclophosphamide and IVIG.

Further reading

Dorr J, Krautwald S, Wildemann B, *et al.*, Characteristics of Susac syndrome: A review of all reported cases. *Nat Rev Neurol* 2013;9(6):307–316.

Jarius S, Kleffner I, Dorr JM, *et al.*, Clinical, paraclinical and serological findings in Susac syndrome: An international multicenter study. *J Neuroinflammation*, 2014;11:46.

Magro CM, Poe JC, Lubow M, *et al.*, Susac syndrome: An organ-specific autoimmune endotheliopathy syndrome associated with anti-endothelial cell antibodies. *Am J Clin Pathol* 2011;136(6):903–912.

Rennebohm RM, Egan RA, Susac JO. Treatment of Susac's syndrome. *Curr Treat Options Neurol* 2008;10(1):67–74.

Susac JO, Hardman JM, Selhorst JB. Microangiopathy of the brain and retina. *Neurology* 1979;29(3):313–316.

Figure 24.1 Top panel: fundus photograph of a patient with Susac syndrome showing multiple BRAOs, the largest of which is identified by the black arrow. Middle panel: saggital FLAIR MRI sequence of a patient with Susac syndrome showing multiple hyperintensities, especially in the corpus callosum, as demonstrated by the white arrow. Bottom panel: saggital T1 MRI sequence demonstrating multiple black holes in the corpus callosum (arrow). MRI photos courtesy of Dr. Robert Rennebohm. For color details, please refer to the color plates section.

PART 4   Inflammatory Vasculopathies

25   SLE, rheumatoid arthritis, and Sjögren's syndrome

Marc Gotkine and Oded Abramsky

Department of Neurology, Agnes Ginges Center for Human Neurogenetics, Hadassah University Hospital, Hebrew University Hadassah Medical School, Jerusalem, Israel

Systemic lupus erythematosus (SLE), rheumatoid arthritis (RA), and Sjögren's syndrome (SS) are rheumatological conditions with clinical features that in their full-blown form leave little room for diagnostic confusion. However, patients may present to neurologists prior to a formal diagnosis, or in the early stages of the disease, making identification and management of neurological sequelae challenging. Even in patients with full-blown disease, the importance of recognizing the neurological manifestations of these systemic conditions is manifold. Both psychiatric and neurological symptoms occur that may signal damage to diverse components of the nervous system, from the brain and spinal cord to the peripheral nerves and muscles. Consequently, a patient with a rheumatological condition presenting, for example, with "difficulty walking" requires a neurologist to provide clinical expertise in order to localize the pathology, as management decisions invariably depend on the neuroanatomical site involved.

Furthermore, when a patient diagnosed with one of these conditions develops neurological involvement such as central nervous system (CNS) vasculopathy, the treatment regimen often involves robust immunosuppressive therapy.

The most challenging patients from the neurological perspective are those who exhibit neurological manifestations at the beginning of or very early in the course of their systemic disease. In these cases recognition of the patterns of neurological involvement as well as knowledge of the non-neurological features of these conditions are critical in order to identify the systemic condition. This chapter will review the clinical and pathophysiological features of SLE, RA, and SS in turn, with a focus on neurological manifestations. A comprehensive review of these complex multisystem disorders is beyond the scope of this chapter. There will be treatment of these disorders as a group later in the chapter.

Systemic lupus erythematosus (SLE)

SLE is a systemic autoimmune disease affecting multiple organ systems. The diagnosis is made on the basis of fulfillment of accepted clinical and paraclinical criteria, summarized in Table 25.1. Neurological and psychiatric symptoms occur in many patients and may reflect damage to various components of the nervous system

from the cerebral cortex to the muscle, although the CNS is usually affected more often than the peripheral nervous system (Table 25.2.)

In SLE only seizures and psychosis among the neurological manifestations contribute to the diagnostic criteria (Table 25.1). However, the distinction between neurological conditions said to be "associated" with SLE (such as immune-mediated myelitis or myasthenia gravis) and those contributing to the diagnosis of SLE (psychosis and seizures) may reflect statistical associations rather than a specific pathogenetic mechanism.

The issue is further complicated by the facts that drugs used to treat SLE and other rheumatological conditions may have a variety of neurological side effects (Table 25.3) and that neurological complications may result from derangements in other organ systems, such as the liver and kidneys.

Epidemiololgy

SLE is most commonly encountered in women of childbearing age. Both geography and race seem to affect the distribution of SLE. The prevalence in the US population is around 40–50 cases per 100,000. Prevalence rates in Europe and Australia are similar. Differences in detection methods worldwide make it difficult to obtain accurate comparative data between countries. In most countries the prevalence rate is considerably lower in Caucasians in comparison to other ethnic groups. While SLE is seen frequently in African Americans, it is rare in black people in West Africa.

Although genetic factors seem to be important, environmental factors play a sizable role in both the frequency and the severity of the disease, and factors such as socioeconomic status often confound epidemiological studies. Exposure to cigarette smoke, crystalline silica, and viruses such as Epstein–Barr may increase the risk of developing SLE.

Pathophysiology

SLE is characterized by the presence of circulating autoantibodies directed against a variety of cellular components, including the plasma membrane, cytoplasm, and nucleus. The neurological features of the disease may be a result of the damaging effects that these antibodies trigger directly on the various tissue components within the nervous system or the blood vessels that supply them.

International Neurology, Second edition. Edited by Robert P. Lisak, Daniel D. Truong, William M. Carroll and Roongroj Bhidayasiri
© 2016 John Wiley & Sons, Ltd. Published 2016 by John Wiley & Sons, Ltd.

Table 25.1 The 1982 revised criteria for classification of systemic lupus erythematosus. Source: Tan 1982. Reproduced with permission of Wiley.

Criterion	Definition
1. Malar rash	Fixed erythema, flat or raised, over the malar eminences, tending to spare the nasolabial folds
2. Discoid rash	Erythematous raised patches with adherent keratotic scaling and plugging; atrophic scarring may occur in older lesions
3. Photosensitivity	Skin rash as a result of unusual reaction to sunlight, by patient history or physician observation
4. Oral ulcers	Oral or nasopharyngeal ulceration, usually painless, observed by a physician
5. Arthritis	Nonerosive arthritis involving 2 or more peripheral joints, characterized by tenderness, swelling, or effusion
6. Serositis	Pleuritis-convincing history of pleuritic pain or rub heard by a physician or evidence of pleural effusion OR Pericarditis documented by ECG or rub or evidence of pericardial effusion
7. Renal disorder	Persistent proteinuria greater than 0.5 grams per day or greater than 3+ if quantitation not peformed OR cellular casts – may be red cell, hemoglobin, granular, tubular, or mixed
8. Neurologic disorder	Seizures OR psychosis in the absence of offending drugs or metabolic derangements known to cause these features
9. Hematologic disorder	Hemolytic anemia with reticulocytosis OR Leukopenia OR Lymphopenia OR Thrombocytopenia in the absence of offending drugs
10. Immunologic disorder	Positive LE cell preparation OR Anti-DNA antibodies OR Anti-Sm antibodies OR False positive serologic test for syphilis
11. Antinuclear antibody	High antinuclear antibody titers in the absence of drugs known to be associated with "drug-induced lupus syndrome"

A diagnosis of SLE is made if any four or more of the criteria are present (not necessarily simultaneously).
It should be remembered that these criteria are intended for designing inclusion criteria for clinical trials and some patients who do not fulfill these criteria may have a partial or "forme fruste" of the condition, which otherwise behaves pathogenetically and clinically like SLE.

For example, the cerebral cortex may be damaged directly by the inflammatory process or alternatively may be damaged by multiple infarcts as the result of "cerebral vasculitis." However, there is little histological support for the pathological diagnosis of "lupus cerebritis" and although cerebral vasculitis in SLE is uncommon, vasculopathy is often seen.

Clinical features

A wide variety of neurological symptoms may occur in patients previously diagnosed with SLE. However, patients ultimately diagnosed with SLE may initially present with neurological symptoms and have no overt systemic involvement on initial clinical evaluation. As a corollary, many patients presenting with neurological syndromes should be screened for clinical and paraclinical parameters associated with SLE (Table 25.1).

Conversely, neurological evaluation of patients with established SLE may not be straightforward, as neurological dysfunction may be a direct consequence of the disease, secondary to other organ involvement or due to therapeutic interventions. The American College of Rheumatology defined 19 neuropsychiatric syndromes (NPS) occurring in SLE. These represent conditions directly associated with SLE, to the exclusion of conditions occurring secondary to other organ involvement or therapy. Table 25.2 summarizes the full range of neurological syndromes associated with SLE, including "secondary associations." While cardiac, renal, and hematological involvement are related to the core diagnostic features of SLE, it should be remembered that SLE and the drugs used to treat it are associated with a multitude of other conditions, such as liver dysfunction, endocrine derangement, and hypertension, which themselves may have neurological ramifications beyond the scope of this chapter.

The antiphospholipid antibody syndrome (APLAS) is a frequent accompaniment to SLE and the frequency of NPS is higher in SLE patients with antiphospholipid antibodies, particularly anticardiolipin antibodies. Furthermore, neuropsychiatric syndromes frequently occur in APLAS in the absence of SLE (see Chapter 22). The significance of serum antibodies to ribosomal P proteins (anti-P) is unclear: they have been proposed as a marker for neuropsychiatric involvement in SLE, particularly psychosis, but many studies have not confirmed an association.

Various NPS may be causally interrelated. For example, cerebrovascular disease may lead to focal deficits, cognitive decline, seizures, and a movement disorder. Similarly, myelitis may be either isolated or a manifestation of more widespread CNS involvement. The fact that these syndromes can occur independently of one another means that they are listed as NPS of SLE in their own right. A possible exception to this is chronic cognitive decline, which is invariably secondary to one or more of the other processes listed. An acute amnestic syndrome due to bilateral hippocampal inflammation known as "limbic encephalitis" may occasionally occur (Figure 25.1); however, the relationship to idiopathic autoimmune limbic encephalitis is not clear.

Of special note is a characteristic form of severe myelitis occurring in SLE. These patients present with an acute flaccid tetraparesis or paraparesis and loss of sphincter control, which usually involves multiple cord segments and is referred to as "acute longitudinal

Table 25.2 Neurological and psychiatric features associated with systemic lupus erythematosus, rheumatoid arthritis, and Sjögren's syndrome.

System	Clinical Features	SLE	Possible pathogenetic relationship with other recognized NPS	Possible relationship with core SLE systemic disorders	Rheumatoid arthritis (RA)	Sjögren's syndrome (SS)	Drug Side effects
Brain	Cognitive	1. Acute confusion (encephalopathy) 2. Dementia Unclear whether this occurs in isolation or only in association with other NPS or drug side effects	1. Meningoencephalitis 2. Strokes 3. Seizures 4. Demyelinating syndrome	Renal dysfunction	No clear association	Associated	Steroids Cyclosporine Methotrexate
	Psychiatric	1. Mood disorder 2. Anxiety disorder 3. Psychosis Psychosis included in SLE diagnostic criteria	1. Stroke 2. Seizures	Increased incidence of affective disorders in chronic systemic disease	Increased incidence of affective disorders in all chronic systemic diseases	1. Affective disorders 2. Psychosis	Steroids
	Seizures	Associated and included in SLE diagnostic criteria	1. Stroke 2. Meningoencephalitis	Renal dysfunction	No clear association	Associated	TNF-a antagonists Cyclosporine Methotrexate Hydroxy-chloroquine Gold salts
	Stroke	Mechanisms include: • Vasculopathy • Hypercoaguable state associated with APLA • Endocarditis with thromboembolism	-	Renal dysfunction Thrombocytopenia may increase susceptibility to brain hemorrhage	Secondary to cervical spine pathology with atlanto-axial dislocation affecting vertebral arteries (rare)	Associated	Methotrexate IVIG Anticoagulant drugs (hemorrhage)
	Movement disorders	Usually chorea occurring almost exclusively in the presence of APLA	Stroke or other focal lesions affecting basal ganglia	Uremia (usually myoclonus)	No clear association	Associated (rare)	Cyclosporine (tremor) Hydroxychloroquine (ataxia)
	Demyelinating syndromes	Includes optic neuritis and myelitis May be related to NMO antibodies	Myelitis included as NPS in own right	-	Possible association	May be difficult to distinguish from MS	TNF-a antagonists
	Headache	Includes migraine with or without aura May be due to idiopathic intracranial hypertension	Meningitis/meningo-encephalitis	Frequent non-specific symptom of systemic/ metabolic derangement	Secondary to cervical spine pathology/ atlanto-axial dislocation	No clear association	Cyclosporine Sulphasalazine Cyclo-phosphamide Steroids Leflunomide Gold salts Hydroxy-chloroquine

System	Clinical Features	SLE	Possible pathogenetic relationship with other recognized NPS	Possible relationship with core SLE systemic disorders	Rheumatoid arthritis (RA)	Sjögren's syndrome (SS)	Drug Side effects
Spinal cord	Meningitis/ meningo-encephalitis	Aseptic meningitis may be related to vasculitis, NAIM	-	-	Pachymeningitis (rare)	Associated	IVIG (aseptic meningitis)
	Myelopathy/ myelitis	May be associated with NMO antibodies	May be part of a "demyelinating syndrome"	No clear association	No clear association	May be associated with NMO antibodies	TNF-α antagonists
	Cord compression	No clear association	No clear association	No clear association	Pannus compression Atlanto-occipital dislocation Vertebral collapse	No clear association	Steroids via osteoporotic fractures
Motor neurons (upper and lower)	Amyotrophic lateral sclerosis	-	-	-	-	Associated (rare)	-
Peripheral nerves	Cranial neuropathy	Trigeminal sensory	Demyelinating disease (fascicular involvement)	No clear association	Secondary to cervical spine pathology with atlanto-axial dislocation (rare)	Trigeminal sensory Oculomotor Vestibulocochlear	No clear association
	Peripheral neuropathy	1. Polyneuropathy (distal SM) 2. MM (vasculitic) 3. GBS-like 4. Plexopathy 5. Autonomic	No clear association	Renal dysfunction Musculoskeletal disorders increase compression neuropathies	1. MM (vasculitic) 2. Polyneuropathy (distal SM) 3. Compression sites	1. Polyneuropathy (distal SM) 2. Posterior ganglionopathy 3. Autonomic 4. MM (vasculitic)	Gold salts Leflunomide
Muscle	Myopathy, myalgia, cramps	Not considered to represent an NPS Myalgia common Myopathy rare	No clear association	Renal dysfunction (cramps, myokymia)	Inflammatory myopathy (rare)	Myalgia common but myopathy rarely noticeable on clinical examination	Steroids Penicillamine Hydroxy-chloroquine Gold salts Cyclosporine Azathioprine
NMJ	Myasthenia gravis	Associated	No clear association	No clear association	Associated	Associated (rare) SS is associated with thymus hyperplasia	Penicillamine (reversible on drug withdrawal)

APLAS = antiphospholipid antibody syndrome; MM = mononeuritis multiplex; NAIM = non-vasculitic autoimmune meningoencephalitis; NPS = neuropsychiatric syndromes associated with SLE; SM = sensorimotor.

Table 25.3 Immunosuppressive drugs may increase the patient's susceptibility to opportunistic infections and increase the rate of malignancy. Both of these phenomena may affect the nervous system and should be borne in mind when any immunosuppressed patient presents with a neurological syndrome. Source: McLaurin 2005. Reproduced with permission of Wolters Kluwer.

Drug	Indication	Neuropsychiatric side effects	Note
Leflunomide	RA	Headache Peripheral neuropathy	
Steroids		Psychosis Cognitive decline (LT) Raised ICP Headache Mood changes Anxiety Insomnia Myopathy (LT)	McLaurin *et al.* note it is unclear whether cognitive decline is associated with steroid dose or disease activity
Azathioprine		Myalgia	
Cyclophosphamide		Headache	
IVIG		Stroke Aseptic Meningitis	
Sulphasalazine	RA	Headache	
Penicillamine	RA	Myasthenia gravis Myopathy Myalgia Neuromyotonia	
TNF-a antagonists	RA	Seizures (rare) Myelitis/ demyelinating disease induction/exacerbation	
Cyclosporine		Encephalopathy Seizures Raised ICP Tremor Headache Myopathy (rare) Leg cramps Paresthesia	
Methotrexate	RA	Encephalopathy Stroke-like episodes Seizures	
Gold salts	RA	Peripheral Neuropathy Myalgia and myokymia Seizures (rare) Hallucinations (rare) Headache	
Hydroxychloroquine Plaquenil	RA SLE	Seizures Visual complaints Ototoxicity Ataxia Headache Neuropathy Myopathy	
Antiepileptic medications		Dealt with elsewhere	

ICP = intracranial pressure; LT = long term; RA = rheumatoid arthritis; SLE = systemic lupus erythematosus.

myelitis" (ALM, Figure 25.2a). This type of myelitis is distinguished from the type that occurs in multiple sclerosis (MS), which is usually limited to fewer than 2–3 spinal segments (Figure 25.3). Acute longitudinal myelitis also occurs in Devic's syndrome, commonly referred to as neuromyelitis-optica (NMO), and antibodies to water channels known as NMO-IgG are often found in these cases (Figure 25.4). NMO may be associated with both SLE and SS, which raises the possibility that the myelitis described in these conditions is closely connected to the spectrum of neuromyelitis-optica–related disorders.

Although headache is often considered to be one of the neurological manifestations of SLE, the association is controversial. Headache prevalence as a whole is probably similar to the general population, while migraine with aura may be more common in SLE sufferers, especially those with anticardiolipin antibodies. In children with SLE, headache may be associated with CNS involvement.

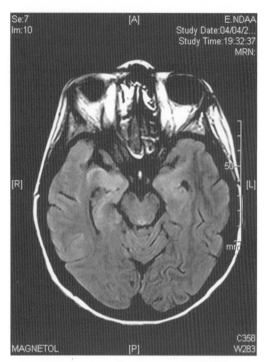

Figure 25.1 FLAIR MRI scan showing bilateral hippocampal inflammation ("limbic encephalitis") in a young woman with systemic lupus erythematosus.

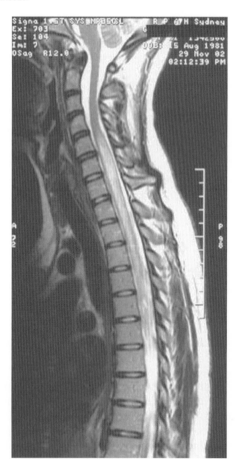

Figure 25.2a T2-weighted MRI scan showing acute longitudinal myelitis spanning more than six spinal cord segments in a young woman with systemic lupus erythematosus. Source: Krishnan 2004. Reproduced with permission of Wolters Kluwer.

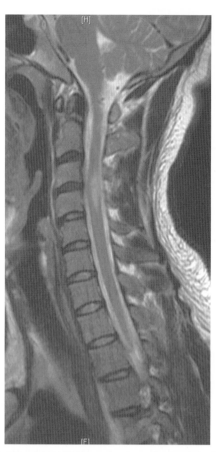

Figure 25.2b T2-weighted MRI scan showing a characteristic plaque of myelitis limited to fewer than three cervical spinal cord segments in a woman with MS.

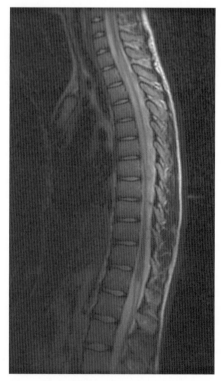

Figure 25.2c T2-weighted MRI scan showing acute longitudinal myelitis spanning more than six spinal cord segments in a young woman with seropositive neuromyelitis-optica.

Rheumatoid arthritis

Rheumatoid arthritis is characterized by a chronic inflammatory arthropathy. There is frequently extra-articular involvement, including the skin, kidney, lung, heart, eyes, and blood components. In contrast to SLE, neurological involvement is almost exclusively confined to the peripheral nervous system, manifesting primarily with peripheral neuropathy (Table 25.2). Neurological evaluation may be very difficult in patients with advanced disease, who may be so severely limited by arthritis that an advanced neuropathy may remain unnoticed by patient and physician alike.

Epidemiology

RA is the most common of the rheumatic diseases, with a prevalence of around 1% worldwide. Some ethnic groups such as certain native American populations have an increased prevalence indicating a genetic component, while the higher rate of RA in urban as compared to rural African areas also confirms a strong environmental influence. The male-to-female ratio is around 2:1 and onset incidence rates peak between 50 and 75 years of age. Rheumatoid factor autoantibodies appear in around 75% of patients during the course of their disease; they are not specific for RA, being found in other system-inflammatory conditions, such as SLE and Sjögren's syndrome.

Clinical features

The most common type of neuropathy is due to vasculitis affecting the vasa nervosum. As with other vasculitic neuropathies, this usually manifests as multiple mononeuropathies (mononeuritis multiplex) occurring during single or multiple episodes. It occurs in roughly 10% of all patients, but the figure rises to 50% in those RA patients with systemic vasculitis. It mainly affects patients with rheumatoid factor seropositivity and long-standing highly manifest disease.

A mild symmetric polyneuropathy is common and is usually asymptomatic, while it is important to differentiate entrapment neuropathies correctly to provide appropriate treatment aimed at decompression rather than immune suppression.

Structural derangement of the cervical spine predisposes to cervical myelopathy and in rare instances the lower cranial nerves, brainstem, and posterior circulation may be distorted by atlanto-axial dislocation. Direct involvement of the CNS and meninges is rare, with coexisting demyelination or pachymeningitis being occasionally observed.

Sjögren's syndrome

Sjögren's syndrome (SS) may occur alone or coexist with SLE, RA, or systemic sclerosis. The core clinical features are due to inflammation of the lachrymal and salivary glands, leading to decreased saliva and tear production. The circulating auto-antibodies, anti-Ro (SS-A) and La (SS-B), are present – either alone or together–in many patients and are associated with extraglandular manifestations of SS. The presence of anti-Ro, when detected by the more specific (less-sensitive) method of immunodiffusion, is strongly associated with sensory neuropathy.

The peripheral and central nervous systems are affected at roughly the same frequency (Table 25.2). A distal polyneuropathy is the most common form of neuropathy, followed by cranial (mainly trigeminal) neuropathy and sensory ganglionopathy. The sensory ganglionopathy or neuronopathy affects all sensory modalities and is associated with lymphocytic infiltration of the dorsal root ganglia. It is frequently painful and asymmetric, affecting proximal as well as distal areas of the body, including the trunk.

This infrequent syndrome also occurs in other situations, such as pyridoxine intoxication and a paraneoplastic syndrome associated with anti-Hu antibodies.

Diffuse CNS symptoms are not uncommon and include seizures, cognitive dysfunction, and occasionally acute encephalopathy. The CNS features are more often focal and include optic nerve and spinal cord involvement. The features may mimic multiple sclerosis both clinically and radiologically, and this should be borne in mind when evaluating patients previously suspected to have MS, especially when atypical features are present. Neuromyelitis-optica may occur in SS even in the absence of SLE.

Treatment of SLE, RA, and SS

Various immune therapies are employed depending on the severity of the disease, type of organ involvement, and individual patient factors. These therapies can be conveniently split into four distinct groups: (1) corticosteroids such as methylprednisolone may be employed for limited periods intravenously during exacerbations or orally as maintenance therapy; (2) immunosuppressive drugs such as azathioprine may allow a decrease in the required steroid dose, while more powerful immunosuppressive agents such as cyclophosphamide are usually reserved for more resistant cases; (3) antibody depleting or neutralizing therapies (plasmapharesis or intravenous immunoglobin) may be used for exacerbations as well as maintenance in some disorders; and (4) monoclonal antibodies directed against proinflammatory cytokines (such as TNF-α in the case of infliximab), lymphocyte subpopulations (such as CD20+ B-cells in the case of rituximab), or TNF-R fusion proteins are being employed more frequently. Belimumab is a relatively recent addition to this group; it inhibits B-cell proliferation by binding to the soluble form of B-lymphocyte stimulator (also known as B-cell activating factor or BAFF). The promising efficacy and tolerability of this group are offset by their prohibitive cost and rare but potentially debilitating side effects, such as progressive multifocal leukoencephalopathy.

While the management of these rheumatological conditions is beyond the scope of this book, it should be emphasized that an accurate neurological assessment is often an essential factor in guiding appropriate therapy. For example, a seizure in a patient with SLE may occur in the context of a metabolic derangement or be due to an acute inflammatory or ischemic insult to the cerebral cortex. The former scenario should prompt correction of the metabolic problem, whereas the latter may signal the need for long-term antiepileptic medication, anticoagulation, more robust immunosuppression, or a combination of these approaches. A similar situation exists in RA in relation to the possible etiologies of peripheral neuropathy. Neurologists should be aware of the potential for neurological side effects of many of the drugs used in these conditions, and the possibility for conditions occurring due to immune compromise, such as opportunistic infections and malignancy.

Further reading

Bertsias GK, Ioannidis JP, Aringer M, et al. EULAR recommendations for the management of systemic lupus erythematosus with neuropsychiatric manifestations: Report of a task force of the EULAR Standing Committee for Clinical Affairs. Ann Rheum Dis 2010;69:2074–2082.

Chamberlain MA, Bruckner FE. Rheumatoid neuropathy: Clinical and electrophysiological features. Ann Rheum Dis 1970;29(6):609–616.

Delalande S, de Seze J, Fauchais AL, et al. Neurologic manifestations in primary Sjogren syndrome: A study of 82 patients. Medicine 2004;83(5):280–291.

Gotkine M, Fellig Y, Abramsky O. Occurrence of CNS demyelinating disease in patients with myasthenia gravis (subsequent correspondence in Neurology 2007;68(16):1326–1327). Neurology 2006;67(5):881–883.

Hochberg MC. Updating the American College of Rheumatology revised criteria for the classification of systemic lupus erythematosus. *Arthritis Rheum* 1997;40(9):1725.

Johnson RT, Richardson EP. The neurological manifestations of systemic lupus erythematosus. *Medicine* 1968;47(4):337–369.

Krishnan AV, Halmagyi GM. Acute transverse myelitis in SLE. *Neurology* 2004;62 (11):2087.

Levine JS, Branch DW, Rauch J. The antiphospholipid syndrome. *N Engl J Med* 2002;346(10):752–763.

McLaurin EY, Holliday SL, Williams P, Brey RL. Predictors of cognitive dysfunction in patients with systemic lupus erythematosus. *Neurology* 2005;64(2):297–303.

Mitsikostas DD, Sfikakis PP, Goadsby PJ. A meta-analysis for headache in systemic lupus erythematosus: The evidence and the myth. *Brain* 2004;127(5):1200–1209.

Mori K, Iijima M, Koike H, *et al.* The wide spectrum of clinical manifestations in Sjögren's syndrome-associated neuropathy. *Brain* 2005;128(11):2518–2534.

Pittock SJ, Lennon VA, de Seze J, *et al.* Neuromyelitis optica and non organ-specific autoimmunity. *Arch Neurol* 2008;65:78–83.

Sofat N, Malik O, Higgens CS. Neurological involvement in patients with rheumatic disease. *QJM* 2006;99(2):69–79.

Tan EM, Cohen AS, Fries JF, *et al.* The 1982 revised criteria for the classification of systemic lupus erythematosus. *Arthritis Rheum* 1982;25(11):1271–1277.

26 Systemic sclerosis

Ho Jin Kim and Jae-Won Hyun

Department of Neurology, Research Institute and Hospital of National Cancer Center, Goyang, Korea

Systemic sclerosis (scleroderma, SSc) is an acquired systemic connective tissue disease characterized by fibrosis of the skin, blood vessels, and visceral organs, including the gastrointestinal tract, lungs, heart, and kidneys, due to the overproduction and accumulation of collagen.

The disorder is referred to as *localized scleroderma* (LSc) when confined to skin, and *systemic sclerosis* (SSc) when the visceral organs are involved. SSc is subdivided into two major forms according to the extent of skin affected. One subtype is *diffuse cutaneous scleroderma*, characterized by a symmetric widespread skin fibrosis affecting distal and proximal extremities and often including the trunk and face. This type of SSc tends to progress rapidly, with early involvement of the visceral organs. The other subtype is *limited cutaneous scleroderma*, characterized by symmetric, but restricted, skin fibrosis affecting distal extremities and face. This type frequently shows features of CREST syndrome (calcinosis, Raynaud's phenomenon, esophageal dysmotility, sclerodactyly, and telangiectasia).

Epidemiology

SSc has a worldwide distribution and affects all races. It affects all ages, but is uncommon in children. The incidence increases with age, peaking in the third to fifth decades. Women are affected about 3–4 times more often than men, and even more often during the childbearing years.

Pathophysiology

The prominent pathological manifestations of SSc are the overproduction and accumulation of collagen and other extracellular matrix proteins, microvascular damage, and inflammation. Arterioles, capillaries, and some small arteries undergo hyalinization with endothelial proliferation. Intimal and adventitial fibrosis results in end-organ hypoperfusion. Although the precise pathogenesis of SSc remains to be elucidated, presumably these pathological findings and their interactions can be regarded as the pathophysiological mechanisms of SSc. Environmental triggers and genetic predisposition interact to produce these features. The widespread pathological process in SSc leads to microvasculopathy and fibrosis, which can decrease the reserve function of many organs.

Clinical features

The initial symptoms of SSc are non-specific, and include Raynaud's phenomenon, fatigue, musculoskeletal complaints, and swelling of the hands. The characteristic skin thickening usually begins as swelling of the skin on the fingers and hands and is associated with tightness, deceased mobility, hyperpigmentation, and eventual atrophy and ulceration of the skin. Patients with systemic involvement frequently develop esophageal dysfunction, resulting in symptoms of dysphagia and reflux. Gastrointestinal involvement results in hypomotility and malabsorption, constipation, and episodic diarrhea. Interstitial fibrosis may cause restrictive pulmonary disease, and cardiac involvement can cause arrhythmia, pericarditis, myocarditis, and myocardial fibrosis with congestive heart failure. Renal failure may result from hypertension due to renal microvascular involvement.

Neurological involvement with SSc is uncommon when compared to other connective tissue diseases and is thought to be coincidental, iatrogenic, or secondary to the involvement of other organs such as the kidney or the gastrointestinal tract, rather than the result of the disease itself. Myopathy is the most common form of neurological problem seen in SSc, usually occurring within the first year or two of the disease. It is usually non-inflammatory and characterized by proximal muscle weakness, mild increase in the level of creatine kinase, and occasionally muscle atrophy. Electromyography may show polyphasic motor unit potentials in the absence of denervation. Muscle biopsy may show histiocyte infiltration and muscle fiber atrophy, but there is no evidence of true inflammatory myositis, nor is there atrophy of the outer portions of the muscle bundles that might suggest dermatomyositis. Although this type of muscle involvement usually tends to be mild, there are some patients who develop severe muscle weakness and atrophy. True inflammatory myositis (sclerodermatomyositis) resembling idiopathic polymyositis is an even less common muscle complication of SSc. Many of these patients have the risk of concurrent cardiac involvement, congestive heart failure, and sudden death.

Peripheral neuropathy has been regarded as uncommon in SSc. In retrospective studies, neuropathy was seen in only 1–2% of patients. However, prospective studies using electrodiagnostic methods revealed that 10–20% of SSc patients develop peripheral neuropathy during the course of their disease. The exact pathogenic mechanism is uncertain, but most neuropathies associated with SSc are thought to be ischemic in origin, resulting from either a chronic non-inflammatory vasculopathy or true vasculitis. Trigeminal sensory neuropathy represents the most common form of neuropathy seen in SSc, affecting 3–17% of patients. As in Sjögren's syndrome, this may be the result of inflammatory ganglionitis of the trigeminal sensory ganglia. Distal axonal polyneuropathy may develop and typically involves motor fibers. Ischemic infarction of different nerves may result in a painful mononeuropathy

International Neurology, Second edition. Edited by Robert P. Lisak, Daniel D. Truong, William M. Carroll and Roongroj Bhidayasiri
© 2016 John Wiley & Sons, Ltd. Published 2016 by John Wiley & Sons, Ltd.

multiplex. Unilateral or bilateral optic neuropathy has also been observed in SSc.

Central nervous system involvement is rare in SSc, possibly because of the paucity of connective tissue and the absence of an external elastic lamina with a sparse media and adventitia in the cerebral arteries. When it occurs, cerebral ischemia is usually associated with renal failure or hypertension. Other rare manifestations described include headache, seizures, depression, and anxiety disorder (Table 26.1). In addition, autonomic nervous system alteration involving cardiovascular and gastrointestinal organs is relatively common. Symptomatic orthostatic hypotension is observed in up to 9% of patients.

Table 26.1 Neurological involvement in systemic and localized scleroderma.

Systemic scleroderma		
Neuromuscular	**Central nervous system**	**Psychiatric**
Myopathy	Headache	Depression
Trigeminal neuropathy	Seizures	Anxiety
Peripheral sensorimotor polyneuropathy	Cognitive impairment	Dysthymia
Carpal tunnel syndrome	Stroke/transient ischemic attack	Suicidal ideation
Ulnar neuropathy Radiculopathy	Mental impairment	Psychoticism
Mononeuritis multiplex		Paranoid ideation
Facial neuropathy	Transverse myelitis	
Other mononeuropathy	Spinal cord compression	
Paraspinal and scapular myopathy	Visual disturbance	
Brachial plexopathy	Unspecific pyramidal signs	
Lumbar plexopathy	Hemiparesis	
8th neuropathy	Aphasia	
6th neuropathy	Subarachnoid hemorrhage	
9th neuropathy	Reversible posterior leukoencephalopathy	
12th neuropathy	Cerebellar ataxia	
Sensory neuropathy		
Chronic progressive ataxic neuropathy	Transient global amnesia	
	Optic atrophy	
	Cerebellar degeneration	
	Spontaneous intracranial hypotension	
Localized scleroderma		
Peripheral nervous system	**Central nervous system**	
Facial neuropathy	Seizures	
Trigeminal neuropathy	Headache	
3rd neuropathy	Hemiparesis/pyramidal signs	
6th neuropathy	Dizziness	
Peripheral neuropathy	Cognitive impairment	
	Vision involvement	
	Expressive aphasia	
	Dysarthria	
	Behavior disorders	

Neurological involvement with LSc was recently reported. Seizures and headache are predominant. Additionally, pyramidal signs and various cranial nerve involvements have rarely been documented.

Patients with SSc may have increased risk for cancer. Recent investigations have revealed a temporal clustering of cancer and subsets of patients with SSc with autoantibodies to RNA polymerase III subunit, but not with autoantibodies to topoisomerase 1 or centromere protein B.

Investigations

Antinuclear antibodies are present in almost all patients. Antinuclear antibodies that are highly specific for SSc are antitopoisomerase 1 (Scl-70), antinucleolar, and anticentromere. Anti-RNA polymerase 1 is found in patients with diffuse cutaneous SSc. Anti-PM-Scl, formerly referred to as anti-PM1, may be found in SSc patients with polymyositis, whereas anti-Jo-1 generally is not found in SSc patients with polymyositis, but is usually found in polymyositis patients with arthritis and alveolitis. Anti-U3 nucleolar ribonucleoprotein (RNP), different from anti-U1 RNP of mixed connective tissue disease, is also highly specific for SSc and is associated with SSc with skeletal muscle disease. SSc patients with anti-U1 RNP antibodies, and probably those with anti-Scl 70 antibodies, seem to be at higher risk of developing neurological complications.

Recent studies using MRI have found white-matter hyperintensities in areas of interface and SPECT studies have observed focal and diffuse cerebral hypoperfusion in more than 50% of asymptomatic SSc patients, suggesting involvement of small and perforating arteries.

The clinical picture of SSc is so distinctive that the diagnosis of SSc is not difficult with the presence of Raynaud's phenomenon, typical skin lesions, and visceral involvement.

Treatment

No curative therapy for SSc exists. Instead, treatments for SSc focus mainly on ameliorating the organ-specific consequences of SSc. Meticulous monitoring and treatment of the pulmonary, gastrointestinal, cardiac, and renal complications are crucial in the management of the disease. Acute myositis is usually responsive to glucocorticoids; these drugs should not be used in the indolent primary form of muscle disease of SSc, because steroids are risk factors for the development of sclerodema renal crisis.

Seizures, which often present in patients with LSc, are usually managed with antiepileptic drugs, with unpredictable response. In contrast, intractable seizures usually required immunosuppressive therapy, with positive results.

Further reading

Amaral TN, Peres FA, Lapa AT, *et al.* Neurologic involvement in scleroderma: A systematic review. *Semin Arthritis Rheum* 2013;43:335–347.

Averbuch-Heller L, Steiner I, Abramsky O. Neurologic manifestations of progressive systemic sclerosis. *Arch Neurol* 1992;49:1292–1295.

Carpentier PH, Maricq HR. Microvasculature in systemic sclerosis. *Rheum Dis Clin North Am* 1990;16:75–91.

Dessein PH, Joffe BI, Metz RM, *et al.* Autonomic dysfunction in systemic sclerosis: Sympathetic overactivity and instability. *Am J Med* 1992;93:143–150.

Harvey GR, McHugh NJ. Serologic abnormalities in systemic sclerosis. *Curr Opinion Rheumatol* 1999;11:490–494.

Hietaharju A, Jaaskelainen S, Kalimo H, Hietarinta M. Peripheral neuromuscular manifestations in systemic sclerosis (scleroderma). *Muscle Nerve* 1993;16:1204–1212.

Joseph CG, Darrah E, Shah AA, *et al.* Association of the autoimmune disease scleroderma with an immunologic response to cancer. *Science* 2014;343:152–157.

LeRoy EC, Black C, Fleischmajer R, *et al.* Scleroderma (systemic sclerosis): Classification, subsets and pathogenesis. *J Rheumatol* 1988;15:202–205.

Nadeau SE. Neurologic manifestations of connective tissue disease. *Neurol Clin* 2002;20:151–178.

Shah AA, Rosen A. Cancer and systemic sclerosis: Novel insights into pathogenesis and clinical implications. *Curr Opin Rheumatol* 2011;23:530–535.

West GS, Killian PJ, Lawless OJ. Association of myositis and myocarditis in progressive systemic sclerosis. *Arthritis Rheum* 1981;24:662–668.

27 Mixed connective tissue disease

Ho Jin Kim and Jae-Won Hyun
Department of Neurology, Research Institute and Hospital of National Cancer Center, Goyang, Korea

Mixed connective tissue disease (MCTD) is an overlap syndrome characterized by the combined features of systemic lupus erythematosus (SLE), systemic sclerosis (SSc), polymyositis (PM), and rheumatoid arthritis (RA), and is associated with high titers of antibody to the U1 nuclear ribonucleoprotein (U1-RNP) antigen. Since it was first described a few decades ago, the concept of MCTD has been highly controversial. Although the original view that it is a relatively benign disease (due to the good response to corticosteroid) was invalidated by subsequent long-term follow-up studies, MCTD remains a useful concept in clinical practice.

Epidemiology

MCTD has been reported in all races and the literature suggests no specific protection or propensity based on race. It affects mainly women in the second and third decades of life. It is estimated to attack women 8–15 times more frequently than it attacks men. Careful epidemiological studies have not been performed, but MCTD appears to be more prevalent than dermatomyositis (1–2 cases per 100,000 population), but less prevalent than SLE (15–50 cases per 100,000 population).

Pathophysiology

As with other immunopathologically mediated connective tissue diseases, the etiology of MCTD remains unknown. A prominent histopathological feature is a widespread proliferative vasculopathy characterized by intimal and medial proliferation, resulting in the narrowing of the lumen of small arteries and large vessels. These lesions may lead to visceral involvement, particularly pulmonary hypertension. Whether MCTD can be widely accepted as a distinct clinical entity awaits the demonstration of common pathogenic events underlying the development of U1-RNP antibodies and their associated clinical features.

Clinical features

As an overlap syndrome, MCTD lacks any unique clinical features. The most common clinical features include a high frequency of Raynaud's phenomenon, arthritis, swollen hands, sclerodactyly, esophageal dysfunction, pulmonary involvement, and polymyositis. Cardiac, cerebral, and renal involvement occur less frequently.

Raynaud's phenomenon affects most patients and is frequently the initial symptom. Sometimes it is severe and associated with digital ulceration, resulting in major morbidity.

Cutaneous features of MCTD include a swollen, sausage-like appearance of the fingers, non-scarring alopecia, lupus-like rashes, heliotrope eyelids, erythematous patches over the knuckles, and periungual telangiectasia. Systemic sclerosis-like changes may be present, but rarely become extensive.

Musculoskeletal abnormalities occur in most patients. Arthritis may resemble the features of RA, but rarely causes deformity. Polymyositis is frequent and may be severe. Rarely, a necrotizing myopathy is associated with MCTD with muscle necrosis and "pipe-stem" vessels.

Esophageal dysfunctions, seen in 80% of MCTD patients, include reduced upper and lower esophageal sphincter pressures and decreased amplitude of peristalsis in the distal two-thirds of the esophagus.

Pulmonary involvement occurs in 85% of patients and often is clinically silent until well advanced. Reduced diffusion capacity for carbon monoxide is the most frequent functional abnormality. Occasionally this is secondary to interstitial pulmonary fibrosis, but more commonly it is a primary consequence of the intimal proliferation of pulmonary arterioles. Pulmonary hypertension is the most frequently observed serious complication and the leading cause of disease-related death.

Nervous system involvement is uncommon. The neurological manifestations tend to be characteristic of the dominant connective tissue disease. Patients with symptoms of predominantly SLE present the approximate frequency of seizures, psychosis, and encephalopathy observed in pure SLE. Trigeminal neuropathy is the most common neurological disorder. It can be a presenting manifestation and occurs in 10–25% of patients with MCTD, observed more commonly in SSc, SLE, and Sjögren's syndrome. The clinical features of this neuropathy include facial numbness and paresthesia; frequent bilateral involvement with the usual sparing of motor fibers is identical to that seen in other connective tissue diseases. The neuropathy does not improve with corticosteroid treatment. Headaches, often with features of migraine, are also common. Aseptic meningitis and transverse myelitis have been reported, but other neurological complications are rare. There are a few reports of symmetric sensory polyneuropathy, acute autonomic neuropathy, carpal tunnel syndrome, and chronic polyradiculoneuropathy similar that seen in chronic inflammatory demyelinating polyneuropathy. The polyradiculoneuropathy responds to corticosteroid treatment, but the sensory polyneuropathy does not.

International Neurology, Second edition. Edited by Robert P. Lisak, Daniel D. Truong, William M. Carroll and Roongroj Bhidayasiri
© 2016 John Wiley & Sons, Ltd. Published 2016 by John Wiley & Sons, Ltd.

Investigations

Almost all patients have high titers of antinuclear antibody with a speckled pattern and very high titers of immunoglobulin G antibodies to U1-RNP. The high titers of circulating U1-RNP antibodies usually persist for years, but antibody levels may decline significantly or become undetectable in those patients with prolonged remission. Rheumatoid factor is found, often at very high titers, in half of patients. Less frequent findings include hypocomplementemia, leukopenia, anemia, and thrombocytopenia (mainly in children).

The diagnosis of MCTD is based on a combination of the typical overlapping clinical symptoms and high titers of circulating antibody to U1-RNP. MCTD usually develops slowly and is rarely obvious on initial evaluation, making it difficult to diagnose. However, MCTD is now being recognized in an earlier phase with minimal symptoms (e.g., Raynaud's phenomenon, arthralgia, myalgia, and swollen hands). In some patients, these mild symptoms may persist for years, but a prospective long-term study showed that the majority of patients with high titers of U1-RNP antibodies and limited clinical manifestations ultimately developed signs and symptoms consistent with MCTD.

Treatment

The therapeutic strategy for MCTD is not fundamentally different from that for the overlapping connective tissue diseases. Because of the lack of controlled studies to guide therapy and the heterogeneous clinical course of MCTD, therapy should be individualized depending on the specific organs involved and the severity of the underlying disease activity. Salicylates, other non-steroidal anti-inflammatory agents, hydroxychloroquine, vasodilators, and low doses of corticosteroids are used to treat mild forms of the disease. If the disease is severe or involves major organ systems, higher doses of corticosteroids (1 mg/kg per day of prednisone) and/or cytotoxic drugs are usually required. In general, the more advanced the disease is, the greater the organ damage and the less effective the treatment will be.

Further reading

Bennett RM, O'Connell DJ. Mixed connective tissue disease: A clinicopathologic study of 20 cases. *Semin Arthritis Rheum* 1980;10:25–51.

Burdt MA, Hoffman RW, Deutscher SL, *et al*. Long-term outcome in mixed connective tissue disease: Longitudinal clinical and serologic findings. *Arthritis Rheum* 1999;42:899–909.

Hagen NA, Stevens JC, Michet CJ. Trigeminal sensory neuropathy associated with connective tissue disease. *Neurology* 1988;38(Suppl1):210A

Klein Gunnewiek JMT, van de Putte LBA, van Venrooij WJ. The U1 snRNP complex: An autoantigen in connective tissue disease. An update. *Clin Exp Rheumatol* 1997;15:549–560.

Nadeau SE. Neurologic manifestations of connective tissue disease. *Neurol Clin* 2002;20:151–178.

Sharp GC, Irvin WS, Tan EM, Gould RG, Holman HR. Mixed connective tissue disease: An apparently distinct rheumatic disease syndrome associated with a specific antibody to an extractable nuclear antigen (ENA). *Am J Med* 1972;52:148–159.

Tani C, Carli L, Vagnani S, *et al*. The diagnosis and classification of mixed connective tissue disease. *J Autoimmun* 2014;48-49:46–49.

28 Behcet's syndrome and nervous system involvement

Ugur Uygunoglu, Sabahattin Saip, and Aksel Siva
Department of Neurology, Istanbul University Cerrahpasa School of Medicine, Istanbul, Turkey

Behçet's syndrome (BS), originally described in 1937 by the Turkish dermatologist Hulusi Behçet as a distinct disease with orogenital ulceration and uveitis known as the "triple-symptom complex," is an idiopathic chronic relapsing multisystem vascular-inflammatory disease of unknown origin. The disease affects many organs and systems, causing mucocutaneous lesions, eye inflammation, and musculoskeletal problems, and major vessels.

Epidemiology

The epidemiology of the disease shows geographic variation: it is seen more commonly along the ancient trade route of the Silk Road that extends from the Mediterranean region to Japan. Its prevalence has been reported to be less than 0.5/100,000 in the United States, between 0.5 and 1/100,000 in Northern and Central Europe, and up to 2.5/100,000 in the northwestern Mediterranean region; it increases further in the eastern Mediterranean region. Prevalence rates of up to 400/100,000 have been found in a population-based study in Turkey and rates of 10–20/100,000 have been reported in Japan, China, and Korea, countries at the other end of the Silk Road. The prevalence among Turkish immigrants living in Germany is lower (21–77/100,000) than that reported in Turkey, but is much higher than among the native German population (0.6/100,000), which may point to the greater significance of genetic compared with environmental factors in the etiology of the disease.

Pathophysiology

The etiology of BS is unknown, but clinical and laboratory data suggest that there is dysfunction of both innate and adaptive immune systems, resulting in an exaggerated response to viral or bacterial insults. It is still controversial whether this hyperreactivity is an autoimmune phenomenon or – as suggested by more recent data – an autoinflammatory phenomenon. The core histopathological phenomenon seems to be a vasculitic involvement in some cases and a low-grade, chronic, non-specific inflammation in others. The human leukocyte antigen (HLA) B51 allele, which is accepted as a genetic risk factor strongly associated with BS, shows 50–80% positivity among BS patients. However, it also shows 20–25% positivity in the general population living along the Silk Road, while in Northern Europe and the United States the prevalence of this allele is 2–8% in the general population and 15% among BS patients.

The cytokine profile (especially interleukin-6), lymphocyte subsets, immune complexes, complement levels, polyclonal activation of B lymphocytes, apoptotic mechanisms, neutrophil chemotactic functions, and aberrant immune responses against self-antigens including heat shock protein, oral mucosal antigens, retinal cells, endothelial cells, myelin, and cardiolipin have been found to be associated with BS; however, the significance of these findings is not clear and the findings vary among patient groups. In a recent study the mitochondrial carrier homolog 1 (Mtch1) autoantibody was found and suggested to be sensitive and specific for neuro-Behçet's syndrome (NBS) and BS.

Clinical features

Due to the lack of specific laboratory, radiological, or histological findings for BS, accurate diagnosis depends on clinical features. According to the International Study Group's classification criteria, a diagnosis of BS requires recurrent oral aphthous ulcerations plus two of the following: genital ulcerations, skin lesions, eye lesions, or a positive pathergy test.

Oral ulcers and other mucocutaneous symptoms

Oral ulcer is the major diagnostic criterion of BS and it must be present at least three times within a 12-month period. Oral ulcers, which may occur in up to 97% of cases, are the most sensitive and, together with genital ulcers, the most specific lesions seen in BS. Papulopustular skin lesions and erythema nodosum-like skin lesions are the other mucocutaneous symptoms of BS.

Ocular involvement

Ocular involvement is a common and serious component of BS. It consists of an acute panuveitis, usually associated with hypopyon. It tends to occur severely, especially in young males with BS, and is associated with significant morbidity.

The pathergy phenomenon

The pathergy phenomenon is a non-specific hypersensitivity reaction of hyperirritable skin seen in BS and is produced by inserting a 20-gauge needle into the dermis of the forearm. The reaction is considered positive if a papule or pustule forms at the site of the puncture within 48 hours. Its sensitivity varies between different ethnic and geographic groups, ranging between 20% and 80%. Minor diagnostic criteria of BS include arthritis or arthralgia, deep venous thromboses, subcutaneous thrombophlebitis, epididymitis, family history, and gastrointestinal, central nervous system (CNS), or vascular involvement.

International Neurology, Second edition. Edited by Robert P. Lisak, Daniel D. Truong, William M. Carroll and Roongroj Bhidayasiri
© 2016 John Wiley & Sons, Ltd. Published 2016 by John Wiley & Sons, Ltd.

Nervous system involvement: Neuro-Behçet's syndrome

Patients with BS may present with different neurological problems related either directly or indirectly to the disease that are suggestive of "neuro-Behçet's syndrome" (NBS; Table 28.1). NBS occurs in approximately 5–10% of all patients with BS. The age of onset of NBS, excluding pediatric cases, is usually later, around age 30 years, with the mean duration between the onset of BS and NBS being about 5 years. NBS is almost three times more frequent in males than in women.

The Cerrahpasa diagnostic criteria for NBS are: "the occurrence of neurological symptoms in a patient that fulfills the International Diagnostic Criteria for BS is not otherwise explained by any other known systemic or neurological disease or treatment, and in whom objective abnormalities consistent with NBS are detected either on neurological examination, neuroimaging studies (magnetic resonance imaging – MRI) and/or abnormal cerebrospinal fluid (CSF) examination." Recently the Cerrahpasa diagnostic criteria were slightly modified by the International Neuro-Behçet's Advisory Group and additional criteria for probable NBS were included too. However, neither of these criteria is validated.

Primary neurological involvement (neurological involvement directly related to BS)

Extra-axial NBS

The second most common form of neurological involvement is cerebral venous sinus thrombosis (CVST), which may be seen in 12–20% of patients with BS who have primary neurological involvement. However, in the pediatric age group with BS, when neurological involvement occurs it is an early event and mostly in the form of CVST and, rarely, as CNS-parenchymal (p-CNS) disease.

Clinical manifestations resulting from thrombosis of the intracranial venous system vary according to the site and rate of venous occlusion and its extent. Our observations suggest that CVST in BS evolves gradually, so that a fulminating syndrome with violent

Table 28.1 The neurological spectrum of Behçet syndrome. Source: Modified from Siva and Saip 2009.

Primary neurological involvement (neurological involvement directly related to BS)

- Cerebral venous sinus thrombosis (extra-axial NBS)
- Central nervous system involvement (intra-axial NBS)
- Arterial NBS
- Neuro-psycho-Behçet syndrome (NPBS)
- Isolated headache syndrome (migraine-like, non-structural)
- Peripheral nervous system involvement
- Subclinical NBS

Secondary neurological involvement (neurological involvement indirectly related to BS)

- Neurological complications secondary to systemic involvement of BS (i.e., cerebral emboli from cardiac complications of BS, increased intracranial pressure secondary to superior vena cava syndrome)
- Neurological complications related to BS treatments (i.e., CNS neurotoxicity with cyclosporine; peripheral neuropathy secondary to thalidomide or colchicine)
- Somatoform neurological symptoms associated with having a chronic disease

Coincidental – unrelated (non-BS) neurological involvement

- Primary headaches and any other coincidental neurological disorders

---

BS = Behçet syndrome; CNS = central nervous system; NBS = neuro-Behçet syndrome.

headache, convulsions, paralysis, and coma is uncommon. Papilledema and sixth nerve paresis are the most common clinical signs reported related to increased intracranial pressure. The superior sagittal sinus is commonly involved; however, a substantial number of these patients also have lateral sinus thrombosis. The extension of the clot into the cerebral veins causing focal venous hemorrhagic infarction is uncommon.

A close association has been reported between CVST and systemic major vessel disease in BS. When the neurological disease is in the form of CVST, it has a better neurological prognosis than the parenchymal type. However, considering the fact that patients with major vessel disease have a higher rate of morbidity and mortality, a diagnosis of CVST in a patient with BS may not always be associated with a favorable outcome.

The two types of intra- and extra-cranial NBS occur in the same individual very rarely, develop in different age groups, and are associated with different systemic manifestations of BS, therefore they presumably have a different pathogenesis.

Intra-axial NBS

The most common form of NBS is due to CNS parenchymal involvement (i.e., intra-axial NBS). The majority of patients (70–80%) with neurological involvement present with parenchymal CNS involvement. This form is due to small vessel disease involving mostly postcapillary venules. The brainstem and diencephalon are commonly affected (Figure 28.1 and 28.2). These patients present with a subacute (or rarely, acute) onset of severe headache, cranial neuropathies, dysarthria, ataxia, and hemiparesis. Cognitive-behavioral changes, emotional lability, a self-limited or progressive myelopathy with urinary sphincter dysfunction, and to a much lesser extent other CNS manifestations such as extrapyramidal signs and seizures have also been reported. There are also a few cases reported with cerebellar degeneration, isolated optic neuritis, or recurrent peripheral facial paresis. Isolated optic neuritis is extremely rare in BS, in which most visual symptoms are due to ocular involvement. Some NBS patients with CNS manifestations may experience a single episode, but most will have a relapsing–remitting course, with a subgroup developing progressive disease.

Arterial NBS

Arterial involvement in NBS is rare, consistent with systemic arterial involvement, which is also uncommon in BS. A limited number of case reports have been published with carotid artery occlusion, vertebral artery thrombosis, vertebral artery dissection, intracranial aneurysms, and intracranial arteritis, with their corresponding neurological consequences in BS. It is noteworthy that the arterial involvement affects mostly large arteries located at the extracerebral sites of the cranio-cervical arterial tree, suggesting that an extra-axial arterial pattern of NBS may exist, as well as an intra-axial arterial NBS pattern related to intracranial arteritis and intra-axial small arterial occlusions, similar to the venous involvement seen in NBS.

Neuro-psycho-Behçet's syndrome (NPBS)

Some patients with BS may develop a neurobehavioral syndrome, which consists of euphoria, loss of insight/disinhibition, indifference to their disease, and psychomotor agitation or retardation, with paranoid attitudes and obsessive concerns not associated with glucocorticosteroid or any other therapy. This is known as "neuro-psycho-Behçet's syndrome." This clinical presentation may occur in the setting of CNS parenchymal involvement, but it may also occur

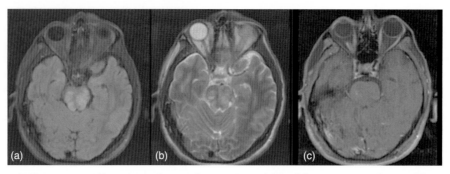

Figure 28.1 A–B: Axial FLAIR-T2 images reveal hyperintense lesion at the pons. C: Axial T1 gadolinium sequence shows gadolinium enhancement at pons.

in isolation without any other neurological manifestation and MRI or CSF changes.

Isolated headache syndrome

Headache is the most common neurological symptom occurring in 70% of BS patients and may be related to different causes, such as p-CNS disease, CVST, ocular inflammation, primary headaches (i.e., migraine, tension-type headache), and isolated headache syndrome, presenting as paroxysmal migraine-like pain occurring with exacerbation of BS systemic features. It may be explained by a vascular headache triggered by immune-mediated disease activity in susceptible individuals and may be seen in 5–15% of BS patients. It is not clear whether isolated headache syndrome is part of NBS or not.

Peripheral nervous system involvement

Peripheral nervous system (PNS) involvement with clinical manifestations is extremely rare in BS. Reported PNS involvement includes mononeuritis multiplex, a distal sensory motor neuropathy, an axonal sensory neuropathy, and myositis.

Subclinical NBS

The incidental finding of neurological signs in patients with BS without neurological symptoms was reported in some case series, with a minority of these patients developing mild neurological attacks later.

Secondary neurological involvement (neurological involvement indirectly related to BS)

Neurological complications secondary to systemic involvement of BS, such as increased intracranial pressure secondary to superior

vena cava syndrome and cerebral emboli secondary to cardiac involvement of BS, are some of the indirect neurological problems seen in BS. CNS neurotoxicity with cyclosporine and peripheral neuropathy secondary to thalidomide or colchicine use are neurological complications related to BS treatments.

Investigations for NBS

Neuroimaging

MRI is the gold standard neuroimaging tool for the diagnosis of NBS. Parenchymal lesions are generally located within the brainstem, occasionally extending to the diencephalon, and less often they are within the periventricular and subcortical white matter (Figures 28.1 and 28.2). The nature of the lesions in acute stages, and their resolution with the occurrence of silent lesions on follow-up studies, are a reflection of the inflammatory nature of CNS MRI lesions seen in NBS. There are also a number of reports of NBS cases in which MRI images have shown mass lesions that mimicked brain tumors, some necessitating histological diagnosis. The presence of brainstem atrophy, particularly in the midbrain tegmentum and pons, has also been reported and correlated with a progressive form of the disease. Heterogenous enhancement with gadolinium may be seen in acute parenchymal lesions. Chronic lesions tend to be iso-intense and smaller, and it is not uncommon to see brainstem atrophy and third ventricular enlargement on follow-up MRIs. The number of lesions detected with susceptibility-weighted imaging (SWI) is larger than with conventional T2*GE. Most of the lesions in intra-axial NBS were found to be hemorrhagic, supporting the proposed venous theory in pathology.

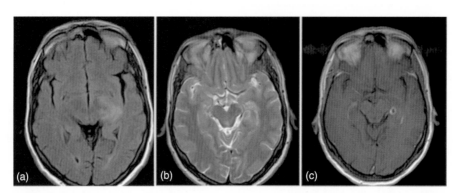

Figure 28.2 A–B: Axial FLAIR-T2 images reveal hyperintense lesion in the left meso-diencephalic region. C: Axial T1 gadolinium sequence shows ring-enhancing lesion in left side of mesencephalon.

Spinal cord involvement is not common, but can be seen. In reported cases, the major site of involvement was the cervical spinal cord, with the myelitis-like inflammatory lesions continuing for more than two segments, and extending to the brainstem in some. We have observed a number of NBS patients presenting with longitudinal extensive myelitis in whom NMO-IgG were negative. In NBS patients with CVST, the thrombosed dural sinuses are often visible on plain MRI and better on magnetic resonance venography (MRV); hemorrhagic venous infarcts are unlikely.

Cerebrospinal fluid

CSF pathology is found in 70–80% of patients with CNS involvement in NBS. An increased number of cells, up to 100 or more per ml, with modestly elevated protein levels is observed in most parenchymal cases. In the acute stage, the increased cells are likely to show a neutrophilic predominance; later, neutrophils decrease and lymphocytes become the prominent cell type. Oligoclonal bands are usually absent, not exceeding 15–20%. Elevated concentrations of IL-6 in the CSF of patients with both acute and chronic progressive NBS in relation to disease activity have also been reported. CSF in patients with CVST will be under increased pressure, but the cellular and chemical compositions are usually normal.

Differential diagnosis

Intra-axial NBS

The differential diagnosis of extra-axial BS includes other diseases in which CVST is seen and will not be listed here separately. The major differential diagnosis of NBS would cover intra-axial disease, as its heterogeneous presentations may cause confusion with many other CNS diseases (Table 28.2).

NBS is often included in the differential diagnosis of multiple sclerosis (MS) and in stroke in the young adult, especially in the absence of its known systemic symptoms and signs. Optic neuritis, sensory symptoms, and spinal cord involvement, which are common in MS, are rarely seen in NBS. MRI findings are clearly different with NBS: more discrete and smaller brainstem lesions are seen in MS, as well as more periventricular and ovoid lesions in the hemispheres. Spinal cord involvement rarely extends more than a few vertebral segments in MS, compared to the more extensive lesions that are reported in NBS, similar to neuromyelitis optica (NMO).

The CSF also reveals different patterns, with a more prominent pleocytosis and low rate of positivity for oligoclonal bands in CNS-NBS compared to MS. An acute stroke-like onset is uncommon in NBS, and MRI lesions compatible with classical arterial territories are also not expected. The absence of systemic symptoms and signs will serve to differentiate primary CNS vasculitis from NBS, and the difference in some of the systemic symptoms and signs, as well as the MRI findings and specific blood tests, will differentiate NBS from secondary CNS vasculitis.

Sarcoidosis can be confused with BS due to uveitis, arthritis, and CNS involvement, but the absence of oral and genital ulcers, and the presence of peripheral lymphadenopathy and bilateral hilar lymph nodes on chest X-ray, as well as pathological examination of the non-caseating granulomatous lesions of sarcoidosis, help in the differential diagnosis. Tuberculosis may resemble BS because of its multisystem involvement and its potential to affect the nervous system. Hilar lymphadenopathy and pulmonary cavities are not expected in BS, whereas its mucocutaneous manifestations are unusual for tuberculosis. Furthermore, CSF and MRI findings are different. Tumefactive lesions have been reported in NBS, but the imaging findings, the response to steroids, and the absence of systemic findings in primary CNS tumors helps to distinguish NBS from brain neoplasms. Due to their ophthalmological and other systemic manifestations, rare diseases such as Vogt–Koyanagi–Harada syndrome, Reiter syndrome, Eales' disease, Cogan's syndrome, and Susac's syndrome are other considerations in the differential diagnosis of BS. All may present with nervous system manifestations and therefore are included in the differential diagnosis of NBS. However, a complete ophthalmological examination by an ophthalmologist will reveal the true nature of eye involvement in each of these syndromes, which is different from the eye involvement seen in BS. Constipation, diarrhea, abdominal pain, and vomiting are common gastrointestinal symptoms, but their frequency varies in different geographic populations. These symptoms are seen relatively frequently in Japan, but not in Turkey and other Mediterranean countries. Due to their common occurrence, oral ulcers are considered separately from the remaining gastrointestinal tract, of which any part, especially the distal ileum and cecum, may also have ulcers. It can be difficult to distinguish inflammatory bowel disease from BS histologically. The rarity of rectal involvement and fistulas in BS can be helpful in differential diagnosis. Eye disease is rare and genital ulcers are absent from inflammatory bowel diseases. The diagnosis can be confirmed by intestinal biopsy. Whipple's disease with its gastrointestinal and various nervous system symptoms may also resemble BS.

Treatment of NBS

Intra-axial (parenchymal) NBS

There are no controlled trials for the management of vascular, gastrointestinal, and neurological involvement, and the task force commissioned by the European League Against Rheumatism (EULAR) concluded that properly designed controlled studies, both new and confirmatory, are needed to guide management of BS. Currently treatment strategies for NBS mostly depend on the clinical experience of neurologists.

High-dose intravenous methylprednisolone (IVMP) pulses for 5–10 days followed by a slow oral tapering is the first choice for treating acute disease or relapses in p-CNS. The dose and duration of steroid treatment can vary among different centers.

Colchicine, azathioprine, cyclosporine, cyclophosphamide, methotrexate, chlorambucil, thalidomide, interferon alfa, and anti-TNF agents are among the drugs used for the preventive treatment of the systemic features of BS, and have been tried for p-CNS disease as well

There is only one randomized controlled trial (RCT) related to the efficacy of azathioprine in BS, in which azathioprine was shown to be effective in decreasing inflammatory eye disease and preserving visual acuity. Azathioprine was shown to improve the long-term outcome of neurological involvement in a large uncontrolled series. Our current approach is to consider starting azathioprine at the first CNS attack, together with high-dose steroid treatment, maintaining with low-dose steroid therapy or on monthly pulses of IVMP for the first 6 months of treatment until the efficacy of azathioprine starts. There are also some reports indicating probable efficacy

Table 28.2   The differential diagnosis of intra-axial (CNS) neuro-Behçet's syndrome with its mimics, including multiple sclerosis.

	Neuro-Behçet syndrome (NBS)	Multiple sclerosis	Neurosarcoidosis	Tuberculosis	Primary angiitis of the central nervous system	Young stroke
Gender	M>F (3–4:1)	F>M (2–3:1)	F>M (1.2:1)	M >F (1.5:1)	M>F (2:1)	M=F
Age (common age range of disease onset), years	30–40	20–40	30–50	15–45	40–60	45
Systemic involvement	Mucocutaneous (oral, genital ulcers, skin lesions) > eye (uveitis) > musculoskeletal (arthralgias) > vascular > CNS > GIS	None	Lungs >lymphatic system> skin> liver> eyes > CNS	Lungs, bone, lymph nodes, GIS, genitourinary paranasal cavities, orbits, or mastoids; CNS	None	Depends on etiology
Probability of CNS involvement	5–10% of patients with BS	100%	5–10% of patients with sarcoidosis	1–5% of patients with tbc	100%	100%
Symptoms at onset						
Common	Headache; brainstem excluding INO; cerebellar; motor; neuropsychiatric symptoms including psychotic behavior	ON; sensory, spinal cord; brainstem including INO; motor; cerebellar symptoms	Facial nerve palsy; optic neuropathy; headache; seizures	Basal meningitis with cranial nerve palsies; headache; neck stiffness; encephalopathy; focal neurological deficit	Headache; cognitive impairment; focal/multifocal neurological deficits; encephalopathy	Acute hemiparesis or other stroke syndromes
Uncommon	ON; sensory; spinal cord; INO	Headache; motor cranial neuropathies; neuropsychiatric symptoms	Sensory; spinal cord, hemiparesis	ON; sensory; spinal cord	Cranial nerve palsies; seizures, ataxia	Neuropsychiatric symptoms, confusion, seizure
MRI						
PF	(+++) Brainstem – large, diffuse, with up/downward extension cerebellar – unlikely	(++) Small, discrete, without extension brainstem > Cblr	(+±)	(±)	(±)	(±)
Optic nerve inv.	(–)	(++)	(+)	(±)	(–)	(–)
Spinal cord	(±) Central, extends three or more segments LETM-like	(++) Peripheral, short segment	(±) Central, extends three or more segments	(±) Spinal cord rare, but arachnoiditis and involvement of vertebral bodies including spondylitis expected	(±) Rarely	(–) Unexpected
Diencephalic structures	(++±)	(+)	(+±)	(+±)	(±)	(±)
Meningeal involvement	(–)	(–)	(+) Involvement of VII & VIII nerves may be seen	(+)	(–)	(–)
PV, SC, JC	(±)	(+++)	(±)	(++)	(+++±)	> Arterial vascular territories
Involvement of vascular territories	(–)	(–)	(–)	(+)	(++) Not classic/anatomical	(+++)
Pattern of gadolinium enhancement	Central nodular or heterogeneous	Nodular, open ring, closed ring	Diffuse or nodular	Diffuse or nodular	Punctate, linear, leptomeningeal, or heterogeneous	Depends on infarct age/mostly cortical
CSF (acute phase)						
Cell count	From a few to hundreds, mostly neutrophilic pleocytosis	5	Mononuclear pleocytosis	Lymphocytic pleocytosis	Lymphocytic pleocytosis	
Protein	Elevated	Normal	Elevated	Elevated	Elevated	
Glucose	Normal	Normal	Hypoglycorrhachia	Hypoglycorrhachia	Normal	
OCB	15%	>90%	20%	–	Unknown	
Significant work-up studies to be conducted (other than CSF and MRI)	Pathergy test, HLA B51	Evoked potentials	ACE, serum and urinary calcium; thorax CT	ESR; tuberculin skin test, polymerase chain reaction (PCR), interferon- γ release assays, thorax CT	MRA/DSA	Hypercoagulable panel tests, hematological panel tests, MRA, duplex USG, TCD, TTE–TEE

ACE = angiotensin-converting enzyme; BS = Behçet's syndrome; Cblr = cerebellum; CNS = central nervous system; CSF = cerebrospinal fluid; DSA = digital subtraction angiography; ESR = erythrocyte sedimentation rate; F = female; GIS = gastrointestinal system; INO = internuclear ophtalmoplegia; JC = juxtacortical; M = male; MRA = magnetic resonance angiography; MRI = magnetic resonance imaging; OCB = oligoclonal bands; ON = optic neuritis; PV = periventricular; SC = subcortical; TCD = transcranial Doppler; TEE = transesophageal echocardiography; TTE = transthoracic echocardiography; USG = ultrasound for the long-term treatment of NBS with mycophenolate mofetil, etanercept, tocilizumab, interferon alpha, and a number of other agents. Cyclosporin is an effective treatment in BS patients who do have eye involvement. However, the higher risk of developing CNS disease under cyclosporin treatment should be kept in mind and should be avoided in patients with established NBS. A growing number of case reports in recent years that have suggested that anti-TNF-alpha agents may be an effective alternative in NBS have also suggested that infliximab may be somewhat effective in controlling relapses and progression in NBS if first-line immunotherapies fail. In our experience, infliximab alone or combined with immunosuppressive therapies could be useful in preventing disease progression and providing clinical improvement in NBS patients who become unresponsive to conventional immunosuppressive treatment, suggesting that infliximab might be a good alternative as a second-line therapy in severe NBS.

Recently anti-IL-6 receptor antibody, tocilizumab, was administered to two patients with NBS who were initially refractory to immunosuppressants and later to anti-TNF therapies. These patients were reported to show improvement both clinically and with inflammatory parameters.

Extra-axial (CVST) NBS

Venous thrombosis of BS is usually treated with either high-dose or medium-dose steroids, because it is accepted that the clot formation in the veins is caused by a low-grade endothelial inflammation rather than hypercoagulability. Nevertheless, anticoagulation is the primary treatment in systemic venous thrombosis and CVST of any etiology. In extra-axial NBS this approach remains controversial. As BS patients with CVST are more likely to have systemic large vessel disease, including pulmonary and peripheral aneurysms that carry a high risk of bleeding, the use of anticoagulation should be considered only after such possibilities have been ruled out.

Recurrences of CVST, although uncommon, are possible in BS, and as these patients are also at higher risk of developing other types of vascular involvement, long-term azathioprine is also recommended in some of these patients with CVST.

Prognosis

Due to the heterogeneity of neurological involvement in NBS, it is difficult to predict its course, prognosis, and response to treatment. Brainstem or spinal cord involvement, frequent relapses, early disease progression, high CSF pleocytosis, and HLA B51 positivity are the poor prognostic features for NBS according to the International Consensus Recommendation (ICR). Initiation with severe disability, primary or secondary progressive course, fever at onset, relapse during steroid tapering, meningeal signs, and bladder involvement may also be associated with poor outcome. Gender, accompanying systemic features, and age onset do not affect the prognosis of NBS.

Further reading

Al-Araji A, Kidd DP. Neuro-Behçet's disease: Epidemiology, clinical characteristics, and management. *Lancet Neurol* 2009;8(2):192–204.

International Study Group for Behçet's Disease. Criteria for diagnosis of Behçet's disease. *Lancet* 1990;335:1078–1080.

Kalra S, Silman A, Akman-Demir G, et al. Diagnosis and management of neuro-Behçet's disease: International consensus recommendations. *J Neurol* 2014;261(9): 1662–1676.

Koçer N, Islak C, Siva A, et al. CNS involvement in neuro-Behçet's syndrome: An MR study. *Am J Neuroradiol* 1999;20:1015–1024.

Saip S, Akman-Demir G, Siva A. Neuro-Behçet syndrome. *Handb Clin Neurol* 2014;121:1703–1723.

Siva A, Saip S. The spectrum of nervous system involvement in Behçet's syndrome and its differential diagnosis. *J Neurol* 2009;256:513–529.

Yazici Y, Yurdakul S, Yazici H. Behçet's syndrome. *Curr Rheumatol Rep* 2010;12: 429–435.

29 Sarcoidosis

Barney J. Stern

Department of Neurology, University of Maryland, Baltimore, MD, USA

Sarcoidosis is a systemic granulomatous inflammatory disease that commonly involves the lungs, lymph nodes, skin, and eyes. Neurological complications occur in approximately 5% of patients with sarcoidosis and can manifest in the central or peripheral nervous system in a variety of ways, some relatively common and characteristic and others quite rare. Thus, neurosarcoidosis is a diagnostic consideration in patients with known sarcoidosis who develop neurological symptoms and signs, and in patients without documented sarcoidosis who present with a spectrum of neurological findings consistent with neurosarcoidosis. Approximately 50% of patients with neurosarcoidosis present with neurological disease at the time sarcoidosis is first diagnosed.

Epidemiology

The prevalence of sarcoidosis is approximately 40 per 100,000 population, although in certain groups the incidence and prevalence can be substantially greater. Sarcoidosis occurs throughout the world and can develop in any racial/ethnic population. Certain areas of the world, such as Sweden, also seem to have a higher incidence of sarcoidosis, whereas it appears to be quite rare in other areas, such as China or Southeast Asia. It most commonly presents in persons in their 20s or 30s, although individuals of any age can be afflicted. Women are affected more often than men. A study of familial risk for sarcoidosis among siblings revealed an odds ratio of 5.8 (95% confidence interval 2.1–15.9), and in a familial multivariate model the adjusted familial relative risk was 4.7 (95% confidence interval 2.3–9.7), indicating that a family history of sarcoidosis is associated with a five- to sixfold greater risk of developing the condition compared to someone without a family history. Reports on the proportion of patients with sarcoidosis who develop neurosarcoidosis range as high as 14%.

Pathophysiology

Non-necrotizing granulomas, the key pathological finding of sarcoidosis, are composed of epithelioid macrophages, lymphocytes, monocytes, and fibroblasts. The inflammation is often perivascular and there can be involvement in the outer aspect of the vascular media and adventitia. With time, fibrosis can develop along with thickening of the intima and media of blood vessels, leading to ischemic injury.

The pathophysiology of sarcoidosis is characterized by an enhanced Th1 immune response, possibly genetically determined, to a circumscribed number of microbial agents. This results in an enhanced production of interferons β and γ and select interleukins. Cytokines, such as tumor necrosis factor alpha, are expressed. With time, a Th2 response can develop and lead to fibrosis. The antigen inciting the inflammatory response remains unknown, although *Mycobacterium* species are implicated. Annexin A11 gene polymorphisms have been associated with an increased disease risk.

Clinical features

The neurological manifestations of sarcoidosis and their approximate frequencies are cranial neuropathies (overall 50–75%; facial palsy 25–50%); meningeal disease including aseptic meningitis and mass lesion (10–20%); hydrocephalus (10%); parenchymal disease (overall 50%), including endocrinopathy (10–15%), mass lesion(s) (5–10%), encephalopathy/vasculopathy (5–10%), seizures (5–10%), vegetative dysfunction (<5%), extramedullary or intramedullary spinal canal disease (<5%), and cauda equina syndrome (very rare); neuropathy (15%), including axonal, mononeuropathy, mononeuropathy multiplex, sensorimotor, sensory, motor, demyelinating, and Guillain–Barré syndrome; and myopathy (15%), including nodule(s), polymyositis, and atrophy.

Sarcoidosis-associated small fiber neuropathy is an increasingly recognized condition. Patients complain of pain and paresthesias in a stocking-glove distribution as well as symptoms involving the face and torso. Associated autonomic manifestations include orthostatic hypotension, gastrointestinal dysmotility, sweating abnormalities, erectile dysfunction, and so on. Symptoms may be quite severe and resistant to conventional treatments for sarcoidosis. The pathogenesis of small fiber neuropathy is thought to be systemic cytokine mediated (especially tumor necrosis factor α) rather than a consequence of local granulomatous inflammation. Therefore, small fiber neuropathy is not a manifestation of neurosarcoidosis in the classic sense, it is rather a "para-neurosarcoidosis" phenomenon.

On rare occasions, stroke syndromes can occur, either from direct inflammation of the intracranial vasculature or secondary to emboli from sarcoidosis-associated cardiomyopathy or arrhythmia. Many of the diverse presentations of neurosarcoidosis can be placed within one of these broad categories.

Headache can be associated with meningeal inflammation (infectious or sterile), hydrocephalus, mass lesion(s), and trigeminal neuropathy.

Neurosarcoidosis can be classified as possible, probable, or definite based on the certainty of the diagnosis of multisystem sarcoidosis, the pattern of neurological disease, and the response to therapy. The following criteria for each classification are adapted

International Neurology, Second edition. Edited by Robert P. Lisak, Daniel D. Truong, William M. Carroll and Roongroj Bhidayasiri
© 2016 John Wiley & Sons, Ltd. Published 2016 by John Wiley & Sons, Ltd.

from Zajicek et al. In *possible* neurosarcoidosis, the clinical syndrome and neurodiagnostic evaluation are suggestive, but infection and malignancy have not been rigorously excluded or there is no pathological confirmation of systemic sarcoidosis. In *probable* neurosarcoidosis, the clinical syndrome and neurodiagnostic evaluation are suggestive and alternative diagnoses, especially infection and malignancy, have been excluded. There is pathological evidence of systemic sarcoidosis. In *definite* neurosarcoidosis, either (1) the clinical presentation is suggestive of neurosarcoidosis, other possible diagnoses are excluded, and there is the presence of supportive nervous system pathology; or (2) the criteria for a "probable" diagnosis are met and the patient has had a beneficial response to therapy for neurosarcoidosis over a 1-year observation period.

Investigations

Patients with known systemic sarcoidosis who develop neurological disease consistent with sarcoidosis should be evaluated for the reasonable exclusion of other disease entities, particularly infection and neoplasia. If the patient does not respond to treatment as expected, the diagnosis should be questioned and a more extensive evaluation pursued.

If a patient without known sarcoidosis develops a clinical syndrome consistent with neurosarcoidosis, the diagnostic challenge can be considerable. Since corticosteroid therapy can mask signs of systemic sarcoidosis or other diseases, treatment should be postponed, if possible, while a search for systemic disease is initiated.

Sarcoidosis most frequently affects intrathoracic structures, followed by lymph node, skin, and ocular disease. If the patient has impaired smell or taste, nasal or olfactory nerve disease might be present. If dry eyes or mouth are noted, lacrimal, parotid, or salivary gland inflammation is possible. Other clues to the presence of systemic sarcoidosis include elevated serum angiotensin-converting enzyme (ACE) activity, hypercalcemia, hypercalciuria, elevated immunoglobulins, and anergy. Patients with possible central nervous system (CNS) disease should be questioned about symptoms relating to neuroendocrinological or hypothalamic dysfunction.

Systemic sarcoidosis can often be demonstrated if a comprehensive, but selective, approach is followed: chest X-ray, thoracic CT scan, pulmonary function tests including diffusing capacity, ophthalmological examination, endoscopic nasal examination, whole-body gallium scan, muscle magnetic resonance imaging (MRI), and fluorodeoxyglucose positron emission tomography imaging.

The preferred imaging technique to evaluate CNS sarcoidosis is MRI without and with contrast enhancement. T1-weighted images depict hydrocephalus, the optic nerves and chiasm, and spinal cord enlargement (Figures 29.1 and 29.2). With T2-weighted and fluid-attenuated inversion-recovery (FLAIR) imaging, areas of increased signal intensity are visualized, especially in a periventricular distribution. Contrast administration can demonstrate leptomeningeal enhancement as well as parenchymal abnormalities and, occasionally, cranial nerve lesions. Spinal MRI can visualize intramedullary disease, which appears as an enhancing fusiform enlargement, focal or diffuse enhancement, or atrophy. Enhancing nodules or thickened or matted nerve roots can be noted with cauda equine imaging.

The cerebrospinal fluid (CSF) pressure can be elevated and analysis can reveal an increased total protein, hypoglycorrhachia, and a predominantly mononuclear pleocytosis. The immunoglobin G (IgG) index can be elevated and oligoclonal bands detected. CSF

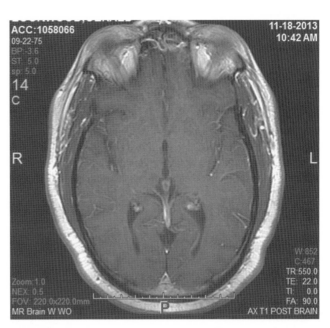

Figure 29.1 A T1-weighted, gadolinium-enhanced brain MRI of a patient with sarcoidosis-associated encephalopathy/vasculopathy demonstrating subtle enhancement in the basal ganglia and frontal lobes.

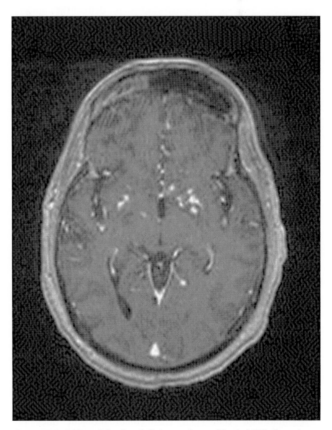

Figure 29.2 A T1-weighted, gadolinium-enhanced brain MRI of a patient with CNS sarcoidosis demonstrating enhancement in the basal ganglia and scattered nodular enhancement of the leptomeninges.

ACE activity can be elevated in patients with CNS sarcoidosis, although abnormalities are also seen in the presence of infection and malignancy. A normal CSF ACE assay does not exclude the diagnosis of neurosarcoidosis.

Nerve conduction studies can be of assistance in evaluating a neuropathy. However, there is nothing specific about the spectrum of findings to suggest the diagnosis of sarcoidosis. Electromyography can demonstrate denervation in appropriate muscles and myopathic changes. Peripheral nerve and muscle samples can be obtained for pathological examination. A skin biopsy for quantitative epidermal nerve fiber analysis, along with quantitative sensory and autonomic testing and confocal corneal microscopy, can document a small fiber neuropathy in patients with neuropathic symptoms and otherwise unrevealing nerve conduction and electromyographic studies.

Differential diagnostic considerations include multiple sclerosis, Sjögren's syndrome, systemic lupus erythematosus, neurosyphilis, neuroborreliosis, human immunodeficiency virus (HIV) infection, Behçet's syndrome, Vogt–Koyanagi–Harada disease, toxoplasmosis, brucellosis, Whipple's disease, lymphoma, germ cell tumors, craniopharyngioma, isolated angiitis of the CNS, primary CNS neoplasia, lymphocytic hypophysitis, pachymeningitis (including IgG4-related disease), cytomegalovirus (CMV) meningoencephalitis, Rosai–Dorfman disease, and low CSF pressure/volume meningeal enhancement.

Treatment

There have been no rigorous studies to define the optimal treatment for neurosarcoidosis. Most authorities recommend corticosteroid therapy as first-line therapy for patients, if there are no contraindications. Increasingly, adjunct therapy with other immunosuppressive and immunomodulatory agents is being utilized. Therapeutic decisions should be guided by the patient's clinical course, the expected natural history of the patient's clinical manifestations, and adverse treatment effects.

Two-thirds of patients have a monophasic neurological illness; the remainder have a chronically progressive or remitting–relapsing course. Patients with a monophasic illness typically have an isolated cranial neuropathy, most often involving the facial nerve, or an episode of aseptic meningitis. Patients with a chronic course usually have CNS disease (parenchymal abnormalities, hydrocephalus, and multiple cranial neuropathies, especially cranial nerves II and VIII), peripheral neuropathy, and myopathy.

A goal of treatment is to diminish the irreversible fibrosis that can develop as well as the tissue ischemia that might result from perivascular inflammation. With time, the inflammatory process can become quiescent, allowing therapy to be decreased, at least temporarily. A peripheral facial nerve palsy usually responds to 2–4 weeks of prednisone therapy. The first week's prednisone dose is 0.5–1.0 mg/kg/day (or 40–60 mg/day), followed by a taper over the following weeks. This approach can also be used as initial therapy for other cranial neuropathies and aseptic meningitis. Patients with a peripheral neuropathy or myopathy can also respond to a short course of corticosteroid therapy; however, prolonged treatment is often necessary.

Asymptomatic ventricular enlargement probably does not require treatment. Mild, symptomatic hydrocephalus can respond to corticosteroid therapy, although prolonged treatment is often required. Life-threatening hydrocephalus or corticosteroid-resistant hydrocephalus requires ventricular shunting. Unfortunately, patients can rapidly evolve from mild hydrocephalus to severe life-threatening disease. Patients and caregivers should be educated as to when to seek emergency care. Shunt placement is not without risk in these patients, which is why "prophylactic" shunting is discouraged. Shunt obstruction from the inflamed CSF and ependyma is common, and placement of a foreign object in the CNS of an immunosuppressed host predisposes to infection.

Corticosteroid therapy can improve the status of patients with a diffuse encephalopathy/vasculopathy or a CNS mass lesion. Seizures occur most commonly in patients with parenchymal disease or hydrocephalus. Control of seizures is usually not difficult if the underlying inflammatory process can be controlled. Corticosteroid treatment for CNS parenchymal disease and other severe neurological manifestations of sarcoidosis usually starts with prednisone 1.0 mg/kg/day. These patients often require prolonged therapy and prednisone should be tapered slowly. The patient might be observed on high-dose prednisone for 2–4 weeks to determine the clinical response. The prednisone dose can then be tapered by 5 mg decrements every 2 weeks as the clinical course is monitored. The disease tends to exacerbate at a prednisone dose approximating 10 mg/day (or 0.1 mg/kg/day). If a low dose of prednisone can be achieved, the patient should be evaluated for evidence of subclinical worsening prior to further tapering by decrements of 1 mg every 2–4 weeks. Patients may require multiple cycles of higher and lower corticosteroid doses. This effort is usually warranted, since the disease can become quiescent and, without attempts at withdrawing medication, patients may be needlessly exposed to long-term side effects of corticosteroids.

A short course of methylprednisolone 20 mg/kg/day intravenously for 3 days, followed by high-dose prednisone for 2–4 weeks, is occasionally warranted for patients with severe acute neurological compromise. Another approach to treating severe disease is the use of infliximab, a monoclonal antibody directed at tumor necrosis factor α.

Alternative or adjunct therapies are increasingly being considered for neurosarcoidosis. Experience in this area is limited and firm recommendations are not available. Indications for the use of alternative treatments include the need to avoid corticosteroids as initial therapy, serious adverse corticosteroid effects, disease activity in spite of aggressive corticosteroid therapy, and an anticipated need for long-term corticosteroid therapy based on the natural history of the patient's disease manifestations.

Immunosuppressive medications to treat sarcoidosis include mycophenolate mofetil, azathioprine, methotrexate, cyclophosphamide, cyclosporine, chlorambucil, and cladribine. Anecdotal experience suggests that these drugs, especially when used in combination with relatively low-dose corticosteroid therapy, can be effective. Patients can incrementally improve beyond that experienced with corticosteroid monotherapy, or the corticosteroid dose can be decreased with the addition of an adjunct therapy. Rarely is it possible to withdraw corticosteroid treatment completely; patients tend to do best on a modest dose of corticosteroid combined with an alternative agent.

Immunomodulatory agents can also be used to treat sarcoidosis and neurosarcoidosis. These agents can be used in conjunction with corticosteroids or corticosteroids and immunosuppressive agents. Hydroxychloroquine, pentoxifylline, thalidomide, minocycline, rituximab, intravenous immunoglobulin (for small fiber neuropathy), infliximab, and adalimumab are reported in case reports and case series to be beneficial. Refractory patients may benefit from combination treatment with a low-dose corticosteroid, an immunosuppressive drug such as mycophenolate mofetil, and infliximab. If a patient with CNS disease fails or cannot tolerate alternative agents, consideration should be given to radiotherapy. Patients may stabilize, although corticosteroids and alternative agents often need to be continued. Patients with small fiber neuropathy can be responsive to tumor necrosis factor α antagonists or intravenous immunoglobulin.

Patients require close attention to their general medical condition. Adverse effects should be managed or treated. Prescribed exercise and dietary programs are often beneficial. Rehabilitation services should be utilized as appropriate. Depression is common and treatable. Hypothyroidism and hypogonadism should be treated. Since patients are often on protracted, low-dose corticosteroid regimens, supplemental corticosteroids are appropriate during surgery or intercurrent illness. Treatment of osteoporosis is often a challenge, since sarcoidosis itself can cause hypercalcemia and hypercalciuria; appropriate consultation is suggested.

Fatigue can be due to a variety of conditions including exercise intolerance, depression, obesity, hypothyroidism, hypogonadism, corticosteroid myopathy, occult neuromuscular disease, sleep apnea, and primary hypersomnia. "Idiopathic" fatigue can be responsive to modafinil or armodafinil therapy. Fatigue may be associated with a sarcoidosis-associated "brain fog"; the cause of both symptoms is unknown, but may be associated with systemic cytokine level elevation.

Further reading

Baughman RP. Therapeutic options for sarcoidosis: New and old. *Curr Opin Pulm Med* 2002;8:464–469.

Hoitsma E, Faber CG, van Santen-Hoeufft M, *et al*. Improvement of small fiber neuropathy in a sarcoidosis patient after treatment with infliximab. *Sarcoidosis Vasc Diffuse Lung Dis* 2006;23:73–77.

Iannuzzi MC, Rybicki BA, Teirstein AS. Sarcoidosis. *N Engl J Med* 2007;357:2153–2165.

Langrand C, Bihan H, Raverot G, *et al*. Hypothalamo-pituitary sarcoidosis: A multicenter study of 24 patients. *QJM* 2012;105:981–995.

Moravan M, Segal BM. Treatment of CNS sarcoidosis with infliximab and mycophenolate mofetil. *Neurology* 2009;72:337–340.

Parambil JG, Tavee JO, Zhou L, *et al*. Efficacy of intravenous immunoglobulin for small fiber neuropathy associated with sarcoidosis. *Respir Med* 2011;105:101–105.

Pritchard C, Nadarajah K. Tumour necrosis factor (alpha) inhibitor treatment for sarcoidosis refractory to conventional treatments: A report of five patients. *Ann Rheum Dis* 2004;63:318–320.

Scott TF, Yandora K, Valeri A, *et al*. Aggressive therapy for neurosarcoidosis: Long-term follow-up of 48 treated patients. *Arch Neurol* 2007;64:691–696.

Stern BJ, Krumholz A, Johns C, *et al*. Sarcoidosis and its neurological manifestations. *Arch Neurol* 1985;42:909–917.

Zajicek JP, Scolding NJ, Foster O, *et al*. Central nervous system sarcoidosis – diagnosis and management. *QJM* 1999;92:103–117.

30 Autoimmune encephalitis with neuronal cell surface antibodies

Josep Dalmau[1] and Myrna R. Rosenfeld[2]

[1] Institució Catalana de Recerca i Estudis Avançats (ICREA) at Institut d'Investigació Biomèdica August Pi i Sunyer (IDIBAPS), University of Barcelona, Barcelona, Spain

[2] Hospital Clínic/IDIBAPS, University of Barcelona, Barcelona, Spain

The autoimmune encephalitis syndromes associated with antibodies to neuronal cell surfaces or synaptic proteins (henceforth referred to as AE with neuronal Abs) are an increasingly recognized cause of complex neuropsychiatric disturbances. In some of these disorders the associated antibodies interfere with the function of the target neuronal/synaptic antigens producing the clinical phenotype. The pathogenicity of the associated antibodies was initially suggested by the similarity of the clinical syndromes to genetic or pharmacological models that resulted in disruption of antigen function, and has since been demonstrated using *in vitro* and *in vivo* models. As in other autoimmune encephalitis, such as postinfectious and paraneoplastic encephalitis, in which an antecedent infection (usually viral) or an underlying tumor is the trigger of the autoimmune response, in AE with neuronal Abs similar triggers appear to be involved in some but not all cases. While largely responsive to antibody-depleting treatments and immunotherapies, not all patients have full recovery and some will have substantial residual deficits. The recent identification of the encephalitis associated with antibodies to IgLON5 that is chronically progressive and associated with pathological signs of tauopathy suggests that the full spectrum of these disorders is evolving.

Antibodies and ancillary tests

The diagnosis of AE with neuronal Abs can be, in many cases, suspected by recognition of the clinical syndrome in an age-appropriate patient, coupled with ancillary tests supporting an inflammatory/immune etiology (Table 30.1). The diagnosis is confirmed by the presence of the associated antibodies in the cerebrospinal fluid (CSF) and serum. It is recommended that all initial evaluations include CSF. A recent study of matched serum and CSF samples from patients with anti-NMDA receptor encephalitis showed that regardless of testing method 100% of the CSF samples were positive, but 13% of the matched serum samples were negative with some testing methods. Ancillary studies can assist in formulating an initial differential diagnosis, but findings are not specific among the different AE with neuronal Abs. The CSF often shows lymphocytic pleocytosis, at times with increased proteins or oligoclonal bands, but it can also be normal. Neuroimaging can be normal or show abnormalities on magnetic resonance imaging (MRI) fluid inversion recovery (FLAIR) and T2 sequences, mostly involving limbic structures. An exception is encephalitis with $GABA_A$ receptor antibodies, in which

Table 30.1 Autoimmune encephalitis syndromes with neuronal cell surface or synaptic antibodies.

Antibody target	Neurological syndrome
NMDA receptor	Characteristic, multistage syndrome with acute onset psychiatric symptoms, seizures, memory deficits, decreased level of consciousness, dyskinesias. Autonomic disturbances leading to central hypoventilation. Partial syndromes can occur. Predominantly affects young women, teenagers and children. Age-related association with ovarian teratoma: present in 45% of all women, but less than 6% in girls younger than 12 years. Almost 80% of cases have full or substantial recovery that can occur slowly over 18–24 months; relapses occur in about 25% (12% within 2 years after initial episode). The associated anti-NMDA receptor antibodies are IgG subtype and target the GluN1 subunit of the NMDA receptor. Anti-NMDA receptor IgM and IgA antibodies or antibodies that target other NMDAR subunits such as the GluN2 are unrelated to anti-NMDA receptor encephalitis and to date have no disease-specific associations.
$GABA_B$ receptor	Limbic encephalitis with prominent and early seizures affecting both men and women. About 50% of patients have an associated cancer, mostly SCLC or other neuroendocrine tumor. Patients with SCLC are older (median age 67 years) than those without (39 years). Almost 75% have full or partial recovery.
AMPA receptor	Subacute onset of limbic encephalitis or rapidly progressive abnormal behavior resembling psychosis progressing to encephalopathy with seizures, dyskinesias, autonomic dysfunction. Frequently affects middle-aged women, and 70% have cancer (breast, thymus, lung). About 70% improve with therapy, but neurological relapses without tumor recurrence are frequent. Relapses lead to cumulative disability.
LGI1	Limbic encephalitis often with hyponatremia, temporal lobe seizures, and less often REM sleep disorder. Brief tonic or myoclonic-like seizures may precede the memory symptoms. Usually affects older men (median age 60 years) and <10% of cases have an associated tumor (usually thymoma). Almost 80% have substantial recovery. Rarely occurs with signs of peripheral nerve hyperexcitability (Morvan's syndrome).
CASPR2	Encephalopathy with seizures and autonomic dysfunction in combination with peripheral nerve hyperexcitability (Morvan's syndrome), and frequent neuropathic pain. The tumor association varies among series; patients with Morvan's often have thymoma. About 70% have full or substantial recovery.

International Neurology, Second edition. Edited by Robert P. Lisak, Daniel D. Truong, William M. Carroll and Roongroj Bhidayasiri.

Antibody target	Neurological syndrome
GABA$_A$ receptor	Rapidly progressive, severe encephalopathy with refractory seizures, status epilepticus, or epilepsia partialis continua. Patients of all ages (reported cases ranged from 3–63 years with median of 22). Extensive MRI FLAIR/T2 cortical–subcortical abnormalities. No cancer association. About 50% have good response to immunotherapy, but have morbidity and mortality from medical complications associated with prolonged seizures.
DPPX	Encephalopathy with agitation, paranoia, tremor, myoclonus, and seizures. Rarely cerebellar signs or hyperekplexia. Neurological symptoms usually preceded by severe diarrhea. Patients have a protracted course with relapses, but many will have partial improvement with immunotherapy.
IgLON5	Chronic or rapidly progressive REM and non-REM sleep disorder with abnormal sleep movements and obstructive sleep apnea. Median age 59 years. No cancer association. Largely unresponsive to immunotherapy and patients usually experience sudden death, likely due to breathing/autonomic dysfunction.
mGluR5 receptor	Encephalopathy with memory loss, depression, hallucinations, bizarre behavior, seizures in association with and often preceding Hodgkin's lymphoma (Ophelia syndrome). Responsive to immunotherapy; one patient responded to treatment of the Hodgkin's lymphoma without immunotherapy.
Glycine receptor	Have been found in association with progressive encephalomyelitis with rigidity and myoclonus, but also with SPS, epilepsy, cerebellar ataxia, inflammatory optic neuropathy, and overlapping with other AE with neuronal Abs.
mGluR1 receptor	Idiopathic or paraneoplastic cerebellar ataxia (Hodgkin's lymphoma). Some patients with or without tumor responded to immunotherapy.
Dopamine-2 receptor	Recently described in the serum of some patients with basal ganglia encephalitis, Sydenham chorea, and Tourette's syndrome.

AMPA = alpha-amino-3-hydroxy-5-methyl-4-isoxazolepropionic acid receptor; Caspr2 = contactin-associated protein-like 2; DPPX = dipeptidyl-peptidase-like protein-6; FLAIR = fluid-attenuated inversion recovery; GABA$_A$ = gamma-aminobutyric acid-A receptor; GABA$_B$ = gamma-aminobutyric acid-B receptor; LGI1 = leucine-rich glioma-inactivated protein-1; mGluR1 = metabotropic glutamate receptor 1; mGluR5 = metabotropic glutamate receptor 5; NMDA = N-methyl-D-aspartate receptor; REM = rapid eye movement; SCLC = small cell lung cancer ; SPS = stiff-person syndrome

patients often have extensive abnormalities on MRI FLAIR and T2 imaging, with multifocal or diffuse cortical–subcortical involvement without contrast enhancement.

In anti-NMDA receptor encephalitis, EEG with video monitoring is very useful to distinguish seizures from non-epileptic complexes, and repetitive orofacial and limb movements. In about 30% of patients with anti-NMDA receptor encephalitis, the EEG has a characteristic pattern that has not been described in other disorders. The pattern, called extreme delta brush, shows rhythmic delta activity at 1–3 Hz and superimposed bursts of rhythmic 20–30 Hz beta activity riding on each delta wave. A few patients with encephalitis and LGI1 antibodies develop brief myoclonic-like or tonic seizures (called also faciobrachial-dystonic seizures). These seizures may occur during the encephalitis or may precede it, and there is some evidence that prompt recognition and treatment may prevent development of memory and cognitive dysfunction.

Clinical spectrum

AE with neuronal Abs affect patients of all ages, although anti-NMDA receptor encephalitis predominantly affects younger adults and children. As noted in Table 30.1, there is a variable association of AE with neuronal Abs and cancer. Anti-NMDA receptor encephalitis is a highly characteristic multistage syndrome, often with a prominent psychiatric component. Many patients or families report a prodromal viral-like illness. Patients with antibodies to AMPA and GABA$_B$ receptors and LGI1 often present with a clinical picture consistent with classic limbic encephalitis. These disorders are distinguished from each other by the presence of prominent psychiatric symptoms and the frequent presence of an associated cancer in anti-AMPA receptor encephalitis, prominent and early seizures with anti-GABA$_B$ receptor antibodies, and the frequent presence of hyponatremia in anti-LGI1 encephalitis.

Patients with antibodies to GABA$_A$ receptors develop a rapidly progressive, severe encephalopathy with refractory seizures, including status epilepticus and epilepsia partialis continua, often preceded by alterations in behavior or cognition. Patients with encephalitis and DPPX antibodies develop a syndrome of CNS hyperexcitability, often with diarrhea. The co-occurrence of limbic encephalitis and peripheral nervous system hyperexcitability (Morvan's syndrome) should raise suspicion for the presence of anti-CASPR2 antibodies, although these antibodies may be associated with isolated central or peripheral syndromes.

In a patient who is recovering or has recovered from AE with neuronal Abs, the possibility of relapse should be kept in mind when evaluating new-onset symptoms. Relapses are well described in anti-NMDA receptor, AMPA receptor, and LGI1 encephalitis and likely occur in the other disorders, although current case series are too small to make any firm conclusions. New-onset memory and behavior disorder in a young adult may be the first symptom of the encephalitis that often predates the diagnosis of an underlying Hodgkin's lymphoma. The combination of the encephalitis and Hodgkin's lymphoma is known as Ophelia syndrome, and is associated with antibodies to the metabotropic glutamate 5 receptor (mGluR5).

Differential diagnoses

The differential diagnosis of AE with neuronal Abs varies with the syndrome. Many patients with anti-NMDA receptor encephalitis are suspected of having viral encephalitis, although viral studies are negative. Prominent and early behavioral symptoms, at times with hallucinations, can result in the initial consideration of a primary psychiatric disorder, malingering, or substance abuse. Older patients tend to present with memory disturbances, leading to a diagnosis of early-onset dementia.

While almost all cases progress within a month to include additional symptoms, these too can be mistaken for other etiologies. The development of stereotypic movements (orofacial and/or limb dyskinesias), rigidity, and catatonia may be interpreted as side effects of recently instituted antipsychotic medication. In this setting, autonomic dysfunction with increased temperature can be confused with neuroleptic malignant syndrome.

A few patients with anti-LGI1 encephalitis develop peripheral nerve excitability, and the combination of rapid decline in memory and behavioral disturbance with myoclonic-like limb movements can lead to a diagnosis of Creutzfeldt–Jakob disease or other rapidly progressive dementia.

Patients with IgLON5 antibodies develop non-REM and REM parasomnias and sleep breathing dysfunction with stridor. These patients may initially be misdiagnosed with isolated obstructive sleep apnea, in part because the stridor is confused with snoring. Video monitoring reveals the abnormal sleep behaviors that do not improve with continuous positive airway pressure.

The neurological symptoms in patients with DPPX encephalitis are often preceded or overlap with severe diarrhea and substantial weight loss, which suggests a primary gastrointestinal disorder. Patients with AE with neuronal Abs have an increased tendency toward the development of autoimmunity, in the form of either additional autoantibodies (e.g., ANA, TPO) or the co-occurrence of other autoimmune disorders that can confuse the clinical picture. Two patients with anti-CASPR2 encephalitis with myasthenia gravis and bulbar weakness and one with progressive bulbar weakness possibly related to undiagnosed myasthenia were initially diagnosed with amyotrophic lateral sclerosis.

Treatment

All types of AE with neuronal Abs can occur in association with cancer and all treatment plans should include prompt cancer identification and treatment. The tumor search should be made according to the autoimmune response; for example, while patients with LGI1 antibodies rarely have an underlying tumor, and when they do it is usually a thymoma, about 50% of patients with $GABA_B$ receptor antibodies have small cell lung cancer (SCLC). In some disorders, other factors such as patient age should be considered; for example, in anti-NMDA receptor encephalitis most young children do not have tumors, while about 45% of young women have teratoma of the ovary. This disorder rarely occurs in the elderly, and the frequency of tumor (carcinomas instead of teratomas) is about 20%.

The pathogenicity of the antibodies and the reversibility of the antibody effects support the use of immunotherapy, although optimal treatment, order of therapy, and risks and benefits of long-term immunotherapy remain to be elucidated. Data from a large retrospective series of patients with anti-NMDA receptor encephalitis demonstrated that just over 50% of patients will respond within

4 weeks to "first-line" immunotherapy (corticosteroids and/or intravenous immunoglobulins or plasma exchange) in association with tumor treatment when indicated. For unresponsive patients, those who received "second-line" immunotherapy (rituximab and/or cyclophosphamide) had better outcomes compared to those who either stayed on first-line treatment or for whom immunotherapy was discontinued. These findings should be interpreted within the context of being derived from a retrospective cohort study in which treatment decisions were not predefined, but they support the early initiation of second-line immunotherapy when there is no clear, early response to first-line treatments. There are many case reports and small case series suggesting the efficacy of rituximab, and this drug is increasingly being used as part of first-line therapy in patients with anti-NMDAR encephalitis. Whether this approach is similarly useful for other syndromes associated with antibodies against cell-surface antigens is unclear.

Determination of improvement should be based on clinical evaluation and should not rest on measurement of antibody titers, which often do not correlate with disease activity. Anti-NMDA receptor antibody titers decline over time, but many patients still have serum and CSF antibodies even after full recovery. If titers are to be studied, especially when trying to characterize new-onset symptoms as possible relapses, change of CSF titers associates better with clinical relapses than do serum titers.

Relapses may occur in any AE with neuronal Abs. Relapsing symptoms should lead to reassessment for an occult or recurrent tumor; symptoms usually respond to immunotherapy.

Further reading
Gresa-Arribas N, Titulaer MJ, Torrents A, et al. Antibody titres at diagnosis and during follow-up of anti-NMDA receptor encephalitis: A retrospective study. *Lancet Neurol* 2014;13:167–177.

Hughes EG, Peng X, Gleichman AJ, et al. Cellular and synaptic mechanisms of anti-NMDA receptor encephalitis. *J Neurosci* 2010;30:5866–5875.

Lancaster E, Dalmau J. Neuronal autoantigens: Pathogenesis, associated disorders and antibody testing. *Nat Rev Neurol* 2012;8:380–390.

Titulaer MJ, McCracken L, Gabilondo I, et al. Treatment and prognostic factors for long-term outcome in patients with anti-NMDA receptor encephalitis: An observational cohort study. *Lancet Neurol* 2013;12:157–165.

31   Epilepsy overview

Andres M. Kanner[1] and Barbara E. Swartz[2]
[1] Miller School of Medicine, University of Miami, Miami, FL, USA
[2] Renown Neuroscience Institute, University of Nevada, Reno, NV, USA

Epilepsy is a neurological disorder characterized by recurrent and unprovoked epileptic seizures. One in 26 people is at risk of experiencing a single epileptic seizure in the course of their life; the lifetime risk of developing epilepsy is 3.2% in North America. The diagnosis of epilepsy is established after the occurrence of at least two unprovoked (or reflex) seizures occurring at least 24 hours from each other, although a diagnosis of epilepsy after a first seizure can be made if the evaluation demonstrates the presence of risk factors associated with recurrent seizures (e.g., epileptiform activity in electrographic [EEG] recordings or an old stroke on brain magnetic resonance imaging [MRI]).

Classification

In 1981, the International League Against Epilepsy (ILAE) introduced a classification that separated seizures into partial (i.e., of focal origin) or generalized. Partial seizures were further classified as either simple partial, complex partial, or partial with secondary generalization, also known as secondarily generalized tonic–clonic (GTC) seizures. Simple partial seizures do not involve an alteration in consciousness, while complex partial seizures do. Simple partial seizures were subdivided into four subcategories: with motor symptoms, with somatosensory or special sensory symptoms, with autonomic symptoms, and with psychic symptoms. Complex partial seizures (CPS) were subdivided into those preceded by simple partial seizures and those with impairment of consciousness at onset. Generalized seizures include both convulsive and non-convulsive events and include absence seizures (typical and atypical), myoclonic, clonic, tonic–clonic, atonic, and unclassified.

In 1989 the ILAE published the classification of the epilepsies: (1) localization-related (focal, local, or partial); (2) generalized; (3) undetermined whether focal or generalized; and (4) special syndromes.

A new proposal has been made to incorporate increased understanding of etiopathogenesis of epilepsy. In this system the etiologies of idiopathic, symptomatic, and cryptogenic have become genetic, structural/metabolic, and unknown, with the understanding that an individual may have more than one etiology. Localization-related epilepsies are "focal" epilepsies. Complex partial and simple partial seizures have been renamed focal seizures "with or without impairment of consciousness or awareness." The term "dyscognitive" has been proposed for the CPS, but is not wholly agreed. Those without

impairment are described as with or without motor and autonomic signs. "Evolving to a bilateral convulsive seizure" replaces "secondarily generalized seizure." Epileptic syndromes are called "electroclinical syndrome," which is a complex of clinical features, signs, and symptoms that together define a distinctive, recognizable clinical disorder. The classification of seizures and electroclinical seizures are presented in tables 31.2 and 31.2, respectively.

Table 31.1 Classification of seizures.

Generalized seizures
Tonic–clonic (in any combination)
Absence
Typical
Atypical
Absence with special features
Myoclonic absence
Eyelid myoclonia
Myoclonic
Myoclonic–atonic
Myoclonic–tonic
Clonic
Tonic
Atonic
Focal seizures with descriptor
Epileptic spasms

Seizures that cannot be clearly diagnosed into one of these categories should be considered unclassified until further information allows their accurate diagnosis.

Table 31.2 Examples of electroclinical syndromes and other epilepsies arranged according to age. Source: Modified from Berg et al. 2010.

Neonatal period
Self-limited neonatal seizures
Self-limited familial neonatal epilepsy
Early myoclonic encephalopathy (EME)
Ohtahara syndrome
Infancy (onset under 2 years)
Febrile seizures
Febrile seizures plus
Epilepsy of infancy with migrating focal seizures
West syndrome
Myoclonic epilepsy in infancy (MEI)
Self-limited infantile epilepsy
Self-limited familial infantile epilepsy
Dravet syndrome
Myoclonic encephalopathy in non-progressive disorders

International Neurology, Second edition. Edited by Robert P. Lisak, Daniel D. Truong, William M. Carroll and Roongroj Bhidayasiri
© 2016 John Wiley & Sons, Ltd. Published 2016 by John Wiley & Sons, Ltd.

Childhood
    Febrile seizures
    Febrile seizures plus (FS+)
    Early-onset childhood occipital epilepsy (Panayiotopoulos type)
    Epilepsy with myoclonic atonic (previously astatic) seizures
    Self-limited epilepsy with centrotemporal spikes (ECTS)
    Autosomal dominant nocturnal frontal lobe epilepsy (ADNFLE)
    Epilepsy with myoclonic absences
    Lennox–Gastaut syndrome
    Epileptic encephalopathy with continuous spike-and-wave during sleep
    (CSWS)
    Landau–Kleffner syndrome (LKS)
Adolescence–Adult
Juvenile absence epilepsy (JAE)
Juvenile myoclonic epilepsy (JME)
Epilepsy with generalized tonic–clonic seizures alone (GTCA)
Autosomal dominant epilepsy with auditory features (ADEAF)
Other familial temporal lobe epilepsies
Familial epilepsy syndromes
Familial focal epilepsy with variable foci (FFEVF)
Genetic epilepsy with febrile seizures plus (GEFS+)

A third axis of classification relates to etiology: (1) genetic; (2) structural; (3) metabolic; (4) immune; (5) infectious; and (6) unknown. The understanding is that these classifications will be expanded as our knowledge increases.

Epidemiology

The worldwide incidence of epilepsy ranges from 50–120 cases per 100,000 per year, with a prevalence rate of 4–10 cases per 1000 people and higher rates in underdeveloped countries and in lower socioeconomic classes. The rates are similar between different ethnic groups, and slightly higher for men than for women. In North America there is a bimodal distribution across age, with higher incidence at the extremes of age, specifically before the age of 1 year and in the elderly. In studies conducted in Rochester, Minnesota, the proportion of incident epilepsy cases in those 65 years of age or older approximately doubled from 14% to 29% over the period 1935–84. With the aging of the US population, this trend is expected to continue. In fact, epilepsy is the third most frequent neurological disorder of elderly people in the United States.

Over half of the 50 million people with epilepsy worldwide are estimated to live in Asia. The median lifetime prevalence overall was 6 per 1000 people in one large study. The age distribution and male/female incidences in these countries differ from those in the United States (Table 31.3) and the treatment gap, defined as the percentage

Table 31.3 Prevalence of epilepsy outside North America and Europe (per 1000 person-years).

Country	Prevalence	Male	Female
China	3.6–76	3.6	2.5
Turkey	7.0	8.7	6.3
Pakistan	10.0	9.2	10.9
India	3.8–5.6	4.4	3.4
Nepal	7.3	6.8	7.9
Singapore	3.5–5	3.5	3.5
Vietnam	5.6–14	–	–
Japan	5.3–8.8	–	–
Russian Federation	3.5	4.5	2.5
China	2.9 (2.3–3.2)	3.8	3.4

of people with 2 or more seizures in the prior year not being appropriately treated in Asian countries, ranges from 38 to >72%. The age distribution has not been reported to be bimodal in most of these countries and the etiologies favor infection and trauma. In the Russian Federation the peak age for epilepsy in the >14-year-old group is 50–59 years. Chinese authors have reported the highest incidence in the 10–19-year-old group, although in an urban Chinese hospital study, newly diagnosed epilepsy was most prevalent in the elderly, likely reflecting difference that occurs with modernization.

The median prevalence of epilepsy in South America is 17.8 per 100,000 person-years, and in Sub-Saharan Africa is 15 per 1000. In Russia it is 3.4.

Age and seizure types

Seizure types vary with age. Patients can experience more than one seizure type, and wide variation in prevalence of the various seizure types is reported in the literature. There is a consensus that generalized seizures account for approximately half of seizures in patients younger than 15 years. The incidence of focal seizures, particularly focal seizures with impairment of consciousness, increases with age. In individuals 35–64 years old, focal seizures with impairment of consciousness have been found to be present in close to 40–50% of new cases of epilepsy. Absence seizures, which account for approximately 13% of seizures in pediatric patients younger than 15 years, are rare after adolescence. In elderly patients, seizures of focal onset account for the most frequent seizures.

In Asia, the range of patients with generalized seizures is 50–69%, and 31–50% have focal seizures, whereas in the Russian Federation 81% have localization-related epilepsy due to trauma and stroke, with one-third having unknown etiology. The other 19% are generalized. In China the overall prevalence by seizure type is 3.1% generalized, 0.57% focal, and 0.23% undetermined.

Mortality

Epilepsy is associated with a high risk of mortality. The standardized mortality ratio (SMR), which expresses the number of observed deaths per number of expected deaths, is two to three times higher in individuals with epilepsy than in the general population. The causes of mortality are related to seizures such as drowning, accidents, aspiration, burns, status epilepticus, and suicide. Nevertheless, the cause of death may often be undetectable, in which case it is referred to as sudden unexpected death in epilepsy (SUDEP). Asphyxia, burns, and poisoning are reported in some series. These do not differ across countries. Predictors of mortality are older age, a delay in starting treatment, status epilepticus due to cerebrovascular disease, and central nervous system (CNS) infection. Complications related to steroid treatment in infantile spasms are an important cause of death in infants.

In North America, SUDEP has been estimated to account for 17% of all deaths in patients with epilepsy. Its incidence ranges between 0.35 and 10 per 1000 patients per year, with patients with persistent seizures having a higher risk of SUDEP.

Pathophysiology

The etiology of epileptic seizure disorders varies with age. Improved genetic testing and neuroimaging have decreased the number of cases of epilepsy of unknown cause. Thus, 70% of seizure disorders are idiopathic among children and young people, while 90% of incident cases in adults have focal epilepsy, with 80% of seizures being of temporal lobe origin. Provoked seizures result from acute, reversible systemic, or neurological conditions, including but not limited to metabolic or toxic disturbances.

Risks and etiology

Any animal and human brain is susceptible to the development of epileptic seizures. Some brains are more susceptible than others and there is a large field of research looking at the contributions of complex inheritance and epigenetics to this susceptibility. Hauser investigated the relative risk (RR) of various causes of epilepsy. A relative risk of 1 implies that the relative risks of exposed and unexposed are equal, while a risk less than 1 suggests a protective effect of the exposure. Relative risks greater than 10 can be considered definite and clinically detectable. Those between 4 and 10 are considered likely risks, those between 2.5 and 3.9 probable, and those between 1.1 and 2.4 possible. Among the variables with relative risks greater than 10, Hauser identified cerebral palsy (RR 17.9–34.4), mental retardation (RR 22.6–31), cerebral palsy with mental retardation (RR 53.7–92.5), severe head trauma (RR 25–580), stroke (RR 22), and CNS infections (RR 10.8), of which viral encephalitis had the highest RR (16.2).

The identified causes of epilepsy vary with the part of the world studied. In the Russian Federation, head trauma and cerebral vascular disease were recognized as the most common causes. In China, etiology varies by age with birth trauma, mesial temporal sclerosis (MTS), focal dysplasia, and infection seen in young patients; head trauma, CNS infections in adults; and stroke and tumors in the elderly being the most likely causes of epilepsy.

Investigations

In the evaluation of patients with an epileptic seizure disorder, clinicians must answer the following questions in order to develop a rational and comprehensive treatment plan: (1) Is it possible that these paroxysmal events may not be epileptic seizures? (2) If they are epileptic seizures, what are the epileptic syndrome and seizure type? (3) Are there comorbid medical, neurological, and psychiatric disorders? (4) Is the patient taking any concomitant medications that need to be factored into the treatment plan? (5) How will the age and sex of the patient influence the choice of pharmacological treatment?

Differential diagnosis

One out of every 4–5 patients referred to an epilepsy center with a diagnosis of epilepsy does not suffer from epilepsy. Paroxysmal events can mimic epileptic seizures and are therefore referred to as non-epileptic events, non-epileptic seizures (NES), or pseudoseizures, although the use of this latter term is discouraged because it is considered to have a pejorative connotation. NES are grouped into two types: physiological and psychogenic. A detailed history is pivotal to reach the proper diagnosis. The following types of physiological or organic events are among the most commonly misdiagnosed as epileptic seizures.

Convulsive syncope

Convulsive syncope is the most frequent type of organic NES (ONES) to be misdiagnosed as epilepsy. The clonic and/or tonic activity associated with the transient drop of blood perfusion in the

CNS accounts for the confusion. The short period of loss of consciousness (<30 seconds) and the rapid reorientation in all spheres on recovery of consciousness are key in differentiating the syncopal episode from a generalized convulsion, in which the ictus can last up to 2 minutes followed by a postictal period of unresponsiveness (several minutes) and confusion (up to several hours duration). In elderly people with an underlying dementia or mild cognitive impairment, the syncopal episode can be longer and may be followed by a prolonged period of confusion. This frequently causes a false positive diagnosis of epilepsy.

Sleep disorders

Sleep disorders include the cataplectic events in narcolepsy, automatic behavior seen in obstructive sleep apnea, and parasomnias.

Complicated migraines and basilar migraines

The transient focal symptoms in the former and the confusional state that is typical of the latter account for the misdiagnosis.

Movement disorders

Acute dystonic reactions, hemifacial spasms, non-epileptic myoclonus, and hyperekplexia are movement disorders misdiagnosed as epileptic seizures. Acute dystonic reactions can present as dystonic movements of cervical, pharyngeal, and cranial muscles or oculogyric crisis, typically triggered by certain drugs 1–4 days after their ingestion (neuroleptics, lithium, trazodone, illicit drugs). Hemifacial spasms typically involve periorbital muscles initially, but may propagate to other facial muscles. Non-epileptic myoclonus may affect any muscle group in the body and usually occurs associated with toxic, metabolic, and degenerative encephalopathies.

Psychogenic NES are the most frequent type of NES identified in patients misdiagnosed as epileptics. These include panic disorders, conversion disorders, dissociative disorders, and malingering. The correct diagnosis requires the recording of a typical event in the course of a video-electroencephalogram (V-EEG) monitoring study. A prolonged study (2–3 days off all antiepileptic drugs) is necessary to rule out the possibility of both real and NES events occurring in the same patient, which is reported in 10–20% of cases.

Treatment/management

The treatment of an initial unprovoked epileptic seizure has been the source of continuous debate among epileptologists. The following principles can be used in guiding the decision of whether or not to treat. (1) Immediate or delayed treatment after a first seizure does not have an impact on the long-term outcome of the seizure disorder. On the other hand, immediate treatment prolongs the time to a first breakthrough seizure and increases the percentage of patients that reach an immediate 2-year remission. (2) The following parameters are suggestive of an increased risk of seizure recurrence: (a) focal seizure; (b) remote symptomatic seizure; (c) any abnormal EEG findings in children and epileptiform activity in adults; (d) first seizure occurring out of sleep; e) abnormal MRI; and f) abnormal neurological examination.

The achievement of seizure remission of antiepileptic drugs (AEDs) varies according to the epileptic syndrome, age of onset of the seizure disorder, and cause of epilepsy. Total seizure remission in the entire population of patients with epilepsy is 60–70%. About 80–90% of patients with idiopathic generalized epilepsy are expected to enter remission with the appropriate AED. In the case of focal epilepsy, about 50%

of patients will become seizure free. However, these expectations vary according to the type of focal epileptic syndrome. For example, almost every child with benign focal epilepsy of childhood is expected to become seizure free, and often these children do not need to be treated with AEDs. Focal seizure disorders beginning after the age of 65 have a significantly better prognosis than those beginning at a younger age. Seizure freedom with AEDs may range from 11–50% when the cause of focal epilepsy is mesial temporal sclerosis and is <5% in the case of double pathology in the temporal lobe (mesial temporal sclerosis and a structural lesion, such as a tumor, hamartoma, or cavernous angioma). Finally, the likelihood of seizure freedom in secondary generalized epilepsy (Lennox–Gastaut syndrome) is virtually zero.

Special populations

Epilepsy in the elderly

Epilepsy in the elderly is the third most frequent neurological disorder, after stroke and Alzheimer's dementia, at least in the Western world. Most patients suffer from a focal epilepsy presenting as focal seizures with and without impairment of consciousness, and secondarily generalized tonic–clonic seizures. The most frequent causes of epilepsy in this age group are stroke, dementia, and head trauma. In fact, stroke increases the risk of seizures by 23-fold within a year, relative to the general population. Conversely, a seizure disorder after the age of 60 increases the risk of stroke (RR 2.89 [95% CI 2.45–3.41]).

Elderly patients have a five- to ten-fold higher frequency of status epilepticus than younger adults, and mortality in this age group is significantly higher, reaching 48% in the elderly group and 35% in the adult group.

Comorbid medical and psychiatric disorders are common in this age group. In a multicenter study, 65% of patients with epilepsy beginning after the age of 60 were being treated for hypertension, 49% for cardiac disease, and 27% for diabetes, and 23% had a history of cancer. The average nursing-home patient on an AED is on five other drugs. The addition of an enzyme inducing AED can result in the loss of efficacy of concomitant medications metabolized in the liver. Slower metabolic rate results in greater toxicity in this population. Thus, the AED should be devoid of any pharmacokinetic interaction with other pharmacological agents, and should be used at the lowest possible dose to avert adverse events.

Epilepsy in women

In addition to identification of the epileptic syndrome and seizure type, planning of the treatment of seizure disorders in women must encompass the following considerations: (1) catamenial occurrence and/or exacerbation of seizures and impact of menopause on seizures; (2) reproductive disorders; (3) contraception; (4) pregnancy, including obstetric aspects and teratogenic risks of AEDs; and (5) breast feeding. Epilepsy per se may affect these functions. For example, women with epilepsy have a significantly higher risk of having polycystic ovaries than the general population. They are more likely to suffer from a variety of menstrual dysfunctions, including anovulatory cycles, which, in turn, have been associated with an increase in seizure frequency. Women with epilepsy have a lower sexual drive and lower birth rate than women in the general population. These menstrual and reproductive disturbances can be worsened with AEDs, particularly the older AEDs (enzyme inducers). Valproic acid facilitates the development of polycystic ovarian syndrome (PCO) in those exposed to this AED between the time of menarche

and the age of 25. Enzyme-inducing AEDs may interfere with sexual drive by decreasing the free fraction of estrogens and testosterone through increased synthesis of binding globulins.

Approximately 30–40% of women experience their seizures around the time of their menstrual cycle or ovulation, in which case they are considered to suffer from catamenial epilepsy. The use of hormone therapy with natural (but not synthetic) progesterone can decrease the seizure frequency in approximately 60% of these women, provided that the majority of the seizures are occurring around the menstrual period.

The use of AED in women of child-bearing age is of concern, as there is no AED that is completely safe to date. A woman with epilepsy on AED has in general twice the risk of giving birth to a baby with major malformations (e.g., 4–8%) compared to a healthy woman. This risk increases with polytherapy, high doses of AED, and family history of genetic disorders. In addition, certain AEDs are known to increase the risk of teratogenic effects, especially valproic acid and phenytoin. Finally, women with epilepsy have twice the risk of experiencing obstetric complications compared to healthy women, and their pregnancy has to be managed by high-risk obstetricians whenever possible.

Epilepsy in individuals with psychiatric comorbidities

Psychiatric disorders can be identified in 25–50% of patients with epilepsy, with higher prevalence among patients with poorly controlled seizures. These disturbances include depression, anxiety, psychotic disorders, and attention deficit disorders, occurring in the interictal periods. Patients with treatment-resistant epilepsy have an increased prevalence of postictal symptoms of depression, anxiety, and to a lesser degree psychosis. In addition, psychiatric symptoms such as panic can be the clinical expression of an aura, and often can be misdiagnosed as panic disorder. The prevalence rates of these major psychiatric disorders are presented in Table 31.4.

Depression and anxiety disorders are among the most frequent psychiatric comorbidities identified in adults. Attention deficit disorders (ADHD) are the most frequently reported in children, but recent studies carried out in pediatric populations have identified a significant prevalence of anxiety and mood disorders that are often misdiagnosed as ADHD. Despite the high prevalence of these psychiatric disorders, they are usually unrecognized and untreated. Only 25–66% of patients with a depressive disorder severe enough

Table 31.4 Prevalence of psychiatric disorders in epilepsy and the general population.

Psychiatric disorder	Prevalence rates	
	Epilepsy	General population
Depression	11–80%	
		3.3% Dysthymia
		4.9–17% Major depression
Psychosis	2–9.1%	1% Schizophrenia
		0.2% Schizophreniform disorder
Generalized anxiety disorder	15–25%	5.1–7.2%
Panic disorder	4.9–21%	0.5–3%
Attention deficit disorders	12–37%	4–12%

to warrant pharmacotherapy are recognized and properly treated early in the course of the condition.

There is evidence of a bidirectional relationship between most psychiatric disorders and epilepsy, including mood and anxiety disorders, ADHD, and psychotic disorders. Thus, patients with a history of major depressive disorders or suicidality (independent of a major depressive disorder) have a 2- to 5-fold greater risk of developing epilepsy, while children with a history of ADHD of the inattentive type have a 3.7-fold higher risk of developing epilepsy. In a study of pre-adolescents and young people with new-onset epilepsy, 45% met the criteria for an axis I diagnosis according to the DSM-IV-TR classification at the time of evaluation of the seizure disorder. In a separate study, children with a psychiatric comorbidity were almost three times more likely to develop epilepsy than those without. Clearly, the relationship between psychiatric disorders and epilepsy is complex: not only are patients with epilepsy at greater risk of developing a psychiatric disorder, but patients with certain psychiatric disorders are at greater risk of developing epilepsy.

Treatment of psychiatric comorbidities has to be incorporated into the overall management of the seizure disorder, as these have negative impacts in the life of patients at several levels, including worse quality of life, worse tolerance of and poor compliance with AEDs, increased suicidal risk, and premature death.

Standardizing care for persons with epilepsy

In developed nations there is a movement to set guidelines for ongoing management for persons with epilepsy. The following are generally agreed:

- The seizure type(s) and epilepsy syndrome, aetiology, and comorbidity should be determined, because failure to classify the epilepsy syndrome correctly can lead to inappropriate treatment and persistence of seizures.
- When a patient with epilepsy receives follow-up care, an estimate of the number of seizures since the last visit and assessment of drug side effects should be documented.
- If a patient is thought to have a diagnosis of epilepsy, the diagnosis should include a best estimation of seizure types.
- All of the new AEDs are appropriate for adjunctive treatment of refractory focal seizures in adults, and some have been found to be effective as monotherapy (e.g., lamotrigine, oxcarbazepine, topiramate, levetiracetam). The choice of AED depends on seizure and/or syndrome type, patient age, concomitant medications, AED tolerability, safety, and efficacy.
- The decision to initiate AED therapy should be agreed by the child, young person, or adult, their family and/or caretakers (as appropriate), and the specialist after a full discussion of the risks and benefits of treatment. This discussion should take into account details of the person's epilepsy syndrome, prognosis, and lifestyle.
- Combination therapy (adjunctive or 'add-on' therapy) should only be considered when attempts at monotherapy with AEDs have not resulted in seizure freedom. If trials of combination therapy do not bring about worthwhile benefits, treatment should revert to the regimen (monotherapy or combination therapy) that has proved most acceptable to the child, young person, or adult, in terms of providing the best balance between effectiveness in reducing seizure frequency and tolerability of side effects.
- Referral to an experienced epilepsy center for consideration of epilepsy surgery should be made in patients who have failed any

two consecutive or combination antiepileptic medications and who are believed to have focal epilepsy.
- Vagus nerve stimulation is indicated for use as an adjunctive therapy in reducing the frequency of seizures in adults who are refractory to antiepileptic medication, but who are not suitable for resective surgery. This includes adults whose epileptic disorder is dominated by focal seizures (with or without secondary generalization) or generalized seizures.

Given the lack of resources in underdeveloped countries, these nations should develop their own guidelines and future goals toward which to work.

Conclusions

Epilepsy is a disorder of the CNS that occurs at all ages and has multiple causes and clinical expressions. Its course is benign in two-thirds of patients. The management of seizure disorder is not limited to the elimination of epileptic seizures, but requires the consideration of comorbid medical, neurological, and psychiatric disorders, some of which may precede the onset of the epilepsy, and of the concomitant medications.

The worldwide burden of epilepsy is severe, with mortality equaling that of lung and breast tumors. In fact, the World Health Organization reported that more people died of epilepsy worldwide than died of AIDS in 2002. In developing countries this burden can be decreased by prevention, by treatment or prevention of indigenous infectious agents, and by improved access to antiepileptic drugs.

Further reading

Berg AT, Berkovic SF, Brodie MJ, *et al.* Revised terminology and concepts for organization of seizures and epilepsies: Report of the ILAE Commission on Classification and Terminology, 2005–2009. *Epilepsia* 2010;51(4):676–685.

Engel J Jr. Epileptic seizures. In: EngelJ Jr (ed.). *Seizures and Epilepsy*. Philadelphia, PA: FA Davis; 1989:137–178.

Engel J, Wiebe S, French J, *et al.* Practice parameter: Temporal lobe and localized neocortical resections for epilepsy: Report of the Quality Standards Subcommittee of the American Academy of Neurology, in association with the American Epilepsy Society and the American Association of Neurological Surgeons. *Neurology* 2003;60:538–547.

French JA, Kanner AM, Bautista J, *et al.* Efficacy and tolerability of the new antiepileptic drugs I: Treatment of new onset epilepsy. Report of the Therapeutics and Technology Assessment Subcommittee and Quality Standards Subcommittee of the American Academy of Neurology and the American Epilepsy Society. *Neurology* 2004;62:1252–1260.

Hauser WA, Hesdorffer DC. Risk factors. In: HawserWA, HesdorfferDC (eds.) *Epilepsy: Frequency, Causes and Consequences*. New York: Demos; 1990:53–100.

Herzog AG, Harden CL, Liporace J, *et al.* Frequency of catamenial seizure exacerbation in women with localization-related epilepsy. *Ann Neurol* 2004;56:431–434.

Kwan P, Arzimanoglou A, Berg AT, *et al.* Definition of drug resistant epilepsy: Consensus proposal by the ad hoc Task Force of the ILAE Commission on Therapeutic Strategies. *Epilepsia* 2010;51:1069–1077.

La France W, Kanner AM. Epilepsy. In: JesteDV, FriedmanJH (eds.). *Psychiatry for Neurologists*. Totowa, NJ: Humana Press; 2006:191–208.

Marson A, Jacoby A, Johnson A, *et al.*; Medical Research Council MESS Study Group. Immediate versus deferred antiepileptic drug treatment for early epilepsy and single seizures: A randomised controlled trial. *Lancet* 2005;365:2007–2013.

National Institute of Clinical Health and Excellence. The epilepsies: The diagnosis and management of the epilepsies in adults and children in primary and secondary care (update). Clinical guideline 137. 2012. https://www.nice.org.uk/guidance/cg137 (accessed November 2015).

Rowan AJ, Ramsay RE, Collins JF, *et al.*; VA Cooperative Study 428 Group. New onset geriatric epilepsy: A randomized study of gabapentin, lamotrigine, and carbamazepine. *Neurology* 2005;64:1868–1873.

32 Structural, genetic and unknown generalized epilepsies and syndromes

Marco T. Medina[1], Antonio V. Delgado-Escueta[2], Luis C. Rodríguez Salinas[3], Marco Medina-Montoya[1], and Barbara E. Swartz[4]

[1] Faculty of Medical Sciences, National Autonomous University of Honduras, Tegucigalpa, Honduras
[2] Department of Neurology, University of California, Los Angeles, CA, USA
[3] Honduras Medical Center, Tepeyac, Tegucigalpa, Honduras
[4] Epilepsy Center and Neurophysiology Laboratory, Renown Neuroscience Institute, University of Nevada, Reno, NV, USA

Structural-metabolic (Symptomatic), Genetic (Idiopathic) and unknown(cryptogenic) epilepsies are common during infancy and childhood. Cryptogenic epilepsies have unknown causes; genetic epilepsies are the direct result of a known or inferred genetic defect(s); and the etiology of structural–metabolic epilepsies is clearly recognized and may include head injury, infection (such as meningitis), brain lesions, and stroke. These are epilepsy categories in transition, for many etiologies may produce similar semiologies and the influence of genetic factors on a broad range of insults, such as trauma, is yet to be understood.

Ohtahara syndrome (EIEE)

Early infantile epileptic encephalopathy with burst suppression (EIEE) is a progressive epileptic encephalopathy currently in the cryptogenic family. The syndrome is characterized by tonic spasms and partial seizures with rare myoclonus, and the electroencephalogram (EEG) pattern of burst-suppression activity. It is an extremely debilitating, progressive neurological disorder, involving intractable seizures and severe mental retardation. No single cause has been identified, although in many cases structural brain damage is present. It is named after the Japanese neurologist Shunsuke Ohtahara, who identified it in 1976.

Pathophysiology

Atrophy is usually present on neuroimaging, thus taking EIEE out of the cryptogenic classification, but some cases of association with a metabolic syndrome have been reported. Genetic abnormalities have been reported on numerous loci – ARX, CDKL5, SLC25A22, STXBP1, SPTAN1, KCNQ2, ARHGEF9, PCDH19, 4PNKP, SCN2A, PLCB1, SCN8A – but no mechanisms have been determined.

Clinical features and investigations

The diagnosis is made by the early presentation of tonic seizures, brain atrophy, and burst suppression on EEG present during the day and night. Bursts of 1–3 s duration alternate with a nearly flat suppression phase of 2–5 s at an approximately regular rate; 5–10 s of burst–burst interval. Some asymmetry in spike bursts is noted in about two-thirds of cases. Ictal EEG of tonic spasms shows principally desynchronization with or without initial rapid activity. The infants are often excessively sleepy and floppy. The natural history is profound retardation and intractable seizures.

Treatment

Treatment of seizures is generally made with adrenocorticotropic hormone (ACTH) or steroids, valproic acid, clobazam, topiramate, rufinamide, or a ketogenic diet. Response is poor. Rarely if the syndrome is associated with hemimegalencephaly or hemiatrophy, hemispherectomy may be used for the seizures.

Prognosis

Evolution to West syndrome with hypsarrhythmia and subsequently to Lennox–Gastaut with slow spike wave on EEG is common. Severe mental retardation and developmental delay are universal.

Severe myoclonic epilepsy in infancy (SMEI) or Dravet syndrome

SMEI or Dravet syndrome is characterized by febrile and afebrile generalized and unilateral clonic or tonic–clonic seizures that occur in the first year of life in an otherwise normal infant. They are later associated with myoclonus, atypical absences, and partial seizures. All seizure types are resistant to antiepileptic drugs. Developmental delay becomes apparent within the second year of life and is followed by definite cognitive impairment and personality disorders. SMEI was once considered cryptogenic, but it is now known that mutations in the SCN1A gene are the major cause, usually occurring de novo.

SMEI is a rare disorder, with an incidence of less than 1 per 40,000. The syndrome affects males more frequently than females. The percentage of SMEI is 3–7% in patients with seizure onset before the age of 3 years.

Pathophysiology

SMEI is not associated with previous significant brain pathology; there is usually no history of abnormal computed tomography (CT) scan or magnetic resonance imaging (MRI). In 25–71% of cases there is a family history of either epilepsy or febrile seizures. Recent

International Neurology, Second edition. Edited by Robert P. Lisak, Daniel D. Truong, William M. Carroll and Roongroj Bhidayasiri
© 2016 John Wiley & Sons, Ltd. Published 2016 by John Wiley & Sons, Ltd.

clinical genetic studies suggest that SMEI is at the most severe end of the spectrum of generalized epilepsy with febrile seizures (GEFS+). 70–80% of SMEI cases have mutations in SCN1A, the gene encoding the α subunit of the voltage-gated sodium channel NaV1.1, many of which are *de novo* mutations. GABRG2, SCN1B, GABRA1, PCDH19, and STXBP1 mutations have been identified in patients with SMEI as well.

Clinical features

Febrile and afebrile generalized and unilateral clonic or tonic–clonic seizures occur in the first year (around 5–8 months of age). These often recur in 6–8-week intervals and may lead to status epilepticus. Generalized tonic–clonic seizures, generalized clonic seizures, alternating unilateral clonic seizures, myoclonic seizures, atypical absences and obtundation status, focal seizures, simple focal motor and complex partial seizures, with or without secondary generalization, and rarely tonic seizures may recur later without fever. Borderline SMEI patients do not experience myoclonic seizures, but nonetheless follow the same clinical course as those who do. Absence seizures are atypical and brief, with rhythmic generalized spike waves on EEG. Status epilepticus is frequent, either convulsive or as obtundation status; obtundation status includes impairment of consciousness with the presence of fragmentary and segmental erratic myoclonias. The disorder progresses to psychomotor retardation in the second year of seizure onset; neurological deficits such as ataxia and corticospinal tract dysfunction develop later.

Investigations

EEG shows generalized spike and polyspike waves. Periodic photic stimulation as well as drowsiness may increase the appearance of EEG paroxysms. Interictal background activity is generally normal at onset, but has a tendency to deteriorate afterward. EEG spikes tend to be absent when the patient is awake and rather marked when the patient is sleeping. CT scan and MRI are usually normal, but diffuse, cerebral or cerebellar atrophy, or increased white-matter signal is occasionally reported.

Treatment

All seizure types are resistant to antiepileptic drugs (AEDs). Valproate, stiripentol, topiramate, levetiracetam, and benzodiazepines are the most useful drugs. The ketogenic diet, when started early, may aid both seizures and cognitive outcomes. See Table 32.1 for other therapies with varying effectiveness. Carbamazepine, lamotrigine, and other sodium channel blockers can aggravate the seizures and should be avoided.

Prognosis

Seizures continue throughout childhood, leading to an unfavorable outcome. There is severe cognitive impairment in 50% of patients, and all have some level of impairment. Many also have behavioral disorders. The mortality rate is high, ranging from 16% to 18%.

West syndrome (WS)

WS is characterized by infantile spasms (IS), mental retardation, and a hypsarrhythmic EEG pattern. While 85–91% of cases are symptomatic, the remaining cases are cryptogenic.

Epidemiology

The incidence of WS ranges from 2.9–4.3 per 10,000 live births worldwide.

Pathophysiology

Symptomatic WS is associated with several prenatal, perinatal, and postnatal factors including prenatal infections, neonatal ischemia, postnatal encephalitis due to herpes virus, several brain dysgenesis, neurocutaneous syndromes, chromosomal abnormalities (Down syndrome, XXY, 22q, 17p 13.3 microdeletion, etc.), or single gene

Table 32.1 Cryptogenic/symptomatic generalized epilepsies and syndromes: Main features.

Epileptic syndrome	Age at onset (latest)	Initial seizure type	Continued seizure type	EEG: wake (W)/ sleep (S)	Therapy	Cognitive prognosis
Ohtahara syndrome	10 days–3 months	Tonic, awake and in sleep	TS, partial, AS, GTCS, rare MS	Suppression burst, W, and S	Steroids, ACTH, VPA, CBZ, KD, TPM, polytherapy	Unfavorable – 100% retardation
Dravet's syndrome	5–8 (18) months	"FS"/ unilateral TCS	GTCS > MS > CS > atyp. AB	W: Theta, sw, poly sw	VPA, TPM, bromide, benzo, stiri, KD	Unfavorable (50% with severe mental retardation)
West syndrome	3–7 (24) months	TS	MS > CS > Aka	W: Hypsa S: Reduced hypsa, s and poly sw	High-dose ACTH, steroids, VPA, NTZ, VGB, surg	75–80% with psychomotor retardation
Lennox–Gastaut syndrome	years	FS, TS	AB > AS > GTCS > mixed types	S: more gen. HSA W: diffuse slsw	Difficult: polytherapy, VPA, CLB, LMT, FBM, TPM, rufinamide, LEV, surg	Mental retardation present in 78–96% of patients
Epilepsy with myoclonic absences	years	MA	TS > GTCS > mixed types	Symmetric slsw at 3 Hz	VPA, Etho, LMT, TPM, LEV, ZNS	Variable, but often unfavorable

AB = absences; ACTH = adrenocorticotropin hormone; Aka = akinetic attack; AS = atonic seizure; CLB = Clobazam; CBZ = carbamazepine; CS = clonic seizure; Etho = ethosuximide; FBM = felbamate; FS = febrile seizure; GTCS = generalized tonic–clonic seizure; HSA = generalized hypersynchronous activity; Hypsa = hypsarrhythmia; KD = ketogenic diet; LEV = levetiracetam; LMT = lamotrigine; MA = myoclonic absences; MS = myoclonic seizure; NTZ = Nitrazepam; poly sw = polyspike wave; s = spikes; slsw = slow spike waves; surg = surgery; sw = slow waves; TCS = tonic–clonic seizure; TPM = topiramate; TS = tonic seizure; VGB = vigabatrin' VPA = valproate; ZNS = zonisamide

(SCN1A, MAG12, CACNA1A, ARX, STK9, etc.) mutations. A family history of epilepsy or febrile seizures is found in 7–17% of patients with WS, although familial incidence of WS ranges from only 3–6%. Several authors have proposed a polygenic mode of inheritance combined with environmental factors. Cerebral malformations are a major cause of West syndrome (abnormal neurogenesis, neuronal migration, dysplasia, microcephaly, hemimegalencephaly, agyria/polygyria, schizencephaly, and heterotopias).

Clinical features

Between 50% and 80% of cases begin between the ages of 3 and 7 months. Previously normal infants may have behavioral regression with the onset of WS. Spasms are often the first manifestation, but loss of milestones may precede the spasms by weeks. Spasms consist of repetitive clusters of sudden, briefly sustained movements of the axial musculature. The flexor spasm, although not the most common, is most characteristic of WS. Extensor spasms involve abrupt extension of the neck and lower extremities with extension and abduction of the arms. Mixed flexor–extensor spasms are exhibited in 40–50% of patients. In some cases no spasms are apparent, although they may be present on polygraphic recording. Myoclonic, clonic, and akinetic seizures also occur. Contraction, which is common during wakefulness and awakenings, is often followed by a cry. Some patients continue to have normal intellectual development. Absence of psychomotor regression is the best prognostic factor of a favorable outcome.

Investigations

EEG during spasms shows either generalized low-amplitude fast activity or a generalized high-amplitude slow wave; however, 13% of patients show no EEG abnormalities during spasms. A hypsarrhythmic pattern, which is most common in the early stages of infancy spasms, involves high-voltage slow waves, spikes, and sharp waves that seem to occur randomly from all cortical regions, giving the impression of chaotic disorganization of cortical electrogenesis. This pattern is almost continuous in the waking state. During drowsiness, spikes increase and polyspikes may appear. In REM sleep, hypsarrhythmia is clearly reduced. Spasms may occur in clusters without hypsarrhythmic pattern, as this represents a refractory subtype of IS. MRI is more sensitive than CT at detecting focal lesions, including abnormal or delayed myelination areas, and cortical dysplasias. In some children with normal or abnormal MRI, positron emission tomography (PET) scans have revealed focal areas of hypometabolism, which often correlate with the dysplastic cortex and white matter.

Treatment

The two major therapeutic approaches are hormonal treatment (ACTH or corticosteroids) and vigabatrin. Vigabatrin is the drug of choice for spasms due to tuberous sclerosis. Valproate and clonazepam control about 25–30% of cases. Clobazem may be used instead of clonazepam for better tolerance and pyridoxine may be useful. Some infants with medically intractable IS and focal lesions or focal hypometabolism may benefit from surgical resection. Persistent spasms are not amenable to focal resection but may benefit from total callosotomy.

Prognosis

Spasms and hypsarrhythmic EEG tend to disappear spontaneously before 3 years of age. However, the majority of survivors suffer from partial epilepsy (10–32%), generalized epilepsy (42–90%), or from various motor, sensory, and mental defects. Only 5–12% of patients have normal mental and motor development. Lennox–Gastaut Syndrome is developed later by 40–60% of patients. Evolution to a completely normal EEG pattern is the least common outcome. After steroid treatment, more than one-third of patients relapse 3–12 months after remission. Different type of seizures, prior neurological and developmental deficits, asymmetric spasms, gross asymmetry on EEG tracings, and abnormal neuroradiological findings prior to steroid treatment all predict an unfavorable outcome. The overall long-term outcome remains grim, with a 20% mortality rate. The risk of death is six times higher in symptomatic cases than in cryptogenic patients.

Lennox–Gastaut syndrome (LGS)

The characteristic features of LGS are (1) generalized seizures, typically tonic, atonic, myoclonic, and atypical absence; (2) interictal EEG characterized by abnormal background, diffuse slow spike-and-wave complexes, and paroxysmal fast rhythms of approximately 10 Hz in sleep; and (3) diffuse cognitive dysfunction and associated personality disorders, which often become apparent only later in the disorder.

Epidemiology

Although the incidence of LGS is low, it accounts for 5% of intractable epileptic patients of all ages and about 10% of epileptic patients under 15 years of age.

Pathophysiology

Approximately 30% of LGS cases are cryptogenic (unknown) in origin. These cases have been reported to have a higher incidence of epilepsy or febrile seizures in families, although there is no evidence of genetic predisposition. The remaining 70% of patients have preexisting brain damage, usually acquired in the prenatal or neonatal period or in infancy. Pre- and perinatal factors include ABO blood group incompatibility, prematurity, prolonged labor, umbilical cord prolapse, respiratory depression, and one or more of several types of cerebral malformations. With the advent of high-resolution MRI, cortical dysplasias, hemimegalencephaly, band heterotopia, lissencephaly or pachygyria resulting from mutations in the doublecortin gene (DCX), bilateral perisylvian polymicrogyrias and polygyrias resulting from a mutation in Xq28, recessive autosomic transmission or 22q11.2 deletion, and bilateral frontoparietal polymicrogyrias resulting from a mutation of the GPR56 gene are being identified as an increasingly common substrate. Postnatal factors include neuroinfections, degenerative or neurometabolic disorders, head injury, anoxic encephalopathy, stroke, and hypoglycemia. Approximately one-third of patients with structural LGS represent an evolution from WS.

Clinical features

LGS usually presents in early childhood, although onset in early adult life has been described in atypical LGS. The first seizure occurs between 1 and 8 years of age, with a peak between 3 and 5 years. Tonic seizures are the most common, particularly in patients with seizure onset at an early age, and have a reported prevalence of between 74% and 90% in sleep EEG recordings. These are often associated with sudden falls and may be difficult to distinguish from astatic episodes. Atypical absence seizures have a gradual onset/offset and are not precipitated by hyperventilation and photic stimulation. Associated myoclonic jerks may be observed. The prevalence of non-convulsive status epilepticus has ranged from 54–97%, with lower rates observed in atypical LGS. Tonic seizures and confusion are the most common ictal manifestations and may be precipitated by intravenous administration of benzodiazepines. EEG during status epilepticus may be difficult to distinguish from interictal EEG. Diffuse cognitive dysfunction may not be evident at seizure onset, but becomes more marked with time. Mental retardation is present eventually in 78–96% of patients, but is less severe in atypical LGS. Behavioral and personality disturbances complicate social adjustment; motor development is less affected.

Investigations

Diagnosis is based on the combination of several types of generalized seizures. Tonic and atypical absences may need ictal EEG recording to be properly identified. Interictal EEG background demonstrates a lower than normal frequency at all ages, as well as an increased amount of slow activity. The waking record is dominated by 2.0–2.5 Hz spike-and-wave and polyspike-and-wave discharges, which are usually diffuse. During slow-wave sleep, discharges are more obviously bisynchronous and are often associated with polyspikes. Paroxysmal fast rhythms (>10 Hz), particularly during slow-wave sleep, are an integral feature of LGS. During tonic seizures, EEG demonstrates bilaterally synchronous (10–25 Hz) activity maximal in the anterior and vertex regions, or attenuation of the background rhythm, which may be preceded by polyspikes. Atypical absence seizures appear as irregular, diffuse, slow spike-wave discharges of approximately 2.0–2.5 Hz that may be difficult to distinguish from the interictal slow spike-wave pattern.

Treatment

Treatment, which includes both seizure control and management of associated cognitive and behavioral issues, has been difficult and disappointing. Antiepileptic drug polytherapy is the most useful approach. Valproate, lamotrigine, benzodiazepines, topiramate, rufinamide, levetiracetam, vigabatrin, zonisamide, and felbamate appear to be the most effective drug therapies. The ketogenic diet may be effective as well. Corpus callosotomy can reduce or abolish drop attacks in many patients, with no major diffuse brain malformation. Total versus anterior callosotomy depends on the age at which the epilepsy started.

Prognosis

Only a minority of patients achieve seizure control. Seizure onset before 3 years of age, a history of WS, symptomatic LGS, severe cognitive dysfunction, and difficulty achieving seizure control are predictive of refractory seizures. Atypical absence myoclonic seizures carry a more hopeful prognosis, as does the coexisting fast and slow spike-wave activity and precipitation of spike-wave activity by hyperventilation.

Epilepsy with myoclonic absences (EMA)

In 1969, myoclonic absences (MA) were recognized as a specific seizure type and proposed as the essential feature of a distinct syndrome. There are two forms of EMA: a pure form in which myoclonic absences are the single or predominant type of seizure, and another form in which MA are associated with other seizure types, particularly with generalized tonic–clonic seizures.

Epidemiology

In specialized centers, MA is an uncommon syndrome, accounting for 0.5–1% of all epilepsies observed in selected populations; 70% of EMA cases are male.

Etiology

The etiology of EMA is unknown. Although a family history of seizure disorders can be found in about one-fourth of cases, specific genetic factors and hereditary mechanisms are not known. Some published cases have been described relating etiological factors such as prematurity, perinatal damage, consanguinity, congenital hemiparesis, and chromosomal abnormalities such as trisomy 12p and Angelman syndrome. Glutamate dehydrogenase (GDH) mutation and glucose transporter type 1 deficiency syndrome (GLUT1DS) have been reported.

Clinical features

The average age of onset of EMA is 7 years (range 11 months to 12.5 years). Approximately half of affected children are cognitively normal and half are mentally retarded prior to the onset of seizures. Manifestations include abrupt onset of absences accompanied by bilateral rhythmic myoclonic jerks of severe intensity. Loss of consciousness during the absence may be complete or partial. Movements may be associated with tonic contraction, which is maximal in shoulder and deltoid muscles. Hyperventilation, awakening, and intermittent photic stimulation may precipitate the attack. During sleep, however, myoclonic seizures decrease in frequency. Episodes of MA status, although rare, have been described. Association with other seizures, such as GTCS, pure absence, and falling seizures, occurs in two-thirds of cases.

Investigations

Ictal EEG shows synchronous and symmetric discharges of spike waves at 3 Hz, similar to that of childhood absences. Polygraphic recording of MA reveals bilateral myoclonias at the same frequency as spikes and waves, followed by a tonic contraction. Interictal EEG findings include normal background activity with superimposed generalized spike waves or, more rarely, focal or multifocal spikes and waves.

Treatment

A combination of valproate and ethosuximide at high doses with appropriate plasma-level control can lead to rapid remission of MA. Lamotrigine, levetiracetam, topiramate, rufinamide, or zonisamide may also be useful.

Prognosis

EMA has a variable but often poor prognosis. MA seizures may persist into adulthood in about half of patients. Patients with "refractory" MA seizures have a high incidence (85%) of associated seizures, mostly tonic–clonic and falling seizures. The duration of MA is likely to play a significant role in the appearance of mental deterioration.

Inflammatory epilepsies

Inflammation has long been recognized as a contributor to ictogenesis, but there is now evidence for its involvement in epileptogenesis. It should be suspected when seizures are highly refractory with no known etiology and normal neuroimaging. Often seizures are accompanied or preceded by personality changes or psychiatric symptomatology. Numerous autoantibodies have been reported in association with such patients, including GABA-B, AMPA, NMDA-R, GAD, mGluR5, VGKC-Complex, paraneoplastic antibodies, LRGI protein Ab, and anti-gliadin Ab. Elevated IgA can be a useful screening tool.

With evidence of an autoimmune serological response, therapy should be initiated with steroids, intravenous immunoglobin, or plasmapheresis. If antibody screening is not possible, a therapeutic trial may be indicated based on clinical symptomatology.

Further reading

Aicardi J, Ohtahara S. Severe neonatal epilepsies with suppression-burst pattern. In: RogerJ, BureauM, DravetCh, et al. (eds.). *Epileptic Syndromes in Infancy, Childhood and Adolescence*, 4th ed. London: John Libbey; 2005:39–52.

Bergen DC, Beghi E, Medina MT. Revising the ICD-10 codes for epilepsy and seizures. *Epilepsia* 2012;53(Suppl 2):3–5.

Bureau M, Tassinari CA. Myoclonic absences: The seizure and the syndrome. In: Delgado-EscuetaA, GuerriniR, MedinaMT, et al. (eds.). *Advances in Neurology: Myoclonic Epilepsies*, Vol 95. Philadelphia, PA: Lippincott Williams & Wilkins; 2005:175–184.

Dravet C, Bureau M, Oguni H, Cokar O, Guerrini R. Dravet syndrome (severe myoclonic epilepsy in infancy). In: BureauM, GentonP, DravetC, et al. (eds.). *Epileptic Syndromes in Infancy, Childhood and Adolescence*, 5th ed. London: John Libbey Eurotext; 2012:125–156.

Dulac O, N'Guyen T. The Lennox-Gastaut syndrome. *Epilepsia* 1993;34(Suppl 7):S7–S17.

Dulac O, Plouin P, Schlumberger E. Infantile spasms. In: WyllieE (ed.). *The Treatment of Epilepsy: Principles and Practice*, 2nd ed. Baltimore, MA: Williams & Wilkins; 1997:540–572.

Elia M, Guerrini R, Musumeci SA, et al. Myoclonic absence-like seizures and chromosome abnormality syndromes. *Epilepsia* 1998a;39:660–663.

Farrell K. Symptomatic generalized epilepsy and Lennox–Gastaut syndrome. In: WyllieE (ed.). *The Treatment of Epilepsy: Principles and Practice*, 2nd ed. Baltimore, MA: Williams & Wilkins; 1997:530–539.

Fusco L, Chiron C, Trivisano M, Vigevano F and Chugani HT. Infantile spasms. In: BureauM, GentonP, DravetC, et al. (eds.). *Epileptic Syndromes in Infancy, Childhood and Adolescence*, 5th ed. London: John Libbey Eurotext; 2012:99–113.

Ohtahara S, Yamatogi Y. Epileptic encephalopathies in early infancy with suppression-burst. *J Clin Neurol* 2003;20:398–407.

Scheffer IE, Wallace R, Mulley JC, Berkovic SF. Clinical and molecular genetics of myoclonic–astatic epilepsy and severe myoclonic epilepsy in infancy (Dravet syndrome). *Brain Dev* 2001;23:732–735.

Vezanni A, Friedman A, Dingledine RJ. The role of inflammation in epileptogenesis. *Neuropharmacology* 2013;69:16–24.

Vigevano F, Bartuli A. Infantile epileptic syndromes and metabolic etiologies. *J Child Neurol* 2002;17:S9–S13.

33 Genetic (primary) idiopathic generalized epilepsies

Afawi Zaid[1] and Altynshash Jaxybayeva[2]

[1] Tel-Aviv Sourasky Medical Center, Tel Aviv, Israel

[2] National Research Center for Maternal and Child Health, Astana, Kazakhstan

Research advances in the last decade show that there is a genetic cause or at least contribution in many human epilepsy syndromes. The number of genes recognized to have a role in epilepsies has dramatically increased. The genes identified are components of neuronal signaling, including voltage-gated ion channels, neurotransmitter receptors, ion channel–associated proteins, and synaptic proteins. These genes have provided useful insights into the molecular basis of epileptogenesis.

Genetic epilepsy means that the fundamental cause is gene mutation. Some gene mutations causing epilepsy may occur *de novo* and thus will lack a pattern of inheritance. Also, most epilepsy that is inherited shows a complex, non-Mendelian pattern, which implies the interplay of multiple genes. Nonetheless, a small number of syndromes do have Mendelian inheritance patterns and have been associated with mutations of single genes that can be identified with genetic testing. Advances in molecular genetics have changed our viewpoint on the genetics of epilepsy. The advent of massively parallel sequencing (MPS), also called next-generation sequencing (NGS), technology such as exome sequencing and whole-genome sequencing, and application of genome-wide association study (GWAS) and comparative genomic hybridization (CGH) chip uncovered more genes in rare Mendelian disorders, complex diseases, and chromosomal disease, dramatically providing new methods and accelerating genomic research in human genetic diseases. We review some of the recent advances in the classification of epilepsy, the molecular genetics in epilepsies, the intervention of modern technology, and neuroimaging.

Advances in the classification of epilepsy

The International League Against Epilepsy (ILAE) Commission on Classification and Terminology revised its terminology and approach to classifying epilepsy. Within these revisions generalized seizures are redefined as "originating at some point within, and rapidly engaging bilaterally distributed networks." These networks are inclusive of both cortical and subcortical structures, but not necessarily the cortex in its entirety. Individual seizure onsets can appear localized; the location and lateralization are not consistent from one seizure to another. Generalized seizures can be asymmetric.

The term idiopathic generalized epilepsy, previously used to describe epilepsy without clear underlying cause other than presumed genetic etiology, has now been replaced by a more strict definition of genetic epilepsy. This term will be used to describe epilepsy that is directly the result of a known or presumed genetic defect that may derive from specific molecular genetic studies (e.g., *SCN1A* and Dravet syndrome) or family studies. All other epilepsies would be categorized as either structural/metabolic or unknown cause.

Advances in molecular genetics

The genes identified are components of neuronal signaling, including voltage-gated ion channels, neurotransmitter receptors, ion channel–associated proteins, and synaptic proteins. These genes have provided useful insights into the molecular basis of epileptogenesis. Thus, it is likely that there are many more epilepsy-related genes yet to be discovered.

Febrile seizure (FS)

Clinical

Febrile seizures occur in childhood, between 3 months and 5 years of age, and are associated with fever. Their pathogenesis is multifactorial. The attacks are accompanied by muscle contractions and reduced consciousness, usually lasting not longer than 5–10 minutes.

Complex febrile seizures have one or more of the following characteristics: (1) the seizures are usually brief and generalized tonic–clonic or last for more than 15 minutes (prolonged) or 30 minutes or more (febrile status epilepticus); (2) there is one or more recurrence within 24 hours (multiple-type febrile seizures); (3) the seizure has partial features, such as a focal onset of the seizure or a postictal Todd paresis of facial muscles or limbs. Seizures are referred to as simple if they last less than 15 minutes.

Males are more frequently affected than females; ratios vary between 1:1 and 1:6. Half of children have their initial seizure at 16–18 months of age. Most electroencephalogram (EEG) manifestations in FS are predominantly delta, either diffuse or posteriorly predominant, disappearing within 1 week of the convulsion.

Genetic

Linkage studies have proposed 11 chromosomal locations responsible for FS attributed to FEB1 to FEB11. Cytokine interleukin 1β (IL-1β) was the most investigated and the genes associated with susceptibility to FS, *SCN1A*, *IL-1β*, *CHRNA4*, and *GABRG2*, were the

International Neurology, Second edition. Edited by Robert P. Lisak, Daniel D. Truong, William M. Carroll and Roongroj Bhidayasiri.
© 2016 John Wiley & Sons, Ltd. Published 2016 by John Wiley & Sons, Ltd.

Table 33.1 Genes associated with genetics generalized epilepsy.

Gene	Associated epilepsy syndrome
ARX	Epileptic encephalopathy
CDKL5	Epileptic encephalopathy
CERS1	Progressive myoclonic epilepsy
CHRNA7	Juvenile myoclonic epilepsy
GABRA1	Juvenile myoclonic epilepsy
GABRG2	Genetic epilepsy with febrile seizure plus Childhood absence epilepsy
KCNQ2	Benign familial neonatal Epileptic encephalopathy
PCDH19	Epileptic encephalopathy Female patient with mental retardation
SCN1A	Genetic epilepsy with febrile seizure plus Dravet syndrome
SCN2A	Genetic epilepsy with febrile seizure plus
SLC2A1	GLUT1 deficiency syndrome
STXBP1	Epileptic encephalopathy

most commonly involved genes in this context. The genetic background of FS involves the regulation of different processes, including individual and familial susceptibility, modulation of immune response, and neuronal excitability and interactions with exogenous agents such as viruses.

Febrile seizures plus (FS+)

Clinical
Genetic generalized epilepsy with febrile seizures plus (GEFS+) is a familial epilepsy syndrome with marked phenotypic heterogeneity, ranging from simple febrile seizure to severe phenotypes, often extending more than 6 years.

No specific EEG changes characterize FS+.

Genetic
Inheritance is autosomal dominant. Mutations in the voltage-gated sodium channel alpha-1, alpha-2, and beta-1 subunit genes (SCN1A, SCN2A, and SCN1B) and the GABA (A) receptor gamma-2 subunit gene (GABRG2) have been identified in families with a clinical subset of seizures termed GEFS+. However, the causative genes have not been identified in most patients with FS or GEFS+ (see Table 33.1).

Severe myoclonic epilepsy of infancy (SMEI)

Clinical
Classic Dravet syndrome, also termed severe myoclonic epilepsy of infancy (SMEI), was first described by Dravet in 1978. In the last ILAE terminology in 2010, Dravet syndrome is now considered genetic epilepsy. Dravet syndrome typically presents in the

first year of life without generalized spikes and waves on EEG with prolonged febrile and non-febrile, generalized clonic or hemiclonic epileptic seizures in children with no pre-existing developmental problems. Other seizure types including myoclonic, focal, and atypical absence seizures appear between the ages of 1 and 4 years. The epilepsy is usually refractory to standard antiepileptic medication and from the second year of life affected children develop an epileptic encephalopathy resulting in cognitive, behavioral, and motor impairment. Seizure types within Dravet syndrome such as status epilepticus may be life threatening, and sudden unexpected death in epilepsy can occur. Despite the phenotypic variability within the typical and borderline forms, they are now all classified as Dravet syndrome.

Genetic
SCN1A-related seizure disorders can be inherited in an autosomal dominant manner, but most are due to *de novo* mutations.

Childhood absence epilepsy (CAE)

Clinical
According to the ILAE 2010 terminology, absence seizures are generalized seizures that occur in school-aged children, usually between the ages of 5 and 9 years. Typical absence seizures consist of sudden cessation of movement, staring, and sometimes blinking. Sometimes there may be a mild loss of body tone, causing the child to lean forward or backward slightly. Unlike other types of seizures, absence seizures occur without an aura or warning. When diagnosing CAE, typical absence seizures need to be differentiated from atypical absence seizures, which can occur at an earlier age. An EEG of a child with CAE will show a typical pattern known as 3 Hz generalized spike-and-wave (GSW) complexes.

Genetic
Genetic studies have shown heterogeneous mutations in ion channels CACNA1H, CHRNA4, CACNG3, and GABRG2 (see Table 33.1).

Juvenile absence epilepsy (JAE)

Clinical
Age of onset is most commonly 9–13 years of age and may be later around puberty, associated with GTCS, with EEG revealing more 3 Hz GSW discharges.

Genetic
Susceptibility mutations are in the EFHC1 and CLCN2 genes.

Juvenile myoclonic epilepsy (JME)

Clinical
Juvenile myoclonic epilepsy appears around puberty and is characterized by seizures with bilateral, single or repetitive, arrhythmic, irregular myoclonic jerks, predominantly in the arms. Jerks may cause some patients to fall suddenly. No disturbance of consciousness is observed. Generalized tonic–clonic seizures occur in more than 90% of patients with JME and, less often, infrequent absences in 30% of patients with JME. The seizures usually occur shortly after awak-

ening and are often precipitated by sleep deprivation. Interictal and ictal EEGs have rapid, generalized, often irregular spike waves and polyspike waves; there is no close phase correlation between EEG spikes and jerks. Frequently, patients are photosensitive. Response to appropriate drugs is good.

Genetic

Mutations have been found in the *GABRA1* gene, a novel *SCN1A* mutation (see Table 33.1) in a cytoplasmic loop in intractable juvenile myoclonic epilepsy without febrile seizures. A mutation of the gene *EFHC1* for myoclonin-1 protein, possibly involved in the spindle apparatus and neuronal migration, has been described by Melina and colleagues. To date there have been five Mendelian genes, three SNP alleles, and three microdeletions associated with the JME phenotype.

Novel progressive myoclonic epilepsy (PME)

Clinical

Impairment of ceramide synthesis causes a novel progressive myoclonus epilepsy, action myoclonus, with onset between 6 and 16 years of age, generalized tonic–clonic seizures, and progressive cognitive deterioration up to dementia. The phenotype is homogenous among affected siblings, with minor differences in progression of deterioration and severity of myoclonus. EEG revealed progressive slowing of background activity and epileptic abnormalities; brain magnetic resonance imaging showed cerebellar and brainstem atrophy in all tested individuals.

Genetic

Mutations occur in *CERS1* (see Table 33.1), the gene encoding ceramide synthase 1.

De novo mutations

De novo mutations in a wide variety of genes appear to be the basis of a significant proportion of the epileptic encephalopathies. Recently it has become clear that *de novo* mutations contribute to epilepsy pathogenesis. In addition to the typical occurrence of *de novo* *SCN1A* mutation in Dravet syndrome, other *de novo* mutageneses in epileptic encephalopathies include mutations in *CDKL5, ARX, STXBP1, PCDH19, KCNQ2, PLCB1, SPTAN1, SCN2A, SLC19A3,* and *SLC25A22.* A novel *de novo* mutation in *GRIN2A* was found in an individual with severe global developmental delay and intractable epilepsy. *De novo* mutations in *GABRB3* have recently been identified as causing epileptic encephalopathies, and a novel *de novo* mutation in *SLC2A1* coding for Glut1 was found.

Advances in technologies

Whole genome sequencing has become affordable, and exome sequencing – that is, the sequencing of large parts of the protein-coding region of the human genome – is established as a standard technology.

Targeting sequencing and epilepsy gene panel

Epilepsy-specific gene panels have become available to test for sequence variants and whole or partial gene deletions and duplications in multiple genes. Available panels can simultaneously screen many potentially relevant genes, and do not require the same degree of pretest correlation of genotype to phenotype as is needed for selection of a single-gene test. The advantage of these panels is being able to detect intragenic deletions below the resolution of chromosomal microarray analysis (CMA) that also might be missed by Sanger sequencing.

Massively parallel sequencing or next second-generation technology

Massively parallel throughput is the ability to process millions of sequence reads in parallel rather than 96 at a time. This may require only one or two instrument runs to complete an experiment. Also, next-generation sequence reads are produced from fragment "libraries" that have not been subject to the conventional vector-based cloning and *Escherichia coli*–based amplification stages used in capillary sequencing. The three available platform sequencers are the 454 GS FLX (Roche), Solexa (Illumina), and SOLiD (Applied Biosystems), and they differ significantly. These methods offer exceptionally high throughput with high accuracy and potentially cheaper analyses. These platforms follow similar processes: (1) The workflow to produce next-generation sequence-ready libraries is straightforward. DNA fragments that may originate from a variety of front-end processes are prepared for sequencing by ligating specific adaptor oligos to both ends of each DNA fragment. (2) Importantly, relatively little input DNA (a few micrograms at most) is needed to produce a library. (3) These platforms also have the ability to sequence the paired ends of a given fragment, using a slightly modified library process. (4) This approach can be used with a *de novo* genome sequence. (5) These platforms produce shorter read lengths (35–250 bp, depending on the platform) than capillary sequencers (650–800 bp), which also can have an impact on the utility of the data for various applications such as *de novo* assembly and genome resequencing. (6) These platforms have high reliability and are cost effective.

Copy number variation (CNV)

Copy number variants (CNVs) play an increasingly recognized role in the genetics of epilepsy. Helbig and colleagues in 2009 reported the first major site containing CNVs that predispose to GGE. Variations of at least 1 kb in length are defined as CNVs, and it has been estimated that there are around 1500 regions of variable copy numbers spread across 360 Mb (~12%) of the human genome. Success in identifying monogenic epilepsy genes relied on traditional genetic mapping in large pedigrees with Mendelian inheritance. The complex etiology of GGE, with multiple genetic and environmental factors contributing to risk, requires larger sample sizes to have sufficient power to detect the responsible genes. Several large studies have identified recurrent genomic "hotspots" that predispose to idiopathic epilepsy, including 1q21.1, 15q11.2, 15q13.3, 15q11–q13, 16p11.2, and 16p13.11. CNVs occur in these regions due to non-allelic homologous recombination between flanking segmental duplications. The specific genes responsible for the susceptibility to epilepsy in these CNVs have not been clearly identified in many instances, although CNVs involving known epilepsy genes (e.g., *SCN1A* or *KCNQ2*) have also been found. Rare, non-recurring CNVs have also been associated with epilepsy. Chromosomal microarrays (CMAs) have been increasingly included in the evaluation of epilepsy when a genetic etiology is suspected. Such suspicions might be raised by the presence of dysmorphic features, developmental delay (DD), autism spectrum disorder (ASD), or a family history of epilepsy.

Whole-exome sequencing (WES)

WES is clinically available, and can provide information about putative pathogenic variants not only in genes already known to be related to specific epilepsy syndrome, but also in genes that might not be expected to harbor mutations, particularly if the epilepsy phenotype differs from that previously observed to be associated with the variant in question. When applied to a trio (the patient and both biological parents), WES provides an efficient approach to the discovery of both *de novo* and inherited mutations in the coding portions of most genes in the human genome. Whole-genome sequencing (WGS), which is widely performed in the research setting, will probably also be available in the clinic shortly and will provide a means to assay both point mutations and copy number variations across the whole genome. As WES (and eventually WGS) becomes more widely used, the same issues will apply. The current practice of applying WES and WGS to a trio, although costly at the outset, provides tremendous efficiency in the analysis of *de novo* variants. These whole-genome approaches will also lead to the identification of many additional variants of unknown significance in patients with epilepsy and the possible identification of novel epilepsy-related genes. The need for iterative re-evaluation of genetic findings, especially variants of uncertain significance, is increasingly recognized in the face of this growing body of publicly available data. Laboratories that currently perform clinical genetic testing for epilepsy are generally willing to re-evaluate the potential pathogenicity of variants, but this step is currently done on an ad hoc basis and only at the request of treating clinicians.

Further reading

Berg AT, Berkovic SF, Brodie MJ, *et al.* Revised terminology and concepts for organization of seizures and epilepsies: Report of the ILAE Commission on Classification and Terminology, 2005–2009. *Epilepsia* 2010;51(4):676–685.

Gallentine WB, Mikati MA. Genetic generalized epilepsies. *J Clin Neurophysiol* 2012;29(5):408–419.

Garofalo S, Cornacchione M, Di Costanzo A. From genetics to genomics of epilepsy. *Neurol Res Int* 2012:876234.

Helbig I, Lowenstein DH. Genetics of the epilepsies: Where are we and where are we going? *Curr Opin Neurol* 2013;26(2):179–185.

Helbig I, Mefford HC, Sharp AJ, *et al.* 15q13.3 microdeletions increase risk of idiopathic generalized epilepsy. *Nat Genet* 2009;41(2):160–162.

Hildebrand MS, Dahl HH, Damiano JA, *et al.* Recent advances in the molecular genetics of epilepsy. *J Med Genet* 2013;50(5):271–279.

Medina MT, Suzuki T, Alonso ME, et al. Novel mutations in Myoclonin1/EFHC1 in sporadic and familial juvenile myoclonic epilepsy. *Neurology* 2008;70(22):2137–2144.

Pittau F, Grouiller F, Spinelli L, *et al.* The role of functional neuroimaging in pre-surgical epilepsy evaluation. *Front Neurol* 2014;5:31.

Poduri A, Lowenstein D. Epilepsy genetics: Past, present, and future. *Curr Opin Genet Devel* 2011;21(3):325–332.

Vanni N, Fruscione F, Ferlazzo E, *et al.* Impairment of ceramide synthesis causes a novel progressive myoclonus epilepsy. *Ann Neurol* 2014;76(2):206–212. doi:10.1002/ana.24170.

34 Localization-related epilepsies

Hirokazu Oguni[1] and Chrysostomos P. Panayiotopoulos[2]

[1] Department of Pediatrics, Tokyo Women's Medical University, Tokyo, Japan
[2] Department of Clinical Neurophysiology and Epilepsies, St. Thomas' Hospital, London, UK

Localization-related epilepsies (LRE; focal, local, partial) are disorders whose seizures originate in a circumscribed locus or within networks limited to one hemisphere regardless of etiology. LRE were believed to develop from an abnormal pathological cortical region giving rise to epileptic seizures (symptomatic or cryptogenic LRE). However, it is now known that idiopathic (presumably genetically determined) and familial syndromes of LRE with gene mutations exist.

Idiopathic LRE

Benign childhood focal seizures are the most common idiopathic LRE, affecting 25% of children with non-febrile seizures. Seizures are infrequent, usually nocturnal, and remit within 1–3 years. Febrile seizures occur in around one-third of patients, particularly in patients of Japanese descent. Affected children have normal physical and neuropsychological development, but some may experience mild and reversible cognitive and linguistic problems during the active stage of the disorder. Brain imaging is normal, as is resting background electroencephalogram (EEG). Severe EEG abnormalities are evidenced as high-amplitude focal spikes that are disproportionate to the frequency of seizures. A normal EEG is rare and should provoke a sleep EEG study. Similar EEG features resolving with age are frequently found in normal school-age children (2–4%) and children having an EEG for reasons other than seizures. The following representative electroclinical syndromes with age-dependent onset and remission have been recognized.

Panayiotopoulos syndrome

Epidemiology
Panayiotopoulos syndrome (PS) is an idiopathic LRE accounting for 6% of all non-febrile childhood epilepsies. The age at onset ranges from 1–14 years, with a peak at 4–5 years.

Etiology
Etiology may be genetically determined, as suggested by its association with Rolandic epilepsy and febrile seizures. A case with *SCN1A* mutation has been reported, without subsequent confirmation.

Clinical features
The cardinal features of PS are infrequent focal seizures, or often a single focal seizure, with autonomic symptomatology and prolonged duration, occurring mostly during sleep. In one-third of cases, the seizures last longer than 30 minutes (autonomic status epilepticus). Typically, the children wake up complaining of nausea, retching, or vomiting followed by deviation of eyes and progressive cloudiness of consciousness. One-third of seizures may evolve to hemiconvulsions or generalized convulsions. Over half of patients at least once experience syncope-like epileptic seizures, characterized by sudden loss of muscle tone in association with unresponsiveness, usually for several minutes and up to 1 hour (the child becomes flaccid and unresponsive). Interictal EEG shows multifocal spikes predominating in the posterior regions. However, EEG foci are not restricted to the occipital regions but frequently shift, multiply, and propagate diffusely with age-related changes, in particular from the occipital region to the fronto-centro-temporal areas. Ictal onsets are unilateral from posterior or anterior regions (Figure 34.1).

Management
The prognosis for patients with PS is excellent, although in rare cases autonomic seizures may cause cardiorespiratory arrest. One-third of patients have only one seizure and most patients experience fewer than five seizures during the clinical course. The other 10–20% may have frequent seizures, especially in the case of children with mild neurobehavioral problems. Antiepileptic drug (AED) treatment is usually not recommended for isolated seizures. Carbamazepine or valproic acid is generally used for recurrent attacks, although any narrow- or broad-spectrum agents may also be effective.

Rolandic epilepsy

Epidemiology
Rolandic epilepsy (RE), officially designated as benign childhood epilepsy with centrotemporal EEG foci, accounts for 15% of all LRE in children 1–15 years of age. The age of seizure onset ranges from 3–14 years and peaks at 5–8 years, with 1.5-fold male predominance.

Etiology
The high incidence of familial antecedents for epilepsy (18–36%) suggests that a genetic trait is playing a major role. Linkage to chromosome 15q14 has been reported, but no responsible gene mutation has been identified.

International Neurology, Second edition. Edited by Robert P. Lisak, Daniel D. Truong, William M. Carroll and Roongroj Bhidayasiri
© 2016 John Wiley & Sons, Ltd. Published 2016 by John Wiley & Sons, Ltd.

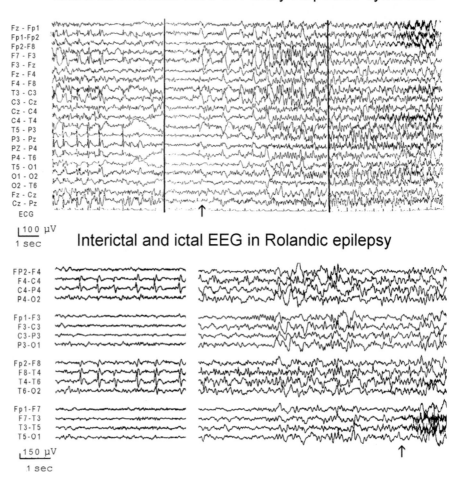

Figure 34.1 Top: Interictal (left) and ictal EEG (right) of a lengthy autonomic seizure of non-occipital onset in a child with Panayiotopoulos syndrome. Interictal EEG showed cloned-like repetitive multifocal spike-wave complexes that were mainly bifrontal, left more than right, midline, and occipital. Clinically, while asleep, he suddenly got up with both eyes open, vomited several times, and then showed a prolonged atonic state with cyanosis and irregular respiration for 3 min. The first EEG change (arrow) consisted of periodic slow waves from the left frontotemporal region (F3) for 3 s followed by rhythmic generalized discharge of mainly monomorphic rhythmic slow waves intermixed with spikes. ECG showed significant tachycardia during the ictus (see the ECG trace). Bottom: Interictal (left) and ictal EEG (right) of a child with Rolandic epilepsy. Interictal EEG showed high-amplitude right-sided centrtemporal spikes. Ictal EEG discharge started in the right centrotemporal region during sleep. The first clinical manifestations (arrow) consisted of contractions of the left facial muscles (note muscle artefacts on the left), progressing to a prolonged generalized clonic seizure, which lasted for 5 min. Source: Panayiotopoulos 2010. Reproduced with permission of Springer Science+Business Media.

Clinical features

The cardinal features of RE are infrequent, often single, focal seizures consisting of unilateral facial sensorimotor symptoms, oropharyngolaryngeal manifestations, speech arrest, and hypersalivation. These sometimes spread to the ipsilateral arm or arm and leg. Consciousness may be retained throughout the seizures. Secondary generalization to convulsions occurs in one-third to two-thirds of patients. Three-quarters of the seizures occur during non-REM sleep, most often soon after sleep onset and just before awakening.

High-amplitude biphasic sharp or sharp–slow wave discharges appear in the centrotemporal regions (Rolandic spikes; Figure 34.1). They are markedly enhanced by sleep, and shift from one side to the other or appear bilaterally. Multifocal epileptic foci including an occipital or frontal spike may appear. Onset of ictal EEG is unilateral from the Rolandic region.

Prognosis and treatment

Seizure recurrence is usually limited to a few times, although around 10–20% of patients may have many seizures. Although the seizures themselves enter into remission in 80% by 2 years, the Rolandic spikes tend to persist up to age 16. Early onset of RE, especially under age 5, is a risk factor for frequent seizure recurrence. On rare occasions, RE may evolve to atypical benign partial epilepsy of childhood, continuous spike and wave during sleep (CSWS), or Landau–Kleffner syndrome (atypical evolution of RE)

through the alterations of the gene encoding the NMDA receptor NR2A subunit (*GRIN2A*). Prophylactic AED treatment may not be needed because of the excellent prognosis. Carbamazepine or oxcarbazepine is a choice of AED for recurrent seizures, although they will respond to any narrow- or broad-spectrum agents.

Idiopathic childhood occipital epilepsy of Gastaut

Epidemiology

This is a pure form of idiopathic occipital epilepsy with an onset at a peak age of 8–9 years (range 3–15 years).

Clinical features

Patients have frequent visual seizures of mainly elementary visual hallucinations, blindness, or both (see symptomatic occipital epilepsy). Spreading to temporal lobe involvement is exceptional and may indicate a symptomatic cause. Interictal EEG shows occipital spikes or occipital paroxysms. Ictal onset with fast spikes is unilateral from the occipital regions.

Prognosis and treatment

Prognosis is unpredictable. Half of patients will remit within 2–4 years from onset. The others will continue having seizures, particularly if not appropriately treated with carbamazepine or other first-line agents for focal seizures.

Monogenic focal epilepsies

Monogenic (single-gene) focal epilepsies have been identified in large families with an epileptic trait segregating in the absence of environmental factors. In these families, phenotypes are determined by mutations in susceptibility genes, some of which have been identified or localized. Most of the genes discovered code for either voltage-gated or ligand-gated ion channel subunits. Genetic polymorphisms have been identified that result in marked ethnic and interindividual differences in response to treatment.

Benign familial neonatal seizures

Etiology

This is an autosomal dominant disorder with 85% degree of penetrance. Mutations in the voltage-gated potassium channel subunit gene *KCNQ2* on chromosome 20q13.3 and *KCNQ3* on chromosome 8q24 produce the same phenotype. However, a recent study demonstrated that the same *KCNQ2* mutations also cause early-onset epileptic encephalopathies.

Clinical features

Seizures mainly start in the first week of life of full-term normal neonates. Seizures are brief, usually 1–2 min, and may be as frequent as 20–30 per day. Most seizures start with tonic motor activity and posturing with apnoea followed by vocalizations, ocular symptoms, other autonomic features, motor automatisms, chewing, and focal or generalized clonic movements. Pure clonic or focal seizures are rare.

Prognosis and treatment

Prognosis is good with normal development. Seizures remit between 1 and 6 months from onset, but 10–14% may later develop other types of seizures. Development occurs. AED may not be needed.

Benign familial infantile seizures

Etiology

Benign familial infantile seizures (BFIS) is probably an autosomal dominant disorder with genetic heterogeneity. Mutations in the prolin-rich transmembrane protein 2 gene (*PRTT2*) have recently been found in 70–80% of BFIS (Zara *et al.*). *PRTT2* mutations are also responsible for infantile convulsions with choreoathetosis syndrome (ICCA) and autosomal dominant paroxysmal kinesigenic dyskinesia (PKD). In the remaining cases, *KCNQ2*, *KCNQ3*, and *SCN2A* may be involved. In case of non-familial infantile seizures, *PRTT2* mutations are found to be low.

Clinical features

The seizures start at 3–20 months (peak at 5–6 months) in otherwise normal infants. They consist of motion arrest, decreased responsiveness, staring, eye and head deviation, simple automatisms, and mild clonic movements. They may progress to generalized convulsions. Alternating from one side to the other is common. Duration is usually short, from 30 sec to 3 min. They occur in clusters of a maximum of 8–10 per day for 1–3 days and may recur after 1–3 months.

Prognosis and treatment

Prognosis is excellent, with normal development and complete seizure remission. In the active seizure period, empirical drug treatment is usually effective.

Autosomal dominant nocturnal frontal lobe epilepsy

Epidemiology

The age at seizure onset ranges from 1–50 years of age, but most cases (85%) start earlier than age 20 (mean age 8–11.5 years).

Etiology

Autosomal dominant nocturnal frontal lobe epilepsy (ADNFLE) is an autosomal dominant disorder with 70% penetrance. Mutations have been identified in three genes encoding neuronal nicotinic acetylcholine receptor alpha 4, alpha 2, or beta 2 protein subunits in approximately 20% of individuals with a positive family history. *KCNT1* mutations are also implicated in severe cases.

Clinical features

Most patients are intellectually and neurologically normal. The clinical seizures are mainly nocturnal and are characterized by brief, less than 1 min motor attacks occurring in clusters. Typically, patients wake up with non-specific aura and manifest with vocalization, grasping or grunting, and hyperkinetic attacks of the extremities or dystonic seizures lasting less than 1 min. Consciousness is usually intact. The attacks are often misdiagnosed as nocturnal parasomnias, night terror, or nightmares. Infrequent secondarily generalized convulsions occur in 60% of cases.

Prognosis and treatment

Seizure frequency and prognosis are different among patients even in the same family. With carbamazepine or other sodium channel blockers, two-thirds of patients become seizure free. The other one-third have poor seizure outcome. In these patients, surgical treatment may be justified if an accurate presurgical evaluation can define the epileptogenic zone.

Familial mesial temporal lobe epilepsy

Epidemiology

Seizures typically start after the age of 10, with a median in the mid-30s.

Etiology

Familial mesial temporal lobe epilepsy (FMTLE) is a genetic disorder with a complex mode of inheritance. The genetic locus was found on chromosomes 4q, 18p, and 3q.

Clinical features

They mainly manifest with déjà vu, other mental illusions and hallucinations, fear, and panic. Consciousness is usually (90%) intact. Ascending epigastric sensation does not occur. Two-thirds of patients also have infrequent secondarily generalized tonic–clonic seizures.

Prognosis and treatment

The prognosis is usually good and seizures are easily controlled with carbamazepine or other narrow- or broad-spectrum AEDs. The phenotype can be variable, however, with some cases becoming refractory, but with good response to surgical therapy.

Familial lateral temporal lobe epilepsy

Etiology

Familial lateral temporal lobe epilepsy (FLTLE) is of autosomal dominant inheritance with high penetrance (about 80%). It is the first non-ion channel familial epilepsy to have been discovered. Mutations have been identified in the leucine-rich, glioma-inactivated 1 (*LGI1*) epitempin gene on chromosome 10q. Autoantibody to *LGL1* protein has also been found to cause limbic encephalitis.

Clinical features

FLTLE and autosomal dominant focal epilepsy with auditory features are the same disorder caused by defects in the same gene. The age at seizure onset ranges from 11–40 years, with an average of 24 years. The seizures are characterized by simple elementary auditory hallucinations arising from the lateral temporal lobe. EEG and SPECT (single photon emission computed tomography) tests indicate epileptic foci in the temporal lobe.

Prognosis and treatment

Prognosis and response to carbamazepine or other AEDs are excellent.

Familial partial epilepsy with variable foci

Epidemiology

Age at onset varies markedly (range from months to 43 years), although the mean age at onset of seizures is 13 years.

Etiology

The syndrome is of autosomal dominant inheritance with 60% penetrance and genetic heterogeneity. A *DEPDC5* (Dishevelled, Egl-10, and Pleckstrin-domain-containing protein 5) gene mutation was found on chromosome 22q, which may be a common cause of familial focal epilepsy.

Clinical features

The defining feature of this syndrome is that different family members have focal seizures emanating from different cortical locations, including temporal, frontal, centroparietal, and occipital regions. Each individual patient has an electroclinical pattern of single-location, focal epilepsy. Seizures are often nocturnal, and there is great intrafamilial variability.

Prognosis and treatment

Severity varies among family members: some are asymptomatic, manifesting with only an EEG spike focus; and most are easily controlled with AEDs, although a few may be intractable to medication.

Symptomatic or cryptogenic LRE

Symptomatic LRE are of known pathology and are largely classified according to anatomical localization into temporal, frontal, parietal, and occipital lobe epilepsies. Cryptogenic epilepsy, a term used for probably symptomatic epilepsy for which the etiology has not been identified, is included in this section. LRE may be further classified into limbic or neocortical epilepsy.

Etiology

Structural causes include malformations of cortical development, hippocampal atrophy, tumors, vascular, traumatic, viral, and other infectious and parasitic disorders, and cerebrovascular disease.

Diagnostic procedures

Magnetic resonance imaging (MRI) provides *in vivo* visualization of the abnormal brain tissue in nearly all patients with symptomatic LRE. The interictal EEG usually demonstrates focal slow-wave activity and EEG spikes. The yield of interictal EEG abnormalities varies from around 30–70% in temporal lobe epilepsy to as little as 5–50% in frontal lobe epilepsy.

Temporal lobe epilepsy (TLE)

Epidemiology

TLE constitutes nearly two-thirds of symptomatic LRE of adolescence and adulthood. It is divided into mesial and lateral TLE. Mesial TLE is the commoner form and includes hippocampal epilepsy.

Clinical features

Most patients have a characteristic clinical course, often starting with febrile seizures during infancy, and developing simple and complex focal seizures (dyscognitive seizures) several years later. The seizures manifest with ascending epigastric sensation and fear followed by oral or gestural automatisms. They usually last 1–2 minutes and leave short-lasting confusional state. Brain MRI reveals unilateral hippocampal sclerosis (Figure 34.2). Lateral TLE manifests with simple and complex focal seizures with auditory hallucinations or illusions, vestibular phenomena, experiential symptoms, or complex visual hallucinations or illusions. Motor ictal symptoms include clonic movements, dystonic posturing, and motor automatisms when the seizure spreads out of the temporal lobe. Impairment of consciousness is not as pronounced as with mesial TLE.

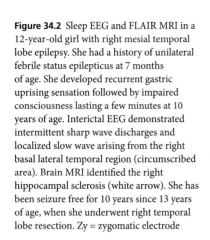
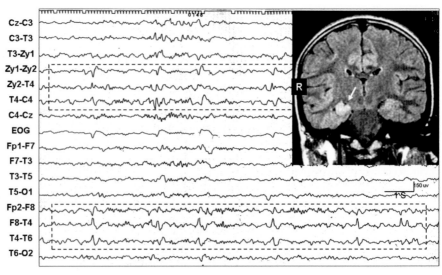

Figure 34.2 Sleep EEG and FLAIR MRI in a 12-year-old girl with right mesial temporal lobe epilepsy. She had a history of unilateral febrile status epilepticus at 7 months of age. She developed recurrent gastric uprising sensation followed by impaired consciousness lasting a few minutes at 10 years of age. Interictal EEG demonstrated intermittent sharp wave discharges and localized slow wave arising from the right basal lateral temporal region (circumscribed area). Brain MRI identified the right hippocampal sclerosis (white arrow). She has been seizure free for 10 years since 13 years of age, when she underwent right temporal lobe resection. Zy = zygomatic electrode

Frontal lobe epilepsy

Epidemiology
Frontal lobe epilepsy (FLE) is the most common LRE following TLE.

Clinical features
The clinical seizure manifestations differ significantly according to the localization of the epileptogenic focus within the frontal lobe, although they tend to show abrupt onset, short duration, rapid secondary generalization, and minimal or no postictal confusional state, and occur in clusters. Nocturnal attacks are relatively common. There are three broad categories of seizure types: focal clonic motor seizures, asymmetric tonic seizures, and frontal lobe complex focal seizures.

The focal clonic motor seizures arise from the motor cortex and involve the orofacial and/or ipsilateral arm or both arm and leg, and at times spread with Jacksonian march. Asymmetric tonic/dystonic seizures arise from the supplementary sensory motor cortex and manifest with one arm being flexed and the other extended, the legs being flexed or extended (see ADNFLE). Consciousness is frequently preserved during the attacks.

Frontal complex focal seizures are associated with screaming or bizarre violent behavior, previously misdiagnosed as hysterical attacks. These are now classified as hypermotor attacks. Vegetative and autonomic symptoms can arise from the insular region or cingulate cortex. Seizures with frontal lobe automatisms can also originate in the cingulate cortex.

Parietal lobe epilepsy

Clinical features
The seizures of parietal lobe epilepsy (PLE) are usually difficult to identify prior to their spreading to adjacent brain areas and manifesting with more overt ictal symptoms there. In PLE, simple focal seizures predominate. Subjective ictal symptoms are somatosensory (paresthetic, dysesthetic, and painful sensations), disturbances of body image, vertiginous, visual illusions, or complex formed visual hallucinations. Medial parietal seizures can propagate anteriorly and be mistaken for supplementary motor seizures, while supramarginal gyrus attacks may be mistaken for an aphasic stroke.

Occipital lobe epilepsy (OLE)

Clinical features
OLE, accounting for 5–10% of all symptomatic LREs, is much easier to locate by symptoms than other symptomatic LREs. Seizures develop in seconds and they are usually brief (seconds to a minute), with elementary visual hallucinations that are mainly circular and multicolored. Postictal headache occurs in half of visual seizures. Blindness may occur from onset. The seizures of OLE are entirely different from the visual aura of migraine, for which they are commonly misdiagnosed. The seizures may spread to temporal or frontal lobes, generating TLE or FLE seizures and secondary generalizations.

Prognosis and treatment
The natural history of TLE is variable, with as many as 30–40% of patients continuing to have seizures despite appropriate medical treatments. In other symptomatic LRE, known cause, congenital neurological deficits, frequent secondarily generalized convulsions, need for multiple medications, and epileptic EEG abnormality all reduce the likelihood of remission. The treatment of symptomatic LRE is independent of etiology or anatomical localization. The first-line AEDs are oxcarbazepine or carbamazepine, levetiracetam, and lamotrigine, followed by topiramate, zonisamide, and phenytoin. Recent progress in epilepsy surgery has enabled 70–90% of patients with mesial TLE to become seizure free. In patients with refractory extratemporal lobe epilepsies, the surgical result is not always satisfactory, especially without well-circumscribed MRI lesions, but some reports (including Swartz *et al.*) find that 75% may be improved. Vagus nerve stimulation may be a good alternative for these difficult cases.

Further reading
Commission on Classification and Terminology of the International League Against Epilepsy. Proposal for revised classification of epilepsies and epileptic syndromes. *Epilepsia* 1989;30:389–399.

Ferrie C, Caraballo R, Covanis A, *et al.* Panayiotopoulos syndrome: A consensus view. *Dev Med Child Neurol* 2006;48:236–240.

Gourfinkel-An I, Baulac S, Nabbout R, *et al.* Monogenic idiopathic epilepsies. *Lancet Neurol* 2004;3:209–218.

Koutroumanidis M, Ferrie CD, Valeta T, *et al.* Syncope-like epileptic seizures in Panayiotopoulos syndrome. *Neurology* 2012;79:463–467.

Lemke JR, Lal D, Reinthaler EM, *et al.* Mutations in GRIN2A cause idiopathic focal epilepsy with rolandic spikes. *Nat Genet* 2013;45:1067–1072.

Neubauer BA, Fiedler B, Himmelein B, *et al.* Centrotemporal spikes in families with Rolandic epilepsy: Linkage to chromosome 15q14. *Neurology* 1998;51(6):1608–1612.

Oxbury JM, Polkey CE, Duchowny M (eds.). *Intractable Focal Epilepsy.* London: WB Saunders; 2000.

Panayiotopoulos CP. *A Clinical Guide to Epileptic Syndromes and Their Treatment,* 2nd ed. London: Springer; 2010.

Panayiotopoulos CP, Bureau M, Caraballo RH, Bernardina BD, Valeta T. Idiopathic focal epilepsies in childhood. In: BureauM, GentonP, DravetC, *et al.* (eds.). *Epileptic Syndromes in Infancy, Childhood and Adolescence,* 5th ed. with video. Montrouge, France: John Libbey Eurotext; 2012:217–254.

Scheffer IE. The role of genetics and ethnicity in epilepsy management. *Acta Neurol Scand Suppl* 2005;181:47–51.

Swartz, BE, Delgado-Escueta AV, Walsh GO, *et al.* Surgical outcomes in pure frontal epilepsies and foci that mimic ehem. *Epilepsy Res* 1998;29:97–108.

Wyllie E, Gupta A, Lachhwani D (eds.). *The Treatment of Epilepsy: Principles and Practice,* 5th ed. Philadelphia, PA: Lippincott Williams & Wilkins; 2011.

Zara F, Specchio N, Striano P, *et al.* Genetic testing in benign familial epilepsies of the first year of life: Clinical and diagnostic significance. *Epilepsia* 2013;54:425–436.

35 Neurodiagnostic tools for the paroxysmal disorders

Barbara E. Swartz

Epilepsy Center and Neurophysiology Laboratory, Renown Neuroscience Institute, University of Nevada, Reno, NV, USA

A careful neurological history and examination is the first key to diagnosing the paroxysmal disorders. Seizures are synonymous with abnormal electrical activity of the brain. Thus, electroencephalogram (EEG) techniques, old and new, are the next diagnostic approach. For other paroxysmal disorders EEG may be used in conjunction with other tests (e.g., tilt-table EEG for syncope evaluation). People with epilepsy also must have a neuroimaging test to search for the etiology of the seizures. Genetic panels are increasingly relied on for syndrome diagnoses, but will not be discussed in this chapter.

Electrophysiology

Although neuroimaging has greatly enhanced our understanding of the epilepsies, electrophysiological techniques remain the gold standard diagnostic tool, simply because they actually measure the brain's electrophysiological function in real time. These techniques are rapidly changing with the almost universal reliance on digital systems.

Electroencephalography

The brain's electrical activity can be directly recorded with proper filtering and amplification. Analogue recording systems have been available commercially since the mid-1900s, but the size of the components limited the number of channels. Nevertheless, using machines with 8 or 12 channels, the early EEG pioneers made contributions to the understanding of brain function that are nearly unparalleled by other disciplines. The filter settings of the standard Grass EEG machine were based on the mechanical characteristics of the pens, amplifiers, and so on. The frequencies that could be detected were divided into delta (0.5–3Hz), theta (3.5–7.5 Hz), alpha (8–12 Hz), and beta 12.5–30 Hz (sometimes broken into low and high beta). These are simply artificial descriptions of a continuum that starts at DC and extends into the 500 Hz range in humans. Today, 32–40 channels of EEG are routine, the 10-10 system proposed by the ILAE in 1994 to replace the 10-20 system has 65 positions, and high-density EEG (128 or more channels) can provide increasingly precise information.

The parameters used to interpret an EEG are space, time, frequency, and amplitude. In diagnosing epilepsy one looks for epileptiform sharps (75–250 msec), spikes (20–75 msec), and spike wave bursts. Focal polymorphic delta slowing or focal rhythmic theta in the temporal area is highly correlated with the seizure focus. The EEG pattern can indicate the epilepsy syndrome: focal spikes in focal epilepsy; multifocal independent spike waves in epileptic encephalopathies; 4–6 Hz frontal maximum polyspike waves in juvenile myoclonic epilepsy; 3 Hz generalized polyspike waves in other generalized genetic epilepsies, and so on. High-frequency continuous spike bursts (CEDS) are highly indicative of cortical dysplasia.

A routine EEG is usually 20 minutes long and has a limited sensitivity of about 30% in focal epilepsy, 50% in generalized epilepsies. Sleep deprivation and prolongation of the record (to 40–60 min) increase the sensitivity greatly. Three routine EEGs will pick up 80–85% of focal epilepsy discharges. Hyperventilation for 3–5 min is used to increase sensitivity, by increasing the chance both of spikes and of focal slowing. Photic stimulation induces epileptiform activity in 20% of cases of genetic, generalized epilepsy, and infrequently in temporal lobe epilepsy. When doubt persists, ambulatory recording can be useful (24–48 hours).

The analysis of EEG has been based on pattern recognition, with some attempt at quantification of the frequencies, amplitudes, and electrical fields done by the reader. Now montages and all other parameters can be changed with a mouse click. Additional analysis of surface current densities, dipole source localization, power spectra, and wave form correlations are readily performed with commercially available systems and a determined reader. These are quite powerful when combined with a neuroimaging tool.

Video EEG

Video EEG (VEEG) is the gold standard for epilepsy diagnosis and should be carried out for at least 72 hours to achieve specificity as well as sensitivity for the location of the seizure focus, and clarification of the epilepsy syndrome, and to avoid false negatives when diagnosing non-epileptiform seizures (NES). Withdrawal of antiepileptic drugs is indicated for subjects with infrequent seizures. Numerous other paroxysmal disorders can be indicated by a VEEG study, including heart block, syncopal convulsions, restless legs, and non-epileptiform seizures. VEEG can be done with the 10-20 placement, the 10-10 system, high-density EEG, or intracranial EEG. The video recording of the behavioral characteristics under consideration (seizure semiology) is time-locked to the digital EEG recording. Detection is by the patient, seizure and spike detection programs, and direct observation by trained staff, which is necessary whenever medications are withdrawn. Numerous researchers are making promising advances in the area of seizure prediction models.

International Neurology, Second edition. Edited by Robert P. Lisak, Daniel D. Truong, William M. Carroll and Roongroj Bhidayasiri
© 2016 John Wiley & Sons, Ltd. Published 2016 by John Wiley & Sons, Ltd.

Intracranial recordings

If EEG is recorded from the surface of the brain during surgery it is called electrocorticography (ECoG). Intracranial EEG recordings can be made on a more prolonged basis, as discussed in Chapter 37. The video is again time-locked to EEG to correlate the seizure semiology with the seizure onset zone. In general, a low-voltage fast pattern associated with high-frequency discharges (up to 500 Hz) can occur at the seizure focus at onset, gradually slowing and increasing in amplitude as spread to neighboring locations occurs. Evaluating the semiology is itself a demanding technique. Several attempts to standardize semiology with epilepsy classification have been published by the International League Against Epilepsy.

Magnetoencephalography

Magnetoencephalography (MEG) is a relatively new technique for analyzing brain function. It measures the tangential magnetic fields that are generated by the radial electrical fields of the brain, and is less affected than EEG by sources of artifact like the skull, other electrical devices in the vicinity, movement of wires, and so on. The best studies comparing MEG, which is always a high-density recording, with high-density recording EEG show comparable but complementary sensitivities. One exciting new application is the ability to do functional mapping with MEG without the need for intracranial EEG recordings. MEG is particularly useful in planning the placement of intracranial grids. A cluster of MEG spikes (≥ 5) within 2 cm is highly correlated with the seizure focus, whereas random scattered MEG spikes are not.

Neuroimaging

Computerized axial tomography and magnetic resonance imaging

These are the work horses of epilepsy imaging. Numerous studies have shown the superiority of magnetic resonance imaging (MRI) to computed tomography (CT), but CT remains in use in many developing countries and is used in most emergency rooms in developed nations. The sensitivity of the CT scan for a lesion leading to epilepsy is approximately 50%, but there are few false negatives with an intracranial bleed, and it is superior to MRI when calcification is present. The sensitivity of an MRI is about 85% in epilepsy. The standard sequences are both T1 and T2 with thin contiguous slices (1–2 mm) sagittal, axial, and coronal, with additional FLAIR axial and coronal studies. Other techniques such as contrast and various sequences (proton density, diffusion/perfusion) can improve detection. Diffusion tensor imaging has emerged as a powerful tool for looking at white-matter pathways (tractography). Surface coils or high Tesla magnet MRI can show areas of cortical dysplasia that are not demonstrated in a routine scan, which has led to a new classification of pathology.

Functional imaging

This usually refers to 18 FDG-PET (18-fluorodeoxyglucose positron emission tomography) or SPECT (single photon emission computerized tomography). The former measures glucose uptake into cells (which has been shown to be highly correlated with synaptic activity), while the latter is a measure of cerebral blood flow. Both are used in the presurgical evaluation of focal epilepsies. FDG-PET is a sensitive interictal test, and spatial resolution is improved by MRI coregistration. Ictal SPECT can be useful for identifying foci and planning intracranial recordings, particularly if performed with subtraction ictal SPECT coregistered to MRI. The latter is more cumbersome to arrange, and therefore less practical than FDG-PET. Some institutions have access to ligand PET. The ligands that appear most useful in epilepsy diagnosis at this time are flumazenil PET and PET that marks presynaptic serotonin receptors.

Functional MRI

Functional MRI is dominating the field for imaging of cognitive brain functions. It takes advantage of the fact that localized cerebral blood flow increases are associated with increased neuronal activity and that this shifts the ratio of oxy- to deoxyhemoglobin, which changes the paramagnetic signal produced by hemoglobin. Functional MRI is quite useful for presurgical mapping of the sensory motor cortex. Mapping of visual cortex and auditory cortex is possible, although rarely used clinically. Mapping of language cortex is possible and quite reliable for lateralization, although it tends to be overly sensitive for localization. Mapping of declarative memory (medial temporal function) is not yet standardized, but will some day replace the Wada test for presurgical evaluation.

MRS

Magnetic resonance spectroscopy produces a spectrum that is unique for any given chemical that has free protons in its outer electron orbit. N-acetyl acetate (NAA), a neuronal marker, and Choline (Cho) and Creatnine (Cr), glial markers, are usually measured and presented as a ratio [NAA/(/Cr, Cr/Cho))]. Glutamine + glutamate are measured in a complex peak called Glx. Abnormalities have been shown (decreased ratio) in scarring, tumors, and dysplasias. Other substances can be measured, but are for research only at this time.

Other techniques

Other techniques such as optical imaging are under investigation.

Conclusion

Multimodal tools exist for the evaluation of epilepsy or its imitators. Increasing use of more complex analytic tools is changing many of our old concepts about epilepsy and its syndromes.

Further reading

Fink R, Pedersen B, Guekht AB, *et al*; Commission on European Affairs: Subcommission on European Guidelines. Guidelines for the use of EEG methodology in the diagnosis of epilepsy. International League Against Epilepsy: Commission report. *Acta Neurol Scand* 2002;106:1–7.

Kuzniecky RI, Knowlton RC. Neuroimaging of epilepsy. *Semin Neurol* 2002;22(3):279–288.

Schomer DL, Lopes da Silva FH. Niedermeyer's Electroencephalography: Basic Principles, Clinical Applications, and Related Fields. Lippincott, William & Wilkins, 2011.

Scherg M, Ille N, Bornfleth H, Berg P. Advanced tools for digital EEG review: Virtual source montages, whole head mapping, correlation and phase analysis. *J Clin Neuorphysiol* 2002;19:91–112.

Swartz, BE, Patell A, Thomas K, *et al*. The use of 18-FDG (PET) positron emission tomography in the routine diagnosis of epilepsy. *J Mol Imaging Biol* 2002;4:245–252.

36 Neuropharmacology of antiepileptic drugs

Paul B. Pritchard, III

Department of Neurosciences, Medical University of South Carolina, Charleston, SC, USA

Although surgical treatment, brain stimulation, and dietary therapy hold promise, antiepileptic drugs (AEDs) remain the cornerstone for the treatment of epilepsy. One may distinguish between the anticonvulsant effect of a drug – the potential to stop epileptic seizures – and the antiepileptic effect – the potential to reverse underlying pathophysiology – but this chapter will simply refer to drugs used in the treatment of epilepsy as AEDs. Dietary therapy, surgical resection, and brain stimulation are discussed in other chapters of this book.

History of antiepileptic drugs

Bromides were the first effective pharmacological agents for epileptic seizures, first touted in 1857 by Charles Locock for the treatment of "hysterical seizures" in women. The premise for the use of bromides was based on the faulty concept that these attacks resulted from the "nervous habit" of masturbation. Dr. Locock's rationale was that bromides would combat underlying nervous tension, diminish one's propensity to masturbate, and thereby combat epilepsy. The demonstration that bromides were effective in the treatment of epilepsy reinforced this misinformed pathophysiology. Ultimately, the inordinate frequency of dermatological reactions to bromides limited their use.

In 1912, Alfred Hauptman in Freiburg serendipitously discovered the antiepileptic qualities of phenobarbital when he prescribed it as a sedative to prevent his psychiatric patients from falling out of bed at night, thereby reducing the number of calls he received as a psychiatric resident on call! Fortunately, he also observed that the patients had a reduction in their seizures after he gave them phenobarbital. The drug reduced and sometimes halted epileptic seizures but, like bromides, also caused sedation.

At the Boston City Hospital, Tracy Putnam used the electroshock method with cats to screen multiple drugs for their antiepileptic effects after they had been found to be ineffective as sedatives. He demonstrated that phenytoin prevented electroshock seizures. Houston Merritt subsequently verified the application of phenytoin as an effective treatment for human epilepsy. Phenytoin was marketed for clinical use in 1935. Serendipity led to the recognition of valproic acid as an AED. While working as a graduate student at the University of Lyon, Pierre Eymard used valproic acid (VPA) as a solvent to dissolve a variety of compounds under investigation. He observed that the animal used in the models under study no longer developed seizures in response to proconvulsant drugs, and he correctly attributed the antiepileptic effect to VPA. Further investigation led to the successful clinical application of VPA and its sodium salt as AEDs in human epilepsy.

For decades the two major models of epileptogenicity were the maximal electroshock-induced seizures and pentylenetetrazol-induced seizures. In general, prevention of electroshock seizures predicts efficacy in partial epilepsies, while effectiveness for pentylenetetrazol-induced seizures favors utility for primary generalized epilepsies. More recently the kindling model has been used to predict efficacy, as with levetiracetam, and the zebrafish embryo model has also been used as the pentylenetetrazol model. *In vitro* investigations of binding capacity, ion channel modulation, and excitability are increasingly used prior to animal models.

Sometimes the spectrum of antiepileptic effects is not predicted by these models. Investigators strive to develop AEDs that are (1) more effective in seizure control; and (2) associated with fewer adverse effects and complications.

Mechanisms of action for antiepileptic drugs

There are numerous mechanisms by which AEDs may modify neuronal excitability. These include (1) decreasing glutamatergic excitation (AMPA receptors, kainate receptors – topiramate); (2) blocking voltage-dependent sodium or calcium channels (oxcarbazepine, valproate, zonisamide); (3) increasing GABAergic inhibition (barbiturates, benzodiazepines, gabapentin); and (4) impairing synaptic vesicle function (levetiracetam).

Other anti-ictal mechanisms are outlined in Table 36.1, but bear in mind that many AEDs have multiple potential mechanisms of action. It is often unclear from which of these mechanisms the clinical benefit is derived. It is possible that multiple mechanisms of action explain the broad-spectrum effectiveness of a given drug. It is worth noting that to date no clinically effective antiepileptic drug has been shown to be antiepileptogenic, with numerous failed trials. Recent data suggest that ethosuccimide may be associated with a more favorable outcome than valproic acid when used as the first agent in primary absence epilepsy.

Table 36.1 Mechanisms of action for antiepileptic drugs.

Mechanism of action	Antiepileptic drugs
Na+ channel blockade (rapid inactivation phase)	CBZ, LMT, OXC, PHT, ZNS
Na+ channel blockage (slow inactivation phase)	LCM
Ca++ channel antagonists	ESX, GBP, LMT, PGB, VPA, ZNS
Enhance GABA inhibitory effects	TGB, VGB
Reduce glutamatergic excitation	FBM, PER, TPM, VPA
Decrease presynaptic transmitter release	LEV
Inhibit carbonic anhydrase	TPM, ZNS
Decrease AMPA glutaminergic sites	PER

CBZ = carbamazepine; ESX = ethosuximide; FBM = felbamate; GBP = gabapentin; LCM = lacosamide; LEV = levetiracetam; LMT = lamotrigine; OXC = oxcarbazepine; PER = perampanel; PGB = pregabalin; PHT = phenytoin; TGB = tiagabine; TPM = topiramate; VPA = valproate; VGB = vigabatrin; ZNS = zonisamide

Rationale for antiepileptic drug selection: Choice of initial drug

There are well over two dozen antiepileptic drugs available. Several factors should be considered in the selection of an initial antiepileptic drug, including spectrum of action, pharmacokinetics, and associated medical illness. We will consider each of these in turn.

Spectrum of action

The choice of the initial AED should be primarily based on the accurate diagnosis of the patient's epileptic disorder and the selection of a drug that has the appropriate spectrum of effective antiepileptic action for that particular case. Some AEDs have a broad-spectrum effective action against primary generalized epilepsies and partial epilepsies. In contrast, ethosuximide has a narrow spectrum of effectiveness and is useful for absence seizures alone. Table 36.2 summarizes the therapeutic spectrum for AEDs in current use.

Certain AEDs appear to exert a proconvulsant effect toward some types of epileptic seizures, in particular absence and myoclonic events. Phenytoin, carbamazepine, and vigabatrin are known to exacerbate myoclonic seizures, while tiagabine, vigabatrin, and carbamazepine may provoke absence seizures. The basis for this paradoxical effect is unclear. However, in general, GABAergic drugs are contraindicated in primary generalized epilepsies. Specific antiepileptic drugs can be harmful to certain epilepsy syndromes, for example sodium channel blockers in Dravet syndrome, and phenytoin in Undvericht–Lundborg syndrome (Baltic myoclonus).

Pharmacokinetics and compliance

The number of medication doses required per day is the best predictor of patient compliance: the degree of compliance is inversely proportional to the number of doses required. This factor confers an advantage to AEDs with more lengthy elimination half-lives, such as zonisamide, phenobarbital, phenytoin, and perampanel, all of which are dosed once daily. Extended-release versions of other AEDs offer similar advantages. AEDs that require three or more doses per day present increased challenges to patient compliance.

Route of administration

The availability of liquid forms as suspensions or elixirs of the AED also has an impact on compliance, particularly in the pediatric population or in adults who find it difficult to swallow tablets or capsules. AEDs that have intravenous formulations (lorazepam,

Table 36.2 Therapeutic spectrum of antiepileptic drugs.

AED	Absence	Myoclonic	Partial seizures (SPS or CPS)	Secondarily generalized Tonic–clonic
CBZ	0	0	+	+
ESX	+	0	0	0
FBM	+	+	+	+
GBP	0	0	+	+
LCM	0	0	+	+
LTG	+	+	+	+
LEV	+	+	+	+
OXC	0	0	+	+
PB	0	0	+	+
PER	0	0	+	+
PGB	0	0	+	+
PHT	0	0	+	+
PRM	0	0	+	+
TGB	0	0	+	+
TPM	+	+	+	+
VPA	+	+	+	+
VGB	-	-	+	+
ZNS	+	+	+	+

CBZ = carbamazepine; CPS = complex partial seizures; ESX = ethosuximide; FBM = felbamate; GBP = gabapentin; LCM = lacosamide; LEV = levetiracetam; LTG = lamotrigine; OXC = oxcarbazepine; PB = phenobarbital; PER = perampanel; PGB = pregabalin; PHT = phenytoin; PRM = primidone; SPS = simple partial seizures; TGB = tiagabine; TPM = topiramate; VGB = vigabatrin; VPA = valproate; ZNS = zonisamide diazepam, phenobarbital, phenytoin, levetiracetam, valproic acid, and pregabalin) provide the advantage of rapid administration for frequent seizures or status epilepticus, and for obtunded patients who are temporarily unable to take the drug orally. Rectal diazepam and intranasal midazolam are also useful to abort seizure clusters or prolonged seizures.

Associated medical illness

Associated medical illness may be a deterrent to the use of AEDs that have the potential for toxic effects on diseased organ systems (Table 36.3). Even though valproate-induced pancreatitis is uncommon, the clinician should be reluctant to use valproate in a patient with pancreatic disease. If weight loss is already an issue, one would avoid topiramate, zonisamide, and felbamate if effective alternatives can be employed. By the same token, AEDs associated with weight gain, such as valproate and gabapentin, are not attractive to patients who are already obese.

On the other hand, associated medical illness can present the opportunity to use a single AED as a dual therapy for epilepsy and the other illness. Dual benefit is most often achieved with other neurological disorders plus epilepsy or with psychiatric disorders. Neurological disorders for which AEDs are effective treatment include neuropathic pain, essential tremor, and migraine. Epilepsy occurs with greater than expected frequency among those suffering from migraine and vice versa. Anxiety disorder and depression also occur with increased frequency among those who have epilepsy.

Other conditions treated with antiepileptic drugs

Essential tremor

Essential tremor (ET) is the most common movement disorder, affecting approximately 4% of the general population. A knockout

model in mice suggests that a deficiency in the alpha-1 subunit in the GABA-A receptor is the basis for the tremor. In humans there is evidence that the loss of inhibitory input through cerebellar Purkinje cell dysfunction causes the tremor. Assuming this to be the case, AEDs that have a GABAergic action have the potential to reduce the tremor. The AED most well supported by clinical trials is topiramate, but there are data that suggest effectiveness for gabapentin and zonisamide as well. While the primary antiepileptic effect of zonisamide is on voltage-gated ion channels, there is also evidence that it enhances GABA release.

Migraine

As with epilepsy, neuronal excitation plays a role in the pathogenesis of migraine. The potential for cortical excitability in migraine consequent to an imbalance between glutamatergic excitation and GABAergic inhibition may be of pathogenic importance. Components of migraine include altered pain sensation, inflammation, and vasodilatation. To the extent that this pathogenesis is valid, AEDs that counter these effects could provide antimigraine prophylaxis. Recently the role of channelopathies in refractory migraine and chronic pain, as well as epilepsy, has suggested possible links between these conditions.

Valproate and topiramate have the most supportive clinical trials and most widespread clinical use as antimigraine agents. There is also favorable evidence from randomized clinical trials that gabapentin, lamotrigine, and levetiracetam are effective for antimigraine prophylaxis. Effects on GABAergic mechanisms could be the basis for the clinical effectiveness against migraine of these drugs, but definitive evidence has been elusive.

Neuropathic pain

Neuropathic pain, whether of central or peripheral origin, is a perplexing clinical problem, the underlying basis for which is injury to sensory neurons, followed by abnormal neuronal sprouting and dysfunctional ion channels in peripheral nerves or the spinal cord. Pathological plasticity of sodium and calcium ion channels is recognized as the basis for the hyperalgesia and allodynia that accompany neuropathic pain.

Multiple clinical trials support the efficacy of carbamazepine, phenytoin, tiagabine, gabapentin, lamotrigine, topiramate, levetiracetam, oxcarbazepine, zonisamide, and valproate for neuropathic pain. Their inhibition of ion channels to decrease excitatory glutamatergic neurotransmission is the likely basis for effective action, but there are variations in the underlying mechanisms of action for these drugs. Gabapentin and pregabalin are considered first-line drugs for neuropathic pain, based on evidence-based guidelines and tolerability.

Psychiatric disorders

Psychiatric disorders that may benefit from AEDs include anxiety and bipolar affective disorder. Disordered GABA transmission has been implicated as the basis for anxiety. The first evidence for the GABAergic mechanism came from the observed efficacy of benzodiazepines, known to enhance GABAergic effect, in treating anxiety. The efficacy and tolerability of tiagabine also have been demonstrated in randomized controlled studies. There is similar evidence to support the use of vigabatrin for anxiety, but the potential of this drug to cause irreversible visual field defects has limited its use.

Table 36.3 Organ toxicity and antiepileptic drugs

Organ system	Antiepileptic drug/effect
Dermatological	PHT (hirsutism), VPA (alopecia, changes in hair color)
Endocrine	VPA (oligospermia, ovarian cysts)
Hematopoietic	CBZ, VPA (thrombocytopenia), FBM (aplastic anemia), CBZ (agranulocytosis)
Hepatic	FBM (hepatic necrosis), VPA (hyperammonemia)
Oral	PHT (gingival hyperplasia)
Pancreatic	VPA, CBZ (pancreatitis)
Renal	TPM, ZNS (nephrolithiasis)
Osseous	PHT, PB, CBZ, VPA (osteoporosis)
Ocular	VGB (concentric visual field defect), TPM (glaucoma)
Neurological	PHT (neuropathy, cerebellar atrophy, choreoathetosis)
Teratogenic	CBZ (spina bifida), PHT (fetal hydantoin syndrome; cardiac anomalies), VPA (cognitive impairment; spina bifida)

CBZ = carbamazepine; FBM = felbamate; PB = phenobarbital; PHT = phenytoin; TPM = topiramate; VGB = vigabatrin; VPA = valproate; ZNS = zonisamide

Bipolar disorder includes two major subtypes: bipolar I (manic and depressive phases) and bipolar II (hypomanic and depressive phases). Dysfunction of dopaminergic neurons, glutamatergic neurotransmission, and inositol signaling have all been theorized as pathogenetic mechanisms for bipolar disorder. The best evidence for AEDs as effective treatment for bipolar disorders rests with valproate, carbamazepine, and lamotrigine.

Failure of initial treatment: Rationale for replacement of initial drug or combination AED therapy

If the patient does not respond to or does not tolerate the initial AED, the clinician must consider an alternative approach and choose another drug. As with the selection of the initial AED, practitioners must select a drug appropriate to the type of epilepsy, and must take factors into account that were considered in the original AED choice.

Should the replacement drug also prove ineffective, a combination of AEDs may be beneficial. In this case, it is common practice to choose drugs that have the potential for complementary effects via different mechanisms of action. Although this is a logical approach, scientific validation of this rationale as a predictor of effectiveness is lacking. Deckers *et al.* reviewed papers in which polytherapy was used in human epilepsy or in animal models. They summarized data to support the choice of AED combinations based on complementary mechanisms of action, but they acknowledged that existing data are not sufficient to make firm decisions on this basis.

Criteria for pharmacoresisant epilepsy have been established through the seminal work of Kwan and Brodie, who demonstrated diminishing returns in seizure control for subsequent AEDs after two or more appropriately chosen, dosed, and administered drugs resulted in treatment failure. Treatment failure warrants (1) reconsideration of the specific diagnosis of seizure/seizure syndrome; (2) consideration of the alternative diagnosis of non-epileptic attack disorder (NEAD) or a combination of epilepsy and NEAD; and (3) consideration of surgical or other non-pharmacological treatment, if applicable.

AEDs in the treatment of status epilepticus

Convulsive status epilepticus

Convulsive status epilepticus (CSE) is a neurological emergency that has continued to carry a high rate of morbidity and mortality, much of it conferred by potentially lethal brain pathologies such as meningitis, cerebral hemorrhage, and intracranial neoplasm. CSE itself has potentially fatal complications, including acute renal failure, pneumonia, and septicemia. The current definition of CSE is a convulsive seizure that (1) involves at least one limb on each side; and (2) exceeds five minutes' duration or includes multiple seizures for which the patient does not return to the neurological baseline.

Refractory status epilepticus

Refractory status epilepticus (RSE) represents ongoing seizures in spite of employing two AEDs that are appropriately selected and dosed. Approximately one-fourth of patients with CSE meet the criteria for RSE.

Super-refractory status epilepticus

A more recent definition, super-refractory status epilepticus (SRSE) was introduced in 2011, defined as continuous or recurrent seizures lasting 24 hours after the initiation of anesthetic drugs. SRSE also includes patients for whom seizure control was attained with anesthetic drugs, but whose seizures recur when weaned off anesthetic agents.

RSE and SRSE are more likely to present as *de novo* status epilepticus caused by acute brain injury. RSE and SRSE impose more severe morbidity and mortality than does CSE caused by pre-existing epilepsy.

A favorable clinical outcome from CSE is inversely related to the time required to control seizures, and the likelihood of seizure control is inversely proportional to the time used to begin appropriate medical therapy. Optimal management of the patient with CSE must include simultaneous efforts directed toward seizure control, identification of the underlying pathology, and avoidance and management of systemic complications of CSE.

Timely and effective treatment to stop ongoing seizures and to avoid the consequences of excitotoxicity-mediated cell death and other complications of CSE is critical. A consensus holds that the first-line drug should be an intravenous benzodiazepine, most often lorazepam, which achieves effective brain levels faster than diazepam. Studies have demonstrated the efficacy and safety of the administration of lorazepam by paramedical personnel prior to arrival at the hospital. A recent large-scale study supported the use of intramuscular midalzolam in the field, which appeared more effective than lorazepam, possibly because the time to administer was shorter. Although intravenous phenytoin or fosphenytoin is most commonly used as the second-line drug, evidence supports intravenous valproic acid as an alternative to phenytoin. If seizures, including electrographic seizures, continue or recur, intubation should be considered, along with the use of propofol, midazolam, or ketamine. It is the goal to monitor with continuous EEG for and abolish electrographic seizures as well.

Non-convulsive status epilepticus

Non-convulsive status epilepticus (NCSE) generally occurs in one of two clinical settings: (1) ambulatory, confused patients who usually have a prior diagnosis of epilepsy; and (2) unresponsive inpatients who have severe brain pathology such as posthypoxic encephalopathy. The former diagnosis is generally benign and responsive to an AED. The latter is often refractory to intensive use of multiple AEDs. Validation of the diagnosis requires a diagnostic EEG and ongoing EEG monitoring in either case. A large study by Classen found that the EEG indicators of poor outcome included periodic epileptiform discharges as well as non-convulsive seizures and non-convulsive status, and that these are seen with significant frequency in other etiologies including infection, metabolic encephalopathy, and acute stroke. Thus, anyone who fails to wake up in the intensive care unit without obvious etiology should be monitored with continuous EEG.

Epilepsia partialis continua

Epilepsia partialis continua (EPC) was originally described by Kojevnikov in patients with Russian spring–summer encephalitis. EPC is most commonly associated with an acute brain lesion and is characterized by continuous muscle twitches in a limited part of the body contralateral to the brain lesion. EPC lasts for hours, weeks, or even years and is notoriously resistant to treatment with AEDs. Given the resistance to treatment and the limited impact on normal function, it is important not to overtreat EPC.

As with refractory epilepsy, refractory status may benefit from surgical intervention when the focus is known, or even vagus nerve stimulation (VNS) therapy and/or the ketogenic diet.

Complications of antiepileptic drug therapy

Most adverse effects of AEDs represent type A reactions: they are predictable, dose dependent, and can be explained by the pharmacological characteristics of the drug. In the majority of type A reactions, symptoms resolve after dosage adjustment of the responsible medication.

Idiosyncratic adverse reactions are type B. They are unpredictable and considered unrelated to the usual pharmacological actions of the drug in question. Although they represent the minority of adverse drug reactions, type B reactions are much more likely to cause significant morbidity and mortality.

Allergic reactions

Virtually all antiepileptic drugs may produce allergic skin eruptions, some relatively benign, others potentially fatal. These reactions are idiosyncratic in nature. Drug reaction with eosinophilia and systemic symptoms (DRESS syndrome) has occurred with a variety of AEDs, and it is more likely to occur among African American men. DRESS may include multiorgan inflammation, such as hepatitis, pericarditis, pneumonitis, and interstitial nephritis.

The most feared AED complications are severe allergic reactions such as Stevens–Johnson syndrome (SJS) and toxic-epidermal necrolysis (TEN), which manifest as extensive and sometimes exfoliative skin eruptions with multiorgan involvement. SJS and TEN most often complicate the use of AEDs or antibiotics, but they may occur in the absence of any pharmacological agents. The Euro-SCAR study demonstrated the strongest AED associations of SJS and TEN with lamotrigine, carbamazepine, phenytoin, and phenobarbital. Typically, SJS and TEN appeared within the first few weeks of exposure to the responsible drug. The introduction of lamotrigine demands a low initial dose and slow dose escalation to limit the risk of serious dermatological complications.

The occurrence of SJS and TEN has been connected to patient ethnicity, and they appear more often in Asian people, particularly among the Thai population. In the case of carbamazepine, multidrug resistance protein 2 (MRP2, ABCC2) is associated with altered carbamazepine metabolism and a greater likelihood of adverse neurological drug reactions among the Asian population. A better understanding of pharmacogenetic principles and influences holds promise for more individualized and effective selection of AEDs in the future. At this time, screening for these genetic markers in a non-Asian population does not appear to be indicated.

Ophthalmic reactions

Vigabatrin (VGB) is an analogue of gamma-aminobutyric acid (GABA), which was introduced in 1979 and provides effective treatment of infantile spasms and adjunctive therapy for partial seizures. Enthusiasm for its use has been muted by the potential for concentric visual field defects secondary to retinal toxicity in patients treated with the drug. There is evidence that this complication is more likely to occur in patients who are simultaneously treated with VGB and other AEDs, but no specific cotreatment drug has been identified. Abnormal visual studies have been reported with other GABAergic drugs, so avoidance of multiple GABAergic agents is reasonable.

The use of VGB requires careful surveillance with electroretinography in younger children and with visual evoked potentials and visual fields in older patients. Electroretinogram is a useful procedure for screening, but is not widely available. Unfortunately, the visual defects are not reversible with discontinuation of the drug. Determination of specific genetic links to this problem has been unfulfilled thus far.

Hepatic reactions

Transient elevation of hepatic enzymes occurs with many AEDs at one end of the spectrum of hepatic injury. Monitoring for more serious hepatic toxicity is essential, especially after the AED is initially ordered.

VPA may lead to fatal hepatic necrosis, primarily in children less than 2 years of age who are taking multiple drugs or who have underlying inborn metabolic disorders. VPA-induced hepatic necrosis is rare in adolescents and adults. There is some evidence that treatment with L-carnitine may mitigate the hepatic damage from VPA. The other AED associated with fatal hepatic necrosis is felbamate (FBM). Typically, serious hepatic disease with FBM occurs within the first 3–4 months of use.

VPA may also cause isolated hyperammonemia in the absence of abnormalities of serum transaminases or bilirubin. Affected patients may be asymptomatic, but impairment of consciousness and decreased seizure control may occur. There is evidence that isolated hyperammonemia is more common when VPA-treated patients take topiramate simultaneously.

Psychiatric reactions

The potential for suicidality associated with AEDs has come into sharper focus within the past few years. The US Food and Drug Administration (FDA) issued a formal warning about this concern in 2009. Since then there has been an ongoing debate as to the validity of AEDs as the basis for suicidality in patients with epilepsy. Much of the discussion has centered around the degree to which epilepsy itself is sufficient to explain increased suicide risk, considering the associated brain dysfunction and the emotional, social, and financial burden of the illness.

A population study of a large cohort in the United Kingdom analyzed suicide-related events among patients with epilepsy who did not receive AEDs versus patients with epilepsy who were administered AEDs. The study found that there was an increased risk of suicidality among patients who were depressed, but not among patients who were treated with AEDs. Studies from Italy and the United States yielded similar outcomes. Other characteristic AED adverse effects are summarized in Table 36.3.

Elective discontinuation of antiepileptic drugs

The use of AEDs entails costs of various types: the financial expense of the drugs and laboratory studies to monitor drug safety, the potential for adverse effects, the expenditure of time to maintain compliance, and the inevitable emotional burden of the illness state. These burdens alone often lead patients to request that their AEDs be discontinued, particularly if seizures have been controlled or if they suffer adverse effects. Pregnant patients may feel compelled to discontinue AEDs out of concern for the potential teratogenic effects.

The clinician should take a cautious and thoughtful approach, particularly in the case of the pregnant patient whose seizures are not under control. Discontinuation of AEDs during pregnancy is often ill-advised because frequent seizures may in themselves be harmful to the fetus. In addition, patients often bring their case for discontinuation of AEDs after the first trimester, a point at which teratogenic risks actually begin to decline.

Cessation of antiepileptic drugs is more often successful in children, because age-related seizure syndromes such as childhood absence epilepsy and Rolandic epilepsy typically go into remission. In addition, the consequences of the loss of employment and driving privileges are not applicable to children.

In the case of the patient whose seizures have been controlled, the decision to discontinue AEDs warrants a thorough and personal analysis of the potential risks and benefits involved, including consideration of the following questions: (1) What is the risk of seizure recurrence? (2) If seizures recur, what is the likelihood that the resumption of AEDs will again achieve seizure control? (3) If seizures recur, what are the patient's risks of physical injury and loss of employment? Braun and Schmidt addressed these issues in their critical review. Most studies do not recommend AED withdrawal until the patient has been seizure free for three years, and there is a suggestion that withdrawing too early may lead to more difficulty with control later.

Herbal treatments as AEDs

Although there is very little scientific evidence to support the practice, a number of herbal preparations have been touted for use in patients with epilepsy. Among others, these agents include blue cohosh (*Caulophyllum thalictroides*), mistletoe (*Viscum sp.)*, skullcap (*Scutellaria laterifolia, S. baicalensis*), valerian (Valeriana officinalis), and betony (*Stachys officinalis*). Apart from anecdotal reports of benefit in the treatment of epilepsy, there is no sound scientific basis for recommending their use.

Beyond the question of efficacy, the possibility of herbal–drug and herbal–herbal interactions complicates their potential utility, as do well-documented adverse effects, including seizures. Many herbal agents have potential teratogenic effects, and they should be especially avoided by pregnant and lactating patients.

Perhaps cannabis has attracted the most recent attention for potential use in epilepsy and other neurological disorders. In fact, cannabinoid receptors have been verified at multiple sites in the human nervous system, including the spinal cord, hippocampus, cerebellum, basal ganglia, and peripheral nerves. Arguments have been made for using marijuana or extracts from the plant to combat pain, muscle spasm, tremor, cervical dystonia, levodopa-induced dyskinesias, Tourette syndrome, and epilepsy.

Preparations tested in controlled studies have included oral cannabis extract (OCE), nabiximols, and tetrahydrocannabinol (THC). In addition, there have been recent anecdotal reports of the use of cannabidiol (CBD) in the treatment of pediatric epilepsy, particular Dravet syndrome. Some strains of marijuana have a relatively high content of CBD and relatively low amounts of THC. CBD is administered as an oil-based extract of the plant.

The Guideline Development Subcommittee of the American Academy of Neurology recently reviewed the subject of medical marijuana as it relates to neurological disorders. It concluded that OCE, THC, and nabiximols are probably useful for spasticity associated with multiple sclerosis (MS) and that OCE is effective for painful spasms that accompany MS. It also found evidence that THC and nabiximols are effective in combating painful MS spasms. It found no evidence to support other use of cannabinoids in neurological disorders, including epilepsy.

Further reading

Arana A, Wentworth CE, Ayuso-Mateos JL, Arellano FM. Suicide-related events in patients treated with antiepileptic drugs. *N Engl J Med* 2010;363:542–551.

Braun KPJ, Schmidt D. Stopping antiepileptic drugs in seizure-free patients. *Curr Opin Neurol* 2014;27:219–226.

Brodie M. Antiepileptic drug therapy – the story so far. *Seizure* 2010;19:650–655.

Claassen J, Mayer SA, Kowalski RG, et al. Detection of electrographic seizures with continuous EEG monitoring in critically ill patients. *Neurology* 2004;52:1743–1748.

Deckers CL, Czuczwar SJ, Hekster YA, et al. Selection of antiepileptic drug polytherapy based on mechanisms of action: The evidence reviewed. *Epilepsia* 2000;41:1364–1374.

Glauser T, Ben-Menachem E, Bourgeois B, et al. ILAE treatment guidelines: Evidence-based analysis of antiepileptic drug efficacy and effectiveness as initial monotherapy for epileptic seizures and syndrome. *Epilepsia* 2006;47:1094–1120.

Hocker S, Tatum W, LaRoche S. Refractory and super-refractory status epilepticus – an update. *Curr Neurol Neurosci Rep* 2014;14:452–458.

Koppel BS, Brust MCJ, Fife T, et al. Systematic review: Efficacy and safety of medical marijuana in selected neurologic disorders. Report of the Guideline Development Subcommittee of the American Academy of Neurology. *Neurology* 2014;82:1556–1563.

Kwan P, Brodie MJ. Early identification of refractory epilepsy. *N Engl J Med* 2000;342(5):314–319.

Landmark CJ. Antiepileptic drugs in non-epilepsy disorders. *CNS Drugs* 2008;22:27–47.

Mockenhaupt M, Viboud C, Dunant A, et al. Stevens–Johnson syndrome and toxic epidermal necrolysis: Assessment of medication risks with emphasis on recently marketed drugs. The EuroSCAR-Study. *J Invest Dermatol.* 2008;128:35–44.

Pearl PL, Drillings IM, Conry JA. Herbs in epilepsy: Evidence for efficacy, toxicity, and interactions. *Semin Pediatr Neurol* 2011;18:203–208.

Piana C, Antunes N, Pasqua OD. Implications of pharmacogenetics for the therapeutic use of antiepileptic drugs. *Expert Opin Drug Metab Toxicol* 2014;10:341–358.

Zaccara G, Franciotta D, Perucca E. Idiosyncratic adverse reactions to antiepileptic drugs. *Epilepsia* 2007;48:1223–1244.

37 Surgical treatment of epilepsy

Ivan Rektor[1] and Barbara E. Swartz[2]

[1] Masaryk University, St. Anne's Hospital, Brno, Czech Republic

[2] Epilepsy Center and Neurophysiology Laboratory, and Renown Neuroscience Institute, University of Nevada, Reno, NV, USA

Epilepsy surgery is the most efficient therapy for patients with pharmacoresistant epilepsy. Patients with epilepsy refractory to pharmacotherapy should receive consultation about the suitability of a surgical solution.

Investigations and indications for epilepsy surgery

Prior to surgery, all relevant information is evaluated by a multidisciplinary team. The diagnostic process leads to the elimination of some candidates as unsuitable for epileptic surgery, or to the determination of the optimal surgical method for those suitable candidates who elect to have surgery. The results of electroencephalography (EEG), especially of ictal video EEG, are compared with those of imaging and metabolic methods as well as neuropsychological findings. All data are considered together with individual anamnesis, including the subjective description of the aura or seizure and psychosocial impact of surgery. The presurgical tests should define the epileptogenic zone (SOZ), the irritative zones (interictal spikes), the functional zones (PET, EEG, neuropsychological tests), and the lesional zones (MRI). Surgical treatment is determined mainly by the detection and location of the seizure onset zone (SOZ; i.e., the brain area that generates epileptic seizures), as well as by the presence or absence of a detectable brain lesion, the biological nature of the lesion, the relation of the SOZ to the lesion and to the location of the eloquent cortex, and, of course, the decision of the patient.

The following questions should be answered:
- Where is the SOZ located and how large is it?
- Is the SOZ the only source of habitual seizures?
- Is there an identified lesion that causes the seizures? Could the lesion be removed entirely or partially?
- What are the risks of removal of the SOZ? What is the relation between the epileptogenic cortex and the localization of brain functions?
- Which operation is more suitable: curative (resection) or palliative?

Semi-invasive and invasive video EEG

The cornerstone of epilepsy diagnostics is video EEG recording of seizures. Intracranial video EEG is necessary in a small portion of epilepsy surgery candidates if scalp and semi-invasive recordings do not yield enough information about the location and extent of the epileptogenic zone. Electrodes are implanted intracranially for 1

or 2 weeks while data are gathered. Electric stimulation via implanted electrodes may provoke seizure activity and also enables precise functional diagnosis of the localization of the eloquent cortex (which must be avoided during surgery). Intraoperative recording (electrocorticography, ECoG) is the main method in some centers; in others, it is complementary to long-term recordings.

The invasive exploration is carried out through surgically inserted intracranial electrodes. There are two main approaches to intracranial recordings: ECoG with intracerebral recording and subdural recording. In the first, thin-depth electrodes with 5–18 contacts are stereotactically inserted into the brain (stereoencephalography, SEEG), providing for exploration of deep structures. SEEG does not require craniotomy. In order to obtain subdural recordings, subdural electrodes in the form of strips or grids (20–128 contacts) are placed on the surface of the brain after craniotomy. This method is less accurate than intracerebral recording, but is easier. The risk for both approaches is similar, and most centers combine methods depending on the targeted structure. Complications are headache and cerebrospinal fluid (CSF) leakage, with infrequent cerebral infection or bleeding (≤5%). Generally, SEEG exploration is used for mesiotemporal structures and deep mesial frontal structures. Extratemporal explorations are carried out subdurally or by SEEG, depending on the location of the lesion and the preference of the center. In some centers, epidural electrodes are also used; foramen ovale electrodes are used for mesial foci (Figures 37.1 and 37.2).

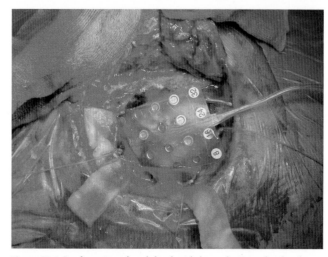

Figure 37.1 Implantation of a subdural grid electrode. For color details, please refer to the color plates section.

International Neurology, Second edition. Edited by Robert P. Lisak, Daniel D. Truong, William M. Carroll and Roongroj Bhidayasiri
© 2016 John Wiley & Sons, Ltd. Published 2016 by John Wiley & Sons, Ltd.

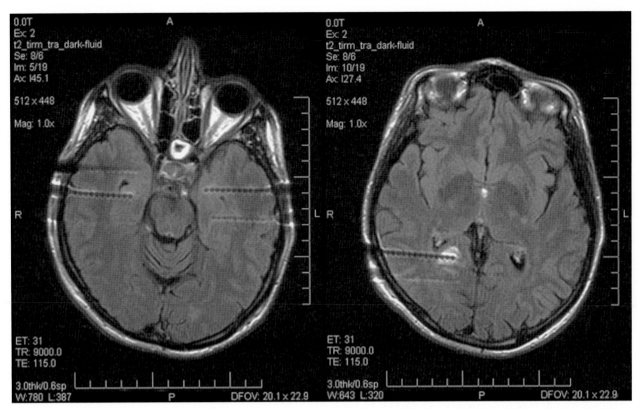

Figure 37.2 Multicontact depth electrodes implanted in a lesion and in the temporal lobes. The postplacement MRI visualized exact localization of individual contacts. The diameter of an electrode (0.8 mm) represents approximately 10% of the diameter of the displayed artifact.

Operations

Epilepsy surgery can be curative or palliative. The goals of surgery are to remove the epileptogenic lesion and epileptogenic zone, to halt disease progression, to prevent the spread of seizure activity, and to inhibit seizures via neuromodulatory techniques.

Curative procedures

Amygdalohippocampectomy/temporal lobectomy

Tissue removal can be limited to mesial structures or extended to the temporal neocortex. In patients with temporal epilepsy with mesial (hippocampal) sclerosis, anteromedial temporal resection (AMTR; i.e., amygdalohippocampectomy with removal of the parahippocampal gyrus and the temporal pole) is the most frequent and most successful surgical method (Figure 37.3). It can be performed on the more active side of the brain for bitemporal epilepsies if memory functions are sufficient on the opposite side. Both AMTR and selective amygdalohippocampectomy (SAH) are effective, and there are cases when SAH should be preferred; that is, in patients with increased risk of postsurgical memory decline. An electrocorticography-based tailored approach can be useful in some cases. For most mesial temporal lobe epilepsy (MTLE) patients, a standard anterior and mesial temporal lobe resection will lead to seizure freedom.

Patients show significant improvement following surgery in 75%, 80% (dominant), and 90% (non-dominant) after temporal lobe surgeries. According to a recent meta-analysis, the median long-term (more than 5 years) seizure-free outcome for patients was 66% in temporal lobe resections, 46% in parietal resections, and 27% in frontal resections. In our center, 75% of patients were seizure free 2 years after surgery, with significant improvement in over 90%. In extratemporal operations, seizure-free outcome was achieved in 63% of patients. The probability of postsurgery seizure freedom is highest in patients with a history of febrile seizures, mesiotemporal sclerosis, tumor, lesion on MRI, EEG/MR concordance, and extensive resection. Negative predictors are postoperative EEG discharges, extratemporal resections, incomplete resections, and multiple recorded ictal patterns.

Complications of surgery are usually minimal; mortality is <0.1%. Hemiparesis, infections, hematomas, and cranial nerve palsies occurred in <5%, and quandrantanopsia in 25–30% of cases.

A meta-analysis of 12 studies concerning temporal lobe surgery indicated a risk of verbal memory decline with left-sided temporal surgery in 44% of patients, twice as high as the rate for right-sided surgery (20%). Gains in verbal memory were relatively rare (7% in left-, 14% in right-sided surgery). For visual memory, the risk of loss was similar for both right- and left-sided surgery (23% and 21%, respectively). Global memory impairment is rare (≤1%). Postoperative memory impairment can be prevented by careful selection of patients (Wada test and and other neuropsychological assessments). Significant dysphasia is seen in 1–3% of patients; transient medication-responsive mood swings occur in 2–20%. Patients continue with medical treatment after surgery for at least 1–2 years. If patients are seizure free, medications can be gradually and carefully reduced over time. Long-term prognosis is good, but patients who are seizure free for the first 5 years remain at risk for relapse.

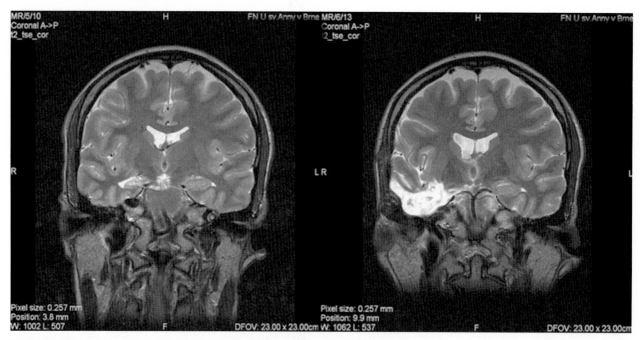

Figure 37.3 Hippocampal sclerosis, before (left) and after (right) anteromesial temporal lobe resection.

Lesionectomy

Removal of an epileptogenic lesion is most frequently performed in dysplasias, low-grade tumors, cavernomas, and other vascular malformations. Even in seemingly simple cases, such as with tumors, it is necessary to carry out an anatomical electroclinical correlation of the seizures, as the SOZ may not be identical with the lesion. Lesionectomy is successful in reducing the majority of seizures in 85% of patients. Freedom from seizures (15–50%) depends on the type of lesion and extent of resection.

Sometimes the lesion itself is epileptogenic – for example, in the case of some dysplasias – while in other cases its surroundings or more distant structures are epileptogenic. Therefore, SEEG may be required to explore the SOZ. In between 50% and 85% of patients, seizure freedom can be achieved after a lesionectomy. Complications vary with the site of surgery and the degree of cortical reorganization. Severe complications such as stroke or aphasia occur in less than 5% of patients. Multiple lesionectomies can sometimes be employed, such as in tuberous sclerosis, through techniques to determine the epileptogenic lesions.

Topectomy/cortectomy of the SOZ

The most common site for this procedure is the frontal lobe. In nonlesional epilepsies, the SOZ identified by prior examination, often including intracranial exploration, is removed. Neuropathological examination of removed tissue often shows malformation of cortical development. Freedom from seizures ranges from 15–50%, with significant improvement in 60–90% of patients. The most frequent complications are due to perioperative ischemia (2.7%) and hemianopsia (2.1%).

Palliative procedures

Multilobar resections

With large lesions, lobar or multilobar resections may be performed. No outcome study has specifically addressed these. Evaluation is the same as in other cortical epilepsies. Complications such as

pyramidal signs or hemianopsia are expected more frequently; however, these large resections are surprisingly well tolerated.

Hemispherectomy

Hemispherectomy is performed in extreme childhood epileptic disorders, as in cases of hemimegencephaly, perinatal common carotid occlusion, Sturge–Weber syndrome, and advanced Rasmussen syndrome. The Wada test should be performed prior to surgery. It is common to remove only the temporal lobe and surgically disconnect the other structures (hemispherectomy); 80–95% of patients with hemispherectomy show significant improvement. Some may become seizure free, although EEG remains malignant in the case of hemispherectomy. Complications depend on the degree of dysfunction in the offending hemisphere and include weakness, speech impairment, and perioperative complications.

Multiple subpial transactions (MSPT)

The epileptogenic cortex is not removed, but is isolated from surrounding tissue to prevent the seizure from spreading, allowing for operations in the eloquent or motor cortex. This is done for palliation or to improve outcome in conjunction with a cortectomy. Outcomes vary, with up to 50% of patients being seizure free, and 30–90% experiencing significant improvement. Complications include monoparesis, visual field defect, sensory loss, and dysphasia; less than 6% of these are persistent.

Callosotomy

In this procedure, one-half to two-thirds of the callosum is transected. The main indications for this surgery are atonic seizures of secondary generalized and multifocal epilepsies. Control depends on the type of seizure: 75–100% decrease in falls; 60–75% in generalized tonic–clonic (GTC); 50% in complex partial seizures; and no change or increase in focal motor seizures. Complications include transient mutism, hemiparesis, and apraxias, which rarely persist but may if the subject has right language dominance.

Neurostimulation methods

Neurostimulation methods is carried out mainly in patients, adults and children, for whom resection is contraindicated for where surgery has failed. An electrode is fixed to the left vagus nerve and a generator is placed under the skin, usually under the collar bone. Patients can block a seizure as it starts by extra stimulation. While in some patients the number of seizures can be reduced by up to 90%, a realistic target is approximately 50% reduction, and 50–60% of patients are responders with at least 50% seizure reduction with a 2-year follow-up. As with other palliative techniques, the character of the seizure may be mitigated. Positive influences on mood and cognitive functions are reported. Complications are minor, including hoarseness and cough.

Deep-brain stimulation (DBS)

DBS therapy intended to be an adjunctive therapy for reducing the frequency of seizures in pharmacoresistemt adult persons with epilepsy. DBS can modulate the remote control systems of epilepsy, such as the thalamus and basal ganglia or directly the epileptic focus in hippocampus. Several subcortical and cortical targets have been tested; the DBS of anterior nucleus of thalamus was approved for clinical use in Europe. DBS may be successful after VNS failure. The efficacy was demonstrated in individuals with a long history of epilepsy who had tried and failed most other treatment options. The safety profile is similar to other DBS therapies, with an additional moderately increased risk of depression and memory impairment.

Responsive brain stimulation (RNS™)

Responsive stimulation aims to suppress epileptiform activity by delivering stimulation directly in response to electrographic activity. The electrodes are implanted intracranially in or over the epileptic focus. The FDA indications are: adjunctive therapy in individuals 18 years or older; partial-onset seizures from no more than two foci; refractory to two or more antiepileptic medications. Optimal treatment candidates have two seizure foci, or foci located in non-resectable zones (for example, perisylvian language and motor areas). Complications are minor. Future studies are necessary to identify optimal stimulation parameters and patient population for whom DBS and RNS would be the optimal treatment. In practice, various operations can be combined (e.g., a lesionectomy with an amygdalohippocampectomy, a subtotal lesionectomy with MSPT) and surgery may be planned in two phases. Other methods are being developed, including gamma knife radiosurgery and thermolesioning using inserted depth electrodes. Several intracerebral targets for chronic electrical stimulation are also under investigation. Novel non-invasive neurostimulation techniques are in development.

Acknowledgments

Supported by the CEITEC – Central European Institute of Technology project (CZ.1.05/1.1.00/02.0068) from the European Regional Development Fund. The authors thank M. Brázdil, J. Christina, P. Daniel, R. Kuba, Z. Novák, J. Hemza, Z. Hummelová, M. Pažourková, I. Tyrliková, and colleagues from the Brno Epilepsy Center.

Further reading

Bancaud J, Talairach J. Séméiloge clinique des crises du lobe temporal. In: *Crises épileptiques et épilepsies du lobe temporal.* Rennes: Documentation médicale LABAZ; 1991.

Bonini F, McGonigal A, Trébuchon A, *et al.* Frontal lobe seizures: From clinical semiology to localization. *Epilepsia* 2014;55(2):264–277.

Chauvel P, Delgado-Escueta AV, Halgren E, Bancaud J (eds.). Frontal lobe seizures and epilepsies. In: *Advances in Neurology*, Vol. 57. New York: Raven Press; 1992.

Hirsch L. Finally a flood of fascinating facts and findings on final outcomes after frontal lobe epilepsy surgery. *Epilepsy Currents* 2013;14:139–142.

Holtkamp M, Sharan A, Sperling MR. Intracranial EEG in predicting surgical outcome in frontal lobe epilepsy. *Epilepsia* 2012;53(10):1739–1745.

Kuba R, Brázdil M, Kalina M, *et al.* Vagus nerve stimulation: Longitudinal follow-up of patients treated for 5 years. *Seizure* 2009;18(4):269–274.

Lüders HO, Noachtar S. *Epileptic Seizures: Pathophysiology and Clinical Semiology.* Cleveland: Churchill Livingstone; 2000.

Rydenhag B, Hans C. Complications of epilepsy surgery after 654 procedures in Sweden, September 1990–1995: A multicenter study based on the Swedish National Epilepsy Surgery Register. *Neurosurgery* 2001;49:51–57.

Sherman E, Wiebe S, Fay-McClymont TB, *et al.* Neuropsychological outcomes after epilepsy surgery: Systematic review and pooled estimates. *Epilepsia* 2011;52:857–869.

Telezz-Zenterno JF, Dhar J, Wiebe S. Long-term seizure outcomes following epilepsy surgery: A systematic review and meta-analysis. *Brain* 2005;128:1188–1198.

Wendling A, Hirsch E, Wisniewski I, *et al.* Selective amygdalohippocampectomy versus standard temporal lobectomy in patients with mesial temporal lobe epilepsy and unilateral hippocampal sclerosis. *Epilepsy Res* 2013;104:94—104.

38   Dementia overview

Murray Grossman

Department of Neurology and Penn Frontotemporal Degeneration Center, University of Pennsylvania, Philadelphia, PA, USA

Dementia is very common. Our goal as physicians is to identify treatable diseases. When considering dementia, it has long been thought that treatable forms of the condition are rare. Nevertheless, we are on the precipice of a sea-change in our approach. There are several important metabolic, infectious, toxic, and immune-mediated causes of dementia that must be recognized. Another frequently cited form of treatable dementia is normal pressure hydrocephalus. It is important to distinguish this from the symptomatically very similar condition of vascular cognitive impairment. Vascular forms of dementia in the modern era are associated less often with multiple large strokes than with small vessel ischemic disease. However, neurodegenerative dementias are much more common, and it is these forms of dementia that are about to become treatable conditions.

Far and away the most common dementing disorder currently is Alzheimer's disease. A major risk factor for Alzheimer's disease is age. There has been an exponential increase in the frequency of Alzheimer's disease – and, indeed, all neurodegenerative forms of dementia – and this is related in no small part to improved survival and the corresponding aging of the population. While this trend is evident in developed countries, it is even more evident internationally in developing countries. Some symptomatic treatments for Alzheimer's disease are available. More importantly, disease-modifying treatments are being developed, and early, accurate diagnosis of this disorder is a crucial first step in the treatment process. It is also valuable to identify factors that hasten or slow the rate of disease progression, since these represent important treatment targets.

Alzheimer's disease is associated with a complex and variable set of histopathological abnormalities. Advances in treating each of these abnormalities must be achieved in order to develop a true cure for Alzheimer's disease. One intense focus of treatment is the clearance of amyloid from the brain. However, amyloid represents only one of several microscopic pathologies, and a cure for Alzheimer's disease is likely to come from the study of the other histopathological abnormalities that are also found in the brains of Alzheimer's patients. Each of these misfolded proteins is associated with a monoproteinopathy that causes a less common form of dementia, with onset typically at a younger age. Examples are tauopathies, TDP-proteinopathies, and synucleinopathies. Tauopathies include progressive supranuclear palsy, corticobasal degeneration, and dementia with Pick bodies; TDP-proteinopathies include amyotrophic lateral sclerosis with cognitive difficulty and the semantic variant of primary progressive aphasia; and synucleinopathies include Parkinson's dementia, Lewy body disease, and multiple system atrophy. While each of these individual conditions may be relatively rare, these pathologically defined categories of dementing disorders are not that infrequent. These conditions are often seen in specialty clinics, where the elementary neurological signs are the most important focus of concern. It is clearly important to manage the risks related to gait difficulty, weakness, and involuntary movement disorders. However, the recognition of cognitive impairment profiles associated with each of these conditions has led to improved diagnosis, better understanding of the pathophysiology of these diseases, and clearer definition of targets for disease-modifying treatment. Ultimately, an etiologically driven treatment for Alzheimer's disease may depend on an individualized cocktail of treatments targeting each of the contributing monoproteinopathies.

This part of *International Neurology* outlines dementia from the perspective that it is a treatable condition. There are some dementing conditions that can be treated easily once identified, either through medical or surgical intervention, as outlined in the comprehensive Chapter 46 by John Ringman and his colleagues. Vascular cognitive impairment is described by Stefanova and Kostić in Chapter 42. The many manifestations of Alzheimer's disease are described in Chapter 39 by Wolk and Vaishnavi, where early diagnosis of mild cognitive impairment is emphasized. Less common forms of dementia are presented in additional chapters, grouped by the underlying histopathological abnormality. There is an overview of the frontotemporal degenerations by Rascovsky and Matallana in Chapter 43; Albert Ludolph in Chapter 45 expertly describes amyotrophic lateral sclerosis and the related cognitive impairment associated with TDP-43; Parkinson spectrum synucleinopathies are characterized by Rektorova and her colleagues in Chapter 40; and akinetic-rigid disorders associated with tau pathology are summarized by Irwin in Chapter 44. This panoramic view of dementia is likely to change dramatically in the next decade as disease-modifying treatments for these conditions are developed.

Acknowledgment

This work was supported by grants from the National Institutes of Health (AG017586, AG038490, NS044266, NS053488, and AG032953), the Wyncote Foundation, and the Arking Family Foundation.

39 Mild cognitive impairment and Alzheimer's disease

David Wolk and Sanjeev Vaishnavi

Department of Neurology, Perelman School of Medicine University of Pennsylvania, Philadelphia, PA, USA

Mild cognitive impairment (MCI) and Alzheimer's disease (AD) are becoming increasingly prevalent as life expectancy increases. Nearly 45% of individuals over the age of 85 have Alzheimer's disease and the estimated lifetime risk of AD is 17.2% in women and 9.1% in men. Prior to the development of dementia, many of these individuals have evidence of cognitive dysfunction with minimal impact on their activities of daily living (ADLs). These individuals in the intermediate stage between normal aging and dementia have been classified as mild cognitive impairment. While initially conceptualized as a prodromal stage for AD, it is clear that MCI is a heterogeneous group with increased risk for progression to AD and other dementias.

Mild cognitive impairment

Mild cognitive impairment is a term used to describe individuals with cognitive deficits that are out of proportion to normal aging, but do not yet meet the criteria for dementia. As initially described, this group of patients required a deficit in the domain of memory in order to meet the criteria for a diagnosis of MCI. Further revisions have expanded MCI to include both amnestic and non-amnestic presentations. MCI is a clinical syndrome and not an etiological diagnosis. Thus, it is a heterogeneous construct in which the presenting cognitive impairment could be due to a number of neurodegenerative or non-neurodegenerative conditions other than AD, including vascular MCI and memory loss due to psychiatric complaints. As described in this chapter, research is being performed with biomarkers to try to differentiate AD-prodromal MCI patients from those with other types of MCI.

Epidemiology

Approximately 10–20% of elderly (over 65 years old) individuals have MCI at any given time. The prevalence of MCI increases with age, to approximately 30% of individuals above the age of 85. There are no significant gender or ethnic differences in the prevalence of MCI, although studies have shown significant variability within and between populations.

As already noted, MCI has been differentiated into amnestic and non-amnestic subtypes, and now also differentiates within those categories based on the number of cognitive domains involved (i.e., single versus multiple domains). The amnestic MCI group probably encompasses approximately two-thirds of all MCI patients and appears to be the group at highest risk of progression to clinical AD.

As a group, patients with MCI often progress to dementia at the rate of 5–15% per year, with 60–80% conversion by 6 years of follow-up, although the greatest risk of progression occurs in the first 2 years after diagnosis. However, these numbers largely reflect data from specialty memory clinics, and community-based samples frequently demonstrate lower rates of conversion and higher rates of "reversion to normal," in which on follow-up testing individuals no longer qualify for the MCI designation. Further, most of the information on progression is focused on the amnestic form and less data are available on non-amnestic individuals. Nonetheless, non-amnestic MCI patients do appear to display an increased risk of conversion to dementia, including but not limited to clinical AD, although often at lower rates than the amnestic form. For example, one study reported that over a period of 30 months, the conversion rate to AD was 48.7% in amnestic MCI and 26.8% in non-amnestic MCI. Identifiable risk factors for progression to AD include the severity of memory deficits, hippocampal volume loss, increased ventricular size, and positive amyloid biomarkers (decreased cerebrospinal fluid [CSF] Ab42, elevated CSF tau, and positive amyloid positron emission tomography [PET]), which will be further discussed in what follows.

Pathophysiology

The pathophysiology of MCI depends on the underlying cause of memory impairment. While a majority of amnestic MCI patients likely have Alzheimer's pathology, there is significant heterogeneity in the etiology of those who meet the core clinical criteria. The heterogeneity is likely to be even greater in those with non-amnestic presentations. Furthermore, application of clinical criteria tends to vary across sites and studies. By the time MCI is identified clinically in those who do indeed have an underlying prodromal AD, there is frequently significant neurodegeneration in various cognitive systems. Postmortem evaluation of brains from MCI patients reveals a pattern of neurodegeneration intermediate between normal aging and AD, with frequent neurofibrillary tangles in the medial temporal lobe and diffuse amyloid in the neocortex, without meeting the pathological criteria for AD.

Clinical features

The most commonly used diagnostic criteria for MCI were first described by Petersen and colleagues and require several clinical characteristics to be present. First (1) there must be a subjective

International Neurology, Second edition. Edited by Robert P. Lisak, Daniel D. Truong, William M. Carroll and Roongroj Bhidayasiri.
© 2016 John Wiley & Sons, Ltd. Published 2016 by John Wiley & Sons, Ltd.

cognitive deficit, identified either by the subject or an informant. This deficit must be (2) demonstrable by neurocognitive testing. However, it is notable that there remains disagreement over the number of tests that should be abnormal in a given domain, whether specific cutoffs should be applied, and what they should be (frequently >1–1.5 standard deviations [SD] below the mean), and the specific psychometric tests that should be administered. Single or multiple cognitive domains may be impaired in MCI, but individuals should (3) not meet clinical criteria for dementia. Consistent with that notion, they should have (4) grossly maintained or minimally impaired activities of daily living (ADLs). As psychometric testing is age adjusted, subjects with "normal" age-related cognitive decline will generally not reach the threshold for objective cognitive impairment on neurocognitive testing.

Investigations

Evaluation of cognitive complaints starts with a detailed history provided by the patient and an informant. Many individuals with early MCI may have very mild or minor complaints, but their informants may have noticed a decline in their cognition. In normal aging, there is frequently decline in retrieval (e.g., difficulty finding words or recalling names on the "tip of the tongue" that, given enough time, will be correctly identified), slowing of cognitive processing, and increased difficulty with multitasking. While these issues make differentiating MCI from normal age-associated decline challenging, by definition MCI patients should perform more poorly compared to normed samples on psychometric evaluation.

Bedside or more formal neuropsychological testing is essential to diagnosing MCI and its subtypes. Most individuals with MCI tend to perform well on tests of global cognitive function, such as the Mini-Mental State Examination (MMSE), making this test insensitive for diagnostic purposes. Furthermore, detailed tests should be performed to assess at least the domains of memory, language, attention/executive function, and visuospatial skills. While no specific battery of tests is recommended, the following are examples of potentially useful measures. (1) Memory: Wechsler Memory Scale, Rey Auditory Verbal Learning Test, California Verbal Learning Test, Grober Bushke Memory Test, or Benton Visual Retention Test. (2) Language: Boston Naming Test, category fluency (naming animals in 1 min). (3) Attention: digit span (forward and reverse). (4) Executive function: lexical fluency (naming words that begin with a particular letter in 1 min), Trail Making Test (A or B), Wisconsin Card Sorting Test, Digit-Symbol Substitution Test, and Stroop Test. (5) Visuospatial skills: Rey-Osterrieth Complex Figure. However, based on clinical history and bedside measures or a screening test such as the Montreal Cognitive Assessment (MOCA), a clinician will often be able to determine whether an individual qualifies for a diagnosis of MCI.

As already noted, MCI can be classified into four subtypes based on neuropsychological testing: (1) amnestic–single domain with only impairment in memory function; (2) amnestic–multiple domain with impairment in memory as well as at least one other domain; (3) non-amnestic–single domain; and (4) non-amnestic–multiple domain. Amnestic MCI patients have the highest risk of progression to AD, while those with non-amnestic MCI may progress to multiple other possible dementias (including posterior cortical atrophy, frontotemporal dementia, Lewy Body disease, and vascular and other subcortical dementias). Nonetheless, non-amnestic MCI patients frequently have AD pathology and can progress to clinical AD. There are also some data to suggest that multiple-domain subtypes

have a higher risk of conversion than single-domain types. A small fraction of patients initially diagnosed with MCI may actually have an underlying psychiatric/affective disorder, medication effect (such as narcotic or alcohol use), or other non-neurodegenerative process, resulting in cognitive impairment that would not be expected to progress to dementia if the underlying etiology is treated.

Alzheimer's disease

Alzheimer's disease (AD) is a progressive neurodegenerative illness clinically diagnosed based on a typical pattern of cognitive impairments involving memory and disruption of ADLs. It is the most common clinical cause of dementia in the elderly population. The underlying pathophysiology (as described shortly) includes the presence of amyloid-beta plaques and tau neurofibrillary tangles in the brain. While the diagnosis of definite AD continues to require neuropathological confirmation, the advent of biomarkers allows for increased certainty in the clinical diagnosis (as will be discussed). The clinocopathological agreement between the original clinical criteria for definite AD and subsequent neuropathology is 64–86%. Typically, Alzheimer's disease presents with difficulty with short-term memory (amnestic impairment) resulting in significant functional impairment (e.g., dementia) over time. Further clinical details about the timeline and progression of this disease are presented later in this section.

Epidemiology

The estimated worldwide prevalence of AD is 11% of those over age 65 and 32% above age 85. As the population ages, the number of individuals living with AD is likely to increase. In the United States, it is estimated that the number of people aged 65 and older with AD will increase from 5 million in 2014 to 13.8 million by 2050. It is also estimated that the global disease burden of AD will double every 20 years, to an estimated 81 million by 2040. There is significant global heterogeneity in AD populations. An estimated 60% of current patients with AD live in developed countries. The rate of growth of AD is highest in developing countries, and is estimated to increase by 300% by 2040. Risk factors for the development of late-onset AD (typically defined as age ≥65) include age (most prominently), sex (women are at a twofold risk compared to men), presence of cerebrovascular disease, head trauma/traumatic brain injury, lower levels of education, and apolipoprotein E4 positivity. In contrast to late-onset AD, a small fraction (<3%) of AD is early-onset, frequently due to autosomal dominant gene mutations. Mutations in the presenilin 1 gene (Chromosome 14) are the most common genetic cause of AD, followed by mutations in amyloid precursor protein (Chromosome 21) and presenilin 2 (Chromosome 1). There is no consensus about the causative role of other environmental and dietary factors in AD.

Pathophysiology

Alzheimer's disease is associated with the pathological hallmarks of accumulation of extracellular amyloid-beta fragments into senile plaques and hyperphosphorylated τ (tau) protein, resulting in intraneuronal paired helical filaments referred to as neurofibrillary tangles (NFT). Neuritic amyloid plaques are also associated with neurites containing τ filaments. The amyloid hypothesis of AD suggests that abnormal cleavage of amyloid precursor protein by β- and γ-secretases (instead of α-secretase) results in the formation of insoluble aggregates of amyloid beta 1-42 into fibrillar amyloid plaques, which are likely associated with an inflammatory response and subsequent cell destruction due to dysregulation of ion flux along neuronal membranes and resultant necrosis or apoptosis. Additionally, soluble, oligomeric forms of beta amyloid may actually be the more toxic species and have been shown to have direct effects on synaptic function, such as the efficacy of long-term potentiation. These neuropathological changes are accompanied by a decrease in cholinergic and other neurotransmitter transmissions, a reduction in synaptic density, and a loss of neurons. The interaction between amyloid plaques and tau neurofibrillary tangles remains a topic of contention, although most data suggest that amyloid deposits can be found up to 20 years prior to clinical symptoms, while tau-mediated neuronal injury appears to more closely map onto neuronal and synaptic dysfunction, as well as the clinical features of the disease.

Clinical features

The core clinical criteria for probable AD dementia (most recently revised in 2011) include (1) insidious onset over months to years; with (2) clear-cut history of progression of cognitive decline by report or observation; (3) typical pattern of cognitive impairment either amnestic or non-amnestic; that (4) cannot be explained by delirium or other major psychiatric disorder; (5) interferes with the function of activities of daily living; and (6) represents a decline from the previous level of functioning. The amnestic presentation is the most common presentation in which learning and recall of recently acquired information are the most salient and earliest deficits. These new criteria incorporate less frequent but well-described non-amnestic presentations, which include a language-predominant form, often referred to as logopenic primary progressive aphasia, a visuospatial form, often referred to as posterior cortical atrophy, and an executive form, often referred to as the frontal variant of AD (see later for further descriptions of these subtypes).

Investigations

The diagnosis of AD requires a detailed clinical and neuropsychological evaluation similar to that already described for mild cognitive impairment. The first step of the evaluation remains obtaining an accurate history. This will require access to collateral information from an informant, given that patients will often not be a reliable source. In particular, questions about early behavioral changes, such as ritualistic behaviors, language changes, prominent visuospatial difficulties, and motor changes, are important to help differentiate typical AD from other types of dementia.

The typical amnestic presentation of AD results from impairment of function of the medial temporal lobe, particularly the entorhinal/perirhinal cortex and the hippocampus, which are areas of prominent NFT pathology. Signs of such dysfunction include impairment of episodic memory or orientation to time and place. Patients have difficulty recalling recently learned information, often without significant improvement after cuing. If offered a list of items from which they are forced to choose the learned material (e.g., multiple choice), they tend to demonstrate performance below normal levels. This can be contrasted with disorders that tend to more significantly affect memory at the encoding or retrieval stage, such as vascular cognitive impairment, in which cuing and recognition memory significantly improve performance relative to free recall. Recent memory is impaired more than remote memory, which deteriorates in the later stages of dementia. As AD progresses, the disease pathology spreads beyond medial temporal dysfunction and involves other domains, including semantic memory, visuospatial, language, and executive functions.

While amnesia is most frequently the earliest domain affected due to tangle pathology within medial temporal structures and, perhaps, the presence of amyloid pathology within the default mode network, which is also closely linked to memory function, atypical presentations have been reported in 5–10% of AD patients. Many of these atypical presentations fall into one of three phenotypic syndromes that are frequently associated with underlying AD pathology: (1) early and prominent language dysfunction marked by poor naming and repetition, which could suggest the logopenic variant of primary progressive aphasia that is often due to AD pathology; (2) prominent visuospatial difficulty out of proportion to memory impairment, which is consistent with posterior cortical atrophy (PCA) – PCA is also often associated with AD, but other etiologies occur as well, including corticobasal degeneration (CBD) and Lewy Body dementia; and (3) early and prominent behavioral changes and frontal disinhibition, which can result from the frontal variant of AD, although it becomes difficult to differentiate this from behavioral variant frontotemporal dementia.

Bedside psychometric testing as already described is particularly valuable at the initial evaluation to characterize the nature of cognitive impairment and to distinguish it from other forms of dementia. Nonetheless, from a practical standpoint for a typical clinical practice, global tests of cognitive function such as the MMSE are likely to be abnormal at the AD stage (<26) and examination of the different domains of cognition captured by such tests is helpful in differential diagnosis. However, the MMSE is relatively dominated by questions that reflect memory function and is somewhat insensitive to non-AD dementias. Other global tests, such as the Montreal Cognitive Assessment (MOCA), may better capture function in multiple domains across neurodegenerative conditions. The Philadelphia Brief Assessment of Cognition has also been validated as accurately identifying the presence and severity of dementia. Another commonly used global measure (in the research setting) is the Clinical Dementia Rating (CDR) scale, which can differentiate very mild (CDR=0.5) to severe (CDR=3) dementia. Ideally, one of these screening instruments combined with more focused testing can be used for effective classification. An annual assessment with a global scale is also useful for tracking disease progression.

Assessment of instrumental (e.g., driving, finances) and basic (e.g., bathing, eating) activities of daily living based on an informant's history is also critical to staging dementia and addressing safety concerns and quality-of-life decisions. A number of formal scales can also be used for this purpose, including the Bristol Activities of Daily Living Scale (Bristol ADL), Functional Rating Scale (FRS), Disability Assessment for Dementia (DAD), and the Instrumental Activities of Daily Living Scale (IADL).

Neuropsychiatric symptoms should also be queried and are frequently present in AD, are usually distressing, and may affect the quality of life of both patients and their caregivers. Standard scales for depression and other psychiatric symptoms include the Geriatric Depression Scale, the Cornell Scale for Depression, and the Neuropsychiatric Inventory (NPI). Neuropsychiatric symptoms also may have diagnostic value, particularly for Lewy body (early hallucinations) and frontotemporal (deliberation, apathy) dementias. Depression may worsen or even mimic dementia (i.e., pseudodementia).

A general neurological evaluation of AD patients is usually normal for age except for the mental status exam, and abnormalities often suggest other etiologies of dementia. At the initial screening visit, routine blood work should be obtained, including tests of vitamin B$_{12}$ levels and thyroid function to evaluate for possible reversible causes of memory loss. In addition, all patients should have some form of neuroimaging, with magnetic resonance imaging (MRI) being the preferred modality. Structural imaging can be helpful to exclude other causes of cognitive dysfunction, including evidence of inflammatory disease, normal pressure hydrocephalus, prior strokes, and significant vascular disease.

Use of biomarkers for MCI and AD

Over the past 15 years, there has been increasing interest in the development of biomarkers (i.e., tools to predict the presence of disease accurately and reliably) to detect Alzheimer's pathology *in vivo* to allow for earlier diagnosis and treatment. These biomarkers can be used to predict the presence of AD pathology in MCI patients or provide additional support in the diagnosis of AD compared to other dementias or psychiatric causes of cognitive changes.

The two major groups of biomarkers used to help diagnose AD pathology include those for amyloid beta deposition (CSF amyloid, amyloid PET) and markers that track neurodegeneration (CSF tau, FDG [fluorodeoxyglucose] PET, volumetric MRI). Based on an extensive literature, Jack and colleagues have described a model of the temporal cascade of biomarker abnormality in the continuum

from normal cognitive function to MCI to clinical AD. Measures of cerebral amyloid are thought to be detectable first in this model, followed by "downstream" markers of neurodegenerative change that are relatively specific to the topographic pattern of AD pathology (e.g., hippocampal volume). Importantly, by the time individuals have the clinical symptoms of MCI, those with prodromal AD are expected to have abnormalities in both of these types of biomarkers (see Figure 39.1).

Consistent with this notion is that both markers of cerebral amyloid and neurodegeneration have been shown to be predictive of conversion to clinical AD across numerous longitudinal studies of MCI. Indeed, buoyed by these data, the National Institute of Aging–Alzheimer's Association (NIA–AA) has proposed a biomarker criterion to grade the likelihood that the MCI syndrome is due to underlying AD pathology. Patients are classified as (1) high likelihood if there are core clinical symptoms and evidence of cerebral amyloid-beta (by CSF or PET) and neuronal damage (by CSF, MRI, or FDG PET); (2) intermediate likelihood if there are core clinical symptoms and a single positive biomarker (either amyloid-beta or neuronal damage); (3) unlikely to be due to AD if there are core clinical symptoms but neither biomarker is positive.

Current recommendations do not advocate the utilization of biomarkers for routine diagnostic purposes in MCI or AD, but

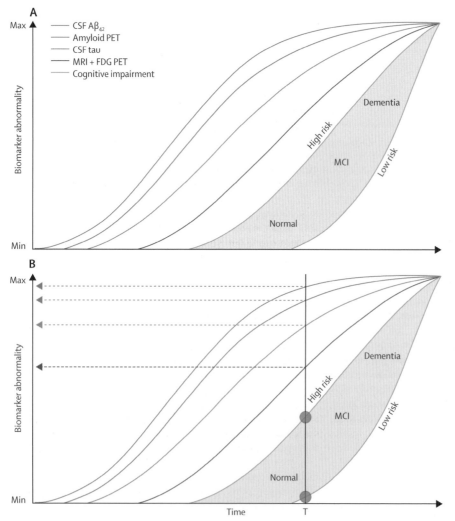

Figure 39.1 Revised model of dynamic biomarkers of the Alzheimer's disease pathological cascade (A and B). Neurodegeneration is measured by FDG PET and structural MRI, which are drawn concordantly (dark blue). By definition, all curves converge at the top right-hand corner of the plot, the point of maximum abnormality. Cognitive impairment is illustrated as a zone (light green-filled area) with low-risk and high-risk borders. (B) Operational use of the model. The vertical black line denotes a given time (T). Projection of the intersection of time T with the biomarker curves to the left vertical axis (horizontal dashed arrows) gives values of each biomarker at time T, with the lead biomarker (CSF Aβ42) being most abnormal at any given time in the progression of the disease. People who are at high risk of cognitive impairment due to Alzheimer's disease pathophysiology are shown with a cognitive impairment curve that is shifted to the left. By contrast, the cognitive impairment curve is shifted to the right in people with a protective genetic profile, high cognitive reserve, and the absence of comorbid pathological changes in the brain, showing that two patients with the same biomarker profile (at time T) can have different cognitive outcomes (denoted by gray circles at the intersection of time T).

Source: Jack 2013. Reproduced with permission of Elsevier.

Aβ = amyloid β; FDG = fluorodeoxyglucose; MCI = mild cognitive impairment; MRI = magnetic resonance imaging.

remain primarily a research tool utilized in investigational studies, clinical trials, and as an optional clinical tool. As more evidence is gained about the stability of these markers in time and how they track underlying physiology and clinical changes, as well as greater standardization, it is likely that future revisions of AD criteria will incorporate these markers, or others that have not yet been developed, in cases in which there is greater uncertainty. Specific biomarkers are described in what follows.

Structural MRI

MRI can reveal evidence of small vessel ischemic disease (SVID) or larger vessel strokes that could suggest vascular dementia, regional atrophy patterns that could suggest particular forms of underlying pathology (hippocampal and temporoparietal in AD, frontal or temporal pole in FTD, unilateral in CBD, occipital-parietal in posterior cortical atrophy), or be completely normal. The presence of mild to moderate vascular changes on MRI (small vessel hyperintensities) does not exclude the diagnosis of AD.

Visual evaluation of atrophy in MCI and AD is not precise given the significant variability in atrophy patterns observed in older individuals, but it can help the clinician gain a general sense of the likelihood of a neurodegenerative process. More quantitative measurement of entorhinal cortex (EC) or hippocampal volume can discriminate between MCI and elderly normal controls and accurately predict future conversion of MCI patients to AD. Additional measures of atrophy, such as cortical thickness, have proven to be relatively sensitive and specific markers for prediction of AD based on the pattern of involvement.

Functional imaging

Functional imaging is currently not used as broadly as structural MRI for all MCI or AD patients. It is often used to provide supporting evidence to the clinical diagnosis of AD in the context of confounding medical or psychiatric comorbidities. The pattern of FDG PET hypometabolism can help to differentiate patterns of AD (temporal and parietal lobes) from frontotemporal degeneration (frontal lobes) or other dementias. FDG PET frequently reveals a typical AD pattern of hypometabolism in the posterior temporal and parietal lobes, as well as the posterior cingulate in MCI patients with likely underlying Alzheimer's pathology. Indeed, FDG PET has demonstrated a relatively high sensitivity (~80%) and specificity (~75%) to predict conversion from MCI to AD in several studies.

Other functional imaging tools remain in the research domain, including task-related and resting state functional MRI (fMRI). Studies using fMRI have reported paradoxical greater activation of the hippocampus in MCI compared to normal controls and AD patients in memory tasks, potentially reflecting compensatory activation. Studies using resting state functional connectivity MRI show early breakdown of large-scale networks (primarily the default-mode network), although there are limited data on the prediction of prodromal AD within MCI patients.

Amyloid imaging

Amyloid imaging (e.g., florbetapir, florbetaben, and flutemetamol PET) is approved by the US Food and Drug Administration (FDA) for use in the detection of beta-amyloid neuritic plaques in individuals being evaluated for AD and other causes of cognitive impairment. These agents have demonstrated high sensitivity (>90%) and specificity (>90%) to underlying neuritic plaques in autopsy and biopsy studies. Approximately 45–65% of MCI patients display elevated amyloid deposition using a variety of amyloid ligands, compared to ~90% of suspected AD patients. This proportion is consistent with the proportions of MCI patients who eventually convert to clinical AD, and longitudinal investigations have revealed a much greater risk of developing clinical AD in those MCI patients with a positive versus negative scan. Nonetheless, despite its prognostic value, its use in AD and MCI is controversial due to concerns about a lack of implication for alteration of management in the context of its expense.

Consensus guidelines of the Amyloid Imaging Taskforce (AIT) provided recommendations for the appropriate use of amyloid imaging in populations in which it may have the greatest utility. In particular, this group suggested that amyloid imaging could be used in the evaluation of patients with "persistent or progressive unexplained MCI" in whom greater certainty of the underlying pathology would result in a change of clinical management. They also suggest utility for the evaluation of patients with core clinical criteria of possible AD in whom there remains uncertainty in the underlying pathology and in patients with young-onset dementia. Amyloid imaging is not recommended in patients with probable AD with typical neurocognitive symptoms, to determine dementia severity, or for screening of asymptomatic patients. These guidelines represent a consensus statement that balances clinical utility and interpretation of both positive and negative biomarker results. In practice, the utilization of amyloid imaging in MCI and AD is limited by the lack of insurance coverage for these agents in the United States.

CSF biomarkers

Similar to imaging markers of amyloid, CSF biomarkers can also help to improve the identification of AD pathology in MCI and AD patients. Combinations of abnormal markers (low Aβ42, elevated phosphorylated tau) have high sensitivity and specificity for predicting AD in a follow-up of 4–6 years for patients with MCI. In addition to providing evidence of cerebral amyloid deposition, CSF measures of tau provide a marker of neurodegeneration that may better track the timing of future conversion to AD in MCI patients. The use of CSF measures has been limited due to its more invasive nature compared to imaging modalities, but it can also be helpful to exclude other causes of cognitive dysfunction (such as infection, vasculitis, inflammatory disease, and normal pressure hydrocephalus).

Generally, combinations of different biomarkers provide the most precise predictive information for conversion to clinical AD in MCI, but the relative gains for each additional study remain unclear, as does consensus on the most appropriate measure in any individual.

Treatment

MCI

There is no proven pharmacological treatment to prevent the development of dementia in patients with MCI. In a single large double-blind, placebo-controlled trial of donepezil in amnestic MCI, there was evidence of a treatment effect of 0.5 points on the MMSE (+/-2) over a 36-month period and a relative risk reduction of progression to AD of 58% at 1 year and 36% at 2 years. This effect was most pronounced in the first 6–18 months of treatment, as subsequently cognitive measures declined in the donepezil group at the same rate as placebo. Other randomized controlled trials have failed to show any significant improvement, and a systemic Cochrane review found little evidence that cholinesterase inhibitors affect progression to dementia or cognitive test scores in MCI. Similarly, trials of memantine in MCI and early AD have not consistently shown any significant improvement in cognition or prevention of conversion from MCI to AD. Likewise, studies of vitamin E, rofecoxib, naproxen, and *Gingko biloba* have shown no benefit in preventing dementia in MCI or a mixed clinical population. Without clear pharmacological treatment for MCI, most patients are followed clinically for signs or symptoms of progression. They are encouraged to maintain physical and mental activity, both of which have been shown in cohort studies and small randomized controlled trials to be protective of future cognitive decline and have other general health benefits with minimal risks.

Alzheimer's disease

Current pharmacological treatment options available worldwide for AD include the cholinesterase inhibitors donepezil, galantamine, and rivastigmine for mild to severe AD and memantine for moderate to severe AD. Cholinesterase inhibitors are thought to augment cholinergic tone, particularly in projections from the basal forebrain that are involved in memory and attention functions. Memantine is an N-methyl-D-aspartate (NMDA) receptor antagonist thought to modulate excitotoxicity, although its exact mechanism remains unclear. The effects of these drugs are relatively modest in terms of benefit for cognitive and functional status and must be weighed in the context of possible side effects. Further, these medicines all appear only to provide symptomatic benefit without modifying the disease course.

Donepezil is a long-acting reversible cholinesterase inhibitor that is the most commonly used medication in AD. It is dosed at 5 mg/day and it can be increased to 10 mg/day after 4 weeks. In moderate to severe disease, a sustained release dose of 23 mg/day has demonstrated some evidence of benefit on cognitive and functional measures. It is recommended that the higher dose be used in individuals treated for 3 months at the 10 mg/day dose.

Rivastigmine is a pseudo-irreversible cholinesterase inhibitor that is available in both an oral formulation and a transdermal patch. The starting oral dose is 1.5 mg twice daily with meals, increased to 3 mg twice daily after 2 weeks. The dose can be further increased every 2 weeks to 4.5 mg and 6 mg twice daily. The transdermal patch is started at 4.6 mg (5 cm^2) per day and increased to one 9.5 mg (10 cm^2) patch per day after 4 weeks and 13.3 mg (15 cm^2) if tolerated. The transdermal patch has less frequent and less severe side effects than the oral preparation.

Galantamine is a reversible competitive cholinesterase inhibitor that also acts as an allosteric modulator of nicotinic receptors. The starting dose is 4 mg twice daily, increased to 8 mg twice daily after 4 weeks. The dose can be further increased to 12 mg twice daily after 4 more weeks. There is also an extended release formulation at 8 mg, 16 mg, and 24 mg once daily.

Most side effects of cholinesterase inhibitors occur early during titration and can be minimized by reducing the dose temporarily and retitrating. Side effects include nausea, vomiting, diarrhea, anorexia, weight loss, fatigue, headache, asthenia, muscle cramps, abdominal pain, dizziness, tremor, and syncope. The rate of anorexia varies widely, from 8–25% at higher doses compared to 3–10% of patients taking placebo. Other general precautions for use of these medications include risk for increased gastric acid secretion and gastrointenstinal bleeding, especially in patients taking anti-inflammatory medications (e.g., non-steroidal anti-inflammatory drugs, NSAIDs), sinus bradycardia, exacerbation of asthma and chronic obstructive pulmonary disease (COPD), urinary outflow obstruction, and reduction of seizure threshold. Side effects are somewhat idiosyncratic across these drugs and some patients may tolerate one better than another.

There is no difference in overall effectiveness between the three cholinesterase inhibitors. They have all demonstrated modest improvement in cognitive performance and measures of daily function. Some individuals will exhibit more significant improvement on these medications than others and they are generally offered to most patients without contraindications.

The efficacy of memantine is limited to subjects with moderate to severe AD (MMSE <15 in trials). A twice daily dosing and extended release formulation are available. The sustained release formulation is started at 7 mg daily and titrated by 7 mg every week until reaching the goal daily dose of 28 mg. The maintenance dose on the shorter-acting version is 10 mg which is titrated in a similar manner. Side effects include headache, dizziness, confusion, somnolence, and infrequent hallucinations. Of note is that diarrhea and gastrointestinal symptoms do not appear to be associated with the agent.

Outside of the medications for AD already mentioned, there have been numerous clinical trials that have failed to show any significant effect on cognitive function of supplements and drugs approved for other purposes such as vitamin E, anti-inflammatory medications, and estrogen replacement. There have been several phase II and III clinical trials for monoclonal antibodies against amyloid, as well as agents with alternative mechanisms of action, which have failed in their primary endpoints. Currently, large-scale clinical trials are being performed using antiamyloid agents in early and presymptomatic AD (identified by the presence of known genetic mutations for early-onset AD or positive amyloid biomarkers). The results of these studies may change the treatment options for AD in the future.

In addition to therapies directed at memory impairment, pharmacotherapy of AD involves management of concurrent neuropsychiatric symptoms, details of which are beyond the scope of this chapter. Briefly, for symptoms of depression, anxiety, and agitation, selective serotonin reuptake inhibitors (SSRIs) are preferred, with some evidence for the use of citalopram for agitation. For more severe agitation, delusions, and hallucinations, atypical neuroleptics are often tried, although there is data that use of any neuroleptics in this population causes increased mortality. The risk–benefit ratio for use of neuroleptics must be discussed with the family and caregivers before prescribing such medications. Non-pharmacological management including cognitive training may provide some improvement in focal cognitive domains, although how effective these strategies are for long-term cognitive outcomes remains unclear. Interventions directed at improving the support system for caregivers show great promise at reducing caregiver burden, as well as providing a positive effect on patient health and delaying time to nursing home admission.

Further reading

Albert MS, DeKosky ST, Dickson D, *et al.* The diagnosis of mild cognitive impairment due to Alzheimer's disease: Recommendations from the National Institute on Aging–Alzheimer's Association workgroups on diagnostic guidelines for Alzheimer's disease. *Alzheimers Dement* 2011;7(3):270–279.

Fargo K, Bleiler L. Alzheimer's Association report. *Alzheimers Dement* 2014;10(2):e47–e92.

Fischer P, Jungwirth S, Zehetmayer S, *et al.* Conversion from subtypes of mild cognitive impairment to Alzheimer dementia. *Neurology* 2007;68(4):288–291.

Hardy JA, Higgins GA. Alzheimer's disease: The amyloid cascade hypothesis. *Science* 1992;256(5054):184–185.

Jack CR, Jr., Knopman DS, Jagust WJ, *et al.* Tracking pathophysiological processes in Alzheimer's disease: An updated hypothetical model of dynamic biomarkers. *Lancet Neurol* 2013;12(2):207–216.

Johnson KA, Minoshima S, Bohnen NI, *et al.* Appropriate use criteria for amyloid PET: A report of the Amyloid Imaging Task Force, the Society of Nuclear Medicine and Molecular Imaging, and the Alzheimer's Association. *Alzheimers Dement* 2013;9(1):e1–e16.

McKhann GM, Knopman DS, Chertkow H, *et al.* The diagnosis of dementia due to Alzheimer's disease: Recommendations from the National Institute on Aging–Alzheimer's Association workgroups on diagnostic guidelines for Alzheimer's disease. *Alzheimers Dement* 2011;7(3):263–269.

Morris JC, Storandt M, Miller JP, *et al.* Mild cognitive impairment represents early-stage Alzheimer disease. *Arch Neurol* 2001;58(3):397–405.

Petersen RC, Parisi JE, Dickson DW, *et al.* Neuropathologic features of amnestic mild cognitive impairment. *Arch Neurol* 2006;63(5):665–672.

Petersen RC, Smith GE, Waring SC, *et al.* Mild cognitive impairment: Clinical characterization and outcome. *Arch Neurol* 1999;56(3):303–308.

40 Parkinson's Disease Dementia, Dementia with Lewy Bodies, and Other Synucleinopathies

Irena Rektorová[1], Marek Baláž[1], Robert Rusina[2], and Radoslav Matěj[3]

[1] First Department of Neurology, Masaryk University and St. Anne's Teaching Hospital, Brno, Czech Republic

[2] Department of Neurology, Charles University, and Thomayer Teaching Hospital, Prague, Czech Republic

[3] Department of Pathology and Molecular Medicine, National Laboratory for Diagnostics of Prion Diseases, Thomayer Teaching Hospital, Prague, Czech Republic

This chapter deals with dementia in Parkinson's disease (PDD), dementia with Lewy bodies (DLB), and cognitive impairment/dementia in multiple system atrophy (MSA) – that is, with neurodegenerative disorders that are also referred to as synucleinopathies. In Parkinson's disease (PD), PDD, and DLB, aggregates of α-synuclein in the cytoplasm of different populations of neurons are present in the form of Lewy bodies (LB) and dystrophic Lewy neurites that constitute the neuropathological hallmarks of these disorders. While cortical LB density is not robustly correlated with either the severity or duration of dementia, extrastriatal dopaminergic and particularly cholinergic deficits play a central role in mediating dementia in both DLB and PD. Compared to PDD, DLB presents with more pronounced visuospatial/visuoconstructive dysfunction and behavioral symptoms, and sometimes with a more pronounced pathology associated with Alzheimer's disease (AD) in addition to extensive cortical and limbic α-synuclein deposits; however, the major difference between PDD and DLB lies in the temporal sequence in which symptoms occur. Dementia develops in fully established PD, but at least 12 months after the onset of parkinsonian features. If dementia develops prior to or within the first 12 months after the onset of parkinsonism, then DLB diagnosis should be considered.

Besides α-synuclein deposits, MSA is characterized predominantly by distinctive glial cytoplasmic inclusions, called Papp–Lantos bodies, which are formed by pathologically changed α-synuclein proteins.

A feature common to all synucleinopathies and encountered frequently in DLB is REM sleep behavior disorder (RBD), often preceding the development of core features of the disease by many years. Patients with RBD have an earlier onset of parkinsonism and hallucinations and a more rapid disease progression than those without.

Parkinson's disease dementia

Dementia occurs in up to one-third of all PD patients. It is characterized by deficits in attention and executive and visuospatial functions, by memory impairment, and by prominent behavioral symptoms such as apathy and hallucinations. It is associated with a twofold increase in mortality rate as well as considerably reduced quality of life and early nursing home placement. Major risk factors for development of dementia associated with PD are higher age, more severe parkinsonism, postural instability with gait difficulty motor phenotype, and mild cognitive impairment at the time of evaluation.

Mild cognitive impairment in PD (MCI-PD) precedes the fully blown dementia and is characterized by subjective and objective deterioration of cognitive functions with retention of normal social life and daily functioning. Other (less conclusive) risk factors for PDD include family history of dementia, male gender, therapy-induced psychiatric disturbances, REM sleep behavioral disorder, and depression.

Epidemiology

The point prevalence of dementia in PD is close to 30%. The incidence rate of dementia in patients with PD is four to six times higher than the rate of dementia in age-matched controls. The cumulative prevalence of PDD is at least 75% of PD patients who survive for more than 10 years after diagnosis.

MCI-PD is seen in about one-quarter of non-demented PD patients. Recent studies have indicated that in particular more posterior cortical dysfunction, increasing age, and the microtubule-associated protein tau (MAPT) gene H1/H1 haplotype predict PDD development.

Neuropathology of cognitive impairment and dementia in PD

LB pathology in cortical and subcortical regions is sufficient to cause MCI-PD/PDD, although AD-related pathology and vascular changes may be present as well. Studies describing clinico-pathological correlations in patients with PDD can be classified into three groups: those studies suggesting a correlation of dementia with nigral and brainstem pathology, those suggesting that limbic and cortical LB-type degeneration is the main correlate, and those suggesting co-incident Alzheimer-type pathology as the main correlate of dementia. On the basis of the recent studies using α-synuclein immunohistochemistry, and assessing several potential pathological correlates simultaneously, the main pathological correlate of dementia in PD seems to be the LB-type degeneration in cerebral cortex and limbic structures (Figures 40.1. and 40.2). AD-type pathology frequently coexists, but it often does not reach a severity to justify a pathological diagnosis of AD. As for neurotransmitter changes, dementia in PD develops particularly due to cholinergic cell losses (in the nucleus basalis of Meynert) projecting to neocortical brain regions. Cortical choline acetyltransferase reductions in PDD correlate with the severity of cognitive deficits.

MCI-PD has been neuropathologically poorly defined and understood so far. Impaired executive functions and particularly posterior cortical deficits may predict dementia development later in the course of the disease. Executive deficits have been related to the dysfunction of the dorsolateral striato-prefrontal loop consequent to the loss of dopaminergic nigral neurons. Extrastriatal dopaminergic systems have also been implicated in the degeneration

---

International Neurology, Second edition. Edited by Robert P. Lisak, Daniel D. Truong, William M. Carroll and Roongroj Bhidayasiri

© 2016 John Wiley & Sons, Ltd. Published 2016 by John Wiley & Sons, Ltd.

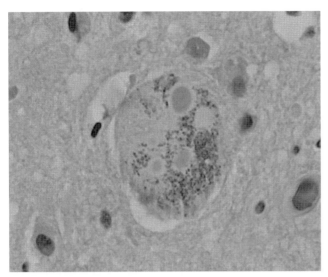

Figure 40.1 Multiple Lewy bodies in the cytoplasm of pigmented neurons in the substantia nigra. Original magnification 400X. For color details, please refer to the color plates section.

of dopamine-producing cells in the ventral tegmental area and in deficient mesocortical projections to the frontal cortex. Cognitive deficits related to posterior temporo-parietal brain regions are probably caused mainly by structural pathology such as LB and/or amyloid deposition and induce an aggressive course of the disease. Cholinergic deficits may be associated with cognitive impairment of both frontal-type and posterior cortical types.

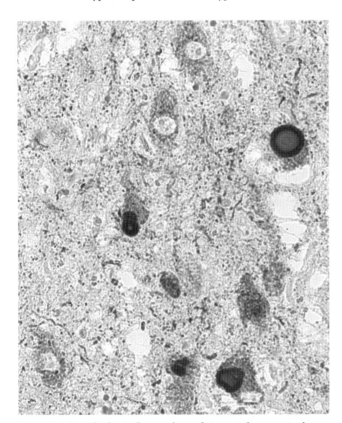

Figure 40.2 Lewy bodies in the cytoplasm of pigmented neurons in the substantia nigra positive in an immunohistochemical reaction using a monoclonal antibody against α-synuclein. Original magnification 400X. For color details, please refer to the color plates section.

Clinical features

PDD typically manifests with a progressive decline in attentional, memory, visuospatial, constructional, and executive functions; behavioral symptoms including hallucinations/psychosis and apathy may also be prominent. Motor slowing and depression may confound testing. The suggested clinical diagnostic criteria for PDD involve four domains that are anchored in core features, associated clinical features, features that make the diagnosis uncertain, and features that are not compatible with the diagnosis of PDD (Table 40.1). When all four criteria are met, probable PDD is diagnosed; when the first and last criteria are met, but clinical characteristics are atypical or uncertainty exists, possible PDD is diagnosed.

Table 40.1 Clinical diagnostic criteria for dementia in Parkinson's disease (PDD). Source: Emre 2007. Reproduced with permission of Wiley.

I. Core features

1. Diagnosis of Parkinson's disease according to Queen Square Brain Bank criteria
2. A dementia syndrome with insidious onset and slow progression, developing within the context of established PD and diagnosed by history, clinical, and mental examination, defined as:
- Impairment in more than one cognitive domain
- Representing a decline from premorbid level
- Deficits severe enough to impair daily life (social, occupational, or personal care), independent of the impairment ascribable to motor or autonomic symptoms

II. Associated clinical features

1. Cognitive features:
- Attention: Impaired. Impairment in spontaneous and focused attention, poor performance in attentional tasks; performance may fluctuate during the day and from day to day
- Executive functions: Impaired. Impairment in tasks requiring initiation, planning, concept formation, rule finding, set shifting, or set maintenance; impaired mental speed
- Visuospatial functions: Impaired. Impairment in tasks requiring visuospatial orientation, perception, or construction
- Memory: Impaired. Impairment in free recall of recent events or in tasks requiring learning new material, memory usually improves with cueing, recognition is usually better than free recall
- Language: Core functions largely preserved. Word-finding difficulties and impaired comprehension of complex sentences may be present

2. Behavioral features:
- Apathy: decreased spontaneity; loss of motivation, interest, and effortful behavior
- Changes in personality and mood, including depressive features and anxiety
- Hallucinations: mostly visual, usually complex, formed visions of people, animals, or objects
- Delusions: usually paranoid, such as infidelity, or phantom boarder delusions
- Excessive daytime sleepiness

III. Features that do not exclude PDD, but make the diagnosis uncertain

- Coexistence of any other abnormality that may by itself cause cognitive impairment, but is judged not to be the cause of dementia, e.g., presence of relevant vascular disease in imaging
- Time interval between the development of motor and cognitive symptoms not known

IV. Features suggesting other conditions or diseases as cause of mental impairment, which, when present, make it impossible to reliably diagnose PDD

- Cognitive and behavioral symptoms appearing solely in the context of other conditions such as acute confusion due to systemic diseases or abnormalities, or due to drug intoxication
- Major depression according to DSM IV
- Features compatible with "Probable Vascular dementia" according to NINDS-AIREN criteria

MCI-PD is characterized by reduced visuospatial, executive, and attentional functions. Single-domain non-amnestic MCI is more common than amnestic MCI. Diagnostic criteria for MCI-PD were published by the Movement Disorders Task Force in 2012. Probable PD-MCI was defined based on comprehensive neuropsychological testing as cognitive decline reported by the patient, carer, or clinician with performance 1–2 standard deviations (SD) below the mean for an age-matched control population on two or more tests from the neuropsychological battery, as well as the lack of a confounding cause for poor test performance such as depression (level II category). Possible MCI-PD may be diagnosed based on abbreviated screening assessment (level I category). Unlike MCI in Alzheimer's disease, MCI-PD is defined within the context of an existing etiology, namely PD, and it includes not just "memory" complaints, but also other cognitive changes.

Investigations

The main differential diagnoses of PDD are DLB (see the later discussion), AD (usually early amnestic syndrome), vascular dementia (usually stepwise cognitive deterioration, pyramidal signs, and relevant cerebrovascular disease changes on brain magnetic resonance imaging [MRI]), Parkinson-plus syndromes (progressive supranuclear palsy, multiple system atrophy, corticobasal degeneration), and Creutzfeldt–Jakob disease (rapid progression of dementia, characteristic electroencephalogram [EEG], MRI, and cerebrospinal fluid [CSF] changes). However, sometimes it is difficult to distinguish between PDD and these other illnesses, particularly in less typical cases. Dopamine transporter imaging (single photon emission tomography or positron emission tomography) may be useful in differentiating AD and DLB/PDD in particular, since they reveal the integrity of presynaptic dopamine neurons. It is also important to distinguish Wilson's disease, the Westphal variant of Huntington's disease, and other conditions such as AIDS-dementia complex, hypoparathyroidism, or carbon monoxide (CO) intoxication. A review of a recent search for diagnostic and prognostic biomarkers is beyond the scope of this chapter.

Treatment of PDD

From a practical point of view, it is important to realize that dementia in PD limits the drug treatment of extrapyramidal motor symptoms, since all antiparkinsonian drugs may trigger or exacerbate hallucinations, psychotic features, and confusion. Anticholinergic drugs in particular should be discontinued, since these agents may lead to a deterioration of memory and executive functions.

In line with the described neurochemical changes in PDD, the positive effects of acetylcholinesterase inhibitors (AChEIs) have been demonstrated by several double-blind placebo-controlled studies. Most of the data are available for rivastigmine, which produced moderate but significant improvements in global ratings for dementia, cognition, and behavioral symptoms; the magnitude of effects was similar to that observed in AD patients treated with AChEIs. The most frequent adverse effects were nausea, vomiting, and tremor. Memantine (N-methyl-D-aspartate receptor antagonist) may have beneficial effects on global status and behavioral symptoms in patients with PDD, but possibly more so in the DLB population.

If AChEIs are ineffective, or if more acute control of behavioral symptoms is required, a cautious trial of atypical antipsychotics is recommended; clinicians should be vigilant to the possibility of a sensitivity reaction. Clozapine is the only drug with proven efficacy

and acceptable tolerability. Adjunctive non-pharmacological interventions such as cognitive behavioral therapy for visual hallucinations have the potential to ameliorate many symptoms, but none has been systematically studied.

There is no recommended treatment for MCI-PD. Preliminary studies suggest that the antidepressant atomoxetine might have a beneficial effect on executive functions in non-dementia cognitive deficits in PD.

Dementia with Lewy bodies

DLB is a neurodegenerative disease with intraneuronal deposits of α-synuclein. The clinical hallmarks of DLB include fluctuating attention and cognition, parkinsonism, and visual hallucinations.

Epidemiology

DLB is a common form of dementia representing 15–20% of cases of dementia in old age and is the second most prevalent cause of neurodegenerative dementia after Alzheimer´s disease. The average onset is 75 years, with a small preponderance for men.

Neuropathology

The core neuropathological features are practically the same as in PDD; it seems likely that the two diseases are phenotypic variants of the LBD/PDD spectrum. A three-stage scoring system according to McKeith and a six-stage scoring system according to Braak distinguish between brainstem-predominant, limbic-transitional, and diffuse neocortical stages, based on the numbers and distribution of LB and Lewy neurites in different brain areas.

Clinical features

Cognitive deterioration is a key feature for DLB diagnosis (Table 40.2). The cognitive profile typically includes early and predominant impairment in visuospatial abilities (constructional apraxia, lack of orientation appraisal) and in attention and executive performance (mainly mental flexibility and a capacity for abstraction). Progressively, bradypsychia and perseverative tendencies with stereotypies develop. Apathy and depression are frequently manifested in DLB.

A typical finding is fluctuation in cognitive performance and/or fluctuating parkinsonism, affecting mainly attention, orientation, psychomotor velocity, communication abilities, akinesia, and gait. This fluctuation, which may be observed in 50–75% of DLB patients, is disease inherent and appears typically without any identifiable external factor. The frequency, duration (hours or days), and severity of fluctuation may be extremely variable, even for the same patient.

Recurrent hallucinations may occur in up to 80% of cases. They are almost purely visual (partially corresponding to α-synuclein deposits in associated visual areas); other sensory modalities are affected more rarely. Visual hallucinations in DLB are often well tolerated and may be more disturbing for the caregiver than for the patient.

Parkinsonism is frequent in DLB, but may be absent in about 20% of patients. Akinesia and rigidity are bilateral, symmetric from the beginning, and predominantly in the lower extremities, with early gait disturbance and instability. Resting tremor is rarely observed, whereas dysarthria is a common feature in DLB.

Dysautonomia may develop with a wide range of manifestations, including orthostatic hypotension, incontinence, and hypersalivation.

Table 40.2 Revised criteria for the clinical diagnosis of dementia with Lewy bodies (DLB). Source: McKeith 2005. Reproduced with permission of Wolters Kluwer.

1. **Central feature: dementia** (deficits on tests of attention, executive function, and visuospatial ability may be prominent)

2. **Core features**
   - Fluctuating cognition (excluding delirium)
   - Recurrent visual hallucinations
   - Spontaneous features of parkinsonism

3. **Suggestive features**
   - REM sleep behavior disorder
   - Neuroleptic sensitivity
   - Low dopamine transporter uptake in the basal ganglia demonstrated by SPECT or PET imaging

4. **Supportive features**
   - Repeated falls and syncope
   - Transient, unexplained loss of consciousness
   - Severe autonomic dysfunctions
   - Hallucinations in other (than visual) modalities
   - Delusions
   - Depression
   - Relative preservation of medial temporal lobe structures on CT/MRI scans
   - Low uptake on SPECT/PET perfusion scan with reduced occipital activity
   - Prominent slow EEG waveforms with temporal lobe transient sharp waves
   - Abnormal meta-iodobenzylguanidine (MIBG) myocardial scintigraphy

Probable DLB
Dementia and at least two core features
or
Dementia and one core feature and one or more suggestive features

Possible DLB
Dementia and one core feature
or
Dementia and one or more suggestive features (even in the absence of core features)

Definite DLB
Neuropathological findings of neuronal loss and α-synuclein deposits in selected brain areas

CT = computed tomography; EEG = electroencephalogram; MRI = magnetic resonance imaging; PET = positron emission tomography; SPECT = single-photon emission computed tomography

The current diagnostic criteria for DLB, summarized in Table 40.2, are based on the association of core features (cognitive and/or motor fluctuations, hallucinations, and parkinsonism) with various suggestive features in a patient with progressive dementia.

Investigations

DLB must be differentiated mainly from AD, PDD, vascular dementia, frontotemporal dementia (FTD), and normal pressure hydrocephalus (NPH). Other disorders causing dementia and parkinsonism should also be ruled out (progressive supranuclear palsy, corticobasal syndrome, multiple system atrophy, Creutzfeldt–Jakob disease, Wilson's disease, Huntington's disease, autoimmune encephalitis, and AIDS-dementia complex), but their manifestations are often more distinct from DLB in its typical course.

Early and prominent visuospatial impairment in association with dysexecutive syndrome in DLB differs from the predominantly amnestic pattern of dementia in AD. At a similar degree of deterioration (the same Mini Mental Score Examination, MMSE), DLB patients have a significantly lower performance in drawing (pentagon-copying items from the MMSE, figural drawing, or the clock test) and perform better in tests of episodic memory. In contrast to FTD, early behavioral and personality changes are absent and disinhibition with compulsivity is uncommon in DLB.

MRI is helpful in excluding significant white-matter lesions, vascular impairment, and ventricular enlargement. DLB differs from AD in the absence of significant supratentorial atrophy, including a preserved hippocampal volume and only a very limited progression rate of atrophy over the disease course.

Dopamine transporter imaging – that is, single photon emission tomography or positron emission tomography with I123 ioflupane (FP-CIT) – shows positive findings in DLB (and PDD), together with other atypical parkinsonian syndromes; negative results in AD are in line with the preserved integrity of presynaptic dopamine neurons.

Cerebrospinal fluid analysis may reveal decreased amyloid beta and α-synuclein and increased total and phosphorylated tau. Decreased CSF α-synuclein may be of diagnostic use in differentiating between DLB and AD; however, CSF analysis is not routinely used in DLB diagnostic management.

Treatment

Patients with DLB have severe cholinergic deficits in both basal forebrain and frontal- parietal cortex. Cognitive and behavioral manifestations in DLB may in part respond to acetylcholinesterase inhibitors, or to memantine in the more advance stages of the disease.

The benefit of levodopa in motor impairment in DLB is less convincing than in PDD; however, up to one-third of DLB patients may show improvement in parkinsonism symptoms. On the other hand, chronic administration of levodopa may induce or exacerbate behavioral symptoms in DLB. REM sleep behavior disorder, a common finding in patients with DLB as well as in PDD, can be treated with low doses of clonazepam; depressive manifestations often respond to antidepressants (serotonin reuptake inhibitors).

Nonselective antipsychotic drugs are unsuitable in DLB as they often aggravate clinical symptomatology (rigidity, sedation, and cognition), even at very low doses; neuroleptic sensitivity is a suggestive feature for DLB. Hallucinations, delusions, and agitation should be treated with caution, using only atypical neuroleptics and at low doses. The most evidence available is for clozapine and quetiapine.

Multiple system atrophy

MSA is an adult-onset, progressive, sporadic neurodegenerative disease clinically characterized by varying severity of parkinsonian symptoms, cerebellar ataxia, autonomic and urogenital dysfunction, and corticospinal signs. Currently, two major types are distinguished: MSA with a predominance of cerebellar symptoms, MSA-C, and MSA presenting mostly with parkinsonian symptomatology, MSA-P (see Chapter 49).

Epidemiology

There are only scarce epidemiological data on the incidence and prevalence of MSA. The incidence rate has been estimated to be 3–4.4 per 100,000. Various data suggest that MSA may account for approximately 5% of those with parkinsonism. In Europe, MSA-P accounts for up to 70% of cases; in Japan, MSA-C is more common.

Neuropathology

The etiology is unknown, but MSA is designated as an α-synucleinopathy. The pattern of neuronal degeneration involves predominantly the striatonigral system in patients with dominant clinical parkinsonism, and the olivopontocerebellar system in those with predominant cerebellar features. However, all the aforementioned brain areas are affected in both MSA types.

There has been only limited study of changes in neurotransmitters in MSA. Dopamine levels appear to be reduced in various parts of the basal ganglia, most probably due to decreased levels of substance P, GABA, and noradrenaline. A significant increase in iron content in the medial putamen, caudate nucleus, and substantia nigra has been observed.

The neuropathological process leading to the development of MSA-related dementia is multifactorial. It appears that amyloid pathology has a limited role in dementia in MSA, although some patients had an increased cortical amyloid burden. Cortical thinning in MSA patients with dementia was observed in areas where cortical thinning was reported in Alzheimer's disease or Parkinson's disease dementia, but its pathological relevance remains unclear. Frontal atrophy was also present in MSA, and frontal lobe-related cognitive deficits were correlated with disease duration. It has been suggested that even in the absence of brain atrophy, changes in the frontal metabolism might account for some of the executive impairment observed in MSA.

Clinical features

The presenting motor disorder most commonly consists of parkinsonism with predominant bradykinesia and rigidity, early gait instability, but often without tremor. Cerebellar ataxia may be the initial motor symptom in a substantial percentage of patients. Autonomous dysfunction is observed almost universally in both motor presentations. The proposed diagnostic criteria for MSA recommend assigning MSA-P diagnosis when parkinsonian signs determine the motor presentation, and MSA-C when cerebellar features determine the motor presentation.

Revised diagnostic criteria (see Table 40.3) define the features and criteria necessary for establishing a diagnosis of MSA. The current criteria retain the distinctions between levels of diagnostic certainty, using the terms *definite MSA* for subjects with autopsy demonstration of typical histological features, *probable MSA* for patients with autonomic failure plus parkinsonism or cerebellar ataxia, and *possible MSA* for people with clinical findings that do not yet clearly represent this disease.

According to older data, the vast majority of patients with MSA do not exhibit clinical signs of dementia or cognitive impairment. Indeed, dementia was an exclusion criterion for this particular diagnosis. Various authors later reported cognitive changes, such as significant deficits in attentional set shifting, spatial working memory, and Tower of London task. Recent reports show that dementia occurs in 5–26% of patients with MSA, with the MSA-P variant being more frequently studied. The severity of motor disability correlates with MMSE scores.

According to various reports, frontal lobe–related functions were impaired in about 40% of patients. Some studies showed no difference in cognitive changes between patients with MSA-P and MSA-C, while other authors report more severe and more widespread cognitive dysfunctions in patients with MSA-P as compared to MSA-C.

Investigations

The differential diagnosis for MSA-P includes other disorders with parkinsonism, including Parkinson's disease and progressive supranuclear palsy. In cases with MSA-C, various cerebellar syndromes

Table 40.3 Revised consensus criteria for the clinical diagnosis of multiple system atrophy (MSA). Source: Gilman 2008. Reproduced with permission of Wolters Kluwer.

Possible MSA: one criterion + two features from other separate domains. When the criterion is parkinsonism, a poor L-DOPA response qualifies as one feature

Probable MSA: criterion for autonomic failure/urinary dysfunction + poor L-DOPA responsive parkinsonism or cerebellar dysfunction

Definite MSA: pathologically confirmed

Autonomic and urinary dysfunction

A. Autonomic and urinary features
1. Orthostatic hypotension
2. Urinary incontinence or incomplete bladder emptying
B. Orthostatic fall in blood pressure or urinary incontinence/erectile dysfunction in men, or both

Parkinsonism

A. Parkinsonism features
1. Bradykinesia
2. Rigidity
3. Postural instability (not caused by primary visual, vestibular, cerebellar, or proprioceptive dysfunction)
4. Tremor
B. Bradykinesia + at least one of items 2 to 4

Cerebellar dysfunction

A. Cerebellar features
1. Gait ataxia
2. Ataxic dysarthria
3. Limb ataxia
4. Sustained gaze-evoked nystagmus
B. Gait ataxia + at least one of items 2 to 4

Corticospinal dysfunction

A. Corticospinal tract features
1. Extensor plantar response + hyperreflexia
B. No corticospinal tract features are used in defining the diagnosis of MSA

A feature (A) is a characteristic of the disease, and a criterion (B) is a defining feature or composite of features required for diagnosis.

associated with neurodegeneration have to be considered, such as spinocerebellar ataxias (SCA). Autonomic dysfunction in MSA has to be differentiated from autonomic neuropathy.

Clinical signs and additional investigations can be of value. These may include autonomic function tests, external sphincter electromyography, neuropsychological assessment, and neuroimaging (Figure 40.3).

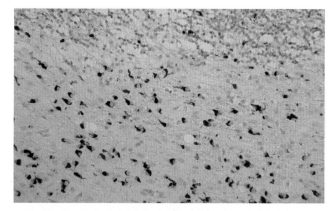

Figure 40.3 Numerous Papp–Lantos oligodendroglial inclusions in the cerebellum positive in an immunohistochemical reaction using a monoclonal antibody against α-synuclein. Original magnification 400X. For color details, please refer to the color plates section.

Brain MRI plays a practical role in demonstrating putaminal, pontine, and cerebellar atrophy and dilatation of the fourth ventricle. A putaminal slit and a hot cross bun sign on MRI have high positive predictive values for MSA.

Treatment

There is no specific treatment for MSA. In contrast to PD, MSA patients show a poor response to dopaminergic drugs, suggesting early postsynaptic dopamine receptor changes and additional involvement of non-dopaminergic systems. Medical treatment is directed toward relieving the parkinsonian and autonomic symptoms of the illness. L-DOPA response is either brief or non-existent. Dyskinesias may appear. Dopamine agonists are no more effective than L-DOPA. Anticholinergic drugs may bring some relief of parkinsonian signs and urinary frequency and urgency. Orthostatic hypotension requires measures such as increased intake of salt, elevation of the head of the bed at night, elastic support garments, and treatment by fludrocortisone or other vasoconstrictor drugs. Urinary retention or incontinence may require catheterization. There are no proven medications for treating MSA-related dementia.

Further reading

Aarsland D, Cummings J, Weintraub D, Chaudhuri KR (eds.). *Neuropsychiatric and Cognitive Changes in Parkinson's Disease and Delated Movement Disorders: Diagnosis and Management.* Cambridge: Cambridge University Press; 2013.

Emre M, Aarsland D, Brown R, *et al.* Clinical diagnostic criteria for dementia associated with Parkinson's disease. *Mov Disord* 2007;22:1689–1707.

Gilman S, Wenning GK, Low PA, *et al.* Second consensus statement on the diagnosis of multiple system atrophy. *Neurology* 2008;71:670–676.

Kim HJ, Jeon BS, Kim YE, *et al.* Clinical and imaging characteristics of dementia in multiple system atrophy. *Parkinsonism Relat Disord* 2013;19:617–621.

Litvan I, Goldman JG, Tröster AI, *et al.* Diagnostic criteria for mild cognitive impairment in Parkinson's disease: Movement Disorder Society Task Force guidelines. *Mov Disord* 2012;27:349–356.

McKeith IG, Dickson DW, Emre M, *et al.* Diagnosis and management of dementia with Lewy bodies: Third report of the DLB Consortium. *Neurology* 2005;65:1863–1872.

Sorbi S, Hort J, Erkinjuntti T, *et al.* EFNS-ENS guidelines on the diagnosis and management of disorders associated with dementia. *Eur J Neurol* 2012;19:1159–1179.

Stankovic I, Krismer F, Jesic A, *et al.* Cognitive impairment in multiple system atrophy: A position statement by the Neuropsychology Task Force of the MDS Multiple System Atrophy (MODIMSA) study group. *Mov Disord* 2014;29:857–867.

Wang HF, Yu JT, Tang SW, *et al.* Efficacy and safety of cholinesterase inhibitors and memantine in cognitive impairment in Parkinson's disease, Parkinson's disease dementia, and dementia with Lewy bodies: Systematic review with meta-analysis and trial sequential analysis. *J Neurol Neurosurg Psychiatry* 2015;86(2):135–143. doi: 10.1136/jnnp-2014-307659

41

Specific vascular syndromes

Elka Stefanova and Vladimir Kostić

Faculty of Medicine, University of Belgrade, and Institute of Neurology, CCS, Belgrade, Serbia

Vascular cognitive impairment (VCI) is usually subgrouped for clinical use, and the subgroups can be characterized by risk factors, mechanisms, pathology, clinical features, neuroimaging, or response to treatment. The most frequent syndromes are presented in this chapter.

Cerebral amyloid angiopathy

In the population-based Honolulu–Asia Aging Study (HAAS), cerebral amyloid angiopathy (CAA) was present in 44% of autopsied brains, which were enriched in pathological findings by the study's targeting of demented subjects. CAA was non-significantly overrepresented in demented (55%) compared with non-demented (38%) brains. In a large population study, severe CAA was identified in 34 of 93 patients with dementia, versus only 7 of 99 of those without dementia, yielding an impressively elevated odds ratio (OR) for dementia of 7.7 (95% confidence interval [CI], 3.3–20.4). A common pathology in the elderly, CAA appears in 10–30% of unselected brain autopsies, and 80–100% when in the presence of accompanying Alzheimer's disease (AD). Although sporadic CAA is most commonly recognized as a cause of spontaneous intracerebral hemorrhage, there is growing evidence that it is an important contributor to age-related cognitive impairment as well. These observations suggest that CAA can cause clinically important vascular dysfunction, a possibility further supported by multiple studies demonstrating potential mechanisms for beta amyloid–induced vascular damage or functional abnormality.

Cognitive impairment has been observed in both familial and sporadic instances of severe CAA, generally in the absence of extensive AD pathology. A notable finding in very severe cases of CAA is cognitive impairment in the absence of major hemorrhagic stroke. Advanced CAA can trigger a series of destructive changes in the vessel wall, including loss of smooth muscle cells, development of microaneurysms, concentric splitting and fibrinoid necrosis, and perivascular leakage of red blood cells. The hallmark of sporadic CAA is deposition of beta amyloid peptide in the walls of penetrating arterioles and capillaries of the leptomeninges and cortex, a well-known common pathology in the elderly.

CAA is most commonly diagnosed by the detection of "hemorrhages confined to cortical or cortico-subcortical ('lobar') brain regions." According to the Boston criteria, the presence of multiple strictly lobar hemorrhages in the absence of other definite causes such as head trauma, brain tumor, or supratherapeutic anticoagulation has been defined as "probable CAA." The key finding for the diagnosis of probable CAA is T2*-weighted gradient-echo MRI sequences, which provide substantially increased sensitivity for the detection of cerebral microbleeds. One prominent feature of CAA was common and severe white-matter abnormalities. White-matter hypodensity was present in 69 of the 88 patients (78%) and severe hypodensity (score of 3–4 on a scale of 0–4) in 34 of 88 patients (39%). The white-matter hypodensity score increased with increasing numbers of MRI-detectable hemorrhages, supporting the possibility that the extent of white-matter injury is a function of the severity of the underlying CAA-related microvasculopathy.

Detection of reduced beta amyloid in cerebrospinal fluid (CSF) or increased retention of the amyloid ligand Pittsburgh Compound B on positron emission tomography imaging is not specific for CAA as opposed to AD, but the two pathologies may be distinguishable in part by the relative occipital predominance of labeling in CAA.

Hereditary small vessel syndromes

The most commonly presented hereditary cause of VCI is cerebral autosomal dominant arteriopathy with subcortical infarcts and leukoencephalopathy (CADASIL). The clinical presentation includes migraines and aura, mood disturbances, recurrent strokes, or cognitive impairment. Characteristic radiographic findings include the appearance of extensive white-matter lesions (WMLs), lacunar infarcts, microbleeds, and brain atrophy.

Nearly all cases of CADASIL are caused by missense mutations of the Notch3 gene that either create or eliminate cysteine residues. The primary method of diagnosis has become the identification of such mutations, which can also occur *de novo* in sporadic cases of CADASIL. Characteristic ultrastructural changes in vessels of the skin and muscle, particularly the deposition of granular osmiophilic material in the arteriolar media, are frequent findings in most CADASIL patients.

Although no treatments have been identified to modify the course of CADASIL, it is notable that cardiovascular risk factors such as hypertension, elevated hemoglobin A1c, and smoking may be associated with a worse clinical and radiographic phenotype.

Other hereditary small vessel syndromes of the brain are rare and have generally not been reported as causes of sporadic disease via *de novo* mutation.

Poststroke dementia

The prevalence of poststroke dementia (PSD) varies in relation to the interval after stroke, definition of dementia, and location and size of the infarct. Among patients who have experienced a first

---

International Neurology, Second edition. Edited by Robert P. Lisak, Daniel D. Truong, William M. Carroll and Roongroj Bhidayasiri
© 2016 John Wiley & Sons, Ltd. Published 2016 by John Wiley & Sons, Ltd.

stroke, the reported prevalence of dementia is 30% immediately after stroke. The incidence of new-onset dementia increases from 7% after 1 year to 48% after 25 years. In general, the risk of dementia increases two-fold after having a stroke. Risk of dementia is higher with increased age, fewer years of education, history of diabetes mellitus and atrial fibrillation, and recurrent stroke. Patients with PSD develop functional impairment and have a high mortality rate. The mortality rate was 19.8 deaths per 100 person-years with dementia compared with 6.9 deaths per 100 person-years without dementia. Even after adjustment for demographic and vascular risk factors, long-term mortality is still 2–6 times higher in stroke patients with PSD than in those without.

Left hemisphere, anterior, and posterior cerebral artery distribution, multiple infarcts, and strategic infarcts have been associated with PSD. Locations considered to be "strategic" have traditionally included (1) the left angular gyrus; (2) inferomesial temporal; (3) mesial frontal; (4) anterior and dorsomedial thalamus; (5) left capsular genu; and (6) caudate nuclei. The concept of strategic infarction, however, needs to be reexamined in larger prospective MRI studies, with the extent and location of stroke defined in relation to cognitive networks. Other neuroimaging findings present in parallel, such as silent cerebral infarcts, white-matter changes, and global and medial temporal lobe atrophy, are associated with increased risk of PSD.

It is not easy to determine to what extent cognitive impairment may be attributable to stroke versus concomitant AD. Estimates of the proportion of patients with PSD with presumed AD vary widely between 19% and 61%. Approximately 15–30% of people with PSD have a history of dementia before stroke, and approximately 33% have significant medial temporal atrophy. According to Gorelick *et al.*, the incidence of dementia 3 years after stroke is significantly greater in those patients with versus those without medial temporal atrophy (81% vs. 58%).

Further reading

Gorelick PB, Scuteri A, Black SE, *et al.* Vascular contributions to cognitive impairment and dementia: A statement for healthcare professionals from the American Heart Association/American Stroke Association. *Stroke* 2011;42(9):2672–2713.

Greenberg SM, Gurol ME, Rosand J, Smith EE. Amyloid angiopathy-related vascular cognitive impairment. *Stroke* 2004;35(11 Suppl 1):2616–2619.

Knudsen KA, Rosand J, Karluk D, Greenberg SM. Clinical diagnosis of cerebral amyloid angiopathy: Validation of the Boston criteria. *Neurology* 2001;56:537–539.

O'Brien JT, Erkinjuntti T, Reisberg B, *et al.* Vascular cognitive impairment. *Lancet Neurol* 2003;2:89–98.

42 Vascular cognitive impairment

Elka Stefanova and Vladimir Kostić

Faculty of Medicine, University of Belgrade, and Institute of Neurology, CCS, Belgrade, Serbia

Recently, the construct "vascular cognitive impairment" (VCI) was introduced to comprise the heterogeneous group of cognitive disorders that share a presumed vascular cause, which includes both dementia and cognitive impairment without dementia. With newer research-based classification systems, the term VCI is now preferred to vascular dementia. The most severe form of VCI is vascular dementia (VaD), and new subtypes with milder cognitive symptoms (e.g., VaMCI) are being defined. A key to defining the spectrum of VCI is neuropsychological testing, bedside or office clinical examination, and neuroimaging.

The use of the VCI classification system may prove to be useful for clinicians in practice. The VCI construct takes into account the fact that in addition to single strategic infarcts, multiple infarcts, and leukoaraiosis, there are other mechanisms of cerebrovascular disease, such as chronic hypoperfusion, that might account for the pattern of cognitive deficits associated with vascular dementia. The VCI construct also enables greater attention to be paid to opportunities for prevention, early intervention, and the coexistence of Alzheimer's disease pathology.

Epidemiology

The prevalence of Alzheimer's disease (AD) doubles every 4.3 years, whereas the prevalence of vascular dementia (VaD) doubles every 5.3 years. VCI is also strongly age related. The prevalence of VaD ranges from 1.0% in a population cohort ≥55 years of age to 4.2% in a cohort of subjects ≥71 years of age. Age-adjusted rates for AD and VaD are 19.2 and 14.6, respectively, per 1000 person-years. Differences in diagnostic criteria may partly explain this variability. Although the differences may have diminished lately, a higher prevalence of VaD (compared to AD) has been reported in East Asia, and men are affected more frequently than women. Recently, Chan *et al.*'s report from China suggested that previous estimates of dementia burden, based on smaller datasets, might have underestimated the burden of dementia in China. Incidence of dementia was 9.87 cases per 1000 person-years, that of AD was 6.25 cases per 1000 person-years, that of VaD was 2.42 cases per 1000 person-years, and that of other rare forms of dementia was 0.46 cases per 1000 person-years.

The mortality of VaD patients exceeds that of AD patients, probably because of the added coronary morbidity. The reported incidence rates of VaD vary between 1.5 and 3.3 per 1000 person-years in elderly populations. Incidence rates are highly dependent on age.

Risk factors

Common risk factors for VaD include hypertension, insulin resistance, hyperlipidemia, hyperhomocystinemia, atherosclerosis, diabetes, and smoking; these are equally common in patients with cortical atherothromboembolism as they are in patients with lacunar stroke. Age is also a risk factor for VaD, suggesting that dementia in patients after the age of 65 increases gradually. However, many patients with small vessel disease (SVD) are not hypertensive. For example, in 70 consecutive autopsies in patients with pathologically verified SVD, vascular risk factors were mostly absent. Many sporadic cases and the monogenetic variants of SVD arise in normotensive patients. Hypertension is a key risk factor for white-matter hyperintensities, but the association between white-matter hyperintensities and blood pressure is rather complex.

Neuropathology and pathophysiology of VCI

The neuropathological criteria for diagnosing either VaD or VCI are not yet established. The types of neuropathological lesions associated with VCI include large and small vessel infarcts, white-matter changes, hemorrhage, gliosis, and, in mixed dementia, the neuropathological changes of AD. In a population-based neuropathological study, in which 13% of participants had pure VaD without major evidence of AD, the requirement that dementia follows a known stroke resulted in high specificity but low sensitivity in autopsy-verified cases.

A simplified mechanistic approach separates VCI associated with (1) large vessel disease; and (2) small vessel disease, including subcortical ischemic vascular disease and non-infarct ischemic changes.

Large vessel disease

One of the clinical archetypes of large vessel disease is poststroke dementia (PSD), a significant cognitive impairment that follows stroke (within 3 months). The association of vascular risk factors, such as hypertension, diabetes, hyperlipidemia, and smoking, with stroke severity has been inconsistent, but the risk factors for PSD dementia include age and low education.

Small vessel disease

Small vessel disease (SVD) is discussed in relation to the white-matter changes seen with neuroimaging, and the term leukoaraiosis is often

International Neurology, Second edition. Edited by Robert P. Lisak, Daniel D. Truong, William M. Carroll and Roongroj Bhidayasiri
© 2016 John Wiley & Sons, Ltd. Published 2016 by John Wiley & Sons, Ltd.

used to describe them. The increased sensitivity of MRI can now detect white-matter disease in more than 90% of older patients. Frank infarction might be rare in leukoaraiosis compared with deep white-matter lesions, and the causal pathway between leukoaraiosis and vascular changes is not well understood. The association with cognitive and functional decline is rather robust, although the cognitive domains affected by leukoaraiosis are not clearly established. In general, patients with confluent lesions have a worse prognosis than those with punctate lesions, but decline in cognition and function are more consistently related to measures of atrophy. There is controversy as to whether periventricular and deep white-matter lesions should be studied independently and whether they are distinct in their etiologies, presentations, or rates of progression.

Subcortical ischemic vascular disease
Subcortical vascular injury due to small vessel infarct or ischemia occurs within the cerebral white matter, basal ganglia, and brainstem. Lacunes are seen in the cortical white matter or, more typically, in the corona radiata, internal capsule, centrum semi-ovale, thalamus, basal ganglia, or pons. Infarcts less than 3 mm in diameter are up to 20 times more prevalent than overt infarcts and occur in 20% of patients older than 65 years.

Non-infarct ischemic changes and atrophy
The neuropathology in VCI does not mean only frank infarctions, but is more probably a continuum of processes related to ischemia. Diffusion tensor magnetic resonance imaging (MRI) can be used to detect abnormalities that extend beyond the visible borders of leukoaraiosis, and these abnormalities show a more robust association with cognition than leukoaraiosis alone.

Neuropathology
The lesion underlying most lacunar strokes is an infarct that is rounded, ovoid, or tubular in shape, and less than 20 mm in axial diameter. Tubular lesions seem to be most common in the basal ganglia or internal capsule. A small proportion (5%) of tubular lesions are caused by a small, deep hemorrhage. Only about 50% of recent infarcts are visible on computed tomography (CT), whereas at least 70% are visible on diffusion-weighted MRI.

Lacunes are small cavities contained cerebral spinal fluid (CSF) located in the deep gray or white matter, typically larger than 3 mm and smaller than 15 mm in diameter. Although lesions larger than 15 mm are sometimes regarded as lacunes, generally the larger the lesion, the more likely that it was caused by mechanisms other than SVD. Many lacunes were never symptomatic but appear silently on brain imaging.

White-matter hyperintensities (Figure 42.1) are rounded areas of decreased attenuation on CT, increased signal on T2-weighted and FLAIR, and often decreased on T1-weighted MRI with respect to normal brain; however, these areas are not as attenuated or intense as the CSF Virchow–Robin spaces or visible perivascular spaces that surround the small, deep perforating arterioles as the arterioles pass through the deep gray and white matter. These spaces are visible on T2-weighted or T1-weighted MRI because they contain increased fluid (in comparison with the surrounding tissue) of similar signal to CSF. Other features of SVD include microbleeds, which are small punctate areas of hypointensity on T2* or susceptibility-weighted imaging that are up to 10 mm in diameter and correspond to small collections of hemosiderin-laden macrophages around small perforating vessels (Figure 42.2).

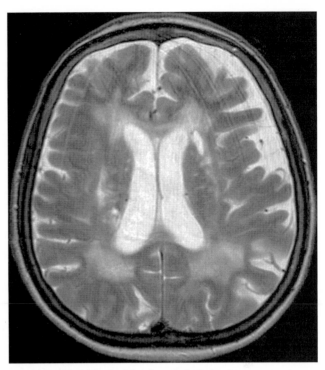

Figure 42.1 T2-weighted axial periventricular ischemic leucoencephalopathy and multiple lacunes. Source: Ivan Nikolić. Reproduced with permission.

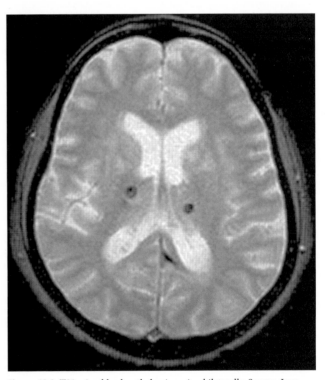

Figure 42.2 T2* microbleeds – thalamic region bilaterally. Source: Ivan Nikolić. Reproduced with permission.

Clinical features

We suggest a practical approach to the classification of dementia and VaMCI (Table 42.1) that is adapted from Gorelick *et al.*, and propose that the term VCI be used for all forms of cognitive disorder associated with cerebrovascular disease, regardless of the pathogenesis (e.g., cardioembolic, atherosclerotic, ischemic, hemorrhagic, or genetic). There are several key considerations for making the diagnosis of VaD or VCI: (1) dementia criteria for the diagnosis

Table 42.1 Vascular cognitive impairment. Source: Adapted from Gorelick 2011. Reproduced with permission of Wolters Kluwer.

1. The term VCI characterizes all forms of cognitive deficits from VaD to MCI of vascular origin.
2. These criteria cannot be used for patients who have an active diagnosis of drug or alcohol abuse/dependence. Patients must be free of any type of substance for at least 3 months.
3. These criteria cannot be used for patients with delirium.

Dementia

1. The diagnosis of dementia should be based on a decline in cognitive function from a prior baseline and a deficit in performance in ≥2 cognitive domains that are of sufficient severity to affect the subject's activities of daily living.
2. The diagnosis of dementia must be based on cognitive testing, and a minimum of 4 cognitive domains should be assessed: executive/attention, memory, language, and visuospatial functions.
3. The deficits in activities of daily living are independent of the motor/sensory sequelae of the vascular event.

Probable VaD

1. There is cognitive impairment and imaging evidence of cerebrovascular disease AND:
    a. There is a clear temporal relationship between a vascular event (e.g., clinical stroke) and onset of cognitive deficits, or
    b. There is a clear relationship in the severity and pattern of cognitive impairment and the presence of diffuse, subcortical cerebrovascular disease pathology (e.g., as in CADASIL).
2. There is no history of gradually progressive cognitive deficits before or after the stroke that suggests the presence of a non-vascular neurodegenerative disorder.

Possible VaD

There is cognitive impairment and imaging evidence of cerebrovascular disease BUT:
1. There is no clear relationship (temporal, severity, or cognitive pattern) between the vascular disease (e.g., silent infarcts, subcortical small vessel disease) and the cognitive impairment.
2. There is insufficient information for the diagnosis of VaD (e.g., clinical symptoms suggest the presence of vascular disease, but no CT/MRI studies are available).
3. Severity of aphasia precludes proper cognitive assessment. However, patients with documented evidence of normal cognitive function (e.g., annual cognitive evaluations) before the clinical event that caused aphasia could be classified as having probable VaD.
4. There is evidence of other neurodegenerative diseases or conditions in addition to cerebrovascular disease that may affect cognition, such as
    a. A history of other neurodegenerative disorders (e.g., Parkinson's disease, progressive supranuclear palsy, dementia with Lewy bodies);
    b. The presence of Alzheimer's disease biology is confirmed by biomarkers (e.g., PET, CSF, amyloid ligands) or genetic studies (e.g., PS1 mutation); or
    c. A history of active cancer or psychiatric or metabolic disorders that may affect cognitive function.

VaMCI

1. VaMCI includes the 4 subtypes proposed for the classification of MCI: amnestic, amnestic plus other domains, non-amnestic single domain, and non-amnestic multiple domain.
2. The classification of VaMCI must be based on cognitive testing, and a minimum of 4 cognitive domains should be assessed: executive/attention, memory, language, and visuospatial functions. The classification should be based on an assumption of decline in cognitive function from a prior baseline and impairment in at least 1 cognitive domain.
3. Instrumental activities of daily living could be normal or mildly impaired, independent of the presence of motor/sensory symptoms.

Probable VaMCI

1. There is cognitive impairment and imaging evidence of cerebrovascular disease and:
    a. There is a clear temporal relationship between a vascular event (e.g., clinical stroke) and onset of cognitive deficits, or
    b. There is a clear relationship in the severity and pattern of cognitive impairment and the presence of diffuse, subcortical cerebrovascular disease pathology (e.g., as in CADASIL).
2. There is no history of gradually progressive cognitive deficits before or after the stroke that suggests the presence of a non-vascular neurodegenerative disorder.

Possible VaMCI

There is cognitive impairment and imaging evidence of cerebrovascular disease but:
1. There is no clear relationship (temporal, severity, or cognitive pattern) between the vascular disease (e.g., silent infarcts, subcortical small vessel disease) and onset of cognitive deficits.
2. There is insufficient information for the diagnosis of VaMCI (e.g., clinical symptoms suggest the presence of vascular disease, but no CT/MRI studies are available).
3. Severity of aphasia precludes proper cognitive assessment. However, patients with documented evidence of normal cognitive function (e.g., annual cognitive evaluations) before the clinical event that caused aphasia could be classified as having probable VaMCI.
4. There is evidence of other neurodegenerative diseases or conditions in addition to cerebrovascular disease that may affect cognition, such as:
    a. A history of other neurodegenerative disorders (e.g., Parkinson's disease, progressive supranuclear palsy, dementia with Lewy bodies);
    b. The presence of Alzheimer's disease biology is confirmed by biomarkers (e.g., PET, CSF, amyloid ligands) or genetic studies (e.g., PS1 mutation); or
    c. A history of active cancer or psychiatric or metabolic disorders that may affect cognitive function.

Unstable VaMCI

Patients with the diagnosis of probable or possible VaMCI whose symptoms revert to normal should be classified as having "unstable VaMCI."

CADASIL = cerebral autosomal dominant arteriopathy with subcortical infarcts and leukoencephalopathy; CSF = cerebrospinal fluid; CT/MRI - computed tomography/magnetic resonance imaging; MCI = mild cognitive impairment; PET = positron emission tomography; VaD = vascular dementia; VaMCI = vascular mild cognitive impairment; VCI = vascular cognitive impairment of VCI or VaD based on memory deficits may not be suitable for the dementia syndrome associated with cerebrovascular disease, in which memory-related structures (e.g., mesial temporal lobe, thalamus) could be intact, resulting in relatively preserved memory functions; (2) it is critical to identify the presence of cortical or subcortical infarcts or other stroke lesions with neuroimaging, and these should be associated with clinical symptomatology; (3) the source of the cardiac or vascular pathology that underlies the cerebrovascular disease associated with VCI should be investigated to provide more specific clinico-pathological relationships; (4) the criterion that the symptoms should appear within 3 months after a stroke is rather arbitrary, and symptoms may develop after this time frame; (5) there are patients who have not had a clinical stroke and in whom severe cerebrovascular disease is evident only in neuroradiological studies; (6) the diagnostic value of white-matter lesions (WMLs) or leukoaraiosis depends on the age of the patients. The present statement proposes to use the term "probable" to characterize the most "pure" forms of VaD, and the term "possible" when the certainty of the diagnosis is diminished or the vascular syndrome is associated with another disease process that can cause cognitive deficits.

Clinical evaluation

VCI is a clinical diagnosis. It requires a detailed account of the cognitive complaint by the patient or caregiver regarding cognitive domains such as memory, speed of thinking or acting, mood, and function. The history should also include details of the acuity of onset, progression, and occurrence of urinary incontinence and gait disturbance. Detailed information about vascular risk factors should be obtained, including history of hypertension, hyperlipidemia, diabetes mellitus, alcohol or tobacco use, and physical activity, and checks for atrial fibrillation, coronary artery bypass surgery, angioplasty and stenting, angina, congestive heart failure, peripheral vascular disease, transient ischemic attacks or strokes, and endarterectomy. Other elements of medical history, including hypercoagulable states, migraine, and depression, may also be helpful.

Physical examination should include blood pressure, pulse, body mass index, waist circumference, and examination of the cardiovascular system for evidence of arrhythmias or peripheral vascular disease. Neurological examination should note focal neurological signs and assess gait initiation and speed.

Cognitive assessment

The neuropsychological profile of VCI is heterogeneous, although the typical expression of VCI is executive dysfunction manifested as impaired attention, planning, difficulties in complex activities, and disorganized thought, behavior, or emotion. The pattern of cognitive deficits in patients with VCI also varies considerably. Subcortical lesions are often associated with abnormalities of information processing speed, executive function, and emotional lability, whereas strategic infarcts can lead to specific cognitive deficits. Because of the heterogeneity and specificity of cognitive deficits and underlying structural abnormalities, global assessments of cognitive impairment provide limited information of clinical use.

Biomarkers

To date, no reliable CSF biomarkers for VaD exist. In general, biomarkers cannot take the place of clinical diagnosis, but they can inform on the relationship between risk factors and disease progression.

Neuroimaging

Although brain imaging methods, particularly CT and MRI, are being used as important tools for supporting the clinical diagnosis of VaD, VCI shows no pathognomonic neuroimaging features. Neuroimaging cannot reliably confirm the chronology of lesions and cannot inform on the relative contribution of neurodegenerative versus ischemic processes to the clinical presentation. Furthermore, the location of the infarct does not always correlate with the pattern of cognitive deficits. The increasing appreciation that VCI might be present in the absence of neuroimaging abnormalities is due to recognition of the importance of incomplete infarction and hypoperfusion.

Although CT is widely available, and in many parts of the world is a pragmatic choice for patients, it is less sensitive than MRI. The new MRI-based neuroimaging techniques continue to advance our knowledge of the pathophysiology of VCI. The main imaging features visible on conventional MRI at 1.5T or 3T include acute lacunar (or small subcortical) infarcts or hemorrhages, lacunes, white-matter hyperintensities (including small deep gray-matter hyperintensities, mostly clinically silent), visible perivascular spaces, microbleeds, and brain atrophy. Other emerging features detectable at higher field strengths include microinfarcts. Additional damage detectable only on advanced MRI (e.g., diffusion tensor imaging and magnetization transfer ratio) includes altered white-matter integrity, disrupted axonal connections, increased brain water content, altered myelination, and secondary focal thinning of the cortical gray matter. The results of diffusion tensor MRI studies have enhanced our understanding of lesion location in relation to clinical presentation, and suggest that such white-matter changes are not necessarily ischemic. Diffusion tensor MRI techniques might eventually enable measurement of the number of fibers per tract and the functional areas connected by white matter.

CSF and serum biomarkers

To date, CSF markers have shown more discriminative ability in patients with VCI than have serum biomarkers. The CSF–albumin index is a measure of blood–brain barrier integrity, which is compromised in many types of dementia, particularly subcortical vessel disease. Matrix metalloproteinases (MMP-2 and MMP-9) are the most studied: MMP-2 is constitutively expressed, whereas MMP-9 is associated with inflammation and has variable specificity in VCI compared with AD. The light neurofilament subunit found in normal myelin has been found in higher concentrations in the CSF of people with subcortical vessel disease compared with people with Alzheimer's disease.

Genetics

Genetic factors for stroke and VaD have not been studied widely. Apolipoprotein E ε 4 (APOE4) is a known risk factor for atherosclerotic disease in general as well as for AD. Surprisingly, it has a negligible effect on stroke and on VaD. However, APOE4 may increase the risk for cognitive decline after stroke. Rare monogenic vascular diseases can all result in stroke as well as in VaD. It is reasonable to perform genetic testing for cysteine-altering mutations in Notch3 in patients with progressive cognitive impairment, characteristic imaging findings, and a family history suggestive of autosomal dominant inheritance. Notch3 testing may also be considered in sporadic patients with suggestive clinical and imaging findings, particularly in the absence of strong cardiovascular risk factors.

Treatment

There is variable but generally limited benefit of treatment in VCI; the results of a meta-analysis concluded that only small benefits of uncertain clinical significance were available from cholinesterase inhibitors or memantine.

Apart from controlling vascular risk factors, the effects of treatment on patients with vascular dementia are modest. The latest reports about primary or secondary prevention in VCI have offered several recommendations and comments:

- There is reasonable evidence that in the middle-aged and young elderly, lowering blood pressure can be useful for the prevention of late-life dementia. The usefulness of lowering blood pressure in people >80 years of age for the prevention of dementia is not well established. In patients with stroke, lowering blood pressure is effective for reducing the risk of poststroke dementia.
- The impact of treatment of hyperlipidemia for prevention of dementia is uncertain. **This is not a recommendation.**
- The effectiveness of antiaggregant therapy for VCI is not well established. **This is not a recommendation.**
- Vitamin supplementation is not proven to improve cognitive function, even if homocysteine levels have been positively influenced, and its usefulness is not well established. **This is not a recommendation.**
- A Mediterranean-type dietary pattern has been associated with less cognitive decline in several studies and may be reasonable.
- Physical activity might be considered for the prevention of cognitive impairment, but the usefulness of other lifestyle modifications is uncertain, e.g., several prospective studies show an increased risk for cognitive decline in smokers compared with non-smokers.

Conclusions

Although VaD was described over a century ago, it remains a difficult and challenging diagnosis. VCI might be preventable, although the evidence for this is not as complete as it is for the prevention of stroke. VCI increases the morbidity, disability, and healthcare costs of the growing elderly population, and decreases their quality of life and survival. Given the substantial health and economic burden of VCI, its prevention and treatment are critical research and clinical priorities. Future studies into specific therapies for VCI will need to consider the clinical features and outcomes carefully.

Further reading

Chan KY, Wang W, Wu JJ, *et al.*; Global Health Epidemiology Reference Group (GHERG). Epidemiology of Alzheimer's disease and other forms of dementia in China, 1990–2010: A systematic review and analysis. *Lancet* 2013;381(9882):2016–2023.

Gorelick B, Scuteri A, Black SE, *et al.* Vascular contributions to cognitive impairment and dementia: A statement for healthcare professionals from the American Heart Association/American Stroke Association. *Stroke* 2011;42(9):2672–2713.

Moorhouse P, Rockwood K. Vascular cognitive impairment: Current concepts and clinical developments. *Lancet Neurol* 2008;7(3):246–255.

Wardlaw JM, Smith C, Dichgans M. Mechanisms of sporadic cerebral small vessel disease: Insights from neuroimaging. *Lancet Neurol* 2013;12(5):483–497.

43 Frontotemporal dementia

Katya Rascovsky[1] and Diana L. Matallana[2]

[1] Department of Neurology and Penn Frontotemporal Degeneration Center, University of Pennsylvania Perelman School of Medicine, Philadelphia, PA, USA

[2] Department of Psychiatry and Institute on Aging, Pontificia Universidad Javeriana, Bogota, Colombia

Frontotemporal dementia (FTD) refers to a spectrum of clinical syndromes characterized by the progressive degeneration of the frontal and anterior temporal lobes. Presentations can range from behavioral impairment to language or motor dysfunction. The present chapter will review the major clinical syndromes within the FTD spectrum and outline some cross-cultural challenges in the diagnosis of FTD.

Epidemiology

Population studies in Europe and the United States estimate the prevalence of FTD at 15–22 cases per 100,000, making it as common as Alzheimer's disease (AD) among people younger than 65 years. FTD typically presents in the sixth decade of life and has a relatively rapid rate of progression, with death occurring 3–4 years from initial diagnosis, and approximately 8 years from symptom onset.

Pathophysiology

Although distinguished by the relatively focal degeneration of frontal and anterior temporal lobes, FTD is histopathologically heterogeneous. Currently, most research groups favor the term frontotemporal dementia for the overall clinical spectrum, and use frontotemporal lobar degeneration (FTLD) when referring to the underlying pathology. In general terms, FTLD can be assigned to one of three major molecular subgroups: FTLD with tau inclusions (FTLD-tau), FTLD with TAR DNA-binding protein inclusions (FTLD-TDP), or FTLD immunoreactive for fused in sarcoma protein (FTLD-FUS).

Genetics

The FTD spectrum appears to be highly familial, with 30–40% of patients reporting a family history of a similar disease, and 15–20% of cases showing an identifiable pathogenic mutation. Most familial FTD cases have mutations in the genes that encode the microtubule-associated protein tau (MAPT) or progranulin (PGRN). Approximately 10% of familial FTD cases have been linked to a hexanucleotide repeat expansion in the *C9ORF72* gene, which is also associated with amyotrophic lateral sclerosis (ALS) with or without FTD.

Behavioral variant frontotemporal dementia

The behavioral variant of frontotemporal dementia (bvFTD) is the most common clinical presentation of FTD, accounting for 56% of cases within the cognitive FTD spectrum (cognitive presentations also include cases with primary progressive aphasia [PPA], discussed later).

The insidious behavioral changes of bvFTD are difficult to recognize; in fact, almost 50% of bvFTD patients are diagnosed with a primary psychiatric illness before their syndrome is identified as a neurodegenerative condition. Early and accurate diagnosis of bvFTD is important, as it allows for appropriate therapeutic and behavioral patient management, as well as tailored family counseling and support.

In the absence of definitive biomarkers, diagnosis of bvFTD should be made on the basis of clinical criteria coupled with diagnostic methods that are practical and easily available. In 2011, the International bvFTD Criteria Consortium (FTDC) developed revised guidelines for the diagnosis of bvFTD (see later and Table 43.1). These guidelines are structured as a diagnostic hierarchy depending on the level of diagnostic certainty.

Possible bvFTD

In order to meet the criteria for possible bvFTD, the patient must show a progressive deterioration of behavior and/or cognition, as manifested by three of the following six clinically discriminating features.

Behavioral disinhibition

Behavioral disinhibition is the hallmark feature of bvFTD and can manifest as socially inappropriate behavior, loss of manners or decorum, or impulsive, rash, or careless actions. BvFTD patients will often engage in inappropriate laughter or cursing, offensive jokes or opinions, or crude or sexually explicit remarks. Patients may also display a general lack of etiquette, loss of respect for interpersonal space, and a lack of response to social cues. As the disease progresses, bvFTD patients may exhibit more extreme violations of social norms, such as inappropriately touching or groping strangers. Disinhibition can also manifest as impulsive behaviors including reckless driving, new-onset gambling, or buying or selling objects without regard for consequences.

International Neurology, Second edition. Edited by Robert P. Lisak, Daniel D. Truong, William M. Carroll and Roongroj Bhidayasiri

I. Possible bvFTD

Patient must show progressive deterioration of behavior and/or cognition as evidenced by three of the following:

1. Behavioral disinhibition
2. Apathy or inertia
3. Loss of empathy
4. Perseverative, stereotyped, or compulsive behavior
5. Hyperorality or dietary changes
6. Dysexecutive neuropsychological profile with relative sparing of memory and visuospatial functions

II. Probable bvFTD

Patient must meet criteria for possible bvFTD and both of the following:

1. Significant functional decline
2. Imaging results consistent with bvFTD (i.e., frontal and/or anterior temporal atrophy on CT or MRI or frontal hypoperfusion or hypometabolism on SPECT or PET)

III. bvFTD with definite FTLD pathology

Patient must meet criteria for possible bvFTD and either of the following:

1. Histopathological evidence of FTLD
2. Presence of a known pathogenic mutation

CT = computed tomography; FTLD = frontotemporal lobar degeneration; MRI = magnetic resonance imaging; PET = positron emission tomography; SPECT = single photon emission computed tomography

Apathy or inertia

Apathy is the most common initial symptom of bvFTD and appears to be more severe in bvFTD than in other dementias. Clinically, apathy is commonly mistaken for depression, but the apathy of bvFTD is rarely accompanied by dysphoric mood. BvFTD patients may cease to engage in important or previously rewarding pursuits such as jobs, hobbies, or household responsibilities. In extreme cases, patients may present with frank inertia, requiring prompts to initiate or continue basic activities of daily living.

Loss of empathy

BvFTD patients can lose their ability to read the emotional expressions of others or imagine their experiences. This loss of empathy is particularly distressing for caregivers, as the patient may appear to be indifferent to the feelings of loved ones and strangers. In day-to-day life, bvFTD patients may engage in hurtful or insensitive comments, or show an inexplicable disregard for others' physical pain or emotional distress. Some patients exhibit a more general decline in social engagement, with emotional detachment, coldness, and lack of eye contact.

Perseverative, stereotyped, or compulsive/ritualistic behavior

BvFTD patients often exhibit simple, stereotyped, or complex compulsive behaviors. Simple repetitive behaviors may include actions such as tapping, rubbing, scratching, or humming. BvFTD patients may also engage in complex compulsive behaviors such as rituals at fixed time intervals, counting, cleaning, checking, collecting, or hoarding. Perseveration may also be evident in language production, as bvFTD patients habitually repeat words, phrases, or entire stories despite the lack of communicative value.

Hyperorality and dietary changes

Hyperorality and changes in eating behavior are common manifestations of bvFTD. Patients often engage in binge eating and continue to eat despite acknowledging satiety. They may also exhibit rigid, stereotyped, or idiosyncratic food preferences such as restricting their intake to a particular kind of food (often sweets or carbohydrates) or demanding unusual food combinations. In extreme cases, hyperorality may manifest as chewing or ingestion of inedible objects.

Dysexecutive neuropsychological profile

While behavioral changes tend to dominate the initial presentation of bvFTD, cognitive deficits appear as the disease progresses. When this cognitive profile emerges, it is characterized by executive and generation deficits in the context of relatively preserved memory and visuospatial functions. BvFTD patients consistently fail verbal fluency tasks that require strategic search (e.g., generating words that start with a particular letter) and show deficits in tests that require planning, mental flexibility, and response inhibition. Interestingly, several studies suggest that the presence of errors in cognitive testing (in the form of perseverations and rule violations) may be particularly helpful in the differential diagnosis of bvFTD. In contrast to patients with AD, bvFTD patients have relatively preserved episodic memory and retain the ability to navigate their environment, copy simple drawings, and assemble objects until late in their disease course.

Probable bvFTD

A diagnosis of probable bvFTD aims to capture patients with a high probability of underlying FTLD pathology and is useful in studies where high diagnostic certainty is important (e.g., clinical trials). This classification is based on the clinical syndrome, plus demonstrable functional decline and frontotemporal imaging findings. Consistent with underlying pathology, structural imaging changes in bvFTD are characterized by disproportionate atrophy in frontal and anterior temporal regions. Atrophy is initially circumscribed to anterior cingulate, frontal insula, and orbitofrontal cortex, but extends to more posterior and lateral aspects of the frontal and temporal lobes as the disease progresses. Functional abnormalities may precede frank structural imaging changes in bvFTD, thus a finding of predominant frontal or frontotemporal hypometabolism or hypoperfusion on positon emission tomography (PET) or single photon emission computed tomography (SPECT) may also aid in differential diagnosis.

BvFTD with definite FTLD pathology

This conclusive classification is limited to patients who exhibit the bvFTD clinical syndrome and have a pathogenic mutation or histopathological evidence of FTLD. At autopsy, roughly 40% of bvFTD cases exhibit FTLD-tau pathology, with most of the remaining cases exhibiting pathology consistent with FTLD-TDP.

Primary progressive aphasia

Frontotemporal degeneration can also present as a progressive deterioration in language, commonly known as primary progressive aphasia (PPA). In order to meet the criteria for PPA, the patient must exhibit a relatively isolated and progressive language disturbance, where language is the predominant deficit and major source of disability early in the disease course. In contrast to the prominent language deficits that define PPA, cognitive skills such as non-verbal episodic memory and visuospatial/constructional abilities may be strikingly preserved.

Recent classification guidelines identify three main subtypes of PPA: non-fluent/agrammatic, semantic and logopenic (see Table 43.2). Although these guidelines provide a common framework for studying and classifying PPA, they are not without controversy. The new guidelines are meant to describe coherent clinical syndromes with common neuroanatomy, but variable underlying pathology. Clinico-pathological studies have linked the majority of non-fluent/agrammatic patients to underlying FTLD-tau pathology, semantic variant to FTLD-TDP pathology, and logopenic variant to underlying AD pathology.

Diagnostic guidelines for the three variants of PPA are described in what follows.

Table 43.2 Diagnosis of primary progressive aphasia (PPA). Source: Gorno-Tempini 2011. Reproduced with permission of Wolters Kluwer.

I. Clinical diagnosis of non-fluent/agrammatic variant PPA (naPPA)

Patient must show progressive deterioration of language as evidenced by one of the following:

1. Agrammatism in language production
2. Effortful, halting speech with speech sound errors

At least 2/3 supportive features:

1. Impaired comprehension of syntactically complex sentences
2. Spared single-word comprehension
3. Spared object knowledge

Diagnosis of imaging-supported naPPA

Patient must meet clinical criteria for naPPA and have imaging results consistent with the syndrome, i.e., left posterior fronto-insular atrophy, hypoperfusion, or hypometabolism.

II. Clinical diagnosis of semantic variant PPA (svPPA)

Patient must show progressive deterioration of language as evidenced by both of the following:

1. Impaired confrontation naming
2. Impaired single-word comprehension

At least 3/4 supportive features:

1. Impaired object knowledge
2. Surface dyslexia
3. Spared repetition
4. Spared speech production

Diagnosis of imaging-supported svPPA

Patient must meet clinical criteria for svPPA and have imaging results consistent with the syndrome, i.e., predominant anterior temporal lobe atrophy, hypoperfusion, or hypometabolism.

III. Clinical diagnosis of logopenic variant PPA (lvPPA)

Patient must show progressive deterioration of language as evidenced by both of the following:

1. Impaired single-word retrieval
2. Impaired repetition of sentences

At least 3/4 supportive features:

1. Speech (phonological) errors
2. Spared single-word comprehension and object knowledge
3. Spared motor speech
4. Absence of clear agrammatism

Diagnosis of imaging-supported lvPPA

Patient must meet clinical criteria for lvPPA and have imaging results consistent with the syndrome, i.e., predominant left posterior perisylvian or parietal atrophy, hypoperfusion, or hypometabolism.

Non-fluent/agrammatic variant of PPA

In order to meet the criteria for the non-fluent/agrammatic variant of PPA (naPPA), the patient must present with either effortful, non-fluent speech or agrammatism in language production (see Table 43.2). Effortful speech refers to hesitant speech production, with markedly reduced rate, altered prosody, and speech sound errors. Some of these errors may be substitutions or mispronunciations related to a disorder of the phonological system, while others appear to involve an articulation planning deficit (i.e., apraxia of speech). Agrammatism in speech production typically manifests as terse, telegraphic sentences with grammatical errors and omissions, as well as simplification of grammatical forms. These core language deficits are often accompanied by impaired comprehension of syntactically complex sentences. In contrast to their profound speech and grammatical deficits, naPPA patients show spared single-word comprehension and object knowledge, thus distinguishing this variant from svPPA (see next section).

Patients with naPPA often have coexisting motor findings, which may eventually develop into concomitant corticobasal syndrome (CBS), progressive supranuclear palsy (PSP), or ALS. Patients with imaging-supported naPPA meet clinical criteria for the syndrome and exhibit consistent imaging abnormalities in left perisylvian regions.

Semantic variant of PPA

In contrast to naPPA, patients with the semantic variant of PPA (svPPA) present with fluent, empty speech, prominent anomia, and difficulty understanding the meaning of words. The characteristic deficits of svPPA stem from a progressive breakdown of semantic memory; that is, the memory system that stores knowledge about objects and concepts. In order to meet the criteria for svPPA, the patient must exhibit impaired confrontation naming and impaired single-word comprehension. These deficits are initially evident for low-frequency words or objects, often leading svPPA patients to ask for the meaning of words in conversation (e.g., "What is a grapefruit?"). As the disease progresses, this semantic breakdown leads to a loss of object knowledge, whereby patients fail to recognize common objects in visual, auditory, or even tactile domains. The progressive breakdown of representational knowledge in svPPA severely limits comprehension and results in empty, circumlocutory speech with frequent use of words that lack a precise reference (e.g., "that" or "thing"). In addition, svPPA patients can exhibit "surface dyslexia," where sight vocabulary words are pronounced as written (e.g., "choir" pronounced as "cho-eere"). In contrast to their profound naming and comprehension deficits, svPPA patients have spared speech production and repetition, helping to distinguish this variant from naPPA and lvPPA (see next section). With disease progression, svPPA patients may exhibit some of the behavioral features of bvFTD. If the right temporal lobe is affected, this may manifest as loss of empathy, lack of social engagement, or complex ritualistic behaviors.

For a diagnosis of imaging-supported svPPA, the patient must meet the clinical criteria for the syndrome and exhibit imaging findings of predominant anterior temporal lobe atrophy, hypoperfusion, or hypometabolism. Although degeneration typically presents in the left hemisphere, right-sided presentations also occur, with predominant non-verbal semantic deficits and concomitant prosopagnosia.

Lopogenic variant of PPA

Although generally associated with underlying AD pathology, the logopenic variant of PPA (lvPPA) is often confused with the non-fluent or semantic PPA variants commonly linked to FTLD. Patients with lvPPA show profound anomia and deficits in sentence repetition. The repetition impairment in lvPPA is thought to reflect a breakdown in phonological working memory, with greater difficulty repeating long sentences versus single words. In addition to these core features, lvPPA patients may present with phonological errors in speech (i.e., phonological paraphasias). In contrast to svPPA, lvPPA is characterized by spared single-word comprehension and object knowledge. Patients with lvPPA also have spared motor speech and absence of clear agrammatism, thus distinguishing this variant from naPPA. For a diagnosis of imaging-supported lvPPA, the patient must meet clinical criteria for the syndrome and exhibit predominant left posterior perisylvian or parietal atrophy on structural imaging, or a similar distribution on functional imaging.

Cross-cultural issues

The diagnosis of FTD can be challenging, particularly in settings where young-onset dementia is underrecognized. In our collaborative work with Latin America, we have found that the stigma of mental illness may prevent caregivers from reporting inappropriate behavior in bvFTD. Furthermore, rating of behavioral features can be difficult and subjective, as classification of "appropriate" behavior depends on culture and situational context. For example, complimenting the opposite sex may be appropriate and expected in certain cultures, but considered inappropriate in others.

Language differences also affect the diagnosis and implementation of specific linguistic tests. For example, the supplementary svPPA feature of surface dyslexia is not applicable in Latin America, as Spanish is a language with transparent letter–sound matching (i.e., it is read as written). Grammatical language differences also pose a challenge, as literal translations of commonly used grammatical tests in the United States can fail to target the intended grammatical demands once translated into Spanish.

Cultural perceptions can also affect the ascertainment of familial FTD in Latin America. For example, a family history of dementia is often minimized due to incomplete knowledge of genetic transmission, fear of rejection by the community, or concerns about a "curse" in the family. These barriers can be reduced by using culturally sensitive training and educational materials for physicians, genetic counselors, and families.

Treatment

Unfortunately, there are currently no known treatments available that alter the course of FTD. Management is therefore directed at minimizing symptoms and helping patients and caregivers cope with the impact of the disease. Pharmacological agents used in the treatment of AD are not indicated in FTD, as they may further aggravate behavioral disturbances. Small studies suggest that selective serotonin reuptake inhibitors may be useful in managing compulsive behaviors and hyperorality in some individuals. Due to the risk of extrapyramidal and cognitive side effects, neuroleptic agents should only be used when behavioral symptoms cannot be managed through other means (e.g., environmental or behavioral interventions). For patients with PPA, speech therapy may identify communication aids that are helpful for a particular individual. These may include picture dictionaries, computer applications with prerecorded words or phrases, or tablets that facilitate written communication. Finally, family education and counseling are crucial in the management of FTD. The personality changes and emotional detachment of bvFTD patients can be psychologically devastating for families, while the patient's impulsive behaviors and lack of judgment may have severe financial and legal consequences. Similarly, language impairment in PPA can limit the patient's ability to communicate and interact with the world, adding to caregiver burden and stress. We hope that increased recognition of FTD syndromes will translate to better diagnosis, management, and care for FTD patients and their families worldwide.

Acknowledgment

This work was supported by AG046499, AG17586, AG32953, NS44266, AG15116, NS53488, and the Wyncote Foundation.

Further reading

Gorno-Tempini ML, Hillis AE, Weintraub S, *et al*. Classification of primary progressive aphasia and its variants. *Neurology* 2011;76:1006–1014.

Grossman M. Primary progressive aphasia: Clinicopathological correlations. *Nat Rev Neurol* 2010;6:88–97.

Mackenzie IR, Neumann M, Bigio EH, *et al*. Nomenclature and nosology for neuropathologic subtypes of frontotemporal lobar degeneration: An update. *Acta Neuropathol* 2010;119:1–4.

Rascovsky K, Grossman M. Clinical diagnostic criteria and classification controversies in frontotemporal lobar degeneration. *Int Rev Psychiatry* 2013;25:145–158.

Rascovsky K, Hodges JR, Knopman D, *et al*. Sensitivity of revised diagnostic criteria for the behavioural variant of frontotemporal dementia. *Brain* 2011;134:2456–2477.

Seeley WW. Frontotemporal dementia neuroimaging: A guide for clinicians. *Front Neurol Neurosci* 2009;24:160–167.

Wood EM, Falcone D, Suh E, *et al*. Development and validation of pedigree classification criteria for frontotemporal lobar degeneration. *JAMA Neurol* 2013;70:1411–1417.

44 Progressive supranuclear palsy, corticobasal syndrome, and other tauopathies

David J. Irwin

Department of Neurology, Frontotemporal Degeneration Center (FTDC), University of Pennsylvania Perelman School of Medicine, Hospital of the University of Pennsylvania, Philadelphia, PA, USA

The cytosolic protein, tau, is found in neurons and glial cells in the central nervous system (CNS) and functions to stabilize the cytoskeleton through binding microtubules. Several age-associated neurodegenerative diseases are associated with intracellular inclusions composed of abnormally modified tau, collectively known as tauopathies. Tauopathies are a major class of frontotemporal lobar degeneration (FTLD) neuropathology (i.e., FTLD-tau) and can present clinically with several forms of frontotemporal dementia (FTD) clinical syndromes including progressive supranuclear palsy syndrome (PSPS) and corticobasal syndrome (CBS). Alzheimer's disease (AD) is considered by some also to be a tauopathy due to the close correlation of neurofibrillary tau pathology with clinical symptoms in AD; however, the exact relationship between amyloid-beta plaques and tau aggregation is still a matter of contention, and as such, this review will focus on primary tauopathies in the FTLD neuropathological spectrum (FTLD-tau) and the resultant clinical phenotypes.

Pathophysiology

The underlying pathophysiology of disease pathogenesis in tauopathies is currently unclear; however, there are several strands of evidence (summarized in this chapter) that suggest that the aggregation and spread of abnormal tau inclusions in neurons and glia are central to the neurodegenerative process. First, several causal pathogenic mutations have been found in the MAPT tau gene for tauopathies. Second, abnormal deposits of tau within neurons and glia are a consistent marker of tauopathies at autopsy and correlate closely to the degree of neuronal loss and gliosis in the brain and clinical symptoms during life. Finally, staging methods of tau pathology performed in AD, as well as animal- and cell-model experiments of tauopathies, suggest that pathological tau aggregates may transmit from cell to cell within an individual. Further work is needed to elucidate the mechanisms of tau unfolding and aggregation, and their association with the neurodegenerative process.

FTLD-tau with MAPT mutation

Over 40 known pathogenic mutations in the *MAPT* tau gene on chromosome 17 result in FTD clinical syndromes accompanied by substantial tau pathology in the CNS found at autopsy. These hereditary cases are collectively known as FTLD-tau with *MAPT* mutation. The tau protein exists in six isoforms based on (1) the presence of 0, 1, or 2 sequence inserts in the amino-terminus of the protein; and

(2) inclusion or exclusion of the second of four microtubule-binding potential repeat domains (MTBD) coded by exon 10. Tauopathies are classified by the predominance of tau isoforms found in cytoplasmic inclusions: those with inclusions predominantly composed of tau with 3 MTBDs (i.e., 3R-tauopathies), those with predominantly 4 MTBDs (i.e., 4R-tauopathies), or those with an equal ratio of 3R:4R tau. Tau normally exists in an equal ratio of 3R:4R tau in non-disease states.

MAPT pathogenic mutations are found worldwide among various ethnicities and these mutations are thought to cause disease by (1) inhibiting the normal microtubule-binding function of tau; or (2) promoting tau protein aggregation; or (3) affecting the splicing of exon 10 to result in imbalances between 3R and 4R tau isoforms. As such, specific neuropathological findings (e.g., tau isoform predominance, inclusion morphology/ultrastructure) vary for each specific mutation, but universally include neuronal and glial tau inclusions together with neurodegeneration throughout the CNS, with a particular propensity for frontal and temporal neocortex and limbic structures. Clinically FTLD-tau with *MAPT* mutations may present with FTD behavioral and language syndromes, as discussed later in the chapter, and often have extra-pyramidal features. The majority of mutations are inherited in an autosomal dominant pattern and usually with a high degree of penetrance. The age of onset varies by specific mutation, but in general disease onset is between the ages 45 and 65 years with a wide variation in disease duration (average ~10 years); however, cases may occur in the second and third decades and also the eighth decade.

Animal models of tauopathies and transmission

In vivo models of tauopathies using mice that harbor a trans-gene for known human *MAPT* pathogenic mutations recapitulate several features of human tauopathies, including pathological deposits of tau inclusions in the CNS, neuronal loss, cognitive/motor deficits, and reduced survival, thereby reinforcing the importance of tau structure and function in the pathogenesis of human tauopathies. Recent data from several research groups demonstrate that tau may undergo a self-templating process to recruit normal soluble tau to form and propagate insoluble tau fibrils between neurons within the CNS. For example, experiments using intracerebral injections of synthetic tau fibrils alone into transgenic mice cause a time-dependent hierarchical deposition of tau in the CNS, and suggest that misfolded tau in isolation is sufficient for the transmission of pathology. Interestingly, the use of different

International Neurology, Second edition. Edited by Robert P. Lisak, Daniel D. Truong, William M. Carroll and Roongroj Bhidayasiri
© 2016 John Wiley & Sons, Ltd. Published 2016 by John Wiley & Sons, Ltd.

injection sites within the CNS of recipient mice results in differing patterns of spread that reflect known trans-synaptic anatomical connections. *In vitro* experiments using transgenic and wild-type murine neuron cultures similarly show the ability of tau fibrils to self-assemble and transmit trans-synaptically between individual cells. Some researchers postulate that varying conformational changes of misfolded tau species (i.e., strains) could contribute to the clinical and underlying pathological heterogeneity of human tauopathies. These observed properties of transmission are similar to human prion disease, where the abnormal PRP^{SC} protein seeds fibrillization of native PRP^{C} to cause the spread of misfolded prion throughout the CNS, accompanied by spongiform degeneration. A key distinction between tauopathies and prion disease is that there is no current definitive evidence of infectivity (i.e., transmission of disease) between humans or non-human primates for AD or FTLD-tau, even in extreme circumstances such as exposure to human CNS tissue.

Transmission of pathogenic tau species may be mediated by axonal transport in donor cell and several mechanisms of cellular uptake at the synapse of recipient neurons. Thus, slowing or halting this process of tau aggregation may be an important strategy for therapeutic developments for tauopathies. Greater understanding of the interplay of tau transmission with other known mechanisms involved with neurodegeneration, such as oxidative stress, protein clearance mechanisms, and neuro-inflammation, is an area of further research.

Progressive supranuclear palsy syndrome
Clinical features

Progressive supranuclear palsy syndrome (PSPS) is an age-associated atypical parkinsonian syndrome. Most patients develop symptoms around the age of 65 years. Key clinical features include a supranuclear gaze palsy for vertical saccades (with early involvement of down gaze) and Parkinsonism with bradykinesia, symmetric rigidity with prominent involvement of axial musculature, and postural instability. Frequent falls are common early in the course of the disorder. Blepharospasm may occur and hypomimia resulting in an "astonished look" is not uncommon. Patients may also develop significant dysarthria and dysphagia with an increased risk for aspiration. Urinary incontinence often emerges later in the course of the disease. Classic Parkinsonian rest tremor is less common, and bradykinesia and rigidity typically have a poor or transient response to dopaminergic therapy. PSPS can be clinically subdivided into classic PSP (i.e., Richardson's syndrome), as already described, and a parkinsonian variant (PSPS-P). PSPS-P more closely resembles idiopathic Parkinson's disease, with prominent asymmetry and rest tremor, and can have a more substantial response to L-DOPA therapy. In addition to the movement disorder, cognitive and behavioral features of PSPS are being increasingly recognized; they may occur at any point during the disease course and may precede motor findings. Features of primary progressive aphasia (PPA) may occur, especially non-fluent, slow, hesitant speech with frank agrammatisms consistent with the non-fluent/agrammatic variant of PPA (naPPA). PSPS patients often have significant executive dysfunction and difficulty with mental planning, organizing, and set shifting. Cognitive impairment has an additive effect, with motor difficulties on functional disability, and can result in an earlier loss of independence. Finally, depression or other mood disorder is not uncommon.

The differential diagnosis includes other age-associated neurodegenerative syndromes with associated parkinsonism, including idiopathic Parkinson's disease, dementia with Lewy bodies, multiple system atrophy, CBS, AD, and Neimann–Pick type C (lysosomal storage disease). Atypical features or rapid progression of symptoms (i.e., ≤18 months) could signify an alternative diagnosis of spongiform encephalopathy or an extensive list of autoimmune/infectious/toxic/metabolic conditions. Cerebrovascular disease and postencephalitic parkinsonism can also have similar clinical features. Neimann–Pick Type C and postencephalic parkinsonism both may have tau inclusions found at autopsy, but these disorders are not considered primary tauopathies.

Epidemiology

There are no established environmental risk factors for PSPS. The prevalence of PSPS is estimated as roughly 5 per 100,000 persons from the few epidemiological studies limited to the United States and Western Europe, and the condition is often underdiagnosed, requiring a formal evaluation at a tertiary academic center. There is no particular gender predominance and PSPS is largely sporadic, but rare *MAPT* mutations may present with a PSPS-like clinical syndrome. Genetic polymorphism in the *MAPT* gene has been linked to increased risk for PSPS; presence of a haplotype of inverted sequence and polymorphisms in linkage disequilibrium (i.e., H1 haplotype) in *MAPT* has been linked to increased risk of PSPS in Caucasian populations. Interestingly, the alternative H2 haplotype is extremely rare in non-European ethnic groups.

A recent genome-wide association study (GWAS) for autopsy-confirmed PSPS in Caucasian patients of European descent found several additional common polymorphisms linked with PSPS. Further research into these and other genetic risk factors will help elucidate the cellular mechanisms of the disease.

Treatment

Treatment is largely supportive; preventive measures for falls and aspiration are critical. Increased supervision is eventually required for patient safety due to cognitive impairment. Diplopia from oculomotor paresis may be aided through use of corrective prisms. Botulinum toxin injections may be useful for dystonia or blepharospasm. As PSPS is progressive, patients eventually succumb to associated illnesses from limited mobility (e.g., infection, aspiration, falls). Symptomatic treatment of associated depression is necessary. Survival varies, although the majority survive <10 years, with ~7-year median disease duration from onset of symptoms. PSPS-P patients may have a slightly longer disease duration on average than those with classic Richardson's syndrome, but there is a need for a detailed longitudinal study of well-characterized patients to identify the prognostic features of the disease.

Clinicopathological correlations

PSPS, especially the findings of a supranuclear gaze palsy and early postural instability/falls, correlates well with underlying tauopathy. Indeed, most large-scale PSPS autopsy studies have found a high frequency of progressive supranuclear palsy neuropathology (i.e., PSP neuropathology). PSP is a 4R tauopathy characterized by globose tau inclusions in the brainstem and subcortical structures, in addition to glial "tufted astrocytes" in gray matter and oligodendrocytic "coiled bodies" in the white matter of the neocortex. Neuroimaging findings also include atrophy of the midbrain with widening of the interpeduncular cisterns. The presence of cognitive symptoms in

PSPS correlates well to the extent of neocortical tau pathology and magnetic resonance imaging (MRI) measures of neocortical gray-matter atrophy. The etiology for varying clinical presentations of PSP tauopathy and heterogeneity of cognitive and motor symptoms are currently unclear.

Corticobasal syndrome

Clinical features

CBS is a heterogeneous clinical syndrome that consists of asymmetric parkinsonism and significant cognitive dysfunction, thus posing a significant diagnostic challenge, as patients may often present to either a movement disorder or cognitive care clinic. Indeed, >50% of patients may have a cognitive presentation in the absence of motor disorder. The key clinical motor features include asymmetric levodopa-resistant parkinsonism, limb dystonia, and myoclonus. Bradykinesia, gait instability, and spread of motor features to the contralateral limb may often occur later in the disease course. Resting, postural, and intentional forms of tremor are less common. Cardinal cognitive features include prominent limb apraxia (i.e., idiomotor, ideational, limb-kinetic, non-representational, or orobuccal), cortical sensory loss (i.e., graphesthesia in absence of primary sensory deficit), and alien limb phenomenon (i.e., intermanual conflict, agnosia of own limb). CBS also incorporates a range of other cognitive symptoms that can include language disturbance, parietal lobe dysfunction, social comportment disorder, and executive impairments of poor planning/organizing, utilization behavior, and perseveration (i.e., frontal-behavioral-spatial syndrome). The language difficulties are often consistent with naPPA, with slow, hesitant speech and grammatical expression/comprehension difficulties. Disorders of social comportment and behavior often include apathy and impulsiveness and can meet criteria for the behavioral variant of FTD (bvFTD). Features of posterior parietal/occipital syndromes (i.e., Gerstmann's and Balint's syndrome), including acalculia, are not uncommon.

The differential diagnosis for CBS is similar to that for PSPS. There is considerable clinical and neuropathological overlap between the two syndromes, as CBS patients can also develop oculomotor difficulties and gait dysfunction.

Epidemiology

There are no established environmental risk factors for CBS and there is minimal epidemiological data on the prevalence of the disorder. Similar to PSPS, CBS risk has also been linked to the H1 haplotype in *MAPT* in Caucasian populations. Age of onset typically ranges from the fifth to seventh decades and the clinical course is variable, with a mean survival of roughly 6 years from onset of symptoms.

Treatment

There is usually a minimal response to dopaminergic therapy and, as with PSPS, supportive treatment strategies are required to prevent falls and aspiration. Occupational therapy and assist devices may help to address difficulties with activities of daily living such as feeding (due to apraxia/dystonia). Physical therapy with a range of motion exercises is an important aspect of care to prevent contractures of a dystonic and rigid limb. Botulinum toxin injections may be useful in the relief of dystonia-related discomfort.

Clinicopathological correlations

CBS was previously referred to as corticobasal degeneration (CBD), but this term is now reserved for the neuropathological findings of 4R tauopathy with large tau-positive diffuse "astrocytic plaques" and "ballooned neurons" in gray matter of limbic and neocortical structures. There is also a large burden of tau-positive "coiled bodies" and astrocytic tau inclusions in white matter for CBD. The basal ganglia and brainstem contain a heavy burden of inclusions as well, and sometimes the morphology is difficult to distinguish from PSP.

This change in nomenclature was necessitated by findings from large-scale autopsy studies in CBS, which found that only ~40% of CBS patients had CBD neuropathology at autopsy, and that CBS could also be associated with several alternative underlying neuropathologies including AD (~25%), TDP-43 proteinopathies (~15%), and PSP pathology (~15%). These discordant clinicopathological relationships have led to the development of clinical research criteria for CBS to help identify CBS due to CBD tauopathy. Conversely, CBD pathology has been linked to four main clinical syndromes (i.e., CBS, naPPA, PSPS, and a frontal-behavioral-spatial syndrome). Neuroimaging findings often include asymmetric perisylvian cortical atrophy and subcortical atrophy in the basal ganglia and thalamus. Implementation of formal clinical criteria for CBS will help further understanding of the natural history and clinicopathological correlations of this complex syndrome.

Other tauopathies (FTLD-tau)

There are several additional forms of tauopathy that are also considered part of the frontotemporal lobar degeneration spectrum disorders (i.e., FTLD-tau), as described in this section. These neuropathologies are associated with a range of FTD clinical syndromes and in some cases associated with amnestic symptoms in elderly patients. Finally, there are patients from geographically isolated regions in the Pacific and West Indies with a clinical phenotype of motor neuron disease and/or parkinsonism with dementia and significant tau and TDP-43 inclusions at autopsy. The direct cause for these atypical cases is currently unclear.

Pick's disease and FTD clinical syndromes

Pick's disease is a 3R-tau predominant tauopathy that is characterized by round tau-positive intraneuronal "Pick bodies" and glial inclusions throughout the limbic and neocortical regions. Pick's disease neuropathology most often presents with a clinical syndrome of bvFTD, but can also be associated with naPPA and CBS. Conversely, the clinical syndrome of bvFTD is associated with roughly equal proportions of patients with tauopathies and TDP-43 proteinopathies. Thus, the term "Pick's disease" is now used exclusively as the neuropathological diagnosis of 3R tauopathy with "Pick body" inclusions. Autopsy studies of PPA variants have also found varying frequencies of tauopathies. NaPPA is more commonly due to tauopathies, while semantic variant (sv-PPA) is largely due to TDP-43 proteinopathies; however, these associations are not absolute. The presence of extrapyramidal features consistent with PSPS or CBS in bvFTD/PPA is a strong indicator of underlying tauopathy. As previously noted, features of naPPA and bvFTD can also occur in PSPS and CBS. Thus, a complex relationship exists between clinical phenotype and underlying neuropathology for tauopathies. These discordant relationships pose a significant problem for accurate diagnosis. Currently, the gold standard is neuropathological examination at autopsy.

Geographically isolated tauopathies with parkinsonism

There is a clustering of patients with a clinical symptomology complex of amyotrophic lateral sclerosis and/or parkinsonism with dementia (ALS-PDC) in two isolated populations in the Pacific (i.e., Chamorro natives of Guam and inhabitants of the Kii peninsula of Japan). At autopsy these patients are found to have widespread tauopathy, including in the lower motor neurons in the spinal cord, along with TDP-43 deposits. The geographic isolation of these cases and high degree of family history indicate a possible genetic etiology, although thus far none has been identified. Numerous environmental factors have been examined with no clear causative agent identified. Interestingly, the prevalence and incidence of ALS-PDC are dramatically declining in Guam, suggesting the loss of an exogenous environmental causative factor.

There is also an abnormally high proportion of atypical parkinsonism patients in the island of Guadalupe in the French West Indies. The majority of patients have key features of PSPS along with atypical symptoms of visual hallucinations, REM sleep behavior disorder, and rest tremor. In the few available autopsies, tau pathology similar to PSPS was found. Guadeloupian PSPS patients are from diverse ethnic backgrounds (African, Indian, Caucasian, and mixed ethnicities) and have minimal positive family history, making a genetic etiology less likely. Epidemiological studies find an association with dietary intake of plants from the *annonaceae* family (e.g., soursop). Further, annonacin, a compound found in high concentration in these plants, is an inhibitor of the mitochondrial respiratory chain and toxic to cultured and *in vivo* murine dopaminergic cells, suggesting a potential mechanism for toxicity; however, the exact mechanism for this clustering of atypical PSPS is not entirely clear.

Other tauopathies

Argyrophilic grain disease (AGD) is a tauopathy characterized by 4R-tau predominant spindle-shaped "grains" in the hippocampus and amygdala. These findings are accompanied by "pre-tangle" tau inclusions in the cornu ammonis of the hippocampus, "coiled bodies" in white matter, and "ballooned neurons" in the amygdala. Less commonly grains and associated tau pathology are more widespread throughout the neocortex. Neurofibrillary tangle pathology in the hippocampus and limbic structures indistinguishable from AD, in the absence of significant amyloid-beta plaque pathology, was formerly known as tangle-predominant senile dementia and has more recently been described as primary age-related tauopathy (PART). PART is largely found in older patients (>80 years) and the distinction between PART and AD pathobiology is currently a matter of debate. Both AGD and TPSD may present with amnestic symptoms similar to AD, and less commonly in patients with FTD spectrum clinical syndromes.

Future directions

The lack of disease-modifying therapies for PSPS, CBS, and other tauopathies is a critical unmet need for these patient populations. With mounting evidence for the central role of tau misfolding and aggregation in disease pathogenesis for tauopathies, many current drug development efforts are directed at preventing pathological tau transmission within the CNS. A major limitation for the implementation of such therapies is the inability to readily detect tauopathies ante mortem, as the gold standard for diagnosis is autopsy. Novel biomarkers for tauopathies will be critical to address this problem.

Neuroimaging studies find that white-matter degeneration in long association tracts may help differentiate tauopathies from TDP-43 proteinopathies. Cerebrospinal fluid (CSF) analysis finds that levels of total-tau (t-tau) and amyloid-beta accurately distinguish autopsy-confirmed patients with AD from FTLD. Further, tauopathies have higher levels of phosphorylated tau (p-tau) in CSF than TDP-43 proteinopathies, and the ratio of p-tau:t-tau may have diagnostic value to distinguish these neurodegenerative conditions. Finally, recent developments of potential neuroimaging radioligands to detect pathological tau deposition *in vivo* are another promising approach to biomarker discovery for tauopathies. These promising initial research findings require replication in large multicenter cohorts before application for widespread clinical use.

In summary, tauopathies are a diverse class of proteinopathies that result in a range of clinical symptoms that reflect the burden and distribution of tau deposits in the CNS. Treatment for PSPS, CBS, and FTD is currently largely supportive, and future work on the underlying biology of tau-mediated disease and improved diagnostics are critical for the development of meaningful therapies for these conditions.

Further reading

Armstrong MJ, Litvan I, Lang AE, et al. Criteria for the diagnosis of corticobasal degeneration. *Neurology* 2013;80:496–503.

Capparros-Lefebvre D, Sergeant N, Lees A, et al. Guadeloupean parkinsonism: A cluster of progressive supranuclear palsy-like tauopathy. *Brain* 2002;125:801–811.

Dickson DW. Sporadic tauopathies: Pick's disease, corticobasal degeneration, progressive supranuclear palsy and argyrophilic grain disease. In: EsiriEM, LeeV M-Y, TrojanowskiJQ (eds.). *The Neuropathology of Dementia*. Cambridge: Cambridge University Press; 2004:227–256.

Forman MS, Farmer J, Johnson JK, et al. Frontotemporal dementia: Clinicopathological correlations. *Ann Neurol* 2006;59:952–962.

Golbe LI. Progressive supranuclear palsy. *Sem Neurol* 2014;34:151–159.

Grossman M. Primary progressive aphasia: Clinicopathological correlations. *Nature Rev Neurol* 2010;6:88–97.

Guo JL, Lee VM. Cell-to-cell transmission of pathogenic proteins in neurodegenerative diseases. *Nature Med* 2014;20:130–138.

Irwin DJ, Cairns NJ, Grossman M, et al. Frontotemporal lobar degeneration: Defining phenotypic diversity through personalized medicine. *Acta Neuropathol* 2015;129(4):469–491. doi:10.1007/s00401-014-1380-1

Lee SE, Rabinovici GD, Mayo MC, et al. Clinicopathological correlations in corticobasal degeneration. *Ann Neurol* 2011;70:327–340.

Murray R, Neumann M, Forman MS, et al. Cognitive and motor assessment in autopsy-proven corticobasal degeneration. *Neurology* 2007;68:1274–1283.

45 Amyotrophic lateral sclerosis and other TDP-43 proteinopathies

Albert C. Ludolph

Department of Neurology, University of Ulm, Ulm, Germany

TDP-43 (43-kDa TAR DNA-binding protein, TARDBP) is a nuclear protein of 43 kDa involved in DNA and RNA binding and transcription, RNA splicing, and RNA metabolism. TDP-43 is seen as one of the molecular markers for neurodegeneration, like tau and ß-amyloid. In 2006, Manuela Neumann discovered phosphorylated TDP-43 as a cytoplasmically displaced marker protein for amyotrophic lateral sclerosis (ALS) and tau-negative frontotemporal dementias (FTDs). Only two years later, TDP-43 was shown to be sufficient to cause ALS when mutations in the gene were found to cosegregate with the phenotype of familial ALS; later, intronic mutations in the most frequent ALS gene among Caucasians, *C9ORF72*, were associated with TDP-43 pathology and the cause of ALS, FTD, and clinical combinations thereof. Beyond the knowledge that TDP-43 was a molecular marker protein in more than 95% of sporadic ALS cases, recently the apparent propagation of neuropathology of TDP-43 in ALS and FTDs has become the basis for the hypothesis that prion-like spreading may not only be the molecular basis of Alzheimer's disease (AD) and Parkinson's disease (PD), but also of ALS and FTDs. This chapter will provide an overview of ALS and other TPD-43 proteinopathies. More detailed information on each of the proteinopathies can be found in their respective chapters of this textbook.

Amyotrophic lateral sclerosis

ALS is one of the most aggressive and disabling neurological diseases and it is universally fatal. It causes progressive muscle wasting and loss of muscle strength that eventually render the patient unable to communicate actively with the environment by speech, mimics, gestures or posture; that is, "deefferentiated." Patients often die of catabolism and severe alveolar hypoventilation resulting in pulmonary infections and respiratory failure. In about 5% of patients, a Mendelian mode of inheritance can be identified.

Epidemiology

In Europe and North America, the incidence of ALS reaches about 3/100,000, with a peak at age 65–70 years. In parts of Asia, most notably China, disease onset may be earlier, at about age 50 years. The male-to-female ratio of ALS approaches 3:2 in the Western world, as compared to 2:1 in other parts of the world, such as East Asia. Whether this difference is only due to differences in demographic development needs to be explored. The life expectancy of patients might also differ in different parts of the world; in the Western world the average life expectancy ranges from 2–4 years. Historically, the disease has been described as more frequent with a younger age of onset in several places of the Western Pacific, including the Kii peninsula, Guam, and Western New Guinea. In these places the disease is associated with L-DOPA unresponsive parkinsonism as well as supranuclear oculomotor deficits and dementia. A similar clinical picture has been described on the Caribbean island of Guadeloupe. The reasons for the occurrence of these clusters are unknown.

Clinical features

Beyond severe progressive paresis, ALS is most often associated with minor deficits on neuropsychological, behavioral, executive, and cognitive tests that are believed to reflect frontal lobe dysfunction. In contrast to this more common ALS presentation, ALS-FTD manifests first with obvious and severe behavioral and cognitive dysfunction, which is followed later by the neuromuscular features and ultimately death from respiratory failure. This "ALS variant" might be better termed FTD-ALS, a clinical observation underlined by recent neuropathological studies. ALS may also present with accompanying parkinsonism-like rigidity or executive and/or cerebellar abnormalities of eye movements.

In the 1990s the El Escorial diagnostic criteria for ALS were developed. Although they were initially very useful, the availability of advanced diagnostic imaging tools has made differential diagnosis of ALS easier and has led to less clinical reliance on the El Escorial criteria; however, the criteria were simplified in 2015 and are now used in the evaluation of patients in early disease for access to clinical trials.

Treatment

The only available pharmacological treatment option for ALS is riluzole. Although the exact mechanism of action of riluzole is unclear, it is known to interfere with the release of glutamate, the major neurotransmitter in corticofugal pathways. Riluzole has been shown to slow disease progression, but only increases survival by 3–4 months in patients with a life expectancy of approximately 1 year.

Neuropathology

Based on the discovery of the primary marker protein TDP-43 by Neumann and colleagues in 2006, Braak, Brettschneider, and collaborators recently performed a postmortem study using

International Neurology, Second edition. Edited by Robert P. Lisak, Daniel D. Truong, William M. Carroll and Roongroj Bhidayasiri
© 2016 John Wiley & Sons, Ltd. Published 2016 by John Wiley & Sons, Ltd.

phosphorylated TDP-43 as a marker for ALS. The study revealed four distinct patterns of neuropathological lesions. Because the study was cross-sectional, it was not possible to determine whether these four patterns reflected four different stages of ALS. Nevertheless, based on the clinical parallels between ALS, PD, and AD in terms of the progressive clinical progression of the disease, and based on the known relationship between the clinical phases of PD and AD and underlying changes in their neuropathology, the investigators proposed a four-stage model of ALS disease progression based on the four patterns of TPD-43 lesions observed. In this conceptualization, ALS affects the cortical association fibers and in parallel consecutive corticofugal tracts, with their monosynaptically connected target neuronal populations most severely affected in the following sequence (i.e., stages):

I.   An initial stage during which only the motor cortex, the bulbar motor neurons, and the anterior horn cells of the spinal cord are affected by TDP-43 neuropathology. As in all stages, loss of neurons is associated with the presence of this marker.

II. A second stage in which TDP-43 neuropathology and associated neuronal damage are evident in precerebellar nuclei, including the olivary nuclei, the reticular neuronal populations, the substantia nigra, and others, and in which there is spread via the cortical association fibers into the gyrus rectus.

III. A third stage in which the entire frontal cortex, including the orbitofrontal areas, shows TDP-43 neuropathology, as do the postcentral gyrus and the medium-sized projection neurons of the striatum.

IV. A fourth stage is characterized by most abundant TDP-43 neuropathology, including the perforant pathway and the hippocampus.

In a second publication that included ventilated late-stage patients, the authors describe an even wider area of TPD-43 neuropathology (i.e., a potential stage V), which included the oculomotor nuclei.

In contrast to the staging of PD and AD, TDP-43 is rarely found in asymptomatic individuals; therefore, the question of whether a neuropathologically defined preclinical stage of ALS exists must remain open. It is interesting to note that not only the neurons but also the oligodendroglia surrounding affected tracts (but not the cortical satellite cells) carry TDP-43 neuropathology. This oligodendroglial pathology seems to occur very early in the disease.

Since there is currently no positron emission tomography (PET) marker for cytoplasmic accumulation of TDP-43, scientists may need to rely on the characteristic pattern of tract damage as observed with diffusion tensor imaging (DTI), with fractional anisotropy of corticofugal tracts as a means to develop a quantitative measure of TDP-43 inclusions.

Although there is currently insufficient evidence to go beyond speculation as to whether these distinct patterns of TDP-43 neuropathology indeed reflect different stages of the illness or different subtypes, it is clear that ALS is not solely a motor neuron disease; rather, it should be viewed as a disease of multisystem degeneration within the central nervous system (CNS). Furthermore, ALS appears to propagate preferentially through monosynaptic connections, both in the CNS and peripherally. Finally, all corticofugal fibers that seem to propagate ALS neuropathology are glutamatergic, which may explain the effects of riluzole on disease progression.

In subtypes of ALS not carrying major TDP-43 cytoplasmic inclusions, in particular those caused by mutations in the fused in sarcoma gene (FUS) and superoxide dismutase (SOD) gene, no attempt at neuropathological staging has been made.

It is currently unknown whether the neuropathology as described by Neumann, Brettschneider, and Braak is the same in non-Caucasians. With regard to the geographic isolates, the disease on Guam and the Kii peninsula is seen as a tauopathy, not a disease characterized by TDP-43 pathology. However, TDP-43 inclusions exist in the Guam disease and some mutations in the *C9ORF72* gene have recently been described in the Kii peninsula patients. The recently discovered ALS cluster on Guadeloupe, which is related to a progressive supranuclear palsy type of presentation, underscores the notion that findings in North American and European autopsies should not automatically be generalized to other parts of the world.

Frontotemporal dementias

The FTDs are a subform of dementias of undetermined prevalence. Most authors estimate that FTDs comprise about 10–15% of all dementias. The principal initial symptoms are behavioral changes, but also aphasias. They are accompanied by pyramidal and extrapyramidal deficits. Treatment strategies are in their infancy.

Epidemiology

The details of the epidemiology of FTDs are far from being clarified; however, this type of dementia is thought to be the third most common after AD and vascular dementias. Up to 50% of patients with FTD have a positive family history. The FTDs affect humans as early as their 50s, a time when they still have major responsibilities such as caring for children and working, which often require them to drive automobiles. Since the clinical hallmark of the most common subtype of FTD, the behavioral variant, is loss of social awareness and impulse control – often associated with apathia – affected individuals and their relatives need social protection and medical care. The primary progressive aphasias (PPAs), a subform of FTDs, are initially characterized by a slowly developing motor aphasia, whereas the initial hallmark of semantic dementias, another subform, is the loss of the meaning of words, progressing to a dramatic loss of knowledge about the world.

Clinical features

FTDs exist in three clinical subtypes: behavioral (bvFTD), semantic (semantic dementia, SD), and primary progressive aphasias (PPAs). The subtypes are defined by their initial, presenting symptoms; in exceptional cases a behavioral deficit is followed by frank ALS (FTD-ALS). This association of FTD with ALS was initially described by Otto Dornblüth in 1889, two years before Pick's first description of a progressive aphasia.

The diagnosis of bvFTD relies on the history of a patient showing behavioral changes, a disorder of social conduct, executive deficits, and beginning features of semantic or motor aphasia. The latter is the initial hallmark of PPA, which later gets features of bvFTD and also often shows symptoms typical of SD. This subform is probably the most dramatic, since the individual loses any understanding of words; in later stages the loss of comprehension goes far beyond this, and the world has no meaning for the patient.

Neuropsychological testing is essential for the diagnosis and yields a typical pattern of deficits for each subform; magnetic resonance imaging (MRI) results may only show typical deficits in later stages, whereas glucose PET shows the characteristic asymmetric metabolism of frontotemporal cortical structures.

Treatment

There are no effective symptomatic or disease-modifying therapies for FTDs. Today, the basis for the future conduct of therapeutic trials is being laid by defining criteria for early diagnosis as well as outcome measures.

Neuropathology

The neuropathology of the TDP-43 positive cases of the behavioral variant of FTD has been thoroughly described; however, the evolving picture is not as clear as that for ALS. Two different patterns of neuropathology have been distinguished based on postmortem studies; both suggest that the neuropathology may sequentially disseminate in stages and propagate along axonal pathways, as is proposed for ALS. In the first, and most frequently observed, pattern, TDP-43 intraneuronal inclusions are located in the cytoplasm (cytoplasmic type, cFTD). In the less frequent pattern, long dendritic aggregates (neuritic type, nFTD) are observed.

Cases with cFTD often involve bulbar somatomotor neurons and the anterior horn cells of the spinal cord. In nFTD autopsy studies, involvement of the cerebral cortex was extensive and frequently reached the occipital areas ("stage IV"). As in ALS, four subtypes or patterns could be distinguished:

I. Autopsies with the lowest burden of pathology – subtype I – were characterized by widespread pTDP-43 aggregates in the orbital gyri, gyrus rectus, and amygdala.

II. In subgroup II, pTDP-43 lesions also emerged in the middle frontal and anterior cingulate gyrus, as well as in the anteromedial temporal lobe areas, the superior and medial temporal gyri, striatum, red nucleus, thalamus, and precerebellar nuclei.

III. In subgroup III, there was involvement of the motor cortex, bulbar somatomotor neurons, and the spinal cord anterior horn cells, in addition to the areas described in subgroup II.

IV. Autopsies with the highest burden of pathology (subgroup IV) were also characterized by pTDP-43 lesions in the visual cortex.</nl>

Based on these patterns, the authors postulated a progressive propagation of pTDP43 pathology from the frontal brain and the amygdala to the occipital cortex. It is interesting to note that the parallel spreading of pathology through the association fibers and corticofugal tracts identified in ALS may also be the underlying principle for bvFTD. Similar neuropathological studies do not exist in PPA and SD.

Although Alzheimer´s disease is not considered a TDP-43 proteinopathy, Josephs and colleagues studied phosphorylated TDP-43 immunohistochemistry in AD. In addition to the plaques and tangles known to be associated with AD, they also detected TDP-43 neuropathology in about 50% of their autopsy samples. They postulated a progression of TDP-43 inclusion pathology in five stages, starting with the amygdala, then affecting the entorhinal cortex and subiculum, invading the dentate gyrus and occipitotemporal cortex, later the inferior temporal cortex, and finally the middle frontal cortex and basal ganglia.

Although these findings and their potential clinical correlation cannot be readily explained, it is remarkable that TDP-43 neuropathology is observed so frequently in AD, particularly given the absence of TDP-43 neuropathology in healthy controls. Therefore

it might be valuable in the future to distinguish between primary TDP-43 proteinopathies such as ALS and FTD and numerous other neurodegenerative diseases mainly associated with tau pathology, but also with TDP-43 neuropathology, such as Guam ALS/PDC and AD.

Nothing has been done yet to elucidate how TDP-43 neuropathology translates to clinical aspects of bvFTD and other dementias. However, comprehensive approaches, including the tract approach, neuropsychological investigations, and other relevant clinical measures, could be informative.

Conclusion

The "primary" TDP-43 proteinopathies, ALS, and tau-negative FTDs are characterized by intracytoplasmic inclusions of phosphorylated TDP-43 proteins. Most interestingly, like synuclein and tau, these proteins propagate along anatomical structures and therefore may support the hypothesis that neurodegenerative diseases of the central nervous system underlie a common and anatomically defined propagation principle. In the case of ALS, these phenomena mirror well-known, hitherto seemingly unexplainable phenotypic characteristics, such as the preferential affection of monosynaptically connected muscles and the characteristic spreading of wasting and paresis. However, in contrast to alpha-synuclein and tau, TDP-43 aggregations are comparatively "fast" and "acute" phenomena, which, in contrast to synuclein, appear first in the CNS and do not cross the neuromuscular synapses.

Further reading

Agosta F, Al-Chalabi A, Filippi M, *et al.* The El Escorial criteria: Strengths and weaknesses. *Amyotroph Lateral Scler Frontotemporal Degener* 2015;16(1–2):1–7.

Braak H, Brettschneider J, Ludolph AC, *et al.* Amyotrophic lateral sclerosis: A model of corticofugal axonal spread. *Nat Rev Neurol* 2013;9:708–714.

Brettschneider J, Del Tredici K, Toledo JB, *et al.* Stages of pTDP-43 pathology in amyotrophic lateral sclerosis. *Ann Neurol* 2013;74:20–38.

Brettschneider J, Del Tredici K, Irwin DJ, *et al.* Sequential distribution of pTDP-43 pathology in behavioural variant frontotemporal dementia (bvFTD). *Acta Neuropathol* 2014;127:423–439.

Josephs KA, Murray ME, Whitwell JL, *et al.* Staging TDP-43 pathology in Alzheimer's disease. *Acta Neuropathol* 2014;127:441–450.

Jucker M, Walker LC. Self-propagation of pathogenic protein aggregates in neurodegenerative diseases. *Nature* 2013;501:45–51.

Kassubek J, Müller HP, Del Tredici K, *et al.* Diffusion tensor imaging analysis of sequential spreading of disease in amyotrophic lateral sclerosis confirms patterns of TDP-43 pathology. *Brain* 2014;137:1733–1740.

Liu MS, Cui LY, Fan DS, *et al.* Age of onset of amyotrophic lateral sclerosis in China. *Acta Neurol Scand* 2014;129:163–167.

Lulé D, Burkhardt C, Abdulla S, *et al.* The Edinburgh Cognitive and Behavioural Amyotrophic Lateral Sclerosis Screen: A cross-sectional comparison of established screening tools in a German-Swiss population. *Amyotroph Lateral Scler Frontotemporal Degener* 2015;16(1–2):16–23.

Neumann M, Sampathu DM, Kwong LK, *et al.* Ubiquitinated TDP-43 in frontotemporal lobar degeneration and amyotrophic lateral sclerosis. *Science* 2006;314:130–133.

Uenal H, Rosenbohm A, Kufeldt J, *et al.*; *ALS Registry Study Group.* Incidence and geographical variation of amyotrophic lateral sclerosis (ALS) in Southern Germany: Completeness of the ALS Registry Swabia. *PLoS One* 2014;9(4):e93932.

Weishaupt J, Brettschneider J, Ludolph AC. Amyotrophic lateral sclerosis. *Curr Opin Neurol* 2014;25:530–535.

46 Metabolic, toxic, infectious, inflammatory, and other dementias

John M. Ringman[1], Arousiak Varpetian[2], and Yu-Wei Lin[3]

[1] Department of Neurology, Keck School of Medicine, University of Southern California, and Alzheimer Disease Research Center, Los Angeles, CA, USA

[2] Department of Neurology, Keck School of Medicine, University of Southern California, and Rancho Los Amigos Rehabilitation Center, Downey, CA, USA

[3] Department of Neurology, Taiwan Adventist Hospital, Taipei City, Taiwan

Relatively isolated cognitive impairment due to normal pressure hydrocephalus or metabolic, infectious, genetic, or inflammatory causes is uncommon. Nonetheless, these entities are important to recognize in order to prognosticate accurately and at times treat effectively. Due to their rarity, a high index of suspicion and a knowledge of appropriate diagnostic tests are crucial. Careful attention to other signs and symptoms that accompany the dementia is key in the differential diagnosis. Diverse types of neurological insults can have generalized cognitive impairment as the ultimate outcome and it is impossible to address them all. It is the purpose of this chapter to describe those conditions in which a dementia syndrome is a common or predominant feature.

Normal pressure hydrocephalus

Normal pressure hydrocephalus (NPH) was first described by the Colombian neurosurgeon Salomón Hakim in the 1960s and is thought to account for about 2–5% of dementia cases. It is an important entity to recognize due its potential reversibility. The classic triad suggestive of its presence includes a gait disorder, urinary incontinence, and cognitive impairment. Gait disturbance is the earliest common symptom, which is present in 94–100% of cases, followed by cognitive impairment (78–98%) and urinary dysfunction (76–83%). The nature of the gait disorder can be helpful in making the diagnosis. It is characterized by reduced speed, decreased step height and stride length, and, when advanced, "en bloc" turning (requiring an abnormally increased number of steps to turn). However, it should be noted that even the classic gait is not specific for the presence of NPH, as it can be seen in the presence of bilateral subcortical ischemia as well. The cognitive deficits are not always dramatic and when present typically take the form of "subcortical" impairment. That is, deficits in tasks of divided attention and psychomotor speed are most evident and recall memory may be impaired, although recognition and other forms of cued memory are relatively intact. Despite the classic triad, NPH can be a challenge to diagnose considering how common these problems are in the elderly, which means that they may coexist by chance. Because of this, the presence of NPH is best judged as an estimate of the degree to which hydrocephalus contributes to an individual patient's disability. Accordingly, a recently published guideline recommended that cases be classified as either *probable* NPH, *possible* NPH, or *unlikely* NPH.

The demonstration of enlarged cerebral ventricles with neuroimaging studies is necessary to make the diagnosis of NPH. The pathophysiology underlying ventricular enlargement is incompletely understood, but it is thought to be due to decreased reabsorption of cerebrospinal fluid (CSF) into the venous sinuses. This might occur as a result of known prior neurological illness (e.g., subarachnoid hemorrhage, trauma, meningitis) as *secondary* NPH, or without a known causative insult as *idiopathic* NPH. The excess of CSF is transmitted to the intracerebral ventricular system, at least transiently increasing the pressure there. "Normal" pressure hydrocephalus is therefore a misnomer and many specialists prefer the term adult hydrocephalus.

Management of NPH is a challenge, as not all persons who have the syndrome respond well to treatment. Enlarged ventricles seen on computed tomography (CT) or magnetic resonance imaging (MRI) are insufficient in predicting who has NPH or who will respond to surgical shunting of the ventricles. Relatively large cerebral ventricles are common in the elderly on an *ex vacuo* basis due to cerebral atrophy from neurodegenerative disease, cerebral ischemia, or nutritional deficiencies. It is common practice for clinicians to attempt to differentiate hydrocephalus from *ex vacuo* ventricular enlargement due to atrophy by estimating the disparity between ventricular size and the extra-axial subarachnoid space. However, this approach has not been validated in a controlled fashion and therefore conclusions based on such an apparent disparity should be drawn with caution. Hydrocephalus may be defined as an Evans index (the ratio of maximum width of the frontal horns of the lateral ventricles to the maximum width of the inner table of the cranium) greater than 0.3. MRI should demonstrate the disappearance of sulci on at least two sequential sections of coronal T1-weighted images. In the Study of NPH on Neurological Improvement (SINPHONI), the majority of patients showed dilation of the sylvan fissure in association with sulcal tightness in the upper convexities, presenting disproportionately enlarged subarachnoid spaces. The presence of one of the triad of symptoms and these MRI features is highly predictive of a positive tap test and shunt responsiveness. The NPH guideline published by the Japan Neurosurgical Society in

International Neurology, Second edition. Edited by Robert P. Lisak, Daniel D. Truong, William M. Carroll and Roongroj Bhidayasiri

2012 shows flowcharts for diagnosing and managing patients suspected of having NPH.

More sophisticated neuroimaging techniques based on ways of measuring CSF flow and hemodynamics are also sometimes employed. These include estimating the rate of CSF flow through the aqueduct of Sylvius with MRI, perfusion imaging with single photon emission computed tomography (SPECT), SPECT/ acetazolamide challenge, resting metabolic imaging with positron emission tomography, and nuclear cisternography. Data supporting their utility is limited, however, and their use cannot be recommended as a standard of practice.

At some point in the evaluation of a patient with suspected NPH, an estimate of intracranial pressure (ICP) should be obtained. Although we have said that "normal" pressure hydrocephalus is a misnomer, ICPs above 240 mm H_2O suggest an alternative diagnosis such as secondary NPH. Such a measurement may be obtained during a lumbar puncture in which CSF is drained in an effort to predict outcome from shunting. Diagnostic lumbar punctures in which a large volume of CSF (40–50 ml) is removed to determine whether a patient's symptoms (usually gait) improve are commonly used in the assessment of NPH. Such an approach has been demonstrated to have specificity for predicting a good outcome to shunt surgery (positive predictive value of 73–100%), but to lack sensitivity. That is, the presence of a response predicted well who would improve with ventricular shunting, but the lack of a response did not adequately rule out the possibility of a subsequent favorable outcome from such an operation. In order to increase the sensitivity with which shunt responders might be detected, continuous external lumbar drainage (ELD) should be employed. Patients are admitted to the hospital and a lumbar catheter is placed, with the goal of removing 10 ml of CSF per hour for 72 hours, during which clinical changes are monitored. This has been demonstrated to improve the sensitivity in identifying shunt responders from 43–62% with lumbar puncture alone to 50–100%. However, the benefits of this procedure must be weighed against the substantial risks of infection, overdrainage with the consequent development of subdural hematomas, and catheter removal in a confused patient, as well as the attendant financial costs of hospitalization. Although a systematic review of existing data by a consensus panel failed to identify standards of practice regarding the diagnosis of NPH, a suggested algorithm (guideline) for the assessment of patients with suspected NPH has been published by Marmarou *et al.*

Depending on the method of patient selection and how a favorable response to shunting is defined, the rate of positive outcomes to ventricular shunting in NPH has been found to be in the range of 61–75%. Even when the presentation is classic and the preoperative assessment is consistent with NPH, it is still difficult to predict which patient will benefit from shunting. Lack of response in such cases can be due to the presence of concurrent illness (e.g., cerebrovascular ischemia) or to operative considerations such as inadequate shunting or complications (e.g., infections, subdural fluid collections). The duration of the condition is also important, as one study indicated that those with symptoms of more than 2 years' duration were less likely to benefit. When the long-term prognosis of patients is considered, a favorable outcome appears to be substantially less common, with one study showing a decrease in persons with improvement from 64% at 3 months to 26% at 3 years. This is due, at least in part, to death and disability from premorbid conditions that are common in this population (e.g., complications of atherosclerosis) and therefore each patient's overall health status needs to be taken into account when considering ventricular shunting.

Toxic and metabolic disorders

Alcohol

Alcohol is by far the most widely available and widely consumed neurotoxin. Although epidemiological studies suggest a mild protective effect of low doses of alcohol (particularly red wine) in relation to the development of dementia and Alzheimer's disease, chronic alcoholism has been repeatedly shown to be associated with cognitive deficits. The pathology underlying these deficits is more controversial, however, as comorbid conditions such as thiamine (see later) and other nutritional deficiencies, hepatic encephalopathy, head injury, cerebrovascular disease, and concurrent Alzheimer's changes may be contributing to varying degrees in a given case. The cognitive deficits associated with chronic alcoholism include amnesia, disorientation, and in some cases emotional lability and perseveration. The underlying neuropathological substrate is controversial, although studies of uncomplicated alcoholism tend to support a more significant decrement in white-matter volume than in neuronal count. As many cases of dementia associated with alcohol consumption may represent Korsakoff's syndrome in which Wernicke's encephalopathy is subclinical, the existence of a distinct category of dementia associated with alcohol consumption per se is contentious.

Wernicke–Korsakoff syndrome

Wernicke's encephalopathy is an acute or subacute syndrome characterized by delirium, ophthalmoplegia, and gait ataxia, and can lead to coma and death. Autopsy series suggest that it is underdiagnosed, possibly due to absence of the classic triad in many cases. Caused by thiamine deficiency, it is most frequently diagnosed in chronic alcoholics, but can occur in any condition in which malnutrition is present. Neuropathology reveals areas of hemorrhagic necrosis in periventricular areas of the diencephalon and mesencephalon. As rapid treatment is essential, parenteral administration of 100 mg thiamine should be routine in the acutely confused patient for whom the etiology is uncertain. As the acute condition resolves with treatment, patients may be left with Korsakoff's syndrome, a dense amnestic disorder in which confabulation is a classic (although variably present) feature. It has been argued that supplementation of food with thiamine is a public health measure that might decrease the prevalence of this problem.

Vitamin B$_{12}$ deficiency

The association of neurological disorders including cognitive impairment, depression, signs attributable to the corticospinal tract and dorsal column pathways (subacute combined degeneration), and peripheral neuropathy with megaloblastic anemia and vitamin B$_{12}$, has an illustrious history and has led to the award of two Nobel prizes. In an English series of 50 patients presenting with megaloblastic anemia, 26% had cognitive decline, 40% had peripheral neuropathy, and 16% had subacute combined degeneration. The syndrome was due to pernicious anemia in 64%, dietary or other gastrointestinal causes in 30%, and unexplained in 6%. Despite its relative rarity, evidence for its presence should be sought in most persons presenting with memory impairment due to the ease with which it can be identified and the potential for reversibility with treatment. Vitamin B_{12} levels in the low normal range are not incompatible with the diagnosis and the presence of deficiency can be confirmed by identifying elevated levels of methylmalonic acid in plasma. The recommendation is 1000 mcg of cyanocobalamin administered intramuscularly (IM) weekly for 3 months, followed by monthly maintenance injections, with the ultimate duration of treatment depending in part on the original cause. With this treatment, 90% of patients will demonstrate significant improvement, with the most advanced cases being less likely to have complete recovery. Lack of a response should lead one to consider alternate diagnoses (e.g., distinct or concurrent folate deficiency, nitrous oxide abuse, an inherited disorder of B_{12} metabolism, multiple sclerosis).

Hypo- and hyperthyroidism

Cognitive impairment can accompany the systemic symptoms of either hypo- or hyperthyroidism. Although rarely if ever a cause of an isolated dementia syndrome, thyroid disorders are common and treatable, and therefore routine screening in a person presenting with a cognitive complaint is recommended by the American Academy of Neurology.

Infectious causes

Infectious disease is a major cause of neurological morbidity worldwide. In the following review we will focus on the most common infectious illnesses for which cognitive or behavioral changes may be a predominant feature.

Dementia associated with human immunodeficiency virus infection

Human immunodeficiency virus (HIV) can cause neurological disease, including cognitive deterioration directly, by way of susceptibility to opportunistic infections, secondarily through damage to other organs, or as an effect of the medications used to treat it. Here we will focus on cognitive decline due to HIV itself, called HIV-associated neurocognitive disorder (HAND).

According to Frascati criteria, HAND includes the subclassifications asymptomatic neurocognitive impairment (ANI), mild neurocognitive disorder (MND), and HIV-associated dementia (HAD, previously called AIDS dementia complex). Dementia is the initial manifestation of the acquired immune deficiency syndrome (AIDS) in 3% of patients and significant cognitive impairment has been found to be present in 15–20% of patients with advanced disease. Milder degrees of impairment on neuropsychological testing have been found in more than 23% of otherwise asymptomatic persons infected with HIV. Encephalitis due to HIV itself (HIVE) is essentially a diagnosis of exclusion during life, but has been found in the brains of approximately 16% of persons who died from HIV disease. The rate of HIVE is thought to have declined since the introduction of zidovudine and more recently with combined antiretroviral therapy (cART). The pathological features of HIVE consist of inflammation, predominantly in subcortical gray- and white-matter structures, consisting of microglia, macrophages, and multinucleated giant cells. The neurological examination is generally non-focal. Cognitively, early impairments in attention, psychomotor speed, and recall memory consistent with a "subcortical dementia" are typical. T2-weighted MRI reveals bilateral and symmetric white-matter hyperintensities in HIVE. Treatment is that

of HIV disease itself and the cognitive impairment is thought to respond to cART.

The picture of HAND has changed since the development of combined cART in 1996. In the post-cART era, about half of all treated HIV patients have cognitive impairment, which seems to reflect little improvement compared with the pre-cART era. However, the prevalence of HAD dropped dramatically in the post-cART era, while ANI is more common than MND and HAD in developed countries. Subcortical dementia with impairment in motor skills, cognitive speed, and verbal fluency was prominent in the pre-cART era, while in the post-cART era, more cortical involvement such as memory deficits and executive dysfunction has been documented.

Magnetic resonance spectroscopy (MRS) may be more sensitive than conventional MRI in detecting HAND and there is evidence that MRS abnormalities can be reversed by cART. In the pre-cART era, a decreased N-acetylaspartate to creatine ratio and an increased choline to creatine ratio were observed, demonstrating neuronal dysfunction and inflammation. The picture might change in the post-cART era. New imaging measures such as diffusion tensor imaging (DTI) and functional MRI (fMRI) may have utility in assessing the efficacy of treatments.

With the higher prevalence of ANI and MND in the post-cART era, developing more reliable and tolerable neurocognitive tests to screen for subtle deficits is important. Neuropsychological testing is the main diagnostic and monitoring tool in HAND. Screening methods include the Mini Mental Status Examination (MMSE), the Montreal Cognitive Assessment (MOCA), and the International HIV Dementia Screen. In the post-cART era, HIV load and CD4 cell counts are no longer closely associated with neuropsychometric performance. A potential serum biomarker is the monitoring of monocyte activation, but additional biomarkers are needed to screen and monitor HAND.

There is controversy regarding the addition of drugs with higher central nervous system (CNS) penetration, so-called CNS-targeted therapy, to treat patients with HAND. To date the trials of CNS-targeted therapy have shown no difference in neurocognitive outcome. More alternative therapeutic strategies such as targeting monocytes activation and application of nanoparticles are under investigation.

Neurosyphilis (syphilitic dementia)

Syphilis is caused by *Treponema pallidum*, with about 12 million new infections worldwide each year. The number of infections in South and Southeast Asia and Sub-Saharan Africa is 40 times that in North America. Syphilis is a sexually transmitted infection and facilitates transmission of HIV. If left untreated, after a 10–20-year incubation period the central nervous system can become affected, leading to dementia, psychiatric disease, and mobility problems. General paralysis of the insane, as dementia due to neurosyphilis was once called, was among the most frequent causes of hospitalization in psychiatric units in the nineteenth and twentieth centuries. Although the prevalence of dementia associated with syphilis is not as high with the use of penicillin, if treatment is not started early penicillin does not restore normal cognitive function in affected persons. The cognitive impairment starts with memory loss and apathy and therefore may be misdiagnosed as Alzheimer's disease. Eventually language and behavior become impaired, with delusions and disinhibition. On neuropathological examination neuronal loss, glial proliferation, and atrophy are observed. Although the American Academy of Neurology no longer recommends serological screening for syphilis in the routine evaluation of persons presenting with dementia, it should be considered in the context of local epidemiological factors.

Progressive multifocal leukoencephalopathy

Progressive multifocal leukoencephalopathy (PML) is a progressive demyelinating disorder of the human brain caused by reactivation of latent infection with the JC virus, a member of the polyomavirus family. PML usually occurs as a late complication of diseases associated with impaired immunity, such as AIDS, and lymphoproliferative disorders, such as Hodgkin's disease and chronic lymphocytic leukemia. PML presents with focal CNS symptoms including limb weakness, visual symptoms, gait ataxia, incoordination, language disturbances, and cognitive impairment in general. Focal non-enhancing hyperintensity of white matter on T2-weighted MRI without swelling or mass effect is characteristic. Currently, mortality from PML is 30–50% in the first 3 months after diagnosis. Starting cART in previously treatment-naïve patients with a CD4 count greater than 100/µl carries a more favorable prognosis. Patients are usually left with neurological sequalae because of oligodendrocyte death. Patients can present with the clinical and radiological findings of PML without detectable JC virus in the CSF by polymerase chain reaction (PCR) if CSF viral load is low. PML has also been associated with use of the medication natalizumab for relapsing–remitting multiple sclerosis, although with proper patient monitoring natalizumab can still be used in this context.

Whipple's disease

Whipple's disease is a systemic infection caused by *Tropheryma whippelei*, a Gram-positive bacillus. Approximately 1000 cases of Whipple's disease have been reported, but its recognition is nonetheless important due to the existence of effective treatment. Whipple's disease commonly affects middle-aged white men with symptoms of diarrhea, weight loss, and arthritis. Neurological symptoms occur in up to 63% of patients and cognitive changes occur in 71% of those with neurological signs. Cognitive symptoms include decreased attention and orientation, and impaired memory and abstract thinking. Aphasia and behavioral changes have also been reported. Other neurological signs include ophthalmoplegia and ataxia. Whipple's disease is diagnosed by detecting periodic acid–Schiff (PAS) positive inclusions in macrophages from small bowel biopsy specimens. Treatment with doxycycline and hydroxychloroquine is recommended. Patients should also be tested for neurological involvement using a polymerase chain reaction (PCR) assay on cerebrospinal fluid, and if positive should also receive high-dose sufamethoxazole or sulfadiazine for 12–18 months. With treatment, two-thirds of those infected recover. Without treatment, the infection is fatal.

Viral encephalitides

The viral encephalitides cause a greater burden of disease in tropical and developing countries. Although they usually present acutely with a general encephalopathy accompanied by various combinations of fever, headache, seizures, and other neurological manifestations, etiological agents that can cause a more indolent form of progressive cognitive decline include measles virus (subacute sclerosing panencephalitis), rubella, arboviruses, and picornaviruses. Encephalitis due to herpes simplex virus usually causes fulminant illness, but should be mentioned here because it is the most common cause of viral encephalitis and treatment is effective, particularly if begun early.

Other infectious agents

CNS infections with other bacteria and fungi usually manifest with focal or other non-cognitive neurological signs and symptoms. Although rarely presenting with isolated cognitive impairment, CNS infections with *coccidioidiomycosis*, *cryptococcus neoformans*, and mycobacteria have been reported to cause a dementing syndrome. Infection with *Borrelia burgdorferi* and related spirochetes (Lyme disease) can cause various neurological manifestations, including meningitis, radiculitis, cranial neuropathies, and even secondary normal pressure hydrocephalus, but whether chronic active infection can cause cognitive impairment is an area of controversy.

Genetic causes

Although illnesses with well-defined genetic bases most commonly manifest in childhood, a number of adult-onset neurodegenerative disorders that feature progressive cognitive impairment have genetic origins. The genetics of Alzheimer's disease (AD) are complex, with rare fully penetrant autosomal dominant forms identified and genes that contribute to the risk of late-onset AD being described. Neither AD, the increasingly understood genetic bases of frontotemporal lobar degeneration, nor the prion diseases will be discussed here, as they are addressed in other chapters of this book.

Huntington's disease

Huntington's disease (HD) is a gradually progressive neurodegenerative condition, classically consisting of the triad of choreiform movements, dementia, and psychiatric changes that is inherited in an autosomal dominant manner. In populations of Western European descent, the frequency is between 3 and 7 per 100,000, and it is more rare in Japan, China, Finland, and in black Africans. Chorea is usually the most obvious manifestation of HD, but rigidity and the attendant impairment in mobility, as well as the cognitive and behavioral changes, have the greatest impact on quality of life and, ultimately, survival. The dementia tends to be of a fronto-subcortical variety, with distractibility and deficits in psychomotor speed and response inhibition being evident. Recall memory is especially impaired and memory for recent and remote material can be equally affected. The behavioral changes can run the gamut from social withdrawal and depression to disinhibited behavior and overt psychosis, and vary more between patients than within a given patient across time. Although the median age of onset is around 40 years, it can begin at any point in the lifespan, with childhood-onset HD being well characterized. Through efforts focused on extended kindred in the Lake Maracaibo region of Venezuela, HD was linked to chromosome 4 in 1983 and the Huntington gene was identified in 1993. An expanded trinucleotide repeat sequence (CAG_X) in an exonic portion of the Huntington gene gives rise to an abnormally long glutamine repeat in the corresponding *huntingtin* protein. There is a negative correlation between the length of the CAG repeat and the age of onset of HD, a feature also seen in other trinucleotide repeat disorders (see later). As the these trinucleotide repeats tend to be unstable and may lengthen from one generation to the next, the age of onset of disease may be younger in successive generations, a phenomenon known as *anticipation*. The exact mechanism through which this causes neurodegeneration is an active area of investigation. In very early disease, hypometabolism in the caudate nuclei can be seen with fluorodeoxyglucose positron emission tomography, and in more advanced disease atrophy of the caudate nuclei can be seen bilaterally with structural imaging. Given the appropriate clinical context, the definitive diagnosis is made through genetic testing. No disease-modifying medications have yet been identified and therefore treatment is symptomatic. Lifespan from the onset of symptoms until death from inanition is typically between 10 and 20 years, although a tremendous amount of variability exists.

Dementia associated with ataxia

The genetic bases of an increasingly large number of conditions that feature progressive ataxia and other neurological signs (e.g., corticospinal tract and peripheral nerve involvement, vision loss) are being revealed. Almost all involve cognitive impairment in their advanced stages, but we will focus on those for which it is a relatively early or predominant feature. Many classifications of these disorders exist, including a distinction between those that are inherited in an autosomal dominant fashion (spinocerebellar ataxias, SCAs), those that are recessively inherited, and those that are maternally inherited.

The SCAs have an incidence of about 1–5 per 100,000 persons. At least 22 different clinical subtypes of SCAs have been defined, with reclassification common as the corresponding gene defects are identified. In a manner similar to that occurring in HD, an abnormally long polyglutamine repeat underlies some of these disorders (SCA1–3, 7, and 17), whereas others are due to alterations in genes encoding for ion channels (the "channelopathies," SCA6), and still others are due to nucleotide repeat expansions occurring in intronic sequences (SCA8, 10, and 12). Intellectual impairment of a subcortical variety is most common in SCA1 (20% of patients) and SCA2 (20–25% of patients), which, worldwide, likely represent the third and fourth most common SCAs after SCA3 and SCA6. Dentato-rubral-pallido-luysian atrophy (DRPLA) is an autosomal dominant progressive neurological syndrome caused by a polyglutamine repeat that is most common in persons of Japanese descent. Also subject to anticipation, the disease is characterized principally by myoclonic epilepsy, mental retardation, and ataxia when the age of onset is early, and by choreoathetosis, psychiatric features, and dementia sometimes indistinguishable from HD with later-onset disease.

Defects in the mitochondrial genome (mitochondrial DNA or mtDNA) account for some instances of maternally inherited neurological disease. Such alterations influence oxidative phosphorylation in mitochondria and therefore can affect diverse organ systems. Neurological manifestations can include myopathy, ophthalmoplegia, ataxia, myoclonus and seizures, headache, stroke, and sensorineural deafness. Cognitive impairment and dementia occur in the later stages of such illnesses, but are not typically presenting features. Testing for common alterations in mtDNA is commercially available.

Recently, a syndrome of ataxia, dementia, and hypogonadotropic hypogonadism was described in 12 patients from 5 consanguinous Middle Eastern families. Mutations of the *RNF216* and *OTUD4* genes were identified, both of which are associated with ubiquitin function. The clinical features included ataxia and hypogonadism, with progressive cognitive dysfunction starting at 20 s. Personality changes and memory loss occurred in the early stage, followed by mutism and uncoordinated movements. Brain MRI showed cerebellar and cortical atrophy, and diffuse foci of hyperintensity in subcortical white matter on T2-weighted and FLAIR imaging. These findings support a relationship between disordered ubiquitination and dementia.

Dementia associated with other movement disorders

Wilson's disease is an autosomal recessive disorder characterized by hepatic, neurological, and psychiatric abnormalities. Onset can be from childhood, but is typically in young adulthood, although onset as late as age 60 has been described. Neurological manifestations are diverse, with dysarthria being present in 97% of patients followed by dystonia, cerebellar signs, tremor, and bradykinesia. Motor impersistence and other elements of frontal lobe dysfunction are present in 19% of affected persons. It is characterized by the deposition of copper in various organs, including the liver and brain, and in 1993 was found to be due to alterations in the *ATP7B* gene, which encodes a protein involved in copper transport. It is an important entity to recognize in light of the efficacy of copper chelation with D-penicillamine in stopping, and in some cases reversing, neurological and other symptoms. The large number of mutations in the *ATP7B* gene that have been described to cause Wilson's, in addition to the possibility of any given patient being a compound heterozygote, precludes simple genetic testing for suspected Wilson's. The diagnosis is therefore supported by the presence of rusty-brown deposition of copper in the outer rim of the iris (Kayser–Fleischer rings), abnormal liver function tests, low serum levels of ceruloplasmin, elevated levels of copper in the urine, or a liver biopsy demonstrating elevated copper content.

Hallervorden–Spatz syndrome is the former name for an autosomal recessive degenerative disorder consisting of progressive and severe dystonia and ridigity, choreoathetosis, and dementia. Intellectual impairment is present at birth in some cases. The identification of genetic alterations in the pantothenate kinase gene (*PANK2*) on chromosome 20 as being causative in some cases has led to a renaming of the syndrome as pantothenate kinase-associated neurodegeneration or PKAN. T2-weighted MRI reveals characteristic bilateral hyperintensities in the globus pallidus (caused by gliosis, demyelination, and axonal swelling), surrounded by hypointensities (from iron deposition), the "eye of the tiger" sign. Treatment of PKAN is symptomatic, with vigilance for myelopathy that can occur as a result of chronic cervical dystonia.

Genetically determined storage disorders

Although typically presenting in childhood, a number of genetically determined storage disorders can present in adulthood with cognitive impairment. Most such illnesses are inherited in an autosomal recessive fashion and are typically accompanied by other neurological (seizures, myoclonus, movement disorders) or systemic signs and symptoms.

Niemann–Pick type C (NPC) disease presents with organomegaly, ataxia, vertical supranuclear ophthalmoplegia, dysarthria, and cognitive deficits (61%). The *NPC1* gene, which accounts for 95% of cases, was identified in 1997 and codes for a protein found in late endosomes and thought to be involved in cholesterol transport.

Neuronal ceroid lipofuscinosis (NCL, or Kuf's disease) presents across the age spectrum with progressive myoclonic epilepsy, cognitive impairment, cerebellar ataxia, and behavioral changes. NCL represents a group of disorders attributed to multiple different genes. Diagnosis is made by the identification of granular osmiophilic deposits on skin or brain biopsies.

Hexosaminidase A deficiency is an autosomal recessive condition more common in Ashkenazi Jews. Complete lack of the enzyme leads to Tay–Sachs disease in infancy, whereas partial deficiency can cause neurological disease of adult onset. Symptoms consist of cerebellar signs, lower motor neuron findings, psychotic episodes, and intellectual deterioration.

Autoimmune disorders

Immunological reactions against self-antigens are the underlying causes of progressive cognitive impairment, usually presenting in an acute or subacute fashion, in a small percentage of cases. Significant cognitive impairment is common in primary autoimmune disease of the CNS, such as multiple sclerosis, but this will not be discussed at length here. Cognitive impairment may also occur in the context of identifiable systemic autoimmune diseases, as distinct illnesses primarily affecting the nervous system that can respond to treatment with corticosteroids, or as paraneoplastic syndromes. As is the case with autoimmune disorders in general, the frequency of autoimmune diseases causing cognitive impairment is higher in females. In addition to mental status changes, other neurological symptoms such as seizures or systemic symptoms (e.g., fever, insomnia, dysautonomia) are frequently present in these disorders.

Systemic autoimmune disorders

Some degree of cognitive impairment is the most common neuropsychiatric manifestation of systemic lupus erythematous (SLE), followed by psychosis and seizures. Only 21% of SLE patients performed within normal limits on neuropsychological testing, with most (42%) having mild impairment and fewer having moderate (30%) or severe impairment (6%). The exact mechanism mediating cognitive impairment in SLE may be difficult to isolate, with the presence of antibodies against CNS antigens, cerebral ischemia due to cardiac emboli, antiphospholipid antibodies, and vasculitis, as well as the effects of the medications used to treat the illness or intercurrent infection, all potentially playing roles.

Sjögren's syndrome is an autoimmune disorder involving the exocrine glands, associated with anti-Ro/SSA or anti-La/SSB antibodies. As a result of angiitis, 20% of all patients with Sjögren's syndrome have central nervous system involvement, including myelitis and dementia. Neuropsychological abnormalities demonstrate deficits of attention and concentration, with better verbal intelligence than non-verbal intelligence, signifying a subcortical dementia. The brain MRI and SPECT findings are characterized by subcortical white-matter lesions and asymmetric hypoperfusion. In one serial study in Japan, patients with Sjögren's syndrome accounted for 7.5% of dementia patients in a memory clinic. Therapy of Sjögren's syndrome includes corticosteroids, azathioprine, cyclophosphamide, and intravenous immunoglobin (IVIG).

Autoimmune encephalitides

The autoimmune encephalitides are a category of illnesses about which we have an increased understanding in recent years. A growing array of antibodies against extracellular epitopes of neuronal cell surface or synaptic proteins have been identified, which cause focal or widespread nervous system dysfunction. The general clinical features include a subacute onset and fluctuating course, sometimes with headache or mild fever, and frequent CSF pleocytosis. Most types of autoimmune encephalitis present as alteration of mood, behavior, memory, consciousness level, and seizures. Abnormal movements include tremor, dyskinesia, myoclonus, and rigidity. The associated symptoms often respond to immunotherapy, and 70–80% of patients have substantial or complete recovery.

Autoimmune dementia, an autoimmune basis for cognitive impairment, is a recognized association of several neuron-specific autoantibodies: NMDA receptor, LGI-1, GABAb receptor, AMPA receptor, and anti-Caspr2. Among patients seropositive for these markers, 33–80% are found to have neoplasms, and therefore detection of these autoantibodies justifies a search for cancer. Here we put emphasis on anti-NMDAR encephalitis, limbic encephalitis, and Morvan's syndrome.

Anti-NMDAR encephalitis

This usually occurs in young adults (18–45 years old), predominantly women. More than one-third of patients have an underlying neoplasm; ovarian teratomas are the most frequent tumors. Prodromal symptoms include headache and fever, followed by rapid onset of psychiatric symptoms such as anxiety, agitation, hallucinations, paranoia, or psychosis. These symptoms are usually followed by abnormal movements. Seizures are more frequent in children and adult male patients. Brain MRI is usually normal, while one-third of patients have non-specific cortical or subcortical FLAIR/T2 abnormalities. The electroencephalogram (EEG) may show a pattern of "extreme delta brush" in some patients. Half of patients respond to first-line immunotherapies (steroids, IVIG, or plasma exchange), and the other half require second-line therapies such as rituximab. About one-fifth of patients have relapses and respond to immunotherapy.

Limbic encephalitis

Three neuronal cell-surface antibodies are associated with limbic encephalitis, including anti-LGI1, anti-GABAbR, and anti-AMPAR. The symptoms include memory deficits, confusion, seizures, and psychiatric features. Brain MRI findings are characterized by increased FLAIR/T2 signal involving one or both temporal lobes, without contrast enhancement. Some patients with anti-LGI1 encephalitis present with fascio-brachial dystonic or tonic seizures and REM sleep behavior disorder. Anti-GABAbR encephalitis is the most frequent cause of limbic encephalitis in patients with small cell lung cancer (SCLC) who are negative for Hu antibodies, and has a better outcome than those with Hu antibodies. Anti-AMPAR encephalitis is associated with thymoma, or cancer of the lung or breast.

Morvan's syndrome

This disorder was previously considered to be associated with VGKC-complex antibodies, but more recently patients with Morvan's syndrome were detected to have Caspr2 antibodies. The clinical features include amnesia, confusion, hallucinations, and sleep and autonomic dysregulation, in associated with neuromyotonia. Morvan's syndrome with Caspr2 antibodies is related to thymomas. These patients respond to immunotherapy.

Other steroid-responsive autoimmune encephalopathies

Steroid-responsive encephalopathy associated with autoimmune thyroiditis (SREAT), also called Hashimoto's encephalopathy, presents subacutely with altered mental status, tremor, myoclonus, and sometimes with transient aphasia. It is associated with the presence of antithyroperoxidase and antithyroglobulin antibodies in the serum. These antibodies are common in the general population, particularly in the elderly, and it is unlikely that they directly cause the CNS symptoms. Non-specific serological evidence of inflammation may be seen, as may elevated liver function tests. Brain MRI is normal or has non-specific changes. In this context empirical treatment with high-dose corticosteroids (1 g methylprednisolone per day) is recommended, as many patients have marked improvement in cognition and other symptoms. Long-term immunosuppression may be required to prevent relapse.

Conclusion

The conditions described in this chapter are only a partial list of the non-degenerative, non-vascular causes of dementia. Despite the vast number of diagnostic tests at our disposal, it is sometimes difficult **to completely rule out** a treatable cause of dementia with confidence. In such a circumstance, brain biopsy may be a useful diagnostic tool. In a retrospective review of 90 brain biopsies undertaken to rule out an inflammatory or infectious process at a major referral center in London, England, 57% of cases were diagnostic, with 11% of biopsies affecting subsequent treatment. The potential benefit of brain biopsy must be weighed against the risks, with institution-dependent factors (e.g., experience of the neuropathologist and neurosurgeon with the procedure) taken into account.

Further reading

Bruzzone R, Dubois-Dalcq M, Grau GE, Griffin DE, Kristensson K. Infectious diseases of the nervous system and their impact in developing countries. *PLoS Pathog* 2009 Feb;5(2).

Clifford DB, Ances BM. HIV-associated neurocognitive disorder. *Lancet Infect Dis* 2013;13:976–986.

Córdova E, Maiolo E, Corti M, Orduña T. Neurological manifestations of Chagas' disease. *Neurol Res* 2010 Apr;32(3):238–244.

Flanagan EP, McKeon A, Lennon VA, *et al.* Autoimmune dementia: Clinical course and predictors of immunotherapy response. *Mayo Clin Proc* 2010;85(10):881–897.

Leypoldt F, Armangue T, Dalmau J. Autoimmune encephalopathies. *Ann N Y Acad Sci* 2014;1–21.

Marmarou A, Bergsneider M, Klinge P, Relkin N, Black PM. The value of supplemental prognostic tests for the preoperative assessment of idiopathic normal-pressure hydrocephalus. *Neurosurgery* 2005;57:S2-17–S2-28.

Mori E, Ishikawa M, Kato T, *et al.* Guidelines for management of idiopathic normal pressure hydrocephalus: Second edition. *Neurol Med Chir.* 2012;52(11):775–809.

Morshed MG, Singh AE. Recent trends in the serologic diagnosis of syphilis. *Clin Vaccine Immunol* 2015 Feb;22(2):137–147.

Nightingale S, Winston A, Letendre S, *et al.* Controversies in HIV-associated neurocognitive disorders. *Lancet Neurol* 2014;13(11):1139–1151.

Prince M, Acosta D, Ferri CP, *et al.* A brief dementia screener suitable for use by non-specialists in resource poor settings—the cross-cultural derivation and validation of the brief Community Screening Instrument for Dementia. *Int J Geriatr Psychiatry* 2011 Sep;26(9):899–907.

Sorbi S, Hort J, Erkinjuntti T, *et al.* EFNS-ENS guidelines on the diagnosis and management of disorders associated with dementia. *Eur J Neurol* 2012;19(9):1159–1179.

Warren JD, Schott JM, Fox NC, *et al.* Brain biopsy in dementia. *Brain* 2005 Sep;128(Pt 9):2016–2025.

PART 7   Movement Disorders

47   Movement disorders: An overview

Roongroj Bhidayasiri[1,2], Jirada Sringean[1], and Daniel D. Truong[3]

[1] Chulalongkorn Center of Excellence for Parkinson's Disease & Related Disorders, Faculty of Medicine, Chulalongkorn University Hospital, Bangkok, Thailand

[2] Department of Rehabilitation Medicine, Juntendo University, Tokyo, Japan

[3] University of California, Riverside, Riverside, CA, USA; The Truong Neuroscience Institute, Orange Coast Memorial Medical Center, Fountain Valley, CA, USA

In the field of neurology, hypokinesia, hyperkinesia, and abnormal execution of movements in the presence of clear consciousness are classified as movement disorders. The term "movement disorders" as it is used today has a different meaning than the term "extrapyramidal disorders," which is a rather old classification referring to disorders of the central nervous system not involving the corticospinal pathway. While many movement disorders are caused by pathology within the basal ganglia (part of the extrapyramidal system), it is now clear that certain forms of movement disorders, such as myoclonus, can arise from other neural structures, such as the spinal cord, or peripheral nerves.

Movement disorders are broadly classified as either a paucity of movements (hypokinesia) or an excess of spontaneous movements (hyperkinesias); see Table 47.1. This simplistic approach recognizes various forms of abnormal movements in which each exhibits characteristic phenomenology. Thus, an appreciation of the pattern of abnormal movements enables clinicians to make an accurate diagnosis and to distinguish their manifestations from other movement disorders that may have similar phenomenology.

Table 47.1 Classification of movement disorders.

Hyperkinesias	Hypokinesias
Tremor	Parkinsonism
Dystonia/athetosis	Catatonia
Chorea/ballism	"Stiff muscles"
Tics	"Freezing"
Myoclonus	
Stereotypy	
Akathisia	
Ataxia	

In clinical practice, individual expressions of movement disorders are generally referenced in two settings: (1) to describe a symptom or sign of a particular abnormal movement, for example tremor defines oscillatory, rhythmic, and regular movements that affect one or more body parts; and (2) to describe a syndrome in which a particular abnormal movement dominates (e.g., tremor syndrome).

Diagnostic recommendations

A systematic approach is recommended when physicians encounter patients who primarily present with abnormal movements. In this chapter, we will illustrate a clinical-based approach that consists of five main questions that need to be addressed consecutively in order to determine the correct diagnosis. These questions are:

1 Are the movements involuntary?
2 Which type(s) of movement disorders is/are present? What is the dominant phenomenology?
3 Where does the abnormal movement disorder originate (i.e., anatomical vs. physiological localization)?
4 What are the associated features? What is the syndrome?
5 What is the differential diagnosis?

The first step in assessing a patient with a movement disorder is to establish whether involuntary movements are present. Certain forms of exaggerated purposeful movements (such as gestures or mannerisms) can be indistinguishable from chorea or akathisia. In general, abnormal involuntary movements are exacerbated by anxiety, and most diminish or disappear during sleep. Moreover, based on the aforementioned operational definition, abnormal motor behaviors accompanied by an alteration of consciousness (e.g., epileptic phenomena) should not be considered movement disorders. This differs from patients with psychiatric disorders, who often exhibit a range of abnormal movements in the presence of abnormal thoughts or contents, but not in a state of altered consciousness.

Once it has been established that the patient has involuntary movements, the next step is to determine the nature of such movements. One should evaluate the main features of the movements, including speed, rhythmicity, duration, pattern, inducibility, suppressibility, and complexity. It is important that the characteristic features of abnormal movements be identified (Table 47.2). Although pattern recognition plays a major role in the identification of abnormal movement, it is also critical for clinicians to have a good understanding of the essential features of each individual type of abnormal movement. For example, oscillatory movements (not rhythmicity) define tremor, and sustained or intermittent muscle contractions causing abnormal movements and/or postures are characteristic features of dystonia.

International Neurology, Second edition. Edited by Robert P. Lisak, Daniel D. Truong, William M. Carroll and Roongroj Bhidayasiri
© 2016 John Wiley & Sons, Ltd. Published 2016 by John Wiley & Sons, Ltd.

Table 47.2 Definitions and characteristic features of different types of movement disorders.

Definitions	Characteristic features
Akathisia: A feeling of inner, general restlessness that is reduced or relieved by moving about	Restlessness
Ataxia: Incoordination in the performance of a motor task	Incoordination
Athetosis: Slow, writhing movements (probably a form of dystonia)	Slow, writhing movements
Ballism: Large-amplitude, irregular, purposeless, non-rhythmic, rapid movements	Unpredictable large-amplitude (usually proximal) movements
Chorea: Irregular, unpredictable, brief, jerky movements, usually of low amplitude	Unpredictable, brief, jerky movements
Dystonia: Sustained or intermittent muscle contractions causing abnormal movements and/or postures	Sustained or intermittent contractions resulting in abnormal postures
Myoclonus: Brief, sudden, shock-like involuntary movements	Shock-like, brief movements
Parkinsonism: A tetrad of bradykinesia, rigidity, tremor, and postural instability	A tetrad of bradykinesia, rigidity, tremor, and postural instability
Stereotypy: Coordinated movements that repeat continually and identically	Stereotypic movements
Tremor: An oscillatory, rhythmic, and regular movement that affects one or more body parts	Oscillatory rhythmic movements

Next, the examiner should observe which body parts are involved to determine if the movements are focal, segmental, hemibody, or generalized. The distribution of movements in the affected body parts helps to determine from which part of the central or peripheral nervous system the movements originate. Many times, the movements may be the result of physiological abnormalities of certain parts of the nervous system, especially in the basal ganglia and its connecting structures. Thus, the source of abnormal movements may not be a fixed lesion as in patients with stroke or demyelinating illnesses, but rather the abnormal functioning of the individual structure in addition to certain networks in the nervous system.

When the movements are complex, consisting of more than one type of abnormal movement, it is particularly important to ascertain the dominant movement type, since this will critically steer the differential diagnosis and investigational pathway. Moreover, original movements can also be masked by drug treatments, disease progression, or secondary complications, as when Parkinson's disease (PD) patients have levodopa-induced dyskinesia. In such situations, collateral history, old video footage, and repeated examinations to capture variability in the condition may help to clarify the situation.

The identification of the clinical characteristics of abnormal movements and of the associated features defines the syndromic pattern. The consideration of the syndrome is a clinically useful approach to assist clinicians in the etiological diagnosis of a particular movement disorder in individual patients. For example, the identification of bradykinesia, rest tremor, and postural instability defines the presence of a parkinsonian syndrome in the patient, which leads to the etiological differential diagnosis of primary, secondary, parkinsonism-plus syndromes, and heredodegenerative disorders. Thus, additional features of orthostatic hypotension, cold hand signs, and jerky myoclonus of the fingers narrow the potential diagnosis to multiple system atrophy or levodopa-treated PD with

autonomic dysfunction. In some instances, certain combinations raise a specific diagnostic suspicion. For example, the combination of dystonia and "lightning" myoclonic jerks strongly suggests myoclonus dystonia. Although sometimes simple pattern recognition can directly lead to the diagnosis, physicians should always ascertain possible differential diagnoses in every case to conform to our practice of carefully considering every possibility before making a final diagnosis, rather than just relying on our diagnostic instincts. Details of the diagnostic workup largely depend on the dominant type of movement disorder and the residual clinical uncertainties with respect to the differential diagnosis. However, these details, although important, are not within the scope of this chapter.

The diagnostic approach to movement disorders remains an art, involving skills in history taking and examinations that are cultivated through years of training and clinical experience. We hope that our application of a proposed diagnostic scheme will assist clinicians in the identification of phenomenologies, associated features, and syndromes, which are the foundations for a differential and the final diagnosis.

Further reading

Abdo WF, van de Warrenburg BP, Burn DJ, Quinn NP, Bloem BR. The clinical approach to movement disorders. *Nature Rev Neurol* 2010;6(1):29–37.

Albanese A, Bhatia K, Bressman SB, *et al.* Phenomenology and classification of dystonia: A consensus update. *Mov Disord* 2013;28(7):863–873.

Bhidayasiri R. Differential diagnosis of common tremor syndromes. *Postgrad Med J* 2005;81(962):756–762.

Bhidayasiri R, Tarsy D. *Movement Disorders: A Video Atlas*, New York: Humana Press; 2013.

Fahn S. Classification of movement disorders. *Mov Disord* 2011;26(6):947–957.

Fahn S, Jankovic J, Hallett M. *Principles and Practice of Movement Disorders*, 2nd ed. Philadelphia, PA: Saunders; 2011.

48 Tremor

Jan Raethjen and Günther Deuschl

Department of Neurology, Christian-Albrechts-University of Kiel, Kiel, Germany

Tremor is the most common movement disorder and denotes a rhythmic involuntary movement of one or several regions of the body. A low-amplitude physiological action tremor can be detected in any healthy subject and may be of functional relevance for normal motor control. Conversely, pathological tremors can be severely disabling and often cause diagnostic problems. In this chapter the clinical appearance, epidemiology, pathophysiology, and management of tremor will be briefly described.

Clinical features

The clinical features are still the most important clues for the correct diagnosis of tremors, and should be documented in a systematic way.

Clinical approach

Tremor *topography* is the first feature that should always be documented. Tremors can occur in any joint or muscle that is free to oscillate. By far the most common locations are the arms and hands, but they can be spared and are often combined with tremor in other regions. The degree of symmetry between the two sides of the body can be an important diagnostic hint (see Table 48.1). Different states of muscle innervation can lead to an *activation* of tremor. *Resting tremor* occurs when the muscles of the affected body part are not voluntarily activated. Tremor amplitude typically increases during mental stress (e.g., counting backward, Stroop test, etc.) and markedly decreases during voluntary activation, especially

Table 48.1 Differential diagnosis of tremor.

Diagnosis	Clinical clues	Helpful investigations
Essential tremor (ET) vs. enhanced physiological tremor (EPT)	Family history (ET) Duration of tremor (ET>EPT) Medical history (ET) Concomitant medication (EPT)	*Neurophysiology* (EMG frequency <8 Hz in early ET)
Essential tremor (ET) vs. orthostatic tremor (OT)	Tremor only during stance (OT)	*Neurophysiology* (polygraphic EMG is pathognomic)
Essential tremor (ET) vs. parkinsonian tremor (type I)	Rest tremor (PD) Unilateral beginning (PD) Other PD symptoms (PD) Alcohol responsivity (ET) Kinetic tremor (ET) Family history (ET) Leg tremor (PD>ET) Face tremor (PD>ET) Head tremor (ET>PD) Voice tremor (ET>PD)	*Neurophysiology* (subclinical low-freq. rest tremor (PD); inhibition (PD) vs. activation (ET) of tremor amplitude during movement) *Neuroimaging* (DaTscan positive in PD)
Essential tremor (ET) vs. dystonic tremor (DT)	Family history (ET) Alcohol response (ET) Geste antagoniste (DT) Focal (DT) Further dystonic symptoms (DT)	*Neurophysiology* (frequency (DT<=ET); geste maneuver in DT) *Neuroimaging* (rarely lesions in DT)
Essential tremor (ET) vs. cerebellar tremor (CT)	Alcohol response (ET) Intention tremor (CT>ET) Ataxia (CT>ET) Eye movements (CT)	*Neurophysiology* (frequency: CT<ET) *Neuroimaging* (MRI lesions/degeneration)
Cerebellar tremor (CT) vs. Holmes' tremor (HT)	Rest tremor (HT) Low frequency (HT) Irregularity (HT) Parkinsonian symptoms (HT) Ataxia (CT>HT)	*Neurophysiology* (frequency: HT<CT) *Neuroimaging* (MRI lesions/degeneration)
Organic tremor (OrT) vs. psychogenic tremor (PsT)	Distractibility (PsT) Variable presentation (PsT>OrT) Selective disabilities (PsT) Entrainment (PsT) Coactivation (PsT>OrT) Somatizations (PsT>OrT)	*Neurophysiology* (entrainment, quantified distractability; left–right coherence, variable frequency)

EMG = electromyography; MRI = magnetic resonance imaging

International Neurology, Second edition. Edited by Robert P. Lisak, Daniel D. Truong, William M. Carroll and Roongroj Bhidayasiri
© 2016 John Wiley & Sons, Ltd. Published 2016 by John Wiley & Sons, Ltd.

when moving the affected limb. *Action tremor* is any tremor that is produced by voluntary contraction of muscles. Its subtypes are *postural tremor,* which occurs while voluntarily maintaining a position against gravity or additional weight, and *kinetic tremor,* which can occur during any voluntary movement. *Simple kinetic tremor* is present during simple voluntary movements that are not goal directed (e.g., slow up and down movements of the hands). *Intention tremor* only occurs during movements directed at a certain target (e.g., target-reaching movements). It increases while approaching the target, but amplitude and velocity may fluctuate from beat to beat. Rare forms of action tremor are present only during certain positions or certain tasks (e.g., *task-specific or position-specific tremor* or *isometric tremor*).

With some experience the three main *frequency ranges* can be distinguished on inspection: high (>7 Hz), medium (4–7 Hz), and low (<4 Hz). Although there is a large overlap between the frequency ranges of different tremors, frequency can be an important diagnostic clue (see Figure 48.1). For exact frequency measurement a signal analysis of accelerometric or electromyographic (EMG) recordings of the affected body part is necessary.

Although not strictly related to the tremor syndrome itself, *additional signs and symptoms* are important to note. For example, a parkinsonian syndrome, cerebellar ataxia, and dystonia in the region of the tremor are important diagnostic and etiological hints.

Types of pathological tremors

Enhanced physiological tremor

Normal physiological tremor is an action tremor and usually not visible on clinical observation. It can only be measured with sensitive accelerometers. An increase of the tremor amplitude leads to enhanced physiological tremor (EPT). The pathological tremor

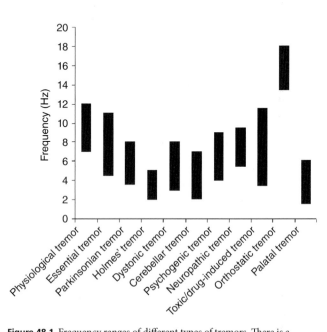

Figure 48.1 Frequency ranges of different types of tremors. There is a large overlap between the frequency ranges. Nevertheless, the frequency of the tremors can be helpful for differential diagnosis. The very low frequencies occurring in patients with Holmes' and cerebellar tremor can be important diagnostic clues and the very high frequencies in orthostatic tremor are pathognomonic.

amplitudes are typically only short lived and are reversible once the cause is removed. Other neurological symptoms or diseases that could cause tremor must be excluded. The majority of *drug-induced or toxic tremors* are assumed to be enhanced physiological tremors.

Essential tremor (ET)

Essential tremor (ET) is a slowly progressive tremor. According to the wide clinical diagnostic criteria, it is believed that a number of different action tremors are under this diagnosis. This may be the reason for many ongoing controversies regarding ET, including the existence of non-motor symptoms or neurodegenerative changes. A new clinical tremor classification is currently under development based on purely clinical and more specifically defined tremor syndromes and avoids any reliance on pathophysiology, pathology, or etiology; these dimensions are separated out into a second axis. This new classification scheme is work in progress.

Because the concept of ET is widely used and has a long-standing clinical tradition, it is necessary to know the currently used clinical definitions of ET that also serve as the basis for future classification schemes. ET is characterized by bilateral tremor of the hands or forearms with predominant kinetic tremor and resting tremor only in advanced stages of the disease, *or* isolated head tremor without evidence of abnormal posture (e.g., dystonic signs; this specific type of focal tremor likely represents a separate entity, and it will not be included in future clinical definitions of ET), *and* absence of other neurological signs with the exception of cogwheel phenomenon and slight gait disturbances. In addition, the following criteria are believed to support the diagnosis, although prospective studies on their diagnostic value are not available: duration longer than 3 years; alcohol responsiveness; and positive family history.

Careful longitudinal studies on ET are rare, but available data suggest that ET evolves over time and may change its phenotype age dependently. It usually starts with a postural and kinetic tremor, which can still be suppressed during goal-directed movements. In advanced stages and with increasing age, tremor frequency decreases, larger amplitudes occur, and an intention tremor can develop. This has been found in roughly 50% of an outpatient population and is accompanied by signs of cerebellar dysfunction of hand movements, like movement overshoot and slowness of movement. In more advanced stages a tremor at rest can develop. Also a mild gait disorder prominent during tandem gait is frequently found. Oculomotor disturbances are found with subtle electrophysiological techniques, but cannot be detected by means of clinical assessment.

The condition may begin during childhood, with a mean onset of 35–45 years. The incidence increases over the age of 40 years and there is an almost complete penetrance by the age of 60 years. The topographic distribution shows hand tremor in 94%, head tremor in 33%, voice tremor in 16%, jaw tremor in 8%, facial tremor in 3%, leg tremor in 12%, and tremor of the trunk in 3% of patients with ET. In some of the topographic regions (e.g., head, voice, and chin) tremor may occur in isolation. Tremor improves with ingestion of alcohol in about 50–90% of patients, which can be useful information to gather as part of medical history in patients with suspected ET.

The disease-related disability varies significantly and is related to the severity of the intention tremor. Up to 25% of patients seeking medical attention must change jobs or retire from work as a result of their symptoms.

For red flags for the diagnosis of ET, see Table 48.1.

Orthostatic tremor

Primary orthostatic tremor (OT) is characterized by a subjective feeling of unsteadiness during stance and rarely during gait. Patients do not have problems when sitting and lying down. Sometimes there is visible but mostly only palpable fine-amplitude rippling of leg muscles. This is the clinical correlate of the pathognomonic 13–18 Hz EMG bursts that can be recorded from the leg muscles in all OT patients.

Parkinsonian tremor

Parkinsonian tremor has been defined as tremor that occurs in Parkinson's disease (PD). Classical parkinsonian tremor (type I) is a tremor at rest that increases in amplitude during mental stress and is suppressed on initiation of a movement and during its course. Tremor frequency typically is 4–6 Hz. It may also be seen in the hands during walking or when sitting as a typical pill-rolling tremor of the hand. The postural/kinetic tremor (with similar frequencies for rest and postural/kinetic tremors) seems to be a continuation of the resting tremor under postural and action conditions ("re-emergent tremor"). Unilateral tremor and leg or face tremor are often seen and are typical for type I tremor.

A clinical variant of parkinsonian tremor is the "monosymptomatic tremor at rest" or "benign tremulous parkinsonism," a classic PD type I tremor with no other symptoms diagnostic of PD. Patients with this type of tremor typically develop further parkinsonian symptoms after a few years. However, the pure tremor at onset can closely resemble other non-parkinsonian tremors that remain clinically isolated over very long periods of time and do not show a dopaminergic deficit in DaTscans (see later discussion).

In some patients a second form of postural and action tremor with a higher (>1.5 Hz) non-harmonically related frequency may occur (type II tremor). In rare cases (<15% of patients with PD) this postural tremor can predominate. A lower-amplitude, high-frequency action tremor is often found in PD (type III tremor). These action tremors are hardly clinically distinguishable from essential tremor or many symptomatic (e.g., drug-induced) tremors.

Dystonic tremor

Typical *dystonic tremor* occurs in patients with dystonia in the same region of the body affected by the dystonia. It is a postural/kinetic tremor usually not seen during complete rest. These are focal tremors with irregular amplitudes and variable frequencies (mostly <7 Hz). Some patients exhibit focal tremors even before they develop overt signs of dystonia. Like dystonia, the tremor can often be inhibited by sensory tricks (geste antagoniste), which is an important clue for differential diagnosis (see Table 48.1).

Tremor associated with dystonia is a more generalized form of tremor at higher frequencies (6–10 Hz) in extremities not affected by the dystonia, and can be difficult to distinguish from other action tremors (e.g., essential tremor).

Cerebellar tremor

The classic *cerebellar tremor* is an intention tremor that may occur uni- or bilaterally depending on the underlying cerebellar abnormality. The tremor frequency is almost always below 5 Hz. Simple kinetic and postural tremor may also be present. Some patients with a mild cerebellar ataxia present with an isolated postural and simple kinetic tremor above 5 Hz, resembling essential tremor. *Titubation* is a low-frequency oscillation (around 3 Hz) of the head and trunk that often occurs in cerebellar disease.

Holmes' tremor

This rare symptomatic tremor is due to a previous lesion (2 weeks' to 2 years' delay) in the region of the midbrain, damaging nigrostriatal and cerebellar pathways. It has been labeled differently in the past (rubral tremor, midbrain tremor, myorhythmia, Benedikt's syndrome). It is often irregular at low frequencies (<4.5 Hz) with resting, postural, and intentional components. The tremor following thalamic damage (*thalamic tremor*) often resembles this type of tremor.

Palatal tremor

These rare tremor syndromes affect the soft palate and can be symptomatic following a brainstem lesion with a variable delay (symptomatic palatal tremor) or due to neurodegeneration and sometimes Alexander's disease. This condition often comes with signs of ataxia, with a pendular nystagmus or extremity tremors. Usually a hypertrophic inferior olive can be shown with magnetic resonance imaging (MRI). Another variant without lesions or progressive course and without olivary hypertrophy is essential palatal tremor. Its most important symptom is a disturbing rhythmic ear click.

Neuropathic tremor

Several peripheral neuropathies regularly present with tremors. These postural and action tremors can be difficult to distinguish from essential tremor. The frequency in hand muscles can be lower than in proximal arm muscles. Abnormal positional sense need not be present.

Psychogenic tremor

Psychogenic tremors have very diverse clinical presentations. Most of them are action tremors, but many also remain during rest and often show very unusual combinations of rest/postural and intention tremors. Typical clinical features are a sudden onset and sometimes spontaneous remissions, decrease of tremor amplitude or variable frequency during distraction, and selective disability. Many patients have a positive "coactivation sign" (tested as with rigidity testing at the wrist). Variable, voluntary-like force exertion can be felt in both movement directions. Others show an entrainment of the tremor rhythm by contralateral rhythmic voluntary movements (tremor assumes the voluntary movement frequency). Some patients have a history of somatizations in the past or additional, unrelated (psychogenic) neurological symptoms and signs.

Epidemiology

Apart from the common short-lived transient *enhanced physiological tremor*, which most people have experienced on stressful or frightening occasions, *essential tremor* is the most common pathological tremor. The broad spectrum of prevalence estimates (1.3–5.1%) indicates that the current clinical definition probably comprises a group of disorders (see earlier). Conversely, *orthostatic tremor* is a rare condition occurring only in patients above 40 years of age. *Rest tremor* is a very common feature of idiopathic Parkinson's disease. The occurrence of classic tremor at rest in a patient with parkinsonism has a likelihood of more than 95% of reflecting idiopathic PD. *Cerebellar tremor* as a whole is relatively common, as it can be caused by cerebellar insults of various etiologies (e.g., demyelination in multiple sclerosis, strokes, hereditary and toxic, including alcoholic degeneration). *Dystonic tremor* is relatively rare, but has been estimated to account for up to 20% of all tremor patients presenting with non-parkinsonian and non-cerebellar tremors. *Neuropathic tremor* occurs in 70–80% of patients with dysgammaglobulinemic polyneuropathy or chronic Guillain–Barré syndrome. It is seen regularly but less commonly in hereditary polyneuropathy (HMSN; 40% of patients). However, it only rarely represents the dominant source of disability in these patients. *Psychogenic tremor* is the most common psychogenic movement disorder (~50%).

Pathophysiology

Physiological tremor mainly emerges from mechanical resonant mechanisms of the oscillating limb. This resonant oscillation can be enhanced by reflex mechanisms likely representing one mechanism of enhanced physiological tremor. Conversely, the majority of pathological tremors are caused by an enhancement or emergence of oscillations within the central nervous system that are transmitted to the peripheral muscles. There is converging evidence that these oscillations originate from several oscillating loops within the motor system rather than one single oscillating structure, whereas subcortical structures (e.g., olivocerebellar circuits in ET, basal ganglia circuits in PD tremor, and brainstem circuits in OT) seem to be important pacemakers of pathological tremors. For ET and PD tremor it has been convincingly shown that the oscillations are projected to the thalamus and (motor) cortex, which in turn transmit the oscillations via fast corticospinal pathways to the spinal motor centers and peripheral muscles. In ET and PD tremor the thalamo-cortical interaction is bidirectional in a closed loop, enabling and amplifying oscillatory activity, in contrast to the mostly unidirectional information flow found in voluntary movements. However, the involvement of the different levels of the motor system seems to be dynamically organized; that is, highly variable over time. Nevertheless, the notion that the oscillations converge in the motor nuclei of the thalamus is clearly supported by the efficacy of thalamic (VIM) surgery in the majority of pathological tremors.

The pathophysiology of the classic cerebellar intention tremor seems to be distinct from the mechanisms underlying most of the other central tremors. It is most likely due to altered characteristics of feedforward or feedback loops. An alteration of peripheral feedback to central tremor-generating structures has also been postulated to be the basis for the tremor enhancement in peripheral neuropathies.

In psychogenic tremor, voluntary-like, yet subconsciously produced rhythmic movements are one physiological mechanism, involuntary oscillations (e.g., clonus-like mechanisms) enhanced by ongoing coactivation of muscles are another.

Investigations

Laboratory blood tests, clinical neurophysiology, and neuroimaging are potentially informative for the differential diagnosis of tremors.

Blood tests play a role in excluding symptomatic tremors in general medical disease (e.g., hyperthyreosis, Wilson's disease, etc.), toxic, and drug-induced tremors. Structural neuroimaging (MRI or computed tomography, CT) is indispensable to diagnosing symptomatic tremor in structural brain lesions (Table 48.1); for example, cerebellar degeneration or lesions in cerebellar tremors or lesions in the midbrain or thalamus in Holmes' and thalamic tremors. The

main functional neuroimaging technique that aids differential diagnosis in pathological tremors is single photon emission computed tomography (SPECT), after radioactive labeling of the dopamine transporter (DaTscan) to detect a dopaminergic deficit in the striatum. As a positive DaTscan is unique to parkinsonian syndromes, it is of great value in distinguishing between tremor-dominant parkinsonism and other types of tremors (Table 48.1).

Clinical neurophysiological evaluation of tremors consists of surface EMG and accelerometric recordings from the affected limbs. Fourier/spectral analysis of these data can determine the exact tremor frequency, which can be an important diagnostic hint (Figure 48.1). In the case of orthostatic tremor, the highly synchronized 13–18 Hz rhythm in both leg muscles appearing when standing up is a pathognomonic finding and the only way to a definitive diagnosis. The pattern and rhythmicity or lack of rhythmicity of EMG bursts can also greatly help to distinguish between myoclonus and tremor. The coupling (coherence) between lower-frequency oscillations in different limbs is unique to psychogenic tremor and is typically absent in lower-frequency organic tremors. The entrainment of the psychogenic tremor rhythm by voluntary rhythmic movements of the contralateral hand (see earlier) or the distraction from psychogenic tremor by such maneuvers can be quantified neurophysiologically.

Treatment

The exact origins of and the neurotransmitter systems involved in pathological tremors are largely unknown and the available medical treatments are mainly symptomatic in nature. Thus the decision regarding appropriate treatment often has to be based on the clinical appearance of the tremor (rest, postural, or intention tremor) and empirical knowledge. The mechanisms of action of most antitremor drugs are often only poorly understood. The allocation of drug treatment according to the clinical characteristics of the tremor is shown in Table 48.2. There is an improvement in 70–80% of patients with parkinsonian disease and essential tremor under adequate drug treatment. The most effective drugs for parkinsonian tremor are dopaminergic agents (levodopa and dopamine agonists) and anticholinergics. In essential tremor, beta blockers and primidone alone or in combination are still regarded as the most efficacious treatments, although some antiepileptic drugs (e.g., topiramate, gabapentin) can be useful alternatives. Benzodiazepines can be helpful in managing primarily kinetic tremors. Utilizing the mathematical relationship between the actual tremor amplitude (as measured, for example, by accelerometry) and tremor rating scales employed in randomized controlled trials, however, it has been shown that beta blockers and primidone remain the most efficacious drugs, producing about a 50–60% reduction in amplitude in ET. The detailed treatment strategies for PD tremors and ET are summarized in Tables 48.3 and 48.4. In focal dystonic tremor the treatment of first choice is botulinum toxin injections. Cerebellar tremor is extremely difficult to treat. Although there are some case reports of successful drug treatments with a number of different substances (cholinergics, 5-HTP, clonazepam, and carbamazepine), hardly any systematic studies are available and no single substance can be recommended as first choice. Treatment of Holmes' tremor is similarly difficult, as only some patients respond to levodopa, anticholinergics, or clonazepam.

Table 48.2 Symptomatic drug efficacy in relation to clinical presentation of tremors.

	Activation of tremor		
	Rest	**Posture**	**Intention**
Beta blockers	–	+	(+)
Primidone	–	+	+
Clonazepam/alprazolam	–	(+)	+
Topiramate/gabapentin	–	+	(+)
Anticholinergics	+	(+)	–
Levodopa	+	–	–
Dopamine agonists	+	–	–
Amantadine	+	–	(+)
Clozapine	+	+	–
Carbamazepine	–	–	(+)

Table 48.3 Drugs and their dosages for essential tremor.

	Drug	**Dosage**	**Remarks**
1st choice	Propranolol	30–320 mg, 3 doses Standard or long-acting	Contraindications: cardiac, pulmonary diabetes, etc. Hand and head tremor
1st choice	Primidone	62.5–500 mg, single dose in the evening	Hand and head tremor Preferentially for patients aged >60 years
1st choice	Combination: propranolol/ primidone	Maximum dosage for each	Try always before using 2nd- and 3rd-choice drugs
2nd choice	Arotinolol	10–30 mg	Cross-over study with propranolol
2nd choice	Gabapentin	1800–2400 mg daily	Conflicting results of three double blind studies: one without, two with benefit
2nd choice	Topiramate	<400 mg	So far small double blind study only
2nd choice	Clonazepam	0.75–6 mg	For predominant kinetic tremor
3rd choice	Botulinum toxin		Double blind study with a significant result, but weakness as a significant side effect
3rd choice	Clozapine	Test: 12.5 mg, 30–50 mg daily	Less well-documented effect than for Parkinson's disease; often ineffective
If drug therapy fails	Surgery		VIM stimulation or thalamotomy

Table 48.4 Treatment strategies for tremors in Parkinson's disease.

Tremor type	**1st step**	**2nd step**	**3rd step**
Classical parkinsonian tremor or monosymptomatic rest tremor	L-DOPA Dopamine agonists Anticholinergics	Amantadine Propranolol Clozapine	STN stimulation
Rest and postural tremor with different frequencies	Propranolol Primidone	Dopamine Dopamine agonists Anticholinergics Clozapine	STN stimulation
Isolated action tremor	Propranolol Primidone Anticholinergics	Amantadine	

STN = subthalamic nucleus

The most effective treatment option in severe tremors is stereotactic surgery. However, the rate of severe complications is as high as 1–2% in bilateral procedures; therefore this option is reserved for severely disabled patients. The ventrolateral thalamus (VIM nucleus) is the surgical target of choice in the majority of tremors. It can be lesioned, but deep brain stimulation (DBS) is currently clearly favored, as it has fewer complications and seems to be more effective; tremor nearly disappears in 80–90% of these mostly drug-resistant patients. In patients with parkinsonian tremor, the subthalamic nucleus is the target of choice, as it has a similar effect on tremor and also alleviates the akinesia. However, lesions in this region are dangerous as they can lead to highly disabling ballism; therefore it is mainly a target for DBS. For essential and parkinsonian tremor, the excellent efficacy of stereotactic surgical procedures is well documented in large studies. In cerebellar tremors this invasive treatment seems to be less successful and careful patient selection is very important. In Holmes', neuropathic, and recently even in orthostatic tremor, there are only relatively small case series and case reports documenting at least some efficacy of thalamic surgery. A new, less invasive, yet accurate lesioning technique with focused transcranial MR-guided ultrasound and completely non-invasive tremor-driven transcranial electrical alternating-current stimulation have been developed, with promising results. These approaches may add to the routine therapeutic options in tremors in the near future.

Further reading

Bain PG, Findley LJ, Thompson PD, *et al*. A study of hereditary essential tremor. *Brain* 1994;117(4):805–824.

Brittain JS, Probert-Smith P, Aziz TZ, Brown P. Tremor suppression by rhythmic transcranial current stimulation. *Curr Biol* 2013;23(5):436–440.

Deuschl G, Bain P, Brin M; Ad Hoc Scientific Committee. Consensus statement of the Movement Disorder Society on Tremor. *Mov Disord* 1998;13(Suppl 3):2–23.

Deuschl G, Raethjen J, Hellriegel H, Elble R. Treatment of patients with essential tremor. *Lancet Neurol* 2011;10(2):148–161.

Elble RJ. Essential tremor frequency decreases with time. *Neurology* 2000;55(10):1547–1551.

Kim YJ, Pakiam AS, Lang AE. Historical and clinical features of psychogenic tremor: A review of 70 cases. *Can J Neurol Sci* 1999;26(3):190–195.

Lipsman N, Schwartz ML, Huang Y, *et al*. MR-guided focused ultrasound thalamotomy for essential tremor: A proof-of-concept study. *Lancet Neurol* 2013;12(5):462–468.

Louis ED, Ford B, Wendt KJ, Cameron G. Clinical characteristics of essential tremor: Data from a community-based study. *Mov Disord* 1998;13(5):803–808.

Marsden CD, Gimlette TM, McAllister RG, Owen DA, Miller TN. Effect of beta-adrenergic blockade on finger tremor and Achilles reflex time in anxious and thyrotoxic patients. *Acta Endocrinol* 1968;57:353–362.

Muthuraman M, Heute U, Arning K, *et al*. Oscillating central motor networks in pathological tremors and voluntary movements: What makes the difference? *Neuroimage* 2012;60(2):1331–1339.

Raethjen J, Govindan RB, Kopper F, Muthuraman M, Deuschl G. Cortical involvement in the generation of essential tremor. *J Neurophysiol* 2007;97(5):3219–3228.

Stolze H, Petersen G, Raethjen J, Wenzelburger R, Deuschl G. The gait disorder of advanced essential tremor. *Brain* 2001;124(11):2278–2286.

Timmermann L, Gross J, Dirks M, *et al*. The cerebral oscillatory network of parkinsonian resting tremor. *Brain* 2003;126(1):199–212.

Zesiewicz TA, Elble R, Louis ED, *et al*. Practice parameter: Therapies for essential tremor: Report of the Quality Standards Subcommittee of the American Academy of Neurology. *Neurology* 2005;64(12):2008–2020.

49 Parkinsonism

Dronacharya Lamichhane[1] and Lisa M. Shulman[1,2]

[1] Department of Neurology, University of Maryland School of Medicine, Baltimore, MD, USA
[2] University of Maryland PD & Movement Disorders Center, University of Maryland School of Medicine, Baltimore, MD, USA

Parkinsonism is a clinical syndrome characterized by various combinations of tremor, bradykinesia, rigidity, and postural instability. It is not a single disease, but a common clinical presentation of a variety of disease processes that cause brain dopaminergic dysfunction. Etiologies include Parkinson's disease (PD), Parkinson's plus syndromes, other neurodegenerative diseases, toxins, vascular disease, and a variety of infections. This chapter reviews parkinsonism, excluding idiopathic PD.

Separating PD from the various causes of atypical parkinsonism (AP) is a common yet challenging task that a neurologist encounters on a routine basis. It is very important to establish a correct diagnosis, because the disease treatment, prognosis, and complications differ accordingly. Once it is determined that someone has parkinsonism, the next step is to look for various clues or disease characteristics pertinent to individual causes of parkinsonism. The distinction is based globally on the following items: rate of progression (relatively slow for PD, more rapid for AP), response to dopaminergic medications (good and sustained in PD, none or limited in AP), presence of "red flags" (symmetric symptoms, early falls, early dysarthria/dysphagia, vertical gaze paresis, square wave jerks, dystonia). Many of these problems become apparent after a year or more of follow-up. Later in the disease course, about 5% of cases are misdiagnosed even in the hands of experts.

Progressive supranuclear palsy

Progressive supranuclear palsy (PSP) was first described in the early 1900s. However, it was not until 1963 that Steele, Richardson, and Olszewski reported a series of patients with pathological confirmation of "heterogeneous system degeneration." The syndrome has been called PSP because of its distinctive clinical finding of vertical supranuclear ophthalmoplegia. However, PSP has been increasingly recognized as a clinically and pathologically heterogeneous condition, since PSP can also less commonly present with apraxia of speech, corticobasal syndrome, or spastic paraparesis. Some other pathologically distinct conditions (e.g., corticobasal degeneration) can also clinically present as a PSP-like phenotype. Patients with PSP-τ pathology can have clinical phenotypes of the Richardson syndrome (RS; classic PSP phenotype or PSP-RS), parkinsonism (PSP-P), pure akinesia with gait freezing (PSP-PAGF), corticobasal syndrome (PSP-CBS), and frontotemporal dementia (PSP-FTD). Each subtype appears to be associated with a somewhat different prognosis and natural history.

Epidemiology

Onset of symptoms is usually in the sixth or seventh decade of life. PSP progresses more quickly than PD. Median survival ranges from 5–9 years and the 10-year survival rate is only 30%. The disease has no gender preference and is sporadic, although there have been reports of cases of familial clustering, with suggestion of an autosomal dominant inheritance pattern. Mutations in *MAPT*, *C9ORF72*, *TDRBP*, and *DCTN1* have been found in these families with PSP-like phenotypes.

Prevalence ranges from 1.39 per 100,000 persons in the United States to approximately 6 per 100,000 in the United Kingdom and in Japan. Annual incidence in Rochester, Minnesota, was 1.1 per 100,000 persons in 1976–90.

Pathophysiology

PSP is characterized by neuronal loss, neurofibrillary tangles, and gliosis in the basal ganglia, brainstem, and cerebral cortex. The neurofibrillary tangles of PSP are primarily "globose" or rounded rather than the "flame-shaped" tangles of Alzheimer's disease (AD). As with AD, the tangles are composed of abnormally phosphorylated 4-repeat τ proteins.

PSP pathology is most prominent in the basal ganglia, diencephalon, and hindbrain. Basal ganglia pathology (especially globus pallidus) is unique, involving extensive astrocytic involvement with inclusions in oligodendrocytes and neurons. The tectum of the midbrain and less so the pons also atrophies. The substantia nigra shows depigmentation as in PD, but the locus ceruleus is relatively preserved. Much of the cortical pathology of PSP is seen in the primary motor strip and the ocular motor association area. The behavioral changes and dementia of PSP are thought to be related to subcortical pathology, leading to secondary cortical dysfunction. Prominent midbrain atrophy is a hallmark of PSP. The gaze palsy is supranuclear and spares the cranial nerve nuclei directly responsible for control of vertical and horizontal gaze.

Clinical features

Gait disturbance with falls is the presenting feature in the majority of people with PSP. This is in stark contrast to PD and should be the first clue that the patient has an atypical parkinsonian syndrome. The gait of PSP is stiff, slightly broad-based, and often accompanied by "unheralded falls," which the patient may ascribe to tripping on uneven ground. In fact, postural instability and personality changes are often present at the time the neurologist evaluates the patient

International Neurology, Second edition. Edited by Robert P. Lisak, Daniel D. Truong, William M. Carroll and Roongroj Bhidayasiri
© 2016 John Wiley & Sons, Ltd. Published 2016 by John Wiley & Sons, Ltd.

Table 49.1 National Institute of Neurological Disorders and Stroke and the Society for PSP (NINDS–SPSP) criteria for diagnosis of progressive supranuclear palsy (PSP).

Mandatory inclusion criteria	Mandatory exclusion criteria	Supportive criteria
Possible PSP	Recent history of encephalitis	Symmetric akinesia or rigidity, proximal more than distal
Gradually progressive disorder	Alien limb syndrome, cortical sensory deficits, focal frontal or temporoparietal atrophy	
Onset at age 40 or later		Abnormal neck posture, especially retrocollis
Either vertical (upward or downward) supranuclear palsy *or* both slowing of vertical saccades and prominent postural instability with falls in the first year of disease onset	Hallucinations or delusions unrelated to dopaminergic therapy	Poor or absent response of parkinsonism to levodopa therapy
	Cortical dementia of Alzheimer's type (severe amnesia and aphasia or agnosia, according to NINCDS–ADRA criteria)	Early dysphagia and dysarthria
No evidence of other diseases that could explain the foregoing features, as indicated by mandatory exclusion criteria		Early onset of cognitive impairment including at least two of the following: apathy, impairment in abstract thought, decreased verbal fluency, utilization or imitation behavior, or frontal release signs
Probable PSP	Prominent, early cerebellar symptoms or prominent, early unexplained dysautonomia (marked hypotension and urinary disturbances)	
Gradually progressive disorder	Severe, asymmetric parkinsonian signs, bradykinesia	
Onset at age 40 or later		
Vertical (upward or downward) supranuclear palsy and prominent postural instability with falls in the first year of disease onset	Neuroradiological evidence of relevant structural abnormality (i.e., basal ganglia or brainstem infarcts, lobar atrophy)	
No evidence of other diseases that could explain the foregoing features, as indicated by mandatory exclusion criteria	Whipple's disease, confirmed by polymerase chain reaction, if indicated	
Definite PSP		
Clinically probable or possible PSP and histopathological evidence of PSP		

NINCDS–ADRA: National Institute of Neurological and Communicative Disorders and Stroke – Alzheimer's Disease and Related Disorders Association.

with PSP-RS. Symmetric rigidity is seen and is often prominent axially, particularly at the neck. Neck posture in PSP may be retrocolic, in contrast to the stooped, flexion posture of PD. In some cases, isolated bradykinesia that predominantly affects the gait, resulting in freezing of gait, may be the only manifestation. Patients are often described as looking "surprised" or "anguished" due to tonic contracture of facial musculature. Accompanying the characteristic facial expression is a unique dysarthria that can be described as "growling."

Vertical supranuclear ophthalmoplegia is not an early finding. Early on, the oculomotor impairment is subtle, consisting of impaired vertical optokinetic nystagmus, slow saccades, and the presence of saccadic intrusions (square wave jerks). There should be an oculocephalic response even if a supranuclear ophthalmoplegia is present.

Frontal lobe dysfunction is the predominant cognitive finding. Patients have decreased verbal fluency, abstract thought becomes concrete, and set switching is severely impaired. Frontal release signs including grasp or palmomental reflex may be present. Motor perseveration is often present, demonstrable as the "applause" sign.

Investigations
Diagnosis is based on clinical findings. There are no available biomarkers. Computed tomography (CT) or magnetic resonance imaging (MRI) may demonstrate midbrain atrophy. MRI of the brain shows the *hummingbird sign* on the midsagittal view and the *morning glory flower sign* on axial views. One study found that midbrain size <9.35 mm had sensitivity and specificity of 95% and 100%, respectively. However, a similar study from Europe concluded that midbrain atrophy only predicts PSP phenotype, not pathology. A focal area of hypometabolism in the brain on fluorodeoxyglucose positron emission tomography (FDG-PET) scanning has been termed the *pimple sign* and is strongly correlated with the clinical phenotype of classic PSP. Clinical diagnosis is based on National Institute for Neurological Disorders and

Stroke–Society for Progressive Supranuclear Palsy (NINDS–SPSP) criteria (Table 49.1). Differential diagnosis includes other neurodegenerative disorders such as PD, corticobasal syndrome (CBS), multiple system atrophy (MSA), dementia with Lewy bodies (DLB), and vascular parkinsonism.

Management
Treatment is supportive, as there is no drug that alters the disease course. All patients with PSP phenotype should be offered levodopa as high as 1000 mg/day, because some patients do respond symptomatically. Adverse effects from dopaminergic therapy, especially visual hallucinations, are common in PSP. A peptide, davunetide, which is purported to increase microtubular stability and to decrease phosphorylation of τ-protein, failed to demonstrate benefit over placebo in a double blind randomized controlled trial. A glycogen kinase synthase inhibitor, tideglusib, also failed to show benefit as measured by the PSP rating scale; however, it reduced the progression of atrophy in the whole brain, particularly in the parietal and occipital lobes. Treatment should include a multidisciplinary approach. Speech pathologists can recommend treatment for dysarthria and dysphagia. Botulinum toxin can be used for the treatment of blepharospasm, apraxia of eyelid opening, and painful dystonic postures of the limbs and neck. Occupational and physical therapy may be helpful in maintaining independence in activities of daily living. Physical therapists are involved in balance and gait training. Most patients eventually require a walker or other assistive devices for safety.

Corticobasal syndrome
The term "corticobasal degeneration" (CBD) refers to a 4-repeat tauopathy with neuronal loss and gliosis primarily found in the cortical region, basal ganglia, and substantia nigra (see Chapter 50). Specific pathological features such as astrocytic plaques differentiate

it from the closely related progressive supranuclear palsy (PSP). One needs to be cautious about the terms CBD, referring to the pathological entity, and corticobasal syndrome (CBS), referring to a classic clinical presentation including motor (asymmetric rigidity, bradykinesia, dystonia, and myoclonus) and higher cortical (apraxia, cortical sensory deficits, alien limb phenomenon, and cognitive impairment) features. It is now recognized that CBS is only one possible presenting phenotype of CBD, with other described phenotypes including Richardson syndrome (CBD-RS), frontotemporal dementia (CBD-FTD), dementia of Alzheimer's type (CBD-DAT), primary progressive aphasia (CBD-PPA), and posterior cortical atrophy (CBD-PCA). Similarly, CBS has been associated with multiple pathologies other than just CBD, including Alzheimer's disease, PSP, and others.

Epidemiology

Symptoms usually begin after age 60 years, but cases have been reported with symptom onset as early as 40 years of age. The disease is progressive, with a survival of 5–10 years. Because only about 25% of clinical cases can be accurately diagnosed with CBD antemortem, the true incidence of the disease is difficult to estimate. About 5% of cases of parkinsonism seen in movement disorder centers represent CBD in the United States. A study in Eastern European and Asian subjects reported an incidence of 0.02 cases per 100,000 people.

Pathophysiology

Pathology of the various clinical CBD subtypes shares similar τ-biochemical and histopathological characteristics, but the neuroanatomical distribution of pathology varies. CBS is characterized by asymmetric atrophy of frontoparietal and perirolandic cortices, basal ganglia, substantia nigra, and thalamus. Often, there is thinning of the anterior corpus callosum, atrophy of the deep white matter, internal capsule, and cerebral peduncles.

"Ballooned" achromatic neurons are found in the atrophied cerebral cortex, particularly in the frontoparietal cortex. Swollen axons, demyelinated axons, and a spongiform appearance to the neuropil are present in the white matter underlying the atrophied cortex. In the substantia nigra, pigmented nerve cell loss and gliosis are seen. Neurofibrillary tangles may be observed in all of the affected areas. Pathological diagnosis of CBD is confirmed by the presence of cortical and striatal τ-positive neuronal and glial lesions.

Clinical features

CBS, the most common clinical phenotype of CBD, is an asymmetric akinetic-rigid syndrome. Rigidity of the affected limb is generally more prominent than in PD. There is usually no response to

dopaminergic therapy. The most common presentation is unilateral loss of dexterity and the sense that the hand has become useless.

Motor symptoms spread to the contralateral side within several years and begin to affect midline structures, with resultant dysphagia, dysarthria, postural instability, and hypomimia. Tremor may be present, but it should not be confused with that of PD. The tremors of CBS are faster (6–8 Hz) and have an irregular, jerky quality. Tremor is more prominent with action and maintenance of posture as opposed to the rest tremor of PD. As the disease progresses, patients may develop stimulus-sensitive and action-induced myoclonus. Other common motor findings include asymmetric limb dystonia, particularly flexion of the upper extremity. Some patients will have pain in the dystonic limb.

Higher cortical functions are eventually impaired. Many CBS patients develop "alien limb" phenomenon, with autonomous movements of the limb such as spontaneous levitation. Cortical sensory loss, including extinction to double simultaneous stimuli and difficulty with two-point discrimination, may be present early. Ideomotor and limb-kinetic apraxias are frequently encountered and can be an early clue to diagnosis.

Language impairment is a common and frequent presenting feature of CBD. Primary progressive non-fluent aphasia is the most common type of aphasia among these patients. Apraxia of speech may accompany aphasia. Over 70% of patients will have cognitive impairment during the disease course. Patients with CBD often have difficulties with learning tasks, word fluency, memory, and cognitive flexibility. Dementia may be present.

Eye movement abnormalities are common. Saccadic eye movements are affected early, with increased latency to the initiation of horizontal saccades, slowing of smooth pursuit movements, and saccadic intrusions. Patients may lose the ability to generate saccades, although spontaneous saccades and optokinetic nystagmus are intact. Blepharospasm and eyelid-opening apraxia have been reported.

Investigations

Diagnosis can be difficult, but there are important clues that distinguish CBD from PD. Lack of response to dopaminergic therapy and the presence of cortical dysfunction in the form of apraxia or cortical sensory loss indicate CBD. No biomarker is available for diagnosis. Neuroimaging with CT or MRI is usually normal, but as the disease progresses, asymmetric frontoparietal cortical atrophy may be apparent. An international consortium of behavioral neurology, neuropsychology, and movement disorder specialists developed new criteria based on consensus and a systematic literature review. Four clinical phenotypes and two diagnostic classifications were proposed in 2013 (Tables 49.2 and 49.3).

Table 49.2 Proposed clinical phenotypes (syndromes) associated with the pathology of corticobasal degeneration.

Syndrome	Features
Probable corticobasal syndrome	Asymmetric presentation of two of: a) limb rigidity or akinesia, b) limb dystonia, c) limb myoclonus, plus one of: d) orobuccal or limb apraxia, e) cortical sensory deficit, f) alien limb phenomenon (more than simple levitation)
Possible corticobasal syndrome	May be symmetric: one of: a) limb rigidity or akinesia, b) limb dystonia, c) limb myoclonus, plus one of: d) orobuccal or limb apraxia, e) cortical sensory deficit, f) alien limb phenomenon (more than simple levitation)
Frontal-behavioral spatial syndrome	Two of: a) executive dysfunction, b) behavioral or personality changes, c) visuospatial deficits
Non-fluent/agrammatic variant of primary progressive aphasia	Effortful grammatical speech plus one of: a) impaired grammar/sentence comprehension with relatively preserved single-word comprehension, or b) groping, distorted speech production (apraxia of speech)
Progressive supranuclear palsy syndrome	Three of: a) axial or symmetric limb rigidity or akinesia, b) postural instability or falls, c) urinary incontinence, d) behavioral changes, e) supranuclear vertical gaze palsy or decreased velocity of vertical saccades

Table 49.3 Diagnostic criteria for corticobasal degeneration.

	Clinical research criteria for probable sporadic CBD	Clinical criteria for possible CBD
Presentation	Insidious onset and gradual progression	Insidious onset and gradual progression
Minimum duration of symptoms, y	1	1
Age at onset, y	>50	No minimum
Family history (2 or more relatives)	Exclusion	Inclusion
Permitted phenotypes (see Table 49.2)	(1) Possible CBS or (2) FBS or NAV plus at least one CBS feature (a–f)	(1) Possible CBS or (2) FBS or NAV or (3) PSPS plus at least one CBS feature (b–f)

FBS = frontal-behavior spatial variant; NAV = non-fluent/agrammatic variant

Management

Early rehabilitation is helpful to maximize function and maintain independence. No effective pharmacological treatment is available, although benzodiazepines may be useful for tremor and myoclonus. Myoclonus in CBD also responds well to anticonvulsants such as levetiracetam and valproic acid, although large class I studies are lacking. Botulinum toxin injections for dystonia in CBS can be used to reduce pain, improve hygiene, and prevent secondary contractures. Anecdotal reports suggest that selected patients with CBS benefit from physical therapy. Therefore, treatment of CBS is largely supportive and symptomatic.

Multiple system atrophy

The term multiple system atrophy (MSA) was introduced in 1969 to encompass the disease entities of olivopontocerebellar ataxia, striatonigral degeneration, and Shy–Drager syndrome, on the basis of similar neuropathological findings in these disorders. MSA is now understood to be a sporadic α-synucleinopathy characterized by autonomic failure, parkinsonism, cerebellar ataxia, and pyramidal dysfunction in various combinations. Two clinicopathological variations have been recognized: MSA-p with prominent parkinsonism and MSA-c with prominent cerebellar signs. Autonomic failure usually manifesting as orthostatic hypotension or urinary incontinence is common to both forms. Since the pathogenic mechanism remains unknown, there is no disease-specific treatment available.

Epidemiology

MSA affects both sexes equally. Median age of onset is 55 years. This progressive disorder results in death in about 9 years. The incidence rate is about 3 per 100,000 in people older than 50 years. MSA-c is more common in North America (63% vs. 13%, 27% undefined) and Europe (63% vs. 34%), whereas MSA-p is more prevalent in Japan (66% vs. 34%). Although MSA is generally a sporadic disease, functionally impaired variants of co-enzyme Q2 were associated with an increased risk of MSA in multiplex families and in patients with sporadic disease. Some case-control studies have suggested that exposure to organic solvents, plastic monomers, and additives, pesticides, and metals carries increased risk of MSA.

Pathophysiology

The systems most consistently and severely affected are the olivopontocerebellar (OPC) and striatonigral (StrN) systems (see Chapter 40). In MSA-c, external examination of the brain shows significant atrophy of the cerebellum, middle cerebellar peduncle, and pontine base. In MSA-p, atrophy and dark discoloration of the putamen are seen, with more pronounced putaminal atrophy posteriorly, resulting in flattening of the lateral border. The neuropathological hallmark of MSA is the presence of α-synuclein immunoreactive cytoplasmic inclusions in oligodendrocytes, termed glial cytoplasmic inclusions (GCIs). They are sometimes referred to as Papp–Lantos inclusions. A neuropathological diagnosis of MSA is established when there is evidence of widespread and abundant central nervous system (CNS) α-synuclein-positive GCIs in association with neurodegenerative changes in StrN or OPC. GCIs are thought to play a central role in the pathogenesis of the disease.

Clinical features

MSA-associated parkinsonism is dominated by a progressive akinetic-rigid syndrome. Rest tremor is uncommon in MSA. Frequent cerebellar features include gait ataxia, limb kinetic ataxia, scanning speech, and eye movement abnormalities. Urogenital dysfunction manifests as urge incontinence, incomplete bladder emptying, and erectile dysfunction in male patients. Although 75% of patients suffer from recurrent orthostatic hypotension (OH), only 15% will have recurrent syncope. The most recent consensus criteria for the diagnosis of MSA were developed in 2008. Although definite MSA requires autopsy confirmation, probable and possible MSA can be diagnosed based on history and physical examination (Table 49.4).

Presence of classic pill-rolling tremor, neuropathy, hallucinations, dementia, and family history of parkinsonism are uncommon in MSA. Orofacial dystonia, camptocormia, inspiratory sighs, severe dysphonia and dysarthria, and new or increased snoring are features that suggest MSA ("red flag" signs). In a European cohort of patients, MSA-p and urinary retention were associated with poor survival. Sometimes it is difficult to differentiate MSA from sporadic adult-onset ataxia, especially when autonomic failure is absent. In practice, MSA is most frequently confused with PD or PSP. Mild limitation of upward gaze alone is non-specific, whereas a prominent (>50%) limitation of upward gaze or any limitation of downward gaze suggests PSP. Before the onset of vertical gaze limitation, slowing of voluntary vertical saccades is usually detectable in PSP and assists in the differentiation of these two disorders.

Table 49.4 Current consensus criteria for multiple system atrophy (MSA).

Definite MSA	Probable MSA	Possible MSA

Autopsy-confirmed case with neuropathological evidence of widespread and abundant CNS α-synuclein–positive glial cytoplasmic inclusions in association with striatonigral and/or olivopontocerebellar neurodegeneration	Sporadic, progressive, adult-onset (age >30 years) disease characterized by:
	
	Autonomic failure involving
	    Urinary incontinence (with erectile dysfunction in males);
	or
	
	    Orthostatic blood pressure drop of at least 30 points systolic or 15 points diastolic within 3 minutes of standing from a recumbent position
	and
	
	One of the following predominant motor features:
	    Poorly levodopa-responsive parkinsonism (defined as bradykinesia with rigidity, tremor, or postural instability); or
	    A cerebellar syndrome consisting of gait ataxia with cerebellar dysarthria, limb ataxia, or cerebellar oculomotor dysfunction
		Sporadic, progressive, adult-onset (age >30 years) disease characterized by:
		
		Parkinsonism (defined as bradykinesia with rigidity, tremor, or postural instability); or A cerebellar syndrome consisting of gait ataxia with cerebellar dysarthria, limb ataxia, or cerebellar oculomotor dysfunction
		
		and
		
		At least one of the following symptoms that suggest autonomic dysfunction, including otherwise unexplained:
		    Urinary urgency
		    Urinary frequency or incomplete bladder emptying
		    Erectile dysfunction in males
		    Significant orthostatic blood pressure drop not meeting the criterion for probable MSA
		and
		
		At least one of the following additional features for MSA-p or MSA-c
		
		Possible MSA-p
		
		    Rapidly progressive parkinsonism
		
		    Poor response to levodopa
		
		    Postural instability within 3 years of motor onset
		
		    Gait ataxia, cerebellar dysarthria, limb ataxia, or cerebellar oculomotor dysfunction
		
		    Dysphagia within 5 years of motor onset
		
		    Atrophy on MRI of putamen, middle cerebellar peduncle, pons, or cerebellum
		
		    Hypometabolism on FDG-PET in putamen, brainstem, or cerebellum
		
		Possible MSA-c
		
		    Parkinsonism (bradykinesia and rigidity)
		
		    Atrophy on MRI of putamen, middle cerebellar peduncle, or pons
		
		    Hypometabolism on FDG-PET in putamen
		
		    Presynaptic nigrostriatal dopaminergic denervation on SPECT or PET

CNS = central nervous system; FDG-PET = fluorodeoxyglucose positron emission tomography; MRI = magnetic resonance imaging; MSA-c = multiple system atrophy with prominent cerebellar signs; MSA-p = multiple system atrophy with prominent parkinsonism; PET = positron emission tomography; SPECT = single photon emission computed tomography

Investigations

Autonomic function tests, external sphincter electromyography, and neuroimaging are used to support the diagnosis of MSA and to assist in ruling out other causes of atypical parkinsonism. To assess a history of urinary retention, bladder catheterization or ultrasound can measure post-void urine. Ultrasound can also measure prostate size. A standard urine analysis should be performed to rule out common causes of urinary symptoms. A tilt table test is a more precise assessment of orthostatic hypotension. In MSA, OH is defined as a drop of at least 30 mmHg systolic blood pressure or 15 mmHg diastolic blood pressure within 3 minutes of standing. Delayed OH (beyond 3 minutes) can also occur. In MSA, OH is the result of degeneration of central autonomic pathways unlike that in PD, where it results from degeneration of postganglionic autonomic nerves. Therefore, cardiovascular autonomic failure can be demonstrated by [123I]meta-iodo-benzyl-guanidine (MIBG) scintigraphy in cases of PD, but it is expected to be normal in MSA. External anal sphincter myography can be used to show degenerative changes in the muscles related to pathological changes of Onuf's nucleus.

MRI of the brain typically shows atrophy of the putamen, pons, and middle cerebellar peduncle. Atrophy of the putamen creates hyperintensity in the dorsolateral margin known as a "putaminal slit." Hypointensity at the mid-pons level appears as a cross, known as the "hot cross bun" sign. This is highly specific, but not very sensitive for the diagnosis of MSA.

Management

Although potential MSA therapies are under study, no definitive treatment is available now. Treatment mainly focuses on the parkinsonism and dysautonomia, since there are no effective therapies for the ataxia of MSA-c. Parkinsonism in MSA-p responds poorly to levodopa therapy and levodopa-induced dyskinesia often develops in the face or jaw. Symptomatic treatment of OH improves quality of life. Non-pharmacological approaches to treat OH include adequate fluid intake, a high-salt diet, and compression stockings. Pharmacological agents including fludrocortisone, midodrine, and pyridostigmine (a cholinesterase inhibitor that improves ganglionic transmission) are first-line options for OH. Droxidopa, a norepinephrine precursor, was recently approved by the US Food and Drug Administration for treatment of neurogenic OH secondary to PD, MSA, and primary autonomic failure. It carries a black-box warning of severe supine hypertension as a serious side effect. Physical, speech, and occupational therapies are critical resources to improve strength, mobility, speech, swallowing, and general quality of life for people with MSA.

Dementia with Lewy bodies

Lewy body dementia encompasses dementia with Lewy bodies (DLB) and Parkinson's disease dementia (PDD). DLB and PDD have similar histopathology with Lewy bodies made of α-synuclein and ubiquitin, and they share major clinical features as well. The difference in diagnosis largely depends on the order of symptom presentation (see Chapter 40). When the movement disorder clearly begins before any cognitive symptoms, it is generally referred to as PDD, and when cognitive symptoms appear in a similar time frame with motor symptoms, it is generally referred to as DLB.

Epidemiology

DLB is the second most common cause of dementia after Alzheimer's disease (AD), with previous studies reporting a prevalence of up to 22% of all cases of dementia. A recent systematic review based on population and clinical studies reported a prevalence of 4.2% in the community setting. Typical onset of symptoms is in the seventh or eighth decade of life, later than the onset of PD. Cognitive decline tends to be more rapid in DLB than in AD; however, life expectancy is similar to that of AD.

Pathophysiology

There is no "gold standard" for the pathological diagnosis of DLB or PDD. The hallmark pathology is α-synuclein in the form of Lewy bodies. Lewy bodies are easily recognizable as large, spherical, highly eosinophilic intracytoplasmic inclusions with a clear halo. Cortical-type Lewy bodies are mostly found in the cingulate gyrus, insula, entorhinal cortex, parahippocampal gyrus, occipitotemporalis gyrus, and amygdaloid nucleus. Presence of brainstem-type and cortical-type Lewy bodies is needed in establishing the diagnosis of DLB. Alzheimer's disease pathology is the most common co-occurring pathology accompanying Lewy body pathology (PDD or DLB).

Clinical features

DLB is a neurodegenerative disease characterized by cognitive impairment, fluctuating alertness, formed visual hallucinations, and parkinsonism. The hallmark feature is the emergence of both cognitive dysfunction and parkinsonism within 1 year, although this timeline is arbitrary. Either may appear first. In contrast, dementia in PD typically occurs many years after the onset of parkinsonism. Tremor is usually absent or minimal in DLB. Cognitive symptoms appear early and are progressive. The main cognitive domains affected are attention, executive functioning, and visuospatial skills. Decline is quicker than that seen in AD. Fluctuations in attention and arousal are common and may span days or even weeks.

Neuropsychiatric symptoms are common in DLB; visual hallucinations occur in 50% of patients. The visions are fully formed, often of people or animals. A majority of DLB patients have other psychiatric disturbances, including depression, apathy, insomnia, anxiety, and paranoid delusions associated with hallucinations. Dysautonomia and rapid eye movement behavioral disorders (RBDs) are also frequently seen. For example, in a series of 174 patients with RBD, the estimated risk of a defined neurodegenerative syndrome (synucleinopathy) from the time of RBD diagnosis was 33% at 5 years, 76% at 10 years, and 91% at 14 years.

Investigations

There is no diagnostic tool to definitively diagnose DLB. MRI of the brain shows atrophy of the dorsal midbrain, striatum, and amygdala, with relatively preserved hippocampus. FDG-PET demonstrates decreased occipital glucose metabolism. Like in PD, cardiac imaging shows decreased cardiac innervation in DLB. So diagnosis of DLB remains clinical, and definitive diagnosis currently depends on postmortem examination.

Management

Treatment of DLB is also symptomatic. Clinically significant parkinsonism can be treated with dopaminergic agents. Given that dopamine agonists are associated with a higher frequency of cognitive impairments, including hallucinations, carbidopa/levodopa is preferable in treating parkinsonism. Cholinesterase inhibitors like donepezil and rivastigmine or memantine have been shown to improve hallucinations, agitation, apathy, and cognition in randomized trials. People with DLB respond poorly to typical neuroleptics, with adverse effects of profound rigidity and mutism ("neuroleptic sensitivity"). Although the available evidence is not favorable, quetiapine is generally used first in the treatment of psychosis from DLB or PDD, mainly to avoid the onerous blood monitoring required for clozapine. Several double blind and open-label trials have demonstrated the efficacy of clozapine in treating not only Parkinson's disease psychosis, but also tremor and drug-induced dyskinesia. Pimavanserin, a pure 5-HT$_{2A}$ inverse agonist, has shown promising results in treating PD-related psychosis, in that it does not require stringent blood count monitoring and also does not cause sedation. Clonazepam is effective in treating RBD, but may exacerbate dementia and alertness. Melatonin can be another option for sleep disturbance.

Frontotemporal dementia

Frontotemporal dementia (FTD) is the second most common type of dementia occurring before the age of 65 years. Three clinical phenotypes have been defined: behavioral variant FTD (bvFTD), semantic dementia, and progressive non-fluent aphasia (see Chapter 45). Cognitive symptoms in amyotrophic lateral sclerosis (ALS) are similar to FTD, with some patients developing clear FTD. With increasing understanding of the common molecular underpinning of ALS and FTD, these two entities are viewed as part of a clinical spectrum where pure FTD and ALS lie at the two ends. ALS patients who do not meet clinical criteria for FTD are said to have ALSCi or ALSBi-ALS with cognitive or behavioral impairment, respectively. FTD patients with some features of motor neuron disease on clinical exam or electromyography are said to have frontotemporal dementia–motor neuron disease (FTD-MND). While mutations in MAPT (microtubule-associated protein T) and progranulin (PGRN) give rise to pure FTD, TDP-43 (TAR-binding protein), FUS (fused in sarcoma), C9orf72, VCP (valosin-containing protein), and p62/sequestosome-1 mutations have been shown to cause either FTD or ALS. SOD1 (superoxide dismutase) mutation causes pure ALS in about 10% of familial cases. Hexanucleotide repeat expansion in the *C9orf72* gene is the most common cause of familial and sporadic ALS and FTD.

Epidemiology

The prevalence of FTD in persons aged between 45 and 64 years is estimated to be between 15 and 22 cases per 100,000 in the United States, 15 per 100,000 in the United Kingdom, and 22 per 100,000 in Italy. Parkinsonism is found in approximately 20–30% of patients with FTD. It is frequently observed in familial FTD linked to chromosome 17q (FTDP-17). In sporadic cases, symptom onset is usually between 45 and 64 years of age. The disease is slowly progressive, with disease duration averaging 10–12 years.

Pathophysiology

BvFTD is associated with symmetric ventromedial frontal, orbital frontal, and insular atrophy and left anterior cingulate atrophy. Microscopic examination of the cerebral cortex shows neuronal loss and microvacuolization. Whitematter changes include loss of myelin and astrocytic gliosis. Neuronal loss in the basal ganglia and substantia nigra may be a prominent feature. With immunohistochemistry, cytoplasmic and nuclear inclusions made of different types of proteins can be identified. FTD-TDP is the most common type of inclusion in familial and sporadic FTD. FTD-τ inclusions are specifically seen in disease related to MAPT mutations, (FTD-MAPT).

Clinical features

The most common subtype of FTD is bvFTD, followed by the two language variants, primary non-fluent aphasia (PnFA) and semantic dementia (SD). The earliest manifestations are often behavioral with disinhibition, poor impulse control, impaired social interactions, or even psychosis. Cognitive impairment follows, affecting judgment and planning, but gradually evolving into a more global dementia. Motor disturbances including bradykinesia, axial and limb rigidity, and postural instability emerge later. In addition to parkinsonism, some patients have upper motor neuron signs. Usually episodic memory and visuospatial abilities remain intact in early FTD, unlike in AD. In comparison to AD, the rate of progression is more rapid in bvFTD. A diagnosis of primary progressive aphasia (PnFA or SD) requires that language impairment is present for at least 2 years before the appearance of other symptoms.

Investigations

In FTD, MRI of the brain shows atrophy of the frontal lobe, anterior temporal lobe, and insula. Frontal anterior temporal and cingulate gyrus show hypometabolism on FDG-PET. Imaging helps to distinguish FTD from other types of dementia such as AD.

Management

Parkinsonism in FTD is unresponsive to levodopa. Treatment of other features of FTD is symptomatic.

Vascular parkinsonism

Vascular parkinsonism is a syndrome characterized by subacute evolution of a levodopa-unresponsive, akinetic rigid syndrome in a patient with vascular risk factors. Clinical features include shuffling gait, tremor, symmetric rigidity with or without cogwheeling, and at times pseudobulbar palsy. Neuroimaging shows severe whitematter disease, often with infarcts in the basal ganglia.

Normal pressure hydrocephalus

The clinical picture of normal pressure hydrocephalus (NPH) is a triad of gait dysfunction, urinary incontinence, and gradual onset of dementia, although all symptoms are not always present. Parkinsonism may accompany this picture. Neuroimaging demonstrates ventricular enlargement out of proportion to cortical atrophy. Clinical improvement should be demonstrable hours to days after lum-

bar puncture with removal of 40–50 ml of cerebrospinal fluid. Surgical shunting is the definitive treatment, although careful patient selection is necessary due to a high complication rate. According to one recent retrospective study, the most common complications associated with shunting were shunt drainage-related subdural hematoma/hygroma, shunt revision, postoperative seizure, shunt infection (2.5%), and symptomatic intracerebral hemorrhage (1.5%). When NPH is confirmed, shunting should be performed soon after the diagnosis. Preliminary reports suggest that low-dose acetazolamide might reduce periventricular whitematter hyperintensities in idiopathic NPH.

Parkinsonism dementia complex of Guam

Parkinsonism dementia complex of Guam (PDC) was first described in 1961 as a fatal neurodegenerative disease characterized by neurofibrillary tangles comprised of τ-proteins. The Chamarro of Guam are at highest risk for the disease. By 1985, the incidence of PDC declined toward rates seen in the continental United States, for reasons that are unclear. To date, no patient born after 1951 has been identified with PDC.

PDC may present with symptoms of symmetric parkinsonism, dementia, or both. Gait disturbance is seen at presentation in most patients. Tremor is rare. Cognitive deficits always develop and begin with difficulty with attention, recent memory, and behavioral changes. PDC patients become severely demented and bedridden.

While there is speculation that PDC is related to a motor neuron disease discovered in Guam in the 1950s known as the Parkinsonism–ALS complex of Guam, the prevalence of the motor neuron disease has markedly declined compared to PDC. This has led to speculation that the former motor neuron disease was caused by an environmental factor. More recent autopsy studies show separate pathology for the two diseases, suggesting that PDC and the motor neuron disease found on Guam are unrelated.

Drug-induced parkinsonism

Drug-induced parkinsonism (DIP) is the most common type of parkinsonism after idiopathic PD. The true prevalence of DIP is unknown, as the condition is often underrecognized and epidemiological studies tend not to separate DIP from other causes of parkinsonism. A community-based study in Brazil estimated that DIP represents up to 37% of all cases of parkinsonism. Risk factors of DIP include older age; female sex; higher dose and longer duration of treatment; type of agent used; cognitive impairment; acquired immunodeficiency syndrome (AIDS); tardive dyskinesia; and preexisting extrapyramidal disorder. One study suggested a 7.16-fold increased risk of DIP in patients with the HLA-B44 haplotype. Use of medications causing DIP can also unmask incidental Lewy body disease or PD.

Antipsychotic drugs cause parkinsonism by either blocking dopamine or depleting dopamine from the presynaptic nerve terminals. Atypical antipsychotics are less inclined to cause parkinsonism than typical antipsychotics, presumably due to the higher affinity of atypical antipsychotics to 5-HT$_{2A}$ than dopamine receptors, although this theory is still debated. Clozapine is the agent least likely to cause parkinsonism. Tetrabenazine causes DIP by depleting dopamine. A meta-analysis of clinical trials revealed parkinsonism as an adverse effect of the treatment with this drug in 27% of patients. Antiemetics such as metoclopramide, levosulpiride,

Table 49.5 Potential drugs causing drug-induced parkinsonism.

Antipsychotic drugs
Typical antipsychotics
Chlorpromazine, perphenazine, fluphenazine, promethazine, haloperidol, pimozide, sulpiride
Atypical antipsychotics
Risperidone, olanzapine, ziprasidone, aripiprazole, quetiapine
Dopamine depleters
Reserpine
Tetrabenazine
Antiemetics
Metoclopramide, levosulpiride, clebopride, itopride
Calcium channel blockers
Flunarizine, cinnarizine
Selective serotonin reuptake Inhibitors
Sertraline, citalopram, fluoxetine, paroxetine
Mood stabilizers
Lithium, valproic acid
Immunosuppressants
Tacrolimus
Antiarrhythmics
Amiodarone, procainamide
Drugs and toxins
MPTP, ecstasy, manganese, pesticides, cyanide, organic solvents, cycas circinalis

and clebopride are well known to cause DIP. However, since domperidone does not cross the blood–brain barrier, it will not cause any extrapyramidal side effects. Although there is no substantial evidence, selective serotonin reuptake inhibitors (SSRIs) can also cause parkinsonism. When paroxetine was assessed for treatment of depression in PD, there was worsening of motor functioning (Table 49.5).

Clinical symptoms of DIP are similar to those of PD and include bradykinesia, rigidity, impaired postural reflexes, and tremor. A typical clinical scenario is that of acute to subacute onset of levodopa-unresponsive parkinsonism with prior history of use of possibly causative drugs. Parkinsonian motor features are often symmetric. Often, DIP is clinically indistinguishable from PD and brain imaging with DaT can help the clinician to determine whether DIP is entirely drug induced. Since DIP is a presynaptically mediated disease, individuals with pure DIP should have normal uptake in the striatum. Autopsy studies of the brains with clinical diagnosis of DIP usually do not show significant pathological changes.

Clinicians should try to minimize the use of medications that have the potential for causing DIP, or use less risky medications if needed. When the symptoms of parkinsonism are already present, discontinuation of the offending drug is suggested, but the disappearance of the symptoms can take a long time. Dopaminergic drugs are not useful in these cases. Anticholinergic drugs and amantadine can provide some improvement, but side effects can be prohibitive, especially in the elderly.

Toxin-induced parkinsonism

Since its discovery, 1-methyl-4-phenyl-1,2,3,6-tetrahydropyridine (MPTP) has been used in animal models of parkinsonism. Humans may be exposed through illicit drug use, as MPTP is sometimes found as a contaminant in intravenous drugs of abuse. Exposure in humans may lead to an acute, moderately severe parkinsonism

in as little as 7 days. Neurological damage is permanent. MPTP is a precursor of MPP+ that selectively kills dopaminergic cells of SNpc by causing failure of cellular respiration through binding with complex I of the chain. Acute ingestion of methanol can lead to bilateral necrosis of putamen, causing parkinsonism. It can also occur as a late complication of cyanide, carbon monooxide, and carbon disulfide poisoning.

Manganese is an essential trace element that can be associated with neurotoxicity. Hypermanganism can occur in a variety of clinical settings. The clinical symptoms of manganese intoxication include non-specific complaints, neurobehavioral changes, parkinsonism, and dystonia. The parkinsonism due to manganese is somewhat unique among toxins associated with parkinsonism, in that these patients may have some clinical features that occur less commonly in PD, such as kinetic tremor, dystonia, specific gait disturbances, and early mental, balance, and speech changes. Chelation with ethylenediaminetetraacetic acid (EDTA) has been attempted, with no apparent benefit. Recently, early-onset generalized dystonia with brain manganese accumulation was described in the United Kingdom resulting from *SLC30A10* gene mutation. Treatment with intravenous disodium calcium edetate led to clinical and radiographic improvement.

Infectious and postinfectious parkinsonism

Parkinsonism can develop within the context of viral encephalitis. During World War I, a peculiar form of encephalitis (von Economo's encephalitis or encephalitis lethargica) appeared and parkinsonism was the major neurological sequela. The exact etiology always remained elusive, but a virus as a causative agent was widely speculated. However, since the emergence of West Nile Virus (WNV) in the United States in 1999, this has become one of the well-known causes of parkinsonism secondary to encephalitis. It seems to have a special predilection for the extrapyramidal system, causing movement disorders like parkinsonian signs and symptoms, postural and kinetic tremors, and myoclonus. West Nile virus neuroinfection can also cause a poliomyelitis-like picture and/or meningitis. St. Louis encephalitis virus can also affect the basal ganglia and substantia nigra, causing tremors, myoclonus, and ataxia. In fact, it was the most important neuroinvasive flavivirus before WNV became widespread. Other viruses that rarely cause transient parkinsonism are Japanese encephalitis, Western equine encephalitis, Epstein–Barr virus, Coxsackie B, and poliomyelitis. Central nervous system Lyme disease deserves a mention here, as many neurological symptoms are ascribed to this infection even when evidence is scant. To date, there are very few case reports of parkinsonism occurring in the setting of CNS Lyme disease.

Further reading

Aerts MB, Esselink RA, Post B, van de Warrenburg BP, Bloem BR. Improving the diagnostic accuracy in parkinsonism: A three-pronged approach. *Pract Neurol* 2012;12:77–87.

Armstrong MJ, Litvan I, Lang AE, *et al.* Criteria for the diagnosis of corticobasal degeneration. *Neurology* 2013;80:496–503.

Bergeron C, Pollanen MS, Weyer L, Black SE, Lang AE. Unusual clinical presentations of cortical-basal ganglionic degeneration. *Ann Neurol* 1996;40:893–900.

Chung EJ, Lee WY, Yoon WT, Kim BJ, Lee GH. MIBG scintigraphy for differentiating Parkinson's disease with autonomic dysfunction from Parkinsonism-predominant multiple system atrophy. *Mov Disord* 2009;24:1650–1655.

Gilman S, Wenning GK, Low PA, *et al.* Second consensus statement on the diagnosis of multiple system atrophy. *Neurology* 2008;71:670–676.

Iranzo A, Fernandez-Arcos A, Tolosa E, *et al.* Neurodegenerative disorder risk in idiopathic REM sleep behavior disorder: Study in 174 patients. *PLoS One* 2014;9:e89741.

Litvan I, Agid Y, Calne D, *et al.* Clinical research criteria for the diagnosis of progressive supranuclear palsy (Steele–Richardson–Olszewski syndrome): Report of the NINDS–SPSP international workshop. *Neurology* 1996;47:1–9.

Rebeiz JJ, Kolodny EH, Richardson EP, Jr. Corticodentatonigral degeneration with neuronal achromasia. *Arch Neurol* 1968;18:20–33.

Simon-Sanchez J, Dopper EG, Cohn-Hokke PE, *et al.* The clinical and pathological phenotype of C9ORF72 hexanucleotide repeat expansions. *Brain* 2012;135:723–735.

Steele JC, Richardson JC, Olszewski J. Progressive supranuclear palsy: A heterogeneous degeneration involving the brain stem, basal ganglia and cerebellum with vertical gaze and pseudobulbar palsy, nuchal dystonia and dementia. *Arch Neurol* 1964;10:333–359.

50 Parkinson's disease

Daniel Truong[1] and Roongroj Bhidayasiri[2]

[1] University of California, Riverside, Riverside, CA, USA; The Truong Neuroscience Institute, Orange Coast Memorial Medical Center, Fountain Valley, CA, USA

[2] Chulalongkorn Center of Excellence for Parkinson's Disease & Related Disorders, Faculty of Medicine, Chulalongkorn University Hospital, Bangkok, Thailand

James Parkinson first described in 1817 in an essay a clinical presentation that consisted of rest tremor, lessened muscular power, abnormal truncal posture, and festinant, propulsive gait. Parkinson's disease (PD) is now recognized to be one of the most common neurological disorders worldwide and a significant cause of disability and reduced quality of life.

Epidemiology

Parkinson's disease affects 7–10 million people worldwide. It is believed to affect approximately 1% of individuals 60 years of age or older. In 2005, it was estimated that the prevalence of PD would more than double by the year 2030. The prevalence of PD increases with age; worldwide the prevalence of PD is 41/100,000 for those aged 40–49, 428/100,000 in those aged 60–69, and 1903/100,000 in those aged 80 and older. PD is 1.5 times more common in men than in women. Approximately 4% of people with PD are diagnosed before the age of 50. The prevalence of PD varies geographically, with rates in Asia lower than rates in Europe, North America, and Australia. A recent meta-analysis of 47 studies from around the world found that, among those aged 70–79, the prevalence of PD in Asia was 646/100,000, less than half that in Europe, North America, and Australia (1602/100,000). Interestingly, the gender difference in PD also appears to be smaller in Asia than in the other countries studied.

Neuropathology

Pathological findings of Parkinson's disease include depigmentation and neuronal loss in the pars compacta of substantia nigra and the presence of Lewy bodies (LBs) and pale bodies. These cells contain neuromelanin and produce dopamine. The hallmark of Parkinson's disease is the deficit of dopamine in the striatum, the site of axonal projection from the substantia nigra. PD develops when the level of dopamine cell loss reaches 80%. Lewy bodies are concentric hyaline cytoplasmic inclusions. They contain accumulation of α–synuclein protein and ubiquitin. In PD, α-synuclein is deposited in neuronal cell bodies and processed as LBs and Lewy neurites. There is growing appreciation for symptoms other than the motor symptoms, and several studies have drawn attention to the involvement of cardiac, gastrointestinal, submandibular gland, cutaneous, and other body regions, all of which have been found to have LB disease with deposition of abnormal α-synuclein.

Braak *et al.* have devised a staging system of LB pathology in PD, with six stages that characterize a progression from the medulla oblongata, through the pontine tegmentum, into the midbrain, and then the basal prosencephalon and mesocortex, and finally through the neocortex. Before the immunohistochemical demonstration of α-synuclein as a component of Lewy bodies, it was commonly assumed that LBs cause neuronal cell death. Recent studies have indicated that LBs may represent a cytoprotective mechanism in PD. There are different hypotheses as to the cause of PD, which include oxidative stress, mitochondrial dysfunction, excitotoxicity, glial cell activation, and apoptosis. The role of toxins in the etiology of PD is not well defined, but MPTP and the pesticide rotenone have been known to cause parkinsonian syndrome.

The majority of PD cases are sporadic. Abnormal gene mutations have been discovered to cause or be associated with the familial form of PD. At least 20 gene loci have been identified for hereditary forms of parkinsonian syndrome. They are named from PARK1 to PARK20, and the list is likely to continue to expand. Different genes have been linked to rare familial forms of disease (encoding α-synuclein, parkin, DJ-1, PINK1, and LRRK2). Additional genes have been identified that seem to affect the risk of developing Parkinson's disease; these are in the early stages of investigation and some have not yet been named.

Rare cases of PD have been identified as occurring in association with gene mutations, but they do not account for the large number of sporadic cases. Abnormal gene mutations have been discovered to cause or be associated with the familial form of Parkinson's disease. A large Italian American family (the Contursi kindred) was discovered to have a PD syndrome linked to PARK1 at the q21–23 region of chromosome 4. Sequence analysis revealed a mutation in the gene that encodes α-synuclein. Different mutations have since been identified and found to be associated with early-onset parkinsonism, moderate response to levodopa, rapid progression, pyramidal signs, frequent psychiatric symptoms, and prominent psychiatric dysfunction. Phenotype analyses showed that the severity of the disease correlated with the copy number, but not with the minimal number of multiplied genes (1–33).

PARK2 or Parkin functions as an E3 ubiquitin protein ligase by targeting misfolded proteins to the ubiquitin proteasome pathway for degradation. The loss of its E3 ligase activity due to mutation leads to autosomal recessive early-onset PD. Other types of autosomal recessive parkinsonism include the phosphatase and tensin homologue–induced putative kinase 1 gene (PINK1), and the DJ-1 gene. These mutations are generally associated with young-onset PD and manifest through good response to levodopa and early development of dyskinesias.

In PARK7 there is a loss of function mutation in the DJ-1 locus, which is associated with rare forms of autosomal recessive early-onset parkinsonism. DJ-1 may function as an antioxidant protein. Overexpression of wild-type DJ-1 protects against a wide variety of toxic injuries resulting from oxidative stress. Familial PD-linked mutations in DJ-1 are considered to cause nigral degeneration through a loss of function mechanism consistent with the recessive inheritance.

PARK6 is caused by mutations in the PINK1 gene and is associated with early-onset familial PD. Little is known about the precise function of PINK1, but it may have a role in mitochondrial dysfunction, protein stability, and kinase pathway. Although early cognitive impairment is uncommon, psychiatric comorbid conditions have been reported to be present in PINK1-associated and DJ-1-associated PD.

PARK8 is associated with mutation in the leucine-rich repeat kinase 2 (LRRK2) and causes autosomal dominant PD. LRRK2 mutations present beyond familial cases and with a high frequency in patients of European descent, Ashkenazi Jews, and those with origins in North Africa. The phenotype associated with LRRK2 mutation is highly variable, but is quite similar to sporadic PD, particularly asymmetric parkinsonism with tremor, but with a decreased risk of cognitive and olfactory impairment, although atypical features such as orthostatic hypotension, dementia, hallucinations, and sleep disturbance have been described in LRRK2 cases. The motor symptoms (e.g., disease severity, rate of progression, occurrence of falls, and dyskinesia) and non-motor symptoms (e.g., cognitive and olfactory dysfunction) of LRRK2-associated PD are more benign than those of idiopathic PD.

Certain environmental and lifestyle associations have been well described in PD for some time. These include coffee consumption and tobacco use, exercise, and particular diets such as those promoting higher urate levels (lower risk), and drinking well water, rural location, certain herbicides, and pesticide (higher risk).

Clinical presentation

The cardinal clinical features of PD consist of slowness, stiffness, rest tremors, and postural imbalance. Initially the postural imbalance may not be obvious, as it is mild at the beginning. The symptoms present mostly in one part of the body and slowly spread to other extremities on the same side before spreading to the other side of the body. Shuffling gait and stooped posture also are characteristic of PD. Besides slowness, there is also a paucity of movements and difficulty in initiating movements. The tremors are present at rest, asymmetric, and disappear with movement. When the tremors are severe, some patients may have action tremors as well. The Parkinson's rest tremors are distal and have a frequency of 3–5 Hz. It is typically a pronation–supination tremor of the forearm or a pill-rolling tremor of the finger. Tremors can occur in the leg or in the chin, but head or voice tremors are rare. Rigidity may occur throughout the body, but is more pronounced on one side. Other symptoms include masked face, decreased blinking, increase drooling, stooped posture, difficulty with walking and getting in and out of a chair, micrographia, and decreased olfaction. Patient speech is hypophonic, rapid, and monotone. Patients often have stammering and palilalia. Drooling is a bothersome feature that results from decreased swallowing rather than increased saliva production.

A variety of non-motor symptoms (NMS) such as sleep disturbances, constipation, mood disorders, autonomic dysfunction, or fatigue can antedate PD motor symptoms by years. REM sleep behavior disorder (RBD) and olfactory dysfunction are the most well-established premotor symptoms, but there is also evidence for constipation and depression. Dementia occurs in PD, more often in patients with older age of onset, the presence of hallucinations, lower Mini Mental Status Examination score at baseline, early appearance of bilateral motor involvement, and the early development of confusional states or psychotic symptoms with levodopa administration. The type of dementia seen in PD represents a combination of cortical and subcortical neuropsychological impairments with dysexecutive, attentional, and visuospatial deficits, and often prominent behavioral disturbances. The memory deficit is typically an impairment of retrieval with relatively preserved mnemonic function. Other cognitive disturbances, such as apraxia, aphasia, or agnosia, are often absent. Constipation is a common symptom and often precedes the diagnosis of PD by many years. The therapeutic interventions used to treat parkinsonian symptoms may further worsen constipation. Anxiety is present in up to 50% of PD patients (see Table 50.1).

After initial smooth response to therapy, the treatment is complicated by the emergence of variations of motor response in a majority of PD patients. These variations can occur in different forms, as early wearing off during the initial stage of motor complications, dyskinesias in the intermediate stage, and complex fluctuations in the advanced stage. In addition to the motor symptoms, many patients also develop non-motor symptoms,

Table 50.1 Prevalence of non-motor symptoms using non-motor questionnaire.

Non-motor symptoms	Mean (%)	Range (%)
Cognitive dysfunction		
Memory	45.8	37.9–62.5
Concentration	38.7	29.6–50.0
Depression		
Sadness	2.5	22.5–56.0
Anxiety	3.	30.7–55.8
Sleep		
Excessive daytime somnolence	30.5	21.2–37.1
Insomnia	40.9	17.6–52.5
REM sleep behavior disorder	34.2	29.6–38.7
Restless leg syndrome	35.8	27.7–41.1
Fatigue	41.5	31.1–58.1
Pain	31.1	18.2–45.9
Gastrointestinal symptoms		
Difficulty swallowing	25.4	16.1–30.3
Constipation	46.5	27.5–71.7
Urinary symptoms		
Urgency	53.4	35.0–61.0
Nocturia	53.8	26.4–66.7

which include depression, anxiety, fatigue, excessive daytime somnolence, insomnia, RBD, restless leg syndrome, apathy, pain, difficulty swallowing, constipation, sexual dysfunction, bowel incontinence, or urinary urgency.

Early-morning "off" (EMO) periods are common and occur in 59.7% of patients across all stages of the disease. EMO periods are often associated with non-motor symptoms. The predominant NMS associated with EMO are urinary urgency, anxiety, dribbling of saliva, pain, low mood, limb paresthesia, and dizziness. Common autonomic dysfunction includes constipation, urinary incontinence, heat or cold intolerance, orthostatic hypotension, sexual dysfunction, and abnormal sweating. Blood pressure may fluctuate with motor impairment in patients with wearing off. Sweating disturbance can be either hyperhidrosis or hypohidrosis. Sweating problems tended to occur predominantly at the beginning of an "off" period or in an "on" period with dyskinesia. Sexual dysfunction is relatively common; some patients suffer from hypersexuality, which is likely to be drug induced. Insomnia, hypersomnia, and parasomnia may all occur and contribute to daytime sleepiness. All Parkinson's medications may cause drowsiness. Dopamine agonists and levodopa can cause sleep attacks. Furthermore, sleep disturbances may take the form of difficulty falling asleep or more commonly fragmentation of nocturnal sleep, with frequent and prolonged awakening. This may be due to PD-specific motor phenomena, such as nocturnal immobility, resting tremor, dyskinesias, or nocturia, as well as coexisting sleep disorders, such as restless leg syndrome, periodic limb movements in sleep, or sleep-disordered breathing. RBD has a strong association with PD and is characterized by excessive nocturnal motor activity that usually represents attempted enactment of vivid, action-filled, and violent dreams.

Depression also occurs in PD, but the presentation is not the same as in patients with primary depression. Distinct features of depression in PD include elevated levels of dysphoria and irritability, but with little guilt or feeling of failure, and a low suicide rate, despite a high frequency of suicidal ideation. Apathy is defined as a loss of motivation, which appears in emotional, intellectual, and behavioral domains. It may affect 30–40% of patients. Apathy and depression are two distinct entities, although it is not always easy to distinguish between the two due to the overlap of symptoms, such as loss of interest, reduced pleasure in activities, fatigue, or apathy itself. Fatigue is also a common complaint and is a premotor symptom in 45% of patients. It is perceived as a sense of exhaustion as opposed to sleepiness.

Impulse control disorders occur in a subset of patients with PD. This spectrum of disorders, characterized by excessive or poorly controlled preoccupations, urges, or behaviors, includes not only punding, pathological gambling, and hypersexuality, but also compulsive shopping and binge eating. In a small percentage of patients, these behavioral abnormalities are associated with overuse of dopamine replacement therapy (DRT) and are referred to as a homeostatic hedonistic dysregulation called dopamine dysregulation syndrome (DDS).

Imaging

Differential diagnosis of parkinsonian conditions can be challenging. Dopamine transporter (DAT) imaging has largely been employed with single photon emission computed tomography

(SPECT), for example using the 123I-FP-CIT ligand (also known as 123I-ioflupane or DaTscan). DAT-SPECT typically reveals normal DAT levels in the caudate and putamen of healthy control participants and patients with essential tremor or with drug-induced or psychogenic parkinsonism. DAT levels are reduced in patients with PD, PD dementia (PDD), multiple system atrophy (MSA), or progressive supranuclear palsy (PSP). However, DAT-SPECT is not efficient for the differentiation of PD from other degenerative parkinsonian syndromes such as MSA and PSP.

Magnetic resonance imaging (MRI) is mostly normal in patients with PD, but may show midbrain atrophy with "hummingbird" or "penguin" sign. Atrophy of superior cerebellar peduncles may be seen in PSP. The MRI in MSA shows a hypointense putamen with hyperintense rim with loss of pontocerebellar fibers ("hot-cross bun" sign).

Transcranial sonography shows hyperechogenic substantia nigra in patients with PD and a hyperechogenic lentiform nucleus in patients with PSP, MSA, or corticobasal degeneration. Two studies have reported reasonable accuracy for transcranial sonography in the clinical diagnosis of PD (82–91% sensitivity, 82–85% specificity) comparable to glucose metabolic positron emission tomography (PET) in the same patients.

123I-metaiodobenzylguanidine (MIBG) myocardial scintigraphy has shown high sensitivity and specificity in the diagnosis of PD, based on evidence that cardiac sympathetic nerve fibers are affected early and commonly in PD. MIBG scintigraphy is moderately sensitive and specific in differentiating PD from other parkinsonian syndromes like MSA or PSP. Conversely, its sensitivity and specificity might be better in cognitively impaired patients, helping in the differential diagnosis between dementia with Lewy bodies (DLB) and Alzheimer's disease.

Differential diagnosis

The differential diagnosis of PD includes other causes of parkinsonism such as essential tremors, MSA, PSP, corticobasal degeneration, DLB, normal pressure hydrocephalus, and other parkinsonism-plus entities. Essential tremor patients have a positive family history in many family members. They have postural tremors, no extrapyramidal symptoms, and no response to levodopa. Patients with PSP have vertical gaze paralysis or slowed vertical saccadic movements, nuchal rigidity, and marked postural rigidity. MSA patients may have other symptoms such as fainting, ataxia, and failure to respond to adequate dose of levodopa. Diffuse Lewy body disease patients have memory problems and hallucinations. Corticobasal degeneration patients have apraxia, aphasia, sensory disorders, dystonia, alien hand, and myoclonus. In alien hand, patients do not recognize their hand as theirs when it rises spontaneously. MRI shows asymmetric atrophy of frontal and parietal regions. Drug-induced parkinsonism has a history of previous use of a causative drug such as an antipsychotic, reserpine, or metoclopramide. Vascular parkinsonism has stepwise progression, with the symptoms fixed from previous events. Normal pressure hydrocephalus patients have ataxia, dementia, and incontinence. MRI would show hydrocephalus. In dementia with Lewy bodies, there is cognitive impairment, hallucinations, and episodes of delirium in addition to parkinsonism. Figure 50.1 provides the diagnostic and treatment algorithm for patients who present with asymmetric parkinsonism.

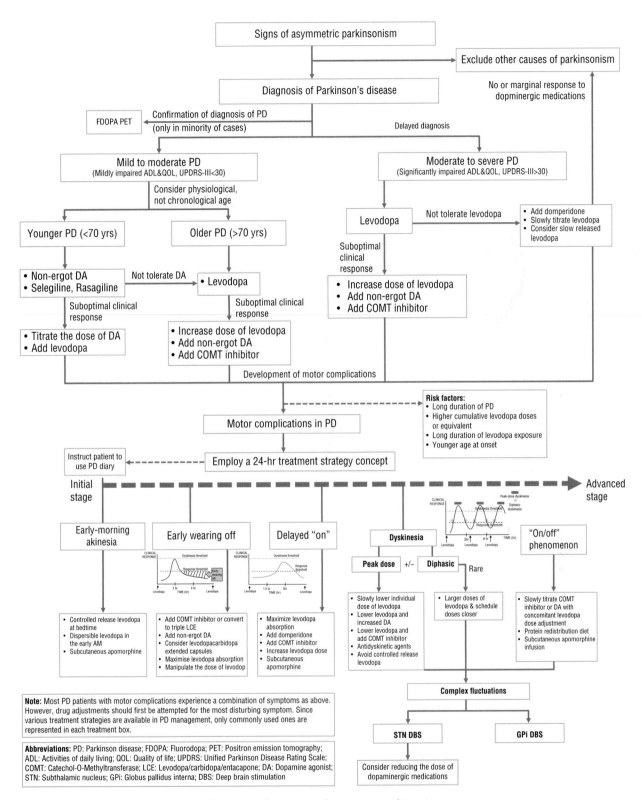

Figure 50.1 Diagnostic and treatment algorithm for patients who present with asymmetric parkinsonism

Treatment

Despite the rapid expansion in knowledge of its neurodegenerative process, the mainstay of treatment of PD remains symptomatic. Neuroprotective or disease-modifying treatment to slow or halt progression does not exist. Therapeutic options, including pharmacotherapy, such as levodopa and other dopaminergic agents (Table 50.2), and surgical approaches such as deep brain stimulation have been markedly improved over the past decades, resulting in better motor function, activities of daily living, and quality of life for PD patients. The principle of PD management should be individualized and the selection of treatments should aim to control symptoms as well as to prevent or delay motor complications.

Management of early Parkinson's disease

Pharmacotherapy for neuroprotection

As previously indicated, no adequate clinical trials have provided definitive evidence for pharmacological neuroprotection. While many agents have appeared promising based on laboratory studies, the symptomatic effects of the study medications commonly confound the clinical neuroprotection end points in clinical trials. Studies in early PD have suggested that the MAO-B inhibitor selegiline postpones the need for dopaminergic treatment by more than 6 months, and may reduce the risk of gait freezing, indicating a delay in disability progression. Similarly, early treatment with another MAO-B inhibitor, rasagiline, for 12 months in the TEMPO study showed less functional decline than delaying dopaminergic treatment for 6 months. In the ADAGIO study, using the delayed-start model, rasagiline was evaluated for potential neuroprotective effects in PD. Rasagiline 1 mg per day met all three primary end points, consistent with the drug having a disease-modifying

Table 50.2 Therapeutic options for motoric symptoms in Parkinson's disease (availability is determined by the time of publication, which may be different between countries).

1. Levodopa
    a. Levodopa/carbidopa
    b. Levodopa/benserazide
    c. Levodopa controlled release
    d. Levodopa/carbidopa/entacapone
    e. Infusible LD
2. Dopamine agonists
    a. Non-ergot derivatives
       - Pramipexole
       - Ropinirole
       - Piribedil
       - Rotigotine
       - Apomorphine
    b. Ergot derivatives
       - Bromocriptine
       - Pergolide
       - Cabergoline
3. Cathechol-O-methyltransferase inhibitors
       - Entacapone
       - Tolcapone
4. Monoamine oxidase B inhibitors
       - Selegiline
       - Rasagiline
5. Adenosine A2A antagonists
       - Istradefylline
6. NMDA receptor antagonist
       - Amantadine
7. Dopamine releaser
       - Zonisamide

effect. However, the 2 mg dose failed to show a difference between early and delayed treatment at the end of the second period. Thus, the results of the study were inconclusive.

Pharmacotherapy for symptom control

Dopamine agonists have diverse physical and chemical properties, but they share the ability to directly stimulate dopamine receptors. This contrasts with levodopa, which needs to be transformed into L-dopamine in presynaptic terminals. This D_2-like receptor agonistic activity of the dopamine agonists produces their antiparkinsonian effect. There are currently five dopamine agonists marketed in the United States: two are ergot derivatives (bromocriptine and pergolide) and the other three are non-ergot derivatives (pramipexole, ropinirole, and rotigotine). Cabergoline and piribedil are two dopamine agonists that are available in Europe and some countries in Asia. With the exception of rotigotine, which is used transdermally, all the aforementioned dopamine agonists are taken orally. The main improvement in dopamine agonists in the last few years has been the introduction of slow-release preparations of oral dopamine agonists and patch formulations.

The efficacy of dopamine agonists used as monotherapy in early PD has been demonstrated in numerous studies involving pramipexole, ropinirole, pergolide, and rotigotine. In the early stage, the clinical benefit from dopamine agonists is usually sufficient, but, when the disease progresses, it becomes necessary to add levodopa, which has a better effect on symptoms. Delaying the introduction of levodopa by using a dopamine agonist postpones and reduces the occurrence of motor fluctuations seen with levodopa treatment. Long-term follow-up studies indicate that approximately 85%, 68%, 55%, 43%, and 34% of PD patients initiated on pramipexole or ropinirole are still controlled on monotherapy at 1, 2, 3, 4, and 5 years, respectively.

There are no data to suggest that one dopamine agonist is more efficacious than another. However, an association has been reported between treatment with pergolide and the development of fibrotic valvular heart disease. Similar findings have also been observed with bromocriptine and cabergoline. Most published studies conclude that treatment with ergot dopamine agonists (pergolide and cabergoline in most cases), particularly at high daily doses and for periods of 6 months or longer, was associated with a substantially increased risk of newly diagnosed cardiac valve regurgitation. As a result, pergolide has been voluntarily withdrawn from the US market and current recommendations suggest that non-ergot derivatives should be considered first when dopamine agonists are indicated.

Levodopa is firmly established as the gold standard in the treatment of PD from over 40 years of use in clinical practice. It remains the most reliable and effective treatment for PD symptoms. A recent placebo-controlled study confirmed a dose-dependent efficacy of levodopa to reduce Unified Parkinson's Disease Rating Scale (UPDRS) scores. Levodopa has also been proven to be better at improving symptoms than dopamine agonists in numerous studies. However, patients will develop motor complications with long-term levodopa therapy. After 5 years of treatment, about 50% of patients taking levodopa develop motor fluctuations, and 30% develop dyskinesias; these numbers may be higher in patients with young-onset PD. Levodopa is now routinely coadministered with a decarboxylase inhibitor, either carbidopa or benserazide, to block peripheral degradation of levodopa to dopamine, allowing more levodopa to cross the blood–brain barrier. The gastric mucosa is another site of action, thus decarboxylase inhibitors also increase duodenal levodopa absorption.

Prevention of motor complications

A number of strategies have been developed to prevent or delay the occurrence of motor complications, including dyskinesias and motor fluctuations characteristic of later stages of the disease. First, the evidence that the early use of dopamine agonists (vs. levodopa) can reduce the incidence of motor complications has influenced most neurologists to start dopamine agonists as symptomatic monotherapy in early PD patients. Second, because the mechanism of levodopa-induced motor complications is probably related to the abnormal, non-physiological, pulsatile stimulation of striatal dopamine receptors, the concept of continuous dopaminergic stimulation (CDS), either by using long-acting dopamine agonists or continuously delivering levodopa, has been proposed as a method of preventing motor complications. Whether employing CDS therapy by continuous levodopa delivery can actually delay dyskinesias or motor fluctuations in early PD patients is unknown.

Management of advanced (complicated) Parkinson's disease

Long-term dopamimetic therapy, not limited to levodopa, is often complicated by variations of motor response in a majority of PD patients. "Advanced disease" is defined as PD with progressive motor impairment despite levodopa therapy and an unstable medication response leading to motor complications. Advanced disease typically develops after 5 years of levodopa treatment in up to 50% of PD patients. Motor complications can be simply divided into motor fluctuations and dyskinesias. Typically, patients may begin to experience a wearing-off (end-of-dose) effect, because the motor improvement after a dose of levodopa becomes reduced in duration over time and parkinsonism reappears. Subsequently, dyskinesias emerge at peak dose levels and are classically choreiform. Eventually, patients may experience rapid and unpredictable fluctuations between "on" and "off" periods, known as the on–off phenomenon.

The medical management of motor complications of PD remains an ongoing challenge. The goal is to maintain dopaminergic stimulation to minimize "off" time while not accentuating dyskinesias. The main approach of oral medications to control motor complications includes modifications of levodopa pharmacokinetics via levodopa dose adjustments, catechol-O-methyltransferase (COMT) inhibition, controlled-release formulations of levodopa, and the adjunctive use of long-acting dopamine agonists (DAs) or MAO-B inhibitors. However, the strategies that accomplish this goal are increasingly more difficult as the disease progresses, requiring both the attention and pharmacological understanding of the treating physicians. In addition, compliance as well as therapeutic adherence is required of the patients, supported by their caregivers. In this section, we aim to provide practical strategies for management by oral medications, with reference to recently published meta-analyses, practical reviews, and evidence-based reviews updated by the Movement Disorders Society (MDS), the report of the Joint Task Force of the European Federation of Neurological Societies (EFNS), and the practice parameter of the American Academy of Neurology (AAN).

Treatment of end-of-dose wearing off

End-of-dose wearing off is the most common and usually the first sign of motor complications. Patients develop a loss of response to a dose of medication before it is time to take the next dose, usually within 4 hours of the earlier dose. If they take their next dose of medication, their symptoms will improve again until the next dose begins to wear off. Treatment depends on the severity of the problem and on how dopaminergic therapy was initiated in the early stage of the disease. The predictability is somewhat reassuring to patients and this may allow simple interventions to be made. Some of the suggested treatment options are as follows.

Add a catechol-O-methyltransferase (COMT) inhibitor. If the patient already takes stable doses of levodopa, this is an option. COMT inhibition increases the peripheral bioavailability of LD and reduces 3-O-methyldopa (3-OMD) formation. The administration of COMT inhibitors with LD ensures a more stable plasma LD level and, consequently, it improves motor fluctuations. Entacapone is a peripheral COMT inhibitor, while tolcapone inhibits both peripheral and central COMT. Several controlled studies have demonstrated that adding a COMT inhibitor is useful and has been shown to reduce "off" time by approximately 1.3 hours per day with entacapone and 2–3 hours per day with tolcapone (another COMT inhibitor available in the United States). Patients should be advised that they may develop dyskinesia within 1–2 days of adding a COMT inhibitor and that a 20–30% reduction in levodopa dose may be required. Side effects of tolcapone include diarrhea in 5–6% of patients and the possibility of developing fulminant hepatitis. Because of the risk of potentially fatal, acute fulminant liver failure, tolcapone should only be used in patients with Parkinson's disease on l-dopa/carbidopa who are experiencing symptom fluctuations and are not responding satisfactorily to other therapies. The patient who fails to show substantial clinical benefit within 3 weeks of initiation of treatment with tolcapone should be withdrawn from the drug. Opicapone, a novel once-daily COMT inhibitor, has been shown in a recent study to achieve significant reductions in absolute "off" time at dose of 50 mg once daily. The drug is currently under review by the European Medicines Agency.

Manipulate the dose of levodopa by shortening the interval between levodopa doses. The next dose should be administered just before the beneficial effects from the previous dose have worn off. Recently, new extended-release levodopa/carbidopa (IPX066 or Rytary$_R$) has been shown to significantly reduce "off" time and increase "on" time without troublesome dyskinesia when compared to levodopa/carbidopa plus entacapone in a 6-week randomized study. Rytary^R achieved initial peak plasma concentration at about 1 hour and can maintained plasma concentration for about 4–5 hours before declining.

Add a dopamine agonist. Dopamine agonists are useful in reducing "off" time because their half-lives are longer than that of levodopa. The dose of levodopa should be maintained until a clinical response to the dopamine agonist is achieved. Later, the levodopa dose can be gradually lowered. Several controlled studies have confirmed the efficacy of dopamine agonists as adjunctive treatment to levodopa in reducing total daily "off" time by about 2 hours, with a reduction of levodopa dose of about 19–25%.

Adenosine A2A antagonists. Adenosine A2A receptors are selectively located on the cell bodies and terminals of the gamma-aminobutyric acid [(GABA)ergic] indirect striatal output pathway, and are functionally linked to dopamine D2 receptor function. Adenosine, via the A2A receptor, may contribute to the overactivity of the indirect pathway in PD by enhancing GABA release in the external globus pallidus. Corticostriatal glutamatergic activity via N-methyl D-aspartate (NMDA) receptor stimulation is increased in PD and results in adenosine release and stimulation of A2A receptors, an action that may further increase the activity of the indirect GABAergic pathway. Istradefylline is a selective A2A antagonist that has been recently approved in Japan and Europe for the treatment of fluctuating PD. In a study in Japan, istradefylline 20 mg/day and istradefylline 40 mg/day reduced daily "off" time. The most common adverse event was dyskinesia.

Zonisamide. In Japan, zonisamide up to 50 mg once a day has been approved as an add-on therapy to levodopa for end-of-dose wearing off with a low incidence of dyskinesia and hallucination. The exact mechanism of zonisamide on PD has not yet been elucidated. Zonisamide has a very long half-life (25 mg; $t_{1/2}$ 90 h).

Safinamide. Safinamide was recently approved in the European Union and modulates dopaminergic and glutamatergic neurotransmission with a unique dual mechanism of action. It improves motor symptoms, motor complications, quality of life, and "on" and "off" time in combination with other PD medications. Safinamide reduces "off" time and extends "on" time without troublesome dyskinesia.

Treatment of dyskinesia

To treat dyskinesia, the pattern of dyskinesia needs to be determined. A patient's history and PD diary are the primary sources of information. It may be important to observe what patients mean by dyskinesia, since they may confuse dyskinesia with tremor, or "off" dystonia. Reviewing patients' video clips of what they claim to be dyskinesia usually provides evidence regarding their ability to report dyskinesia versus tremor. If dyskinesia is mild and non-troublesome, there is no need to treat it, but patients should be advised to observe signs of disabling dyskinesia, which tend to occur late in the afternoon or early evening. While caregivers appear to consider dyskinesia as debilitating, most PD patients prefer to be "on" with dyskinesia than to be "off." Therefore, in advanced PD patients, the balance between reductions in dyskinesia and deteriorating parkinsonism is critical to management. It is also important for advanced PD patients to be aware that it is often difficult to delineate a dose of medication that provides stable "on" time without inducing dyskinesia. A compromise to achieve the "balance" is probably the goal of management. The following steps are recommended for treating patients with disabling dyskinesias.

(1) For peak-dose dyskinesias:

Review the patient's drug regimen. Determine whether there are any drugs that may alleviate dyskinesia without reducing the antiparkinsonian effect. Examples of options are selegiline and anticholinergics.

Examine other adjunctive therapies. If the patients are receiving sustained-release levodopa, better symptom control may be achievable if they are switched to an immediate-release preparation, particularly if dyskinesia occurs late in the day. A trial of switching to the new extended-release levodopa/carbidopa (IPX066) may also be considered. If a COMT inhibitor is used, dose reduction may be necessary. Alternatively, a reduction in levodopa dose may be considered, but this may result in the inability to induce an "on" response in some patients. Some authors suggest that the addition of a dopamine agonist coupled with a reduction in the levodopa dose may reduce dyskinesia while sustaining motor benefit.

Add amantadine or clozapine. Amantadine is the only agent that suppresses dyskinesia through its action at the NMDA receptor. The antidyskinetic effect of amantadine is effective at 300 mg per day. The efficacy is generally retained in the long term despite common concerns about tachyphylaxis. Alternatively, the atypical antipsychotic clozapine may be considered. However, it lacks definite evidence in reducing dyskinesia, and its potential toxicity, such as agranulocytosis, has limited its use.

(2) For diphasic dyskinesias: this type of dyskinesia can be difficult to treat, since it goes against the usual principle of lowering the levodopa dose in peak-dose dyskinesia and has not been specifically studied in large clinical trials. Therefore, the recommendation is based on smaller studies with different pooled outcomes. Utilize larger doses of levodopa and schedule the doses closer together with the hope of providing a more continuous "on" state. It should be noted that this strategy often precipitates peak-dose dyskinesia.

Treatment of "off" dystonia

Dystonia can be caused by levodopa or PD itself, so it can occur during both the "on" and "off" states. Therefore, a careful history, noting the relationship between the timing of dystonia and the timing of levodopa administration, is critically important. Generally, "off" dystonia is much more common than "on" dystonia and frequently occurs in the morning, manifested as painful dystonic cramping of the toes and feet on wakening. This symptom, termed early-morning dystonia, occurs as a result of the wearing off of the levodopa overnight. Several treatment options are available, as follows:

- Add rotigotine patch or slow-release pramipexole or ropinirole.
- Add a bedtime dose of sustained-release levodopa to increase plasma concentrations of levodopa throughout the night and early morning.
- Have the patient take the first dose of levodopa before rising from bed. This strategy can be used with water-soluble levodopa, which has an onset of action of between 10 and 15 minutes.
- Use apomorphine injection.
- Botulinum toxin injections for focal dystonia can be effective without changing dopaminergic medications.

Treatment of dose failures or no "on" response and delayed "on"

In some patients with advanced PD, taking a dose of levodopa may not result in any improvement in symptoms; this is known as a dose failure. If the occurrence of dose failure is not related to a reduction in levodopa dose or appears suddenly after additional medication has been prescribed, drug interactions should be suspected. Certain medications have been reported to reduce levodopa bioavailability, including oral iron, aluminium/magnesium-containing antacids, pyridoxine, and cholesterol-lowering drugs. Recently, PD patients who received *Helicobacter pylori* eradication therapy showed a significant increase in levodopa absorption, which was coupled with a significant reduction of clinical disability and a prolonged "on" time duration. If drug interactions are excluded, it is likely that these symptoms are due to inadequate absorption of levodopa, whether as a result of an inadequate dose, slowing of gastrointestinal transit time, or competition for levodopa absorption from dietary protein. The following strategies are recommended to augment levodopa absorption:

- Withdraw anticholinergic agents.
- Relieve constipation using laxatives, for example high-fiber, fruit diet, lactulose, linaclotide, or lubiprostone.
- Instruct the patient to take the medication sufficiently in advance of meals. A high-protein meal may reduce levodopa absorption due to large neutral amino acids competing with levodopa for transfer across the intestinal mucosa and the blood–brain barrier. If this option fails, reducing any fat intake close to the time medication is taken may be helpful.

- Add domperidone (not available in the United States). Domperidone is a prokinetic D2 receptor antagonist that does not cross the blood–brain barrier. Therefore, the incidence of extrapyramidal symptoms is rare. Domperidone therapy significantly reduces upper gastrointestinal symptoms and accelerates gastric emptying of a solid meal, and does not interfere with response to antiparkinsonism treatment.
- Switch to water-soluble levodopa or immediate-release levodopa to help shorten the delay in "on" response. The sustained-release formulation often results in a more delayed "on" response and is generally not recommended in this particular situation. Dissolving immediate-release levodopa in an ascorbic acid solution or fizzy drink may improve uptake from the gut.
- Use apomorphine. This is available in two formulations – apomorphine intermittent injection and apomorphine continuous infusion – intended for different types of problems with PD. In this case, subcutaneous intermittent injection is the appropriate approach. These formulations are administered via a multidose pen, the APO-go Pen (Britannia Pharmaceuticals), or a similar device marketed in the United States. The European product is a portable subcutaneous injection device containing 30 mg apomorphine hydrochloride in 3 mL solution. In the United States, the concentration and formulation of apomorphine are the same, although the cartridge contains 20 mL. The antiparkinsonian benefits from this treatment are close to those observed with levodopa, but with a much shorter onset of effect. Apomorphine rescue injections can reliably revert "off" periods even in patients experiencing complex "on–off" motor fluctuations.

Random "on–off" (unpredictable "on–off") or "yoyoing"

As PD progresses, patients may develop an unpredictable "on–off" response to medication, such that motor function does not follow levodopa dosing cycles. The typical example is that the medication may kick in, but well before the time of the next dose there is an abrupt "off" period (without warning), unlike the gradual "off" time that develops in the wearing-off response. There is a complete loss of predictability and, therefore, patients will not know when they will be able to perform activities. Usually, they have severe akinetic "off" periods, accompanied by severe dyskinesias during the "on" stage.

This is one of the most difficult fluctuations to treat. Patients at this stage are very sensitive to manipulations of even small doses of levodopa. The fine tuning of medications at this stage has to be individualized. However, sustained-release formulations are best avoided because their bioavailability is unpredictable. Other approaches to consider are as follows:

- Add a COMT inhibitor. It is recommended that a COMT inhibitor be gradually titrated, for example initially 100 mg of entacapone, to avoid disabling dyskinesias.
- Try a different dopamine agonist if the current one is not helpful.
- Implement a protein-redistribution diet. Because patients at this stage have a decreased capacity to store dopamine centrally, a minor reduction in levodopa transport into the brain can lead to a dramatic reduction in striatal dopamine levels, resulting in an "off" episode.
- Consider Duodopa. Recently, a novel formulation of infusible levodopa (LD) has been developed in which the drug is embedded in a carboxymethylcellulose gel, providing a concentration of LD/CD (carbidopa) of 2.0/0.5 g in only a single 100 mL infusion (Duodopa). A 100 mL cassette contains 2 g of LD for a full day's coverage. It is delivered through a portable pump that has programmable delivery rates between 10 and 200 mg of LD/h intrajejunally through a percutaneous endoscopic gastrostomy tube in which the tip is positioned below the Treitz band in the proximal jejunum. Duodopa has been shown to produce a clear improvement in motor fluctuations and dyskinesias. The main problems related to Duodopa treatments are severe gastrointestinal complications and peripheral neuropathy.
- Consider surgical procedures such as deep brain stimulation (DBS). Both the globus pallidus interna (GPi) and the subthalamic nucleus (STN) are common surgical targets for DBS. However, STN has been proposed as the preferred surgical target site for treating motor complications. Bilateral STN DBS has been shown to provide patients with a full range of antiparkinsonian benefits, including improvements in tremor, bradykinesia, and rigidity. In addition, stimulation of the STN may allow levodopa doses to be lowered, thereby reducing the severity of levodopa-related dyskinesias.
- Use apomorphine. Continuous subcutaneous apomorphine infusion is administered via a pump device using a subcutaneous catheter (Britannia Pharmaceuticals). It is usually worn on a belt or around the neck. The apomorphine dose can be adjusted for continuous delivery over a period ranging from 12–24 (usually 16) hours a day. Continuous administration over 24 hours may result in tolerance. This phenomenon tends to resolve rapidly. Thereafter, the infusion period should be reduced by at least 2–4 h per day.

Treatment of Parkinson's disease psychosis

More than 50% of patients with PD have psychosis at some time. This psychosis includes both delusions and hallucination. Best practice treatment guidelines include initial consideration of comorbidities and reduction of dopaminergic therapy. Atypical antipsychotics are commonly used and include quetiapine, risperidone, and olanzapine. The latter two drugs are poorly tolerated. Quetiapine is more often used, mostly in small doses, despite failure in the four largest randomized controlled trials. Clozapine has shown antipsychotic benefit without worsening motor symptoms in several randomized controlled trials. However, clozapine is associated with increased risk of agranulocytosis. Recently pimavanserin has been shown to be effective in Parkinson's psychosis at dose of 40 mg once a day.

Treatment of non-motor symptoms

Non-motor symptoms may have a bigger impact on quality of life than motor symptoms in some circumstances. Some of the symptoms can precede the diagnosis, but they become more frequent as the illness progresses. Depression may improve with the selective serotonin reuptake inhibitor paroxetine (20–40 mg/day), the serotonin-noradrenaline (norepinephrine) reuptake inhibitor venlafaxine (75–100 mg), and the tricyclic antidepressants desipramine (up to 100 mg/day) and nortriptyline (up to 150 mg/day).

Case reports and small series have suggested positive effects of methylphenidate, levodopa and selegiline as well as mixed noradrenergic–serotonergic reuptake inhibitors. Given that the mechanism of apathy in PD is multifactorial, treatment strategies should also include psychotherapy and related non-pharmacological techniques. Methylphenidate (5 mg twice a day) reduces apathy in the early stage of the disease. Apathy occurs in PD patients following STN stimulation after tapering of dopaminergic medication is relieved by the administration of dopamine agonist.

Fatigue could be treated with methylphenidate or modafinil.

Dementia in Parkinson's patients improves with rivastigmine or donepezil, but memantine and galantamine are also used.

Sleep disorders are present in most Parkinson's patients. Treatment of excessive daytime sleepiness (EDS) involves regular daytime exercise and regular hours of sleep at night. Furthermore caffeine, modafinil (Provigil®), and armodafinil (Nuvigil®) improve excessive daytime sleepiness, but modafinil has a shorter half-life. Sodium oxybate (Xyrem®; Jazz Pharmaceuticals) is a unique compound approved by the US Food and Drug Administration for the treatment of cataplexy and EDS in patients with narcolepsy. It is a metabolite of γ-aminobutyric acid with a very short half-life and short clinical effect, usually 2.5–4.0 hours. Therefore, two doses are used to achieve a typical full night of sleep, one at initiation of sleep and the other 4 hours later. Nocturnal sodium oxybate improves excessive daytime sleepiness and fatigue in PD patients.

Insomnia could be treated with the short-acting benzodiazepines, zopiclone, zaleplon, eszopiclone, and amitriptyline. Night-time apomorphine infusion or rotigotine patch may help in cases of insomnia due to severe nighttime rigidity, restless legs syndrome, and "off" periods.

For REM sleep behavior disorder clonazepam is usually the first line of treatment, but treatment may include melatonin, rotigotine patch, or pramipexole.

Orthostatic hypotension requires both non-pharmacological and pharmacological therapies. Non-pharmacological therapies include increased salt and water intake, waist-high support stockings, physical counter-maneuvers, and avoidance of volume-depleting drugs (diuretics, antihypertensives).

Pharmacological therapy includes fludrocortisone 0.1 mg/day or midodrine (10 mg twice a day). Pyridostigmine is a cholinesterase inhibitor that improves ganglionic neurotransmission in the sympathetic baroreflex pathway. Because this pathway is activated primarily during standing, this drug improves orthostatic hypotension and total peripheral resistance without aggravating supine hypertension. The pressor effect is modest; it is most adequate for patients with mild to moderate orthostatic hypotension. Dosing is started at 30 mg 2–3 times a day and is gradually increased to 60 mg 3 times a day. The drug's effectiveness can be enhanced by combining each dose of pyridostigmine with 5 mg of midodrine without occurrence of supine hypertension. Mestinon Timespan®, a 180 mg slow-release pyridostigmine tablet, can be taken once a day and may be a convenient alternative. The main side effects are cholinergic (abdominal colic, diarrhea). L-threo-3,4-dihidroxyphenylserine (Northera®) is used for refractory orthostatic hypotension. The drug is slowly titrated from 100 mg 3 times a day to the maintenance dose of 600 mg 3 times a day.

Drooling occurs in many Parkinson's patients, mainly due to decreased clearance. Pharmacological intervention includes oral atropine drops (2–3 times a day), botulinum toxin A or B into the parotid and submandibular injections, glycopyrrolate (1–4 mg/day), and ipratropium bromide spray (Atrovent) 1–2 doses per day sublingually.

Conclusion

Due to the improvement of medical and surgical treatments for PD, there are several therapeutic options for physicians to consider for their patients. However, the most important principle in the management of PD is to customize therapy to the needs of individual patients. The selection should be based on scientific rationale and evidence-based data. The aim should be not only to control motoric symptoms, but also to prevent or delay motor complications if possible. There are no proven neuroprotective drugs, but several agents have been found to have at least a levodopa-sparing effect or to reduce the risk of freezing. Surgical interventions should be reserved for patients with intractable motor complications. Because certain symptoms, for example dysarthria, dysphagia, and axial symptoms, may not respond to dopaminergic therapy, other neurochemicals may be involved and could be targets of future research.

Further reading

Bhidayasiri R., Truong DD. Motor complications in Parkinson disease: Clinical manifestations and management. *J Neurol Sci* 2008;266(1–2):204–215.

Braak H, Del Tredici K, Rub U, *et al*. Staging of brain pathology related to sporadic Parkinson's disease. *Neurobiol Aging* 2003;24:197–211.

Goetz CG, Poewe W, Rascol O, Sampaio C. Evidence-based medical review update: Pharmacological and surgical treatments of Parkinson's disease: 2001 to 2004. *Mov Disord* 2005;20:523–539.

Horstink M, Tolosa E, Bonuccelli U, *et al*. Review of the therapeutic management of Parkinson's disease. Report of a joint task force of the European Federation of Neurological Societies and the Movement Disorder Society – European Section. Part I: Early (uncomplicated) Parkinson's disease. *Eur J Neurol* 2006;13:1170–1185.

Horstink M, Tolosa E, Bonuccelli U, *et al*. Review of the therapeutic management of Parkinson's disease. Report of a joint task force of the European Federation of Neurological Societies (EFNS) and the Movement Disorder Society – European Section (MDS-ES). Part II: Late (complicated) Parkinson's disease. *Eur J Neurol* 2006;13:1186–1202.

Miyasaki JM, Shannon K, Voon V, *et al*. Practice parameter: Evaluation and treatment of depression, psychosis, and dementia in Parkinson disease (an evidence-based review): Report of the Quality Standards Subcommittee of the American Academy of Neurology. *Neurology* 2006;66:996–1002.

Pahwa R, Factor SA, Lyons KE, *et al*. Practice Parameter: Treatment of Parkinson disease with motor fluctuations and dyskinesia (an evidence-based review): Report of the Quality Standards Subcommittee of the American Academy of Neurology. *Neurology* 2006;66:983–995.

Suchowersky O, Gronseth G, Perlmutter J, *et al*. Practice Parameter: Neuroprotective strategies and alternative therapies for Parkinson disease (an evidence-based review): Report of the Quality Standards Subcommittee of the American Academy of Neurology. *Neurology* 2006;66:976–982.

Suchowersky O, Reich S, Perlmutter J, *et al*. Practice Parameter: Diagnosis and prognosis of new onset Parkinson disease (an evidence-based review): Report of the Quality Standards Subcommittee of the American Academy of Neurology. *Neurology* 2006;66:968–975.

Truong DD, Bhidayasiri R, Wolters E. Management of non-motor symptoms in advanced Parkinson disease. *J Neurol Sci* 2008;266(1–2):216–228.

Verstraeten A, Theuns J, Van Broeckhoven C. Progress in unraveling the genetic etiology of Parkinson disease in a genomic era. *Trends Genet* 2015;31:140–149.

51 Dystonia

Stanley Fahn

Department of Neurology, Columbia University Medical Center, New York, USA

Dystonia is the second most common movement disorder seen by neurologists after parkinsonism. The most recent definition of dystonia agreed to by a consensus committee is: "Dystonia is a movement disorder characterized by sustained or intermittent muscle contractions causing abnormal, often repetitive, movements, postures, or both. Dystonic movements are typically patterned, twisting, and may be tremulous. Dystonia is often initiated or worsened by voluntary action and associated with overflow muscle activation." "Patterned" as used here indicates that the involuntary movements affect the same muscles repeatedly and do not travel in a random fashion to involve other muscles, as with choreic movements.

Limb, axial, and cranial voluntary muscles can all be affected by dystonia. When the dystonic movements are present only during voluntary movements, it is called *action dystonia*. If the dystonic contractions appear only with a specific action, it is referred to as *task-specific dystonia* (e.g., writer's cramp and musician's cramp). Dystonic movements that appear while the affected body part is at rest are considered a more advanced stage of dystonia. Sustained abnormal postures may be the eventual outcome.

Dystonic movements tend to be suppressed with relaxation, hypnosis, and sleep; they tend to increase with fatigue, stress, and emotional states. Dystonia often disappears during deep sleep. A characteristic and almost unique feature of dystonic movements is that they can be diminished by tactile or proprioceptive "sensory tricks" (gestes antagonistes). For example, patients with cervical dystonia (torticollis) often place a hand on the chin or side of the face to reduce nuchal contractions, and orolingual dystonia is often helped by touching the lips or placing an object in the mouth. Lying down or sitting may reduce truncal dystonia; walking backward or running may reduce leg dystonia.

Epidemiology

A number of epidemiological studies in dystonia have been carried out, particularly on primary focal dystonia and a few studies on generalized dystonia. In a study on the Mayo Clinic population, the prevalence of generalized dystonia was found to be 3.4 per 100,000 population, and the prevalence of focal dystonia to be 30 per 100,000. The frequency of primary dystonia in the Ashkenazi Jewish population is much higher, around 1 per 6000. The high prevalence in that population is due to the occurrence of the DYT1 mutation in an individual in the historic Jewish Pale of settlement (Lithuania and Byelorussia), approximately 400 years ago. Focal dystonia is more common than segmental dystonia, which is much more common than generalized dystonia. The prevalence rate of focal dystonias varies in different countries, being slightly lower in Japan (between 6 and 14 per 100,000) than in Western Europe (between 11 and 14 per 100,000).

Pathobiology

Pathology

Dystonia is a disorder of the central nervous system that can occur either without obvious structural lesions or with damage in the putamen or its connections (including thalamus and cerebral cortex) caused by environmental insults or heredodegenerative diseases. Environmental causes include encephalitis, trauma, strokes, toxicants, and antipsychotic drugs (resulting in acute dystonic reactions and tardive dystonia). Heredodegenerative forms of dystonia include Wilson's disease and neurodegenerations with brain iron accumulation. Some environmental dystonias (e.g., due to antipsychotic drugs) and some hereditary dystonias (e.g., dopa-responsive dystonia, Oppenheim dystonia) cause no known structural damage.

Etiology

Dystonia can be caused by genetic mutations (inherited dystonia) and environmental insults (acquired dystonia), but by far the most common are focal dystonias without any known cause (idiopathic dystonia). The last group makes up the majority of patients with dystonia. The major inherited and acquired dystonias are listed in Table 51.1.

Genetics

A large number of gene mutations have been discovered to cause both primary (non-structural) dystonia and degenerative dystonia. The heredodegenerative dystonias are listed in Table 51.1. These are divided into autosomal dominant, autosomal recessive, X-linked, and mitochondrial disorders. Typically these diseases result in progressive degenerative changes in the basal ganglia and their connections. These can usually be detected by magnetic resonance (MR) neuroimaging and a metabolic workup. Neurodegenerations with brain iron accumulations (NBIAs) are clinically detected by the presence of high iron content in the globus pallidus and other brain regions, manifested by decreased signal intensity in T2-weighted images.

The majority of patients with dystonia are without structural lesions in the brain. These so-called primary dystonias can be genetic or idiopathic. The genetic forms are classified with a DYT label. One heredodegenerative dystonia and the paroxysmal dyskinesias are

International Neurology, Second edition. Edited by Robert P. Lisak, Daniel D. Truong, William M. Carroll and Roongroj Bhidayasiri
© 2016 John Wiley & Sons, Ltd. Published 2016 by John Wiley & Sons, Ltd.

Table 51.1 Principal dystonic disorders by etiology.

A. Inherited, no structural lesions, isolated dystonia
1. Oppenheim dystonia (also called DYT1)
   Autosomal dominant inheritance of mutated *TOR1A* gene.Early onset (< age 40), affecting limbs first
   All populations affected, with highest prevalence in the Ashkenazi Jewish population
2. Childhood and adult onset, familial cranial and limb (DYT6)
   Autosomal dominant inheritance of mutated *THAP1* gene on 8p11.21
   Childhood- and adult-onset affecting all populations, especially the Mennonite and Amish populations
3. Adult-onset familial torticollis (DYT7)
   Autosomal dominant inheritance mapped to 18p
4. Adult-onset familial cervical-cranial predominant (DYT13)
   Autosomal dominant inheritance mapped to 1p36
5. Other DYT disorders listed in Table 51.2
6. Sporadic, usually adult-onset, usually focal or segmental

B. Inherited, no structural lesions, isolated dystonia
1. Dystonia with parkinsonism
   a. Dopa-responsive dystonia (DRD) (DYT5)
      1. GTP cyclohydrolase I deficiency
         Autosomal dominant inheritance located at 14q22.1
         Childhood onset with leg and gait disorder, may be diurnal
         Adult onset with parkinsonism
      2.Tyrosine hydroxylase deficiency
         Autosomal recessive inheritance
         Infantile onset
   b. Rapid-onset dystonia-parkinsonism (RDP) (DYT12)
      Autosomal dominant inheritance of mutated Na-K-ATPase gene (ATP1A3)
      Adolescent and adult onset progresses over hours to a few weeks,then plateaus
2.Dystonia with myoclonic jerks that respond to alcohol
   Myoclonus-dystonia with childhood, adolescent, and adult onset
   Autosomal dominant inheritance of the epsilon-sarcoglycan gene on chromosome 7q21 (DYT11)
   Autosomal dominant inheritance on 18p11 (DYT15)

C. Inherited, degenerative dystonia (typically **not** pure dystonia)
1. X-linked recessive
   a. Lubag (X-linked dystonia-parkinsonism) (DYT3)
      TAF1 gene, Filipino males, steadily progressive -> disabling
      Parkinsonism can appear at onset and be only feature or develop after and replace dystonia
      Pathology: mosaic gliosis in striatum
2. Autosomal dominant
   a. Juvenile parkinsonism (presenting with dystonia)
   b. Huntington disease (usually presents as chorea)
      Gene: IT15 located at 4p16.3 for huntington protein
   c. Neurodegeneration with brain iron accumulation type 3 (neuroferritinopathy),
      FTLI mutation at 19q13.33
3. Autosomal recessive
   a. Wilson's disease
      Gene: Cu-ATPase located at 13q14.3
   b. Niemann–Pick type C (dystonic lipidosis) (sea-blue histiocytosis)
      defect in cholesterol esterification; *NPC1*gene at 18q11.2
   c. Juvenile neuronal ceroid-lipofuscinosis (Batten disease)
   d. GM1 gangliosidosis
   e. GM2 gangliosidosis
   f. Metachromatic leukodystrophy
   g. Lesch–Nyhan syndrome
   h. Homocystinuria
   i. Glutaric acidemia
   j. Neurodegeneration with brain iron accumulation Type 1, pantothenate kinase-associated neurodegeneration (PKAN)
   k. Neurodegeneration with brain iron accumulation Type 2, infantile neuroaxonal dystrophy (PLAN) (*PLA2G6* mutation) (PARK14)
   l. Other neurodegeneration with brain iron accumulation (MPAN, C19orf12 mutation at 19q12; CoPAN, *COASY* mutation at 17q21.2; Aceruloplasminemia, CP mutation at 3q24-q25; FAHN, *FA2H* mutation at 16q23.1)
   m. Neuroacanthocytosis
4. Mitochondrial
   a. Leigh disease
   b. Leber disease

D. Acquired, no structural lesions, dystonia
   Drug-induced – levodopa, dopamine D2 receptor blocking agents
   Psychogenic
E. Acquired, static lesions, dystonia
1. Perinatal cerebral injury
2. Encephalitis, infectious, and postinfectious
3. Head trauma
4. Basal ganglia, thalamus or cortical lesions
5. Hypoxia
6. Peripheral injury
7. Toxins – Mn, CO, cyanide
8. Metabolic-hypoparathyroidism
9. Immune encephalopathy: Sjögren's syndrome, Rasmussen's syndrome
F. Dystonia present in other neurological syndromes
1. Parkinsonism – Parkinson's disease, progressive supranuclear palsy, multiple system atrophy, cortical-basal ganglionic degeneration
2. Tourette syndrome (dystonic tics)
3. Paroxysmal dyskinesias

Source: Adapted from Fahn 2011. Reproduced with permission of Elsevier.

also classified with a DYT label, which makes the DYTs a complicated mixture of disorders. In fact, these disorders should have been classified as a separate entity. Table 51.2 lists the DYT classification disorders.

Pathophysiology

The pathophysiology of primary dystonia remains unclear, but recent studies imply that both the basal ganglia and the cerebellum are involved. Positron emission tomography (PET) has identified a range of changes, including increased resting glucose metabolism in the premotor cortex and lentiform nucleus and decreased D2 dopamine receptor binding in the putamen. Standard MRIs have not revealed structural pathology, but diffusion tensor imaging has shown subtle abnormalities in sensorimotor circuitry of dystonia patients. Human and animal models of DYT1 dystonia reveal that a cerebellar outflow tract disruption between cerebellum and thalamus is associated with disease manifestation, provided that the remainder of the cerebellothalamocortical pathway is intact. In contrast, non-manifesting DYT1 gene carriers have an additional disruption in this pathway between thalamus and cerebral cortex.

Electromyography (EMG) in the dystonias shows co-contraction of agonist and antagonist muscles, with prolonged bursts and overflow to extraneous muscles. Physiological studies are consistent with a decrease in inhibitory control and an increase of brain plasticity. Spinal and brainstem reflex abnormalities, including reduced reciprocal inhibition and protracted blink reflex recovery, indicate a reduced presynaptic inhibition of muscle afferent input to the inhibitory interneurons as a result of defective descending motor control. Because primary dystonia is etiologically heterogeneous, there are probably several different (possibly converging) pathways that lead to these changes, producing a common clinical picture of dystonic muscle contractions.

Classification

A recent revision of the classification of torsion dystonia utilizes two major axes: Clinical Features and Etiology. The Clinical Features axis has five sections, and the Etiology axis has two sections (Table 51.3). The five sections of the Clinical Features axis are age at onset, body distribution, temporal pattern, presence of other movement disorders, and presence of systemic manifestations. Prognosis of primary dystonia correlates with age at onset. As a general rule, the younger the age at onset, the more likely that the dystonia will

Table 51.2 DYT gene nomenclature for the dystonias.

Name	Locus	Inheritance pattern	Phenotype	Gene, product
DYT1	9q34.11	AD	Early onset, limb onset (Oppenheim dystonia)	*TOR1A*, TorsinA
DYT2	Unknown	AR	Early onset	Unknown
DYT3	Xq13.1	XR	Filipino, X-linked dystonia-parkinsonism (Lubag)	*TAF1*
DYT4	19p13.3	AD	Generalized dystonia with spasmodic dysphonia	*TUBB4A*, Beta-tubulin 4a
DYT5a	14q22.2	AD	Dopa-responsive dystonia (DRD) (Segawa disease)	*GCH1*, GTP cyclohydrolase 1
DYT5b	11p15.5	AR	DRD, infantile parkinsonism	TH, tyrosine hydroxylase
DYT6	8p11.21	AD	Mixed type, onset often with spasmodic dysphonia, Mennonite/Amish and others	*THAP1*
DYT7	18p	AD	Adult cervical	Unknown
DYT8	2q35	AD	Paroxysmal non-kinesigenic dyskinesia (Mount–Rebak)	Formerly called myofibrillogenesis regulator 1, now *PNKD*, PNKD protein
DYT9	1p34.2	AD	Paroxysmal choreoathetosis with episodic ataxia and spasticity	(Now known to be the gene for GLUT1; same as DYT18)
DYT10	16p11.2	AD	Paroxysmal kinesigenic dyskinesia (PKD) (EKD1)	*PRRT2* gene, proline rich transmembrane protein 2
DYT11	7q21.3	AD	Myoclonus-dystonia	*SGCE*, epsilon-sarcoglycan
DYT12	19q13.2	AD	Rapid-onset dystonia-parkinsonism (RDP)	*ATP1A3*, Na+/K+-ATPase alpha 3 subunit
DYT13	1p36	AD	Cervical–cranial–brachial	Unknown
DYT15	18p11	AD	Myoclonus-dystonia	Unknown
DYT16	2q31.2	AR	Early-onset dystonia-parkinsonism	*PRKRA*
DYT17	20p11.2-q13	AR	Juvenile onset with torticollis, spreading to segmental and generalized dystonia	Unknown
DYT18	1p34.2	AD	Paroxysmal exertional dyskinesia (PED)	*SLC2A1*, glucose transporter 1 (GLUT1)
DYT19	16q13-q21	AD	Paroxysmal kinesigenic dyskinesia without epilepsy (EKD2)	Unknown
DYT20	2q31	AD	Paroxysmal nonkinesigenic dyskinesia (PNKD2)	Unknown
DYT21	2q14.3-q21.3	AD	Adult-onset mixed dystonia, only in Sweden so far	Unknown
DYT23	9q34.11	AD	Cervical dystonia	*CIZ1* (CDKN1A-Interacting Zinc Finger Protein 1)
DYT24	11p14.2	AD	Cervical-cranial-brachial dystonia (jerky torticollis)	*ANO3* (anoctamin 3)
DYT25	18p11.21	AD	Cervical-cranial dystonia	*GNAL* (guanine nucleotide-binding protein alpha-activating)

Genetic nomenclature is presented in the chronological order given. The DYT1 gene has a deletion of one of a sequential pair of GAG triplets. DYT2 is designated for any possible autosomal-recessive forms of primary dystonia. DYT3 is associated with X-linked dystonia-parkinsonism, also known as Lubag, and encountered in Filipino males. It appears to be caused by mutations that lead to reduced expression of the transcription factor TATA-box binding protein-associated factor 1. It is the only disorder in this table that is a neurodegenerative disease. The other conditions in the table have not been associated with degeneration. DYT4 was labeled for an Australian family with dystonia, including a whispering dysphonia. DYT5a is for the GTP cyclohydrolase I gene mutations causing autosomal-dominant dopa-responsive dystonia (DRD). DYT5b is for autosomal-recessive DRD and infantile parkinsonism associated with mutations in the gene for tyrosine hydroxylase. DYT6 is the gene causing an adult- and childhood-onset dystonia of cranial, cervical, and limb muscles (mixed), initially discovered in a large Mennonite/Amish kindred, but now known to exist worldwide. DYT7 denotes familial torticollis in a family from northwest Germany. DYT8–10 are for paroxysmal dyskinesias: 8 is for non-kinesigenic type (PNKD), known as the Mount–Rebak syndrome; 9 is for a family with episodic choreoathetosis and spasticity, now recognized to be the same as DYT18; 10 is for paroxysmal kinesigenic dyskinesia (PKD) on chromosome 16. The same gene mutation can cause episodic ataxia and hemiplegic migraine. DYT11 has been named for mutations in the epsilon-sarcoglycan gene that causes myoclonus-dystonia. DYT12 is for the Na+/K+-ATPase alpha3 subunit gene mapped to chromosome 19q causing rapid-onset dystonia-parkinsonism. Speech is often involved. This gene mutation also can cause alternating hemiplegia of childhood. DYT13 is for gene mapped to 1p36 causing cervical–cranial–brachial dystonia in a family in Italy. DYT15 is for a myoclonus-dystonia family mapped to 18p11. DYT16 is for the stress-response gene *PRKRA*, which encodes the protein kinase, interferon-inducible double-stranded RNA-dependent activator identified in Brazilian families with early-onset dystonia-parkinsonism. DYT17 is for juvenile-onset cervical dystonia that can become generalized. DYT18 is paroxysmal exertional dyskinesia (PED) due to a gene mutation in the glucose transporter. DYT19 causes another form of PKD without epilepsy. DYT20 causes a second form of PNKD. DYT21 was found in a Swedish family with dystonia. DYT23 causes familial cervical dystonia. DYT24 causes jerky torticollis. DYT25 results in cervical-cranial segmental dystonia.

AD = autosomal dominant; AR = autosomal recessive; DRD = dopa-responsive dystonia; M-D = myoclonus-dystonia; RDP = rapid-onset dystonia-parkinsonism; XR = X-linked recessive

become severe and spread to multiple parts of the body. In contrast, the older the age at onset, the more likely that dystonia will remain focal. Onset with leg involvement is the second most important predictive factor for a more rapidly progressive course.

Dystonia usually begins in a single body part, and either remains focal or spreads to other body parts. When a single body part is affected, the condition is referred to as *focal dystonia*. Common forms of focal dystonia are spasmodic torticollis (cervical dystonia), blepharospasm (upper facial dystonia), and writer's cramp (hand and arm dystonia). Involvement of two or more contiguous regions of the body is referred to as *segmental dystonia*. *Generalized dystonia* indicates involvement of trunk plus at least two other parts of the body. *Multifocal dystonia* involves two or more non-contiguous regions, not conforming to segmental or generalized dystonia. *Hemidystonia* refers to involvement of the arm and leg on the same side and is usually symptomatic in causation.

Table 51.3 Classification of torsion dystonia.

Clinical features	Etiology
1. Age at onset	1. Neuropathology
Infancy (birth to 2 yrs)	Degenerations
Childhood (3–12 yrs)	Static lesions
Adolescence (13–20 yrs)	No structural lesion
Early adulthood (21–40 yrs)	2. Inherited or acquired
Late adulthood (>40 yrs)	Inherited
2. Body distribution	Acquired
Focal (single body region)	Idiopathic
Segmental (2 or more contiguous regions)	
Multifocal (2 or more non-contiguous regions)	
Generalized (trunk + 2 or more other regions)	
Hemidystonia (unilateral arm + leg ± face)	
3. Temporal pattern	
Persistent	
Action induced	
Diurnal	
Paroxysmal	
4. Associated features (presence of other movement disorder)	
Isolated dystonia (dystonia is the only motor feature, with the exception of tremor)	
Combined dystonia (dystonia is combined with other movement disorders such as myoclonus, parkinsonism, etc.)	
5. Other neurological or systemic manifestations	
e.g., presence of cognitive impairment or psychiatric symptoms	

Source: Albanese 2013, Reproduced with permission of Wiley.

The temporal pattern distinguishes between the great majority of dystonias that are continual. A diurnal pattern is sometimes seen in dopa-responsive dystonia, being mild or absent in the morning and worsening as the day goes on. Paroxysmal dystonia belongs to a separate movement disorder, paroxysmal dyskinesias.

The section of associated features separates those dystonias that are isolated (no other movement disorder present, with the exception of tremor) and those dystonias that are combined with other movement disorders, the most common being parkinsonism and myoclonus.

The second axis in the current classification is the Etiology axis. It includes pathology as well as etiology. Both pathology and etiology have been discussed earlier and are summarized in Tables 51.1 and 51.2.

Clinical features

Some clinical features of dystonia were described at the beginning of the chapter. The speed of dystonic contractions can be slow or fast, even reaching the speed of myoclonus. Dystonic contractions are of relatively long duration compared to myoclonus and chorea, and dystonic contractions usually result in a twisting of the affected body part (rather than simply flexion or extension). The dystonic movement usually is activated or made worse when the involved body part moves voluntarily. For example, a child with DYT1 dysto-

nia may manifest twisting and elevation of a leg when walking forward, but not when walking backward or running (or when sitting or lying). As the disorder worsens, there is less selectivity, and the muscles can be involved even while at rest. Whereas primary dystonia often begins as action dystonia and may persist as the kinetic form, secondary dystonia often begins as fixed postures.

Body position is another important factor. Dystonia may be absent when the patient is sitting and appear when the patient stands up. Dystonic tremor is usually not completely rhythmic compared to parkinsonian tremor or essential tremor. Cervical dystonia is often associated with arrhythmic tremor of the neck; the tremor is always in the horizontal plane. Some patients with primary dystonia may manifest tremor of the arms and hands that resembles essential tremor.

When evaluating a patient with dystonia, the first question is: "Is dystonia present, or is the involved muscle tight because of guarding from pain, or is it rigidity?" Then determine whether it is isolated dystonia (no other movement disorder present) or combined dystonia (another movement disorder is present, often parkinsonism or myoclonus). This step will then point to the diagnosis to a considerable degree. The presence or absence of other neurological signs would direct one into considering an acquired or neurodegenerative diagnosis. Other features, such as age at onset, family history, rate of progression, body parts involved, and MRI results will also guide the evaluator to a diagnosis. Some genes are commercially available for testing, and this should be pursued when those gene mutations are within the differential diagnosis. There are specific syndromes of various types of dystonia, and recognizing their features will help lead one to the correct diagnosis. These are discussed next.

Adult-onset focal dystonias

These are the most common forms of dystonia. Their appearance varies depending on which body part is affected. Although most cases remain focal, dystonia can spread to a contiguous, neighboring segment, thus becoming segmental myoclonus. The most common focal dystonia involves the neck musculature, known as *spasmodic torticollis* or *cervical dystonia*. The head can turn (rotational torticollis), tilt, or shift to one side, or bend forward (antecollis) or backward (retrocollis). Any combination of head positions can be found in individual patients. About 10% have a remission within a year, but relapses usually occur, even many years later. The average age at onset is between 20 and 50 years. The muscles involved are innervated by cranial nerve (CN) XI and the upper cervical nerve roots. Some cervical dystonias are manifested as a static pulling of the head into one direction, but many have a jerky, irregular rhythmic feature. In this situation, the main differential diagnosis is essential tremor. Some patients try to fight the pulling of the neck muscles and the physician can be misled by seeing or feeling contracted muscles, thinking that these are the dystonic muscles, when in fact they could be the compensatory muscles contracting. To distinguish between involuntary and compensatory/voluntary contractions, the patient should be told to let the movements occur without trying to overcome them. Then the true direction of which muscles are involved by the dystonia is revealed. This is especially important when deciding which muscles to inject with botulinum toxin (see Treatment section). Common sensory tricks to reduce dystonia are touching the face or the back of the head. Mechanical devices to place cutaneous pressure on the occiput can sometimes be used to advantage.

Blepharospasm usually occurs in older individuals, women more often than men. It begins as excessive blinking, and many patients complain of eye irritation or dryness, although dry eyes from Sjögren's syndrome are usually ruled out. This blinking phase then leads to some longer closing of the eyes, even for very long durations. Usually there is a combination of eyelid closing and blinking. The muscles involved are the orbicularis oculi innervated by CN VII, and the movements are symmetric in the two eyes, quite distinct from hemifacial spasm, which is unilateral. One interesting difference is that in blepharospasm the eyebrows come down, while in hemifacial spasm the eyebrow elevates with contraction of the ipsilateral frontalis muscle. In ptosis the eyebrow may elevate because the patient is trying to open the eyelids by simultaneously contracting the frontalis muscles.

Dystonia can spread from upper face blepharospasm to the lower face with movements around the mouth. Common sensory tricks to reduce blepharospasm are touching the corner of the eye, coughing, and talking. Bright light notoriously aggravates blepharospasm and patients have difficulty being in sunlight or bright light, and they often wear sunglasses most of the time. Driving at night is very difficult because of oncoming headlights.

Oromandibular dystonia (OMD), which affects jaw muscles innervated by CN V, is often associated with lingual dystonia (tongue muscles by CN XII), and is less frequent than blepharospasm. Jaw-opening dystonia is where the jaw is pulled down by the pterygoids; in jaw-clenching dystonia the masseters and temporalis muscles are the prime movers. The jaw can also be moved laterally. It is important to distinguish the latter from facial muscle pulling of the mouth to one side, which is of psychogenic etiology. OMD can markedly affect chewing and swallowing. Some OMDs appear only with action and are not present at rest. Such actions can involve talking or chewing. Often a patient attempts to overcome jaw-opening and jaw-closing dystonias by purposefully moving the jaw in the opposite direction. This maneuvering has frequently led to misdiagnosis of tardive dyskinesia, because the movements superficially appear rhythmic. To distinguish between OMD and tardive dyskinesia, the patient should be told to let the movements occur without trying to overcome them. In this manner, the true direction of where the dystonia wants to take the jaw is revealed, and the rhythmic movements stop in OMD. Sensory tricks that have been useful are the placing of objects in the mouth or biting down on an object, such as a tongue blade or pencil. Dental implants have sometimes helped by the physical application of a continual sensory trick.

Embouchure dystonia is an action dystonia involving the muscles around the mouth (embouchure) that may develop in professional musicians who play woodwind and horn instruments. More common are *musician's cramps* involving the fingers in instrumentalists such as pianists, guitarists, violinists, and those playing other stringed instruments. This is a form of occupational cramp, the most common being *writer's cramp*. These are task-specific dystonias. In writer's cramp, only the action of writing brings out the dystonic tightening of the finger, hand, forearm, and arm muscles, such as the triceps. If the dystonia progresses, other actions of the arm, like finger-to-nose maneuver, buttoning, and sewing, bring out the dystonia. Ultimately, dystonia at rest can develop, but usually does not. In about 15% of patients with writer's cramp the dystonia will spread to the other arm. Otherwise, the patient can learn to write with the uninvolved arm. Sensory tricks that have been useful are placing the pen/pencil between other fingers, using larger writing implements, and placing the non-writing hand on top of the writing hand.

Dystonia of the vocal cords has two presentations: adduction and abduction of the cords with speaking. The former is much more common and produces a tight, constricted, strangulated type of voice with frequent pauses breaking up the voice, and it takes longer to complete what the patient is trying to say. The latter produces a whispering voice. With dystonic adductor dysphonia, the patient is still able to whisper normally, and may present this way to the physician, who needs to be aware that this is a compensating mechanism. A major differential diagnosis is vocal cord tremor, seen fairly commonly in patients with essential tremor.

Focal trunk dystonia can present in adults, both as primary dystonia and as tardive dystonia. The dystonia is usually absent when the patient is lying or sitting, and appears on standing and walking. This is an uncommon form of adult-onset focal dystonia.

Oppenheim dystonia

Oppenheim dystonia was named after Hermann Oppenheim, who coined the term dystonia in 1911 to describe Jewish children with what he called dystonia musculorum deformans. More recently, following genetic studies, it is now more commonly known as DYT1 dystonia. The gene (*TOR1A*) codes for the protein torsinA, found in neurons in the endoplasmic reticulum. The abnormal torsinA becomes more prominently located in the nuclear envelope, which is continuous with the endoplasmic reticulum. The universal mutation in this disorder, most common in the Ashkenazi Jewish population due to a founder effect introduced about 370 years ago, is a deletion of one of an adjacent pair of GAG triplets (codes for glutamate) near the functional domain. The disorder usually begins in childhood, but sometimes in adults, and it almost always starts in either an arm or a leg. It tends to spread contiguously and in many cases (especially if it begins in a leg) becomes generalized and disabling. TorsinA is an ATPase of the heat-shock type that functions in restoring damaged proteins, particularly in membranes. The abnormal protein loses ATPase activity, with a resultant decrease as a chaperone protein. The penetrance rate is only 30%. The *TOR1A* gene can be tested commercially for the mutation, which is recommended for all patients with onset of primary dystonia below the age of 26.

Dopa-responsive dystonia (DRD)

DRD usually begins in childhood with a peculiar gait (walking on toes). Adult-onset cases tend to resemble Parkinson's disease. Even in childhood, one can detect parkinsonian features of bradykinesia and loss of postural reflexes, a feature that distinguishes this from Oppenheim dystonia. It can therefore resemble childhood-onset Parkinson's disease with dopamine nigrostriatal neuronal degeneration. The latter condition shows a depletion of F-DOPA uptake or dopamine transporter in PET and single photon emission computed tomography (SPECT) scanning, whereas these studies are normal in DRD, which does not show neuronal degeneration. The disorder is due to a mutation in the gene for guanosine triphosphate (GTP) cyclohydrolase 1, which is the rate-limiting step for synthesis of tetrahydrobiopterin, the cofactor for tyrosine hydroxylase and other hydroxylases, required for the synthesis of biogenic amines, such as dopamine. The dopamine deficiency in the striatum accounts for the symptoms, and the patients respond extremely well to low doses of levodopa. They can respond after years of no treatment, and they usually do not develop the fluctuations or dyskinesias so commonly seen in patients with Parkinson's disease. Interestingly, these patients also respond to low dosages of anticholinergic medications, such as trihexyphenidyl. Some patients show a diurnal pattern of symptoms, being almost normal in the morning and markedly dystonic at the end of the day. These patients obtain benefit from sleep.

Acquired and heredodegenerative dystonias

In examining patients with dystonia, features of a neurological insult in the medical history, such as exposure to drugs, toxins, trauma, or presence of neurological abnormality on examination, would suggest that the patient's dystonia is secondary (acquired) rather than primary. Table 51.1 lists the major causes of acquired and heredodegenerative dystonias. The most common causes of acquired dystonias seen in a busy movement disorder center are the drug-induced dystonias, especially tardive dystonia, induced by dopamine receptor blocking agents. Tardive dystonia can affect all ages, but as in classic tardive dyskinesia, older people are most susceptible. In children and adolescents, it can manifest as generalized dystonia, but it is usually reversible after a long period of being without the offending drugs. Older people are more likely to have a focal form of tardive dystonia, usually OMD, cervical dystonia, or blepharospasm. Tardive dystonia resembles primary dystonias unless there is an accompanying tardive akathisia or classic tardive dyskinesia, which allows the diagnosis to be made quite readily. When these other forms of the tardive syndromes are not present, one clinical feature of tardive dystonia that is fairly common to allow this diagnosis is the posture of hyperextension of the neck and trunk with pronated arms, extended elbows, and flexed wrists. Also the diagnosis of tardive dystonia may be suspected if the patient has had a recent exposure to dopamine receptor blocking agents.

Treatment

Treatment of the dystonias continues to evolve. Certain principles remain fundamental. Although there are agents that can often reduce the severity of dystonia, it is most important to identify specific disorders that are treatable, such as Wilson's disease, drug-induced dystonia, and infectious causes, and to treat them. Of course, as in all diseases, one needs to educate the patient and family, and provide genetic counseling. The focal dystonias of eyelids, vocal cords, jaw, neck, and limbs are more easily treated with botulinum toxin (BTX), and this is the preferred approach. Segmental and generalized dystonias require systemic pharmacological therapy, but residual focal involvement can be treated with BTX. Surgical therapy is reserved for disabling dystonia resistant to medications and/or BTX injections. However, because of successful outcomes with deep brain stimulation (DBS), surgery is started sooner now, before the patient develops fixed dystonic postures. The usual surgical target is the internal segment of the globus pallidus, and stimulation by implanted electrodes has replaced ablative surgery. The surgery usually does not provide immediate relief. Rather, improvement develops after several weeks and steadily continues until a plateau of benefit is reached. This delay in response suggests that a plastic change is taking place in the brain. The abnormal firing pattern in the pallidum is affected and modified by the stimulation, and that supposedly leads to the gradual benefit. Other targets besides the pallidum are being explored.

Pharmacological therapy, as applied in generalized dystonia, should start with a trial of levodopa to make sure that DRD is not overlooked. If that fails, the drugs with the most success are high dosages of anticholinergics (e.g., trihexyphenidyl and benztropine), baclofen, and benzodiazepines. The sooner treatment is started, the better the chance of avoiding progressive disabling dystonia. Other medications with some reported benefit are carbamazepine, a dopamine depletor (tetrabenazine or reserpine), dopamine receptor blockers, and a combination of dopamine depletor, dopamine receptor blocker, and anticholinergic medication. Because these drugs can produce intolerable side effects, they should be started at low doses and built up gradually until either therapeutic benefit or intolerable side effects are seen. Work with one drug first to determine what it can accomplish. If there is some benefit, a second drug could be added when the final dosage of the first drug is reached. Adding multiple drugs this way may provide benefit not seen with just a single drug. Peripheral side effects of anticholinergics can usually be controlled by employing pilocarpine eye drops (for blurred vision due to dilated pupils), pyridostigmine for urinary hesitation and constipation, and artificial saliva for dry mouth. Central side effects, like impaired memory, are the major limitation to reaching the high therapeutic doses needed for benefit, particularly in adults, who cannot tolerate these drugs as well as children.

DBS is helpful not only for generalized dystonia, but also for focal dystonias. DBS is increasingly being utilized when these focal dystonias fail to get adequate relief from BTX or medications. Even secondary and heredodegenerative dystonias have improved with DBS, particularly tardive dystonia, but also those in which the pallidum shows neurodegeneration, such as neurodegeneration with brain iron accumulation. In general, though, the primary dystonias, including Oppenheim dystonia, have a more favorable result. These surgical procedures are best performed at specialty centers with an experienced team of a neurosurgeon, a neurophysiologist to monitor the target during the operative procedure, and a neurologist to program the stimulators. The patient needs close follow-up to adjust the stimulator settings to their optimum. Patients with cognitive decline should not have DBS because cognition can be further impaired. Adverse effects include surgical complications (especially cerebral hemorrhage), mechanical problems with the stimulator and leads to the electrodes, infections attacking any of the inserted hardware, and neurological and behavioral changes, such as troubles with speech.

Further reading

Albanese A, Bhatia K, Bressman SB, *et al.* Phenomenology and classification of dystonia: A consensus update. *Mov Disord* 2013;28(7):863–873.

Charlesworth G, Bhatia KP, Wood NW. The genetics of dystonia: New twists in an old tale. *Brain* 2013;136(7):2017–2037.

Fahn S, Jankovic J. Hallett M. *Principles and Practice of Movement Disorders*, 2nd ed. Edinburgh: Saunders Elsevier; 2011.

Lohmann K, Klein C. Genetics of dystonia: What's known? What's new? What's next? *Mov Disord* 2013;28(7):899–905.

52 Chorea and related disorders

Roongroj Bhidayasiri[1,2], Onanong Jitkritsadakul[1], and Daniel D. Truong[3]

[1] Chulalongkorn Center of Excellence for Parkinson's Disease & Related Disorders, Faculty of Medicine, Chulalongkorn University Hospital, Bangkok Thailand

[2] Department of Rehabilitation Medicine, Juntendo University, Tokyo, Japan

[3] University of California, Riverside, Riverside, CA, USA; The Truong Neuroscience Institute, Orange Coast Memorial Medical Center, Fountain Valley, CA, USA

Chorea is characterized by irregular, flowing, non-stereotyped, random, involuntary muscle contractions. When chorea is proximal and of large amplitude, it is called *ballism*. Current neurophysiological studies confirm this overlapping of chorea and ballism. Chorea is usually exacerbated by anxiety and stress and subsides during sleep. Many patients attempt to disguise chorea by incorporating it into purposeful activities. *Athetosis* refers to sinusoidal, slow movements affecting distal limbs, particularly the arms. Therefore, the term *choreoathetosis* is often employed to describe the pattern of generalized chorea that involves the whole body, particularly distal extremities. *Pseudoathetosis* refers to slow, writhing movements in the distal limbs, caused by a lack of proprioception.

In this chapter, we summarize the current understanding of the pathophysiology of chorea, its classification, an overview of common causes of chorea in different regions of the world, and principles of diagnosis and management.

Classification

Chorea is a manifestation of a number of diseases, both acquired and inherited. Although it is not completely understood, current evidence suggests that chorea results from an imbalance in the direct and indirect pathways. The disruption of the indirect pathway causes a loss of inhibition on the pallidum, allowing hyperkinetic movements to occur. In addition, enhanced activity of dopaminergic receptors and excessive dopaminergic activity are proposed mechanisms for the development of chorea at the level of the striatum. Based on current knowledge, it is possible to understand chorea and ballism as manifestations of a common pathophysiological chain of events, so that classification of choreic syndromes are increasingly based on etiology, while phenomenologically based distinctions between chorea and ballism are becoming less important.

Chorea is characterized as primary when it is idiopathic or genetic in origin and secondary when related to infectious, immunological, or other medical causes (Table 52.1). Huntington's disease is a prototypic choreic disorder of inherited origin. Other inherited causes are also discussed in more detail later in this chapter. In secondary, or sporadic, chorea, stroke and tardive syndromes are among the most common causes. A number of metabolic conditions, particularly non-ketogenic hyperglycemia, have been increasingly recognized causes of chorea, especially in Asian people. Choreiform movements can also result from structural brain lesions, mainly in the striatum, although most cases of secondary chorea do not demonstrate any specific structural lesions.

Table 52.1 Classification of chorea (only common causes listed).

Primary chorea	Secondary chorea	Others
Huntington's disease	Sydenham's chorea	Metabolic disorders
Neuroacanthocytosis	Drug-induced	Vitamin B_1 or B_{12}
Dentatorubral pallidoluysian	chorea	deficiency
atrophy	Immune-mediated	Toxin exposure
Benign hereditary chorea	chorea	Paraneoplastic
Wilson's disease	Infectious chorea	syndromes
Pantothenate kinase-associated	Vascular chorea	Post-pump
neurodegeneration (PKAN or	Hormonal disorders	choreoathetosis
formerly Hallervorden–Spatz		
syndrome)		
Paroxysmal choreoathetosis		
Senile chorea		

Hereditary causes

Huntington's disease

Huntington's disease (HD), the most common cause of hereditary chorea, is an autosomal dominant disorder caused by an expansion of an unstable trinucleotide repeat near the telomere of chromosome 4. Each offspring of an affected family member has a 50% chance of inheriting the fully penetrant mutation. According to the first description of the disease by George Huntington in 1872, there are three marked peculiarities: (1) its hereditary nature; (2) a tendency for insanity and suicide; and (3) manifestation as a grave disease only in adult life. However, Huntington failed to mention cognitive decline, which is now recognized as a cardinal feature of the disease.

Epidemiology

HD has a worldwide prevalence of 4–8 per 100,000 with no gender preponderance. HD has the highest prevalence rate in the region of Lake Maracaibo in Venezuela, with approximately 2% of the population affected, and the Moray Firth region of Scotland. HD is notably rare in Finland, Norway, and Japan, but data for Eastern Asia and Africa are inadequate. It is believed that the mutation for HD

International Neurology, Second edition. Edited by Robert P. Lisak, Daniel D. Truong, William M. Carroll and Roongroj Bhidayasiri

arose independently in multiple locations and does not represent a founder effect. New mutations are extraordinarily rare.

Genetics

Although the familial nature of HD was recognized more than a century ago, the gene mutation and altered protein (huntingtin) was described only recently. HD is a member of the growing family of neurodegenerative disorders associated with trinucleotide repeat expansion. The cytosine-adenosine-guanidine (CAG) triplet expansion in exon 1 encodes an enlarged polyglutamine tract in the huntingtin protein. In unaffected individuals, the repeat length ranges between 9 and 34 with a median normal chromosome length of 19. Expansion of a CAG repeat beyond the critical threshold of 36 repeats results in disease, and forms the basis of the polymerase chain reaction–based genetic test. This expanded repeat is somewhat unstable and tends to increase in subsequent offspring, termed *anticipation*. Expansion size is inversely related to age at onset, but the range in age at onset for a given repeat size is so large (with a 95% confidence interval of +/− 18 years for any given repeat length) that repeat size is not a useful predictor for individuals. It is likely that other genetic or environmental factors have a significant role in determining age of onset. With the exception of juvenile-onset cases, there has been a poor correlation between phenotype and CAG repeat length. Because of meiotic instability with a tendency of increasing the expansion size during spermatogenesis, juvenile-onset cases with very large expansions usually have an affected father. Predictive genetic testing of asymptomatic at-risk relatives of affected patients is currently available and governed by international guidelines.

Clinical features

HD is a progressive disabling neurodegenerative disorder characterized by the triad of movement disorders, dementia, and behavioral disturbances. Illness may emerge at any time of life, with the highest occurrence between 35 and 40 years of age. Although the involuntary choreiform movements are the hallmark of HD, it is the mental alterations that often represent the most debilitating aspect of the disease. There is also a large variability in the clinical presentation and some of this variability is predictable; for example, the juvenile-onset form may present with parkinsonism (the so-called Westphal variant), while the late-onset form may present with chorea alone.

Chorea is the prototypic motor abnormality characteristic of HD, occurring in 90% of affected patients. Chorea usually starts with slight movements of the fingers and toes and progresses to involve facial grimacing, eyelid elevations, and writhing limb movements (Figure 52.1). Motor impersistence is another important associated feature, whereby individuals are unable to maintain tongue protrusion or eyelid closure. Other motor manifestations also common in HD include eye movement abnormalities (slowing of saccades and increased latency of response), parakinesias, rigidity, myoclonus, and ataxia. Dystonia tends to occur when the disease is advanced or is associated with the use of dopaminergic medications. While dysarthria is common, aphasia is rare. Dysphagia tends to be the most prominent in the terminal stage and aspiration is a common cause of death.

Cognitive impairment seems to be inevitable in all HD patients. Typically, the impairment begins as selective deficits involving psychomotor, executive, and visuospatial abilities and progresses to more global impairment, although higher cortical language tends to be spared.

A wide range of psychiatric and behavioral disturbances is recognized in HD, with affective disorders among the most common, thought to be secondary to the disruption of the frontal-subcortical neural pathway. Depression occurs in up to 50% of patients. The suicide rate in HD is five-fold that of the general population. Psychosis is also common, usually with paranoid delusions. Hallucinations are rare. Apathy and aggressive behavior are commonly reported by caregivers.

Differential diagnosis

A variety of hereditary and acquired neurological disorders may mimic HD (Table 52.2). Benign hereditary chorea is a condition that is clinically distinct from HD. Although inherited in an autosomal dominant fashion, the symptoms are non-progressive with no alterations in cognitive or behavioral functions. The onset is usually before the age of 5 years. The presence of sensorimotor neuropathy may suggest an alternative diagnosis of neuroacanthocytosis. The diagnosis is supported by the presence of acanthocytes on a peripheral blood smear in the context of appropriate clinical presentation.

Spinocerebellar ataxias are distinguishable from HD by the prominent cerebellar dysfunction.

Wilson's disease should be considered in all patients with movement disorders who are less than 40 years of age, although patients with Wilson's disease rarely exhibit chorea.

Dentatorubral pallidoluysian atrophy (DRPLA) is a triplet repeat polyglutamine disorder with profound clinical heterogeneity. It is rarely reported in North America and Europe, but is more common than HD in Japan. Symptoms vary and may include chorea, myoclonus, ataxia, epilepsy, and dementia. Although its pathology is reminiscent of HD, the involvement of the dentate nucleus of the cerebellum differentiates the disorder.

Several other distinct genetic disorders have been identified that can present with a clinical picture indistinguishable from that of HD, referred to as Huntington's disease-like (HDL) syndromes. So far, four conditions have been described, namely disorders attributable to mutations in the prion protein gene (*HDL1*), the junctophilin 3 gene (*HDL2*), the gene encoding the TATA box-binding protein (*HDL4/SCA17*), and a recessively inherited HD phenocopy in a single family (*HDL3*) for which the genetics are still poorly understood. While the list of HDL genes is expected to grow, these disorders still account for only a small proportion of cases with the HD phenotype.

Neuropathology

The HD brain shows significant atrophy of the head of caudate (as evidenced on brain magnetic resonance imaging [MRI], Figure 52.2) and putamen, and to a lesser extent the cortex, globus pallidus, substantia nigra, subthalamic nucleus, and locus coeruleus. Microscopically, medium spiny neurons are the vulnerable population in HD. Indirect projections to the external globus pallidus are the first to degenerate. The cytopathological hallmarks of HD are intranuclear inclusions consisting of amyloid-like fibrils that contain mutant huntingtin, ubiquitin, synuclein, and other proteins.

Treatment

Current treatments in HD are largely symptomatic, aimed at reducing the motor and psychological dysfunction of individual HD patients. In general, treatment of chorea is not recommended unless it is causing disabling functional or social impairment. Clozapine, an

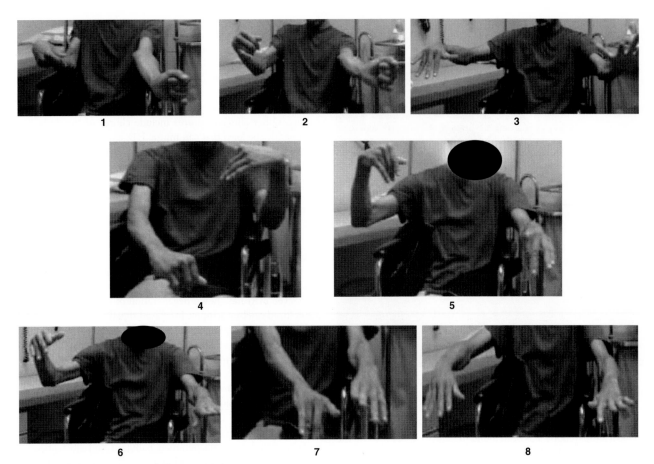

Figure 52.1 Chorea in a patient with Huntington's disease.

Table 52.2 Comparison of clinical features of Huntington's disease, Chorea-acanthocytosis, tardive dyskinesia, and benign hereditary chorea.

	Huntington's disease	Chorea-acanthocytosis	Tardive dyskinesia	Benign hereditary chorea
Movement disorders	Generalized chorea	Orofacial chorea, tongue and lip biting, or feeding dystonia, axial chorea or rubber-man syndrome	Orobuccolingual dyskinesia (fly-catching tongue, bon-bon tongue) with stereotypic pattern	Generalized chorea
Age at onset	30–40	30–40	Any age (more common in the elderly)	Early childhood
Genetic transmission	Autosomal dominant	Autosomal recessive	None	Autosomal dominant
Gene and chromosome	Huntingtin gene Chromosome 4p16.3	*VPS13A* gene Chromosome 9q21	None	*TITF1* gene Chromosome 14q13.1–q21.1
Dementia (subcortical)	Yes (early presentation)	Yes (late presentation)	No	No
Acanthocytes on PBS	No	Yes	No	No
Elevated CPK	No	Yes	No	No
Evidence of peripheral neuropathy	No	Yes	No	No
Progression	Yes	Yes	No	No (stable)
Suspect lesion in MRI brain	Bilateral caudate atrophy	Bilateral caudate atrophy	Normal MRI	Normal MRI
Management	Antipsychotic drugs, tetrabenazine, antidepressants	Antipsychotic drugs, levodopa	Stop DRBAs	–

CPK = creatine phosphokinase; DRBA = dopamine receptor blocking agent; MRI = magnetic resonance imaging; PBS = peripheral blood smear

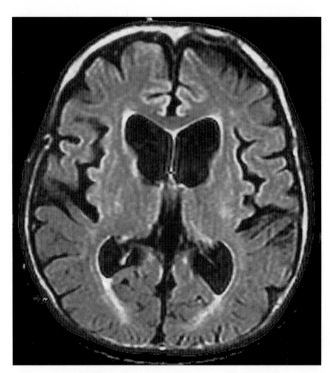

Figure 52.2 MRI of the brain in a patient with Huntington's disease disclosed predominant caudate atrophy.

atypical antipsychotic, has been found to reduce chorea without the extrapyramidal side effects of the typical agents. Other agents including tetrabenazine and amantadine have been shown to improve chorea. Traditional neuroleptics such as haloperidol can improve chorea, but are associated with increased risk of tardive dyskinesia, dystonia, difficulty swallowing, and gait disturbances, and should not be considered as first-line agents.

The selective serotonin reuptake inhibitors (SSRIs) have become the first-line agents in the treatment of depression in HD. SSRIs may also suppress chorea and reduce aggression in HD. A brief course of benzodiazepines may be useful for co-occurring anxiety. The atypical antipsychotic agents, such as clozapine, quetiapine, and olanzapine, are often required to treat psychosis in HD. Valproic acid may be useful in the long-term management of aggression and irritability.

Neuroacanthocytosis

Clinical features
Neuroacanthocytosis is a rare, multisystem, degenerative disorder of unknown etiology that is characterized by the presence of deformed erythrocytes with spicules known as acanthocytes, and abnormal involuntary movements. The term *neuroacanthocytosis* is used to describe autosomal recessive chorea–acanthocytosis (ChAc) and X-linked McLeod syndrome, but there are other movement disorders in which erythrocyte acanthocytosis may also be seen, such as Huntington disease-like 2 and pantothenate kinase-associated neurodegeneration. Disorders of serum lipoproteins such as Bassen–Kornzweig disease form a distinct group of neuroacanthocytosis syndromes in which ataxia is observed, but movement disorders are not seen. In classic ChAc cases, the mean age of onset is around 30 years. ChAc is caused by mutations in

a large gene on chromosome 9 (*VPS13A*; 73 exons), which codes for chorein. The disease tends to be progressive, with death occurring within 15 years of diagnosis. Involuntary choreic and dystonic movements of the orofacial region, as well as tongue and lip biting, are virtually diagnostic, although a full spectrum of movement disorders may be seen. Feeding dystonia is another characteristic feature. Other clinical features include chorea of the limbs (predominantly the legs) that can mimic HD, axonal neuropathy (50% of cases), areflexia, and elevated plasma creatine kinase (CK) level. Seizures are also common and can be a presenting feature. Psychiatric symptoms are typical and include apathy, depression, anxiety, and obsessive-compulsive syndrome. However, in contrast to HD, mental deterioration is minimal.

Treatment is largely supportive.

Diagnosis
Diagnosis is usually made on the basis of family history, morphological analysis of erythrocytes, and an elevated plasma creatine kinase level. MRI has shown degeneration of the caudate and more generalized cerebral atrophy. Increased signal on T2-weighted MRI in the caudate and putamen is a common feature. However, these findings are non-specific. The diagnosis of ChAc can be confirmed by the detection of mutations in the *VPS13A* gene or western blot detection of chorein, the protein encoded by the *VPS13A* gene. In patients with the McLeod RBC phenotype from serological studies, the diagnosis may be confirmed by analysis of the *XK* gene on chromosome Xp21. The most consistent neuropathological finding is extensive loss of predominantly small and medium-sized neurons and gliosis in the caudate, putamen, pallidum, and substantia nigra, with relative sparing of the subthalamic nucleus and cerebral cortex.

Dentatorubral pallidoluysian atrophy
Dentatorubral pallidoluysian atrophy (DRPLA) is a triplet repeat polyglutamine disorder with the gene defect localized to chromosome 12. Development of clinical phenotypes is associated with CAG repeat lengths exceeding 53. Atrophin-1 is a mutant protein and its function is not known. The condition is rarely reported in North America and Europe, but is more common in Japan. It is inherited in an autosomal dominant fashion and clinical features include chorea, myoclonus, ataxia, epilepsy, and cognitive decline. Neuroimaging studies have revealed atrophy of the cerebellum, midbrain tegmentum, and cerebral hemispheres with ventricular dilatation. Pathologically, there is neuronal loss and gliosis in the dentate nucleus, red nucleus, globus pallidus, and subthalamic nucleus.

Treatment is largely supportive.

Benign hereditary chorea
Benign hereditary chorea (BHC) or essential chorea is another disorder inherited in an autosomal dominant fashion and characterized by choreiform movements. In contrast to HD, the onset of choreiform movements in BHC is in early childhood; severity of symptoms peaks in the second decade and the condition is non-progressive. Life expectancy is normal and some reports have suggested that the disease improves with age. The condition is not associated with other neurological deficits, although some investigators believe that BHC is a heterogeneous syndrome that may have a variety of causes. BHC is considered to be a distinct disease of early-onset, non-progressive, uncomplicated chorea with a locus on 14q.

Senile chorea

It is not clear whether "senile chorea" (SC) is a distinct clinical entity or the late manifestation of HD. Critchley's criteria for diagnosis of SC are: (1) late-onset (>50 years), generalized chorea in the absence of dementia, psychiatric disorders or behavioral abnormalities; (2) no family history compatible with HD; (3) no previous intake of dopamine receptor blocking drugs; (4) no other identifiable cause of chorea. Although the presence of a cognitive deficit may be suggestive of chorea related to heredodegenerative causes such as HD, the patient with senile chorea usually has mild cognitive impairment. Thus, a genetic study is necessary to differentiate SC from late-onset HD.

Others

There are other inherited neurological disorders that can present with prominent chorea. These conditions are rare and the details are not included in this chapter. Examples include paroxysmal choreoathetosis, familial chorea-ataxia-myoclonus syndrome, pantothenate kinase-associated neurodegeneration (PKAN or Hallervorden–Spatz syndrome), intracerebral calcification with neuropsychiatric features, Wilson's disease, multisystem degeneration, olivopontocerebellar atrophy, and spinocerebellar degeneration (Sanger–Brown type).

Parainfectious and autoimmune causes

Sydenham's chorea

Sydenham's chorea (SC) is a delayed complication of group A ß-hemolytic streptococcal infections and is one of the major criteria of acute rheumatic fever. It is characterized by chorea, muscular weakness, and a number of neuropsychiatric symptoms. It is considered to be an autoantibody-mediated disorder, with the evidence suggesting that patients with SC produce antibodies that cross-react with streptococcus caudate, and subthalamic nuclei. However, documented evidence of previous streptococcal infection is found in only 20–30% of cases. The age of presentation is usually between 5 and 15 years, with female preponderance. Chorea is usually generalized, consisting of finer and more rapid movements than those seen in HD. It occurs at rest or with activity, but remits during sleep. The condition is self-limited within 5–16 weeks, but recurs in up to 50% of patients. However, symptomatic treatment with antipsychotics, tetrabenazine, or valproic acid can be considered in severe cases with generalized chorea. Previously affected females are at increased risk of developing chorea during pregnancy (chorea gravidarum) and during sex hormone therapy. Evidence of striatal dysfunction in SC is supported by MRI revealing lesions in the caudate and putamen in some patients, and reversible striatal hypermetabolism on brain single photon emission computed tomography during the acute illness.

Chorea gravidarum

Chorea gravidarum, chorea occurring during pregnancy, is an increasingly rare disorder. Affected patients usually have had previous episodes of chorea associated with the use of oral contraceptives or a history of rheumatic fever. The movements usually remit after delivery, but may recur in subsequent pregnancies.

Systemic lupus erythematosus and antiphospholipid syndrome

Although central nervous system involvement in systemic lupus erythematosus (SLE) is common, chorea has been reported in less than 2% of these patients. It usually appears early in the course of the disease and is characteristically generalized. Although many etiologies have been proposed, such as vascular damage, neuronal injury, or glial injury, the exact pathogenesis of SLE-associated chorea is still unclear. However, antiphospholipid antibodies are frequently identified in SLE patients with chorea. These antibodies may play a role in neuropsychiatric manifestation of SLE and likely are related to emerging chorea. It is often difficult to recognize chorea as a manifestation of a systemic autoimmune disease, because it can simulate Sydenham's and Huntington's choreas and not infrequently appears in childhood long before other manifestations of SLE or the antiphospholipid syndrome have emerged. The use of estrogen-containing oral contraceptives or pregnancy may precipitate the appearance of chorea. In addition, chorea can occur not only in patients with well-defined SLE, but also in patients with "probable" or "lupus-like" SLE and in patients with primary antiphospholipid antibody without clinical features of SLE. Some reports suggested that steroid therapy can lead to resolution.

Paraneoplastic syndrome

Chorea is a rare manifestation of paraneoplastic syndrome. Anti-Hu and anti-CRMP5 are the most commonly identified antibodies that are usually associated with small cell lung carcinoma. However, patients with these antibodies are less likely to present with chorea alone, as it usually develops with extensive encephalomyelitis, sensory neuropathy, and cerebellar degeneration. After the paraneoplastic antibodies are identified, the urgent management for depleting antibodies such as plasmapheresis or intravenous immunoglobulin should be implemented and tumor screening should be done as soon as possible.

Drug-related causes

Drug-induced chorea may be an acute phenomenon or the consequence of long-term therapy. Multiple drugs including dopamine agonists, levodopa therapy, oral contraceptives, and anticonvulsants have been implicated in acute chorea (Table 52.3). The details of drug-induced chorea are not covered in this chapter (see Chapter 56).

Vascular causes

Chorea is the most common movement disorder following stroke, but is a rare complication of acute vascular events. The subthalamic nucleus is the most commonly reported location of ischemic or hemorrhagic damage in patients with poststroke chorea, especially when the chorea is severe and proximal (called *hemiballismus*). However, many patients with chorea or ballism associated with stroke may have lesions in other basal ganglia structures and some of them appear normal on imaging. Chorea can also occur in polycythemia vera, although it manifests in less than 1% of cases.

Metabolic causes

Metabolic alterations including hyperglycemia, hypoglycemia, hypernatremia, hyponatremia, hypomagnesemia, hypocalcemia, and hepatic and renal failure have been implicated in the development of various movement disorders, including chorea. Recently, a combination of chorea, non-ketotic hyperglycemia, and

Table 52.3 Drugs known to cause chorea (in addition to antipsychotic medications).

1. Anticonvulsant medications: Common causative agents include:
   a. Phenytoin
   b. Carbamazepine
   c. Valproate
   d. Gabapentin
2. CNS stimulants
   a. Amphetamines
   b. Cocaine
   c. Methylphenidate
3. Benzodiazepines
4. Estrogens
5. Lithium
6. Levodopa
7. Dopamine agonists
8. COMT inhibitor in conjunction with levodopa
9. Antihistamines: H1 and H2
10. Others, e.g., baclofen, cimetidine, aminophylline, etc.

CNS = central nervous system; COMT = catechol-O-methyl transferase

a high-signal basal ganglia lesion on the T1-weighted brain MRI has been recognized to affect predominantly elderly Asian women. Characteristically, the T1-weighted brain MRI shows hyperintense basal ganglia lesions (Figure 52.3), but T2-weighted MRI findings are vary. The clinical course is usually benign and most patients gradually recover with medical treatment, particularly correction of hyperglycemia.

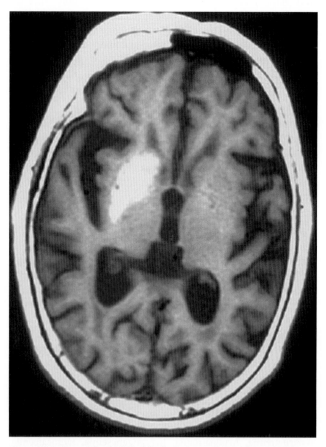

Figure 52.3 T1-weighted MRI of the brain in a patient with non-ketotic hyperglycemia chorea revealed high signal intensity lesions in the right basal ganglia, especially the putamen.

Infectious causes

Multiple infectious agents that affect the central nervous system (CNS) have been associated with chorea. Chorea can occur in the setting of acute bacterial meningitis, encephalitis, tuberculous meningitis, or aseptic meningitis. Movement disorders are also encountered in 2–3% of all patients with acquired immunodeficiency syndrome (AIDS). In the setting of AIDS, hemichorea and hemiballism are relatively common due to toxoplasmosis abscess; however, direct human immunodeficiency virus (HIV) invasion and injury to the basal ganglia resulting in chorea can occur. Less commonly, Lyme's disease has been reported to cause chorea. Interestingly, chorea may be found as a rare manifestation of prion protein infection, especially in the variant Creutzfeldt–Jakob disease.

Diagnosis

Although there are numerous causes of chorea, careful history and a concomitant neurological and psychiatric review of systems will guide the individual workup. A detailed past medical history is very important to rule out in particular prior streptococcal infections or rheumatic fever. As previously mentioned, a past history of rheumatic fever predisposes individuals to the development of a paroxysmal movement disorder under the influence of different agents. A family history of choreic or degenerative illness should be noted as well as a medication history of potential causative agents. Genetic testing, neuroimaging, and laboratory investigations will help to confirm the suspected diagnosis. Despite careful workup in most patients, causes are unidentified in 6% of cases.

Treatment

For primary chorea, dopaminergic antagonists such as antipsychotic medications are effective in treating chorea; however, their use is limited due to the side effects of parkinsonism and tardive syndromes. Moreover, clozapine is associated with an increased risk of agranucocytosis, and some atypical antipsychotics may predispose certain patients for metabolic syndromes. Dopamine-depleting agents such as tetrabenazine, which inhibit presynaptic dopamine release and block postsynaptic dopamine receptors, show favorable results compared with other medications used to treat chorea, especially in HD, and have been reported to have synergistic effects when used in combination with the dopamine antagonist pimozide. For secondary chorea, the treatment objective should be to address the primary causative factor. If chorea is due to an exogenous agent, the offending agent should be withdrawn. The infectious process should be treated accordingly. Drugs used to treat primary chorea can be used symptomatically to treat secondary chorea.

Conclusion

Chorea is a relatively common movement disorder that can be caused by a number of structural, autoimmune, neurodegenerative, pharmacological, and metabolic disturbances of basal ganglia function. Focal or hemichorea is usually suggestive of focal structural lesions, while the phenomenology of generalized chorea is rarely diagnostic. Clues to diagnosis may be found in the family or medical history, on neurological examination, or in laboratory testing and neuroimaging. Iatrogenic causes or tardive syndromes can be prevented by cautious use of antipsychotics, particularly in those at risk. While most therapies are largely supportive, correct diagnosis is essential for appropriate genetic counseling, preventing future recurrences, and therapies for disabling symptoms.

Further reading

Bhidayasiri R, Truong DD. Chorea and related disorders. *Postgrad Med J* 2004;80(947): 527–534.

Bhidayasiri R, Fahn S, Weiner WJ, Sullivan KL, Zesiewicz TA. Evidence-based guideline: Treatment of tardive syndromes: Report of the Guideline Development Subcommittee of the American Academy of Neurology. *Neurology* 2013;81(5):463–469.

Cardoso F. Chorea: Non-genetic causes. *Curr Opin Neurol* 2004;17(4):433–436.

Dalmau J, Rosenfeld M. Paraneoplastic syndrome of the CNS. *Lancet Neurol* 2008;7:327–340.

Fernandez M, Raskind W, Matsushita M, *et al.* Hereditary benign chorea: Clinical and genetic features of a distinct disease. *Neurology* 2001;57(1):106–110.

Harper PS. The epidemiology of Huntington's disease. *Hum Genet* 1992;89(4):365–376.

Huntington's Disease Collaborative Research Group. A novel gene containing a trinucleotide repeat that is expanded and unstable on Huntington's disease chromosomes. *Cell* 1993;72:971–983.

Koide R, Ikeuchi T, Onodera O, *et al.* Unstable expansion of CAG repeat in hereditary dentatorubral-pallidoluysian atrophy (DRPLA). *Nat Genet* 1994;6(1):9–13.

Oh S-H, Lee K-Y, Im J-H, Lee M-S. Chorea associated with non-ketotic hyperglycemia and hyperintensity basal ganglia lesion on T1-weighted brain MRI study: A meta-analysis of 53 cases including four present cases. *J Neurol Sci* 2002;200:57–62.

Schneider SA, Walker RH, Bhatia KP. The Huntington's disease-like syndromes: What to consider in patients with a negative Huntington's disease gene test. *Nat Clin Pract* 2007;3:517–525.

Schrag A, Quinn NP, Bhatia KP, Marsden CD. Benign hereditary chorea: Entity or syndrome? *Mov Disord* 2000;15(2):280–288.

Vidakovic A, Dragasevic N, Kostic V. Hemiballism: Report of 25 cases. *J Neurol Neurosurg Psychiatry* 1994;57:945–949.

Vital A, Bouillot S, Burbaud P, Ferrer X, Vital C. Chorea-acanthocytosis: Neuropathology of brain and peripheral nerve. *Clin Neuropathol* 2002;21(2):77–81.

Walker RH, Jung HH, Danek A. Neuroacanthocytosis. *Handb Clin Neurol* 2011;100: 141–151.

53 Myoclonus

John N. Caviness[1] and Daniel D. Truong[2]

[1]Department of Neurology, Mayo Clinic, Scottsdale, AZ, USA

[2] University of California, Riverside, Riverside, CA, USA; The Truong Neuroscience Institute, Orange Coast Memorial Medical Center, Fountain Valley, CA, USA

Myoclonus is defined as sudden, brief, shock-like, involuntary movements caused by muscular contractions (positive myoclonus) or inhibitions (negative myoclonus). It refers to a *symptom or sign* and it does not constitute a diagnosis. Myoclonus may have a variety of etiologies and physiological mechanisms. Accurate characterization of the individual patient presentation of myoclonus has strong implications for diagnosis and treatment.

The only study of myoclonus epidemiology in a defined population is from Olmsted County, Minnesota. The average annual incidence of pathological and persistent myoclonus between 1976 and 1990 was 1.3 cases per 100,000 person-years. The lifetime prevalence of myoclonus, as of January 1, 1990, was 8.6 cases per 100,000 population. Little information is available about diseases that commonly manifest myoclonus in specific regions of the world. The incidence of idiopathic progressive myoclonic epilepsy (Unverricht-Lundborg, EPM1) in Finland is 5 in 100,000 births.

Classification

Characterization of the type of myoclonus present in a given patient is based on three types of classification methods: exam findings, neurophysiology, and clinical etiology. These methods complement one another.

Exam findings

The basic parts of a myoclonus exam should include distribution, temporal profile, and activation characteristics of the movement. The distribution can be focal, multifocal, segmental, or generalized. A multifocal myoclonus distribution may have bilaterally synchronous movements as well. The temporal profile can be continuous or intermittent, as well as rhythmic or irregular. If intermittent, the myoclonus can occur sporadically or in trains. The activation of the myoclonus may be at rest (spontaneous), induced by various stimuli (reflex myoclonus), or induced by voluntary movement (action myoclonus), or some combination of these. These activation characteristics should be noted as absent or present. Patients may exhibit more than one pattern of myoclonus and all distributions and temporal patterns should be described.

Clinical neurophysiology

Clinical neurophysiology yields information about myoclonus pathophysiology. These findings support a source for the origin of the myoclonus, which in turn assists with both diagnosis and treatment. The methods employed should include multichannel surface electromyography (EMG) recording with testing for long latency EMG responses to nerve stimulation, electroencephalography (EEG), EEG-EMG polygraphy with back averaging, and evoked potentials (such as median nerve stimulation somatosensory evoked potential [SEP]). Positive and negative findings from these methods can then be used to provide evidence for determining the physiological type of myoclonus. For example, a back-averaged focal cortical EEG transient, enlarged cortical SEP, and enhanced long EMG responses suggest cortical-origin myoclonus. The main physiological categories for myoclonus classification are:

- *Cortical*: most common; has been reported for various neurodegenerative diseases, toxic-metabolic conditions, posthypoxic state (Lance–Adams syndrome), storage disorders, and other conditions.
- *Cortical-subcortical*: corresponds to the myoclonus in myoclonic and absence seizures. The physiology is believed to involve interactions of cortical and subcortical centers, such as the thalamus.
- *Subcortical*: seen in essential myoclonus and reticular reflex myoclonus, among others.
- *Segmental*: arises from segmental brainstem (palatal) and/or spinal generators.
- *Peripheral*: except for hemifacial spasm, peripheral myoclonus is rare.

Clinical etiology classification

The major categories of the myoclonus etiological classification scheme are physiological, essential, epileptic, and symptomatic (secondary). Each of the major categories is associated with different clinical circumstances. Physiological myoclonus occurs in neurologically normal people. Physical exams do not reveal relevant abnormalities and there is minimal to no associated disability present. Jerks during sleep are the most familiar examples of physiological myoclonus. Essential myoclonus refers to idiopathic myoclonus that progresses slowly or not at all, and the jerks represent the most prominent or only clinical finding. Epileptic myoclonus refers to the presence of myoclonus in the setting of epilepsy, a chronic seizure disorder. Myoclonus can occur as only one component of a seizure, the only seizure manifestation, or one of multiple seizure types within an epileptic syndrome. Symptomatic (secondary) myoclonus manifests in the setting of an identifiable, underlying disorder – neurological or non-neurological. Most cases of myoclonus are in the symptomatic category, followed by the epileptic and essential categories.

International Neurology, Second edition. Edited by Robert P. Lisak, Daniel D. Truong, William M. Carroll and Roongroj Bhidayasiri

© 2016 John Wiley & Sons, Ltd. Published 2016 by John Wiley & Sons, Ltd.

Features of major myoclonic disorders

Posthypoxic myoclonus

Myoclonus is known to occur in posthypoxic patients after anesthesia incidents, cardiac arrest, near drowning, pulmonary embolism, or respiratory failures. Not all patients develop myoclonus after hypoxic incidents. The duration of hypoxia often has to reach a certain threshold before posthypoxic myoclonus develops. Spontaneous, action-induced, and stimulus-induced myoclonus may occur. Action myoclonus dominates the clinical picture. Action jerks can spread to involve other body parts early on (bilateral or generalized jerks) and later become multifocal. Myoclonus can present in facial muscles, affecting speech and swallowing. Some patients also have cerebellar ataxia and negative myoclonus, which lead to sudden falls. Epilepsy is normally not a striking feature and seizures most often are generalized tonic–clonic. Most patients have some improvement in the myoclonus with time. Recently, an animal model of posthypoxic myoclonus has been developed based on systematic prolongation of cardiac arrest. In this model, meaningful myoclonus persists only after duration of hypoxia of about 7 minutes, although transient myoclonus may occur in animals with as little as 3 minutes of hypoxia.

Progressive myoclonus epilepsy

Various storage diseases fall under the clinical syndrome of progressive myoclonic epilepsy (PME). PME is a chronic, progressive, neurological syndrome that manifests as some combination of myoclonus, seizures, ataxia, and dementia. These disorders usually affect individuals less than 30 years of age and are often fatal. Several clinical differences exist between individual storage diseases as to their age of onset, rate of progression, details of clinical expression, other clinical manifestations, and patterns of stimulus sensitivity. The neuropathology in the brain is widespread. Tissue biopsy and enzyme activity measurements are useful for diagnosis. There has been a dramatic increase in the genetic mutations described for PME etiologies. For example, the *EMP2A* mutations are a worldwide cause of Lafora disease, but *NHLRC1* mutations causing Lafora disease are particularly common in Japan.

Essential myoclonus

Cases of sporadic essential myoclonus are very heterogeneous with regard to distribution, what exacerbates the jerks, and other examination findings. Sporadic essential myoclonus probably consists of various heterogeneous, yet undiscovered causes of myoclonus, and cases with false-negative family histories. Hereditary-essential myoclonus is associated with dominant inheritance and variable severity. The myoclonus is usually distributed throughout the upper body, exacerbated by muscle activation, and dramatically decreased with alcohol ingestion. The term "myoclonus-dystonia syndrome" has been introduced because of the common occurrence of dystonia in these cases. Mutations in the ε-sarcoglycan gene have had the strongest association with the myoclonus-dystonia syndrome. Recent evidence shows that myoclonus-dystonia cases with the ε-sarcoglycan mutation have EMG discharges that are more variable and of longer duration than cortical myoclonus cases (e.g., posthypoxic, PME causes).

Neurodegenerative disorders

Multiple system atrophy manifests as varying degrees of parkinsonism, ataxia, and autonomic dysfunction, but a stimulus-sensitive distal limb myoclonus was found in 31% of patients in one series. Myoclonic jerks, both action- and stimulus-sensitive, commonly occur in corticobasal degeneration. The distribution of the myoclonus in corticobasal degeneration is either asymmetric or focal, and is similar to the other clinico-pathological manifestations of the disease. The usual presentation of myoclonus in Alzheimer's disease is small multifocal distal jerking, although more widespread or generalized jerks can be seen. The myoclonus in Creutzfeldt–Jakob disease is a clinical hallmark of the disorder and can occur at rest and/or be exacerbated by action or stimuli. When the myoclonus in Alzheimer's disease is large and widespread, it may be confused with Creutzfeldt–Jakob disease. Cortical myoclonus occurs across the spectrum of Lewy body disorders. The myoclonus in Parkinson's disease is less common than in dementia with Lewy bodies, where it occurs in at least one-third of cases. The myoclonus in dementia with Lewy bodies is of larger amplitude and much more likely to occur at rest than the myoclonus in Parkinson's disease. An idiopathic syndrome of "primary progressive myoclonus of aging" has been described. The clinical course of these patients resembles a chronic neurodegenerative syndrome, but the cause is unknown.

Metabolic disorders

In metabolic conditions, myoclonus often occurs in the hospital setting, frequently with mental status changes. The myoclonus may be multifocal and subtle, or generalized and almost constant, as in the entity "myoclonic status epilepticus." Prognosis in such cases depends on the severity and reversibility of the underlying process. Asterixis, which is known as "negative myoclonus," is a well-known characteristic of toxic and metabolic encephalopathies. It is characterized by brief lapses in postural tone and is particularly common in kidney and liver failure. Usually, the effects are improved or reversed when use of the agent is discontinued or the metabolic condition is reversed.

Drugs

The literature on drug-induced myoclonus continues to grow. Such myoclonus is potentially fully treatable, since it is almost always reversible on withdrawal of the offending agent(s). It must be emphasized that all drugs, either in isolation or combination, must be scrutinized for a potential causative role in myoclonus. A spectrum of lithium-induced myoclonus exists with regard to different clinical manifestations of motor cortex hyperexcitability. At therapeutic levels, or mild lithium toxicity, isolated cortical action myoclonus can be associated with EEG background rhythm changes. Instances of greater lithium toxicity can demonstrate motor seizures and/or generalized convulsions. The synergistic relationship between myoclonus-causing drugs in the setting of polypharmacy in complex psychiatric cases has become very apparent. Organ failure, especially from the liver or kidney, may elevate the levels of certain myoclonus-causing drugs or their metabolites and thereby contribute to myoclonus.

Autoimmune disease

Opsoclonus-myoclonus syndrome presents with progressive opsoclonus (irregular, rapid eye movements) and multifocal or generalized myoclonus. Opsoclonus-myoclonus in adults may be due to infectious, autoimmune, or paraneoplastic etiology. Idiopathic opsoclonus-myoclonus occurs in younger adult patients, and the clinical evolution is more benign. Neuroblastoma is a major paraneoplastic etiology consideration in children. There are a growing number of recently described idiopathic autoimmune disorders associated with myoclonus and a variety of antibodies. An example is anti-N-methyl-D-aspartate (NMDA) receptor encephalitis, which can be seen in children and adults. Antibodies to voltage-gated potassium channels have been discovered in patients with myoclonus. This syndrome may present similar to Creutzfeldt–Jakob disease, but it is important to diagnose because response to therapy may be seen. In all idiopathic cases, a comprehensive search for possible antibodies and cancer is needed.

Psychogenic jerks

Jerks that mimic the "shock-like" speed of myoclonus may have a psychogenic etiology. Such movements are often variable in duration and can hold a position somewhat longer than myoclonus. Nevertheless, such jerks may prove difficult to distinguish from non-psychogenic myoclonus. Underlying psychopathology may or may not be obvious, posing a further challenge to diagnosis. Clinical neurophysiology can be helpful in some cases, showing a Bereitschaftspotential before the jerks or a prolonged response to stimulation. Despite challenges, an accurate psychogenic diagnosis facilitates proper treatment of the underlying psychological issues.

Evaluation

The evaluation of myoclonus etiology begins with a thorough neurological history and examination. From this information, it is useful to clinically classify the case into one of the four etiological categories: physiological, essential, epileptic, and symptomatic. The presence of the myoclonus and the other aspects of the clinical presentation determine what type of testing should be done, in addition to minimal testing if the myoclonus etiology is still unknown. For example, if an infectious or inflammatory syndrome is present, a cerebrospinal fluid exam should be done. Knowledge of the various diagnostic entities will facilitate the proper diagnostic confirmation. The following minimal testing should be done in all unexplained cases of myoclonus:

Electrolytes	Drug and toxin screen
Glucose	Brain imaging
Renal function tests	Electroencephalography
Hepatic function tests	

If these basic tests do not reveal the diagnosis, then more advanced testing should be considered. Additional testing may include clinical neurophysiology testing, cerebrospinal fluid examination, enzyme activity, paraneoplastic testing, and other metabolic testing. In some cases, genetic testing may be considered. Before genetic testing is begun, the patient should be fully aware of the implications of both positive and negative results. If appropriate, genetic counseling is recommended.

Treatment

The best strategy for the management of myoclonus is treatment of the underlying disorder; however, this is not always possible. Some causes of myoclonus can be reversed partially or totally, such as an acquired abnormal metabolic state, a medication or toxin, or an excisable lesion. The general principle of the treatment of myoclonus is to control the myoclonus to the level that is tolerable by the patient. The treatment of myoclonus can be effective, but is often unsatisfactory and mostly empirical (Table 53.1).

Table 53.1 Appropriate dose of agents for the treatment of myoclonus.

Drug	Dosage (mg/day)
Baclofen	15–100
Benztropine	15–100
Carbamazepine	up to 2000
Clonazepam	up to 15
Diazepam	5–30
γ–Hydroxybutyric acid	6.125[1]
5-Hydroxytryptophan	up to 3[1,2]
Levetiracetam	3000
Phenobarbital	50–100
Phenytoin	250–325
Piracetam	2.4–16.8[1]
Primidone	500–750
Tetrabenazine	50–200
Trihexyphenidyl	up to 35
Valproic acid (sodium valproate)	1200–2000

[1] g/day.
[2] In combination with a peripheral aromatic amino acid decarboxylase inhibitor (such as carbidopa 100–300 mg/day).

Some of the drugs used to treat myoclonus are anticonvulsants. Unlike in epilepsy, antimyoclonic agents are usually used in combination. Rarely can one agent achieve complete control of myoclonus. The treatment is ideally dictated by the underlying diagnosis. For symptomatic therapy, the best treatment effect will depend on the physiology/origin of the myoclonus. Side effects are common in myoclonus therapy, so the side effect profiles of the antimyoclonic agents is an important consideration. Levetiracetam, piracetam, valproic acid, and clonazepam are commonly used agents for the treatment of cortical myoclonus. The epileptic myoclonus (cortical-subcortical physiology) of juvenile myoclonic epilepsy and similar syndromes best responds to valproic acid. Clonazepam can be used for multiple types of myoclonus, but may yield the best response for subcortical myoclonus cases.

Levetiracetam

Levetiracetam is effective in patients with cortical myoclonus, especially with posthypoxic myoclonus. The standard initial dose for epilepsy is 500 mg twice daily; as drowsiness may occur, it is wise to begin initially with 250 or 500 mg/day with gradual titration upward. The maximum recommended dose is 3000 mg/day. Pediatric doses are 20–40 mg/kg/day. Levetiracetam is minimally protein-bound and excreted in the urine. It has virtually no interactions with other drugs. It is considered the drug of choice in the treatment of myoclonus.

Valproic acid

Valproic acid is effective in cortical and subcortical myoclonus. It is usually begun at 125 mg twice daily, and titrated to clinical response. For the treatment of myoclonus, doses of 750–1000 mg/day are usually required. It is contraindicated in patients with significant hepatic dysfunction and urea cycle disorders. It may cause neural tube defects, craniofacial defects, and cardiovascular malformations if taken during pregnancy. Valproic acid may increase levels of warfarin, lamotrigine, phenobarbital, and phenytoin. Fatal hepatic failure and pancreatitis may occur in patients taking valproic acid, and they require frequent monitoring.

Clonazepam

Clonazepam is used in cortical, subcortical, and spinal myoclonus. It is the drug of choice for spinal myoclonus. Clonazepam is typically begun at 0.5 mg three times a day and titrated until there is control of symptoms or side effects appear. Doses of at least 3 mg/day are generally required. The most common side effect is drowsiness, but ataxia and personality changes may also occur. Clonazepam is contraindicated in patients with narrow angle glaucoma or with hepatic dysfunction.

Other drugs

Other drugs that may also be used in myoclonus are primidone, piracetam, and γ–Hydroxybutyric acid (GHB). Piracetam is available in Europe and many other parts of the world. The usual dosage for myoclonus is 16–24 mg/day. It is contraindicated in patients with renal insufficiency and hepatic dysfunction. GHB has been approved in the United States for the treatment of cataplexy in patients with narcolepsy. It is used in other countries for the treatment of alcohol withdrawal and for maintaining its abstinence. A dose of 6.125 g/day has been reported to be effective in alcohol-sensitive myoclonus-dystonia.

Botulinum toxin

Botulinum toxin therapy has had some reported success in treating segmental or peripheral myoclonus. For segmental palatal myoclonus, it is recommended that an ear, nose, and throat surgeon perform the injections, which vary between 5 and 10 units. However, many authors consider this therapy to be unproven as effective or safe, so caution is advised.

Deep brain stimulation

Patients with medically refractory hereditary myoclonus-dystonia syndrome have seen positive results with globus pallidus interna deep brain stimulation. It is not clear what factors predict success, however, so caution is advised.

Further reading

Andrade DM, Hamani C, Minassian BA. Treatment options for epileptic myoclonus and epilepsy syndromes associated with myoclonus. *Expert Opin Pharmacother* 2009;10:1549–1560.

Baizabal-Carvallo JF, Jankovic J. Movement disorders in autoimmune diseases. *Mov Disord* 2012;27:935–946.

Caviness JN. Epileptic myoclonus. In: Sirven JI, Stern JM (eds.). *Atlas of Video-EEG Monitoring*. New York: McGraw-Hill Medical; 2011:309–328.

Caviness JN. Segmental myoclonus. In: Albanese A, Jankovic J (eds.). *Hyperkinetic Movement Disorders: Differential Diagnosis and Treatment*. Chichester: Wiley-Blackwell; 2012:221–235.

Caviness JN. Treatment of myoclonus. *Neurotherapeutics* 2014;11:188–200.

Kinugawa K, Vidailhet M, Clot F, *et al.* Myoclonus-dystonia: An update. *Mov Disord* 2009;24:479–489.

Tai KK, Bhidayasiri R, Truong D. Myoclonus: Post-hypoxic animal model of myoclonus. *Parkinsonism Relat Disord* 2007;13:377–381.

Van der Salm SMA, de Haan RJC, Cath DC, van Rootselaar AF, Tijssen MAJ. The eye of the beholder: Inter-rater agreement among experts on psychogenic jerky movement disorders. *J Neurol Neurosurg Psychiatry* 2013;84:742–747.

54 Tics and Tourette syndrome

Valerie Suski[1] and Mark Stacy[2]

[1] Department of Neurology, University of Pittsburgh Medical Center, Pittsburgh, PA, USA
[2] Department of Neurology, Duke Institute for Brain Sciences, Duke University, Durham, NC, USA

Tourette syndrome (TS) is a childhood neurological disorder characterized by the presence of motor and phonic tics, which can be associated with neuropsychiatric comorbidities such as obsessive-compulsive disorder (OCD), learning disabilities, and attention deficit hyperactivity disorder (ADHD). This disorder was named after the French neurologist Dr. Georges Gilles de la Tourette, who first described this syndrome after observing one of his patients in 1885. Over the years, the diagnostic criteria for TS have changed and expanded to describe a wide variety of presentations and severity. Nevertheless, the diagnosis remains challenging at times. TS may be unrecognized in many children with mild symptoms or with suppressible tics. Early recognition and diagnosis with appropriate treatment for those with debilitating symptoms can improve quality of life for these children.

The clinical hallmark of TS is tics. Tics are sudden, rapid, stereotypic, non-rhythmic motor movements (motor tics) or sounds (phonic tics). The current diagnostic criteria for TS, according to the American Psychiatric Association's *Diagnostic and Statistical Manual of Mental Disorders* (DSM-V), are: (1) the presence of at least two or more motor tics and at least one phonic tic but not necessarily at the same time; (2) the occurrence of multiple tics nearly every day through a period of more than 1 year without a tic-free period of more than 3 consecutive months; (3) symptoms not being due to medications or drugs and not related to another medical condition; and (4) the age of onset prior to 18 years.

Epidemiology

TS has been reported worldwide in all religious, ethnic, and socio-economic groups. The general population has an estimated prevalence of up to 1% worldwide, with the average age of onset between 2 and 15 years. There is a lower prevalence of TS in African Americans in the United States and it is rare in the sub-Saharan black African group. China also has a reported lower prevalence rate of TS. Simple tics, which involve one group of muscles, occur in between 0.4% and 1.76% of children aged 5–8 years old and in as high as 28% of children in the special education setting.

The etiology of TS remains unknown. Few genes have been implicated in a limited number of TS cases through molecular genetic studies (e.g. SLITRK1, DRD3, and histidine decarboxylase mutations); however, commercial testing is not available at this time. Initially, familial studies suggested an autosomal dominant disorder with variable penetrance; however, recent studies show that the pattern of inheritance may be more complex, including possible bilineal transmission theories. Males are more commonly affected than females, with a predominance of 3:1. If OCD is included as an alternative expression of TS, the gender ratio is nearly equal.

Besides gender, environmental factors (e.g., maternal smoking exposure and prenatal stressors) also affect tic severity and neuropsychological function.

There does not appear to be a familial association in 10–15% of TS cases. Some studies suggest that increased numbers of dopamine or serotonin neurotransmitters can cause tics in areas of the brain responsible for voluntary movements. Non-genetic risk factors evaluated include prenatal (maternal smoking, drug use, or toxin exposure) and perinatal events (jaundice, infections). Most of the studies show that these factors may not necessarily cause TS, but may correlate with the severity of symptoms. Differential diagnoses for TS are outlined in Table 54.1.

Table 54.1 Differential diagnoses for tics.

Toxicities	Neuroleptics
	Stimulants (e.g., cocaine, amphetamines)
	Carbon monoxide
	Levodopa
	Opiate withdrawal
	Anticonvulsants
	Antidepressants
Genetic disorders	Huntington's disease
	Wilson's disease
	Rett syndrome
	Hyperekplexias
	Neurodegeneration with brain iron accumulation
Infectious	Sydenham's chorea
	Subacute sclerosing panencephalitis (SSPE)
	Pediatric autoimmune neuropsychiatric disorders associated with streptococcal (PANDAS)
	Lyme disease
	Postencephalitis (herpes, varicella zoster)
	HIV infections of central nervous system
Chromosomal abnormalities	XYY
	XXY
	Fragile X syndrome
	Down syndrome
Prenatal/perinatal insults	Birth defects
	Congenital central nervous system defects
Systemic illness	Neuroacanthocytosis
	Behçet's disease
Other	Head trauma
	Hemifacial spasms
	Seizures (e.g., focal motor and complex partial)
	Mannerisms
	Akathisias
	Transient strokes
	Autism/Asperger's syndrome
	Stereotypies
	Psychogenic

International Neurology, Second edition. Edited by Robert P. Lisak, Daniel D. Truong, William M. Carroll and Roongroj Bhidayasiri
© 2016 John Wiley & Sons, Ltd. Published 2016 by John Wiley & Sons, Ltd.

Pathophysiology

The pathophysiology of tics and TS is not well understood, although functional imaging has helped to advance our knowledge. Single photon emission computed tomography (SPECT) studies demonstrating an increase in striatal dopamine reuptake sites suggest that there is presynaptic dopaminergic dysfunction in TS. One positron emission tomography (PET) study found increased action for the cerebellum, insula, thalamus, and putamen during the time of tic release. These functional studies have shown increased activation in the frontal cortex–striatum–thalamus–cortex pathway, which is also affected in various other movement disorders.

Clinical features

Tics are abrupt, intermittent, and repeated movements or sounds that occur in the background of normal behavior. The severity of these symptoms often fluctuates throughout the day. Tics have been categorized as "semi-voluntary," because certain patients have the ability to suppress the tic; however, this is usually temporary. Tics can interfere with normal behavior or movements. There is often a warning or premonitory urge associated with tic performance. This is usually a sensation or feeling, which can worsen with tic suppression. These premonitory stimuli are frequently vague, difficult to define, and may not be recognized for years. They have been described as a brief or prolonged "urge to move," "tension," "itch-like," or "uncomfortable" sensations. The execution of a tic, whether it be phonic or vocal (e.g., humming, coughing, throat clearing) or motor (e.g., blinking, head jerking, or shoulder shrugging), can temporarily relieve the premonitory urge to tic. Not every tic is preceded by an associated urge. Recognition of this phenomenon is important, since these sensory symptoms may be more troublesome to the patient than the actual tic performance itself.

Tics are classified as simple or complex. Simple motor tics consist of a single movement involving a limited number of muscle groups, lasting seconds or less, such as eye rolling, facial grimacing, or shoulder shrugging. Complex motor tics involve multiple muscle groups, are coordinated into a sequence of movements, and may be slower and more deliberate than simple motor tics. Examples include punching oneself, jumping, or copropraxia (performing obscene gestures). Simple vocal or phonic tics are described as meaningless sounds or noises, such as throat clearing, yelping, and sniffing. Complex phonic tics are usually meaningful words, phrases, or sentences (i.e., uttering words or phrases out of context) and stuttering. More dramatic complex phonic tics are coprolalia (uttering obscene words), palilalia (repeating oneself), or echolalia (repeating others' words). Severity for any of the above tics may worsen with associated physical or emotional distress.

In addition to the categories of simple or complex, tics may also be classified by the duration of the symptoms. The diagnosis of provisional tics is made in patients less than 18 years old with one or more motor or vocal tics lasting less than 12 consecutive months. Chronic or persistent tic disorder occurs in patients less than 18 years old with either one or more motor or phonic tics, but usually not both. Persistent tics can occur many times a day, almost daily, or on and off throughout a period of greater than one year. Both provisional and persistent tics cannot be secondary to other etiologies (e.g., medications, infections, or neurodegenerative diseases) and do not meet the criteria for TS.

Although motor and phonic tics are the predominant feature of TS, these symptoms may be accompanied by a variety of neuropsychiatric comorbidities. Almost half of TS patients report symptoms of obsessive-compulsive disorder (OCD). Children with OCD will often describe a system of rituals associated with retiring to bed, playing sports or musical instruments, or collecting objects. Common examples of such symptoms include compulsive checking, counting, touching surfaces, and obsessive worrying. Symptoms of attention deficit hyperactivity disorder (ADHD) are reported in 15–80% of TS patients, and include impulsivity, inattention, distractibility, and hyperactivity. Although not as prevalent as OCD and ADHD symptoms, some patients with TS may also manifest common behavioral comorbidities, such as mania, affective/personality disorders, learning disabilities, and self-injurious behavior.

Investigations

There are no confirmatory tests for TS. The diagnosis is made from clinical observation, determining potential triggers, and assessing comorbidities. Secondary etiologies should be considered when making the diagnosis of TS. Given the semi-voluntary suppressibility and the fluctuating nature of the disorder, tics may be absent at the time of an examination. It may take several visits before the tics may be witnessed by the physician.

Secondary causes of tics, referred to as tourettism, and tics may accompany other medical conditions, such as Huntington's disease, neuroacanthocytosis, Wilson's disease, and Sydenham's chorea. Acquired causes of tics include medication side effects, head trauma, postviral encephalitis, stroke, and carbon monoxide poisoning. Tics can be associated with chromosomal disorders (Down syndrome, Klinefelter's syndrome, XYY syndrome, and Fragile X syndrome) and other conditions such as developmental disorders, autism, and stereotypic movement disorders. Medications including stimulants, caffeine, carbamazepine, and corticorsteroids can exacerbate tics. Group A beta-hemolytic streptococcal infection is an extremely rare form of tourettism with sudden onset of an autoimmune neuropsychiatric disorder.

Treatment

There are several options, pharmacological and non-pharmacological, for treatment of tics and TS. Most children with mild tics can avoid pharmacological treatment. One-third of children have tics or TS that remit or greatly improve as they approach adulthood. Educating teachers about TS can potentially lead to earlier identification and diagnosis in the school system. Diagnosis and general education regarding the nature of their symptoms is often a highly effective, non-pharmacological therapy for patients. In many instances, neuropsychological evaluations may identify ways to reconfigure the patient's learning environment and provide supportive counseling.

Medications are considered if symptoms of TS are functionally disabling and not improved with non-pharmacological interventions. Dopamine receptor antagonists (i.e., neuroleptic or antipsychotic) medications are most useful for suppressing tics. The most frequently used typical neuroleptic medications include fluphenazine, haloperidol, pimozide, sulpiride, and tiapride. Frequently used atypical neuroleptics for TS include risperidone, aripiprazole, ziprasidone, quetiapine, metoclopramide, and olanzapine, with the newest being paliperidone and sertindole. Common side effects of dopamine receptor antagonists include sedation, cognitive difficulties, dysphoria, depression, dystonia, weight gain, and social phobias. Before beginning any neuroleptic drug, the patient and family should be warned of the potential for the development of tardive dyskinesias and the rare potential for acute dystonic reaction.

Other medications with different mechanisms of action may suppress tics in certain TS patients. Clonidine and guanfacine (α-receptor agonists) may be useful medications for children with mild tics and ADHD. Clonazepam, reserpine, tetrabenazine, calcium channel blockers, and anticonvulsants (topiramate) also have tic-suppressing effects. Treatment of TS with stimulants remains controversial due to exacerbation of tics in some patients (in 25%), but may be tolerable if symptoms of inattention and hyperactivity are improved. A combination of clonidine plus stimulant may have an additive benefit on ADHD symptoms without worsening tics.

Antidepressant medications, particularly serotonin reuptake inhibitors, may alleviate OCD symptoms in TS. Currently available drugs include selective serotonin reuptake inhibitors (fluoxetine, fluvoxamine, paroxetine, sertraline) and tricyclic antidepressants (clomipramine, desipramine). With the overlap of complex tics and OCD, these drugs may be particularly useful in this setting, avoiding the potential risk associated with neuroleptic agents.

Alternative therapies are emerging. Habit-reversing training is the substitution of one tic for a more socially acceptable tic. Cognitive behavioral therapy helps with poor impulse control. Relaxation techniques and biofeedback alleviate stress, reducing tics. Botulinum toxin injections in muscles that are responsible for particular movements or vocalizations (trapezius for shoulder shrugging, vocal cords for coprolalia) may be effective. Botulinum toxin may benefit symptoms by weakening the muscle or changing proprioceptive feedback, modifying the premonitory urge for movement.

Deep brain stimulation surgery has been attempted for refractory TS in a small number of cases. The surgical target is still controversial; however, the most commonly studied site is the thalamus (centromedian-parafascicular complex or CM) and less so the globus pallidus interna (GPi), globus pallidus externa (GPe), and the anterior limb of the internal capsule.

Tourette syndrome is not neurodegenerative; therefore, patients have a normal life span. In general, 10% of TS patients will have severe tics, 30% will experience a decrease in frequency and severity, 30–40% will completely resolve by late adolescence, and the other 30–40% will continue to exhibit moderate to severe symptoms in adulthood. Patients with severe tics and comorbidities appear to be more likely to become socially isolated. However, most patients develop strategies with medication, social support, and behavioral compensation that allow for management of the most difficult of symptoms, and with time the disabling components of the disorder are minimized.

Further reading

Jankovic J, Kurlan, R. Tourette syndrome: Evolving concepts. *Movement Disorders* 2011;26:1149–1156.

Kadesjo B, Gillberg C. Tourette's disorder: Epidemiology and comorbidity in primary school children. *J Am Acad Child Adolesc Psychiatry* 2000;39:548–555.

Lerner A, Bagic A, Boudreau EA, *et al.* Neuroimaging of neuronal circuits involved in tic generation in patients with Tourette syndrome. *Neurology* 2007;68:1979–1987.

Mueller-Vahl KR, Berding G, Brucke T, *et al.* Dopamine transporter binding in Gilles de al Tourette syndrome. *J Neurol* 2000;247:514–520.

Robertson MM. The prevalence and epidemiology of Gilles de la Tourette syndrome. Part 2: Tentative explanations for differing prevalence figures in GTS, including the possible effects of psychopathology, aetiology, cultural differences, and differing phenotypes. *J Psychosom Res* 2008;65(5):473–486.

55   Ataxia

Sergey N. Illarioshkin

Research Center of Neurology, Russian Academy of Medical Sciences, Moscow, Russia

From the historical viewpoint, the term "ataxia" means "disarray" – that is, any unspecified motor clumsiness. However, our present understanding of this term refers to poorly coordinated movements resulting mainly from lesions of the cerebellum and/or cerebellar connections. In addition to cerebellar ataxia (accounting for the vast majority of all ataxic cases seen in clinical practice), there are also cases of sensory and vestibular ataxia caused, respectively, by lesions of spinal proprioceptive pathways and the vestibular system. Some authors also distinguish so-called frontal ataxia, a specific syndrome caused by lesions of the frontal lobe and disintegration of frontopontocerebellar pathways.

Clinical features

Cerebellar ataxia

Clinically, cerebellar ataxia manifests by imbalanced stance and unsteady, broad-based gait, as well as by limb incoordination, clumsy movements, slurring dysarthria (scanning speech, staccato), and saccadic ocular dysmetria and oscillations. Patients stand with the legs farther apart than is normal, they sway or fall in an attempt to stand with the feet together, and, because of poor balance, they need support or want to hold onto objects in the room. Mild gait ataxia may be exaggerated when patients attempt tandem walking in a straight line. Ataxia may be generalized or affect predominantly gait, upper or lower extremities, speech, or eye movements. It may be unilateral or spread to both sides of the body. Ataxic patients display improper initiation and termination of their movements (dysmetria) and experience problems with the execution of fast rhythmic movements (dysdiadochokinesis).

Ataxia is accompanied frequently by muscle hypotonia, slowness of movements, intention tremor (action tremor with increased amplitude of oscillations on approaching the target), abnormal control of multijoint movements (asynergia), exaggerated postural reactions, and nystagmus (usually horizontal in cerebellar disease). Cerebellar patients may have some alterations in mental processes and cognitive functions (so-called cerebellar cognitive-affective syndrome), usually caused by large and acute ischemic lesions of the posterior lobe. One should stress that motor problems in ataxic patients typically are not related to muscle weakness, hyperkinesias, spasticity, and so on, although all these and other additional symptoms may complicate the clinical phenotype. Severe ataxia may become an important cause of physical disability and social maladjustment.

Relatively isolated trunk ataxia with abnormal stance and gait is seen when the disease is restricted to the vermal portions of the cerebellum; patients tend to sway or fall forward with rostral-vermal lesions and backward with caudal-vermal lesions. Limb ataxia is usually attributed to diseases of the cerebellar hemispheres. Saccadic ocular dysmetria is seen with dorsal vermis involvement. With a unilateral cerebellar hemisphere lesion, ipsilateral disturbances of gait, posture, and movement are evident: such patients stand with the shoulder on the affected side lower than the other, they stagger and deviate to the side of the lesion on walking, and the affected extremities show marked ataxia in all tests of motor coordination. Although in humans there is no strict correspondence between cerebellar hemisphere subregions and locomotion of particular segments of the body, it is believed that diseases of anterosuperior parts of hemispheres manifest predominantly as lower limb ataxia (the pattern frequently seen in alcoholic cerebellar degeneration), while lateral-posterior parts of the cerebellum are responsible for ataxia of the upper limbs, face, and speech. Ataxia also may be caused by lesions in cerebellar pathways. These disorders are sometimes manifested by very characteristic phenotypes, such as coarse high-amplitude "rubral" tremor (Holmes' tremor) seen in attempts to hold hands in the upright position, a feature typical of lesions in the dentatorubral loop, for example in multiple sclerosis or Wilson's disease.

Sensory ataxia

Compared to cerebellar ataxia, sensory ataxia is relatively rare. It usually results from disease of the posterior columns (Friedreich's ataxia, deficiency of vitamins E and B_{12}, neurosyphilis) leading to proprioceptive deafferentation. Sensory ataxia can be diagnosed in the presence of clear proprioceptive deficit in the "ataxic" body part and a significant worsening of clumsiness with eye closure. In addition, a phenomenon of pseudoathetosis (abnormal slow writhing movements, usually of the fingers, resulting from loss of proprioception) is occasionally seen in affected limbs, with eye closure.

Vestibular ataxia

Vestibular dysfunction may cause a rare syndrome designated as vestibular (or "labyrinthine") ataxia. This syndrome may be regarded as a specific subtype of sensory ataxia. Patients with vestibular ataxia exhibit serious stance and gait difficulties (vestibular disequilibrium), but no incoordination of limbs or speech. With a unilateral labyrinthine lesion, "flank walking" in the direction of the lesion side is a predominant feature. This type of ataxia is frequently associated with dizziness, vomiting, and hearing loss.

International Neurology, Second edition. Edited by Robert P. Lisak, Daniel D. Truong, William M. Carroll and Roongroj Bhidayasiri
© 2016 John Wiley & Sons, Ltd. Published 2016 by John Wiley & Sons, Ltd.

Frontal ataxia

Frontal ataxia (frontal dysbasia) is manifested as apraxia of gait and inability to stand, with festination on unnaturally straightened legs and difficulties with initiation of gait. Motor problems are mostly evident in the leg contralateral to the frontal lesion. Gait problems are typically accompanied by "frontal" cognitive and behavioral symptoms, such as mental slowness, perseveration, decrease in verbal fluency, and dysphoria.

This chapter will focus on cerebellar ataxia as a major type of ataxia.

Pathophysiology

Pathophysiologically, cerebellar ataxia represents failure to maintain normal anti-inertia mechanisms that ensure smoothness, evenness, and accuracy of movements.

Any normal voluntary movement is regarded as the result of precisely coordinated, "orchestrated" activity of a variety of antagonistic and synergistic muscles. This temporally and spatially ordered interplay between different muscles is realized through extensive bilateral connections of the cerebellum, with structures of the central nervous system participating in motor functions at different levels (motor cortex, basal ganglia, brainstem nuclei, reticular formation, spinal motor neurons, proprioceptive neurons, and pathways). The cerebellum as the main "motor coordinator" receives advance information about any changes of muscle tone and posture of body segments, as well as about any intended movement. Using this advance information, the cerebellum "prepares" the correct activity of voluntary muscles, organizes fine motor control, and ensures accurate execution of the movement.

While under normal conditions cerebellar functional circuitry consisting of many feedback and feedforward connections is preserved, cerebellar disorders lead to malfunctioning of this circuitry and result in desynchronization of muscle contractions. Handicaps in cerebellar motor control clinically manifest as confused, irregular "jolts" leading to scanning speech, intention tremor, dysmetria, body titubation (a coarse fore-and-aft tremor of the trunk), and other cerebellar phenomena. The existence of some corticopontocerebellar projections representing the dorsal stream of cognitive processing suggest that the cerebellum also may play a role in spatial awareness and attentional functions.

Cerebellar ataxic disorders

The cerebellum and cerebellar pathways are affected in a variety of acute and chronic conditions that can cause ataxia (Table 55.1).

Acute ataxia

Acute ataxia is typically seen in ischemic (lacunar, cardioembolic, and atherothrombotic infarcts) or hemorrhagic stroke affecting cerebellar hemispheres, as well as in multiple sclerosis, head trauma, infectious cerebellitis or cerebellar abscess, parasitic invasion, MELAS (mitochondrial myopathy, encephalopathy, lactic acidosis, and stroke-like episodes) syndrome, acute drug toxicity and poisonings (ethanol, neuroleptics, anticonvulsants), Arnold–Chiari malformation, and other conditions. In these disorders ataxia is frequently associated with headache, vomiting, vertigo, brainstem signs, and cranial nerve involvement. One should remember that even small cerebellar infarcts and hemorrhages are regarded, due to the limited volume of the posterior fossa, as potentially life-threatening conditions in view

Table 55.1 Etiologies of acute and chronic ataxia.

Acute ataxia	Chronic ataxia
Stroke: • ischemia • hemorrhage	Multiple sclerosis Cerebellar tumors Chronic cerebral ischemia
Multiple sclerosis Head trauma Infections: • cerebellitis • cerebellar abscess • neurosyphilis • HIV • parasitic invasion	Normal pressure hydrocephalus (Hakim–Adams syndrome) Paraneoplastic cerebellar degeneration Cerebellar dysgenesis or hypoplasia (congenital ataxia, usually non-progressive) Prion disease (ataxic form) Chronic alcoholism Hypothyroidism
Acute drug toxicity and poisonings: • ethanol • antipsychotics • antidepressants • anticonvulsants • lithium • soporific medications • chemotherapeutic medications • thallium • methylmercury • bismuth • zinc	Vitamin B_{12} deficiency Hyperthermia (heat shock) Abuse of medications with anxiolytic, soporific, and anticonvulsant action Gluten ataxia Autoimmune syndrome with antibodies against glutamic acid decarboxylase-65 (GAD65) Hereditary ataxias with autosomal dominant, autosomal recessive, and X-linked recessive inheritance
MELAS, Leigh disease and other mitochondrial encephalomyopathies with acute onset Tumors and malformations with acute and subacute manifestations Thiamine deficiency (Wernicke's encephalopathy) Periodic ataxias Paraneoplastic cerebellar degeneration Hyperthermia (heat shock) Hypoglycemia (insulinoma) Electrolyte imbalance Kidney disease Inborn metabolic abnormalities: • maple syrup disease • Hartnup disease • mevalonic aciduria and other acidurias • hereditary hyperammonemias	Sporadic idiopathic degenerative ataxias: • parenchymatous cortical cerebellar atrophy • olivopontocerebellar atrophy Genetic metabolic diseases: • mitochondrial encephalomyopathies with chronic ataxic symptoms (NARP, etc.) • Refsum disease • Gaucher disease type III • Niemann–Pick disease • Tay–Sachs disease • hexosaminidase B deficiency • neuraminidase deficiency • vitamin E deficiency (AVED) • adrenoleukodystrophy and other leukodystrophies • Wilson's disease • neuroacanthocytosis • cerebrotendinous xanthomatosis

of the high risk of obstructive hydrocephalus on the development of brain edema and remote pressure effects. Therefore, in patients with acute cerebellar ataxia, emergency neuroimaging examinations (computed tomography [CT] or magnetic resonance imaging [MRI]) must be performed and decompression surgery (ventriculostomy or posterior craniectomy) must be promptly undertaken. The same is true for any other disorders characterized by large, acute cerebellar lesions with rapidly progressive edema of the posterior fossa structures. Because of the risk of herniation in these patients, lumbar puncture is strongly contraindicated.

Repeated paroxysms of acute ataxic symptoms are seen in periodic (episodic) ataxias. These hereditary diseases are caused by genetic defects of calcium or potassium ion channels, which result in abnormalities of neuronal membrane excitability. Some patients with ataxic paroxysms may benefit from administration of acetazolamide (acetazolamide-responsive forms of periodic ataxias). Periodic ataxias belong to a group of so-called channelopathies.

Chronic ataxia

Chronic ataxia may be caused by a number of different disorders (see Table 55.1), both genetic and non-genetic in origin. Chronic or subacute cerebellar ataxia, especially at a young age, is a typical manifestation of multiple sclerosis, for which a relapsing–remitting course and the presence of multiple demyelinating lesions on brain and spinal MRI facilitate the diagnosis. One should always remember that chronic or subacute cerebellar ataxia may result from tumors (typical cerebellar tumors are cerebellopontine schwannoma, medulloblastoma, and hemangioblastoma), normal pressure hydrocephalus (Hakim–Adams syndrome), and paraneoplastic cerebellar degeneration (lung cancer and other systemic malignancies); all these conditions require appropriate and timely surgery. Cerebellar degenerative disorders also may be caused by chronic alcoholism, hypothyroidism, gluten disease, autoimmune disease with antibodies against glutamic acid decarboxylase-65 (GAD65), vitamin B_{12} deficiency, heat shock, and abuse of some medications with anxiolytic, soporific, and anticonvulsant action.

Chronic progressive ataxia is a key feature of idiopathic degenerative ataxic syndromes, both hereditary and sporadic.

Hereditary ataxias

Hereditary ataxias are a clinically and genetically heterogeneous group of disorders transmitted, most frequently, as autosomal dominant or autosomal recessive traits; each of these major subtypes of hereditary ataxias also demonstrates striking genetic heterogeneity. There are nearly 70 distinct genetic forms of "pure" hereditary ataxias and nearly 300 additional genetic conditions manifesting, among others, by ataxic symptoms. The differential diagnosis between these conditions represents a serious challenge owing to significant phenotypic overlap.

For autosomal dominant spinocerebellar ataxias (SCAs), at least 40 loci have been mapped to different chromosomes, and 28 causative genes and their protein products have been identified. In a number of autosomal dominant SCAs, mutations represent pathological expansions of intragenic trinucleotide repeats or other repeats ("dynamic" mutations). Most frequently, coding CAG repeat expansion leads at the protein level to proportional expansion of the polyglutamine chain (the so-called polyglutamine disorders with a very specific mechanism of neurodegeneration). There is an inverse correlation between the copy number of trinucleotide repeats in the mutant gene and the age at disease onset. Moreover, the longest expanded alleles are associated with the most severe phenotypes. In addition to dynamic mutations, autosomal dominant SCAs can be caused by point mutations in several genes encoding for protein kinase gamma, fibroblast growth factor, beta-3 spectrin, inositol 1,4,5-triphosphate receptor, potassium channel KCND3, and many other essential proteins. The frequencies of particular forms of autosomal dominant SCAs in different populations are strikingly different. For example, in Russia more than 40% of the autosomal dominant SCA families have the *ATXN1* gene mutation on chromosome 6p (SCA1), while in the majority of Western Europe countries the *ATXN3* gene mutation is most prevalent (SCA3 or Machado–Joseph disease).

Among autosomal recessive and X-linked recessive ataxias, the most common form is Friedreich's ataxia caused by GAA repeat expansion in the non-coding region of the *FRDA* gene on chromosome 9q. A protein product of this gene, frataxin, is thought to be involved in the homeostasis of mitochondrial iron, and Friedreich's ataxia thus represents a Mendelian form of mitochondrial cytopathy. Typically, the disease presents with early onset (before the age of 20 years), "mixed" sensory/cerebellar ataxia, dysarthria, muscle weakness, cardiomyopathy, skeletal deformities, diabetes, and a relentlessly progressive course. There is strong correlation between the length of the GAA repeat chain and the type of clinical presentation of Friedreich's ataxia, with the oldest and relatively "benign" cases being associated with mild GAA repeat expansion. Other clinically important recessive ataxias include ataxia-telangiectasia, ataxia with oculomotor apraxia, several forms of spastic ataxia, and several forms of congenital non-progressive cerebellar hypoplasia.

Sporadic (idiopathic) degenerative ataxia

Sporadic (idiopathic) degenerative ataxia is a heterogeneous entity comprising parenchymatous cortical cerebellar atrophy and olivopontocerebellar atrophy. The latter is now regarded as a form of multiple system atrophy, a severe neurodegenerative disorder characterized by involvement of many cerebral and spinal systems (cerebellum, basal ganglia, brainstem, spinal autonomic nuclei, and motor neurons) and the presence of specific α-synuclein-positive glial cytoplasmic inclusions.

Diagnosis

The diagnosis of patients with ataxic disorders is based, first of all, on neuroimaging (CT, MRI) and neurophysiological examinations (evoked potentials, nerve conduction studies, etc.), which provide important information about structural and functional characteristics of the central and the peripheral nervous system. In many cases of hereditary ataxias, DNA diagnosis is available both for affected individuals and for clinically healthy relatives from the "risk group." Genetic counseling and prenatal DNA testing may be offered to prevent new cases of the disease in affected families. Recently, a new technology of exome sequencing made it possible to perform genome-wide analysis for genetically heterogeneous disorders, such as hereditary ataxias, which may greatly facilitate the search for mutations in a variety of genes. This technology is poised to be integrated soon into routine clinical algorithms.

In patients with sporadic ataxia, a detailed search is needed for possible somatic disorders that may cause cerebellar dysfunction (malignancies, endocrine and hepatic disorders, etc.). Since ataxia may be a major presentation of a variety of metabolic diseases (see Table 55.1), appropriate biochemical screening should be undertaken in unclear cases.

Management

Management and prognosis of ataxic syndromes rely on the primary cause of ataxia. If radical therapy is possible (such as surgery of cerebellar tumor or vitamin supplementation in specific vitamin deficiency), one can expect complete or partial recovery, or at least cessation of further disease progression.

There is no therapy uniformly beneficial for ataxia itself. Limited positive effect has been reported in degenerative ataxias with amantadine, buspirone, L-5-hydroxy tryptophan, thyrotropin-releasing hormone, pregabalin, and several other medications, but this has not been confirmed in randomized studies. Cerebellar tremor was reported to be successfully treated with isoniazid and some anticonvulsants (clonazepam, carbamazepine, and topiramate). Stereotaxic thalamic surgery, including deep brain stimulation, may also be a good option in some cases.

In Friedreich's ataxia, treatment options have been mostly directed at protection against mitochondrial damage or chelating excessive mitochondrial iron. For instance, the mitochondrial antioxidant idebenone was shown to reduce cardiac hypertrophy and, at higher doses, to improve neurological function, while iron-chelating therapy with deferiprone and other agents has been shown to have some positive effect in pilot clinical studies and cell model experiments. However, further large controlled clinical trials are still needed.

Physical therapy is important in the management of ataxic patients. It is directed at preventing various complications such as contractures or muscle atrophy, maximizing strength and conditioning, and improving coordination and gait. Special complexes of "cerebellar" or "sensory" exercises, as well as biofeedback with stabilography, are strongly recommended.

A number of new molecular strategies for the treatment of different forms of hereditary ataxias are currently under development. They include the administration of small molecules increasing frataxin gene transcription in Friedreich's ataxia, oligonucleotide-based strategies for "gene silencing" in polyglutamine-type auto-

somal dominant ataxias, and other approaches. Hopefully, in the future these technologies will offer significant advantages over any traditional therapy.

Further reading

Brice A, Pulst S-M (eds.) *Spinocerebellar Degenerations: The Ataxias and Spastic Paraplegias*. Philadelphia, PA: Elsevier; 2007.

Diener HC, Dichgans J. Pathophysiology of cerebellar ataxia. *Mov Dis* 1992;7:95–109.

Durr A. Autosomal dominant cerebellar ataxias: Polyglutamine expansions and beyond. *Lancet Neurol* 2010;9:885–894.

Fogel BL, Lee H, Deignan JL, et al. Exome sequencing in the clinical diagnosis of sporadic or familial cerebellar ataxia. *JAMA Neurol* 2014;71:1237–1246.

Ruigrok THJ. Role of the cerebellum. In: Wolters ECh, van Laar T, Berendse HW (eds.). *Parkinsonism and Related Disorders*. Amsterdam: VU University Press; 2007:55–80.

Santos R, Lefevre S, Sliwa D. Friedreich ataxia: Molecular mechanisms, redox considerations, and therapeutic opportunities. *Antioxid Redox Signal* 2010;13:651–690.

Taroni F, DiDonato S. Pathways to motor incoordination: The inherited ataxias. *Nature Rev Neurosci* 2004;5:641–655.

56 Drug-induced movement disorders

Rick Stell

Western Australian Neuromuscular Research Institute, Sir Charles Gairdner Hospital, Perth, WA, Australia

Drugs are a frequent, although underrecognized, cause of movement disorders, and the list of potential agents is steadily increasing. The most common drugs are those that block or stimulate dopamine receptors (DBA). Although movement disorders related to antipsychotic medication were probably seen earlier, the causative effects of these drugs were not recognized until 1956, when the first report of chlorpromazine-induced movement disorder was made by Hall. While initially thought to be rare, it is now estimated to occur in up to 20% of patients exposed to these drugs. The extrapyramidal side effect (EPS) with dopamine-blocking drugs seems to depend on the degree of D2 receptor antagonism and the speed of dissociation. Drugs with less D2 affinity and more rapid dissociation are less likely to produce EPS.

Clinical presentations may be acute, subacute, or delayed for months, and may mimic virtually every known hyper- and hypokinetic movement disorder, either alone or in combination.

This chapter focuses on several movement disorders caused by commonly prescribed drugs, excluding the neuroleptic malignant syndrome.

Acute syndromes

Acute dystonic reactions

The incidence of acute dystonic reactions (ADR) has been reported to range between 2.3 and 63%, the wide range probably indicating that it is often not recognized or is misdiagnosed. Most (90%) acute dystonic reactions occur within 5 days of exposure, and usually within 2–24 hours, lasting from hours to days. Clinical manifestations vary with age: children often develop generalized spasms, sometimes with an axial emphasis (e.g., opisthotonos), whereas adults' involvement is usually segmental with a craniocervical emphasis, such as blepharospasm, oculogyric crises, trismus, and torticollis.

Dystonic spasms and postures tend to have an abrupt onset and are frequently painful and fluctuating in their distribution. Proposed risk factors include male sex, age <30 years, high neuroleptic dosage, potency of the drug, and possibly a familial predisposition – several families have been reported to include a number of affected individuals. Another risk factor is the condition for which the DBA was prescribed. Patients treated with DBAs for their first episode of psychosis have a reported 34–60% risk of developing drug-induced acute dystonia. In addition to high-potency neuroleptics, ADR may also be seen with the benzamide antiemetic metoclopramide, as well as domperidone and sulpiride.

The pathophysiology of ADR has been linked to a sudden imbalance between striatal dopamine and cholinergic systems, causing a relative preponderance of acetylcholine. ADR resolves spontaneously on drug withdrawal, but this may take hours.

Acute dystonia responds well to parenteral anticholinergics (biperiden, benztropine), antihistamines (diphenhydramine), or benzodiazepines (diazepam or lorazepam), although repeated doses may be necessary over a few days. The response to anticholinergics is so consistent that a lack of effect should raise the possibility of phencyclidine-(PCP) induced dystonia.

Acute akathisia

Acute akathisia (from the Greek meaning "inability to sit") is a very common and early dose-related side effect of neuroleptics and other dopamine receptor blocking drugs, although it is less frequently seen with atypical neuroleptics. There have been reports of cases in association with selective serotonin reuptake inhibitors (SSRIs), antiepileptics (carbamazepine, ethosuximide), antidepressants (lithium), calcium channel blockers (flunarizine, diltiazem), and dopamine depleters (tetrabenazine). Patients present with an aversion to keeping still and a subjective sensation of restlessness, accompanied by complex or stereotyped movements, including pacing, marching on the spot, picking at clothes, rocking, and crossing/uncrossing legs. The prevalence varies widely between studies, but acute akathisia is estimated to affect 40% of exposed patients, although this may be an underestimate. Half (50%) of affected individuals develop the condition within the first month, and 90% within 3 months of drug exposure.

The pathophysiology of acute akathisia is not well understood, but it may result from a blockade of the mesocortical dopamine receptors.

Treatment should comprise dose reduction, switching to a less potent drug, or, if possible, drug withdrawal, as this is the most effective treatment. If this is not possible or not effective, the addition of various drugs including anticholinergics, amantadine, propranalol, clonidine, benzodiazepines, and, more recently, opioid agonists (such as propoxyphene) has been reported to be effective. Traditionally, beta-adranergic blockers such as propranolol have been used as first-line agents to treat akathisia. Their use is supported by studies demonstrating subjective and objective benefit. Anticholinergics are probably not as effective and are limited by dose-related anticholinergic side effects. Several placebo-controlled trials have demonstrated benefit from benzodiazepines, including clonazepam (0.5–1 mg/day) and diazepam (1–2 mg/day). $5-HT_{2A}$

International Neurology, Second edition. Edited by Robert P. Lisak, Daniel D. Truong, William M. Carroll and Roongroj Bhidayasiri
© 2016 John Wiley & Sons, Ltd. Published 2016 by John Wiley & Sons, Ltd.

antagonists such as mirtazapine, mianserin, and cyproheptadine have also been shown to be antiakathisic, as a result of their capacity to increase dopaminergic transmission.

Acute choreoathetosis

A wide variety of commonly used drugs have been reported to cause choreoathetosis, raising the question of individual susceptibility as a consequence of prior basal ganglia damage. Individual susceptibility has been well established for contraceptive-induced chorea, as affected women often present a past history of Sydenham's chorea or rheumatic fever. By blocking presynaptic dopamine reuptake and also by altering postsynaptic receptor sensitivity, cocaine may cause or trigger chorea and other hyperkinetic movements. Choreoathetosis and, less frequently, tremor, asterixis, and myoclonus have also been reported with phenytoin and anticonvulsants such as carbamazepine, felbamate, and gabapentin.

Acute tics

Drug-induced tics are indistinguishable from those seen in Tourette syndrome and are caused by drugs that enhance dopaminergic transmission (e.g., amphetamines, SSRIs, and cocaine). Because tics are not always exacerbated or caused by central stimulants, undefined predisposing factors may also be important to this drug effect.

Subacute syndromes

Drug-induced parkinsonism (DIP)

Of the subacute drug-induced movement syndromes, DIP is the most common. Related to dopamine blocking agents, it occurs in 10–15% of exposed patients; however, if subtle signs are included, the incidence may be as high as 90%. Of these patients, 50–70% develop signs or symptoms within 1 month and 90% by 3 months, although symptoms may occur after long-term drug exposure when the dose of the drug is increased, and may coexist with typical tardive dyskinesias. Most cases of DIP follow exposure to dopamine receptor blockers, especially the piperazine class of phenothiazines and butyrophenones. The risk is smaller for atypical neuroleptics, olanzapine and clozapine, the latter almost only occurring at doses above 250 mg. Other classes of drugs may also cause DIP, including dopamine depleting agents (reserpine), calcium channel blockers (amiodarone, verapamil, diltiazem), immunosuppressants (cyclophosphamide, cyclosporine), valproic acid, and antidepressants (SSRIs, lithium). The role of the SSRIs fluoxetine and, to a lesser extent, paroxetine and fluvoxamine in DIP is controversial, as in most reports there has been concomitant use of other potentially relevant drugs. The only consistent susceptibility factors for DIP are the dose and potency of the neuroleptic used.

A diagnosis of DIP requires a history of neuroleptic or other potentially relevant drug exposure and cannot be entertained otherwise. The clinical features of DIP are often indistinguishable from Parkinson's disease (PD). While it is said that some patients present symmetric akinetic rigid parkinsonian syndrome without tremor, these represent the minority. Other clues to the diagnosis include early age of onset, presentation with gait disturbance, dominant postural or kinetic tremor, and the coincidence of other well-recognized drug-related movements; in particular, the presence of orobuccolingual dyskinesia in the absence of levodopa response is more supportive of DIP than PD.

Prognosis in DIP is uncertain. Klawans and colleagues reported that patients may take 18 months or more to recover. Other authors have suggested that up to 20% never recover, or recover only later to develop typical PD. This suggests that certain drugs may unmask subclinical PD in a significant proportion of patients. In support of this assertion is the report of Rajput, in which two patients whose DIP resolved within 3 weeks of stopping neuroleptics were later found to have pathological evidence of PD. Additionally, Burn and colleagues found that 30% of DIP patients showed abnormal F-DOPA positron emission tomography (PET) scans, 75% of whom went on to develop PD.

The best treatment of DIP has not been established. In most cases, it is reversible once the offending drug is withdrawn, although as mentioned this may take 18 months or more. If withdrawal of the offending drug is not possible, it may be replaced by an atypical neuroleptic such as clozapine or quetiapine. Mild DIP may be left untreated. If symptomatic treatment is necessary, levodopa may help in up to 30% of cases, although at the risk of aggravating the underlying psychiatric disorder. Some patients respond well to anticholinergics and amantadine, but these may worsen psychotic symptoms or result in confusion in elderly patients. Other options include dopamine agonists, propranolol, and electroconvulsive therapy.

Chronic or tardive syndromes

Chronic or tardive syndromes are those that occur after long-term exposure to drugs, requiring exposure of at least 3 months and usually 1–2 years, and persist for at least 1 month after cessation of the offending drug. They have been reported most often in association with drugs that interfere with dopaminergic transmission, although seldom with drugs that act presynaptically, such as reserpine or tetrabenazine. Prevalence rates vary widely, probably reflecting the differences in patient samples and diagnostic criteria. A meta-analysis of 56 surveys indicates an average prevalence of 20%.

Risk factors for tardive dyskinesia (TD) include advanced age, duration of drug exposure, and duration of the psychiatric disease. There are several clinical subtypes of tardive dyskinesia, which may occur alone or in combination. The orobuccoliguomasticatory syndrome is the most common and first described subtype, representing 40% of patients in one study. It is characterized by stereotyped movements of tongue twisting and protrusion, along with facial grimacing. The clue to the diagnosis (apart from the history of drug exposure) is the not infrequent coexistence of other typical tardive movement syndromes, such as tardive tics, myoclonus, and tremor. Risk factors for developing tardive dyskinesias include chronic neuroleptic therapy (especially polypharmacy), age greater than 40, chronic schizophrenia, female sex, and the indiscriminate use of anticholinergic medication.

Large-scale prospective studies indicate an average yearly incidence of developing TD of approximately 5% per year for the first several years with typical neuroleptics and a cumulative 5-year incidence of 20–26%. Glazer et al. have suggested that the risk increases in a linear fashion with continued exposure, with a 25-year risk estimated at 68%. Having said this, with the advent of the second-generation, prevalence of both acute EPS and TD has declined over months of treatment in patients switched from traditional neuroleptics. A study of approximately 2700 patients with an average duration of over 300 days indicates that the risk of TD is significantly lower (by two- or three-fold) with most modern neuroleptics than with older neuroleptics of higher potency. On the other hand, the newer atypicals have a higher risk of producing metabolic syndrome.

The pathophysiology of tardive dyskinesias is only partly understood. The most enduring hypothesis is that of denervation blockade. This leads to dopamine receptor supersensitivity, in which amounts of dopamine normally too small to induce dyskinesias are able to do so.

Prevention remains the best treatment. Dopamine receptor blockers should be used for as short a time as possible and in the lowest dosage possible. Once tardive dyskinesia has developed, the offending drug should be withdrawn, although this is often not possible without relapse of the psychiatric illness. Improvement occurs in most cases, but complete and persistent resolution is seen in only 2%. The switch to atypical dopamine receptor blockers such as clozapine has been proposed as a desensitization technique and

may be helpful in up to 40% of cases based on uncontrolled studies (controlled studies are lacking). Withdrawal of anticholinergics is recommended for orofacial dyskinesias, although they may help in the treatment of tardive dystonia.

Further reading

Burn DJ, Brooks DJ. Nigral dysfunction in drug-induced parkinsonism: An 18F-dopa PET study. *Neurology* 1993;43:552–556.

Glazer WM. Managing risk of tardive dyskinesia. *Behav Healthc* 2006;26(12):27–32.

Kane JM, Smith JM. Tardive dyskinesia: Prevalence and risk factors, 1959 to 1979. *Arch Gen Psychiatry* 1982;39:473–481.

Klawans HL, Gegen D, Bruyn GW. Prolonged drug-induced parkinsonism. *Confin Neurol* 1973;35:368–377.

Rajput AH, Rodzilsky B, Hornykiewicz O, *et al*. Reversible drug-induced parkinsonism: Clinicopathologic study of two cases. *Arch Neurol* 1982;39:644–646.

57 Paroxysmal movement disorders

Sopio Sopromadze[1] and Alexander Tsiskaridze[2]

[1] Department of Neurology, N. Kipshidze Central University Clinic, Tbilisi, Georgia
[2] Department of Neurology, Ivane Javakhishvili Tbilisi State University, Tbilisi, Georgia

Paroxysmal movement disorders are a heterogeneous group of rare conditions characterized by episodic dyskinesias with sudden onset and brief duration. These disorders affect both adults and children and may be inherited or acquired. Paroxysmal dyskinesias (PxDs) can occur spontaneously or may be precipitated by sudden movements, prolonged exercise, caffeine and alcohol consumption, emotional stress, or fatigue. Abnormal movements can present with dystonic, choreic, ballistic, and other presentations, or a combination of these hyperkinesias. The current classification of PxDs by Demirkiran and Jankovic from 1995 is based on the precipitating events (Table 57.1) and includes: (1) paroxysmal kinesigenic dyskinesias (PKD); (2) paroxysmal non-kinesigenic dyskinesias (PNKD); and (3) paroxysmal exercise-induced (exertion-induced) dyskinesias (PED).

Initially hypnogenic paroxysmal dyskinesia, a fourth form of paroxysmal disorder, was included in the PxD classification. However, recently it has become clear that hypnogenic paroxysmal dyskinesia is a form of frontal lobe epilepsy in which dyskinesias occur only at night during sleep. Besides these three forms of PxDs, which are of genetic origin, occur without loss of consciousness, and are characterized by normal cerebral imaging, symptomatic PxDs have been described in patients with multiple sclerosis, stroke, trauma, encephalitis, metabolic disorders, cerebral neoplasms, and migraine.

Historical aspects

The first description of a patient with PxD was made in 1940 by Mount and Reback and the term "paroxysmal choreoathetosis" appeared in the literature for the first time. The patient was a 23-year-old man who had episodes of "choreo-dystonia that could last several hours." Over the years, more cases were described and the disorder became known as "paroxysmal dystonic choreoathetosis" (PDC). Later, in 1967, Kertesz described a new episodic disorder termed "paroxysmal kinesigenic choreo-athetosis," in which episodes were very brief and induced by sudden movements. As more families and cases were described, it became clear that this disorder, where the attacks were brief and responded well to antiepileptic drugs (AEDs), was different from PDC. In 1977, Lance described a third form of attacks lasting between 5 and 30 minutes and provoked by prolonged exercise but not by sudden movements, which was further classified as "paroxysmal exercise-induced dyskinesia."

Epidemiology

PKD is the most frequent among the paroxysmal dyskinesia syndromes, but it remains a rare disease, with prevalence estimated as 1/150,000. It is considered a familial disorder with autosomal dominant inheritance and incomplete penetrance, but sporadic cases often occur. PKD is more prevalent in males than females, usually as high as 3.75:1. The prevalence of PNKD is estimated to be 1/1,000,000 worldwide. A male preponderance is observed (1.4:1). PED is the rarest paroxysmal dyskinesia subtype.

Pathophysiology

The pathophysiology of PxDs is controversial. Whether these conditions are of an epileptic origin or represent a basal ganglia disorder is as yet unknown. The primary pathophysiological process

Table 57.1 Idiopathic paroxysmal dyskinesias.

(PxDs) Classification	Age of onset	Triggering factors	Duration	Frequency	Treatment	Gene/protein
Paroxysmal kinesigenic dyskinesia (PKD)	Early childhood	Sudden movements	Very brief	Several per day	Carbamazepine Phenytoin Topiramate Levetiracetam Lamotrigint Valproate Oxcarbazepine Phenobarbital Lacosamide	Proline-rich transmembrane protein 2 (PRRT2)
Paroxysmal non-kinesigenic dyskinesia (PNKD)	Childhood	Alcohol, caffeine, stress, excitement, or fatigue	1–4 h	1/day–1/year	Benzodiazepines Gabapentin L-DOPA	Myofibrillogenesis regulator 1 (MR-1)
Paroxysmal exercise-induced dyskinesia (PED)	Childhood, adolescence	Sustained exercise, walking, swimming, or running	5–30 min	1/week–1/year	Benzodiazepines Carbamazepine Ketogenic diet	Glucose transporter 1 (SLC2A1)

International Neurology, Second edition. Edited by Robert P. Lisak, Daniel D. Truong, William M. Carroll and Roongroj Bhidayasiri
© 2016 John Wiley & Sons, Ltd. Published 2016 by John Wiley & Sons, Ltd.

may be that of epilepsy due to the paroxysmal nature of the disorder, prodromic aura-like symptoms, short duration of attacks, and response to AEDs. However, paroxysmal movement disorders do not have typical epileptic features: consciousness is preserved during attacks and electroencephalography (EEG) is normal in most cases. Involvement of the basal ganglia is supported by the observation that secondary PKD occurs in conditions affecting the basal ganglia, and response to levodopa has been described; as supportive evidence, ictal single photon emission computed tomography (SPECT) studies found increased perfusion of the contralateral basal ganglia in cases of unilateral attacks. One interictal SPECT study showed decreased perfusion of the posterior region of the caudate nuclei.

Concerning cellular mechanisms, channelopathy has been considered the main pathophysiological hypothesis for a rather long time. Indeed, paroxysmal dyskinesias have many clinical similarities to other episodic disorders of the nervous system, such as episodic ataxias and periodic paralysis. For instance, there are common features shared by PKD and an ion channel disorder, episodic ataxia type 1(EA1). Like PKD, episodes of ataxia in EA1 are often triggered by movement, are brief, and can occur several times a day. Both conditions have an early age of onset and there is a tendency for both to abate in adulthood. EA1 responds to AEDs. Dysfunction of the basal ganglia might be secondary to the ion channel disorder. Response to AEDs such as carbamazepine, oxcarbazepine, phenytoin, or lacosamide, which are voltage-gated sodium channel blockers, could even point to possible sodium channel disorder. However, the discovery of the proline-rich transmembrane protein 2 (*PRRT2*) gene mutations has led to these speculations being abandoned.

Recently genetic causes of various forms of paroxysmal dyskinesias have been elucidated. The three major types of PxDs (PKD, PNKD, and PED) have been related to mutations in *PRRT2*, myofibrillogenesis regulator 1 (*MR-1*), and glucose transporter 1 (*SLC2A1*) genes, respectively. However, there is marked pleiotrophy of mutations in such genes, which expands the spectrum of clinical manifestations. It is also noteworthy that not all patients with a clinical picture of PxDs have mutations in these genes.

PRRT2 is the major gene accounting for PKD. This gene encodes a protein expressed throughout the nervous system. In the Chinese population, three different studies have identified *PRRT2* mutations in a total of 16 out of 17 families and 10 out of 29 sporadic cases. In a European population of 34 index cases, *PRRT2* mutations were reported in 65%, including 13 out of 14 familial cases (93%) and 9 out of 20 sporadic cases (45%). Further studies in other populations have confirmed the predominance of *PRRT2*. As already noted, the pathophysiology of PKD remains largely unknown. Whether PKD has a subcortical or cortical origin is debatable. Brain imaging is normal during PKD.

The gene responsible for PNKD is the myofibrillogenesis regulator 1 (*MR-1*) gene. Mutation in this gene causes paroxysmal dystonic choreoathetosis. The function of *MR-1* is not fully understood. The *MR-1* gene is homologous to the hydroxyacyl glutathione hydrolase (*HAGH*) gene. It catalyzes the detoxification of methylglyoxal, which is reported to be neurotoxic. This compound is present in coffee and alcoholic beverages and is produced as a byproduct of oxidative stress, which may be a possible mechanism whereby coffee, alcohol, and stress precipitate attacks in PNKD.

The pathophysiology of PED is still unknown, but some familial cases have been found to be associated with mutations in the *SLC2A1* (facilitated glucose transporter) gene. *SLC2A1* encodes the glucose transporter *GLUT1*. All mutations in this gene responsible for PED have been found to affect the ability of *GLUT1* to transport glucose. It has thus been proposed that an energy deficiency on exertion caused by a reduced glucose transport rate is a cause of this paroxysmal movement disorder in *SLC2A1*-related cases. Glucose transporter member 1 (*SLC2A1*) encoding facilitates glucose entry into the brain and across the astrocyte membrane.

Clinical features

PxDs represent a group of episodic abnormal involuntary movements manifested by recurrent attacks of dystonia, chorea, athetosis, or a combination of these disorders. PKD, PKND, and PED are distinguished clinically by precipitating factors, duration and frequency of attacks, and response to medication.

Paroxysmal kinesigenic dyskinesia

PKD is the most common type of PxD, with brief dyskinetic episodes precipitated by a sudden movement (e.g., standing up), continuous exercise, hyperventilation, or startle. Onset is in early childhood and it is more common in males. A preceding "aura-like" sensation in the limbs has been reported in 63% of cases. PKD attacks are very brief, with many attacks per day. The movements can be any combination of chorea, athetosis, ballism, and/or a dystonic posture. Some patients manage to suppress the attack during the aura by holding the affected limb tightly, by moving slowly, or by crossing the legs. Attacks usually are unilateral. Dystonic spasms of the jaw or face may lead to dysarthria. Consciousness is always preserved, and there is no postictal change. Most cases are idiopathic and apparently sporadic. Family history is present in 27% of cases and usually follows an autosomal dominant pattern of inheritance. Overall prognosis for the idiopathic form is good and the disease often abates in adulthood, as the attack frequency decreases with age.

Paroxysmal non-kinesigenic dyskinesia

PNKD is idiopathic, with onset in childhood or early teens. As with PKD, more males than females are affected. In PNKD, attacks are longer, less frequent, and precipitated not by sudden movements or physical exertion as in PKD, but rather by alcohol, caffeine, stress, excitement, or fatigue. Episodes typically last 1–4 hours, and the frequency of episodes ranges from several per day to one per year. In some affected individuals episodes occur less often with increasing age. Patients often have a combination of involuntary dystonic, choreatic, athetotic, and ballistic movements, mainly affecting the limbs, often unilateral or asymmetric. Neurological findings, EEG, and brain imaging are normal in the idiopathic cases.

Paroxysmal exercise-induced dyskinesia

PED is less common than PNKD and PKD. Onset is in childhood or adolescence. Involuntary movements occur after continuous exercise such as walking, swimming, or running. Dystonic episodes last 5–30 minutes, and the frequency of episodes ranges from several per week to one per year. In some cases the attacks are triggered by exposure to cold. Dystonic movement affecting lower limbs, often bilaterally, is the most common feature.

Investigations/diagnosis

The diagnosis is based primarily on history and clinical observation, confirmed by normal imaging and laboratory workup for metabolic disease, including thyroid disease, hypoglycemia or hyperglycemia, and electrolyte disturbance (hypocalcemia).

The following diagnostic evaluations are recommended:

- Brain and spine imaging, preferably MRI, to rule out secondary causes of PxDs.
- EEG, including continuous video-EEG monitoring, should be considered to rule out seizures as a cause of the dyskinesias.
- Medical genetics consultation and testing for mutations.

Treatment

PKD responds well to AEDs, with a particular sensitivity to carbamazepine (1.5–15 mg/kg/day) and phenytoin (5 mg/kg/day). If they are contraindicated or not effective, other anticonvulsants can be tried, such as topiramate, levetiracetam, lamotrigine, valproate, oxcarbazepine, phenobarbital, and lacosamide.

PNKD patients usually do not benefit from antiepileptic drugs like carbamazepine, although clonazepam (2–4 mg/day) may be helpful. Many patients learn to avoid precipitants. Some patients may respond to gabapentin and levodopa. A few patients have been treated successfully with deep brain stimulation of thalamic nuclei or globus pallidus.

Avoiding precipitating events, like prolonged physical exercise, may prevent PED attacks. Anticonvulsants, such as clonazepam and carbamazepine, have been found to be of limited benefit. In patients with PED secondary to GLUT1 mutations, a ketogenic diet has been found to be fairly effective.

Conclusion

PxDs are rare neurological disorders characterized by a sudden onset of dystonic, choreatic, athetotic, and ballistic movements. Three main groups of PxDs can be distinguished, mainly based on the precipitating events. Treatment depends on the type of PxD, where patients with PKD have the best chance of benefiting from anticonvulsant treatment. A number of other disorders that manifest with motor disturbance are important to be considered in the differential diagnosis. Causative genes have been found, but further studies are needed to determine the possible effect of a modifier gene. Correct diagnosis of the paroxysmal dyskinesia often leads to an appropriate and effective treatment.

Further reading

Bhatia KP. Paroxysmal dyskinesias. *Mov Disord* 2011;26:1157–1165.

Bhatia KP, Griggs RC, Ptácek LJ. Episodic movement disorders as channelopathies. *Mov Disord* 2000;15:429–433.

Bruno MK, Hallett M, Gwinn-Hardy K, *et al*. Clinical evaluation of idiopathic paroxysmal kinesigenic dyskinesia: New diagnostic criteria. *Neurology* 2004;28:2280–2287.

Demirkiran M, Jankovic J. Paroxysmal dyskinesias: Clinical features and classification. *Ann Neurol* 1995;38:571–579.

Erro R, Sheerin UM, Bhatia KP. Paroxysmal dyskinesias revisited: A review of 500 genetically proven cases and a new classification. *Mov Disord* 2014;29:1108–1116.

Houser MK, Soland VL, Bhatia KP, Quinn NP, Marsden CD. Paroxysmal kinesigenic choreoathetosis. *J Neurol* 1999;246:120–126.

Ko CH, Kong CK, Ngai WT, Ma KM. Ictal (99m)Tc ECD SPECT in paroxysmal kinesigenic choreoathetosis. *Pediatr Neurol* 2001;24:225–227.

Mehta SH, Morgan JC, Sethi KD. Paroxysmal dyskinesias. *Curr Treat Options Neurol* 2009;11:170–178.

Méneret A, Gaudebout C, Riant F, *et al*. PRRT2 mutations and paroxysmal disorders. *Eur J Neurol* 2013;20:872–878.

Méneret A, Grabli D, Depienne C, *et al*. PRRT2 mutations: A major cause of paroxysmal kinesigenic dyskinesia in the European population. *Neurology* 2012;10:170–174.

58   Acute bacterial meningitis

Sudesh Prabhakar

Department of Neurology, Fortis Hospital, Mohali, Chandigarh, India

Acute bacterial meningitis (ABM) is a neurological emergency requiring prompt evaluation and treatment. It is a fulminant purulent infection of the meninges, characterized by fever, headache, and meningismus. The associated inflammatory reaction of the central nervous system (CNS) may result in altered sensorium, seizures, and raised intracranial pressure (ICP), usually within a few hours or days. The causative organisms vary in developing as compared to developed countries, depending on the use of vaccination against *Haemophilus influenzae*. Despite the availability of potent newer antibiotics, the mortality rate in ABM remains high (6–32%) in developing countries.

Epidemiology

The etiological agent for ABM depends on the age of the patient, their immunological status, and the country in which they reside. The epidemiology of bacterial meningitis has changed significantly in recent years, with almost complete elimination of *H. influenzae* type b in developed countries due to vaccination against *H. influenzae*. *Streptococcus pneumonia* and *Neisseria meningitidis* are the most common causative organisms of community-acquired bacterial meningitis in adults and are responsible for 80% of cases of meningitis. Other common organisms include *Listeria monocytogenes* and group B Streptococci. Depending on the immune status of the patient, the mortality still is very high (around 20%). Patients in the extremes of age are most vulnerable. Recently, *H. influenzae* type b was still found to be the predominant cause of bacterial meningitis in young children in diverse geographic locations in India. Bacterial meningitis following neurosurgical procedures is usually due to Staphylococci, Gram-negative bacilli, or anaerobic pathogens. Since the introduction of a vaccination program for the three most common pathogens of acute bacterial meningitis (*H. influenzae*, *N. meningitidis*, *Streptococcus pneumoniae*), the epidemiology of acute bacterial meningitis has changed considerably throughout the world. These three agents accounted for more than 75% of all cases of acute bacterial meningitis prior to the introduction of effective vaccination programs. After the introduction of *H. influenzae* vaccine in 1980s, the incidence of meningitis decreased dramatically in the United States (from 48% of cases of bacterial meningitis to about 7%). There was a marked reduction in the incidence of acute bacterial meningitis in general and *H. influenzae* meningitis in particular. This highlighted the importance of vaccination programs in the prevention of acute bacterial meningitis. A heptavalent pneumococcal vaccine and a tetravalent meningococcal vaccine were licensed for use in the United States in 2000 and 2005, respectively. Subsequent to that, the incidence of pneumococcal and meningococcal meningitis has further decreased. Studies from Northwest and Southern Europe, Canada, Brazil, and Israel showed trends similar to those seen from the United States. The most common agents in these countries now are *S. pneumonia* and *N. meningitides*, as vaccination has virtually eliminated *H. influenzae* type b–related meningitis.

Bacterial meningitis is a more significant problem in the developing world. In most of Africa and Asia, *H. influenzae* continues to be a major cause of meningitis due to lack of widespread immunization. Although the incidence of pneumococcal meningitis is declining in the developed world, it continues to be a major cause of meningitis in the developing world

The impact of meningitis is less striking in the developing world, although the vaccination program has affected the epidemiological profile of acute bacterial meningitis there as well. Due to the widespread use of meningococcal vaccination, the epidemics of meningococcal meningitis in the meningitic belt of Africa (from Ethiopia to Senegal) are decreasing in frequency as well as severity. The epidemiology of meningococcal meningitis has changed in these regions too. While the initial epidemics used to be due to *N. meningitides* serogroup A (NmA), current epidemics are usually due to other meningococcal serogroups (e.g., NmW, Nmx, and NmC).

Etiology

Bacterial meningitis due to *S. pneumoniae* is usually associated with pneumonia and sinusitis. The predisposing factors include head injury with basal skull fractures, and cerebrospinal fluid (CSF) leaks, complement deficiency, diabetes, thalassemia major, and multiple myeloma. *Neisseria meningitides*, a common organism seen in the nasopharynx, is responsible for almost 25% of cases of meningitis in all age groups. The risk of invasive disease is mainly dependent on the immune status of the individual and the virulence of the organism. In some cases the colonization leads to an asymptomatic

International Neurology, Second edition. Edited by Robert P. Lisak, Daniel D. Truong, William M. Carroll and Roongroj Bhidayasiri
© 2016 John Wiley & Sons, Ltd. Published 2016 by John Wiley & Sons, Ltd.

carrier state. Deficiency of any of the components of complement makes the individual highly susceptible to meningococcal infection. The relative incidence of meningitis caused by *H. influenzae*, *S. pneumoniae*, and *N. meningitides* is lower in Southeast Asia compared to Western countries. Gram-negative bacilli such as *Klebsiella pneumoniae* and *Pseudomonas aeruginosa* are increasingly being recognized as important sources of community-acquired bacterial meningitis (CABM) as well as nosocomial meningitis. Most Indian studies report *S. pneumonia* as the most common etiological agent of CABM. However, the commonly held view of *H. influenzae* as being rare in Asia has been challenged in a study published by the World Health Organization (WHO), and large-scale vaccination for *H. influenzae* type b has been recommended for Asian countries as well.

Coagulase negative staphylococci and *Staphylococcus aureus* are common pathogens causing CSF shunt infections. Meningitis associated with other neurosurgical procedures is usually due to Gram-negative bacilli and staphylococci. Patients with defective cell-mediated immunity secondary to hematological malignancies, organ transplantation, cancer, and HIV infection may develop *Listeria monocytogenes* meningitis. Patients with defective humoral immunity, on the other hand, are unable to control the infection due to polysaccharide-encapsulated bacteria such as *S. pneumonia* and *N. meningitidis*. *Listeria monocytogenes* has become an increasingly important cause of meningitis in neonates, pregnant women, and the elderly. Food-borne human *Listeria* infection has been reported from contaminated milk, soft cheese, and so on. Recurrent meningitis usually occurs in association with head trauma, fracture of the base of the skull, and CSF rhinorrhea. It may also occur with meningomyelocele, parameningeal focus of infection, and post-splenectomy cases.

Pathophysiology

Both *S. pneumoniae* and *N. meningitidis*, the common bacteria producing meningitis, colonize in the nasopharynx. They are transported across epithelial cells into the bloodstream. Localized infections like sinusitis, ear infections, and mastoiditis can reach the meninges through emissary veins. Blood-borne bacteria reach the intraventricular choroid plexus, directly infecting the epithelial cells and CSF. The organisms, especially *S. pneumoniae*, migrate between the epithelial cells to reach the CSF, where they multiply due to lack of host immune defense. The inflammatory reaction produced by the bacteria is mainly responsible for the neurological manifestations of bacterial meningitis. The invasion of bacteria in the subarachnoid space (SAS) produces inflammation and release of tumor necrosis factor (TNF) and interleukins 1, 2, 6, and 8, causing significant reduction of cerebral blood flow. Later there is increased permeability of the blood–brain barrier, causing vasogenic edema. Microvascular thrombosis, vasculitis, and neuronal apoptosis produce cytotoxic edema. The edema leads to increased ICP.

Pathology

The meninges over the cerebral convexities in bacterial meningitis are usually yellowish-green in color. The exudates spread to basal cisterns and the posterior surface of the spinal cord. The exudate is very thick and localized to basal cisterns in *H. influenzae* infection, whereas in pneumococcal infection the exudates are thinner and more extensive over convexities (Figure 58.1). In acute

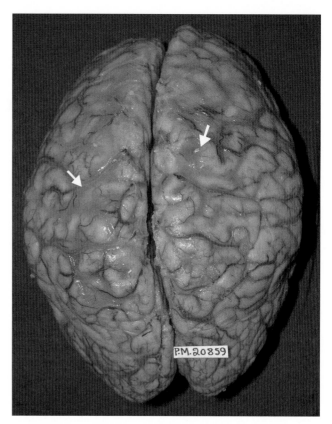

Figure 58.1 Gross photograph of brain showing exudates over the superolateral surface of bilateral cerebral hemispheres (arrows).

fulminant meningococcal meningitis, there may occasionally be no inflammatory exudate; however, there is significant interstitial edema. Microscopically, the exudates show neutrophils and bacteria in the early stage. In case of early treatment, these changes may vary. Within a week, the neutrophilic response may change to a lymphocytic response. If the treatment is not adequate, it may produce a picture that mimics chronic meningitis, such as tuberculous meningitis. The infection can also spread to veins, leading to cortical venous thrombosis. As the exudates increase, the subarachnoid space is reduced and CSF flow may be compromised. Obstruction of the foramina of Luschka and Magendie may result in communicating hydrocephalus (Figure 58.1).

Clinical features

The clinical presentation of bacterial meningitis may be fulminant (overnight or within a few hours) or relatively subacute (over a few days). The presenting symptoms vary depending on the age of the patient. Children usually present with fever, lethargy, altered sensorium, irritability, vomiting, respiratory symptoms, and headache, whereas adults may have fever, headache, confusion, nausea, vomiting, photophobia, lethargy, or coma. Elderly persons may present with fever, progressing to confusion and coma. Nuchal rigidity, headache, and fever are seen in more than 90% of cases. Seizures, either as initial presentation or later in the illness, may occur in 40% of cases. All adult patients, with the exception of the elderly, and the majority of children present with signs of meningeal irritation; that is, nuchal rigidity, Brudzinski's sign, and Kerning's signs. Presence of a diffuse erythematous maculopapular rash suggests meningococcemia or enterovirus infection. In meningococcal meningitis, the rash becomes purpuric or petechial with the passage of time.

Investigations

ABM is an emergency. Once the diagnosis of ABM is suspected, blood culture is taken and empirical treatment started before CSF examination or computed tomography (CT) scan reports are available.

Imaging

CT scan prior to lumbar puncture is recommended in cases of focal neurological deficit, new-onset seizures, papilledema, unconsciousness, or immune compromised state. Magnetic resonance imaging (MRI) is preferred over CT scan, as it better delineates ischemia and edema. Contrast MRI shows evidence of meningeal enhancement, but it is not of specific diagnostic value.

Lumbar puncture (LP) and blood tests are recommended on an urgent basis; the generic recommendation about starting antibiotics without first doing an LP in a patient with suspected meningitis should be clarified, as per guidelines.

In an emergency setting, a brain CT scan is readily available in majority of hospitals in developing countries and could be done quicker than an MRI.

Cerebrospinal fluid

The CSF abnormalities characteristic of bacterial meningitis include an opening intracranial pressure of >180 mm of water, polymorphonuclear leucocytosis (>100 cells/μl), decreased glucose concentration (<40 mg/dL, CSF/serum glucose ratio of <0.4), and increased protein concentration (>45 mg/dL). CSF bacterial culture is positive in more than 80% of patients and Gram's stain is positive in more than 60%. The latex agglutination (LA) test for detecting antigen of N. meningitidis, S. pneumoniae, H. influenzae, or Streptococcus agalactiae is very helpful in making a rapid diagnosis, especially in patients pretreated with antibiotics. Polymerase chain reaction (PCR) can detect a small number of viable and non-viable organisms in CSF and is a very helpful test in expert hands.

Differential diagnosis

Meningitis due to other causes

The differential diagnosis of a suspected case of ABM includes viral meningoencephalitis, particularly herpes simplex virus (HSV) encephalitis, fungal meningitis, tuberculous meningitis, carcinomatous or lymphomatous meningitis, meningitis associated with sarcoidosis, systemic lupus erythematosus (SLE), and lupus. CSF findings, electroencephalogram (EEG) changes, and neuroimaging can distinguish ABM from HSV encephalitis. However, in 20–25% of patients with viral meningitis, CSF may show polymorphonuclear pleocytosis, which changes to a lymphocytic reaction within 24 hours.

Fungal meningitis can present acutely in immune compromised patients and CSF may show polymorphonuclear pleocytosis. The CSF should always be subjected to fungal smear and culture examination. Tubercular meningitis is usually a chronic infection with a history of a few weeks. Only occasionally in acute cases may initial polymorphonuclear leucocytosis be evident, which changes to a lymphocytic response within a few days. Evidence of extracranial

tuberculosis clinically or radiologically and CSF PCR examination are helpful in reaching a diagnosis.

Subarachnoid hemorrhage

Subarachnoic hemorrhage (SAH) is a major differential diagnosis in an acute-onset illness with headache, vomiting, and fever. Hemorrhagic CSF with leucocytosis clinches the diagnosis.

Subdural empyema

Subdural empyema and epidural abscess may mimic bacterial meningitis. The CSF shows normal sugar and mild mononuclear pleocytosis. Neuroimaging is diagnostic (Table 58.1).

Treatment

Empirical antibiotic treatment

The treatment for ABM must start immediately after diagnosis is made. The emergence of penicillin- and cephalosporin-resistant S. pneumoniae has made these drugs useless for initial therapy. Ceftriaxone or cefotaxime provide good coverage for the S. pneumoniae group, group B streptococci, and H. influenzae, and adequate coverage for N. meningitidis. Vancomycin is added in patients older than 3 months but less than 55 years of age, and those with hospital-acquired infections. Ampicillin should be added for coverage of L. monocytogenes in children less than 3 months and adults more than 55 years of age. In hospital-acquired meningitis, a combination of ceftazidime and vancomycin should be given to cover Gram-negative organisms and staphylococci. Ceftazidime is the only drug effective for CNS infections with Pseudomonas aeruginosa.

Specific treatment

Penicillin G is the antibiotic of choice for susceptible strains of N. meningitidis. Hence, if the organism is sensitive or moderately sensitive, penicillin G should be initiated. A 7-day course of intravenous therapy is sufficient for a routine, uncomplicated case of meningococcal meningitis. In resistant cases, the empirical treatment can be continued, depending on sensitivity. The same is the case for S. pneumoniae. Sensitivity should be tested for penicillin and cephalosporin. Usually CSF is sterile within 24–36 hours of therapy. Failure to sterilize suggests antibiotic resistance. The treatment should be continued for 10–14 days for meningitis due to S. pneumoniae, H. influenzae, and group B streptococci. Meningitis due to L. microcytogenes and Enterobacteriaceae needs treatment for 3–4 weeks. Meropenem is the preferred drug for meningitis due to P. aerugenosa. Linezolid is a newer antibiotic with activity against S. pneumoniae, S. aureus, and Enterococcus faecalis (Table 58.2).

Table 58.1 Antibiotics used in empirical therapy for acute bacterial meningitis.

Indication	Antibiotics
Age of patient 3 months to 55 years	Cefotaxime or ceftriaxone + vancomycin
Age <3 months or >55 years	Cefotaxime + ampicillin
Comorbid chronic illness, organ transplant, pregnancy, malignancy, and immunosuppression	Ceftriaxone + vancomycin
Hospital-acquired infections; meningitis following neurosurgery	Ceftazidime + vancomycin + ampicillin

Table 58.2 Antibiotic dose schedule in acute bacterial meningitis.

	Infants and children	Adults Dosing	interval
Penicillin G	0.3 mU/kg/day IV	24 mU/day	4‡6 hours
Ampicillin	300 mg/kg/day IV	12 g/day	4 hours
Ceftriaxone	100 mg/kg/day IV	4 g/day	12 hours
Cefotaxime	100‡150 mg/kg/day IV	8‡12 g/day	4 hours
Nafcillin	200 mg/kg/day IV	9‡12 g/day	4 hours
Oxacillin	200 mg/kg/day IV	9‡10 g/day	4 hours
Cefepime	150 mg/kg/day IV	6 g/day	8 hours
Meropenem	120 mg/kg/day IV	6 g/day	8 hours
Vancomycin	60 mg/kg/day IV	2‡3 g/day	6 hours

However, some cases of resistance have been reported in *E. faecium* and *S. aureus*.

Role of steroids and glycerol

Early use of dexamethasone has been shown to improve the outcome in adults with ABM. It reduces unfavorable outcomes such as hearing loss and neurological sequelae, as well as death. Treatment for a period of 4 days is sufficient and effective. Dexamethasone should be used in both pneumococcal and meningococcal meningitis at the initiation of therapy, either before or along with the first dose of antibiotic. The mechanism of action is by inhibiting the synthesis of the inflammatory cytokines and by decreasing CSF outflow resistance. There is no role of adjunct glycerol in either adults or children with ABM.

Prevention

Hemophilus influenzae type b (Hib) conjugate vaccine has decreased the incidence of Hib meningitis in children in developed countries. Polyvalent vaccine containing a polysaccharide capsule of groups A, C, Y, and W135 is recommended for high-risk children over 2 years of age. Vaccinations are available against pneumococci and meningococci as well and are recommended in high-risk children. All those coming into intimate contact with patients with meningococcal meningitis should be given prophylactic rifampicin at a dosage of 10 mg/kg in children and 600 mg/day in adults for 2 days. In case of any contraindication for the use of rifampicin, a single intramuscular injection of ceftriaxone may be given.

Prognosis

Bad prognostic signs in ABM include obtunded sensorium at admission, seizures within 24 hours of admission, signs of raised ICP, extremes of age, delay in start of treatment, and associated immune deficiency. Very low CSF glucose levels (40 mg/dL) and very high protein (>300 mg/dL) are observed in patients with poor outcome. Third, sixth, seventh, and eighth cranial nerves may be involved in the course of ABM, but can recover. Deafness, however, may be permanent, especially in children.

Complications

The spread of infection can lead to focal cerebritis and subsequent abscess formation. Focal signs such as hemiparesis usually imply complications, for example abscess, cerebritis, arteritis, or cerebral venous sinus thrombosis, and require urgent imaging. Subdural effusion and empyema are other important complications in *H. influenzae* and Gram-negative meningitis, particularly in children. These patients manifest with persistent fever, focal neurological deficit, and enlarging head circumference in the absence of hydrocephalus, and may require surgical management. Hydrocephalus may be an important complication in ABM, especially with *H. influenzae* infection, because of thick basal exudates, and may require drainage.

Further reading

Heckenberg SGB, Brouwer MC, van de Beek D. Bacterial meningitis. In: BillerJ, FerarroJM (eds.). *Handbook of Clinical Neurology*, Vol. 121 (3rd series) Neurological Aspect of Systemic Diseases (Part III). Philadelphia, PA: Elsevier; 2014:1361–1375.

Invasive Bacterial Infections Surveillance (IBIS) Group of the International Clinical Epidemiological Network. Are *H. influenzae* infections a significant problem in India? A prospective study and review. *Clin Infect Dis* 2002;34:949–957.

Mani R, Pradhan S, Nagarathna S, Wasiulla R, Chandermukhi A. Bacteriological profile of community acquired bacterial meningitis: A ten year retrospective study in a tertiary neuro care center in south India. *Indian J Med Microbiol* 2007;25:108–114.

Ramachandran P, Fitzwater SP, Aneja S, *et al*. Prospective multi-centre sentinel surveillance for *Haemophilus influenzae* type b and other bacterial meningitis in Indian children. *Ind J Med Res* 2013;137:712–720.

van de Beek D, de Gans J, Tunkel AR, Wijdicks EF. Community acquired bacterial meningitis in adults. *N Engl J Med* 2006;354:44–53.

59 Brain abscess

Gagandeep Singh

Department of Neurology, Dayanand Medical College & Hospital, Ludhiana, Punjab, India

Brain abscess, a suppurative process involving the cerebral parenchyma, was recognized as early as 460 BCE by Hippocrates. More recently, several pioneering neurosurgeons, including Paul Broca, Victor Horsley, and William Macewen, optimized surgical approaches to brain abscess, which until the middle of the nineteenth century were the only options in the successful management of this condition. In the 1950s, the introduction of penicillin had a dramatic impact on its management and outcome. The next major advance was the introduction of computed tomography (CT), which led to early and straightforward diagnosis. Finally, a shift in the microbiological spectrum of brain abscesses has recently been noted with increasing frequencies of fungal and tubercular etiologies, owing to the emergence of acquired immunodeficiency syndrome (AIDS) and the widespread use of immunosuppressive drugs in cancer and transplant patients.

Brain abscesses are less common in developed countries; only about two to three cases may be seen among non-immunocompromised subjects in a year, even in tertiary-care hospitals. In resource-poor countries, however, these may represent up to 8% of all intracranial space-occupying lesions.

Table 59.1 Relationship between predisposing conditions, microbial organisms responsible for brain abscess, and empirical choice of antibiotics.

Predisposing conditions	Microbial organism isolated	Empirical antimicrobial treatment
Otitis media	Mixed flora, *Streptococcus*, and anaerobic organisms	Cefotaxime or ceftriaxone and metronidazole
Infective endocarditis	*Streptococcus Sp.*	Cefotaxime or ceftriaxone and metronidazole; vancomycin if staphylococcal endocarditis suspected
Penetrating brain injury	*Staphylococcus aureus*, Gram-negative bacteria	Vancomycin plus cefotaxime or ceftriaxone and metronidazole
Post neurosurgery	*Staphylococcus aureus*, Gram-negative bacteria	Vancomycin plus cefotaxime or ceftriaxone and metronidazole
HIV infection	*Toxoplasma gordii, Mycobacterium Tuberculosis, Nocardia*	Pyremethoprim and sulfadiazine, antitubercular treatment in addition to ceftriaxone and metronidazole
Post organ transplant	*Nocardia, Actinomycetes, Candida, Aspergillus*	Cefotaxime or ceftriaxone and metronidazole and vancomycin plus voriconazole

Pathophysiology

A brain abscess results from either contiguous spread from infected paranasal sinuses, middle ears, and mastoid bones, or remote spread from dental abscesses, lungs, infected heart valves, or mechanical introduction by penetrating wounds and neurosurgical procedures. Over the years, a shift in the spectrum of the underlying conditions from otitic and sinus infections to abscesses resulting from trauma and neurosurgical procedures has been noted. The causative micro-organism(s) and hence appropriate antibiotic treatment are largely determined by the predisposing condition (Table 59.1). *Streptococci sp.* and *Bacteroides fragilis* are the usual infectious organisms in abscesses arising from paranasal sinus, otitic, and dental infections and in patients with congenital cyanotic heart disease. When infection develops from the lungs, a mixed flora is usually encountered, but exotic organisms such as *Nocardia*, *Actinomycetes*, and *Mycobacterium sp.* may also be isolated from abscesses, complicating trauma and neurosurgical procedures. With stringent microbiological technique, pathogens can be isolated in up to 85% of cases; multiple pathogens are found in up to 20% of cases.

The location of the abscess is also determined by the source of infection: abscesses originating from sinus infections are frontal in location, otitic and mastoid infections seed in the temporal lobe or cerebellum, and hematogenous infections are distributed to various lobes in proportion to cerebral blood flow.

From the pathogenic standpoint, a series of well-defined stages characterize the development of a parenchymal abscess: early cerebritis (days 1–5), late cerebritis (days 6–10), early capsule formation (days 11–15), and late capsule formation (more than 16 days). The pathological stages have a bearing on the imaging diagnosis of the brain abscess. Throughout all stages, the abscess is hypointense on T1- and hyperintense on T2-weighted sequences on magnetic resonance imaging (MRI) and is surrounded by variable degrees of edema (Figure 59.1a). Ill-defined gadolinium enhancement characterizes the early cerebritis stage and transforms to irregular ring-like enhancement in the late cerebritis stage, and to smooth ring-like enhancement in the capsular stage (Figure 59.1b). In the capsular stage the abscess wall forms a hypointense rim on T2 images (Figure 59.1a).

International Neurology, Second edition. Edited by Robert P. Lisak, Daniel D. Truong, William M. Carroll and Roongroj Bhidayasiri
© 2016 John Wiley & Sons, Ltd. Published 2016 by John Wiley & Sons, Ltd.

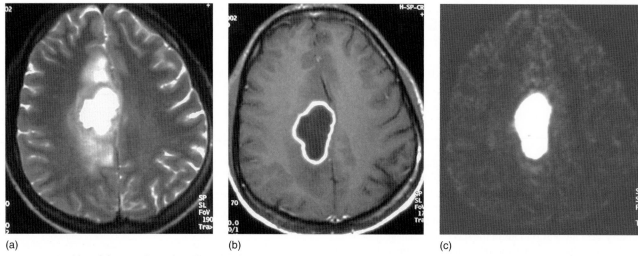

(a)   (b)   (c)

Figure 59.1 T2 (a), gadolinum-enhanced T1 (b), and diffusion-weighted (c) magnetic resonance images of a brain abscess in an individual with bronchiectasis.

Clinical features

In keeping with the pathological evolution of brain abscess already described, the clinical course is often subacute. Symptoms consist of fever, headache (due to increased intracranial tension), and focal neurological deficits. However, this symptom triad might be missing, with headache and alternation in consciousness as the only presenting features. Other symptoms include seizures, malaise, photophobia, and neck stiffness. During bedside examination attention should be directed toward detecting evidence of raised intracranial tension and the originating site of infection (e.g., lungs, heart, oral cavity).

Investigations

A common diagnostic dilemma is the differentiation of brain abscess from high-grade glioma with a necrotic center. Diffusion-weighted imaging (DWI) using echo planar spin echo sequences and perhaps *in vivo* proton magnetic resonance spectroscopy are exquisitely sensitive in the differentiation of brain abscess from malignant glioma. Pyogenic abscesses demonstrate hyperintensity on DWI (Figure 59.1c) as well as reduced apparent diffusion coefficients due to restricted water diffusion. Tumors do not exhibit these characteristics, although false positives can occur due to epidermoids, chordomas, and lymphomas.

Treatment

The management of brain abscess depends on the stage, location, number, and comorbid factors (Table 59.2). During the early cerebritis stage, or in the presence of multiple abscesses without evidence of raised intracranial tension, medical management is indicated. When capsule formation and central necrosis ensue, particularly in an abscess greater than 2.5 cm in size, surgical management, usually stereotactic aspiration of the abscess cavity, is the preferred initial management. A stereotactic approach is advantageous inasmuch as it allows histological distinction from neoplastic conditions, provides material for microbiological identification and antibiotic sensitivity, and is considerably less damaging to neural tissue. Open excision might be undertaken in the case of an abscess located in an

Table 59.2 Treatment options in brain abscess.

Treatment options	Indications
Antibiotics alone	• Deep-seated (brainstem or basal ganglionic), small abscess
	• Single or multiple abscess(es), in which the microbial organism can be isolated from the primary site of infection (e.g., lungs)
	• Abscess in early cerebritis stage
	• Underlying immunocompromised state
Dexamethasone	• Transient use in event of raised intracranial tension
	• Profoundly altered sensorium
Anticonvulsants	• Usually administered except in deep-seated abscesses
Stereotactic aspiration	• To obtain material for microbial isolation
	• Biopsy to differentiate from tumors
	• Abscesses in eloquent areas
Open excision	• Abscesses that recur despite repeated aspiration
	• Multiloculated abscess(es)
	• Abscess associated with a sinus tract (usually complicating trauma)

eloquent area or one that does not respond to multiple aspirations, multiloculated abscess(es), and the presence of a sinus tract that allows refilling of the abscess.

Antibiotic treatment is administered for several weeks irrespective of whether surgical treatment is undertaken. The choice of antibiotic regimen is dictated by the underlying predisposing condition and the suspected organism. Initial empirical treatment comprised of a third-generation cephalosporin (either cefotaxime, 6–9 g/day in divided doses, or ceftriaxone, 4 g/day in divided doses) and metronidazole (2 g/day in divided doses), but should also include vancomycin (2 g/day in divided doses) in the case of an abscess-complicating trauma and neurosurgical procedures. Treatment should continue for 6–8 weeks, although there is recent evidence to suggest that 1–2 weeks of intravenous therapy followed by oral antibiotics (ciprofloxacin, metronidazole, and amoxicillin) can be beneficial in selected cases.

Mortality due to brain abscess remains as high as 10–20% despite advances in diagnosis and treatment. A dreaded complication is rupture of the abscess into the ventricles, leading to ventriculitis. Treatment is in the form of external ventricular drainage. In addition, long-term neurological sequelae such as epilepsy and persistent focal neurological deficits are encountered in as many as 60% of cases.

Further reading

Bonfield CM, Sharma J, Dobson S. Pediatric intracranial abscesses. *J Infect* 2015;71(Suppl 1):S42–S46. doi 10.1016/jinf.2015.04.012

Brouwer MC, Coutinho JM, van de Beek D. Clinical characteristics and outcome of brain abscess: Systematic review and meta-analysis. *Neurology* 2014;82:806-813.

Brouwer, MC, Tunkel AR, McKhann GM, van de Beek D. Brain abscess. *N Engl J Med* 2014;371:447–456.

Carpenter J, Stapleton S, Holliman R. Retrospective analysis of 49 cases of brain abscess and review of the literature. *Eur J Clin Microbiol Infect Dis* 2007;26:1–11.

Muccio CF, Caranci F, D'Arco F, *et al.* Magnetic resonance features of pyogenic brain abscesses and differential diagnosis using morphological and functional imaging studies: A pictoral essay. *J Neuroradiol* 2014;41:153–167.

Sharma BS, Gupta SK, Khosla VK. Current concepts in the management of pyogenic brain abscess. *Neurol India* 2000;48:105–111.

60 Subdural empyema

Sandi Lam[1,2] and Eric Momin[1]

[1] Department of Neurosurgery, Baylor College of Medicine, Houston, TX, USA

[2] Division of Pediatric Neurosurgery, Texas Children's Hospital, Houston, TX, USA

Subdural empyema is a focal purulent infection between the dura and arachnoid mater, with few anatomic barriers to spread. More than 95% of subdural empyemas occur intracranially rather than in the spinal neuraxis. Subdural empyemas comprise 15–22% of focal intracranial infections, with historically high mortality prior to the widespread availability of antibiotics. Between 70% and 80% of cases occur over the cerebral convexities; they also occur parafalcine, on the tentorium, and infratentorially.

Epidemiology

The male:female ratio is 3:1. Most cases of subdural empyema occur as a result of direct extension of infection rather than by hematogenous spread. In contrast, most subdural empyemas in infants result from infection of subdural effusions from meningitis.

Among studies of North American patients, intracranial subdural empyema is most often a complication of sinusitis and, less frequently, otitis or neurosurgical procedures. The causative source varies in other parts of the world: a retrospective analysis of 65 pediatric cases of subdural empyema from India showed an otogenic source as the most common identifiable etiology, followed by postmeningitic and rhinogenic sources. A retrospective series of 36 patients with subdural empyema from Australia showed that the most common source of infection was a neurosurgical procedure, followed by sinusitis and otogenic sources. *Streptococcus milleri* group (also known as *anginosus*) is most commonly isolated. Multiple organisms, including Gram negatives such as *Escherichia coli*, and anaerobes such as *Bacteroides* may be present. In patients with previous neurosurgical procedures, one must also suspect *Pseudomonas aeruginosa* or *Staphylococcus species* as the causative organism.

Pathophysiology

Local infection can spread into the intracranial compartment and subdural space from the frontal, sphenoid, or ethmoid sinuses from osteomyelitis or through retrograde thrombophlebitis of the valveless diploic veins. Most cases of complicated sinusitis occur in otherwise healthy men of ages 20–40 years. There may be chronic otitis media, mastoiditis, cranial traction devices, neurosurgical postoperative infections, compound skull fractures, or penetrating head trauma. Meningitis and infections of pre-existing subdural fluid collections are also associated with subdural empyemas. Pulmonary or hematogenous etiologies are rare; tuberculous infections can also occur. This suppurative process can lead to intracranial venous thrombosis, which can compound neurological morbidity beyond infection or mass effect from the subdural space.

Clinical features

Patients may present with neurological symptoms due to mass effect, inflammation of the brain and meninges, and cerebral cortical vein thrombosis or dural sinus thrombosis. Focal deficits and seizures develop with disease progression.

Common presenting features of subdural empyema include fever, headache, meningismus, altered mental status, hemiparesis, nausea/vomiting, sinus tenderness, local swelling/inflammation, seizures, speech difficulty, homonymous hemianopsia, and papilledema. Raised intracranial pressure occurs with mass effect or with cerebral thrombophlebitis. Cranial nerve palsies and visual changes may be apparent on examination.

Investigations

Imaging studies

While magnetic resonance imaging (MRI) is recognized to be more sensitive in showing morphological detail, detecting intraparenchymal abnormalities, and delineating the extent of infection, computed tomography (CT) is usually first obtained because of availability; as such, it fulfills the need for timely diagnosis. In cases associated with sinusitis, CT of the head will show sinus opacification, air-fluid levels, or bony erosion.

CT is most helpful when obtained with and without intravenous (IV) contrast, allowing differentiation from chronic subdural hematoma or postoperative changes. CT findings (Figure 60.1) include a hypodense subdural lesion, enhancing especially along the medial border at the pial surface, inward displacement of the gray-white junction, and effacement of the ventricles, cortical sulci, and/or basal cisterns. Mass effect is often caused by edema rather than the empyema itself. Edema is more prominent in cases of subdural empyema complicated by cortical venous thrombosis (with or without venous infarction), cerebritis, or associated cerebral abscess.

International Neurology, Second edition. Edited by Robert P. Lisak, Daniel D. Truong, William M. Carroll and Roongroj Bhidayasiri
© 2016 John Wiley & Sons, Ltd. Published 2016 by John Wiley & Sons, Ltd.

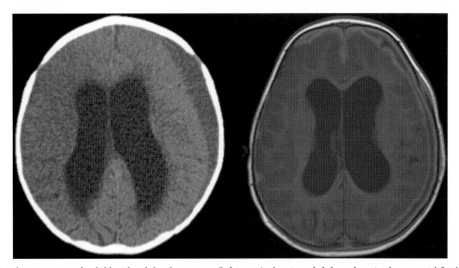

Figure 60.1 Head CT without contrast of a child with subdural empyema (left image), showing a left frontal-parietal extra-axial fluid collection and midline shift. This child presented to the emergency room with seizures and a one-week history of fever and lethargy. A stroke from cortical venous thrombosis is evident with hypodensity in the contralateral hemisphere, consistent with diffuse subdural empyema with bilateral involvement. MRI with contrast of the same patient shows rim enhancement of the left holohemispheric subdural lesion, indicative of subdural empyema (right image). Leptomeningeal enhancement is visible over the right hemisphere along with ischemic changes in the underlying cortex.

On MRI, subdural empyemas generally appear hypointense on T1-weighted images with rim enhancement following gadolinium administration, hyperintense on T2-weighted images, and with high signal on diffusion-weighted images (DWI); see Figure 60.2.

Early in the disease course, imaging may be unrevealing. If the initial head CT is normal yet clinical suspicion of subdural empyema persists, a repeat CT or MRI is warranted.

Laboratory studies

Complete blood count shows leukocytosis with predominance of polymorphonuclear neutrophils. Erythrocyte sedimentation rate and C-reactive protein are elevated, but generally <100 mm/h.

Blood, urine, and sputum should be cultured to identify potential organisms. Additional preoperative workup should include screening for electrolyte abnormalities and metabolic dysfunction.

Lumbar puncture is not recommended given the potential risk of cerebral herniation. Cerebrospinal fluid (CSF) findings, when obtained, are typically non-specific, showing sterile pleocytosis with predominant polymorphonuclear neutrophils, elevated protein, and normal to low glucose levels. Gram stain and CSF cultures are negative in >85% of cases. Normal and sterile CSF samples do not rule out the diagnosis of subdural empyema.

Causative organisms vary with the source of primary infection (Table 60.1). Sterile intraoperative cultures are reported in up to half of cases, presumably as a result of preoperative administration of antibiotics.

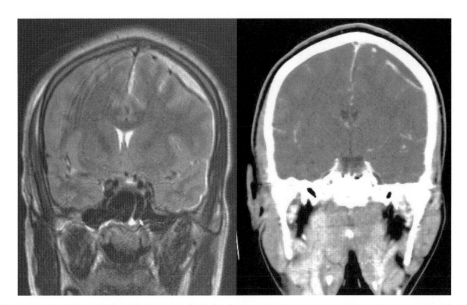

Figure 60.2 MRI of the brain of a patient with frontal sinusitis and subdural empyema, demonstrating T2 hyperintensity at the left convexity (left image) and T1 hypointensity with rim enhancement on the cortical surface in the subdural empyema (right image).

Table 60.1 Common causative organisms in cases of subdural empyema.

Associated etiology	Common organisms
Paranasal sinusitis	Alpha-hemolytic streptococci Staphylococci Anaerobic/microaerophilic streptococci Aerobic Gram-negative bacilli Bacteroides species
Otitis media, mastoiditis	Alpha-hemolytic streptococci *Pseudomonas aeruginosa* Bacteroides species Staphylococci
Trauma or postsurgical infection	Staphylococci Aerobic Gram-negative bacilli
Meningitis (neonate)	Group B streptococci *Enterobacteriaceae* *Listeria monocytogenes*
Meningitis (child)	*Streptococcus pneumoniae* *Hemophilus influenzae* *Neisseria meningitidis* *Escherichia coli*

Treatment

Broad spectrum antibiotic therapy should be started as soon as possible with coverage for aerobic and anaerobic organisms. Recommended empirical therapy for adult patients includes penicillin, a third-generation cephalosporin, and metronidazole. Antibiotics may be tailored according to Gram stain, bacterial culture, and sensitivity results. Antibiotic therapy is recommended for 4–6 weeks, and a longer course of 6–8 weeks in patients with osteomyelitis. In subdural empyemas following neurosurgical procedures or trauma, vancomycin should take the place of penicillin as part of the initial empirical antibiotics. For neonates and children, empirical antibiotic choices are the same as for meningitis treatment, which varies by local rates of microbial drug resistance. Anticonvulsants are recommended prophylactically, and are necessary if seizure activity occurs.

Surgical management is indicated in almost all cases of subdural empyema. There is no consensus on the optimal surgical approach between burr hole drainage or craniotomy for debridement and drainage. The purulent material tends to be in fluid state early in the disease process, and loculations develop over time. Repeat procedures may be required. Definitive surgical management of infected sinus disease should also be undertaken. A limited number of subdural empyema cases managed non-surgically have been reported, but this treatment strategy is not considered except in cases with very limited extension, no mass effect, no neurological symptoms, and early favorable response to antibiotics.

Unfavorable prognostic indicators include age over 60 years, poor neurological status at time of presentation, rapidity of disease progression, delay in starting antibiotics, and subdural empyema resulting from trauma or surgery. Mortality with treated cases of subdural empyema ranges between 5% and 20%. Up to half of patients have neurological deficits at the time of discharge from hospital, 15–35% with hemiparesis, and up to 30% with persistent seizures.

Further reading

Adame N, Hedlund G, Byington CL. Sinogenic intracranial empyema in children. *Pediatrics* 2005;116(3):e461–e467.

Banerjee AD, Pandey P, Devi BI, Sampath S, Chandramouli BA. Pediatric supratentorial subdural empyemas: A retrospective analysis of 65 cases. *Pediatr Neurosurg* 2009;45(1):11–18.

Dill SR, Cobbs CG, McDonald CK. Subdural empyema: Analysis of 32 cases and review. *Clin Infect Dis* 1995;20(2):372–386.

French H, Schaefer N, Keijzers G, Barison D, Olson S. Intracranial subdural empyema: A 10-year case series. *Ochsner J* 2014;14(2):188–194.

Greenberg, MS. *Handbook of Neurosurgery*, 5th ed. New York: Thieme; 2001.

Jim KK, Brouwer MC, van der Ende A, van de Beek D. Subdural empyema in bacterial meningitis. *Neurology* 2012;79(21):2133–2139.

Osborn MK, Steinberg JP. Subdural empyema and other suppurative complications of paranasal sinusitis. *Lancet Infect Dis* 2007;7(1):62–67.

61 Epidural abscess

Sandi Lam[1,2], Humphrey Okechi[3], and Jared Fridley[1]
[1] Department of Neurosurgery, Baylor College of Medicine, Houston, TX, USA
[2] Division of Pediatric Neurosurgery, Texas Children's Hospital, Houston, TX, USA
[3] Department of Neurosurgery, Kijabe Hospital, Kijabe, Kenya

Epidural abscess develops between the skull and the dura mater. In general, the adherence of the dura to the skull limits the expansion of intracranial epidural abscesses; however, a parameningeal focus of infection involving the dural venous sinuses can cause a septic thrombophlebitis. Autopsy studies reveal that up to 80% of epidural abscess cases have evidence of associated subdural abscess formation.

Epidemiology

The incidence of intracranial epidural abscess is estimated to be at least 9 times less common than spinal epidural abscess. There is a male predominance, with the incidence being highest in males in their second and third decades of life.

Pathophysiology

Intracranial epidural abscesses arise from direct extension in association with sinusitis, cranial osteomyelitis, direct penetrating trauma, or postoperative infection.

The pathophysiology of epidural abscess in the spine differs from that of intracranial epidural abscesses. The etiology of these spinal infections can be hematogenous or from direct extension of a contiguous local infection. In the spine, there is a relatively large potential space in the epidural compartment between the dura and the vertebral bodies, allowing significant extension and enlargement of spinal epidural abscesses. The focus of this chapter will be limited to intracranial epidural abscesses.

Clinical features

Patients with intracranial epidural abscess generally present with signs and symptoms of infection and an expanding intracranial mass lesion, such as fever, headache, altered mental status, malaise, nausea, vomiting, focal neurological deficits, seizures, sinus tenderness/local swelling, and evidence of wound infection in more than 90% of patients who have undergone craniotomy. Pott's puffy tumor may be seen on clinical examination, which is a subperiosteal abscess of the frontal bone with underlying osteomyelitis associated with frontal sinusitis. The clinical presentation of patients with intracranial epidural abscess is generally described as more indolent when compared to subdural empyema, although individual cases may vary.

Investigations

Complete blood count reveals leukocytosis with an elevated percentage of polymorphonuclear neutrophils and possibly band forms. Erythrocyte sedimentation rate is usually elevated, but represents a non-specific finding. Blood, urine, and sputum should be cultured to identify potential organisms and sources. Other tests should include electrolytes, blood urea nitrogen, creatinine, blood glucose, liver function tests, coagulation panel, chest X-ray, and electrocardiogram for preoperative evaluation, for correction of electrolyte abnormalities, and to screen out underlying metabolic dysfunction while directing the choice of antibiotics for medical treatment.

Lumbar puncture is not recommended in the setting of intracranial epidural abscess, since there is the potential risk of brain herniation due to increased intracranial pressure. It is known that cerebrospinal fluid (CSF) studies often show moderate pleocytosis with predominantly polymorphonuclear neutrophils, with moderately elevated protein and normal to low glucose levels. Gram stain and CSF cultures are negative in >75% of cases. Normal and sterile CSF samples do not rule out the diagnosis of intracranial epidural abscess.

Computed tomography (CT) of the head is usually the most widely available and quickly accessible imaging modality, and should be obtained with and without contrast (to help differentiate from chronic epidural hematoma and postoperative changes). It demonstrates a hypodense enhancing extra-axial lesion, often crescentic or lenticular in shape. However, subdural empyema may also have a similar radiological appearance. Magnetic resonance imaging (MRI) of the brain with and without gadolinium enhancement has higher sensitivity and may provide more detail in delineating the extent of infection. The signal of an intracranial epidural abscess on MRI is hyperintense on T2-weighted imaging (T2WI), variable signal on T1-weighted imaging (T1WI), and enhancing with gadolinium administration, especially along the periphery of the lesion (Figure 61.1). It is also expected to show restriction on diffusion-weighted imaging (DWI) sequences. This lesion may be contiguous to an area of skull osteomyelitis, sinusitis, skull fracture, or craniotomy defect.

International Neurology, Second edition. Edited by Robert P. Lisak, Daniel D. Truong, William M. Carroll and Roongroj Bhidayasiri
© 2016 John Wiley & Sons, Ltd. Published 2016 by John Wiley & Sons, Ltd.

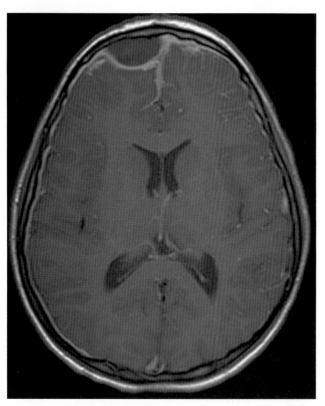

Figure 61.1 Epidural abscess. MRI T1-weighted image with gadolinium showing a left frontal extra-axial peripherally enhancing lenticular lesion in a patient with frontal sinusitis.

Causative organisms vary with the primary etiology of infection (Table 61.1). In the authors' experience, in developing countries up to 90% of intraoperative Gram stain and cultures are sterile, presumably as a result of preoperative empirical antibiotic administration.

Table 61.1 Common causative organisms in cases of intracranial epidural abscess.

Associated etiology	Common organisms
Paranasal sinusitis	Alpha-hemolytic streptococci Staphylococci Anaerobic/microaerophilic streptococci Aerobic Gram-negative bacilli Bacteroides species
Otitis media, mastoiditis	Aerobic and anaerobic streptococci Pseudomonas aeruginosa Bacteroides species Enterobacteriaceae Staphylococci
Penetrating trauma	Staphylococci Aerobic Gram-negative bacilli Clostridium species
Postoperative	Staphylococci Enterobacteriaceae Pseudomonas aeruginosa Proprionibacterium species

Treatment

Empirical broad spectrum antibiotics should be started as soon as possible, and may be subsequently tailored according to Gram stain, culture, and sensitivity results. Initial empirical therapy should provide coverage for Gram-positive cocci, Gram-negative bacilli, and anaerobes. The usual recommended empirical antimicrobial therapy includes a penicillin, metronidazole, and a third-generation cephalosporin. In cases of penetrating trauma or postoperative infection, the penicillin should be substituted with vancomycin. The course of antibiotic therapy is usually at least 6 weeks, and extended to 8 weeks or longer in the presence of osteomyelitis.

Prophylaxis for seizures is recommended, and anticonvulsants are mandatory if seizure activity occurs.

Burr holes or craniotomy for decompression, debridement, and drainage of epidural abscess is warranted in the vast majority of cases. Delay in surgical intervention has been associated with significant morbidity and mortality. A drain may be left in the epidural space perioperatively. Reoperation may be necessary in cases of persistent or recurrent suppurative infection.

The neurological status at time of presentation is generally a good predictor of neurological outcome. Delays in diagnosis or treatment are associated with increased morbidity and mortality. Mortality is estimated at 10–20% from treated intracranial epidural abscess.

Further reading

Hlavin ML, Kaminski HJ, Fenstermaker RA, *et al*. Intracranial suppuration: A modern decade of postoperative subdural empyema and epidural abscess. *Neurosurgery* 1994;34:974–981.

Idowu OE, Adekoya VA, Adeyinka AP, Beredugo-Amadasun BK, Olubi OO. Demography, types, outcome, and relationship of surgically treated intracranial suppurative otitis media and bacterial rhinosinusitis. *J Neurosci Rural Pract* 2014;5(Suppl 1):S48–S52.

Krauss WE, McCormick PC. Infections of the dural spaces. *Neurosurg Clin N Am* 1992;3:412–433.

Salomao JF, Cervante TP, Bellas AR, *et al*. Neurosurgical implications of Pott's puffy tumor in children and adolescents. *Child Nerv Syst* 2014;30(9):1527–1534.

Tunkell, AR. Subdural empyema, epidural abscess, and suppurative intracranial thrombophlebitis. In: Mandell GL, Bennet JE, Dolin R (eds.). *Mandell, Douglas, and Bennett's Principles and Practices of Infectious Diseases*. Philadelphia, PA: Churchill Livingstone; 2005:1165–1168.

62 Septic cerebral venous sinus thrombosis

Ismail A. Khatri[1] and Mohammad Wasay[2]

[1] Department of Neurology, King Saud bin Abdulaziz University for Health Sciences and King Abdulaziz Medical City, Riyadh, Saudi Arabia
[2] Division of Neurology, The Aga Khan University, Karachi, Pakistan

Cerebral venous and sinus thrombosis (CVT) is an uncommon disease and accounts for <1% of all strokes. Multiple predisposing factors have been associated with CVT, among which only a few are reversible. Some of the transient conditions associated with CVT include pregnancy, dehydration, and infection. Cerebral venous thrombosis varies widely in its presentation, predisposition, neuroimaging, outcomes, and prognosis. The exact incidence and prevalence of CVT are unknown due to lack of population-based data. Although no age is exempt from cerebral venous thrombosis, in the pediatric population neonates are most affected, and in adults the highest incidence is in the third decade, with female preponderance.

Infection-related/septic cerebral venous sinus thrombosis

Infection-related/septic cerebral venous sinus thrombosis has decreased dramatically in incidence after the widespread use of antibiotics for infections. Infection used to be the main cause of CVT before the era of antibiotics. Due to its rarity of occurrence, septic CVT may be misdiagnosed or remain undiagnosed, which can result in treatment delay in this potentially life-threatening condition. It is more common in children compared to adults. Cavernous sinuses are the most commonly involved sinuses in septic CVT, and usually follow the infection of paranasal sinuses, dental abscesses, otitis media, and orbital infections.

Anatomy and pathophysiology

The dural sinuses and cerebral veins lack valves. This lack of valves make the blood flow pressure dependent, and blood can flow in either direction depending on the pressure gradient. The cavernous sinuses, which are the most commonly affected sinuses in septic CVT, are located in the base of the skull, separated from sphenoid air sinuses by a thin membrane, or sometimes only by soft tissue, if the bone is not fully formed. The oculomotor, trochlear, and the superior two divisions of the trigeminal nerve travel adjacent to the cavernous sinus, while the abducens nerve and carotid artery pass through the cavernous sinus. The cavernous sinuses receive most of the venous return from the face via ophthalmic veins, and drain into the internal jugular veins through superior and inferior petrosal sinuses. These anatomic peculiarities make the cavernous sinuses susceptible to infections involving the facial structures, and adjacent paranasal sinuses. Middle ear, pharynx, and teeth can be other sources of septic CVT. Lateral sinus thrombosis is mostly associated with middle ear infection or mastoiditis. Superior sagittal sinus is uncommonly involved in septic CVT and is mostly in relation to meningitis. Orbital infections are rarely complicated by septic thrombosis of cavernous sinuses, despite the direct drainage of ophthalmic veins in the cavernous sinuses. In the preantibiotic era, the majority of septic CVT resulted from facial infections. With the significant decrease in overall incidence, most of the recent reports are related to ear infections, orbital infections, and paranasal sinusitis.

The exact mechanism of septic thrombosis is as yet unclear. Infection may trigger thrombosis directly by causing septic thrombosis, or indirectly by precipitating thrombosis in patients already at risk of thrombosis due to predisposing thrombophilia. The infection may spread within veins (thrombophlebitis) or as septic emboli that get trapped within the trabeculations of cavernous sinuses. Bacteria are potent inducers of thrombosis, and thrombus in turn is a great growth medium for bacteria. Bacteria trapped in the deeper layers of thrombus may be protected from antibiotic penetration and can become a source of infection. Intracranial infections like meningitis, subdural abscess, and empyema can be a source of the direct spread of micro-organisms to the cerebral venous sinuses.

Microbial etiology

Bacterial infections are by far the most common cause of septic CVT; however, viral, parasitic, and fungal etiologies have been well described. *Staphylococcus aureus* is the most commonly identified organism, followed by streptococcal species, Gram-negative organisms, and anaerobes. Cytomegalovirus, herpes simplex, measles, hepatitis, and human immunodeficiency virus (HIV) all have been attributed to the development of CVT. It is probable that the combination of coagulopathy and opportunistic infections is the main culprit for septic CVT in HIV patients rather than the

International Neurology, Second edition. Edited by Robert P. Lisak, Daniel D. Truong, William M. Carroll and Roongroj Bhidayasiri
© 2016 John Wiley & Sons, Ltd. Published 2016 by John Wiley & Sons, Ltd.

HIV itself. Fungal infections including aspergillus, mucormycosis, and coccidioidomycosis all have been reported to contribute to septic CVT. Despite affecting the central nervous system (CNS) frequently in the form of meningitis and CNS tuberculosis (TB), tuberculosis has rarely been reported in association with septic CVT, mostly affecting patients with disseminated disease. Parasitic infections including malaria, trichinosis, and toxoplasmosis have also been reported.

Thrombophilia and septic CVT

Septic CVT is frequently associated with thrombophilic or prothrombotic states. Infection is a common trigger of CVT in previously healthy children. Almost two-thirds of children screened for thrombophilia can have one or more prothrombotic conditions. The vast majority of children who have septic CVT in association with otitis media or mastoiditis have also been shown to have prothrombotic conditions. Whether prothrombotic states increase the risk of septic CVT is not clear.

Clinical presentation

The illness is usually acute and patients are commonly very sick, toxic, and febrile. The latent period between primary infection of face or nose and the development of septic CVT is usually less than a week. Patients with more fulminant disease manifest most of the symptoms and signs early in its course. Fever is almost always present. In patients with cavernous sinus thrombosis, eyelid swelling, proptosis, and chemosis are common, and present in 80–100% of cases. Lethargy, headache, papilledema, and cranial nerve palsies are present in 50–80% of cases, whereas nuchal rigidity, seizures, and hemiparesis are less common and present in less than 25% of patients. Decreased visual acuity, internal ophthalmoplegia, and periorbital sensory changes due to involvement of the trigeminal nerve are less common. Spread to the opposite eye through intracavernous spread occurs usually within 24–48 hours. Infrequently, the cavernous sinus thrombosis may present in a more indolent form with isolated gaze palsy. A high level of suspicion is important in making a timely diagnosis and initiation of management. If the involved sinuses are other than cavernous sinus, the symptoms and signs may differ. Lateral sinus thrombosis is usually a complication of middle ear infection or mastoiditis, and patients usually present with the features of primary site infection along with symptoms and signs of raised intracranial pressure and focal neurological signs.

Differential diagnosis

Orbital cellulitis can mimic septic cavernous sinus thrombosis, although it is usually unilateral and is not associated with papilledema, pupillary changes, and marked systemic toxic effects. Other conditions that can cause painful ophthalmoplegia include preseptal cellulitis, orbital apex syndrome, myeloproliferative disorders or metastases, post-traumatic aseptic thrombosis, chronic granulomatous infections, and Tolosa–Hunt syndrome. Ophthalmic migraine can sometimes be mistakenly diagnosed if the headache is predominantly unilateral. Aseptic thrombosis of cavernous and other dural sinus thrombosis usually does not have such dramatic manifestations. Rarely, carotid cavernous fistula and other vascular anomalies may be confused with cavernous sinus thrombosis.

Radiological findings

Modern radiological techniques including computed tomography (CT) and magnetic resonance imaging (MRI) have made the diagnosis of septic CVT more precise, rapid, and detailed. On the contrasted high-resolution CT scan, filling defect in the cavernous sinus along with expansion in the dimensions were the most common findings in one study. CT scan also helped confirm the suspected location of underlying infection, as well as the integrity of bony structures. The authors in this study found contrast-enhanced MRI studies complementary to CT findings and added little additional information except soft tissue identification.

Diagnosis of cavernous sinus thrombosis may be challenging. The bony changes are better appreciated on CT scan. Most experience for the diagnosis of septic CVT is reported with the high-resolution CT scan using 3 mm or smaller slice thickness. In addition to the filling defect and expansion/bulging of the lateral walls, other abnormalities seen on CT scan include heterogenous enhancement within the cavernous sinus, with intensive enhancement of lateral wall, densification of retro-orbital fat, and exophthalmos. MRI may make the greatest contribution in patients with non-conclusive CT scans or if the involvement of meninges and brain parenchyma is to be evaluated. Postcontrast MRI with dedicated pituitary views may be helpful in identifying cavernous thrombosis (Figure 62.1).

Other investigations

In addition to radiological studies, other diagnostic evaluations should include complete blood count, blood cultures, and cerebrospinal fluid (CSF) studies, including CSF culture in suspected cases of septic CVT. Blood culture is more often positive (approximately 70% of cases) in septic CVT than CSF cultures (20% of cases). CSF often shows granulocytic pleocytosis and elevated proteins. Low CSF glucose may be seen in 35% of cases. Conventional angiography is rarely used in the presence of high-resolution CT and MRI. Orbital venography has been used in the past to confirm the diagnosis, although it was associated with complications and may have increased the risk of dissemination or extension of thrombosis or infection.

Management

The mainstay of treatment is the management of underlying infection and systemic stabilization of the patient. The initial choice of intravenous antibiotics should be made keeping in view the most common organisms involved in the suspected site of origin of septic CVT. A reasonable initial combination may include ceftriaxone, vancomycin, and metronidazole to cover the broadest spectrum. Blood and CSF cultures should direct the specific therapy. For toxic patients, the dose for ceftriaxone should be 2 g intravenously every 12 hours, vancomycin 750–1000 mg intravenously every 12 hours, and metronidazole 7.5 mg/kg intravenously every 6 hours. Another suggested regimen is a combination of a third-generation cephalosporin, nafcillin, and metronidazole. The total duration of therapy is not clearly established, and should depend on the clinical response, the primary site of infection, and associated complications, but a minimum of 3–4 weeks of intravenous therapy is required. The role of steroids is not well established in the management of septic CVT. They may help in decreasing the inflammation and swelling, although this use is not well supported by evidence.

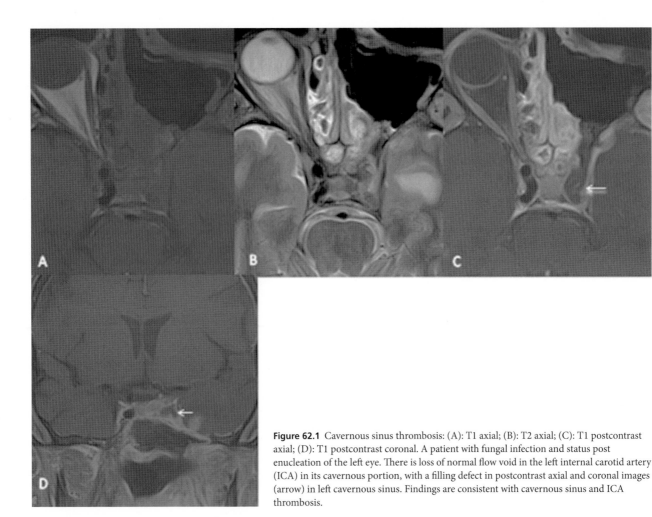

Figure 62.1 Cavernous sinus thrombosis: (A): T1 axial; (B): T2 axial; (C): T1 postcontrast axial; (D): T1 postcontrast coronal. A patient with fungal infection and status post enucleation of the left eye. There is loss of normal flow void in the left internal carotid artery (ICA) in its cavernous portion, with a filling defect in postcontrast axial and coronal images (arrow) in left cavernous sinus. Findings are consistent with cavernous sinus and ICA thrombosis.

Although standard for care in cases of aseptic CVT, the role of anticoagulants in the management of septic CVT is controversial. The theoretical advantage of anticoagulation therapy is prevention of the propagation of thrombus, as well as possible inhibition of platelet function and anti-inflammatory effect through various mechanisms. The potential risk is of intracranial as well as systemic hemorrhage. Another argument against the use of anticoagulants has been the assumption that the thrombus confines the infection and hence prevents the dissemination of infection. Anticoagulation may allow further extension of the infectious process. However, the reported incidence of hemorrhage in the setting of septic CVT and use of anticoagulants is extremely low. Anticoagulation therapy was first used in cavernous sinus thrombosis in the 1940s and there have been no controlled clinical trials to address the efficacy or safety of their use in septic CVT. Most of the literature is based on retrospective data analyses and reviews. The number of patients included in the reviews is too small to draw definitive conclusions. The mortality associated with septic CVT has not been convincingly shown to be reduced with the combined use of antibiotics and anticoagulants, although there was a trend toward decreased morbidity when anticoagulants were used early along with antibiotics. The current available evidence favors the use of anticoagulants along with antibiotics early in the course of septic CVT; however, no clear protocols or target values of anticoagulation have been established. Intravenous heparin should be used initially, followed by oral anticoagulants. The optimal duration of treatment is not known.

Surgical drainage of the cavernous sinus is almost never performed. Surgical treatment is reserved for the primary site of infection, which may require drainage of the primary focus, particularly if the focus is in a non-draining site.

Outcome and prognosis

In the preantibiotic era, septic CVT was almost always fatal. With the introduction of antibiotic treatment, both the mortality rate and the incidence have markedly declined, likely due to early treatment of facial and sinus infections. Despite all the advances in diagnosis and treatment, the mortality rates are still reported at around 30%, with significant morbidity in survivors. The residual deficits in survivors include partial or complete visual loss, cranial nerve abnormalities, pituitary dysfunction, seizures, hemiparesis, facial disfigurement, as well as personality changes. Full recovery is achieved in less than 50% of patients.

Early recognition, aggressive treatment with high-dose intravenous antibiotics, judicious use of anticoagulation therapy early in the course, and surgical consideration in select cases are keys to the management of septic cerebral venous/cavernous sinus thrombosis.

Fortunately, this potentially lethal condition has become rare. Since it is not seen frequently in practice, it is even more critical for clinicians to be aware of the condition, and to have a high index of suspicion for it, as early recognition and aggressive treatment can prevent both morbidity and mortality.

Further reading

Bhatia K, Jones NS. Septic cavernous sinus thrombosis secondary to sinusitis: Are anticoagulants indicated? A review of the literature. *J Laryngol Otol* 2002;116(9):667–676.

DiNubile MJ. Septic thrombosis of the cavernous sinuses. *Arch Neurol* 1988;45(5):567–572.

Ebright JR, Pace MT, Niazi AF. Septic thrombosis of the cavernous sinuses. *Arch Intern Med* 2001;161(22):2671–2676.

Ghosh PS, Ghosh D, Goldfarb J, Sabella C. Lateral sinus thrombosis associated with mastoiditis and otitis media in children: A retrospective chart review and review of the literature. *J Child Neurol* 2011;26(8):1000–1004.

Kojan S, Al-Jumah M. Infection related cerebral venous thrombosis. *J Pak Med Assoc* 2006;56(11):494–497.

Levine SR, Twyman RE, Gilman S. The role of anticoagulation in cavernous sinus thrombosis. *Neurology* 1988;38(4):517–522.

Saadatnia M, Fatehi F, Basiri K, Mousavi SA, Mehr GK. Cerebral venous sinus thrombosis risk factors. *Int J Stroke* 2009;4(2):111–123.

63 Encephalitis due to bacterial infections

Karen L. Roos and Jennifer Durphy

Department of Neurology, Indiana University School of Medicine, Indianapolis, IN, USA

Encephalitis is a syndrome of fever and headache with either an altered level of consciousness, a focal neurological deficit, or seizure activity. Cerebrospinal fluid (CSF) analysis typically demonstrates an increased number of white blood cells and an increased protein concentration. Electroencephalography (EEG) and FLAIR and diffusion-weighted magnetic resonance imaging (MRI) may demonstrate focal abnormalities. Encephalitis is distinguished from encephalopathy, which is an altered or depressed level of consciousness with EEG evidence of diffuse slowing and an absence of a CSF inflammatory response. Although herpesviruses and arthropod-borne viruses are frequently the etiological agents of encephalitis, bacteria may also cause encephalitis. Bacteria do not cause an isolated meningitis. All bacteria cause a meningoencephalitis. For the more common etiologies of bacterial encephalitis, please see Chapter 58.

Mycoplasma pneumoniae

Mycoplasma pneumoniae is the causative organism of 7–30% of cases of community-acquired pneumonia, but an uncommon cause of encephalitis. In a review of all published reports on patients with *M. pneumoniae* childhood encephalitis in the English-language literature from 1972–2003, there were only 58 well-defined cases. *Mycoplasma pneumoniae* is more likely to cause a delayed or postinfectious immune-mediated neurological disorder than an acute encephalitis due to direct invasion of brain parenchyma by the pathogen. The clinical presentation of encephalitis includes fever, headache, vomiting, an altered level of consciousness, and seizure activity.

Diagnosis is made by a combination of a positive CSF culture or polymerase chain reaction (PCR) or both, with or without acute and convalescent serological tests demonstrating a four-fold increase in *M. pneumoniae* IgG, or by detection of *M. pneumoniae* in throat specimens by culture or PCR or both with confirmatory serological tests. The diagnosis cannot rely exclusively on a single elevated IgM or IgG titer, as there are many false-positive serological results. A history of preceding flu-like or respiratory symptoms prior to the onset of neurological disease, and chest radiograph evidence of a pulmonary infiltrate, is supportive evidence of encephalitis due to this bacteria. Spinal fluid analysis demonstrates a lymphocytic pleocytosis in the majority of patients, but a pleocytosis of polymorphonuclear leukocytes has been reported as well. A CSF lymphocytic pleocytosis would be expected in an immune-mediated disorder, whereas a pleocytosis of polymorphonuclear leukocytes is more suggestive of acute bacterial infection of the CNS. Bickerstaff's brainstem encephalitis, which is a syndrome of progressive ophthalmoplegia and ataxia with disturbance of consciousness or hyperreflexia, has also been report-

ed associated with *Mycoplasma pneumoniae* infection. *Mycoplasma pneumoniae* was detected by PCR analysis of a throat swab and anti-GQ1b antibodies were detected in serum. Anti-GQ1b ganglioside antibodies have been detected in other immune-mediated neurological syndromes following bacterial infections, including Miller Fisher syndrome and Guillain–Barré.

Antimicrobial therapy should be initiated for the patient with signs and symptoms of encephalitis with a positive CSF culture or PCR for *M. pneumoniae*, and/or a CSF pleocytosis of polymorphonuclear leukocytes. The recommended therapeutic agents are either a macrolide (erythromycin or azithromycin), tetracycline, chloramphenicol, or a fluoroquinolone. Patients with respiratory symptoms and chest radiograph evidence of a pulmonary infiltrate should also be treated with antimicrobial therapy. A delay between respiratory symptoms and the neurological disorder, and evidence of a CSF lymphocytic pleocytosis, is suggestive of an immune-mediated encephalitis, and treatment with high-dose intravenous corticosteroid therapy, intravenous immunoglobulin or plasma exchange is recommended. In these patients, *M. pneumoniae* is often detected by PCR in throat swabs, but not CSF specimens.

Listeria monocytogenes

Listeria monocytogenes is a Gram-positive bacillus that contaminates food and infection is acquired from coleslaw, hot dogs, Mexican-style cheese that contains unpasteurized milk, soft cheeses (Brie, Camembert), and processed lunch meats. Once in the gastrointestinal tract, the organism can directly invade the intestinal epithelium. *L. monocytogenes* is an intracellular parasite with a unique ability to infect neighboring cells without ever becoming extracellular. The organism uses host cell actin filaments to form filopodial projections that are engulfed by neighboring phagocytic cells. *Listeria* is then able to escape the lysosome of its new cell and repeat the process. Portal circulation carries the pathogen from the gut to the liver, where *Listeria* becomes concentrated in the reticuloendothelial cells. A bacteremia then ensues. The central nervous system is infected during the bacteremia or by intra-axonal spread. *Listeria monocytogenes* can gain access to cranial nerves through the oral mucosa and via retrograde axonal spread infect cranial nerve nuclei in the brainstem.

The T-cell-mediated immune response of the host is important in determining the risk for disease. Individuals with impaired cell-mediated immunity due to pregnancy, organ transplantation, acquired immunodeficiency syndrome (AIDS), cancer, chemotherapy, and other immunosuppressive therapies are at increased risk

---

International Neurology, Second edition. Edited by Robert P. Lisak, Daniel D. Truong, William M. Carroll and Roongroj Bhidayasiri
© 2016 John Wiley & Sons, Ltd. Published 2016 by John Wiley & Sons, Ltd.

for disease. In addition to immune status, age (neonates and individuals over the age of 50) and underlying medical conditions (diabetes and alcoholism) increase the risk for listeriosis and CNS infection. Healthy individuals can develop *Listeria* infections as well.

Listeria monocytogenes may cause a meningoencephalitis characterized by fever and headache and an altered level of consciousness. Nuchal rigidity, focal neurological signs, and seizures are less common. The organism may cause a brainstem encephalitis, also referred to as a rhombencephalitis. There may be a prodromal phase consisting of headache, nausea, vomiting, fever, and malaise. This is followed by the onset of cranial nerve palsies, cerebellar deficits, and long-tract motor or sensory deficits. A prodromal phase is not mandatory, as brainstem signs can develop without fever or headache.

Diagnosis is made by demonstrating the organism in blood cultures and examination of the cerebrospinal fluid. The majority of patient with *Listeria monocytogenes* meningoencephalitis have a CSF pleocytosis with a predominance of polymorphonuclear leukocytes. Approximately 25% have a lymphocytic pleocytosis. The glucose concentration may be normal or decreased. In the majority of cases the organism can be cultured from CSF. In *Listeria* brainstem encephalitis, there is a high signal intensity lesion on T2-weighted, diffusion, and FLAIR MR imaging. Spinal fluid analysis demonstrates a lymphocytic or monocytic pleocytosis. The absence of a CSF pleocytosis has also been reported.

There are a number of features particular to *L. monocytogenes* meningoencephalitis as compared with meningoencephalitis due to the other bacterial etiologies: (1) the presentation is typically acute but may be subacute; (2) nuchal rigidity is less common; (3) the presentation may be characterized by brainstem signs and symptoms; (4) blood cultures are often positive (75% of cases); (5) spinal fluid analysis may demonstrate a lymphocytic pleocytosis or be normal; and (6) the CSF glucose concentration may be normal.

Ampicillin is the recommended antimicrobial agent for the treatment of *L. monocytogenes* CNS infections. The dose of ampicillin is 150 mg/kg/day for neonates (in an 8-hour dosing interval), 300–400 mg/kg/day for infants and children (in a 4–6-hour dosing interval), and 12–15 g/day for adults (in a 4–6-hour dosing interval). The duration of treatment is 2–3 weeks. Gentamicin is added to ampicillin in patients who are severely ill. Trimethoprim-sulfamethoxazole can be used in patients who are allergic to penicillin.

The more common bacteria to cause a meningoencephalitis are *Streptococcus pneumoniae*, *Neisseria meningitidis*, *Staphylococcus aureus*, and Gram-negative bacilli, including anaerobes. These are discussed in Chapter 58.

Whipple's disease

Whipple's disease is caused by the bacteria *Tropheryma whipplei*, and was first described by George H. Whipple in 1907. Whipple's disease is characterized by two stages. There is a prodromal stage of chronic intermittent non-specific symptoms, primarily migratory arthralgias, diarrhea, and fever. This is followed over the course of several years by a steady-state stage of weight loss, abdominal pain, fever of unknown origin, and diarrhea, with symptoms reflecting the involvement of other organs in addition to the gastrointestinal tract.

The pathognomonic neurological sign of Whipple's disease is oculomasticatory, or oculofacial-skeletal myorhythmia. Oculomasticatory myorhythmia consists of pendular horizontal convergent–divergent oscillations of both eyes synchronous with involuntary contractions of the jaw and tongue. There is a vertical gaze palsy at presentation in 50% of patients. Myoclonus and cerebellar ataxia have also been reported. Cognitive changes are common, affecting 71% of patients with neurological involvement, and take the form of dementia, delirium, memory loss, somnolence, apathy, depression, and/or anxiety. *T. whipplei* has a predilection for the hypothalamus and brainstem. MRI may demonstrate atrophy of the hippocampus, focal or multifocal ring-enhancing lesions with edema, or multifocal white-matter hyperintensities on T2-weighted imaging. Patients with supranuclear vertical gaze palsies may have rostral brainstem lesions or normal MRI.

Whipple's disease may be diagnosed by periodic acid–Schiff (PAS) staining of small bowel biopsy specimens. The organism may be identified by PCR in CSF or jejunal tissue obtained by biopsy. Spinal fluid analysis is usually normal, but a low-grade pleocytosis and a mild elevation of the protein concentration have been reported. The CSF PCR test to detect nucleic acid of *T. whipplei* is a useful test, although the sensitivity of this assay has not been determined.

The recommended treatment is two weeks of parenteral streptomycin (1 g/day) with penicillin G (1.2 million U/day) or ceftriaxone (2 g every 12 hours). This is followed by the oral administration of 160 mg of trimethoprim and 800 mg of sulfamethoxazole twice per day for 1–2 years. There have been reports of CNS relapse when tetracycline or penicillin was used alone.

Cat-scratch disease

Cat-scratch disease is caused by the Gram-negative bacillus *Bartonella henselae*. The disease was first described in 1950. Its "typical" presentation is that of fever, an erythematous papule at the inoculation site, and a regional lymphadenopathy that develops 2–3 weeks after a cat scratch or bite. Cat-scratch disease is considered a benign, self-limited disease in an immunocompetent individual and usually resolves in a few months. In approximately 10% of patients, there will be an "atypical" disease, such as encephalitis, neuroretinitis, endocarditis, or Parinaud oculoglandular syndrome (POS).

The pathogenesis of cat-scratch disease encephalitis has not yet been defined. It is not clear whether encephalitis is due to direct invasion of the brain by bacilli, as has been demonstrated in histopathological examination of brain tissue at autopsy, a vasculitis, or a parainfectious immune-mediated process, such as an acute disseminated encephalomyelitis.

Cat-scratch encephalitis occurs from within a few days to up to two months following the presentation of "typical" cat-scratch disease. The most common symptoms of encephalitis are convulsions and status epilepticus. Other symptoms include persistent headache, lethargy, malaise, combative behavior, and ataxia. Aphasia, transient hemiplegia, and hearing loss may also occur.

The diagnosis of cat-scratch disease encephalitis is based on the detection of *B. henselae* antibodies in a single serum titer of ≥1:64, which has both sensitivity and specificity approaching 100%. Seroconversion may not occur until the third week of illness. PCR of lymph node tissue and culture are also used in diagnosis, but are less widely available. In approximately one-third of patients with cat-scratch disease encephalitis, there is a CSF pleocytosis with a lymphocytic predominance and an increased protein concentration; 50% of patients have an elevated erythrocyte sedimentation rate and 25% an elevated peripheral leukocytosis.

Electroencephalography in a majority of patients will show diffuse background slow wave activity indicative of encephalopathy.

Findings on MRI and CT imaging studies are either negative or non-specific, demonstrating focal or diffuse white- and gray-matter abnormalities.

The preferred treatment for "typical" cat-scratch disease is supportive therapy only. A number of antibiotics have been shown to be efficacious, including rifampin, doxycycline, ciprofloxacin, trimethoprim-sulfamethoxazole, and azithromycin. Antimicrobial therapy with intravenous doxycycline 200 mg twice daily is recommended for patients with cat-scratch encephalitis. One study showed dramatic clinical improvement with the use of high-dose corticosteroids.

Prognosis is generally good, with full recovery in most patients within a month and the remainder within a year. There are, however, anecdotal reports of patients with persistent disability and partial seizures requiring long-term treatment.

Brucellosis

Infection with Brucella is acquired through the inhalation of infected aerosolized particles through contact with animal parts and through the consumption of unpasteurized dairy products. Four species of brucella cause human disease: *B. melitensis*, *B. abortus*, *B. suis*, and *B. canis*. Brucellae are small, Gram-negative coccobacilli. Consider this organism as the causative agent of encephalitis in veterinarians, farmers, abattoir workers, individuals who work in microbiology laboratories, and the household contacts of individuals with these occupations.

Brucella invades the mucosa, after which a bacteremia occurs. Initial symptoms are fever, headache, sweats, and malaise. A malodorous perspiration is pathognomonic. On physical examination, there may be evidence of lymphadenopathy, hepatomegaly, or splenomegaly. Central nervous system involvement in brucellosis can present as a meningitis, an encephalitis, a brain abscess, or demyelinating disease. Examination of the CSF demonstrates an increased number of white blood cells, an increased protein concentration, and a decreased glucose concentration. Diagnosis is made by isolation of the organism from blood culture, a positive indirect enzyme-linked immunosorbent assay (ELISA), isolation of the organism from CSF, evidence of *Brucella* agglutinating antibodies in CSF, or identification of bacterial nucleic acid by PCR.

Treatment guidelines are based on the recommendations of the World Health Organization. Doxycycline 100 mg twice daily for 6 weeks is used in combination with either streptomycin or rifampin. Monotherapy is not recommended due to the risk of relapse with a single antibiotic.

Legionnaires' disease

Legionnaires' disease was first described in 1976 during an epidemic of pneumonia in Philadelphia that resulted in 34 deaths. The recognition of the disease was followed by a number of anecdotal reports and small case series in the 1980s of encephalopathy, cranial nerve palsies, cerebellar dysfunction, myelopathy, peripheral neuropathy, and myositis. Since then, only a rare case of Legionnaires' disease with neurological complications has been reported, and few physicians today include *Legionella pneumophilia* in a differential diagnosis of bacterial etiologies of encephalitis. Diagnosis depends on serology, isolation of the organism by culture, or evidence of

Legionella pneumophila by direct fluorescent antibody (DFA) test of a specimen obtained by bronchoalveolar lavage.

Historically, treatment of encephalitis associated with *Legionella pneumophilia* pneumonia has been with rifampin and erythromycin or rifampin and azithromycin. Rifampin monotherapy is not recommended as resistance may develop.

Recommendations

Encephalitis may be caused by a bacteria or occur as a parainfectious immune-mediated process following a bacterial infection. Every patient with encephalitis should have at least three specimens of blood sent for Gram's stain and culture and should have examination of cerebrospinal fluid. Cerebrospinal fluid should be sent for Gram's stain and bacterial culture, and 16S rRNA bacterial PCR to detect bacterial nucleic aid.

When *Mycoplasma pneumoniae* is the suspected causative organism because of a history of preceding flu-like or respiratory symptoms prior to the onset of neurological disease, obtain a chest X-ray, send CSF for culture and PCR for *M. pneumoniae*, and obtain acute and convalescent serology to demonstrate a fourfold increase in *M. pneumoniae* IgG. A delay between respiratory symptoms and the neurological disorder in association with evidence of a CSF lymphocytic pleocytosis is suggestive of an immune-mediated encephalitis. Send serum for anti-GQ1b ganglioside antibodies.

Whipple's disease causes a clinical presentation of a subacute encephalitis. The organism may be identified by PCR in CSF or jejunal tissue obtained by biopsy.

For cat-scratch disease encephalitis, inquire about a new kitten and a scratch or bite. Look for an inoculation site and examine the patient for lymphadenopathy. The diagnosis of cat-scratch disease encephalitis is based on the detection of *B. henselae* antibodies in a single serum titer of ≥1:64. Seroconversion may not occur until the third week of illness.

Encephalitis due to a species of *Brucella* should be considered in the patient who has contact with animals or who has ingested unpasteurized dairy products. The diagnosis requires isolation of the organism from blood or CSF, a positive ELISA, evidence of *Brucella* agglutinating antibodies in CSF, or identification of bacterial nucleic acid by PCR.

Legionnaires' disease associated with acute encephalitis is rarely reported today. In a patient with pneumonia and encephalitis in whom the causative organisms cannot be identified by sputum, blood, and CSF culture, consideration can be given to bronchoalveolar lavage for a direct fluorescent antibody test for *Legionella pneumophila*.

Further reading

Dalton MJ, Robinson LE, Cooper J, *et al.* Use of Bartonella antigens for serologic diagnosis of CSD at a national reference center. *Arch Intern Med* 1995;155(15):1670°1676.

Daxboeck F, Blacky A, Seidl R, Krause R, Assadian O. Diagnosis, treatment and prognosis of *Mycoplasma pneumoniae* childhood encephalitis: Systematic review of 58 cases. *J Child Neurol* 2004;19:865–871.

Lorber B. Listeriosis. *Clin Infect Dis* 1997;24:1–11.

Fenollar F, Puechal X, Raoult D. Whipple's disease. *N Engl J Med* 2007;356:55–66.

Kimmel DW. Central nervous system Whipple's disease. In: Noseworthy JH (ed.). *Fifty Neurologic Cases from Mayo Clinic.* Oxford: Oxford University Press; 2004:39–40.

64 Mycobacterium tuberculosis and avium

Einar P. Wilder-Smith

Department of Medicine, National University of Singapore, Singapore

Tuberculosis (TB) re-emerged as a major health problem at the end of the 1980s due to the emergence of the human immunodeficiency virus (HIV) and the development of drug-resistant *Mycobacterium*. Compounding this are the often inadequate resources available to screen and investigate those at risk of TB. Prompt diagnosis and treatment are crucial to reduce the number of people dying from TB, which the World Health Organization (WHO) estimated at 1.3 million in 2012 alone.

Achieving a diagnosis can be challenging, particularly in view of the non-specificity of many of the clinical presentations and the constraints on investigative methods often encountered in countries with high incidence rates. This contributes to delayed onset of recognition and treatment, explaining at least in part the often poor clinical outcomes. Drug resistance to TB has steadily increased, with multidrug-resistant TB detected in about 5% of all patients globally and in virtually all countries surveyed. Nevertheless, the majority of deaths from TB still occur in drug-sensitive disease, highlighting the importance of early disease recognition and treatment as well as preventive measures.

This chapter focuses on TB infection of the nervous system, which mainly affects the brain and the spinal cord. *Mycobacterium tuberculosis* is nearly always the infecting agent and other non-tuberculous mycobacteria are only rarely pathological, apart from opportunistic infection in immunosuppressed (predominantly HIV/AIDS) patients.

Epidemiology

As estimated by the WHO, 8.6 million new TB cases occurred in 2012. Of these, 4.8 million were in Asia, accounting for 60% of all new cases globally. Nearly 1 million people died of TB in that, excluding 0.32 million patients infected with HIV. A disproportionate amount of TB-related mortality is related to its effects on the central nervous system.

The peak incidence occurs in individuals aged 2–4 years and mortality in childhood TB meningitis is 20%; survival with neurological sequelae occurs in 54%. The majority of new TB cases (more than 85%) involve the lungs, and 1% of all TB cases have nervous system involvement, mainly in the form of meningitis and meningoencephalitis.

The most important risk factor for TB of the nervous system is immune suppression, when there is failure to contain mycobacterial spread beyond the lung. This explains why one-third of nervous system TB occurs in children and patients infected with HIV.

As *M. tuberculosis* is ubiquitous, the majority of people are exposed to TB during their lifetime. The number of TB mycobacteria and an intact immune response determine whether disease will develop or not. Other important determinants of a successful immune response are age, nutritional status, diabetes, HIV, and treatment with immunosuppressive drugs such as steroids and chemotherapy. One of the undisputed benefits of BCG (Bacillus Calmette-Guérin) vaccination is effective protection against TB meningitis.

Pathophysiology

All tuberculosis starts with the inhalation of TB bacilli and their subsequent multiplication within the alveoli. From here there is spread to other organs via the bloodstream.

Central nervous system (CNS) TB develops from "Rich foci," which are subependymal or subpial accumulations of bacilli that within the brain are most commonly located in the Sylvian fissure. Here, with growth they rupture into the subarachnoid or ventricular space to cause meningitis. The accumulation and subsequent growth of TB bacilli in other locations result in tuberculomas or abscesses. Extracerebral sites that result in neurological disease are the spinal vertebrae, where the hematogenously spread bacillus preferentially lodges in the anterior or inferior angle of the vertebral body. From here the disease spreads to the intervertebral disc, which is typically destroyed and spreads to the adjacent vertebral body.

Tuberculosis meningitis

In tuberculosis meningitis (TBM), typically a thick exudate of the leptomeninges develops predominantly over the basal regions of the brain with involvement of the basal cisterns. This process predisposes to cerebrospinal fluid (CSF) obstruction and not infrequently results in communicating (70%) or obstructive (30%) hydrocephalus. As the disease progresses, ependymitis develops and spread to other CNS sites occurs. The exudate is composed of a network of mononuclear cells, red blood cells, neutrophils, lymphocytes, and varying numbers of tubercle bacilli. With disease progression, the predominant cell type is lymphocytic. One of the consequences of the exudate is irritation of the bystanding brain vessels, which may occlude, leading to stroke either through direct participation in the inflammatory process or through reactive vasoconstriction.

In childhood, TBM often manifests several weeks after the primary infection, explaining why the majority of cases of TBM show evidence of an active primary complex.

International Neurology, Second edition. Edited by Robert P. Lisak, Daniel D. Truong, William M. Carroll and Roongroj Bhidayasiri
© 2016 John Wiley & Sons, Ltd. Published 2016 by John Wiley & Sons, Ltd.

Tuberculomas

Tuberculomas and abscess tuberculomas consist of Langerhans' cells, epithelioid cells, and lymphocytes. Typically the center contains caseous material in which TB bacilli can be demonstrated.

In children, tuberculomas of the brain are more frequent infratentorially, whereas in adults there is supratentorial preference. Liquefaction of the caseous core of a tuberculoma results in the formation of abscesses, which are often larger and multilobulated in immune-compromised individuals.

Abscesses are made up of large numbers of neutrophils and numerous TB bacilli. Neurological deficits depend on the site of the tuberculomas and cause symptoms and signs as a result of arachnoiditis, vasculitis, and compression.

Clinical features

Co-infection with HIV does not alter the clinical presentation of TB, but increases the number of complications.

Tuberculous meningitis

Fever, headache, and anorexia are the most frequent presenting symptoms of TBM. The most common clinical sign is meningism (40–80%), followed by coma (30–60%) and cranial nerve palsies (30–50%), of which sixth nerve palsy is by far the most common (30–40%). Seizures (generalized or partial) occur in 50% of children, but in only 5% of adults. Hemiparesis is noted in 10–20% of cases. Physicians should be aware that fever may be absent and that neurological signs can rapidly progress to coma.

In about 75% of cases of TBM and more frequently in children than adults, extrameningeal TB – mostly seen over the lungs – is present.

TBM is classified into three grades with increasing severity predicting increased mortality. A fully oriented patient with no focal neurology is graded 1. Grade 2 is scored with a Glasgow Coma Scale of 10–14 with or without focal neurology, and Grade 3 with a Glasgow Coma Scale of less than 10.

Tuberculomas

In the brain, tuberculomas produce signs through their irritative and space-occupying characteristics. India has a particularly high incidence of intracerebral tuberculomas, which often present with seizures.

Tuberculosis of the spine (often termed Pott's disease) frequently results in a tender spine prominence or angulation (gibbus) with neurological deficit at the lower thoracic motor and sensory level. About half of those with spinal disease manifest paraparesis. In countries with a high standard of living, those affected are usually elderly; in countries where TB is common, those affected are predominantly younger than 20 years of age. Pott's disease often occurs without evidence of other TB foci. Early manifestations are back pain and stiffness.

In about 50% of cases, a paraspinal cold abscess develops that follows along ligamentous tracks, draining into distant regions such as the iliac crest, groin, or buttock. Spread along the spine may sometimes skip several spinal levels.

Investigations

Tuberculous meningitis

Diagnosis depends on a high index of suspicion. Examination of the CSF is essential and identification of acid-fast bacilli clinches the diagnosis. Meticulous microscopic technique and use of more than

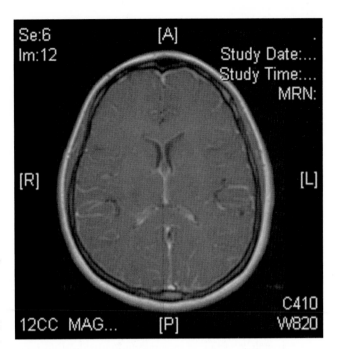

Figure 64.1 Gadolinium-enhanced axial MRI using T1-weighted sequence showing diffuse leptomeningeal enhancement with periependymal enhancement of the lateral ventricles.

5 ml of CSF results in detection in 60% of cases. Cultures take 6 weeks and are positive in approximately 70% of cases. Characteristic is a lymphocyte-predominant CSF cell count of less than 1500 cells/mm^3, low glucose (less than 0.5 CSF to blood ratio), and moderately elevated protein levels. In early disease, cells may be predominantly polymorphonuclear. Staining for acid-fast bacilli shows poor sensitivity. Polymerase chain reaction (PCR) has no better bacteriological diagnostic accuracy than staining for acid-fast bacilli in untreated CSF samples, but may be superior when treatment has already commenced. The typical neuroradiological triad accompanying TBM is basal meningeal enhancement (the most consistent), hydrocephalus, and, less commonly, supratentorial ischemia. These changes are, however, non-specific, and can also be seen with other diseases such as viral meningoencephalitis, cryptococcal disease, metastasis, sarcoidosis, and lymphoma. Figure 64.1 shows leptomeningeal and ependymal enhancement in a patient with TBM.

Tuberculomas, abscesses, and other complications

Tuberculomas, stroke, and hydrocephalus generally occur in the first 3 months of meningitis. Verification of tuberculomas and abscesses ultimately remains histological and should if possible be attempted prior to initiation of treatment, mainly to exclude differential diagnoses.

Treatment

Medication

Since delay of treatment can be fatal, treatment should be initiated when clinical and laboratory findings are compatible with a diagnosis of TB. The recommendation is 9–12 months of multidrug therapy, although a recent review suggested that 6 months of treatment may be sufficient in areas with low levels of bacterial resistance. The first 2 months of intensive treatment require quadruple therapy with isoniazid (10 mg/kg/day), rifampicin (10 mg/kg/day), and pyrazinamide (30 mg/kg/day), with the addition of one of the following: ethambutol (15–20mg/kg/day), streptomycin (15 mg/kg/day; maximum 1 g), or ethionamide (15–20 mg/kg/day). Isoniazid – which has excellent CSF penetration – should be given together with rifampicin for the continuation phase of treatment from months 3 to 9. Intolerance to one or more of the medicines during the intensive phase of treatment necessitates prolonged treatment with the remaining medications in the regimen. Pyridoxine therapy (100 mg/day) should be given with isoniazid therapy to prevent the development of peripheral neuropathy.

Adjunctive corticosteroids (prednisone 1–3 mg/kg/day or dexamethasone 0.3–0.5 mg/kg/day in a taper-down dose regimen) significantly reduce mortality across all severity grades, irrespective of co-infection with HIV. For this reason, steroids should be administered in all cases from day 1 of treatment, in a tapering dose for the first 1–2 months.

Despite increasing resistance to antituberculous drugs worldwide, implications for treatment are not yet clear. Although bacilli resistant to isoniazid and rifampicin show worse clinical outcomes, the clinical implications of single drug resistance are as yet unclear. Currently, detection of resistance to isoniazid should result in prolonged treatment with a regimen that includes pyrazinamide. Identifying patients with multidrug resistance can be difficult, as the time for bacteriological sensitivities to manifest is 6 weeks. Therefore, when standard treatment fails to halt disease progression, drug resistance should be considered and at least three previously unused drugs should be prescribed, of which one should be a fluoroquinolone.

Neurosurgery
The best treatment for hydrocephalus remains unclear, as there have been no trials comparing available treatment options. Serial lumbar punctures and ventriculoperitoneal or atrial shunting have all been used successfully. Conservative treatment (acetazolamide and furosemide) normalizes intracranial pressure in 80% of children with communicating hydrocephalus within a month, with most showing normal lumbar CSF pressure (<15 cm H_2O) after a week of treatment. As CSF circulation and reabsorption can be lastingly abnormal, permanent approaches of CSF drainage in the form of shunting are currently considered preferable, but need to be weighed against complications seen in up to 30% of cases.

Mycobacterium avium
Mycobacterium avium (MA) only rarely infects the human nervous system and then only in severe immunosuppression syndromes, most commonly that accompanying HIV infection, and

uncommonly as part of the immune reconstitution syndrome, or in non-HIV patients where there is a failure of CD4 cells to activate macrophages.

Central nervous system disease can result from the disseminated form of MA, which may occur when CD4 counts drop below 100/mm^3. Disseminated MA has been reported more frequently in developed countries (United States and Europe) and is particularly rare in Africa. Mycobacterium avium has recently been observed to result in chronic pulmonary infections in otherwise healthy elderly persons, and under these circumstances occasionally invades the brain with abscess formation. Systematic review has shown that the incidence of opportunistic illnesses including MA has decreased over the past 30 years of the HIV epidemic, most markedly after antiretroviral therapy availability.

The initial MA infection is via the gastrointestinal tract or the lung, with subsequent hematogenous spread to the brain, where disease mostly presents as one or multiple ring-enhancing space-occupying lesions. Diagnosis can only be achieved with specialized histological analysis and bacterial culture. Differential diagnosis includes cryptococcus, bartonella, cytomegalovirus, syphilis, and toxoplasmosis. Surgical removal combined with a combination of ethambutol, clarithromycin, and rifampicin has been effective in some cases, although side effects often form a considerable or absolute barrier to persistent antibiotic treatment. More recently, treatment cocktails including macrolides (clarithromycin, azithromycin) have shown improved results in disseminated MA. Clofazimine appears safe and may be considered as a salvage therapeutic option in solid organ transplant recipients with MA infection who are intolerant or unresponsive to ethambutol, clarithromycin, and rifampicin.

Further reading
Begley C, Amaraneni A, Lutwick L. Mycobacterium avium–intracellular brain abscesses in an HIV-infected patient. *ID Cases* 2015;2(1):19–21. doi:10.1016/j.idcr.2014.11.002

Bernaerts A, Vanhoenacker FM, Parizel PM, *et al.* Tuberculosis of the central nervous system: Overview of neuroradiological findings. *Eur Radiol* 2003;13:1876–1890.

Davies PDO, Gordon SB, Davies G. *Clinical Tuberculosis*, 5th ed. Boca Raton, FL: CRC Press; 2014.

Fortin C, Rouleau D. Cerebral mycobacterium avium abscesses: Late immune reconstitution syndrome in an HIV-1-infected patient receiving highly active antiretroviral therapy. *Can J Infect Dis Med Microbiol* 2005;16(3):187–189.

Gordin FM, Horsburgh CR. Mycobacterium avium complex. In: MandallGL, BennettJE, DolinR. (eds.). *Principles and Practice of Infectious Diseases*, 6th ed. Philadelphia, PA: Elsevier/Churchill Livingstone; 2005:2897–2909.

Thwaites GE, van Toorn R, van Loenhout-Rooyackers JS, *et al.* Tuberculous meningitis: More questions, still too few answers. *Lancet Neurol* 2013;12:999–1010.

van Loenhout-Rooyackers JH, Keyser A, Laheij RJ, Verbeek AL, van der Meer JW. Tuberculous meningitis: Is a 6-month treatment regimen sufficient? *Int J Tuberc Lung Dis* 2001;5:1028–1035.

World Health Organization. *Global Tuberculosis Report 2013*. http://apps.who.int/iris/bitstream/10665/91355/1/9789241564656_eng.pdf (accessed 14 October 2014).

65 Leprosy

Minh Le[1] and Minh Hoang Van[2]

[1] Department of Neurology, University Medical Center, Ho Chi Minh City, Vietnam

[2] Department of Dermatology, University of Medicine and Pharmacy, Ho Chi Minh City, Vietnam

Leprosy (Hansen's disease) is a result of chronic infection by *Mycobacterium leprae*. It affects mainly the skin, peripheral nerves, upper respiratory airways, anterior eye segments, and testes. There are various forms of the disease, which depend on the person's cell-mediated immune response to the infection.

Bacteriology

Mycobacterium leprae, measuring 0.5 μm × 4.0 μm, is an acid-fast bacillus (AFB) stained by the Ziehl–Neelsen method in smears and by the Fite–Faraco method in tissue sections. Acid fastness is related to mycolic acid in the cell wall of the micro-organism. The staining properties of *M. leprae* in skin smears or biopsy specimens are important in assessment of the therapeutic efficacy of antileprotics: viable organisms stain solidly; degenerate organisms stain irregularly and eventually become non-acid fast. The carcasses of non-viable organisms in tissues or in smears can be detected by silver staining methods. *M. leprae* is an obligate intracellular parasite with a preference to infect cooler body areas. It has the longest doubling time (13–14 days) of all known bacteria and has never been cultured in the laboratory without a surrogate host. Despite this, it is possible to grow *M. leprae* in nine-banded armadillos and on the foot pads of mice. The incubation period of the disease is about 5 years. Symptoms can take as long as 20 years to appear.

Epidemiology

The prevalence of leprosy has recently reduced globally. According to the World Health Organization (WHO), in 1985 Hansen's disease was endemic in 122 countries; in 1995 there were 1.83 million people in the world affected by active leprosy compared to 12–15 million in the previous decade. Prevalence rates vary geographically, with 75% of leprosy occurring in Southern Asia, 12% in Africa, and 8% in the Americas. Official reports recently received from 115 countries and territories indicate that the global registered prevalence of leprosy at the end of the first quarter of 2013 stood at 189,018 cases, while the number of new cases detected during 2012 was 232,857 (excluding the small number of cases in Europe). Most countries that were previously highly endemic for leprosy have eliminated it at the national level. Leprosy today prevails in the poor areas of the world, particularly in the tropical regions.

The most important source of leprosy is infected humans, but armadillos, chimpanzees, and monkeys are other reservoirs of leprosy.

Pathogenesis

The two portals of entry seriously considered are the upper respiratory tract and the skin, in which transmission through secretions from the nasal mucosa of untreated patients is thought to be the main route of infection.

Bacteremia is present in up 15% of paucibacillary patients and is common in multibacillary patients. *M. leprae* invades peripheral nerves via the blood vessels of the perineurium, and causes infection of endothelial cells leading to ischemia of the nerves. *M. leprae* has a tendency to bind to laminin-2 in the basal lamina of the Schwann cell-axon unit, and ultimately activates α-dystroglycan receptors of this cell.

Immunity

The characteristics of host cell-mediated immunity determine the clinical manifestation of disease, as described by the Ridley–Jopling classification. Lepromatous Hansen's disease is characterized by a strong proliferation of AFB, anergy to lepromin, minimal inflammatory response, and disseminated nerve and skin lesions. Tuberculoid Hansen's disease is characterized by intense cell-mediated immunity, delayed hypersensitivity response to lepromin, intense inflammatory lesions that cause local destruction of infected nerves, and, rarely, AFB detected in skin and nerves. Borderline forms share the characteristics of the two extremes. Table 65.1 shows the clinical and histopathological classification of leprosy based on the Ridley–Jopling classification.

International Neurology, Second edition. Edited by Robert P. Lisak, Daniel D. Truong, William M. Carroll and Roongroj Bhidayasiri

Table 65.1 Clinical and histopathological classification of leprosy.

Clinical features	Histopathological features
Tuberculoid form (TT) Few well-defined anesthetic macules or plaques; neural involvement common	Granulomas with or without giant cells; rare bacilli; nerve damage; no subepidermal free zone
Borderline forms Borderline tuberculoid (BT) More lesions, borders less distinct; neural involvement common	Similar to TT but with occasional bacilli, usually in nerves; subepidermal free zone
Midborderline (BB) More lesions than BT, borders vague; neural involvement common	Epithelioid cells and histiocytes; focal lymphocytes; increased cellularity of nerves; bacilli readily found, mostly in nerves; subepidermal free zone
Borderline lepromatous (BL) Numerous lesions, borders vague; less neural damage than in BB	Histiocytes, few epithelioid cells, some foamy cells; bacilli plentiful in nerves and histiocytes; subepidermal free zone
Lepromatous form (LL) Multiple macules, nodules, or diffuse infiltrations; symmetrically neural lesions develop late	Foamy histiocytes with large numbers of bacilli; few lymphocytes; numerous bacilli in nerves; minimal intraneural cellular infiltration; subepidermal free zone
Indeterminate form (I) Vaguely defined, hypopigmented, or erythematous macules	Small lymphocytic infiltrates around nerves and appendages; rare bacilli, usually in nerves

The WHO classification of leprosy for field workers, which is based on the burden of AFB in tissues and the number of skin lesions, determines two main forms of leprosy: paucibacillary (PB) leprosy, in which patients have skin smears negative for AFB or five or fewer cutaneous lesions; and multibacillary (MB) leprosy, in which patients have positive skin smears for AFB or more than five skin lesions. "Single-lesion" paucibacillary is the third category of the WHO classification. The WHO classification under PB would include I, TT, and BT of the Ridley–Jopling classification; MB would include BB, BL, and LL. Single-lesion paucibacillary would include I and TT.

Clinical features

Skin lesions with associated sensory loss and enlarged peripheral nerves are the cardinal symptoms and signs of leprosy. Sensory disturbances are the outstanding features of Hansen's disease, and include anesthesia or hypesthesia to pain and temperature, and sometimes paresthesias or dysesthesias. Often sensory abnormalities precede paralysis, with impaired temperature and touch frequently linked.

Tuberculoid (TT) patients have single or few macules or indurated skin lesions that are hypopigmented, hypoesthetic, and anhydrotic. Cutaneous nerves and superficial peripheral nerve trunks are often enlarged in the region of lesions. The commonly involved nerves that present indurated hypertrophy are the great auricular, ulnar, radial, fibular, and sural nerves. Cold nerve abscesses due to intense response to bacilli within nerves can occur in larger nerve trunks of TT patients. Calcifications of nerves in long-standing cases of PB leprosy may be sufficiently intense to appear on X-ray. Acrodystrophy and autoamputation are the common late complications of neuropathy, in which loss of pain is predominant.

Lepromatous leprosy (LL) is characterized by the infiltration of nearly the entire skin with a predilection for cooler areas of the body including the ears, central portion of the face, and extensor surfaces of the thighs and forearms. Some regions such as scalp, palms, soles, and midline of the back are, however, not involved. Skin lesions include macules, nodules, papules, ulcerations, and diffuse myxedema-like involvement. Sensory loss is commonly first distributed to the ear helices, nose, malar regions, dorsal surface of the hands, forearms, feet, and dorsolateral surfaces of the lower legs. Other areas are the upper respiratory tract from the nasal mucosa to the larynx, the eye, lymph nodes, and testes. Commonly affected nerves are the ulnar, posterior tibial, common peroneal, and the median and facial nerves. The preservation of tendon reflexes is one particular aspect of the clinical findings of neuropathy associated with leprosy that should be mentioned, as this can help differentiate from length-dependent neuropathies where tendon reflex loss is a hallmark.

Borderline leprosy is the intermediate group in which patients' resistance to the micro-organism varies from weak to strong. This group includes three subgroups: borderline tuberculoid (BT), midborderline (BB), and borderline lepromatous (BL). This area of the spectrum is unstable, and such borderline patients can swing back and forth toward the two extremes of TT and LL. The essential characteristics of these subgroups are shown in Table 65.1, and the BT subgroup is illustrated in Figure 65.1.

Indeterminate leprosy (I) usually presents as hypopigmented, or slightly erythematous, poorly defined macules. Texture, the amount of hair, sensation, and sweating in the affected area are, at the most, only slightly changed. Because of this vague and non-specific feature, indeterminate lesions can be diagnosed only with close cooperation between clinician and pathologist.

Lucio's leprosy is a particular form of the disease in which there is highly anergic and very diffuse infiltration of skin. Obstructive vasculitis causes massive dermal infarcts, and ulcers can later supervene as this form of leprosy progresses.

Pure neural leprosy affects peripheral nerves in the absence of skin lesions.

(A)
(B)

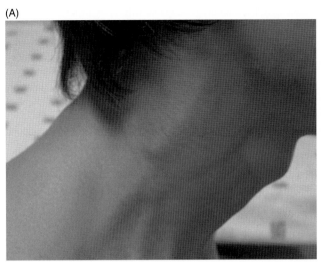
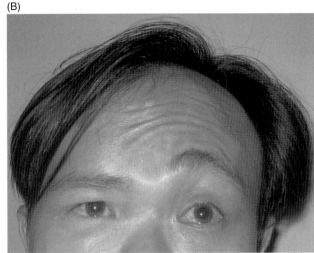

Figure 65.1 (A) Enlargement of the right great auricular nerve in borderline tuberculoid (BT) leprosy. (B) Borderline tuberculoid (BT) leprosy. Same patient with facial paralysis on the right side, and macular lesions of the upper and middle right hemiface.

Leprosy reactions

Inflammatory immune reactions that occur during the progression and the treatment of leprosy should also be taken into account because of their harmful effects on the patient. There are two main reactions: type 1, or reversal reactions, and type 2, or erythema nodosum leprosum reactions (Table 65.2). Reversal reactions (type 1) can occur in any leprosy subtype, although they are most prevalent in the borderline forms (BT–BB–BL), and represent an episodic upgrading of cell-mediated immunity. There is exacerbation of previous lesions, with associated negative skin smears for AFB and good response to anti-inflammatory therapy. Clinical findings include aggravation of previous skin lesions, new skin lesions, and neuritis, which usually appears during the first few months following initiation of chemotherapy. By way of repeated reversal reactions, borderline lesions may gradually change toward tuberculoid leprosy or tuberculoid lesions toward scar tissue. Permanent neurological deficits may result unless anti-inflammatory treatment is quickly initiated.

Erythema nodosum leprosum (ENL) occurs in approximately half of all lepromatous patients, though it may also occur in borderline lepromatous patients. These type 2 reactions often arise after several months or more of therapy, but may also develop in untreated patients. The clinical findings of ENL include malaise, fever, painful indurated cutaneous nodules, painful peripheral nerve lesion, iridocyclitis, orchitis, and arthritis. Hepatomegaly and splenomegaly can also rarely occur. ENL is the result of antigen-antibody complex deposition and results in complement fixation with subsequent cell lysis (Table 65.2).

Diagnosis

The cardinal signs of leprosy are hypoesthetic lesions of the skin, enlarged peripheral nerves, and AFB in skin smears.

A careful physical examination of the entire skin surface and superficial peripheral nerves to look for skin lesions, sensory changes, peripheral nerve enlargement, and motor deficit (e.g., facial paresis, claw hand, foot drop) is crucial for diagnosis. Sensory changes are the most important criteria for clinical diagnosis of leprosy. While leprosy can be diagnosed clinically, histopathological evaluation is useful to confirm the diagnosis, for classification and the

identification of pure neural leprosy. Biopsy specimens should be taken from the edges of the lesions, and stained with the Fite–Faraco method. Skin smears should be obtained from multiple sites, frequently at two sites, including the edges of macules or plaques, or nodules, and earlobes. The Ziehl–Neelsen staining method is used for skin smears.

The histopathological features of TT leprosy and LL leprosy differ. Destruction of the architecture of cutaneous nerves by granulomatous inflammation is the main histopathological finding in TT leprosy. Large numbers of AFB are detected in Schwann cells, macrophages, and axons of involved nerves in LL leprosy, together with a combination of Wallerian degeneration and segmental demyelination.

Diagnosis of leprosy is most commonly based on the clinical signs and symptoms. Only in rare instances is there a need to use laboratory and other investigations to confirm a diagnosis of leprosy. In an endemic country or area, an individual should be regarded

Table 65.2 Comparison of type 1 and type 2 reactions. Source: http://emedicine. medscape.com/article/1165419-overview 2015. Reproduced with permission from Medscape Drugs & Diseases (http://emedicine.medscape.com/).

Features	Type 1 (reversal) reaction	Type 2 (ENL) reaction
Leprosy type at risk	BB, BT, BL	LL, BL
Onset	Gradual, over a few weeks	Sudden
Clinical symptoms and signs	Malaise	Fever, malaise, arthritis, edema, hepatosplenomegaly, lymphadenopathy, orchitis, iridocyclitis
Skin lesions	Increased erythema, induration of pre-existing lesions, appearance of new lesions	New erythematous lesions or tender nodules on face, extremities, and trunk
Nerve involvement	Frequent, often severe	Frequent, often severe

BB = midborderline; BL = borderline lepromatous; BT = borderline tuberculoid;
LL = lepromatous leprosy

as having leprosy if he or she shows one of the following cardinal signs: (1) skin lesion consistent with leprosy and with definite sensory loss; (2) enlarged and sensitive peripheral nerve, accompanied by signs of nerve damage such as paralysis, loss of sensation, skin dystrophy; or (3) a positive skin smear.

A person presenting with skin lesions or with symptoms suggestive of nerve damage, in whom the cardinal signs are absent or doubtful, should be called a "suspect case" in the absence of any immediately obvious alternate diagnosis. Such individuals should be told the basic facts of leprosy and advised to return to the center if signs persist for more than six months or if at any time worsening is noticed. Suspect cases may be also sent to referral clinics that have more facilities for diagnosis.

Other investigations

The lepromin test consists of the intradermal inoculation of 0.1 mL of lepromin (a suspension of heat-killed *M. leprae*) and is used to test the patient's immune response toward *M. leprae*. Evaluation of this response is based on the measurement of the diameter of induration at the injection site 3–4 weeks post inoculation (Mitsuda reaction). This skin test is never used as a diagnostic test of leprosy, as many people in the general population are reactive. The Mitsuda reaction is only useful for classifying Hansen's disease: a strong response is seen in TT and BT (>5 mm); intermediate reactions in BL and BB (3–5 mm); and a weak or non-reactive response in LL (0–2 mm).

Motor and sensory nerve conduction velocity studies can be helpful in demonstrating abnormality in the nerve trunks and branches, which often predates clinical characteristics. It can also be useful to monitor nerve function.

Differential diagnosis

The differential diagnoses of leprosy are extensive and include sarcoidosis, syphilis, yaws, granuloma annulare, leishmaniasis, lupus erythematosus, superficial mycoses, lymphoma, psoriasis, pityriasis rosacea, neurofibromatosis, syringomyelia, lead toxicity, diabetes mellitus, primary amyloidosis, sensory polyneuropathies, other mononeuropathies, and familial hypertrophic neuropathy.

Antileprotic treatment

Specific leprosy treatment and prevention and treatment of deformities are the main objectives for the management of leprosy. Optimum management of this chronic disease should be comprehensive and requires the cooperation of internists, neurologists, orthopedic surgeons, ophthalmologists, and physical therapists.

Because of known drug-resistant strains of *M. leprae* toward dapsone, rifampicin, and other antibiotics, monotherapy with any antileprotic is

discouraged. The multidrug therapeutic (MDT) regimen recommended by the WHO is based on the classification of leprosy into PB and MB. The paucibacillary regimen includes rifampicin 600 mg given once monthly under supervision, plus dapsone 100 mg daily for 6 months. The treatment regimen for single skin lesion paucibacillary leprosy includes rifampicin 600 mg, ofloxacin 400 mg, and minocycline 100 mg.

The multibacillary regimen includes rifampicin 600 mg and clofazimine 300 mg given once monthly under supervision, plus dapsone 100 mg/day and clofazimine 50 mg/day for 12 months. Prothionamide, ethionamide, or minocycline may be used as a substitute for clofazimine when there is hyperpigmentation of the skin from clofazimine. Ofloxacin, clarithromycin, and minocycline are currently used in clinical trials and may be used as an alternative regimen when patients are allergic to rifampicin.

Treatment of leprosy reactions

Reactions in leprosy are considered a medical emergency. Immobilization by splint, analgesics, and prednisone are the mainstay of the treatment of acute neuritis in reversal reaction. Prednisone up to 80 mg daily is given initially, then tapered off over 2–3 months to a minimally effective level as long as neuritis persists. Long-term corticosteroid therapy may be given, preferably in an alternated-day regimen. The efficacy of clofazimine in reversal reactions has not been established. Specific treatment of *M. leprae* by antileprotic agents is continued during management for reversal reactions.

Mild analgesics are required for milder forms of ENL. Severe forms of ENL require more vigorous treatment with steroids or thalidomide. Thalidomide is used at the initial dose of 100 mg 3–4 times daily, then gradually tapered to the minimum effective level. Thalidomide is prescribed only for males and females without reproductive potential. Increasing the dosage of clofazimine up to 300 mg/day is another treatment alternative, but the effects are only apparent after 4–6 weeks. Prednisone is often used when thalidomide cannot be used. Iridocyclitis should be managed aggressively by combined systemic anti-inflammatory treatment and local corticosteroids. Sometimes surgical measures are needed to control increased intraocular pressure.

Further reading

Meyers WM. Leprosy. In: Guerrant RL, Walker DH, Weller PF (eds.). *Tropical Infectious Diseases: Principles, Pathogens, and Practice*, 2nd ed., vol. 1. Philadelphia, PA: Elsevier/Churchill Livingstone; 2006:436–447.

Orlova M, Cobat A, Huong NT, *et al*. Gene set signature of reversal reaction type I in leprosy patients. *PLoS Genet* 2013;9(7):e1003624. doi:10.1371/journal.pgen.1003624

Ramaratnam S. Leprosy neuropathy. *Medscape*. May 30, 2013.

Sabin TD, Swift TR, Jacobson RR. Neuropathy associated with infections – leprosy. In: Dyck PJ, Thomas PK (eds.). *Peripheral Neuropathy*, 4th ed., vol. 2. Philadelphia, PA: Elsevier-Saunders; 2005:2081–2108.

Spierings E, De Boer T, Zulianello L, Ottenhoff THM. Novel mechanisms in the immunopathogenesis of leprosy nerve damage: The role of Schwann cells, T cells and *Mycobacterium leprae*. *Immunol Cell Biol* 2000;78:349–355.

World Health Organization. *WHO Expert Committee on Leprosy: Seventh Report*, WHO Tech Rep Ser No. 874. Geneva: WHO; 1998.

66 Neurosyphilis

Jonathan Carr

Division of Neurology, University of Stellenbosch, Stellenbosch, South Africa

Neurosyphilis is seen predominantly in two major socioeconomic spheres. In the developed world, the manifestations of neurological syphilis appear largely to be associated with ongoing localized epidemics among men who have sex with men (MSM). The developing world probably recapitulates the circumstances seen in the developed world over a century ago, with conditions of urban crowding and poor access to healthcare. Overlapping these two extremes are the marginalized populations of the developed world, for whom access to healthcare providers is limited as a result of historical or social factors such as drug abuse.

Epidemiology

The prevalence of syphilis and neurosyphilis mirrors that of human immunodeficiency virus (HIV) infection. Currently, the burden of syphilis is likely to be greatest in the developing world, and is causally related to a high frequency of unprotected sex with multiple partners. In the developed world unprotected sexual behavior is likely responsible for the high prevalence in MSM and other high-risk populations.

Pathophysiology

The primary stage of syphilis is typically characterized by a chancre, although this may be absent or not visible to the patient. The secondary stage is characterized by a skin rash and lymphadenopathy, but may additionally be complicated by uveitis and meningitis. Secondary syphilis is also the period in which invasion of the nervous system occurs, and although abnormal cerebrospinal fluid (CSF) findings are common, they do not represent neurosyphilis. The definition of tertiary syphilis varies widely, but is typically assumed to include cardiovascular and neurological complications.

Neurosyphilis shares the major features of other chronic meningitides, including findings of a meningo-encephalitis with a chronic inflammatory cell infiltrate of the leptomeninges and superficial cortex. Involvement of the leptomeninges is associated with changes in the vessels, with subintimal proliferation as seen in other forms of chronic meningitis, such as tuberculous meningitis. However, there is a unique involvement of the parenchyma with loss of neurons and gliosis with neurosyphilis. The clinical correlates of the two major pathological processes, vascular occlusion and involvement of cortex and white matter, are varied. Classically, the syndromes were described in neuropathological terms, and were made up of acute syphilitic meningitis, meningovascular neurosyphilis, general paresis of the insane, and tabes dorsalis. The notion that these represent an orderly progression of events with a defined time course is unlikely to be accurate. Few reliable studies of the natural history of neurosyphilis exist, and all are hampered (including modern studies) by the great difficulty in establishing the latency from primary to tertiary neurosyphilis. Currently, the most common manifestations of neurosyphilis are acute syphilitic meningitis, stroke, and neuropsychiatric syphilis. Tabes dorsalis is an extremely rare entity, as are gummata.

Clinical features

Given that the clinician may be faced with weak laboratory data to support a clinical diagnosis of neurosyphilis, it is important to emphasize that atypical forms of neurosyphilis or formes frustes of neurosyphilis are controversial entities with little evidence to support their existence. Reports on atypical presentations of neurosyphilis have tended to be small series, in which the majority of case descriptions have been compatible with standard forms of neurosyphilis, or else arose as a result of inclusion criteria that were overinclusive and therefore included patients who were unlikely to have neurosyphilis. Although neurosyphilis may be rare in developed countries, the presentations are likely to be similar to those seen in developing countries.

The decision to investigate for neurosyphilis with lumbar puncture is usually made in the setting of positive serum serology associated with a clinical presentation compatible with neurosyphilis. Lumbar puncture is therefore not advised in syphilis of unknown duration or in latent syphilis. The following syndromes represent the majority of presentations.

Neuropsychiatric

This is usually a combination of delirium superimposed on dementia, frequently associated with behavioral change that gradually worsens over months. Dementia is global and has a guarded prognosis for recovery. Although they occur, hallucinations and delusional behavior are not common. Physical examination usually reveals hyperreflexia, prominent reflexes, and tremor. Argyll Robertson pupils are an uncommon finding. This presentation is likely to correspond to that known traditionally as general paresis, a form of parenchymal neurosyphilis. The latency of onset of this condition is unlikely to be decades as is sometimes reported, and there is likely to be moderate overlap with meningovascular disease.

International Neurology, Second edition. Edited by Robert P. Lisak, Daniel D. Truong, William M. Carroll and Roongroj Bhidayasiri
© 2016 John Wiley & Sons, Ltd. Published 2016 by John Wiley & Sons, Ltd.

Stroke

Large and small vessel involvement may occur. Large vessel involvement may give rise to strokes in middle cerebral artery territory. Strokes of varying ages in different vascular territories are also seen. Disease of the posterior circulation occurs as well, giving rise to small infarctions of the brainstem. Radiologically, evidence of diffuse small vessel disease may also be present.

Encephalopathy with seizures

This group overlaps with neuropsychiatric neurosyphilis. Patients may present with generalized tonic–clonic or complex partial seizures, and either of these may present with status epilepticus. A common electroencephalographic (EEG) correlate is the presence of periodic lateralized epileptiform discharges. Patients are often noted subsequently to have a global cognitive impairment.

Spinal cord stroke

A common presentation is acute stroke of the spinal cord, resulting in spinal shock or a Brown–Séquard syndrome. Gradually progressive spastic paraparesis is also seen, possibly on an ischemic basis, and a diffuse syphilitic myelitis has been reported, of presumptive autoimmune etiology.

Meningitis

Two forms of meningitis are seen. Acute meningitis associated with fever and neck stiffness is a manifestation of secondary syphilis and may be associated with a rash. A more chronic condition associated with cranial nerve palsies (sometimes multiple) also occurs, and is likely to represent a relatively pure form of meningovascular neurosyphilis.

Tabes dorsalis

Tabes has become extremely uncommon. Classically, tabes is associated with loss of reflexes, usually the ankle, sometimes with Argyll Robertson pupils and bladder dysfunction, and with loss of posterior column function. The latter results in Charcot joints, characterized by joint destruction and sclerosis, commonly in the knee.

HIV and neurosyphilis

Multiple reports were published in the late 1980s on the unexpectedly high frequency (and possibly novel) presentations of syphilis associated with HIV infection, proposing that neurosyphilis had become a more aggressive disease in the setting of immunosuppression. The major syndromes were those of acute meningitis, stroke, and uveitis. Many of the presentations were associated with secondary syphilis, and it is likely that the epidemic of syphilis that was taking place in the United States at the time was responsible for the increased number of cases seen. The descriptions of the manifestations of neurosyphilis in HIV-positive patients match those of well-described syndromes in the pre-HIV era, and the latency from infection to development of neurosyphilis is unlikely to have been reduced. It is appropriate to reiterate that the reported aggressiveness of neurosyphilis associated with HIV infection is based on an assumption of predictable development of neurosyphilitic syndromes; however, the information in both the pre- and post-HIV era concerning latency from acquiring syphilis to the development of specific syndromes of neurosyphilis is poor.

Ocular syphilis

The place of ocular syphilis in the classification of the complications of syphilitic infection is uncertain. Although classified as a form of neurosyphilis, it is unclear whether ocular syphilis should receive the same treatment. However, there is unlikely to be clear evidence indicating what course the clinician should follow, and the most conservative course of assuming that ocular syphilis should be treated as neurosyphilis should probably be followed. Common manifestations include uveitis, interstitial keratitis, and optic neuritis.

Investigations

Treponema pallidum can only be cultured with difficulty, and for the diagnosis of neurosyphilis, serological testing together with neuroimaging represents strong surrogate markers. Polymerase chain reaction (PCR) is becoming increasingly available, and is sensitive and specific in most studies; at present its role is complementary to standard serological testing. In a significant proportion of cases, neither the clinical presentation nor the special investigations allow the clinician to diagnose the presence of neurosyphilis with absolute certainty, and there is no gold standard test for ruling the disease in or out.

In general, screening tests in the serum such as rapid plasma regain (RPR) and Venereal Disease Research Laboratory (VDRL) are sensitive. It is likely that a negative result from a highly sensitive test such as the fluorescent treponemal antibody test (FTA) in serum excludes the possibility of neurosyphilis (that is, has a high negative predictive value; Table 66.1). In the CSF, a sensitive serological test that would indicate the potential presence of neurosyphilis is important. In CSF, the VDRL is specific but lacks sensitivity (false negatives can occur), whereas the FTA is sensitive (but is associated with false positives). Approximately, 20–50% of cases of neurosyphilis will have a negative VDRL in CSF. As in the serum, a negative FTA in CSF is highly likely to exclude neurosyphilis. Usually, features of disease activity such as elevated lymphocyte count, protein, and IgG index will be found in CSF. All tests of this nature are likely to have higher predictive values when applied to populations where the prevalence of the disease is relatively high, whereas if the prevalence is low, the predictive values of the tests decline. The most frequent finding on magnetic resonance imaging (MRI) in cases with neuropsychiatric presentations is cerebral atrophy. It is now well established that temporal lobe hyperintensity on T2-weighted imaging is a feature of neurosyphilis. Patients presenting with stroke will not uncommonly have evidence of previous events, and both large and small vessel disease may be seen. Recommendations to investigate HIV-positive patients on the basis of CD4 counts of less than 350 and RPR titers of >1:32 are not supported by the US Centers for Disease Control and Prevention (CDC).

Treatment

Treatment of HIV-negative patients with neurosyphilis

The current CDC treatment regimen is aqueous crystalline penicillin G (benzyl penicillin) 18–24 million units per day, administered as 3–4 million units intravenously (IV) every 4 hours or continuous infusion, for 10–14 days. Patients allergic to penicillin may be treated with ceftriaxone 2g daily for 10–14 days.

Treatment of HIV-positive patients with neurosyphilis

HIV-positive patients should receive the same treatment as non-HIV-positive patients.

Table 66.1 Characteristic of laboratory test in syphilis. In the CSF, a sensitive serological test that would indicate the potential presence of neurosyphilis is important. In CSF, the VDRL is specific but lacks sensitivity (false negatives can occur), whereas the FTA is sensitive (but is associated with false positives). Approximately, 20-50% of cases of neurosyphilis will have a negative VDRL in CSF.

CSF Tests		
VDRL		**Associated problems**
CSF-Syphicheck:Treponemal immunochromatographic strip tests (ICSTs):	**All characterized by high specificity.**	Prozone Effect
TRUST (Toluidine Red Unheated Serum Test):		Prozone Effect
FTA-ABS (Fluorescent Treponemal Antibody absorbed)		High false positive rate
TPHA T. pallidum hemagglutination test	**All characterized by high Negative Predictive Value**	High false positive rate
EIA assays		
Line immunoassay INNO-LIA Syphilis test:		
TPPA T. pallidum particle agglutination test		High false positive rate
PCR assay	**Variable sensitivity and specificity**	
Serum Tests		
RPR (Rapid Plasma Reagin)	Screening Test	False positive results Prozone Effect Concerns about sensitivity in early and late syphilis
TRUST (Toluidine Red Unheated Serum Test)	Screening Test	False positive results Prozone Effect
FTA (Fluorescent Treponemal Antibody)	Largely serves as confirmatory test	False positive results

CSF = cerebrospinal fluid; EIA = enzyme immunoassay; PCR = polymerase chain reaction; VDRL = Venereal Disease Research Laboratory

Follow-up

The principal issues in terms of follow-up are when repeat examination of the CSF should be obtained, and how to interpret the results. The available information is scant and recommendations vary widely, from follow-up at 6 months or less to follow-up at 1–2 years. Of the CSF parameters, cell count will respond most rapidly, and protein levels and IgG index more slowly. Although the cell count will tend to fall substantially by 6 months, it is unlikely that in all cases the cell count will be normal by that time. Regarding serology in CSF, the VDRL is insensitive and typically has low titers, giving rise to a floor effect. There is potentially a 1–2 dilution margin of error in determination of VDRL titers, and unfortunately the results of CSF serology may sometimes have low utility in determining response to treatment. Given that improvement in the CSF picture will be slow to occur, early monitoring of CSF is unlikely to be of great value, but the decision of when to monitor CSF is largely one of clinical judgment. Currently, CDC recommendations are that HIV-infected persons should be clinically evaluated and undergo serological testing at 3, 6, 9, 12, and 24 months after therapy. The CDC recommends "repeat CSF examination if CSF pleocytosis present initially, at six-month intervals until normal." Given the CSF lymphocytosis associated with HIV infection itself, determination of a successful treatment response will inevitably be difficult in some cases.

Further reading

Adams RD. *Principles of Neurology*, 6th ed. New York: McGraw-Hill; 1997:722–728.

CDC. Syphilis module. STD Curriculum for Clinical Educators. Atlanta, GA: Centers for Disease Control and Prevention. http://www2a.cdc.gov/stdtraining/ready-to-use/Manuals/Syphilis/syphilis-notes-2013.pdf (accessed November 2015).

CDC. Neurosyphilis. 2010 Treatment Guidelines. Atlanta, GA: Centers for Disease Control and Prevention. http://www.cdc.gov/std/treatment/2010/qanda/syphilis.htm#neuro (accessed November 2015).

67 Lyme disease

Patricia K. Coyle

Department of Neurology, Stony Brook University Medical Center, Stony Brook, NY, USA

Lyme disease (Lyme Borreliosis) is the most common tick-borne infection in the United States, Europe, and Northern Asia. It is caused by a bacterial spirochete, *Borrelia burgdorferi*. Similar to other human spirochetal infections (e.g., syphilis, leptospirosis, relapsing fever), Lyme disease targets specific body organs and causes clinical syndromes associated with early local, early dissemination, and late stage infection.

Epidemiology

This global infection is restricted to areas that contain the tick vector. Most cases occur in the United States and Europe, with limited cases from Asia and North Africa. In the United States 95% of reported cases occur in 15 states. Areas of geographic risk are the Northeast, followed by the upper Midwest and Northern West Coast. About 25–30,000 cases are reported in the United States annually, but it is estimated that there are likely 300,000 infections each year. Annual cases in Europe may be three-fold higher than what is formally reported in the United States.

Demographics

Lyme disease affects both sexes and all ages, with bimodal peaks in children aged 5–14 years, and middle-aged adults aged 40–50 years. It is slightly more common in males in the United States, and females in many areas of Europe. A major risk factor is time spent out of doors, either on a recreational or vocational basis. In temperate climates cases peak during warmer weather. In the United States this is from May through October.

Tick vector

Virtually all infections occur via a bite from black-legged hard shell Ixodid ticks. In the United States the specific vectors are *Ixodes scapularis* (deer tick) and *I. pacificus* (in the West). In Europe it is *I. ricinus*, and in Asia *I. persulcatus*. These ticks have a two-year life cycle involving three stages (larva, nymph, adult). Each stage has one blood meal, with the tick feeding over days to repletion. Questing nymphs are believed responsible for most human infections. Infected ticks need to feed for longer than 24 hours before the spirochetes can be inoculated. This emphasizes the value of daily tick checks.

Organism

Borrelia burgdorferi sensu lato is a group of spirochetes belonging to the genus *Borrelia* in the family Spirochaetaceae, which also includes *Leptospira* and *Treponema*. *Borrelia burgdorferi* is a Gram-negative bacterium with an outer membrane surrounding a protoplasmic cylinder, and motile flagella. There is one small linear chromosome and up to 21 linear and circular plasmids that vary among strains and species. There are 20 Lyme disease–associated *Borrelia* species, but three major genospecies. Species and strains differ based on genetic characteristics. *B. burgdorferi* sensu stricto is the only genospecies in North America, while *B. afzelii* and *B. garinii* are additional major genospecies that also cause infections in Eurasia (Table 67.1). *B. garinii* is typically associated with neurological disease.

Clinical expression

Target organs

Lyme disease targets the skin, joints, heart, and nervous system. Based on 154,405 US cases reported from 2001–10, 70% had the

Table 67.1 Global considerations for neurological Lyme disease

Features	United States	Eurasia
Major genospecies	*B. burgdorferi* sensu stricto neurotropic subtypes	*B. garinii*, occ *B. afzelii*
Neurological involvement	Less common; 15%	More common; >35%
Major neurological syndrome	Facial nerve palsy	Acute painful radiculoneuritis; most chronic encephalomyelitis cases
Cerebrospinal fluid findings	Mildly inflammatory Intrathecal anti-*B. burgdorferi* antibodies in ≤60% Oligoclonal bands, intrathecal immunoglobulin production ≤20%	Very inflammatory Intrathecal anti-*B. burgdorferi* antibodies in close to 100% Oligoclonal bands, intrathecal immunoglobulin production in most
Antibiotic responsiveness	Intravenous cephalosporin (ceftriaxone) preferred; generally for 4 weeks	Oral doxycycline reported as effective as intravenous antibodies

International Neurology, Second edition. Edited by Robert P. Lisak, Daniel D. Truong, William M. Carroll and Roongroj Bhidayasiri
© 2016 John Wiley & Sons, Ltd. Published 2016 by John Wiley & Sons, Ltd.

erythema migrans (EM) local infection skin rash, 31% had arthritis, 14% had neurological disease (i.e., 9% peripheral facial palsy, 4% radiculoneuritis, 1% meningitis/encephalitis), and 1% had cardiac issues. In Europe neurological disease is more common than arthritis.

Disease stages

Early local infection involves EM, an expanding red rash that starts out as a papule at the tick bite site. It occurs within 1–30 days of the bite. The skin site is filled with spirochetes. Summertime flu-like illness (with seroconversion) can also represent early clinical infection.

After proliferation within skin, spirochetes briefly disseminate hematogenously. Early dissemination syndromes (within 3 months of inoculation) involve multifocal EM, non-specific arthralgias/myalgias, cardiac disease, and nervous system involvement. Early local and disseminated infections spontaneously improve.

Late stage infection syndromes, which occur any time after 3 months, involve arthritis, skin, or nervous system involvement. They do not spontaneously improve without antibiotics.

Extraneural manifestations

EM is a pathognomonic clinical marker for Lyme disease that requires no supportive laboratory data. Since it occurs so early in the infection, Lyme serology is frequently negative. The rash occurs at the tick bite site, cannot occur within the first 24 hours (this is an allergic reaction), and should enlarge over days. Although the classic EM involves a painless large bull's-eye lesion, it can be atypical (i.e., small, rectangular, pruritic, ecchymotic, or painful). Any suspicious skin lesion during summertime in Lyme-endemic areas may be EM. Multifocal EM documents dissemination. Lymphocytoma (a bluish red nodular lesion on the earlobe or nipple) is a dissemination lesion of *B. afzelii* and *B. garinii*. *B. afzelii* is also associated with acrodermatitis chronica atrophicans, a late stage persistent skin infection that typically affects the lower leg of elderly women. This is not seen in the United States.

Lyme carditis can occur during early dissemination. Classically it involves acute second- or third-degree heart block. Males are at higher risk. Recently three cases of sudden death associated with Lyme carditis were reported in the United States (two men and one woman ranging in age from 26–38 years).

Joint syndromes involve arthralgias and myalgias during dissemination, and frank arthritis during late stage infection. Classically this is a symmetric oligoarticular swelling (such as the knee). Temporomandibular pain is suggestive. Small joints are spared.

Neurological Lyme disease

Both the central (CNS) and peripheral nervous systems (PNS) can be targeted. *B. burgdorferi* may disseminate and spread to the CNS very quickly, even during the early local infection stage. Concomitant neurological complaints should be investigated.

Dissemination is associated with cranial (especially VII) neuropathy, acute painful radiculoneuritis (Bannwarth syndrome), and meningitis/encephalitis. Facial nerve palsy occurs during summertime, is generally associated with a multisymptom complex (arthralgias, myalgias, fatigue, headache, stiff neck, cognitive issues), and may be bilateral in up to one-third of patients. It is the most

common neurological manifestation in the United States. Other cranial nerve involvement is unusual (e.g., III, IV, or VI; VIII; V; rarely II). In Europe the most common neurological syndrome is a striking acute painful radiculoneuritis with pronounced radicular (dermatomal, myotomal) features. It frequently starts with severe interscapular spine pain, and may be present with EM and facial nerve palsy, but without headache or stiff neck. These patients show the most inflammatory cerebrospinal fluid (CSF) changes. Dissemination is also associated with aseptic meningitis, encephalitis, acute cerebellar, and transverse myelitis syndromes.

Late stage neurological syndromes are unusual. In the United States the most common is late Lyme encephalopathy, characterized by typically mild chronic cognitive issues (in attention, memory, processing speed). Often these patients received oral non-penetrating antibiotics for extraneural disease. There is also a very mild chronic axonal polyneuropathy with occasional paresthesias and shock-like pains, and finally an extremely rare parenchymal neurological chronic encephalomyelitis that can mimic brain tumor, multiple sclerosis, or parkinsonian syndrome. Other reported neurological syndromes have included chronic meningitis, myopathy, stroke, or vasculitis, and postinfectious encephalomyelitis.

Diagnosis

Clinical diagnosis is based on endemic area exposure, time of year, likelihood of tick exposure, and suggestive syndrome. However, at least 50% of patients will not recall a tick bite. The only syndrome that does not require any laboratory investigation is EM. A major limitation is the fact that there is no useful laboratory test for active infection. Culture of the organism is impractical. DNA detection by polymerase chain reaction (PCR) is helpful in skin and synovial fluid, but not very sensitive in CSF or serum/plasma. Yield in CSF is increased by examining a pelleted sample. There is no available antigen assay. Therefore, the most important laboratory diagnostic test is detection of specific antibodies. This documents exposure, but not active infection. Following serology is useless to verify antibiotic responsiveness. IgG antibodies may persist for years in successfully treated patients. IgM antibodies also persist in a minority of successfully treated patients, and are not viewed as indicating persistent infection.

Antibody testing involves a two-tier system. The rapid screening test, typically direct or indirect enzyme-linked immunosorbant assay (ELISA), uses spirochetal sonicate preparations or rarely recombinant proteins. *B. burgdorferi* contains a number of shared proteins with other organisms (p41 flagellin, heat shock proteins). There are also oral spirochetes (*Treponema denticola*) that cross-react with *B. burgdorferi*. Therefore there is a built-in false positive rate as high as 20–25% for most first-tier tests, but typically these titers are low positive. Borderline or positive first-tier tests are confirmed by second-tier qualitative western immunoblots that involve an individualized subjective interpretation. Very rarely the more specific immunoblot is positive, despite a negative screening ELISA. The only true standardization of serological assays comes from the Centers for Disease Control and Prevention (CDC), and involves criteria for a positive immunoblot. IgM immunoblot requires two of three discrete bands (23-, 39-, 41-kDa); IgG immunoblot requires five of ten discrete bands (18-, 23-, 28-, 30-, 39-, 41-, 45-, 58-, 66-, 93-kDa). The earliest positive test is IgM immunoblot, followed by ELISA and then IgG immunoblot. The CDC has recommended ignoring positive IgM immunoblots, when clinical symptoms are longer than

4–6 weeks, as likely false positives. However, it would be concerning to ignore such a result in a symptomatic individual with endemic-area exposure.

The Lyme IgG C6 peptide antibody test uses a recombinant peptide, a 25 amino acid sequence from the unique VlsE surface protein. This assay offers good specificity but not sensitivity, and is not in wide use.

Seronegative cases of Lyme disease do occur, but probably account for less than 10% of infections. Only half of EM cases are seropositive, and following antibiotics (which when given early can interfere with the developing humoral response), 20–30% of patients never seroconvert.

CSF should be evaluated in any suspected neurological infections, and is typically abnormal. European cases show much more inflammatory CSF than US cases. CSF is more abnormal in disseminated neurological syndromes than late stage syndromes. Non-specific abnormalities involve mononuclear pleocytosis and increased protein. Oligoclonal bands and intrathecal immunoglobin production, both IgG and IgM, are routine findings in European cases, but are very unusual in US cases. This likely reflects genospecies and strain differences. Intrathecal anti-*B. burgdorferi* antibody production is the single most helpful CSF test to provide indirect evidence of CNS infection. It is often required in European neurological cases, but not in the United States, where even Lyme meningitis cases show only 60% intrathecal antibody positivity. There have been examples of spirochetes isolated from normal CSF, so that does not absolutely exclude neurological Lyme disease. Intrathecal antibodies may persist for months to years after treatment, but should slowly decrease over time.

Other helpful diagnostic tests involve electrophysiological testing to document a polyradiculoneuropathy, median nerve entrapment, or myopathy, and cognitive function tests to document objective abnormalities. Brain magnetic resonance imaging (MRI) is only abnormal in 25% of neurological Lyme disease infections; the most common pattern involves small, subcortical, vasculitic-type lesions, but a variety of MRI lesions have been described. Brain single photon emission computed tomography (SPECT) shows an abnormal blood flow pattern in late Lyme encephalopathy, but is a very non-specific pattern. All these objective laboratory abnormalities improve following therapy.

Treatment

Lyme disease is a bacterial infection that responds to appropriate antibiotic treatment. The best response is seen with early therapy.

Three oral antibiotics treat EM. Doxycycline is used at 100 mg twice a day (pediatric dose 2 mg/kg twice a day). Amoxicillin is used at 500 mg three times a day (pediatric dose 50 mg/kg/day in three divided doses). Cefuroxime axetil is used at 500 mg twice a day (pediatric dose 30 mg/kg divided twice a day). Treatment duration is 14–21 days. Doxycycline treats Ehrlichia (which can be a tick co-pathogen infection). It is not used in patients under the age of 8, or in pregnant or lactating women, because of concerns about dental effects.

Neurological Lyme disease is treated with a penetrating regimen. The preferred agent is intravenous ceftriaxone at 2 g once a day for 14–28 days (the pediatric dose is 50–75 mg/kg daily). It should not be given intramuscularly. For very significant parenchymal infections, treatment may be extended out to 6–8 weeks. This is an outpatient regimen. Patients typically have a peripherally inserted central catheter (PICC) line or midline, so it can be used the entire time. They are advised to take acidophilus, to decrease risk for pseudomembranous colitis.

About 5–15% of people with penicillin allergy are also allergic to cephalosporins. This can be evaluated, and desensitization protocols can be employed. Alternative regimens are doxycycline (typically 200 mg twice a day), given intravenously or by mouth, and penicillin (at 18–24 MU intravenously daily, divided over every four hours).

Prevention

Preventive strategies involve avoiding tick-infested areas, daily tick checks, personal protective measures (protective clothing, insect repellants and sprays, impregnated clothing), and environmental steps (pesticides, landscaping techniques). After tick bite a single dose of 200 mg doxycycline given within 72 hours prevents EM in 87% of cases. No human Lyme disease vaccines are currently marketed.

Tick co-pathogens

The Ixodid tick can contain a number of pathogens, including multiple distinct strains of *B. burgdorferi*, *Babesia microti* (a parasite that causes babesiosis), *Anaplasma phagocytophilum* (an *Ehrlichia* agent that causes human granulocytic anaplasmosis, HGA), *B. miyamotoi*, an *Ehrlichia muris*-like agent, *Rickettsia* species, *Bartonella henselae*, tick-borne encephalitis virus in endemic Eastern Europe and Asia, and Powassan deer tick virus in the United States, Canada, and the Russian Far East. It is possible to get dual infections, and optimal antimicrobials may differ. The two major tick co-pathogens are often assessed by checking serology for *Babesia* and HGA.

Pathogenesis

Pathology

Typical neuropathology shows very few spirochetes that are always extracellular. There is little overt destruction. The CNS shows mild meningeal and perivascular mononuclear inflammation; occasional organisms; microglial nodules; and mild spongiform changes. Rarely there may be obliterative vasculopathy, demyelination, or granulomatous changes. The PNS shows axonal injury; inflammation in the epineural, perineural, perivascular, and vasa nervorum; and angiopathy. Muscle has shown focal myositis, interstitial inflammation, focal necrosis, and rare spirochetes. Lack of neuropathological damage suggests that immunological and inflammatory factors may mediate many of the symptoms in neurological patients.

Pathophysiology

Different strains of *B. burgdorferi* show different virulence and tissue tropism properties. This factors into disease expression. Except during early infection, spirochete numbers are very limited within infected tissue. *B. burgdorferi* can persist for years undetected. It produces inflammation out of proportion to its numbers. Spirochetal lipoproteins are known to activate the host immune system. At least 132 genes encode a variety of *B. burgdorferi* lipoproteins that show differential expression in culture, tick, and mammalian host. They can activate endothelial cells, immune cells, and chemokines/cytokines. Spirochetes are extracellular but tissue tropic, and bind to endothelial cells, platelets, and most mammalian cells. They are often associated with extracellular matrix collagen fibers. *B. burgdorferi* also generates cross-reactivity to a number of autoantigens.

Chronic Lyme disease/post-treatment Lyme disease syndrome

There is no universally recognized definition for this syndrome, which refers to persistent problems lasting more than 6 months after adequate antibiotic treatment for Lyme disease. Perhaps 10–20% of treated patients have continuing complaints, and in some patients these persist for over 6 months. The problems most often involve non-specific and subjective pain (e.g., headache, arthralgias, myalgias), fatigue, paresthesias, and cognitive issues. This diagnosis has also been given to patients with these non-specific complaints, and no evidence of *B. burgdorferi* infection. Morphological variants (L-form or cyst-form *B. burgdorferi*) have been suggested to result in chronic infection. Patients are often treated with unusual and prolonged courses of antibiotics, as well as odd combinations.

There are a number of possibilities to explain these chronic symptomatic patients. First, they could have a persistent infection that was inadequately treated. This would be most likely an issue when unsuspected CNS infection occurred in a patient treated for extraneural disease. However, in several randomized trials no convincing response to antibiotics could be demonstrated. Second, patients could have an undiagnosed co-pathogen infection, but this has not proved to be the case. Third, patients could have a comorbid condition, such as a vascular headache, triggered by the prior infection. Fourth, patients could be reinfected; that is possible if there are not sufficient protective cytotoxic antibodies. Fifth, patient complaints could represent anxiety, hypochondriasis, or conversion disorder. Finally, patients could have a postinfectious (presumed immune or inflammatory) disorder, such as fibromyalgia syndrome. Chronic Lyme arthritis occurs in up to 10% of Lyme disease patients. It is not antibiotic responsive, and appears to be an immune-mediated syndrome linked to specific HLA-DR4 alleles. It is characterized by a strong systemic and synovial immune response to the OspA *B. burgdorferi* protein.

In a single informative patient with persistent neurological complaints, CSF contained a T-cell clone responsive to both spirochetal and autoantigen epitopes. Other studies have implicated increased T_H17 responses and elevated interleukin-23, autoantibodies, and increased interferon-α activity. Further studies are clearly needed to clarify this cohort of ill-defined heterogeneous patients.

Further reading

Borchers AT, Keen CL, Huntley, AC, Gershwin, ME. Lyme disease: A rigorous review of diagnostic criteria and treatment. *J Autoimmun* 2015;57:82–115. doi:10.1016/j.jaut.2014.09.004

Marques AR. Lyme Neuroborreliosis. *Continuum* 2015;21(6):1729–1744.

Shapiro ED. Lyme disease. *N Engl J Med* 2014;370:1724–1731.

68 Introduction to protozoans of the central nervous system

Marylou V. Solbrig

Departments of Internal Medicine (Neurology) and Medical Microbiology, University of Manitoba, Winnipeg, MB, Canada

Apex predators try to kill and eat you right there on the prairie, savannah, or *veldt*, while parasites try to infect but keep you alive. Protozoans are obligate intracellular parasites. Generally, they cause mild or persistent, subacute infections, and protozoan diseases are among the most common and successful parasitic diseases of humans. However, when protozoans access an immunoprivileged site such as brain or eye, or spread to an immunocompromised host, these organisms produce severe infections.

Protozoans pathogenic for humans are found in rich and poor countries, in both tropical and temperate climates. Their numbers of infected hosts, plus the low success rates and high central nervous system (CNS) toxicities of the best available treatments for some, render protozoan diseases significant contributors to the global burden of infectious diseases. The medical needs related to pathogens in this group, especially their neurological complications, remain challenging and incompletely met.

For malaria, there are 99 endemic countries. Malaria is the most important of the parasitic diseases of humans, affecting – that is, placing at risk – approximately 3.4 billion people worldwide and causing 1–3 million deaths per year, many from cerebral malaria. The World Health Organization (WHO) estimated 207 million malaria cases worldwide in 2012. Malaria, transmitted by the bite of infected *Anopheles* mosquitoes, poses a heavy burden in tropical communities, threatens non-endemic countries, and presents a danger to travelers. Drug resistance has evolved and despite efforts, successful vaccines have not been developed.

The genus *Trypanosoma* contains many species of protozoans. *Trypanosoma cruzi*, the cause of Chagas' disease in the Americas, and the two trypanosome subspecies that cause human African trypanosomiasis, *Trypanosoma brucei gambiense* and *T. brucei rhodesiense*, are the only members of the genus that cause disease in humans.

In South America where an estimated 8% of the population is seropositive, *T. cruzi* is spread by infected assassin bug bite, transfusion, transplant, or *in utero* exposure. American trypanosomiasis (Chagas' disease) is a significant cause of cardiovascular and thromboembolic disease and there is no specific therapy to treat chronic disease.

Human African trypanosomiasis is associated with complex public health and epizootic problems, such that eradication has not been possible. The tsetse fly is the vector and infection reservoirs are present in cattle and other animals. In humans, once nervous system treatment is required, therapy can be unsatisfactory due to poor tolerance and high toxicity of medications.

Amoebae species are global pathogens. *Entamoeba histolytica* occurs in fecally contaminated water, food, or hands. Free-living amoebas of genera *Acanthamoeba*, *Naegleria*, and *Balamuthia* have been isolated from fresh and brackish water throughout the world. Any part of the body may be affected by Entamoeba via hematogenous dissemination from colon or liver. Acanthamoeba cause corneal, systemic, or cerebral disease. Naegleria causes a meningoencephalitis that is usually fatal.

Toxoplasmosis is a worldwide pathogen, spread from contaminated hands, foods, water, or acquired *in utero* or via transplant. Seropositive populations are found in many temperate zones, and seropositive populations approaching 100% are reported in some moist tropical climates. A known cause of congenital infections and retinochoroiditis, toxoplasmosis had been a rare opportunistic infection of immunocompromised patients until the time of acquired immune deficiency syndrome (AIDS). Early in the AIDS epidemic, cerebral toxoplasmosis was the most frequent cause of focal cerebral lesions in human immunodeficiency virus (HIV) disease.

The protozoans of neurological importance in humans are presented in the chapters that follow. Their diagnosis is considered when evaluating neurological illness in residents in endemic regions, in travelers to endemic areas, in individuals who are immunosuppressed due to medication or concurrent disease, in recent recipients of transfusions or transplants, in neonates who acquired infection *in utero*, or in others with pertinent exposures. Diagnostics, prognostics, therapeutics, biomarkers of drug resistance, ecology and elimination studies, vaccines, and metabolomics (the study of chemicals in biosystems with measures of >20,000 compounds with the latest analytic methods) to understand host–pathogen biology are lines of investigation that will have an impact on poorly controlled pathogens. The generation of systems biology datasets based on clinical infections around the world, particularly for malaria, can be a unique global resource. For now, Chagas' disease and toxoplasmosis, along with cysticercosis, toxocariasis, and trichomoniasis, have been designated Neglected Parasitic Infections by the US Centers for Disease Control and Prevention, and targeted as priorities for public health action, based on the number of people infected, severity of diseases, and ability to prevent and treat.

International Neurology, Second edition. Edited by Robert P. Lisak, Daniel D. Truong, William M. Carroll and Roongroj Bhidayasiri
© 2016 John Wiley & Sons, Ltd. Published 2016 by John Wiley & Sons, Ltd.

69 Amoebic disease of the central nervous system

Melanie Walker

Departments of Neurology and Neurological Surgery, University of Washington School of Medicine, Seattle, WA, USA

Free-living amoebic *Acanthamoeba* species, *Balamuthia mandrillaris*, *Entamoeba histolytica*, and *Naegleria fowleri* cause extremely rare and sporadic central nervous system (CNS) infections. *Sappinia pedata* has also been identified in patients with CNS disease, but its pathogenicity has not yet been established. Typically, *N. fowleri* produces primary amoebic meningoencephalitis (PAM), which is clinically indistinguishable from acute bacterial meningitis. Infection by other amoebas causes granulomatous amoebic encephalitis (GAE), which presents as subacute or chronic infection. Signs and symptoms of GAE can result from brain abscess, aseptic or chronic meningitis, or CNS malignancy. While *Entamoeba* species are the least likely to invade the CNS, they deserve mention because they are the most common human amoebic pathogens. Due to complex life cycles, free-living amoebas may also harbor intracellular bacteria that complicate or contribute to the clinical picture.

Epidemiology

Although these one-celled protozoa are simple in form, amoebas are found abundantly in a variety of habitats all over the world. Amoebas thrive in aquatic environments (freshwater as well as ocean), and in upper layers of the soil. A few adopt a parasitic lifestyle on the body surface of aquatic animals or in the internal organs of both aquatic and terrestrial animals. Few animals escape invasion by some type of amoeba, and humans are no exception. Some are harmless, but others are pathogenic and can impart serious disease burden: amoebic dysentery affects hundreds of millions of people worldwide, causing mortality second only to malaria.

While amoebic CNS disease is rare, cases have been reported worldwide, which reflects the ubiquity of the organisms. Warmer climates (and warmer seasons of the year) tend to harbor a higher number of *reported* cases. While most reports come from the United States, Australia, and Europe, this is likely secondary to identification and/or reporting bias such as co-infection with a more commonly recognized pathogen or in the setting of moribund immune status. Implications of climate change on disease burden and areas of geographic clustering are concerning but not yet clear.

With the exception of cases limited to the optic anatomy, amoebic CNS infections are almost uniformly fatal and may go unrecognized. Only a handful of survivors of PAM have been reported, and it is unclear whether or not early detection and aggressive management correlate to better outcomes. The high mortality rate is multifactorial: diagnosis is difficult, response to therapy is poor to

marginal, and the disease burden is greater in immunosuppressed patients. In most individuals with PAM or GAE, a diagnosis is not made until after death. PAM has been reported in infants as young as 4 months of age, but it is most common in the first 3 decades of life. Although persons of any age can be affected by GAE, infection occurs more commonly in individuals at the extremes of age. *Acanthamoeba* antibodies may be present in up to 80% of healthy human populations, suggesting that subclinical infections might also be possible in healthy individuals. Immunosuppression can contribute to CNS dissemination and also primary infection in GAE, but does not appear to play a role in PAM.

Pathophysiology

PAM secondary to *N. fowleri* is an exceptionally uncommon result of CNS invasion of the healthy host, following the very common exposure to the amoeba during routine activities of daily living. Infection develops over a period ranging from a few hours to 2 weeks after swimming, diving, bathing, or playing in warm, usually stagnant, freshwater. The *N. fowleri* is believed to migrate through the cribriform plate near the site of entry in the nasopharynx, along the fila olfactoria and blood vessels, and into the anterior cerebral fossa. Extensive inflammation, necrosis, and hemorrhage develop rapidly into meningoencephalitis. For unknown reasons, not all individuals who harbor the amoeba develop disease, but reclassification of *Naegleria* from Amoebozoa to Excavata is starting to shed light on the organism's origins and behavior.

In contrast, GAE appears to result from either acanthamebic keratoconjunctivitis, which is the uncommon spread of the amoeba from the cornea into the CNS, or from hematogenous spread of all of these ubiquitous organisms (e.g., *Acanthamoeba* or *Balamuthia* species) from primary inoculation sites in the lungs or skin into the CNS. Abscesses and focal granulomatous infections result and, consequently, it is not uncommon to see bilateral intracranial pathology.

Entamoeba histolytica is the most common pathogen responsible for amoebic dysentery. The organism is transmitted in cyst form from feces-contaminated food or water by way of food handlers (usually asymptomatic carriers), flies, cockroaches, and from sexual contact. The infective cyst stage develops into a trophozoite in the small intestine. Trophozoites readily die outside the body, but while inside, they release an enzyme that dissolves tissue, which allows them to penetrate beyond the intestinal mucosa. If the disease

International Neurology, Second edition. Edited by Robert P. Lisak, Daniel D. Truong, William M. Carroll and Roongroj Bhidayasiri
© 2016 John Wiley & Sons, Ltd. Published 2016 by John Wiley & Sons, Ltd.

disseminates beyond the gastrointestinal tract, abscesses may develop on the brain, lungs, heart, or other tissues, and death can result.

Clinical features

As with all neurological disease, signs and symptoms typically refer to the anatomic location more than the underlying disease mechanism. As such, it is difficult to make a definitive diagnosis based on clinical findings. Amoebic CNS disease presents a number of diagnostic challenges; however, there may be some clues for the astute healthcare provider. PAM presents with severe headache and other meningeal signs, fever, vomiting, and focal neurological deficits, and tends to evolve quickly (<10 days). Initial symptoms are typically not recognized as dangerous by many patients, since they may be vague. Rapid progression to coma and death is the most common clinical scenario with PAM. *Acanthamoeba* species cause mostly subacute or chronic GAE, with a clinical picture of headaches, altered mental status, seizures, and focal neurological deficit, which generally progresses to death over a period of several weeks. Additionally, *Acanthamoeba* species can cause granulomatous skin lesions, keratitis, and corneal ulcers following corneal trauma or in association with contact lens use – which may provide an early opportunity for treatment. Poor contact lens hygiene and exposure to contaminated water may increase the risk among contact lens users. The mechanism of infection in contact lens wearers with safe lens care practices or those who do not wear lenses is unclear; however, bacterial endosymbionts may cloud the clinical picture, as up to a quarter of *Acanthamoeba* isolates harbor intracellular bacteria or viruses. *Balamuthia* species may also cause cutaneous lesions or follow sinus infections, but unlike in the case of *Acanthamoeba*, patients are typically immunocompetent. *Sappinia* species have not definitively been linked to primary

CNS pathology or as lethal to humans, but a single case of encephalitis and brain abscess post sinus infection has been reported in the literature.

Investigations

While amoebic disease can be difficult to diagnose, mindful clinical history and laboratory evaluation offer the highest likelihood of pathogen identification. Light microscopy is accessible in almost every medical setting around the world, but more sophisticated testing should be attempted where possible. Neuroimaging with computed tomography (CT) or magnetic resonance imaging (MRI) can be helpful in managing acute treatment; however, imaging alone will not provide a definitive diagnosis. Cerebrospinal fluid (CSF) may be difficult to obtain in GAE, as lumbar puncture is generally contraindicated for patients who present with elevated intracranial pressure secondary to a focal lesion. Imaging and pathological findings in amoebic CNS disease are discussed in Table 69.1.

Treatment

Rapid diagnosis is essential to patient survival with amoebic CNS disease. Identification of the organism allows more appropriate selection of medication, but there are other considerations. If the lesion(s) are discrete, surgical resection should be considered whenever possible. In all cases of disease, the clinician must first provide supportive management. This often requires treatment of increased intracranial pressure using steroids, osmolar therapy, or even mechanical decompression or drainage in severe cases. Symptomatic and supportive care should be aggressive and careful to avoid neuroactive medications that might complicate evaluation of mental status, especially where neuroimaging is not readily available. In

Table 69.1   Imaging and pathological findings in amoebic central nervous system disease

	Laboratory diagnosis	CT scan	MRI scan
Granulomatous amoebic encephalitis (GAE)			
Acanthamoeba species, Balamuthia mandrillaris, Entamoeba histolytica, Sappiknia spp.	Microscopic examination of stained smears of biopsy specimens (brain tissue, skin, and cornea) may detect trophozoites and cysts Confocal microscopy or cultivation of the causal organism, and identification by direct immunofluorescent antibody PCR-based techniques (conventional and real-time PCR) have been described for detection and identification of free-living amoebic infections Because *Entamoeba* spp. disseminate from the intestinal tract to the brain, wet mounts and permanently stained preparations (e.g., trichrome) of fresh stool samples should be used for diagnosis *Such techniques may be available in selected reference diagnostic laboratories*	Multiple bilateral enhancing lesions involving the cerebral cortex and underlying white matter, with mild mass effect Hemorrhage commonly seen within the lesion(s) May also appear as solitary space-occupying lesions associated with mass effect	Multifocal lesions showing T2 hyperintensity and a heterogeneous or ring-like pattern of enhancement Hemorrhage within the lesion can be confirmed with gradient echo imaging May present as a mass lesion with linear and superficial gyriform pattern of enhancement
Primary amoebic meningoencephalitis (PAM)			
Naegleria fowleri and other spp.	A wet mount of CSF may detect motile trophozoites, and a Giemsa-stained smear will show trophozoites with typical morphology	May be normal in early disease Later findings include evidence of generalized edema and basilar meningeal enhancement	Edema can be visualized on T2 sequence even early in the course of disease Obliteration of vessels secondary to edema can lead to infarction Basilar meningeal enhancement can be seen subacutely

CSF = cerebrospinal fluid; CT = computed tomography; MRI = magnetic resonance imaging; PCR = polymerase chain reaction

Table 69.2   Recommendations for management in amoebic central nervous system disease.

Granulomatous amoebic encephalitis (GAE)			
Pharmacotherapy	**Surgical therapy**	**Prognosis**	**Comment**
The treatment of choice for GAE is ketoconazole alone or combined with amphotericin B and sulfadiazine. *Balamuthia* has been reported to respond to miltefosine, fluconazole, and albendazole. *Acanthamoeba* has also been successfully treated with trimethoprim-sulfamethoxazole (TMP-SMZ), fluconazole, pentamidine, and miltefosine.	Brain biopsy may facilitate diagnosis; Excision of solitary or multiple lesions often required; Shunting may be required for hydrocephalus.	Poor, often diagnosed post-mortem; *Sappinia* species Insufficient information from single case report	Hyperbaric oxygen has been reported as a useful adjunct.
Primary amoebic meningoencephalitis (PAM)			
The treatment of choice for PAM is amphotericin B, at maximally tolerated doses (including intrathecal), with adjunctive rifampin and doxycycline. Sulfisoxazole, artemisinin, and phenothiazine have also shown benefit as has azithromycin as an adjunct to amphotericin B. Miltefosine, chlorpromazine, and an experimental drug rokitamycin remain unproven.	Intrathecal catheter placement in some cases; Steroids may be helpful in the management edema, but shunting may be required for hydrocephalus	Fair if diagnosed within days, otherwise fatal	

the case of *Balamuthia* infection, prognosis is most favorable when surgery and medical management are adjunct measures. Treatment for amoebic disease of the CNS is outlined in Table 69.2, but challenges treating specific pathogens and updated dosing recommendations should be researched in the current literature. In conjunction with the US Food and Drug Administration (FDA), the Centers for Disease Control and Prevention (CDC) has an expanded-access investigational new drug (IND) protocol in an effect to make miltefosine available directly from the CDC for treatment of free-living amoebae in the United States.

Further reading

CDC. DpDx: Laboratory identification of parasites of public health concern. Atlanta, GA: Centers for Disease Control and Prevention. http://www.cdc.gov/dpdx/ (accessed November 2015).

Chappell CL, Wright JA, Coletta M, Newsome AL. Standardized method of measuring *Acanthamoeba* in sera from healthy human subjects. *Clin Diagn Lab Immunol* 2001;8:724–730.

Fritsche TR, Gautom RK, Seyedirashti S, *et al.* Occurrence of bacterial endosymbionts in *Acanthamoeba* spp. isolated from corneal and environmental specimens and contact lenses. *J Clin Microbiol* 1993;31(5):1122–1126.

Fritsche TR, Horn M, Wagner M, *et al.* Phylogenetic diversity among geographically dispersed chlamydiales endosymbionts recovered from clinical and environmental isolates of *Acanthamoeba* spp. *Appl Environ Microbiol* 2000;66:2613–2619.

Gelman BB, Rauf SJ, Nader R, *et al.* Amoebic encephalitis due to *Sappinia diploidea*. *JAMA* 2001;285(19):2450–2451.

Singh P, Fau-Kochhar R, Kochhar R, *et al.* Amoebic meningoencephalitis: Spectrum of imaging findings. *AJNR* 2006;27(6):1217–1221.

The Medical Letter. Drugs for Parasitic Infections. http://secure.medicalletter.org/TG-article-132b (accessed November 2015).

Walker MD, Zunt JR. Neuroparasitic infections: Cestodes, trematodes, and protozoans. *Semin Neurol* 2005;25(3):262–277.

70 Toxoplasmosis of the central nervous system

Marylou V. Solbrig

Departments of Internal Medicine (Neurology) and Medical Microbiology, University of Manitoba, Winnipeg, MB, Canada

Toxoplasmosis is infection by *Toxoplasma gondii*, a microscopic protozoan, so named because the organism was first identified in North African rodents called gondis.

Epidemiology

T. gondii is an obligate intracellular protozoan infecting humans, other mammals, and birds. Present in migratory birds, the parasite is worldwide, known on every continent but Antarctica.

Humans can be infected at any time during life. Almost all infections of humans are acquired by mouth, by ingestion of oocysts or tissue cysts. The exceptions are infections acquired *in utero* and after tissue transplant. Oocysts can be present in cat feces, and tissue cysts may be found in undercooked meat. Contact with soil was identified as a risk factor in a European study, and contaminated water and soil may act as vehicles for the transfer of oocysts to vegetables and fruits for human consumption.

The sexual part of the life cycle occurs in the intestine of domestic cats and other felines, called definitive hosts, which shed infectious oocysts in their feces. Small vertebrates such as rodents and birds feeding on the ground become infected. Toxoplasma cysts form in muscle and brain, where the parasite remains, waiting to be eaten by cats to complete the life cycle. Other ground-feeding animals, cattle, pigs, sheep, and deer can become infected and are sources of infection for humans. Dogs, after rolling in cat excrement, can transmit oocysts on their fur to the hands of petting children. Unfiltered municipal drinking water and well water have been implicated in Toxoplasma transmission.

In utero infection occurs when the fetus is infected via the bloodstream from a mother who developed primary infection during pregnancy. Primary infection may also be acquired from a Toxoplasma-infected tissue or organ donor. The risk is highest for hearts and bone marrow, less for lung and kidney.

In the normal host the risk of developing encephalitis during primary Toxoplasma infection is low: 10–50% of adults in North America and up to 80% in Central America have antibodies to Toxoplasma and no history of disease. Roughly 20% of populations studied in Europe are seropositive, and over 60% in tropical areas of Asia and Africa. In moist tropical areas of South America, close to 100% of the population over age 40 years may have antibodies. While the percentage of seropositive individuals is lowest in dry desert areas, oocytes may survive in areas of flooded or irrigated land and account for foci for acquiring disease. Only approximately 10% of acutely infected individuals (normal hosts) have clinical signs and symptoms, which are usually mild.

The risk of intrauterine infection is highest if maternal infection is acquired shortly before delivery. Infants infected in the first half of gestation have the highest rates of encephalitis. In acquired immune deficiency syndrome (AIDS) patients with Toxoplasma antibody, the risk of recrudescence of active toxoplasmosis is at the time CD4 cell counts fall below 200 per mm^3. Sulfonamides and clotrimazole used for Pneumocystis prophylaxis have anti-Toxoplasma activity and decreased risk of recrudescence.

Toxoplasma accounts for 30–40% of retinochoroiditis in the United States.

Pathophysiology

Toxoplasma infections are common in humans, and usually asymptomatic, because immunity is acquired quickly to tachyzoites multiplying in cells.

The exceptions to asymptomatic diseases are those in immature fetuses, immunocompromised patients, or when infection involves immunologically privileged or sequestered sites, such as brain or eye. Delay in developing effective immunity leads to a higher burden of organisms. As immunity develops, encysted bradyzoites develop in tissue. Cysts then rupture, leaving necrotic tissue and foci for hypersensitivity reactions. In immunocompromised patients, freed bradyzoites will transform into tachyzoites that multiply and injure tissue.

Clinical features

Signs of systemic infection include macular rash, fever, muscle pain, adenopathy, and headache. Central nervous system (CNS) toxoplasmosis occurs after acute generalized infection in children and adults, after intrauterine infection, in immunocompromised patients, and as reactivated encephalitis or retinochoroiditis years after primary infection.

Primary toxoplasmosis

Primary infection in children or adults can be a mononucleosis-like syndrome with encephalitis or ocular disease. The patients develop a febrile syndrome with lymphadenopathy, splenomegaly, macular rash, muscle pain, myocarditis, headache, and encephalitic syndrome characterized by seizures, tremors, varying degrees

International Neurology, Second edition. Edited by Robert P. Lisak, Daniel D. Truong, William M. Carroll and Roongroj Bhidayasiri
© 2016 John Wiley & Sons, Ltd. Published 2016 by John Wiley & Sons, Ltd.

of impaired consciousness, and inflammatory spinal fluid. Diffuse encephalitis occurs in transplant patients with primary infection.

Congenital toxoplasmosis

Toxoplasmosis in the newborn varies from asymptomatic to a progressive, fatal illness. Rash, jaundice, and hepatosplenomegaly can occur in the neonatal period.

Neurological signs include seizures, hydrocephalus, microcephaly, retinochoroiditis, small cerebral calcifications, increased cerebrospinal fluid (CSF) protein, and inflammatory cells. Aqueductal occlusion is a complication of protracted encephalitis. There is periventricular vasculitis and necrosis of the lateral and third ventricular walls consistent with antigen-antibody reaction. Mild cases may have isolated chorioretinal scars.

Immunocompromised patients

Although Toxoplasma infection is almost always followed by chronic infection, acquired immunity keeps the infection controlled. Breakdown of this immunity by corticosteroids, AIDS, malignancies such as Hodgkin's disease, or in cases of heritable immunodeficiencies such as X-linked hyperIgM syndrome causes encephalitis.

Toxoplasma encephalitis (TE) has been the most frequent cause of focal CNS infection in patients with AIDS, with TE and primary CNS lymphoma the leading causes of CNS lesions in patients with advanced AIDS. Cerebral abscesses are found in patients with human immunodeficiency virus (HIV) infection, with focal signs developing over several weeks. Lesions are commonly in the basal ganglia or at the corticomedullary junction. Patients with AIDS and hemiballism or chorea probably have cerebral toxoplasmosis.

AIDS patients may also develop a diffuse, subacute encephalitis with CSF mononuclear pleocytosis, elevated protein, and low or normal glucose. In this form of toxoplasmosis, usually limited to the brain, proliferating Toxoplasma kill their host cells, namely astrocytes and neurons, and migrate to the next viable cell where the process repeats. Tissue necrosis and high parasite burdens spread to eventually involve vessel walls with Toxoplasma, which leads to hypertrophic arteritis, thrombosis, infarction, and retrograde hemorrhage.

Cerebral toxoplasmosis in immunosuppressed patients can manifest as lesions with no enhancement, nodular enhancement, and ring-like enhancement, and can occur at the corticomedullary junction and/or basal ganglia. A magnetic resonance imaging (MRI) feature highly suspicious for CNS toxoplasmosis is the "eccentric target sign," a ring-shaped zone of peripheral enhancement with a small eccentric nodule, which may represent focal invagination or folding of a cyst wall into itself or a leash of inflamed leaky vessels entering the lesion through a sulcus.

Retinochoroiditis

Toxoplasmosis is the most common cause of posterior uveitis in immunocompetent subjects and is associated with congenital or acquired infection. Retinochoroiditis in immunocompetent adults is accompanied by serological evidence of long-standing chronic, usually asymptomatic infection.

Retinochoroiditis involves the *retina posteri* and secondarily spreads to choroid and vitreous. Patients have a painless blurred vision, usually in one eye. On ophthalmological exam there is yellowish necrotic retinal focus with indistinct margins with vitreous haze if acute, and whitish scars and peripheral hyperpigmentation if old. Often, multiple lesions at various stages of inflammation and

healing are seen, as well as frosted branch angiitis. Progressive intraocular infection, panophthalmitis, and orbital cellulitis can occur.

Examples of ocular and cerebral toxoplasmosis are shown in Figure 70.1.

Investigations

Strategies for diagnosis of toxoplasmosis vary according to the immune background of the patient and the clinical setting. For the immunocompetent patient/transplant recipient or pregnant woman in the setting of either primary infection or need to determine immune status, the approach is IgG/IgM, or dye test serology. Serological tests for antibody are used to support a clinical diagnosis of toxoplasmosis, measuring antibody with the dye test, direct Toxoplasma agglutination test, indirect immunofluorescent antibody, or enzyme-linked immunosorbent assay (ELISA). Diagnosis of acute infection can be made by detection of both IgG and IgM antibodies to Toxoplasma in serum. IgM, IgA, and IgE measure a more recent antibody response than IgG, and are useful for diagnosing congenital toxoplasmosis when passively transferred IgG maternal antibody could obscure diagnosis in the neonate.

For the immunocompromised patient in the setting of cerebral or disseminated toxoplasmosis, the diagnostic approach is parasite detection by polymerase chain reaction (PCR) from blood; or PCR, cell culture, mouse assay, or histology from CSF, bronchiolar lavage, or tissue specimens. While antibody titers can be high with active toxoplasmosis in the CNS, they may be low with active chorioretinitis and in AIDS patients. In AIDS cases, antibodies may be non-diagnostic, low, or may not reliably distinguish recent, remote, or inactive infection. As such, serological tests may not be dependable in AIDS patients and a diagnosis of toxoplasmosis is based on identification of the agent, its antigens, DNA, or response to empirical antibiotic treatment within 2 weeks.

Treatment

The combination of sulfadiazine (1–1.5 g every 6 hours by mouth) and pyrimethamine (200 mg loading dose, then 50–75 mg per day by mouth) is the classic and probably best means of treating active disease. The addition of folinic acid avoids hematological toxicity without interference with antibiotic efficacy.

Recommended drug therapies for cerebral toxoplasmosis are pyrimethamine+sulfadiazine+leucovorin or pyrimethamine+sulfadiazine+folinic acid for at least 6 weeks, followed by suppressive regimens with the same agents in AIDS patients. Trimethoprim (TMP)/sulfamethoxazole(SMX) – TMP 5 mg/kg and SMX 25 mg/kg intravenously (IV) or orally twice per day – appears to be equivalent to pyrimethamine/sulfadiazine in patients with AIDS. Atovaquone with or without pyrimethamine can also be considered. Individuals who have completed initial therapy for toxoplasma encephalitis should continue treatment indefinitely unless immune reconstitution with a CD4+ T-cell count greater than 200/μL occurs as a consequence of HAART (highly active antiretroviral therapy). Periodic MRI scans are beneficial for following patients. Maintenance therapy (secondary prophylaxis) is half doses of the same regimen used in the acute phase. As one example, prophylaxis of toxoplasmosis encephalitis TE in Toxoplasma-seropositive AIDS patients is a daily dose of TMP-SMX, the double-strength tablet (160 mg–800 mg), when the CD4 T-cell count falls below 100 cells/μL. Clindamycin is an alternative in cases of sulfadiazine allergy. Although spiramycin

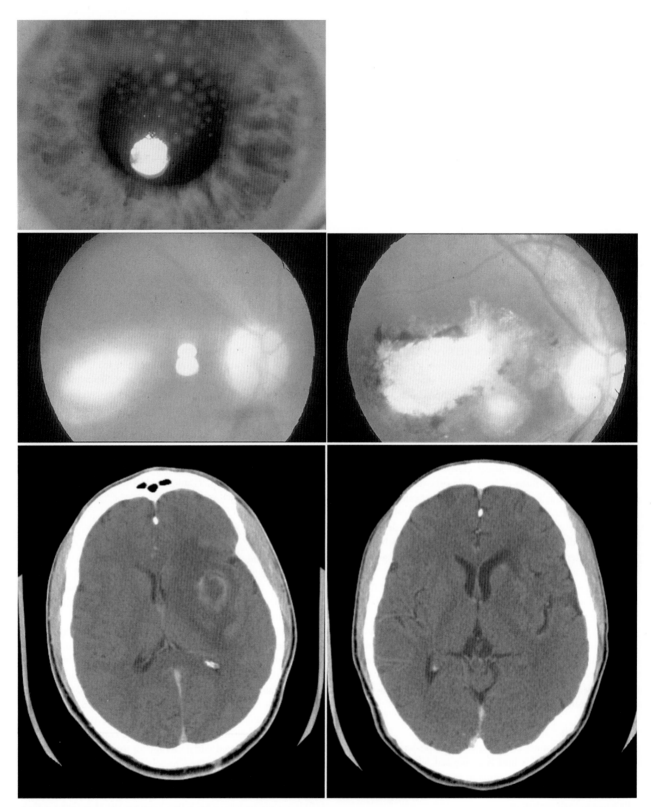

Figure 70.1 Ocular and cerebral toxoplasmosis.

Anterior uveitis with mutton-fat keratic precipitates (top). Source: Courtesy of Caygill Ophthalmic Library, Department of Ophthalmology, University of California, San Francisco. Toxoplasmosis retinochoroiditis after 6 months (middle left) and after 2 years (middle right). The central exposed white area of each image is the sclera, seen after necrosis of the retina and choroid. Proliferation of pigmented layer at margins of lesion is noted with more advanced disease, and the healed lesion is densely pigmented with irregular borders and central atrophy (middle right). Source: Courtesy of Caygill Ophthalmic Library, Department of Ophthalmology, University of California, San Francisco.

Toxoplasmosis cerebral abscess. CT scans with contrast from an AIDS patient presenting with seizures, aphasia, contrast-enhancing CT lucency, and toxoplasma titers that were positive (lower left). During treatment, 25 days later, there is resolution of the abscess (lower right). Source: Courtesy C. Jay, Department of Neurology, University of California, San Francisco.

has poor CNS penetration, it concentrates in placenta and can treat toxoplasmosis during pregnancy. Congenital infection is treated with oral pyrimethamine and sulfadiazine daily for 1 year. An alternative regimen of spiramycin plus prednisone has been shown to be efficacious.

Patients with ocular toxoplasmosis should be treated for 1 month with pyrimethamine plus either sulfadiazine or clindamycin. Primary prophylactic regimens use pyrimethamine–sulfadoxine (Fansidar) with folinic acid, dapsone–pryimethamine, or trimethoprim–sulfamethoxazole (Cotrimoxazole, Bactrim). Toxoplasma-seropositive patients who have CD4 counts <100 cells/μL should receive prophylaxis against toxoplasma encephalitis. The TMP-SMX double-strength tablet daily dose is also *Pneumocystis jirovecii* pneumonia (PCP) prophylaxis.

Further reading

Frenkel JK. Toxoplasmosis. In: Connor DH, Chandler FW, Schwartz DA, Manz HJ, LackEE (eds.). *Pathology of Infectious Diseases*, Vol. 2. Stamford, CT: Appleton & Lange; 1997:1261–1278.

Frenkel JK. Toxoplasmosis. In: Aminoff MJ, Daroff RB (eds.). *Encyclopedia of the Neurological Sciences*, Vol. 4. San Diego: Academic Press; 2003:544–549.

Kaplan JE, Masur H, Holmes KK. Guidelines for preventing opportunistic infections among HIV-infected persons – 2002. Recommendations of the US Public Health Service and the Infectious Diseases Society of America. *MMWR Recomm Rep* 2002;40:4499–4503.

Montoya JG, Liesenfeld O. *Toxoplasmosis. Lancet* 2004;363:1965–1976.

Panel on Opportunistic Infections in HIV-Infected Adults and Adolescents. Guidelines for the prevention and treatment of opportunistic infections in HIV-infected adults and adolescents: Recommendations from the Centers for Disease Control and Prevention, the National Institutes of Health, and the HIV Medicine Association of the Infectious Diseases Society of America. https://aidsinfo.nih.gov/contentfiles/lvguidelines/Adult_OI.pdf (accessed November 2015).

Ramsey RG, Gean AD. Neuroimaging of AIDS. I. Central nervous system toxoplasmosis. *Neuroimaging Clin N Am* 1997;7(2):171–186.

Remington JS, McLeod R, Thulliez P, Desmonts G. Toxoplasmosis. In: Remington JS, Klein JO, Wilson CB, Baker CJ (eds.). *Infectious Diseases of the Fetus and Newborn Infant*, 6th ed. Philadelphia, PA: Elsevier Saunders; 2006:947–1091.

Robert-Gangneux F, Darde M-L. Epidemiology of and diagnostic strategies for toxoplasmosis. *Clin Microbiol Rev* 2012;25:264–296.

Sharath Kumar GG, Mahadevan A, Guruprasad AS, *et al.* Eccentric target sign in cerebral toxoplasmosis: Neuropathological correlate to the imaging feature. *J Magn Reson Imaging* 2010;31:1469–1472.

71 Cerebral malaria

Polrat Wilairatana[1], Srivicha Krudsood[2], and Noppadon Tangpukdee[1]
[1] Department of Clinical Tropical Medicine, Mahidol University, Bangkok, Thailand
[2] Department of Tropical Hygiene, Mahidol University, Bangkok, Thailand

Cerebral malaria may be defined strictly as unarousable coma (i.e., non-purposeful response or no response to a painful stimulus) during malaria infection. Although cerebral malaria is generally the result of infection by *Plasmodium falciparum*, it can uncommonly be caused by *P. vivax*.

Epidemiology

Malaria is the most important parasitic infection in the world. There were an estimated 207 million malaria cases worldwide in 2012. Most of the estimated cases (80%) were found in sub-Saharan Africa. About 9% of estimated cases globally are due to *P. vivax*, although the proportion outside Africa is 50%. There were an estimated 627,000 malaria deaths worldwide in 2012. Most deaths occurred in sub-Saharan Africa (90%) and in children under 5 years of age (77%), many of whom succumbed to cerebral malaria. In most developed countries, malaria is seen in migrants or people returning from travels in malaria-endemic areas.

Pathology

Although six *Plasmodium* species (*P. falciparum*, *P. vivax*, *P. malariae*, *P. ovale curtisi*, *P. ovale wallikeri*, and *P. knowlesi*) are known to cause human malaria under natural transmission, *P. falciparum* is the most common cause of severe malaria, including cerebral malaria. *P. vivax* patients, predominantly found in Asia, may have cerebral malaria. Severe vivax malaria is associated with multiple organ failure. The inclusion of *P. vivax* as an etiological agent of cerebral malaria is controversial, as the contribution of respiratory and renal failures to the patient's impaired consciousness is difficult to separate from the primary central nervous system effects of the parasite.

The hallmark histopathological feature of cerebral malaria is engorgement of cerebral capillaries and venules with parasitized (PRBC) and non-parasitized (NPRBC) red blood cells. Sequestration of PRBCs in cerebral microvessels is significantly higher in the brains of cerebral malaria patients than those with non-cerebral malaria. Cerebral edema is not a major pathological process.

Pathophysiology

Sequestration

Red blood cells containing mature forms of parasites sequestering in deep vascular beds of vital organs may be responsible for the major organ complications. In cerebral malaria, sequestration is maximal in the brain. The prognosis of severe malaria is thought to be related to sequestered parasite biomass. Sequestration is found in *P. falciparum* but not *P. vivax* malaria.

Cytoadherence

P. falciparum is the only species of human malaria that induces cytoadherence of PRBCs to vascular endothelium. Cytoadherence causes sequestration of PRBCs in capillary and venules.

Cytokines

In severe malaria, blood concentration of both proinflammatory cytokines and anti-inflammatory Th2 cytokines is elevated, but there is an imbalance in patients with fatal diseases. The cytokines promote cytoadherence of PRBCs and mechanical obstruction in the brain microcirculation. Nitric oxide (NO) production is increased via inducible NO synthase (iNOS) in severe malaria.

Other factors

Both PRRBCs and NPRBCs have reduced deformability (RD) and are associated with poor outcome. Impaired RD promotes destruction of red blood cells and impairment of microcirculatory flow.

Pathogenesis of coma

Consciousness can be impaired by various interacting mechanisms. Inhomogenous obstruction of cerebral microcirculation by sequestered PRBCs causes hypoxia and net lactate production in the brain, but without infarction of the brain tissue. Local overproduction of NO or other cytokines may impair neurotransmission. However, the relative contributions of these mechanisms may differ in adults and children. Seizures are an important cause of impaired consciousness in children. Coma in malaria is not caused by raised increased intracranial pressure.

Cerebral malaria caused by P. *vivax*

Major organ dysfunction is rarely reported in *P. vivax* malaria. If a patient with *P. vivax* exhibits severe malaria (commonly associated with *P. falciparum*), the infection is presumed to be mixed. Although "pure" *P. vivax* could cause cerebral malaria, the pathogenesis of cerebral malaria in *vivax* malaria remains unknown.

International Neurology, Second edition. Edited by Robert P. Lisak, Daniel D. Truong, William M. Carroll and Roongroj Bhidayasiri
© 2016 John Wiley & Sons, Ltd. Published 2016 by John Wiley & Sons, Ltd.

Clinical features

Clinical manifestations of malaria differ considerably depending on the intensity of malaria transmission. In low transmission settings, symptomatic malaria occurs at all ages and cerebral malaria occurs both in adults and in children. Pregnant women are at greater risk of developing severe disease. In high transmission settings, severe malaria is confined to the first few years of life. Cerebral malaria is the major presentation of severe malaria in low and medium transmission settings, but when malaria transmission is very intense, it is less common, and occurs almost exclusively in infants and young children.

The clinical hallmark of malaria is fever. Cerebral malaria is a clinical syndrome characterized by coma at least 1 hour after termination of a seizure or correction of hypoglycemia, detection of asexual forms of *P. falciparum* or *P. vivax* in blood smear, and exclusion of other encephalopathy causes. This definition is useful for comparisons of different studies. There are different clinical features of cerebral malaria in African children and Southeast Asian adults (Table 71.1). It remains unclear whether these differences are associated with age or immunity.

The common presentation of severe malaria in children is coma with convulsions, severe anemia, respiratory distress (acidosis), and hypoglycemia. The earliest symptom of cerebral malaria in children is usually fever. Depth of coma may be assessed by using the Glasgow Coma Scale for adults and the Blantyre Coma Scale for children. The scales can be used repeatedly to assess either improvement or deterioration. In Southeast Asia, where malaria transmission is much lower than in Africa and protective immunity is not acquired, all age groups can get severe malaria, but young adults are the most affected group. The main complications of severe malaria in adults include cerebral malaria, renal failure, jaundice, and pulmonary edema. In both high and low transmission areas, pregnant women are vulnerable to hypoglycemia, pulmonary edema, and severe anemia.

In cerebral malaria, the onset of coma may be sudden, often following a generalized seizure, or gradual, with initial drowsiness, confusion, disorientation, delirium, or agitation, followed by unconsciousness. Extreme agitation is a poor prognostic sign. The length of prodromal history is usually several days in adults, but can be as short as 6–12 hours in children. A history of convulsions is common. Focal signs are relatively uncommon. The febrile patient has no signs of meningismus, although passive resistance to neck flexion is not uncommon and hyperextension of the neck may occur in severely ill patients. Abnormal posturing including decorticate, decerebrate rigidity, and opisthotonos may be found; when it occurs it signifies raised intracranial pressure and recurrence of seizures.

In some children, extreme opisthotonos may lead to a mistaken diagnosis of tetanus or meningitis. The eyes may show a divergent gaze (Figure 71.1), with normal oculocephalic reflexes. Pupil and corneal reflexes are usually normal. However, in children with profound coma, corneal reflexes may be absent and "doll's eyes" may be negative. Malarial retinopathy is better than any other clinical or laboratory feature in distinguishing malarial from non-malarial coma (Figure 71.2). Retinal hemorrhage can be seen in about 15%

Table 71.1 Clinical features of cerebral malaria in children and adults. Source: Idro 2005. Reproduced with permission of Elsevier.

	Children	Adults
Coma	Rapidly develops after convulsion	Gradually develops in 2–3 days or after generalized convulsion
Convulsions	>80% of cases with history of convulsions,60% occurs during admission;	20% of cases, mostly generalized tonic clonic, status epilepticus is rare
	>50% of cases with recurrent focal motor, 34% with tonic–clonic, 14% with partial with secondary generalization, 15% with subtle or electrographic; status epilepticus is common	
Neurological signs	>30% of cases have brainstem signs and associated with increased intracranial pressure; retinal abnormalities in 60%; brain swelling by CT scan in 40%	Symmetrical upper motor-neuron signs are common; brainstem signs and retinal abnormalities are less common
Conscious recovery	Rapid, 1–2 day(s)	Slower, 2–4 days
Mortality	18.6–75% of deaths occur within 24 h of admission	20%; 50% occur within 24 h
Neurological sequelae	11% of cases	<5% of cases

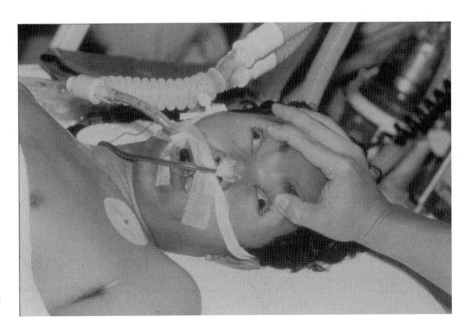

Figure 71.1 Dysconjugate gaze in a man with cerebral malaria; the optic axes are not parallel in horizontal plane. Source: © Polrat Wilairatana.

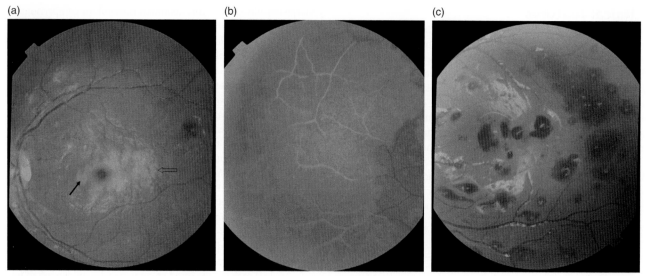

Figure 71.2 a Severe macula whitening (solid arrow) completely surrounding the foveola of a child with cerebral malaria. Papilledema is present as well as a white-centered hemorrhage temporal to the macula and cotton-wool spots above superior temporal arcade. The open arrow indicates glare. Figure 71.2b. White retinal vessels in an area of confluent peripheral retinal whitening. Figure 71.2c. Large number of retinal hemorrhages in a child with cerebral malaria. For color details, please refer to the color plates section.
Source: Beare 2006. Reproduced with permission of *American Journal of Tropical Medicine and Hygiene*.

of cases. Patients with papilledema have increased risk of death. Cranial nerve involvement is rare. Muscle tone and tendon reflexes are often increased, but can also be normal or reduced. Abdominal reflexes are absent and the plantar reflexes are extensor in approximately half of cases.

Post-malaria neurological syndromes (PMNS)

Neurological sequelae occur in less than 5% of adults recovering from cerebral malaria. In children, residual neurological abnormalities are more common, with approximately 11% still having symptoms at the moment of discharge, including hemiplegia, cortical blindness, diffuse cortical damage, tremor, isolated cranial nerve palsies, and aphasia. In children, these are associated with profound and protracted coma, anemia, and prolonged convulsions. Symptoms completely resolve over 1–6 months in over half of children, but a quarter of them will be left with major residual neurological deficits.

More subtle cognitive impairments in children as late neurological sequelae are common, particularly in comatose patients with concomitant multiple seizures, deep/prolonged coma, hypoglycemia, and clinical features of intracranial hypertension. Other late neurological complications, including psychosis, encephalopathy, parkinsonian rigidity and tremor, fine tremor, and cerebellar dysfunction may occur following recovery from cerebral malaria.

There appears to be a strong interaction between mefloquine and cerebral malaria, such that 5% of patients who receive mefloquine after severe malaria develop PMNS (a risk 10–50 times higher than following mefloquine treatment of uncomplicated malaria). Mefloquine should not be used following cerebral malaria.

Poor prognostic factors

In adults, depth of coma, agitation, oliguria, jaundice, and shock are important clinical predictors of poor outcome. Metabolic acidosis,

raised plasma, or cerebrospinal fluid lactate are useful prognostic markers. Non-immune patients with ≥4% parasitemia are associated with malaria complications or death.

In children, the presence of leukocyte pigment and/or mature parasites in blood smear, hypoglycemia, impaired consciousness, and respiratory distress predict 84% of deaths among African children. Other features associated with fatal outcome include hypoglycemia, increased plasma lactate or acidosis, increased cerebrospinal fluid lactate concentration, and mature parasites (>20% with visible malaria pigment).

Diagnosis

Cerebral malaria should be considered in comatose patients with history of fever who have been in malaria-endemic areas or have been exposed to other risks of malaria infection (e.g., blood transfusion). The diagnosis should be confirmed by thick and thin blood films or rapid diagnostic tests, such as dipstick detection of *P. falciparum* antigens *Pf*HRP2 and *p*LDH, which have a diagnostic sensitivity similar to that of microscopy, but do not require an experienced microscopist. Although *P. vivax* uncommonly impairs consciousness, patients with *P. vivax* malaria and altered consciousness should be considered as cerebral malaria. Cerebral malaria should be considered in any patient with coma and asexual malaria parasitemia, until proven otherwise.

Differential diagnosis of cerebral malaria includes hypoglycemia and bacterial or viral meningoencephalitis.

Sudden unexplained deterioration may result from hypoglycemia or sepsis. It is extremely unusual for a patient with falciparum cerebral malaria to have a negative blood smear. When it does happen, it is the result of previous antimalarial treatment, but in such cases *Pf*HRP2 tests are still positive. If the smear and *Pf*HRP2 tests are negative for *P. falciparum*, the patient has another cause of coma apart from *P. falciparum*.

Treatment

Resuscitation

Because most cerebral malaria patients die within 24 hours of admission, emergent or intensive care unit (ICU) care with attention to treatment of shock, severe metabolic acidosis, respiratory failure, and seizures is needed.

Antimalarial treatment

In cerebral malaria, an effective parenteral antimalarial drug should be given. Oral antimalarial drugs may have erratic absorption from the gastrointestinal tract during severe malaria. In general, chloroquine should not be used because most *P. falciparum* infections are resistant to chloroquine. Infusion can be given in normal saline or 5% or 10% dextrose. Oral treatment should be started as soon as the patient can swallow reliably enough to complete a full course of treatment.

Option 1: Artesunate

Artemisinins are active at both early and late stages, whereas quinine takes effect during the later stages of parasite development. Intravenous artesunate is significantly superior to quinine in the treatment of severe malaria. The dose of intravenous or intramuscular artesunate is 2.4 mg/kg given over 3 minutes on admission, followed by the same dose after 12 and 24 hours, and then 2.4 mg/kg daily until the patient is able to take oral medication. All cases of cerebral malaria should be followed with a full course of an oral, locally effective artemisinin-combination therapy (ACT) once they are able to take oral medication and after at least 24 hours of parenteral therapy have been completed. Oral ACT include artemether-lumefanthrine 1.5/9 mg/kg twice daily for 3 days with food *or* dihydroartemisinin-piperaquine 3/16 mg/kg once daily for 3 days *or* artesunate 4 mg/kg/day for 3 days + mefloquine 25 mg/kg divided in 2–3 days *or* artesunate 4 mg/kg/day for 3 days + sulphadoxine 25 mg/kg + pyrimethamine 1.25 mg/kg (SP) single dose *or* artesunate 4 mg/kg/day for 3 days + amodiaquine 10 mg base/kg/day for 3 days.

Option 2: Artemether

A loading dose of artemether 3.2 mg/kg is given intramuscularly as a single dose on day 1. However, intramuscular artemether should not be given to patients in shock because absorption is unreliable. The maintenance dose is 1.6 mg/kg once a day starting on day 2 until the patient is able to tolerate oral medication. All cases of cerebral malaria should be followed with a full course of an oral, locally effective artemisinin-combination therapy (ACT) once they are able to take oral medication and after at least 24 hours of parenteral therapy have been completed. Choices of oral ACT are the same as in Option 1.

Option 3: Quinine

Quinine, a loading dose of 20 mg salt/kg of quinine dihydrochloride over 4 hours should be given followed by 10 mg salt/kg every 8 hours (each given over 4 hours). If there is a history of mefloquine or quinine administration within 24 hours before admission, the loading dose of quinine should not be given. Maintenance dose 10 mg salt/kg is given by infusion over 4 hours every 8 hours. Doses should be reduced by 30–50% after the third day of treatment to avoid accumulation of the drugs in patients who remain seriously ill. However, a minimum of 3 doses of intravenous quinine should be given before changing to oral treatment. Quinine may also be given intramuscularly into the anterior thigh (not the buttock) after dilution to 60–100 mg/mL. Intravenous quinine can cause hypoglycemia, and blood glucose should be monitored every 4 hours. Quinine is safe for fetuses. Once the patient is able to tolerate oral medication, treatment should be completed with a full course of oral ACT (as mentioned in Option 1) or oral quinine 10 mg salt/kg every 8 hours to complete the remainder of a total 7 days of quinine treatment. In areas of multidrug-resistant malaria, quinine should be combined with oral clindamycin 5 mg/kg 3 times a day for 7 days. If clindamycin is unavailable, use doxycycline 3 mg/kg once a day for 7 days, or oral tetracycline 4 mg/kg 4 times a day for 7 days. Doxycycline and tetracycline should not be given to children under 8 years old or to pregnant women. However, clindamycin can safely be given to these groups. Survival outcome of the patients treated with quinine or artemether is similar.

Antimalarial treatment for asexual blood stages of "cerebral malaria" from *P. falciparum* and *vivax* malaria is similar. Although most *P. vivax* is chloroquine sensitive, chloroquine is not recommended for treatment in this severe form of *vivax* malaria. Antimalarial drugs that kill asexual blood stages of *P. falciparum* can also kill asexual blood stages of *P. vivax*, but not any hypnozoites in the liver following *vivax* infection. Radical cure of *vivax* infection requires treatment with primaquine 0.25 mg base/kg daily (0.375–0.5 mg base/kg in Oceania) together with food for 14 days if pregnancy and G6PD deficiency have been excluded. In mild G6PD deficiency, intermittent therapy with reduced-dose primaquine 0.75 mg base/kg once weekly for 6 weeks to eradicate hypnozoites may be given. Primaquine should not be given in severe G6PD deficiency.

Supportive treatment

Many cerebral malaria patients have multiple organ failure. If patients have renal failure, metabolic acidosis, or respiratory failure, hemofiltration/dialysis or ventilation, respectively, is life saving and should be started early. Convulsions are very common in children with cerebral malaria; however, choice and dose of a seizure-prophylactic drug have not been well established and this is currently not recommended. The common drugs for treatment of convulsions in cerebral malaria are intravenous benzodiazepines (diazepam, midazolam, or lorazepam). If a seizure episode persists for longer than 10 minutes after the first dose, give a second dose of a benzodiazepine. In status epilepticus despite the use of two doses of these drugs, give intravenous phenytoin 18 mg/kg or intravenous/intramuscular phenobarbitone 15 mg/kg if it is the only available option.

A number of ancillary treatments that, in the past, may have benefited select groups of patients presently cannot be universally recommended. These are listed in Table 71.2.

Table 71.2 Non-recommended ancillary treatments in cerebral malaria.

Corticosteroids
Other anticerebral edema agents (mannitol, urea)
Oxpentifylline
Prostacyclin
Other anti-inflammatory agents
Iron chelating agents
Dichloroacetate
Low molecular weight dextran
Antitumor necrosis factor antibodies
Hyperimmune serum
Cyclosporin A
Adrenaline
Heparin
Hyperbaric oxygen

Further reading

Adhikari B, Tangpukdee N, Krudsood S, Wilairatana P. Factors associated with cerebral malaria. *Southeast Asian J Trop Med Public Health* 2013;44:941–949.

Beare NAV, Taylor TE, Harding SP, Lewallen S, Molyneux ME. Malarial retinopathy: A newly established diagnostic signs in severe malaria. *Am J Trop Med Hyg* 2006;75:790–797.

Idro R, Newton CRJC. Pathogenesis, clinical features, and neurological outcome of cerebral malaria. *Lancet Neurol* 2005;4:827–820.

White NJ. Malaria. In: CookGC, ZumlaAI (eds.). *Manson's Tropical Diseases*, 22nd ed. London: WB Saunders; 2009:1201–1300.

World Health Organization (WHO). *Management of Severe Malaria*, 3rd ed. Geneva: WHO; 2012.

72 Trypanosomiasis

Francisco Javier Carod-Artal

Universitat Internacional de Catalunya, Barcelona, Spain, and Neurology Department, Raigmore Hospital, Inverness, UK

American trypanosomiasis

Trypanosomes are parasitic protozoa that infect millions of poor people in tropical regions. American trypanosomiasis or Chagas' disease (CD) is an acute or chronic infection caused by the flagellate protozoan *Trypanosoma cruzi*.

Humans become involved when infected vectors infest the cracks and holes in poor housing in endemic areas. Infection is acquired by the transmission of *T. cruzi* via the bite of the kissing bug of the family *Reduviidae*. The entry of trypanosome through the wound of skin or mucous membrane is facilitated by the sleeping victim scratching the bite. Sylvatic vertebrates and several domestic animals are reservoirs for *T. cruzi*.

Trypanosome can also be transmitted through infected blood (transfusion, drug abusers), transplant donation, and rarely by oral ingestion. Congenital transmission affects 1–10% of babies born from infected mothers.

Epidemiology

CD has been a neglected tropical disease in Latin America for many years. *T. cruzi* infection is widespread from Southern Chile, Argentina, and Brazil throughout South and Central America. More than 14 million people have chronic infection, with approximately 14,000 deaths each year. Up to 8% of the South American population is seropositive, but only 10–30% have symptomatic disease. The number of acute cases has been reduced substantially due to the implementation of vector control programs in endemic countries.

In recent years, epidemiological changes have occurred and the disease has spread to non-endemic countries in Europe and North America. CD has reached areas outside the traditional geographic boundaries due to population migrations from endemic countries toward developed countries. In the United States, approximately 2% of Latin American immigrants may be infected with *T. cruzi*. In Europe, blood transfusion and congenital cases have been reported. Prevalence of *T. cruzi* infection among Latin American pregnant women ranges from 2% (Geneva) to 3.4% (Barcelona).

Clinical features

Acute *T. cruzi* infection occurs most often in childhood. It is usually asymptomatic, but can present with cutaneous lesions (chagoma; orbital edema or Romaña's sign), fever, lymphadenopathy, and hepatosplenomegaly. Severe cases of myocarditis and meningoencephalitis can occur in 5% of patients, with a 2–10% mortality rate.

Most infected persons remain asymptomatic in a latent stage that may last years. Only positive antibodies for CD can be detected in this indeterminate form of the disease.

Cardiac and gastrointestinal involvement is the most frequent clinical feature of chronic CD. Megaesophagus and megacolon provoke dysphagia and constipation, respectively. Chronic cardiomyopathy affects 30% of patients between 10 and 30 years of age after initial infection. Chagasic cardiomyopathy is characterized by congestive heart failure, sudden death, cardiac arrhythmias, and thromboembolism.

Chagasic myocardiopathy is independently associated with ischemic stroke. Apical aneurysm, mural thrombus, congestive heart failure, and cardiac arrhythmias are risk factors in chagasic stroke. Prevalence of apical aneurysm in CD stroke patients is around 37%. However, stroke may be the first manifestation of CD in patients with mild or undetected systolic dysfunction. Chagasic patients without associated vascular risk factors and no clinical evidence of heart failure are also at risk of stroke. One-third of chagasic patients who suffer a stroke may have an asymptomatic *T. cruzi* infection. In central Brazil, around 40% of CD patients are diagnosed as having CD after their first stroke.

CD reactivation can occur in the chronic stage of the disease. Acute exacerbation of chronic *T. cruzi* infection has been described in patients with acquired immune deficiency syndrome (AIDS), transplant-associated immunosuppression, and lymphoreticular neoplasias. Neurological involvement occurs in most cases, and meningoencephalitis and space-occupying cerebral lesions (called chagomas) are common.

Pathophysiology of chronic Chagas' disease

Parasite persistence and autoimmune responses explain part of the spectrum of chronic CD. *T. cruzi* antigens and DNA have been detected in host tissues during the chronic stage. Persistent low-grade parasitism and unbalanced immunological response seem to be the most important pathogenic mechanisms.

Myocardial fibrosis in the chronic disease results from several factors: (1) myocardial cell destruction due to direct tissue damage by *T. cruzi*; (2) inflammatory response responsible for progressive neuronal damage and microcirculation alterations; and (3) neuronal involvement with selective parasite destruction of postganglionic parasympathetic neurons in the heart.

The reduction of cellular immunity can favor reactivation of CD in the chronic stage in the central nervous system (CNS).

Investigations

T. cruzi may be observed by direct examination of fresh blood (thick smear) during the acute phase. Parasitological techniques (microhematocrit and other concentration techniques) also permit

International Neurology, Second edition. Edited by Robert P. Lisak, Daniel D. Truong, William M. Carroll and Roongroj Bhidayasiri.
© 2016 John Wiley & Sons, Ltd. Published 2016 by John Wiley & Sons, Ltd.

direct visualization of trypomastigotes in both acute CD and its reactivation in immunosuppressed patients.

Diagnosis of chronic and indeterminate CD relies on serological methods. Screening assays include indirect immunofluorescence antibodies, indirect hemagglutination test, and enzyme-linked immunosorbent assay (ELISA). Positive titer indicates only infection at some unknown time in the past.

Polymerase chain reaction (PCR) based assays are useful in the diagnosis of congenital CD, in acute reactivation in immunosuppressed patients, and to examine tissue samples from infected organ donors. However, PCR standardization and validation studies in CD are still needed.

The cerebrospinal fluid (CSF) of patients with acute CD encephalitis may show moderate lymphocytic pleocytosis, low glucose levels, and raised protein levels. *T. cruzi* trypomastigotes can be detected in CSF on direct examination.

Abnormalities in electrocardiogram (ECG), such as left anterior fascicular block, right bundle-branch block, and atrial fibrillation, are common in the chronic cardiac form of CD. Arrhythmias may be detected in patients with normal ejection fraction. Frequently observed echocardiography features are decreased left ventricular dysfunction, diminished ventricular ejection fraction, systolic wall motion abnormalities, apical aneurysm, and left ventricular thrombosis.

Brain embolism should be suspected in cases of occlusion of the middle cerebral artery (MCA) or its branches (Figure 72.1). The MCA territory is the most common recipient site for cardiac embolism, as observed in at least 70% of CD stroke patients.

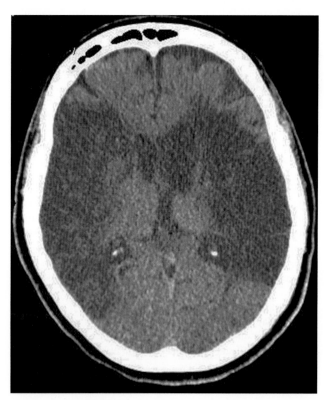

Figure 72.1   Computed tomography (CT) scan showing bilateral middle cerebral artery infarction in a Chagas' disease stroke patient.

Treatment

Treatment is available for acute disease (including congenital and transfusion transmission) and for reactivation of chronic infection. Trypanocide drugs are useful mainly against circulating trypomastigotes, and decrease parasitemia and mortality. Nifurtimox (8–10 mg/kg, for 30–120 days) and benznidazole (5–10 mg/kg, for 30–60 days) are drugs of choice. Common side effects include nausea and vomiting, headache, dermatitis, and paresthesias. Polyneuritis, leukopenia, and bone marrow suppression can occur less frequently.

Although recent clinical trials have reported high rates of parasitological cure in children with early chronic *T. cruzi* infection, no specific therapy is still effective in the chronic stage of the disease.

Management of chronic chagasic cardiomyopathy involves use of anti-arrhythmic drugs and diuretics. Some patients may require a pacemaker due to severe atrioventricular conduction block. Secondary prevention with oral anticoagulants should be considered in CD patients with stroke and heart failure, atrial fibrillation, or apical aneurysm.

Prevention of the disease may be achieved by vector control and improvement in basic housing conditions in endemic areas.

Human African trypanosomiasis

Human African trypanosomiasis (HAT), also called sleeping sickness, is a neglected tropical disease caused by *Trypanosoma brucei*. This protozoan parasite is transmitted to humans by the bite of the blood-sucking tsetse fly (*Glossina* genus).

East African HAT is caused by *Trypanosoma b. rhodesiense*, whereas the West African form is provoked by *T.b. gambiense*. These HAT subtypes differ in their tempo of infection as a result of the greater adaptation of *T.b. gambiense* to the human host. *T.b. gambiense* represents more than 97% of reported cases and causes a chronic infection. *T.b. rhodesiense* causes a more acute and severe illness, and it has been reported in European and American travelers returning from East African game parks.

Epidemiology

HAT occurs in no fewer than 36 African countries. Tsetse fly infestation covers about 10 million km2 of African landmass and 60 million people who live mainly in rural parts of sub-Saharan Africa are at risk of contracting the disease. The prevalence of HAT has declined substantially over the past two decades due to considerable progress in reducing the number of people infected and the development of better treatment options. HAT annual incidence was estimated at 70,000 cases in 2006, and the number of reported new cases fell below 10,000 in 2009.

Pathophysiology

The tsetse fly bite erupts into a red sore and within 1–3 weeks the person can experience the first stage of the disease, called the hemolymphatic stage. As the disease progresses, the trypanosomes multiply in subcutaneous tissues, blood, and lymph. This process provokes specific organ dysfunction such as myocarditis, skin lesions, and hepatosplenic involvement.

The late or encephalitic stage occurs when the parasites cross the blood–brain barrier to infect the CNS. This process can take years with *T.b. gambiense*. In contrast, *T.b. rhodesiense* infection develops rapidly and invades the CNS after a few months or weeks.

Clinical features

The early stage (hemolymphatic) is characterized by non-specific symptoms such as intermittent fever, headache, painful chancre, and aching muscles and joints. Cardiac features (congestive cardiac failure), endocrine dysfunction, ophthalmic disturbances (iritis, keratitis), and infertility can also occur. A typical feature of *T.b. gambiense* infection is a posterior cervical lymphadenopathy known as Winterbottom's sign. Clinical presentation in travelers may be atypical, with febrile illness, diarrhoea, hepatomegaly, or jaundice.

Late-stage symptoms can develop over many months and years and, if not treated, the disease is invariably fatal. The most common neurological features are (1) behavioral disturbances including changes in personality, irritability, violent behavior, agitation, confusion, delusions, hallucinations, and delirium; (2) alteration of the circadian rhythm and sleep disturbances, including reversal of sleep/wake cycle with daytime hypersomnolence and nocturnal insomnia; (3) focal impairment including motor weakness, dystonia, paresthesias, abnormal movements, tremor, slurred speech, and seizures; and (4) peripheral involvement, including polyneuropathy and muscle fasciculation.

Investigations

Screening of people at risk helps identify patients at an early stage. Diagnosis should be made as early as possible and before the advanced stage.

Persistent parasitaemia is common in *T.b. rhodesiense*, and diagnosis can be made by identifying trypanosomes in peripheral blood (thick smear) or tissues (lymph node aspirate, bone marrow). *T.b. gambiense* parasitemia is usually cyclical due to the greater adaptation to the host; serological tests (card agglutination trypanosomiasis test) can help in the diagnosis, although they have limited sensitivity.

CSF analysis is mandatory to rule out late-stage disease. Lymphocytic pleocytosis (>20 white blood cells/μL), raised CSF protein (50–200 mg/mL), increased intrathecal IgM synthesis, and the presence of trypanosomes can be detected. However, there is no universal consensus as to how late-stage disease should be diagnosed using CSF criteria in HAT.

Differential diagnosis includes malaria (both diseases may coexist), leishmaniasis, typhoid fever, viral encephalitis, AIDS, brucellosis, toxoplasmosis, and chronic tuberculosis meningitis.

Treatment

Pentamidine administered intramuscularly is the first-line therapy to treat the early stage of *T.b. gambiense* infection, whereas intravenous suramine is the drug of choice for *T.b. rhodesiense*. Side effects include renal failure, skin lesions, anaphylaxis, and peripheral neuropathy for suramine; and hypo/hyperglycemia, hypotension, gastrointestinal symptoms, and QT interval prolongation for pentamidine.

Treatment of late-stage HAT is more problematic, as the drugs used are more toxic. Late-stage disease in both types of HAT is treated by the trivalent arsenical melarsoprol (Mel B). It is the only drug effective at present to treat late-stage *T.b. rhodesiense*. Accurate staging of the disease is essential because of the potentially fatal complications of melarsoprol treatment. Mel B has many undesired effects, the most important of which is a severe post-treatment reactive encephalopathy (PTRE) with coma, seizures, status epilepticus, and cerebral edema. PTRE occurs in about 10% of cases and may prove fatal in up to 50% of these. Melarsoprol injections are also very painful.

The use of steroids in HAT remains controversial. In a large study, a combination of melarsoprol and prednisolone reduced the incidence of PTRE and fatalities in *T.b. gambiense* disease.

A more recently available alternative drug for late-stage *T.b. gambiense* disease is the eflornithine plus nifurtimox combination, which has now become the first-line treatment for late-stage *T.b. gambiense* HAT, reserving Mel B for second-line treatment.

The main approach to controlling HAT is to reduce the reservoirs of infection and the presence of the tsetse fly. Poor surveillance, wars, and increasing parasite resistance are some of the reasons that may explain the re-emergence of HAT in some areas.

Further reading

Carod-Artal FJ. American trypanosomiasis. *Handb Clin Neurol* 2013;114:103–123.

Carod-Artal FJ, Gascon J. Chagas disease and stroke. *Lancet Neurol* 2010;9:533–542.

Carod-Artal FJ, Vargas AP, Falcao T. Stroke in asymptomatic Trypanosoma cruzi-infected patients. *Cerebrovasc Dis* 2011;31:24–28.

Carod-Artal FJ, Vargas AP, Horan TA, Nunes LG. Chagasic cardiomyopathy is independently associated with ischemic stroke in Chagas disease. *Stroke* 2005;36:965–970.

Kennedy PG. Clinical features, diagnosis, and treatment of human African trypanosomiasis (sleeping sickness). *Lancet Neurol* 2013;12:186–194.

Oscar H. Del Brutto

School of Medicine, Universidad Espíritu Santo, and Department of Neurological Sciences, Hospital-Clínica Kennedy, Guayaquil, Ecuador

Cestodes (tapeworms) inhabit the intestine of vertebrates and require two or more hosts to complete their complex life cycles. Humans may act as either definitive or intermediate hosts of these parasites. Most human cestode infections are benign conditions. However, severe disease may occur when humans accidentally become the intermediate hosts of these parasites and tissue invasion occurs. Of the four cestode infections relevant to humans, coenurosis, sparganosis, cysticercosis, and equinococcosis, this chapter will deal with the two latter as more common and cosmopolitan.

Neurocysticercosis

Neurocysticercosis (NCC) is defined as the infection of the central nervous system (CNS) and its meninges by the encysted larval stage of *Taenia solium*, and occurs when a human becomes the intermediate host of this cestode after ingesting its eggs by direct contagion from a Taenia carrier. Ingestion of contaminated pork as a cause of human cysticercosis is a common misconception, since the role of pigs is to perpetuate the infection cycle only by causing human Taeniasis (Figure 73.1).

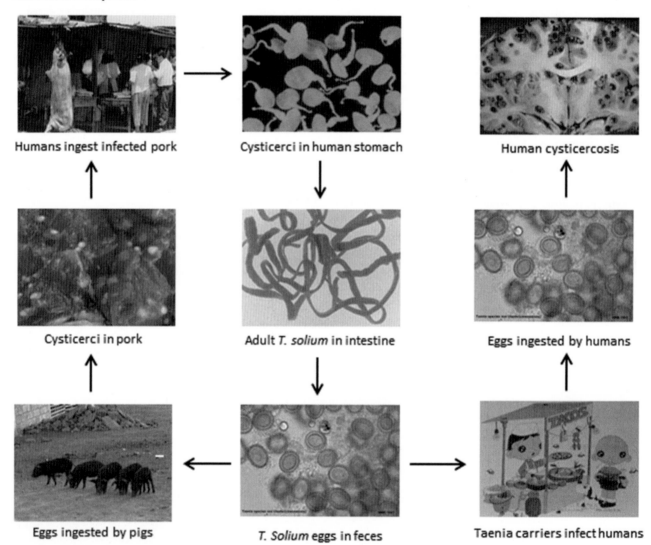

Humans ingest infected pork

Cysticerci in human stomach

Human cysticercosis

Cysticerci in pork

Adult *T. solium* in intestine

Eggs ingested by humans

Eggs ingested by pigs

T. Solium eggs in feces

Taenia carriers infect humans

Figure 73.1 Major steps in the normal and aberrant life cycle of Taenia solium.

International Neurology, Second edition. Edited by Robert P. Lisak, Daniel D. Truong, William M. Carroll and Roongroj Bhidayasiri
© 2016 John Wiley & Sons, Ltd. Published 2016 by John Wiley & Sons, Ltd.

Epidemiology

NCC is the most common helminthic infection of the nervous system, affecting millions of people in the developing world where conditions favoring the transmission of this disease, including inadequate pig farming, poverty, and illiteracy, are common. The disease has also become a health problem in the United States, Western Europe, and even in some Muslim countries, due to mass immigration of people from disease-endemic areas. Human cysticercosis is potentially eradicable. To be effective, however, eradication programs must be directed to all the interrelated targets for control, including human carriers of the adult tapeworm, infected pigs, and eggs in the environment.

Pathophysiology

Cysticerci are vesicles containing an invaginated scolex similar to adult *T. solium*. Parasites can be located in brain parenchyma, ventricular system, subarachnoid space, and spinal cord. Parenchymal cysts usually lodge in the cerebral cortex or basal ganglia. Subarachnoid cysts are located in the Sylvian fissure or in the cisterns at the base of the brain. Ventricular cysticerci may attach to the choroid plexus or float in the ventricular cavities. Spinal cysticerci are found either in the cord parenchyma or in subarachnoid space.

After entering the CNS, cysticerci are in a vesicular stage and elicit few inflammatory changes in surrounding tissues. Parasites can remain in this stage for years or may enter, as the result of the host's immune attack, into a process of degeneration. The three stages of involution through which cysticerci pass are the colloidal, the granular, and the calcified stages. Through this process of degeneration, cysticerci are associated with inflammation that induce pathological changes in the CNS. Within brain parenchyma, the inflammatory reaction is associated with edema and reactive gliosis. In the subarachnoid space, the leptomeninges thicken, causing entrapment of cranial nerves and blood vessels. Luschka and Magendie's foramina are occluded by the thickened leptomeninges, with subsequent development of hydrocephalus. Ventricular cysticerci also elicit a local inflammatory reaction if attached to the choroid plexus or to the ventricular wall. In such cases, ependymal cells proliferate and may block cerebrospinal (CSF) transit at the cerebral aqueduct or Monro's foramina, causing obstructive hydrocephalus.

Clinical features

Epidemiological surveys conducted in endemic countries have shown that most individuals with NCC are asymptomatic and only have serological or imaging evidence of the disease. This finding differs from those based on data from hospital-based registries, where up to 80% of NCC patients present with recurrent seizures. Seizures may occur at any stage of cysticerci involution, from viable cysts to calcifications, and mechanisms involved in epileptogenesis vary according to the stage of parasites. Viable cysts most likely induce seizures due to compressive effects on the brain parenchyma, while degenerating cysts induce seizures as a result of the inflammatory reaction associated with the attack of the host immune system to the parasites. In calcified lesions, the gliosis that develops around dead parasites, exposure of antigenic material to the brain parenchyma, or even the development of hippocampal sclerosis may account for their epileptogenic activity (Figure 73.2).

Up to 15% of symptomatic NCC cases develop focal neurological signs, which often follow a subacute or chronic course resembling that of other intracranial expansive lesions. Focal signs are most often seen in patients with large subarachnoid cysts compressing the brain. In addition, acute stroke syndromes have been described; these are often related to subcortical infarctions related to occlusion of blood vessels affected by cysticercotic angiitis. Cognitive decline has also been observed in some patients with NCC and its prevalence might be more common than suspected.

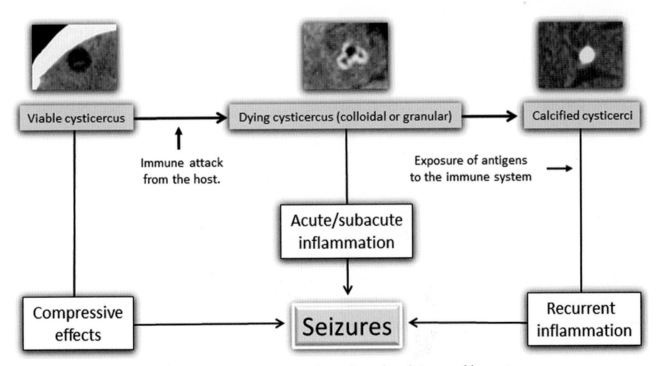

Figure 73.2 Proposed mechanisms of epileptogenesis in neurocysticercosis according to the evolutive stage of the parasite.

Many patients with extraparenchymal NCC – and some with the parenchymal form of the disease – may develop intracranial hypertension, which may be related to hydrocephalus due to arachnoiditis, granular ependymitis, ventricular cysts, or to cysticercotic encephalitis or large cysts growing within the brain parenchyma (rare). Other rare forms of NCC present with ophthalmological and endocrinological manifestations (intrasellar NCC), root pain and weakness of subacute onset (spinal NCC), and decreased visual acuity due to vitreitis, uveitis, or endophthalmitis (intraocular cysticercosis).

Diagnosis

Despite important advances in neuroimaging and immune diagnostic tests, the diagnosis of NCC is a challenge. Clinical manifestations are non-specific, immune diagnostic tests have poor specificity and sensitivity, and neuroimaging findings are not pathognomonic, with the single exception of the so-called hole-with-dot finding that is seen in some parenchymal brain cysts in the vesicular stage (Figure 73.3).

A set of diagnostic criteria provides the elements needed to diagnose patients with suspected neurocysticercosis based on the integrated evaluation of clinical, radiological, immunological, and epidemiological data. The set includes four categories of diagnostic criteria – absolute, major, minor, and epidemiological – stratified according to their individual strength. Absolute criteria allow unequivocal diagnostis of neurocysticercosis, major criteria strongly suggest the diagnosis but cannot be used alone to confirm the disease, minor criteria are frequent but non-specific manifestations of the disease, and epidemiological criteria refer to circumstantial evidence favoring the diagnosis of cysticercosis. Interpretation of these criteria results in two categories of diagnostic certainty – definitive and probable – according to the likelihood that neurocysticercosis is present in a given patient (Table 73.1).

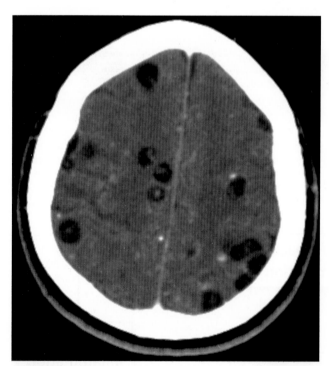

Figure 73.3 Contrast-enhanced computed tomography showing the pathognomonic "hole-with-dot" imaging of parenchymal brain cysticerci in the vesicular stage.

Treatment

For a rational therapeutic approach, NCC must be categorized in terms of location and number of lesions within the central nervous system, viability of lesions, and severity of the host's immune response to the parasite (Table 73.2). The first line of management includes the use of symptomatic drugs for the control of clinical manifestations (seizures, headache) and the mechanisms underlying their occurrence (brain edema, mass effect). Cysticidal drugs – albendazole, praziquantel – have improved the prognosis of many patients with parenchymal NCC, and several double blind, placebo-controlled studies have shown that their use is associated with the resolution of lesions and clinical improvement in most of these cases.

Table 73.1 Diagnostic criteria and degrees of diagnostic certainty for neurocysticercosis (NCC)

DIAGNOSTIC CRITERIA

Absolute Criteria (allow unequivocal diagnosis of NCC):
- Histologic demonstration of the parasite from biopsy of a brain or spinal cord lesion.
- Evidence of cystic lesions showing the scolex on neuroimaging studies (hole-with-dot imaging).
- Direct visualization of subretinal parasites by fundoscopic examination.

Major Criteria (strongly suggest the diagnosis but cannot be used alone to confirm the disease):
- Evidence of lesions highly suggestive of NCC on CT/MRI (cystic lesions without scolex, ring or nodular enhancing lesions, small parenchymal brain calcifications). Note: the presence of two different lesions should be considered as two major diagnostic criteria.
- Positive serum immunoblot for the detection of anticysticercal antibodies (conformation-sensitive immunoassay may be of value in patients with a single cerebral cyst and a negative immunoblot).
- Resolution of intracranial cystic lesions after therapy with albendazole or praziquantel.
- Spontaneous resolution of small (less than 20mm) single enhancing lesions in the brain parenchymal.

Minor Criteria (frequent but non-specific manifestations of NCC):
- Evidence of lesions suggestive of NCC on CT/MRI (hydrocephalus, meningeal enhancement).
- Presence of clinical manifestations suggestive of NCC (mainly recurrent seizures).
- Positive CSF ELISA for detection of anticysticercal antibodies or cysticercal antigens (use Quick ELISA for detection of cysticercal antibodies or ELISA using a monoclonal antibody for detection of cysticercal antigens in serum as alternatives).
- Evidence of cysticercosis outside the central nervous system (subcutaneous nodules, cigar-shaped calcifications in striated muscles, and cysticerci in the anterior chamber of the eye).

Epidemiologic Criteria (circumstantial evidence favoring the diagnosis of NCC):
- Individuals coming from or living in an area where cysticercosis is endemic.
- History of frequent travel to disease-endemic areas.
- Evidence of a household contact with *T. solium* infection.

DEGREES OF DIAGNOSTIC CERTAINTY

Definitive Diagnosis:
- Presence of one absolute criterion.
- Presence of two major plus one minor or one epidemiologic criteria.

Probable Diagnosis:
- Presence of one major plus two minor criteria.
- Presence of one major plus one minor and one epidemiologic criteria.
- Presence of three minor plus one epidemiologic criteria.

CSF = cerebrospinal cluid; CT = computed tomography; ELISA = enzyme-linked immunosorbent assay; MRI = magnetic resonance imaging

Table 73.2 Guideliness for therapy of neurocysticercosis (Level 1 of evidence favor the use of cysticidal drugs in patients with parenchymal brain vesicular and colloidal cysts. For other forms of the disease, guideliness are based on Levels II and III of evidence).

PARENCHYMAL NEUROCYSTICERCOSIS

Vesicular cysts:

- **Single cyst:** Albendazole 15 mg/kg/day for three days or single-**day** therapy with praziquantel 30 mg/kg in 3 doses every 2 hours. Corticosteroids rarely needed. Antiepileptic drugs (AED) for seizures.
- **Mild to moderate infections:** Albendazole 15 mg/kg/day for one week or praziquantel 50mg/kg/day for 15 days. Combined albendazole and praziquantel therapy may be used. Corticosteroids when necessary. AED for seizures.
- **Heavy infections:** Albendazole 15 mg/kg/day for one week (repeated cycles of albendazole or combined therapy with albendazole and praziquantel may be needed). Corticosteroids are mandatory before, during, and after therapy. AED for seizures.

Colloidal cysts:

- **Single cyst:** Albendazole 15 mg/kg/day for 3 days or single-day therapy with praziquantel 30 mg/kg in 3 doses every 2 hours. Corticosteroids may be used when necessary. AED for seizures.
- **Mild to moderate infections:** Albendazole 15 mg/kg/day for one week. Corticosteroids are often needed before and during therapy. AED for seizures.
- **Cysticercotic encephalitis:** Albendazole and praziquantel are contraindicated. Corticosteroids and osmotic diuretics to reduce brain swelling. AED for seizures. Decompressive craniectomies in refractory cases.

Granular and calcified cysticerci

- **Single or multiple:** No need for albendazole or praziquantel therapy. AED for seizures. Corticosteroids for patients with recurrent seizures and perilesional edema surrounding calcifications.

EXTRAPARENCHYMAL NEUROCYSTICERCOSIS

Small cysts over the convexity of cerebral hemispheres:

- **Single or multiple:** Albendazole 15 mg/kg/day for one week. Corticosteroids may be used when necessary. AED for seizures.

Large cysts in Sylvian fissures or basal CSF cisterns:

- **Racemose cysticercus:** Albendazole, 15 to 30 mg/kg/day for 15 to 30 days (repeated cycles of albendazole may be needed). Corticosteroids are mandatory before, during, and after therapy.

Other forms of extraparenchymal neurocysticercosis:

- **Hydrocephalus:** No need for albendazole or praziquantel. Ventricular shunt. Continuous administration of corticosteroids (50 mg three times a week for two years) may be needed to reduce the rate of shunt dysfunction.
- **Ventricular cysts:** Endoscopic resection of cysts. Albendazole may be used only in small lesions located in lateral ventricles. Ventricular shunt only needed in patients with associated ependymitis.
- **Angiitis, chronic arachnoiditis:** No need for albendazole or praziquantel. Corticosteroids are mandatory.
- **Cysticercosis od the spine:** Surgical resection of lesions. Anecdotal use of albendazole with good results.

Treatment of extraparenchymal neurocysticercosis is more complicated, as many patients do not respond to the first trial with cysticidal drugs. In these cases, repeated administration of the drugs or surgical interventions may be needed. Some other forms of the disease, like cysticercotic encephalitis, must not be treated with cysticidal drugs, as the use of these exacerbates the inflammatory reaction against parasites and may cause seizures or intracranial hypertension. Patients with calcifications should not receive cysticidal drugs, but it must be remembered that these are not completely inert lesions, as they represent permanent epileptogenic foci that may reactivate to cause recurrent seizures. Long-term therapy with antiepileptic drugs is needed in most of these cases.

Echinococcosis

Echinococcosis (hydatid disease) is caused by infection with the larval forms of *Echinococcus spp.* There are two main forms of the disease: cystic echinococcosis caused by *E. granulosus*, and alveolar echinococcosis caused by *E. multilocularis*. In addition, infection by *E. vogeli* may rarely cause cystic echinococcosis. Canids are definitive hosts of these cestodes and sheep, rodents, or humans may be intermediate hosts. Humans become infected by ingesting water or food contaminated with dog feces containing eggs of these tapeworms. After entering the body, eggs transform into cysts that grow in the CNS or other organs.

Epidemiology

E. granulosus infections have been mainly reported in Eastern Europe, Mediterranean countries, the Middle East, Southeast Asia, and South America. *E. multilocularis* is restricted to the Northern Hemisphere, including the Arctic, Canada, Europe, countries of the former Soviet Union, Japan, and China. There are no reliable estimates on the number of infected persons.

Pathophysiology

E. granulosus cysts are spherical and well demarcated from surrounding tissues. Cysts can be located in the brain parenchyma, ventricular system, subarachnoid space, epidural space, and spinal canal. In contrast, *E. multilocularis* cysts are small, group in clusters, elicit a severe inflammatory reaction from the host, and tend to metastasize both locally and distantly. These cysts are usually located within the brain parenchyma.

Hydatid disease of the heart may cause a cerebral infarct. Hydatid cysts may subsequently grow within the necrotic brain tissue, suggesting that the infarct is caused by embolic occlusion of an intracranial artery by fragments of a cyst broken off within the heart.

Clinical features

Cystic echinococcosis of the brain is characterized by seizures or increased intracranial pressure. Focal neurological deficits result from strategically located cysts or a cerebral infarct caused by a cardiogenic brain embolism of cystic membranes. Cranial nerve palsies are common in patients with parasellar cysts due to involvement of the cavernous sinus. In patients with alveolar echinococcosis, clinical manifestations include intracranial hypertension, seizures, and focal neurological deficits. Manifestations progress more rapidly and are more severe than in cystic hydatid disease. Spinal cord involvement associated with root pain and motor or sensory deficits may be observed in both forms of echinococcosis.

Diagnosis

There are no pathognomonic neuroimaging findings for CNS echinococcosis and, in the absence of systemic (lung or liver) involvement, definitive diagnosis usually relies on histological confirmation. Cystic echinococcosis presents on neuroimaging studies as a single, large, non-enhancing lesion (Figure 73.4). Some lesions show calcifications. Cysts located in the subarachnoid space may be multiple and confluent. Epidural cysts have a bi-convex shape or a multilocular appearance, and may be associated with bone erosion. In alveolar echinococcosis, lesions are often multiple, surrounded by edema, and show ring-like enhancement. Computer tomography

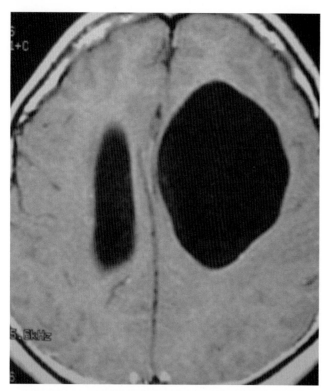

Figure 73.4 T1-weighted magnetic resonance imaging showing cystic echinococcosis in the brain, characterized by a large and round hydatid cyst that displaces midline structures.

(CT) best demonstrates bone erosion in vertebral bodies in patients with echinococcosis of the spinal canal.

Immunological diagnosis is not accurate due to cross-reactions with other parasitic diseases or due to false-negative results in patients with intact cystic hydatid lesions. Nevertheless, serology is more reliable for the diagnosis of alveolar than cystic echinococcosis, particularly to assess response to treatment during the follow-up.

Treatment

There is no level I of evidence favoring any therapeutic regimen for CNS echinococcosis and guidelines are based only on level II or III evidence. Cystic echinococcosis of the brain usually requires surgery. Accidental rupture of the cyst may cause allergic reactions or recurrent hydatid disease due to spillage of the cyst's contents. Experience with albendazole for cerebral cystic echinococcosis is scarce. Albendazole at daily doses of 10–15 mg/kg per day can be given before surgery to prevent hazards of transoperative rupture of cysts or postoperatively to treat recurrent cystic echinococcosis. Clinical deterioration may occur during therapy due to an intense inflammatory reaction surrounding the dying cyst. Concomitant administration of corticosteroids is advised to reduce the risk of such complications.

Treatment of patients with cystic echinococcosis of the spine includes decompressive laminectomy, removal of cysts, excision of involved bone, and stabilization of the spine. Albendazole is advised to reduce the risk of recurrent cystic echinococcosis after surgery.

Surgical removal of alveolar cysts of the brain usually requires resection of adjacent tissue. Albendazole administration should follow or even precede the surgical procedure or may be used as primary therapy for patients with inoperable alveolar echinococcosis. With this approach, 90% of lesions regress or remain static.

Further reading

Baird RA, Zunt JR, Halperin JJ, Gronseth G, Roos KL. Evidence-based guideline: Treatment of parenchymal neurocysticercosis. Report of the Guideline Development Subcommittee of the American Academy of Neurology. *Neurology* 2013;80:1424–1429.

Del Brutto OH. Clinical management of neurocysticercosis. *Expert Rev Neurother* 2014;14:389–396.

Del Brutto OH, Rajshekhar V, White AC, Jr., *et al.* Proposed diagnostic criteria for neurocysticercosis. *Neurology* 2001;57:177–183.

Fleury A, Carrillo-Mezo R, Flisser A, *et al.* Subarachnoid basal neurocysticercosis: A focus on the most severe form of the disease. *Expert Rev Anti-Infect Ther* 2011;9:123–133.

Garcia HH, Nash TE, Del Brutto OH. Clinical symptoms, diagnosis, and treatment of neurocysticercosis. *Lancet Neurol* 2014;13:1202–1215.

Luo K, Luo DH, Zhang TR, Wen H. Primary intracranial and spinal hydatidosis: A retrospective study of 21 patients. *Pathog Glob Health* 2013;107:47–51.

Mahanty S, Garcia HH. Cysticercosis and neurocysticercosis as pathogens affecting the nervous system. *Progress Neurobiol* 2010;91:172–184.

Stojkovic M, Junghanss T. Cystic and alveolar echinococcosis. In: Garcia HH, TanowitzHB, Del Brutto OH (Eds.). *Handbook of Clinical Neurology*, Vol. 114 (3rd series). Amsterdam: Elsevier; 2013: 327–334.

74 Trematodes: Schistosomiasis

Manjari Tripathi

Department of Neurology, All India Institute of Medical Sciences, New Delhi, India

Trematodes are flatworm parasites, otherwise known as flukes. Their life cycle of sexual reproduction occurs in mammalian and other vertebrate definitive hosts. They also undergo asexual reproduction in snails, who are the intermediate hosts. It is important to be able to recognize these as a cause of symptoms, as it is possible to prevent and control infections by preventing egg-containing excreta from contaminating water sources, and controlling and eradicating the snail population by the use of molluscicides. Schistosomiasis is a trematode and is the second most common parasitic infection after malaria. Five species, *S. haematobium, S. mansoni, S. japonicum, S. mekongi*, and *S. intercalatum*, may infect humans. Eggs of the organism have been discovered in Egyptian and Chinese mummies. Today, schistosomiasis affects the lives of millions of people in the developing world.

Epidemiology

According to the 2002 World Health Organization (WHO) Expert Committee report, 79 countries are endemic for *Schistosoma*, with the organism being most abundant in South America, sub-Saharan and Southern Africa, and the Middle East. Additional areas are added to the list every year as a result of international travel and migration.

Pathogenesis

The eggs or parasite can reach the spinal cord retrogradely from portal venous systems through Batson's vertebral plexus (see Figure 74.1). Aberrant migration of parasites, dissemination of eggs via portal-systemic shunts, and emboli from the heart can carry the infection to the brain. Neuroschistosomiasis is produced by a predominantly cellular inflammatory response to antigenic products released by parasite eggs. Infection rates increase in patients co-infected with human immunodeficiency virus (HIV).

Clinical features

The early phase of infection is manifested by a hypersensitivity reaction to schistosomula (aka Katayama fever), characterized by fever, fatigue, malaise, myalgia, right upper quadrant pain, bloody diarrhea, non-productive cough, eosinophilia, and pulmonary infiltrates. Rarely, aseptic meningitis can develop. In the chronic phase, presentation varies depending on the location of the parasite.

Neurological complications can occur during all phases of schistosomiasis, the most common of which is transverse myelitis. In broad terms, neurological involvement can be classified into either cerebral or spinal schistosomiasis.

Cerebral schistosomiasis

Patients with the cerebral form of schistosomiasis may present with acute or subacute onset of headache, altered sensorium, seizures, and focal neurological deficits. Space-occupying lesions with significant mass effect, multiple focal lesions spanning the cerebral hemispheres, as well as non-specific granulomas with surrounding edema are the underlying pathology in most cases. Neurological deficits may be in the form of hemiparesis, visual impairment, dysphasia, or ataxia, depending on the location of these lesions.

In some cases, the picture may resemble that of a malignant cerebral neoplasm with progressive evolution of symptoms and features of raised intracranial pressure.

Rarely, multiple strokes can result from small vessel vasculitis or cardiac embolism due to associated endomyocardial fibrosis. Focal seizures may be the sole manifestation in some cases and are more common with *S. japanicum* infection.

Severe parasitic infection in undernourished children can lead to cognitive impairment. Asymptomatic infection of the brain is also prevalent in endemic regions.

Spinal schistosomiasis

The acute spinal form presents with progressive ascending weakness with bladder, bowel, and/or sexual dysfunction. Lumbar and radicular pain radiating down the legs precedes weakness in the majority of cases. Cauda equina syndrome can also be a typical manifestation of spinal schistosomiasis. Systemic features are usually lacking.

Atypical presentations include progressive myelopathy resembling spinal cord tumor, and anterior spinal artery infarction. A large proportion of patients with myelopathy develop significant disability.

Investigations

Histopathological examination with identification of larva is the gold standard for diagnosis of neuroschistosomiasis. Short of this,

International Neurology, Second edition. Edited by Robert P. Lisak, Daniel D. Truong, William M. Carroll and Roongroj Bhidayasiri
© 2016 John Wiley & Sons, Ltd. Published 2016 by John Wiley & Sons, Ltd.

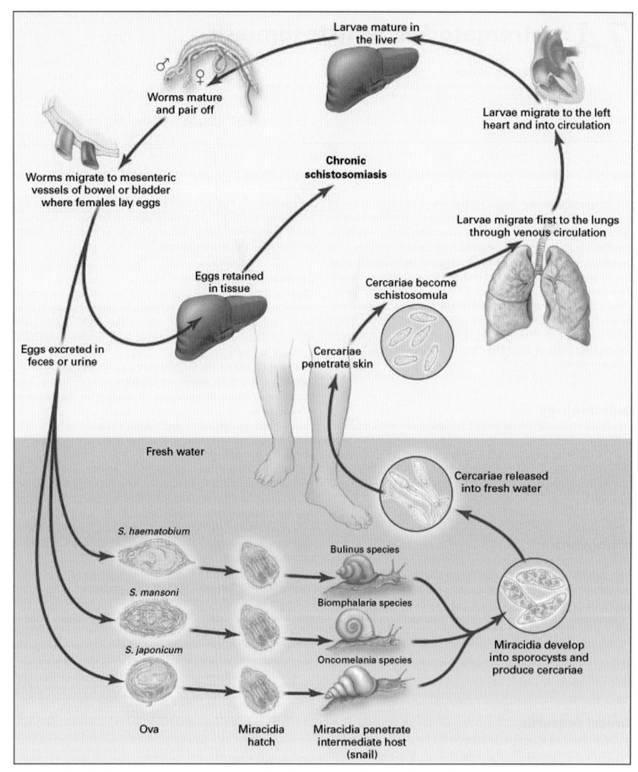

Figure 74.1 Life cycle of *Schistosoma*. Source: Ross 2002. Reproduced by permission of QIMR Berghofer Medical Research Institute.

diagnosis can be made on clinical grounds supported by imaging and laboratory data.

Cerebral lesions may be single or multiple, involving the cerebral hemispheres and occasionally the cerebellum. On magnetic resonance imaging (MRI), lesions appear hyperintense on T2, with surrounding vasogenic edema. Cord lesions are usually isointense on T1 and hyperintense on T2 with cord expansion. Central linear enhancement, surrounded by multiple enhancing punctate nodules, is specific, but peripheral enhancement is equally common.

Table 74.1 Etiology of eosinophilic meningitis.

Infectious	Non-infectious
Parasitic	Malignancy
Angiostrongylus cantonensis	Hodgkin's disease
Gnathostoma spinigerum	Non-Hodgkin's lymphoma
Baylisascaris procyonis	Eosinophilic leukemia
Other helminthes	Medications
Neurocysticercosis	Ciprofloxacin
Cerebral paragonimiasis	Ibuprofen
Neurotrichinosis	Intraventricular vancomycin
Cerebral toxocariasis	Intraventricular gentamicin
Cerebral/spinal schistosomiasis	Intraventricular iophendylate dye
Fungi	Ventriculoperitoneal shunts
Coccidioides immitis	Hypereosinophilic syndrome
Bacteria, rickettsiae, viruses	

Several serological techniques, including enzyme-linked immunosorbent assay (ELISA), indirect hemagglutination, and recently recombinant peptide antigen assay, are used in the diagnosis of *Schistosoma* infection. A positive test is only indicative of prior exposure and hence finds limited use in endemic zones. The other problems encountered in neuroschistosomiasis are delayed seroconversion and cross-reactivity with other helminthic antigens. Cerebrospinal fluid (CSF) examination may reveal elevated protein with mildly reduced glucose, as well as lymphocytes and eosinophils on microscopy. Other specimens, such as urine and stool, rarely show ova with characteristic morphology.

Differential diagnosis (see Table 74.1) includes other causes of eosinophilic meningitis and space-occupying lesions, such as tuberculoma, toxoplasma, neoplasms, abscess, and cysticercosis. Spinal schistosomiasis should be differentiated from transverse myelitis, spinal cord tumors, cysticercosis, tuberculosis, and angiostrongyliasis.

Biopsy of brain and spinal cord lesions reveals granuloma formation with extensive inflammation and vasogenic edema. There can be perilesional gliosis and necrotizing granulomas, with deposits of helminth ova in the center of these granulomas. The granulomas may have multinucleated giant cells around the ova, and a refractile shell with the pathognomonic acentric spine. Mixed inflammatory infiltrates comprised of eosinophils, plasma cells, and lymphocytes are also seen. Calcification and arteritis may also occur.

Treatment

Praziquantel is the drug of choice; a single dose of 40 mg/kg or 60 mg/kg is effective in most cases. However, the doses vary from a single dose to 3–6 days. Treatment does not affect the developing schistosomula and thus may not clear an early infection. Therapeutic failures are not uncommon, but could also be due to reinfection or drug-resistant strains.

Stool examination should be carried out after 3–6 months of treatment. When egg excretion has not decreased, a repeat treatment is needed.

Side effects are mild and include nausea, vomiting, malaise, and abdominal pain. Resistance to praziquantel is an emerging problem in endemic countries, where the drug has been used for several years. Concurrent administration of albendazole may control coexistent helminths, but does not have any impact on the trematode. Corticosteroids (preferably dexamethasone) can be combined with antihelminthics in the spinal and cerebral forms.

A ventriculoperitoneal shunt is required in cases of obstructive hydrocephalus, especially in those caused by posterior fossa lesions. In spinal schistosomiasis, decompressive laminectomy with surgical resection of the lesion and liberation of the roots is indicated in severe cases not responding to medical therapy. However, the real efficacy of surgery is indeed controversial.

Artemether, when given with praziquantel, controls the secondary infection rate. Artemether can also be used as a prophylactic agent for high-risk groups such as flood relief workers, tourists, and fishermen in endemic regions. Vaccines developed against the target antigen glutathione S-transferase are being investigated.

The importance of neurorehabilitative measures in paraplegic patients cannot be overemphasized. However, to make these treatment options available in developing countries is a challenging public health issue.

Further reading

Ferrari TC, Moreira PR. Neuroschistosomiasis: Clinical symptoms and pathogenesis. *Lancet Neurol* 2011;10(9):853–864.

Ferrari TC, Moreira PR, Cunha AS. Spinal cord schistosomiasis: A prospective study of 63 cases emphasizing clinical and therapeutic aspects. *J Clin Neurosci* 2004;11:246–253.

Gryseels B, Polman K, Clerinx J, Kestens L. Human schistosomiasis. *Lancet* 2006;368(9541):1106–1118.

Ross AG, Bartley PB, Sleigh AC, *et al. Schistosomiasis. N Engl J Med* 2002;346:1212–1220.

Szekeres C, Galletout P, Jaureguiberry S, *et al.* Neurological presentation of schistosomiasis. *Lancet* 2013:18;381(9879):1788.

75 Nematodes

Manjari Tripathi

Department of Neurology, All India Institute of Medical Sciences, New Delhi, India

Nematodes are popularly and commonly known as roundworms. They have elongated and symmetric bodies. They have an intestinal system and a large body cavity. These infections are often endemic and present in the developing world. Trichinosis can cause life-threatening manifestations, including myocarditis, central nervous system (CNS) involvement, and pneumonitis, hence a high index of suspicion and early treatment are a must.

Trichinosis

Trichinosis is a parasitic disease caused by infection with *Trichinella spiralis*.

Epidemiology

Humans are infected with trichinosis by consuming contaminated pork or wild game. The disease is common in Africa, Central and South America, Asia (China, Japan, Korea, and Thailand), and Eastern European countries. The life cycle of trichinosis is shown in Figure 75.1.

According to a World Health Organization (WHO) report in 2005, the prevalence rate is 4–20%.

Pathophysiology

The life cycle is maintained by two hosts. Ingestion of the infected flesh of a host is responsible for the infection. Animals associated with trichinosis are rats and pigs. Others are bears, polar bears, cats, walruses, seals, wolves, foxes, and raccoons. After ingestion of raw or partly cooked meat that contains viable larvae, the wall (nurse cell) is digested by the acids in the host's stomach and causes a release of the larvae. The free larvae then move to the small intestine and penetrate the mucosa at the base of villi. They enter the lymph circulation and migrate to vascular, metabolically active skeletal

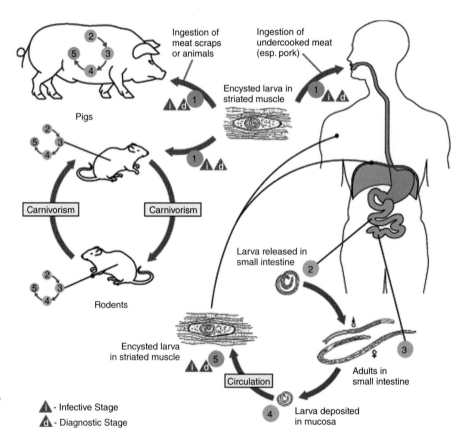

Figure 75.1 Life cycle of Trichinella spiralis.
Source: http://www.cdc.gov/parasites/trichinellosis/biology.html. Reproduced with permission of CDC-DPDx.

International Neurology, Second edition. Edited by Robert P. Lisak, Daniel D. Truong, William M. Carroll and Roongroj Bhidayasiri
© 2016 John Wiley & Sons, Ltd. Published 2016 by John Wiley & Sons, Ltd.

muscles. The most frequently affected muscles are the tongue; diaphragmatic, intercostal, masseter, laryngeal, extraocular, nuchal, intercostal, and pectoral muscles; deltoid, gluteus, biceps, and gastrocnemius. In other tissues, like the myocardium and brain, the larvae disintegrate, resulting in inflammation.

The larvae grow over 3 weeks until they reach a size of 400 × 260 µm; however, they can be double this size too. They may persist for 6 months to several years before calcification and death. The life cycle is complete when a host ingests the infected muscle.

Clinical features

Severity of infection ranges from asymptomatic to fatal. Initial symptoms may include nausea, diarrhea, fever, headache, maculopapular rash, periorbital and facial edema, chemosis, trismus, and dysphagia. Myalgia is common, particularly in the calf and forearm, and is often associated with edema and spasm. Myocarditis may occur in severe infection.

CNS involvement is seen in 10–20% of cases, usually in patients with severe Trichinella infection. Such cases present with agitated behavior, delirium, and headache. Cranial nerve deficits, paresis, aphasia, convulsions, and cerebellar syndromes may occur. Venous infarction and intracerebral bleed are rare.

Investigations

The eosinophil count is often above 300/mm³ and increases 10–12 days after infection. Absence of eosinophilia may indicate a poor prognosis. The erythrocyte sedimentation rate (ESR) and creatine phosphokinase (CPK) may be elevated.

Electromyography findings are myopathic, with muscle irritation presenting as fibrillation potentials. Muscle biopsy, which may yield false-negative results if performed in the first 2 weeks of infection, is necessary to confirm diagnosis. Microscopically, specimens reveal motile larvae coiled within a connective tissue pseudocyst.

Enzyme-linked immunosorbent assay (ELISA) is specific for the excretory–secretory product of muscle larvae and for the tyvelose antigen. Cerebrospinal fluid (CSF) shows mildly elevated protein, occasional eosinophilia, and, rarely, larvae. Brain computed tomography (CT) may show multiple small hypodense lesions in the cerebral cortex and white matter. Small intracerebral bleeds and infarcts have been reported on magnetic resonance imaging (MRI).

Myalgia with extraocular muscle involvement can be seen in thyrotoxic ophthalmopathy, pseudotumor oculi, or extra-ocular infiltration due to other causes.

Differential diagnosis of trichinosis infection includes myositis and a wide range of CNS syndromes and infections. Positive results from at least two screening tests are required to confirm diagnosis.

Treatment

Albendazole at 800 mg/kg in 4 divided doses for 7 to 14 days is the recommended treatment. Steroids may be needed in severe infection to prevent a Jarisch–Herxheimer-like reaction. Symptomatic treatment includes analgesics and antipyretics.

Gnathostomiasis

Gnathostomiasis is caused by several species of Gnathostoma, particularly *Gnathostoma spinigerum*.

Epidemiology

Humans are infected by eating raw or undercooked fish, poultry, or pork. Infection is most prevalent in Thailand, followed by Japan, Mexico, Myanmar, China, India, the Philippines, Malaysia, Sri Lanka, Indonesia, Australia, Laos, Cambodia, Vietnam, and Ecuador.

Pathophysiology

The definitive hosts are dogs, cats, tigers, leopards, lions, mink, opossums, raccoons, and otters. Adult worms live in them as a tumor in the stomach wall. Eggs are shed from this into the feces. After one week, the eggs turn into larvae, which hatch and are ingested by the first intermediate host, *Cyclops*. The copepods are then ingested by the definitive hosts (e.g., fish, snakes, frogs, chicken, pigs), in whom they penetrate the gastric wall, migrate to muscles, and mature to third-stage larvae before getting encysted.

Human infection occurs when persons eat third-stage larvae in raw and undercooked meat, or if they drink or bathe in water contaminated with larvae or infested copepods. The larvae may migrate in the body for as long as 10–12 years.

Symptoms result from mechanical destruction of tissues caused by the migration, by toxins that resemble acetylcholine, protease, hemolysin hyaluronidase, and host response.

Clinical features

Eosinophilic myeloradiculitis and eosinophilic meningitis are the main neurological syndromes associated with gnathostomiasis.

Patients with eosinophilic myeloradiculitis present with severe radicular pains involving limbs, trunk, cervical, and perianal regions, accompanied by motor, sensory, and autonomic dysfunction. Meningeal symptoms may be associated. Cranial nerve palsies, headache, visual impairment, and altered sensorium may be seen in high cervical cord lesions.

Patients with eosinophilic meningitis present with headache, vomiting, photophobia, and nuchal stiffness. Fever is uncommon. Seizures, altered sensorium, and cranial nerve palsies can occur. Intracerebral and subarachnoid hemorrhages are not uncommon and the usual presentation is agonizing neuritic bursting headache followed by stroke or decreased sensorium over a few days. Mortality is seen in 7–25% of cases (see Table 75.1). Neurological sequelae are common in 30–40% of cases.

Investigations

In CSF, white blood cell count (WBC) greater than 500 cells/µL and eosinophilia (>10%) with raised protein and normal or mildly

Table 75.1 Differentiating features between gnathostomiasis and angiostrongyliasis.

Feature	Gnathostomiasis	Angiostrongyliasis
Root pain	Prominent	Rare
Illness	Severe	Less severe
Complications	Coma with respiratory failure	Coma without respiratory failure
Cerebrospinal fluid	Clear/xanthochromic, with red blood cells	Clear/turbid, no red blood cells
White blood cell count	<500/µL	500–2000/µL
Eosinophilia	60% of cases	>95% of cases
Magnetic resonance imaging	Focal lesions and large hemorrhagic tracts	Small hemorrhagic tracts
Other	Intracerebral/subarachnoid hemorrhage and bleeding in brainstem	

reduced glucose, red blood cells (RBC), and xanthochromia may be observed.

Fuzzy white-matter hyperintensities, multiple intracerebral hemorrhages, basal ganglia hyperintensities, and nodular enhancement are noted on brain MRI. Hyperintense intramedullary lesions with cord expansion are seen on spine MRI.

CT scan is helpful to detect subarachnoid blood in the acute setting. CT may also reveal obstructive hydrocephalus, or meningeal inflammation.

Leucocytosis with eosinophilia (exceed 50% of the circulating WBC) may be present, particularly during the active phase of larval migration. Microscopic hematuria may be present.

In terms of serology, ELISA and Western blot are promising diagnostic tests. Immunoblot testing for neurological disease has been described. Surgical resection may help in making the diagnosis by revealing larvae in the skin, subcutaneous tissue, gingivae, or wounds. Tissue will show eosinophils, with fibroblasts, histiocytes, and foreign-body giant cells, and an eosinophilic granuloma. Migratory tracts may be present, with perivascular infiltration of eosinophils, plasma cells, and lymphocytes. No CNS granuloma or parasite fragments are seen.

Differential diagnosis for the cerebral form includes tuberculoma, toxoplasma, neoplasms, abscess, and cysticercosis; the spinal form includes other causes of transverse myelopathy.

A quick protein microarray is available for the rapid screening of patients suspected of infection.

Treatment
Corticosteroids can produce symptomatic relief and must be used when giving albendazole, as even a single use of albendazole may increase intracranial pressure and inflammatory reaction. Treatment failures may need ivermectin.

Angiostrongyliasis
Angiostrongyliasis, caused by the parasite Angiostrongylus cantonensis, is the most common cause of eosinophilic meningitis.

Epidemiology
Humans become infected by ingestion of raw or undercooked terrestrial snails and slugs, or via transport hosts such as freshwater prawns, frogs, fish, and planarians, and, rarely, contaminated lettuce. Major outbreaks have been reported in Thailand, Taiwan, Hawaii, Vietnam, Malaysia, Indonesia, the Philippines, Japan, Papua New Guinea, and the United States. The disease is most common in young adults and children, with male predominance seen in some reports.

Pathophysiology
The nematode is present in the pulmonary arteries of rodents; it is thus known as the rat lungworm. Snails and slugs are the intermediate hosts for larvae development. Humans are incidental hosts and become infected by ingestion of larvae in raw or undercooked snails and from contaminated water and vegetables. The larvae then migrate via the blood to the CNS. The pathogenesis of symptoms can occur due to direct mechanical damage to the CNS by the worms' motion, toxic products like nitrogenous waste, and antigens released by the parasite.

Clinical features
The typical neurological syndrome is eosinophilic meningitis. Patients present with headache, retro-orbital pain, nuchal stiffness, photophobia, and visual blurring. Systemic features include fatigue, malaise, myalgia, paresthesias, abdominal pain, vomiting, and rash. Fever has been reported in some outbreaks. Cranial nerve palsies, behavioral disturbances, seizures, myeloradiculitis, and persistent cognitive impairment may also occur. The disease usually takes a benign course with neurological sequel. Coma and mortality are rare (see Table 75.1).

Investigations
CSF is clear or mildly turbid. WBC is 150–2000 cells/µL. Eosinophils are greater than 10%. Protein is elevated. Glucose may be normal or reduced. Peripheral blood eosinophilia may be observed.

MRI shows multiple hyperintense signals in the cerebral hemispheres, white matter, and cerebellum. Enhancing lesions in the cisterns, stick-like pial enhancement, basal ganglia hyperintensities, prominent Virchow–Robin spaces, and linear tracks are also seen.

Immunoblot ELISA confirms the diagnosis. Recently, an ELISA for IgG1 antibodies has been developed. The intrathecal synthesis pattern of IgG1+IgG2 and IgE can also contribute to the diagnosis. The sensitivity of ELISA tests may approach 100%. The dot-ELISA is also promising. For antigen detection, immunodot, a rapid and simple test, has been developed using specific *A. cantonensis* monoclonal antibody (AW-3C2). The diagnostic specificity approaches 100%, and the sensitivity is around 60%. A more sensitive method for antigen detection, the immuno-PCR, detects circulating 204-kDa AcL5 antigen in patients with 100% specificity and 98% sensitivity.

Treatment
Albendazole administered for 2 weeks may reduce headache. Corticosteroids produce symptomatic relief.

Further reading
Chen JX, Chen MX, Ai L, *et al.* A protein microarray for the rapid screening of patients suspected of infection with various food-borne helminthiases. *PLoS Negl Trop Dis* 2012;6(11):e1899.

Eamsobhana P, Yong HS. Immunological diagnosis of human angiostrongyliasis due to *Angiostrongylus cantonensis* (Nematoda: Angiostrongylidae). *Int J Infect Dis* 2009;13(4):425–431.

Lo Re V, III, Gluckman SJ. Eosinophilic meningitis. *Am J Med* 2003;114(3):217–223.

Pozio E, Gomez Morales MA, Dupouy-Camet J. Clinical aspects, diagnosis and treatment of trichinellosis. *Expert Rev Anti Infect Ther* 2003;1:471–482.

Punyagupta S, Juttijudata P, Bunnag T. Eosinophilic meningitis in Thailand. Clinical studies of 484 typical cases probably caused by *Angiostronglus cantonensis*. *Am J Trop Med Hyg* 1975;17:551–561.

76 Fungal infections of the central nervous system

Thomas Cesario

School of Medicine, University of California Irvine, Orange, CA, USA

Fungal infections of the central nervous system (CNS) are less common than bacterial infections, but can be devastating and difficult to treat. While they can exist in nature as primary pathogens, particularly in certain cases such as coccidioidal meningitis, they are often pathogenic agents that prey on compromised patients. This chapter will discuss fungal infections of the CNS in humans.

Candidiasis

Among the most commonly encountered fungi are members of the Candida genus. These include agents such as *Candida albicans, Candida glabrata, Candida parapsilosis,* and *Candida tropicalis.* These are organisms that can be found on the normal host, especially after antibiotic therapy, or they may exist in patients predisposed to colonization by these organisms, such as individuals with diabetes mellitus. These agents are well-known pathogens in patients with acquired immune deficiency syndrome (AIDS), transplant patients, and patients receiving chemotherapy. Additionally, they may be encountered in neonates and individuals suffering from congenital immune deficiency diseases. Candida organisms exist worldwide and thus can be found virtually anywhere.

One of the largest reviews of *Candida* meningitis described 18 cases of chronic meningitis, including 3 infants and 15 adults, 9 of whom had underlying disease. Headache was common, as was fever, and the sensorium was altered in some patients as well. Symptoms often existed for long periods prior to diagnosis and in one case as long as 21 months. Cerebrospinal fluid (CSF) findings typically showed a pleocytosis, but in some cases polymorphonuclear cells predominated, while in others there was a lymphocytic predominance. Cultures of the CSF grew *Candida* but with some difficulty, often requiring repeated taps and special efforts. Amphotericin plus flucytosine was the preferred treatment and eight patients were ultimately cured of infection.

Candida meningitis has also been reported in neonates in association with disseminated infection, prematurity being a risk factor. The clinical features are similar to those of other systemic infections, although CSF findings seem somewhat inconsistent. Similarly, *Candida* meningitis has been reported in both children and adults with cancer and in individuals infected with human immunodeficiency virus (HIV). This infection may occur in adults as either an isolated CNS infection or as part of disseminated candidiasis. It has also been reported in neurosurgical patients, especially those with CSF shunts in place. Several authors have commented on the relatively prolonged course of the disease, and

in general about half the patients died. The best prognosis seems to be in patients with CSF shunts when the device is removed and the patients treated as noted earlier. The diagnosis is often made by culture of the CSF, although more than one lumbar puncture may be needed to find the organism. There may also be other inflammatory CNS changes. Authors agree that patients at least initially should be treated with amphotericin and flucytosine, but newer antifungals like micafungin and anidulafungin may turn out to be equal or better alternatives.

Aspergillosis

Aspergillus species may also infect the CNS. This is typically due to *Aspergillus fumigatus.* These organisms are ubiquitous in nature, being found in soil, water, and organic materials. They typically do not pose a threat for the immunocompetent patient, even though they are occasionally cultured from sites in the body, particularly after broad spectrum antibiotic therapy. In contrast, they may induce disease in compromised individuals, including cancer patients, especially those with hematological malignancies, transplant patients, HIV-infected patients, individuals receiving high-dose steroid therapy, or other people in immunocompromised states. The organisms may produce a meningitis or localized aspergillomas. In many cases, *Aspergillus* tends to invade blood vessels and as such may induce vascular obstruction with downstream consequences, including stroke. Typically patients have disease due to this organism in one or more organs, especially including the lungs. The findings in patients with CNS aspergilloma are typically those associated with mass lesions, including focal neurological deficits and mental status changes. Seizures are common clinical manifestations of CNS aspergillosis. Meningitis occurs in a similar setting and may be manifest by fever, mental status changes, seizures, and focal deficits. Meningeal signs are uncommon. Attempts to culture the organism can be met with frustration, but *Aspergillus* may be cultured from other organs, since it typically is part of a disseminated infection, with the brain being a key site for spread. Galactomannan and 1,3-b-D-glucan may be found in the serum or CSF of patients with aspergillosis of the central nervous system. Where lesions are localized, surgical intervention plus antifungal therapy may be critical, but where the disease involves the meninges or is diffuse, antifungal therapy, including typically either voriconazole, posaconazole, itraconazole, or caspofungin, should be instituted as soon as possible. Prognosis is guarded at best.

International Neurology, Second edition. Edited by Robert P. Lisak, Daniel D. Truong, William M. Carroll and Roongroj Bhidayasiri
© 2016 John Wiley & Sons, Ltd. Published 2016 by John Wiley & Sons, Ltd.

Cryptococcosis

Unlike *Candida* or *Aspergillus,* which may be found colonizing in patients, *Cryptococcus* and the fungi described subsequently are typically not found as passive agents growing along with other flora. These agents are encapsulated yeasts that can be detected in nature. There are two distinct types of *Cryptococcus* that are known to be pathogenic. These include *Cryptococcus neoformans* (especially variant *grubii*) and *Cryptococcus gattii.* Cryptococci are found throughout the world in areas where bird droppings are common, especially around areas frequented by pigeons or chickens, particularly if rotting vegetation is in the vicinity. The *gatii* variety is cultured from river red gum trees and forest red gum trees, which are common to Australia. They have also been found in other areas, particularly if the trees have been exported to these locations. Thus the *gatii* variant has been found in California.

CNS infection with cryptococci is a threat to the immunocompromised; however, occasional cases have occurred in immunocompetent individuals, especially due to *C. gatti.* While infection of the lung can be seen in individuals without apparent underlying disease, this is usually not the case with infection in the nervous system. HIV/AIDS is the main predisposing factor in cryptococcal meningitis, accounting for 95% of cases in low- and middle-income countries and 80% in high-income countries. It is estimated that the annual burden of cryptococcal meningitis is almost a million cases, primarily in sub-Saharan Africa and Southeast Asia. The cellular immune system is critical in controlling this organism. When this system is intact, the organism tends to be confined to the lung, where it is initially inhaled. Thus cryptococcal pneumonia, lung nodules, or lung abscesses may be seen in otherwise normal patients. These may resolve on their own. On the other hand, when underlying disease like hematological malignancies, AIDS, or severe pharmacological immune suppression is present, as in organ transplantation, this organism may escape the lung and target other organs for metastatic infections. The preferred extrapulmonary site in these patients is the meninges, although prostate, skin, and bones are targeted to a lesser extent. In the years before effective AIDS treatment was available, 5–10% of AIDS patients developed cryptococcal meningitis in the United States and as many as 30% of African AIDS patients acquired this disease. Typically, 300–500 cases of non-AIDS cryptococcal meningitis will be seen annually among the US population of 300 million.

The manifestations of disease in AIDS patients are slightly different than in other immune-suppressed patients, but in general the signs and symptoms of cryptococcal disease in the CNS are similar. Typically, the most significant findings are those associated with chronic meningitis. The incubation period is often weeks and can be longer than a month. Generally, in the more immune-suppressed patients this period will be shorter. Disease onset is typically associated with headache and there may also be altered consciousness, focal neurological signs, and indications of increased intracranial pressure like papilledema when obstruction to the flow of the CSF occurs. Fever and meningismus may or may not be present. Signs and symptoms of CNS cryptococcal infection may be gradually progressive over many months and indeed even over years, but invariably if the disease is left untreated the ultimate result is death. Complications may, however, occur. These include blindness and intracranial hypertension.

In addition to meningitis, cryptococci in the brain may produce mass lesions that typically present as other space-occupying masses.

Diagnosis of the CNS infection is made typically by examination of the CSF. The cryptococcal latex agglutination test (LACT) and more recently the cryptococcal lateral flow immunoassay have become major diagnostic aids. In addition to its use in the CSF, indirect diagnostic assistance is often offered by the serum LACT. Thus the serum test is positive in 70% of non-AIDS patients and over 90% of AIDS patients if infection of the CNS is present. The organism is also cultured in many cases on ordinary bacterial culture media. Besides the CSF, the organism may be cultured from other sites in the body such as the bone marrow, blood, or urine. The CSF, in cases of cryptococcal meningitis, also commonly will have 10–100 cells/mL, usually with a lymphocytic predominance, but this is not invariable. Low CSF glucose and higher CSF protein concentrations may be present and likely correlate with the disease duration and burden of the fungi. The LACT needs to be titered in the CSF, as it is a therapeutic index and has significant prognostic implications. Culture of the CSF is important. If examination of the CSF is precluded because of severe intracranial hypertension or mass effect, attempts to culture the organisms from other sites and the serum LACT may be useful as indirect aids to diagnosis. Radiological examinations including computed tomography (CT) and magnetic resonance imaging (MRI) have no diagnostic abnormality specific to cryptococcal disease, but may have changes similar to those seen in other cases of chronic meningitis or mass lesions.

It is generally agreed that therapy should be initiated with amphotericin (0.7–1.0 mg/kg/day) plus flucytosine (100–150 mg/kg/day in four divided doses) for the first 2 weeks, followed by oral fluconazole (400 mg/day) if the patient improves. If the patient fails to improve or has poor prognostic indicators, a repeat lumbar puncture should be performed to ensure response, although many agree that regular lumbar punctures are important, at least in HIV/AIDS cryptococcal meningitis patients, to decrease intracranial pressure or to follow both the inflammatory and microbiological course of the disease. The amphotericin/flucytosine combination should be continued if the initial response to therapy is poor until cultures are negative. Antifungal treatment including fluconazole should be continued until the cultures are negative and the LACT titer falls to levels <1–8. Other CSF abnormalities are expected to return to normal during treatment. AIDS patients in particular should receive continuous suppressive treatment with fluconazole at 200 mg/day when patients have completed the course of therapy as already outlined.

Patients do need to be continuously followed after treatment to ensure that relapse does not occur, and retreatment is necessary. This includes repeat lumbar puncture at periodic intervals until the patient has been normal without evidence of relapse for at least 1 year. The majority of patients will do well, but bad prognostic indicators include the severity of the underlying disease, very high CSF LACT titers, and failure to respond to treatment.

The course of treatment outlined generally yields good results and has reduced the mortality rate to between 9 and 55%, dependent in part on the population being studied and availability of effective pharmacological interventions.

Coccidioidomycosis

Coccidioides immitis and *Coccidioides posadasil* are dimorphic fungi that grow in semiarid regions of the world. This includes certain parts of the southwestern United States, northern Mexico, areas in Guatamala and Nicaragua in Central America, and places in Bolivia, Paraguay, Venezuela, Argentina, and Columbia in South America. Current environmental and demographic factors have allowed for an increase in the number of cases in the southwest of the United States. The organisms grow in their saprobic states a few inches below the surface. They form small regions on their filaments called arthroconidia, which are prone to break free. When the dry season comes they are often aerosolized, particularly when disturbances like windy conditions occur. These are the infectious units for humans. Arthoconidia can be carried long distances if winds are severe. When inhaled, within 2 days the arthroconidia are converted to the parasitic form, which is a spherule. These enlarge and ultimately contain multiple endospores. While inhalation from the soil has been the almost exclusive means by which humans acquire the fungus, rare reports of alternative means have occurred. The organism is quite infectious and individuals living in endemic areas have a skin test conversion rate of 3% per year.

When inhaled, *Coccidioides* initially becomes an infection of the lung. Most patients with this early infection remain without symptoms and those that are symptomatic usually have mild symptoms that do not precipitate a visit to a physician. The incubation period for the pulmonary symptoms is 7–21 days. While up to half of patients may have some radiographic evidence of infection in the lung, only 5–10% of patients develop pulmonary residuals, including cavitary lesions. Erythema nodosum and erythema multiforme are also seen during the infection. While the organism may escape the lung, patients with intact cellular immune systems rarely develop complications from dissemination. However, there are certain ethnic groups prone to develop disease from dissemination and these include Filipinos, Mexicans, and black people. In addition, pregnant women, especially in the third trimester, patients receiving immunosuppressant drugs including steroids, those with diabetes, patients with hematological malignancies, and particularly those with AIDS may experience severe problems from dissemination.

Less than 1% of patients develop disseminated disease that requires medical attention. The usual sites where the presence of the fungus becomes evident include the meninges, bone – particularly the vertebrae and joints – skin, and components of the genitourinary system. The meninges, however, are among the most important and most frequent of these. Patients who develop coccidioidal meningitis have headache, which is often one of the first signs, and as the disease progresses will develop other signs and symptoms that may include gait disturbances, focal findings, altered consciousness, cranial nerve signs, and papilledema as evidence of basilar meningeal inflammation. Fever and weight loss are common and meningismus may be seen in about half the cases. Left untreated the disease will inevitably progress to death within 2 years. Complications include hydrocephalus in 30–50% of patients, and infarction of the brain can occur if an infectious vasculitis results from the inflammatory process.

The diagnosis of coccidioidal meningitis rests largely on the examination of the CSF. The cell count is usually between 100 and 1500 cells per mL^3, most of which will be lymphocytes in the typical case. In addition, especially as the disease progresses, the glucose level in the CSF will fall and the protein level will rise to concentrations in the range of 250 mg percent. Higher concentrations occur with obstruction to the flow of the CSF. The organism may be cultured from the CSF, but only in about 15% of cases. The specific diagnosis is usually made by detection of antibodies in the CSF, often using the complement fixation method. Repeated examinations, however, are sometimes necessary to find the antibody in spinal fluid, but it is usually detectable within 3 weeks after the onset of symptoms.

Reasonably effective treatment exists. Fluconazole in doses of 400–800 mg/day is recommended. Patients should begin to experience symptomatic relief after the onset of treatment, but if they continue to progress and show evidence of failing to respond, intrathecal amphotericin should be initiated. This may be delivered intracisternally or through an Ommaya reservoir. Doses are adjusted beginning with 0.01 mg and increasing as tolerated, with a maximum dose of 1.5 mg. The dosing interval may also be adjusted from daily to even weekly as needed and as tolerated. With this regimen it can be expected that 75–80% of patients will respond. Other agents may also be effective, including itraconazole, posaconazole, and lipid encapsulated amphotericin. There is less experience with these other agents.

Mucormycosis (zygomycosis)

The Phycomycetes are an order of fungi that includes both the Mucorales and the Entomophthorales, which are agents responsible for nasal diseases. The Mucorales include three species of filamentous agents that are largely responsible for the disease of mucormycosis. These are ubiquitous agents found in the environment and frequently encountered by humans through the aerosol route, but only immunocompromised patients are at serious risk of consequences from these fungi. Thus those with diabetes, especially when acidotic, patients on steroids, individuals with hematologic malignancies, transplant patients, AIDS patients, those with renal or hepatic failure, malnourished patients, or individuals with immune deficiencies face a significant threat from these agents. Rarely, people who have no underlying disease encounter problems from these organisms.

The most common form of nervous system infection with the Phycomycetes is rhinocerebral mucormycosis. This begins in the sinuses and nasal cavities and gradually erodes through tissues and in blood vessels to invade intracranial structures and cause infarction of cerebral tissue. The symptoms often include nasal stuffiness, purulent nasal discharge, sinus pain, and headache. Signs include fever, black eschars in the nose and sometimes on the hard palate, periorbital edema, proptosis, and eventually blindness. These signs and symptoms relate to the route by which the fungus spread. Cavernous sinus thrombosis may occur and when the frontal lobes become involved, obtundation may result. Less common instances of isolated metastatic lesions to the brain have also been reported, with the findings related to the mass effect and location of the lesion.

Diagnosis is established by demonstration of the fungal filaments in tissue sections. Current therapy includes amphotericin and extensive surgical debridement. Experimentally there is some evidence that posaconazole may be useful. With maximal therapy the mortality rate ranges from 25–75%, depending in part on the underlying disease and the stage at which diagnosis is established and treatment undertaken.

Histoplasmosis

Histoplasma capsulatum is a dimorphic fungus whose physical state is related to the temperature of its environment. In nature it is in the mycelial state and in humans it is generally in the yeast phase. Moist, shady soil, fertilized with bird or bat droppings in moderate climates, is the favored environment for the organism. *Histoplasma* has been found in the United States in the Mississippi and Ohio river valleys. It has also been found in Latin America and along the St. Lawrence river. In addition, cases have been identified in Europe and Asia, but the specific location of the organism in those regions is less well known.

Humans acquire *Histoplasma* by inhaling the infectious microconidia. The vast majority of infections are without symptoms and only about 5% will develop a self-limited flu-like illness. Most problematic cases evolve into subacute pulmonary infections with focal infiltrates and hilar or mediastinal nodes. Cavities may result. Nodular lung lesions may go on to calcify. It is the immunocompromised who fail to contain the organism and allow dissemination to become a serious disease for the host. This can become a systemic disease with multiorgan involvement, including mucous membranes, liver, spleen, and bone marrow. Of these cases, 5–25% will develop CNS disease. This may be either solid intracerebral lesions or basilar meningitis. The solid lesions will present as mass lesions and the basilar meningitis may have the typical meningeal array of signs and symptoms, including fever, meningismus, and abnormal CSF. Diagnosis is established by culture (25–50% positive) or detection of antigen or antibody in the CSF. Often it is necessary, however, to establish a diagnosis by culture of the organism from other sites, particularly bone marrow, detection of antigen especially in urine or serum, or identification of antibody in serum. Treatment consists of amphotericin (1.0–1.5 g total dose given over 30–40 administrations) or lipid encapsulated amphotericin (3–5 mg/kg/day to a total dose of 100–150 g) daily for 6–12 weeks, followed by suppression with itraconazole (200 mg twice or three times per day) or fluconazole (600–800 mg/day). With this regimen there is a 20% failure rate, but the relapse rate can be as high as 40%.

Blastomycosis

Blastomyces dermatitidis is another dimorphic fungus that has been reported from North and South America, Europe, Africa, and Asia. There is insufficient information about the environment in which it exists, but it appears to be a soil organism that exists along riverbeds, particularly in areas with organic matter as a part of the soil. The pathogenesis of the disease is very similar to histoplasmosis, with the organism entering the lung and primary disease being pulmonary in nature. Dissemination can occur, but in contrast blastomycosis is primarily a disease of the immunocompetent and can affect skin, bone, genitourinary tract, and CNS. Approximately 10% of cases involve the CNS. Less is known of blastomycosis in the CNS because there have been fewer reports of this entity, but it appears to cause either nodular lesions in the brain or a basilar meningitis. The CNS disease has the same features as histoplasmosis, but is more difficult to diagnose, as culture from the CSF appears harder and serologies are less reliable. Besides culturing multiple sites in the body, particularly bone marrow, involved tissue, and urine, serologies should be done and biopsies with histological examination for the organism carried out. The only treatment known so far is amphotericin followed by long-term azole therapy.

Fungal infections associated with contaminated steroid injections

In 2012 the first case of CNS infection with an unusual fungal species was detected in Tennessee in the United States. Within a short time it became apparent that there was a large-scale outbreak associated with contaminated methylprednisolone used to reduce inflammation in various joints, including those in the spine. Ultimately, 749 cases of infection were reported in 20 states and 265 had infection of the CNS or related tissues. The syndromes included meningitis, stroke, arachnoiditis, epidural or intradural abscesses, and paraspinal bone, disc, or facet joint infection. The responsible organism was found to be *Exserohilum rostratum*. Of 328 patients for whom analysis was possible, 26 died.

Further reading

Friedman JA, Wijdicks FM, Fulgham J, Wright AJ. Meningoencephalitis due to Blastomyces dermatitidis. *Mayo Clin Proc* 2000;75:403–408.

Johnson R, Einstein H. Coccidioidal meningitis. *Clin Infect Dis* 2006;42:103–107.

Kleinschmidt-Demasters BK. Central nervous system aspergillosis: A 20 year retrospective study. *Human Pathology* 2002;33:116–124.

Mathiesen G, Shelub A, Truong J, Wigen C. Coccidioidal meningitis: Clinical presentation and management in the fluconazole era. *Medicine* 2010;89:251–84.

Shih CC, Chen YC, Chang SC, Luh KT, Hsieh WC. Cryptococcal meningitis in non HIV infected patients. *Q J Med* 2000;93:245–251.

Sloan D, Parris V. Cryptococcal meningitis: Epidemiology and therapeutic options. *Clin Epidemiol* 2014;6:169–182.

Smith R, Schaefer M, Kainer M, et al. Fungal infections associated with contaminated methylprednisolone injections. *N Eng J Med* 2013;369:1508–1609.

Sundaram C, Mahadevan A, Laxmi V, et al. Cerebral zygomycosis. *Mycoses* 2005;48:396–340.

Voice RA, Bradley SF, Sangeorzan JA, Kauffman CA. Chronic candidal meningitis: An uncommon manifestation of candidiasis. *Clin Infect Dis* 1994;19:60–66.

Wheat LJ, Musial CE, Jenny-Avital E. Diagnosis and management of central nervous system histoplasmosis. *Clin Infect Dis* 2005;40:844–852.

77 Rickettsial disease

Kelly J. Baldwin[1] and Narendra Rathi[2]

[1] Department of Neurology, Neuro-Infectious Disease, Geisinger Medical Center, Danville, PA, USA
[2] Rathi Children Hospital, Akola, India

The classification of the Rickettsiaceae family has undergone important changes over the past 20 years due to the generalization of the use of gene sequencing and genetic phylogeny. In this chapter, we will focus on Rickettsiae that are pathogenic for humans. Rickettsiae are intracellular alpha proteobacteria associated with eucaryotic hosts (arthropods or helminthes). Based on antigenic and genetic data, Rickettsiae are divided into three groups: (1) the spotted fever group (SFG), which accounts for most tick-borne rickettsioses; (2) the typhus group (TG), which includes *Rickettsia prowazekii*, the agent of epidemic typhus, transmitted by body louse, and *Rickettsia typhi*, the agent of murine typhus, transmitted by rat and cat fleas; and (3) *Orientia tsutsugamushi*, the agent of scrub typhus, transmitted by mites.

Until recently, the diagnosis of rickettsioses was confirmed almost exclusively by serological methods. Serology does not allow discrimination between rickettsiae belonging to the same group. As all these tests detect antibodies, they would be able to make a diagnosis only after 5–7 days of disease onset and hence play no role for initiation of therapy in a suspected case. The recognition of multiple distinct rickettsioses during the last 20 years has been greatly facilitated by the broad use of cell culture systems, molecular methods for the identification of rickettsiae, and polymerase chain reaction (PCR). As a consequence, over a dozen additional rickettsial species or subspecies have been identified as emerging rickettsioses. Another consequence is that there are multiple species of rickettsiose in each country. Several new species were identified in arthropod vectors prior to being isolated in humans. Description of the known rickettsioses could have included these new emerging rickettsioses, which can explain variable clinical descriptions of the first described rickettsioses.

Symptomatic evidence of central nervous system (CNS) involvement is a frequent feature in rickettsial infections. In a large clinical case series of patients with rickettsial disease, abnormal neurological finding (28%) was the most common complication of rickettsial diseases and included encephalopathy (15%), meningitis (5%), meningoencephalitis (5%), and encephalitis (3%). CNS involvement is a result of the systemic nature of these infections and their propensity for invasion of endothelial cells. The degree of insult to the CNS varies according to the various rickettsial infections.

Epidemiology

The geographic and temporal distribution of rickettsioses is mainly determined by their vectors (Table 77.1, Figure 77.1). Louse-transmitted diseases occur worldwide. Lice parasitize poor people, preferentially in cold places and during wars. Common fleas such as dog, cat, and rat fleas are reported worldwide, as are their transmitted diseases, murine typhus and flea-borne spotted fever (caused by *Rickettsia felis*). Tick species are highly dependent on their environment; very few are found worldwide, with the exception of *Rhipicephalus sanguineus*, the dog tick, vector of *Rickettsia conorii* (in the Old World). Therefore, tick-transmitted diseases are usually restricted to parts of the world where they can be fed by the local fauna.

Table 77.1 Main clinical and epidemiological features of Rickettsiae infection.

Group	Organism	Arthropod vector	Main clinical features	Prominent neurological features
Spotted fever group				
Rocky Mountain spotted fever	*Rickettsia rickettsii*	Tick	No eschar. Rash often purpuric. High fever, 2–5% fatality rate.	Headache (>80%), stupor (20%), meningitis (>20%), ataxia (20%), coma (20%), seizures (10%), decreased hearing (10%), papilledema (<10%)
Mediterranean spotted fever Kenya tick typhus	*Rickettsia conorii*	Tick	Single eschar or popular rash. High fever, 2–5% fatality rate	Encephalitis, meningitis, meningoencephalitis Deafness, central nerve palsies, Guillain–Barré polyneuropathy
Israeli spotted fever	*Rickettsia conorii israelensis*	Tick	Eschar rare, rash, high fever	Encephalitis, meningitis, meningoencephalitis
Astrakhan fever	*Rickettsia conorii astrakhan*	Tick	Eschar rare, maculopapular rash (100%), high fever	Hearing loss (14%)
Indian tick typhus	*Rickettsia conorii indica*	Tick	Rash usually purpuric. Eschar rarely found. No lymphadenopathy.	
Siberian tick typhus	*Rickettsia sibirica*	Tick	Rash (100%), eschar (77%), high fever	Encephalitis. Rare, usually mild

(Continued)

International Neurology, Second edition. Edited by Robert P. Lisak, Daniel D. Truong, William M. Carroll and Roongroj Bhidayasiri
© 2016 John Wiley & Sons, Ltd. Published 2016 by John Wiley & Sons, Ltd.

Lymphangitis associated rickettsioses	*Rickettsia sibirica mongolitimonae*	Tick	Eschar (75%) may be multiple, rash (63%), lymphangitis (25%), and adenopathy. Ropelike lymphangitis between eschar and lymph node	Meningitis, cerebellitis (2 unreported cases)
Japanese spotted fever	*Rickettsia japonica*	Tick	Eschar (91%) and rash (100%)	Meningoencephalitis
African tick-bite fever	*Rickettsia africae*	Tick	Outbreaks and clustered cases common (74%). Eschars (95%), which are often multiple (54%), maculopapular or vesicular rash (50%) and lymphadenopathy, apthous stomatitis	Subacute neuropathy
Queensland tick typhus	*Rickettsia australis*	Tick	Rash (100%) sometimes vesicular, eschar (65%), high fever, and lymphadenopathy	Confusion, transient visual hallucinations, seizures, rare
Flinders Island spotted fever	*Rickettsia honei*	Tick	Rash (85%), eschar (25%), and lymphadenopathy (55%)	Not reported
Scalp eschar and neck lymphadenopathy (SENLAT), tick-borne lymphadenopathy (TIBOLA)	*Rickettsia slovaca* *Rickettsia raoultti*	Tick	Typical large eschar on the scalp with painful cervical lymphadenopathy. Fever and rash rare	Meningoencephalitis, very rare
Far Eastern spotted fever	*Rickettsia heilongjiangensis*	Tick	Rash, eschar, and lymphadenopathy	Not reported
Rickettsial pox	*Rickettsia akari*	Mouse mite	Vesicular rash, eschar, high fever	Headache
Flea-borne spotted fever	*Rickettsia felis*	Flea	Vescicular rash	Not reported
	Rickettsia helvetica	Tick	No rash, fever, or lymphadenopathy. Sudden death	
	Rickettsia aeschlimannii	Tick	Rash, eschar, lymphadenopathy, high fever	
American boutonneuse fever	*Rickettsia parkeri*	Tick	Rash, eschar, lymphadenopathy	
Spotted fever	*Rickettsia massiliae*		Rash, eschar common, no lymphadenopathy	
	Rickettsia philipii	tick	No rash. Eschar, lymphadenopathy, and high fever	
Typhus				
Epidemic typhus	*Rickettsia prowazekii*	Human louse	Rash (40%)	Encephalitis, frequent
Murine typhus	*Rickettsia typhi*	Flea	Rash (20–40%)	Encephalitis, less frequent than in epidemic typhus (<5%). Subacute meningitis or meningoencephalitis
Scrub typhus	*Orientia tsutsugamushi*	Chigger (thrombiculide mite)	Eschar, generalized lymphadenopathies. Rash rare	Encephalitis, meningitis, deafness, cerebellitis, papilledema

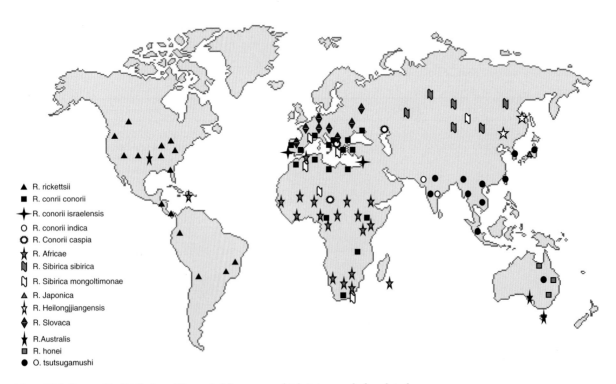

Figure 77.1 Geographic distribution of the spotted fever group of rickettsioses and of scrub typhus.

Tick behavior may determine the targeted human population and the seasonality. It may also influence the clinical presentation. For example, *Amblyomma* ticks are aggressive hunting ticks. They frequently attack in groups. This behavior explains clustered cases and several inoculation eschars in African tick-bite fever.

Pathophysiology

Rickettsiae are intracellular parasites of phagocytes that invade the CNS as part of a systemic infection. Rickettsiae can be divided into two categories according to their targets during natural infection: (1) organisms that parasitize vascular endothelial cells (*Rickettsia rickettsii*, *R. conorii*, TG Rickettsiae); and (2) organisms that parasitize both endothelial cells and phagocytes (*O. tsutsugamushi*). In terms of their intracellular niches, *O. tsutsugamushi* and the Rickettsiae lyse the phagosome and replicate, predominantly in the cytoplasm of host cells. The central pathophysiological event of Rickettsia infection, including CNS infection, has been identified as parasitism of vascular endothelial bacteria by blood-borne bacteria. Histological studies have confirmed rickettsial invasion of vascular endothelial cells in the brains of humans and experimentally infected mice. Rickettsiae invade and multiply at focal points in these small blood vessels, causing necrosis and proliferation of endothelial cells and development of platelet-fibrin thrombi at the site of damage, resulting in partial or even complete occlusion of the vascular lumen. These changes are associated with a perivascular inflammatory response, initially consisting of polymorphonuclear and monocytic cells, with the subsequent appearance of lymphocytes, macrophages, and plasma cells. This is the late phase of vascular damage, in which the immune response plays a major role. The classically described "typhus nodules" in the brain show similar pathology. Vasculitis is responsible for skin rash, microvascular leakage, edema, tissue hypoperfusion, and end-organ ischemic injury.

Clinical features

Early diagnosis of these infections from clinical features is a difficult task due to the non-specificity of early symptoms and signs – often resembling benign viral illness – symptomatology varying from mild to severe, low index of suspicion, absence of rash in the initial 2–3 days, and rash as a clinical feature of Rickettsia being neither sensitive nor specific. Fever, rash, and headache were considered for years the diagnostic clues for rickettsial diseases. Indeed, this remains a major triad, but a spotless phenotype of Rocky Mountain spotted fever (RMSF) has been identified, and many of the newly described rickettsial diseases have no rash. Major findings in rickettsioses include fever in a patient with exposure to a potential vector that may be associated with rash, inoculation eschar, or localized lymphadenopathy. Table 77.1 shows major clinical symptoms with specificities for different species of Rickettsiae.

Spotted fever group rickettsioses

Rocky Mountain spotted fever

In the early phases of the disease, most patients have non-specific signs such as fever, headache, malaise, arthromyalgias, and nausea. Abdominal signs, especially in children, are often prominent, leading sometimes to erroneous diagnosis such as acute appendicitis. Only approximately 60% of patients recall a tick bite. The rash appears late in the course of the disease (3–5 days) and may be absent in 10% of patients. In contrast with most other SFG rickettsioses, *R. rickettsii* does not generally elicit an eschar at the tick-bite site. As a result, when only non-specific symptoms dominate the clinical presentation, misdiagnosis and treatment delay can occur.

The frequency and severity of neurological signs depend on the severity of illness. Headache is frequent (79–91%) and is one of the most consistent clinical findings in RMSF. Neurological complications are frequently the cause of death. Serious CNS complications include stupor, delirium, seizures, ataxia, papilledema, focal neurological deficits, and coma. Coma is more likely to occur in fatal than in non-fatal cases. Cranial and peripheral nerve palsies can occur, of which hearing loss is the most frequent. The incidence of meningeal signs is >20% and among them about 60% are accompanied by abnormalities of the cerebrospinal fluid (CSF). The white blood cell (WBC) count in the CSF is rarely more than 100/mm^3. Polymorphonuclear cells may predominate, but more commonly lymphocytes predominate. CSF glucose is decreased in 8% of patients and protein is elevated in 35% of patients. Abnormalities in neuroimaging studies are not common in patients with RMSF, and when present they are often subtle. Since RMSF may present without rash, this illness must be considered in the differential diagnosis of every patient with encephalitic manifestations in endemic countries, especially if an appropriate epidemiological history is present. In general, the CNS manifestations resolve in parallel with the fever if adequate treatment is begun early in the course of illness. However, neurological sequelae are common following RMSF. They include learning disabilities, behavioral disturbance, depression, transverse myelitis, aphasia, and deafness.

Mediterranean spotted fever

After an average asymptomatic incubation of 6 days (range of 1–16 days), the onset of Mediterranean spotted fever (MSF) is abrupt and typical cases present with high fever (>39 °C), flu-like symptoms (i.e., headache, chills, arthromyalgia), and a black eschar (tache noire) at the tick-bite site. Eschar is indolent and is usually localized on the trunk, the legs, and the arms. Usually the rash follows the fever within 2–3 days. It is rarely delayed until the 5th day and is almost never absent entirely (1–4% of cases). Gastrointestinal symptoms may be present in about 30% of patients and are more likely to be present in children. Headache is a common sign in MSF and is usually intense. Neurological complications occur in 10–15% of MSF cases. Hearing loss is the most frequent complication. Meningitis can occur, but is less common than in RMSF. Serious CNS complications include stupor, delirium, seizures, ataxia, focal neurological deficits, and coma and are usually associated with other organ failures representing the "malignant form" of MSF. This very severe form accounts for 5–6% of MSF cases and with a high mortality rate.

Other spotted fever group rickettsioses

Table 77.1 summarizes the main clinical signs of other SFG rickettsioses and identifies which of them can manifest with neurological symptoms.

Typhus group rickettsioses

Epidemic typhus

Typhus is transmitted by the human body louse, which lives in human clothing and thrives in areas of low socioeconomic status, owing largely to poor hygiene and close living quarters of multiple people and animals. Humans are the reservoirs and lice are the vectors. The organism multiplies in the gut and can survive for weeks in human feces. Patients who recover can have latent reactive infections. The majority of patients with epidemic typhus experience the abrupt onset of fever, malaise, and coughing. A severe headache is nearly invariably present in patients with typhus and has been used as a key clinical criterion for identifying suspected cases in epidemics; severe leg myalgias have also been used in this way. Infected patients may also complain of a number of other non-specific symptoms, including abdominal pain, nausea, and diarrhea.

The rash of epidemic typhus classically begins several days after the onset of symptoms, appearing as a red macular or maculopapular eruption on the trunk that later spreads centrifugally to the extremities. Rash occurs in 20–80% of people, and is rarely observed on dark skin. The majority of patients with epidemic typhus manifest one or more abnormalities in CNS function. Common neurological symptoms include confusion and drowsiness. Coma, seizures, and focal neurological signs may develop in a minority of patients. Delirium and coma have been reported in 35% and 39% of fatal cases, respectively.

Murine typhus

Murine typhus is common in hot and humid climates such as Northern Africa, Southern Europe, and Southeast Asia. Murine typhus is typically a mild illness associated with rat and opossum fleas. The onset of illness is usually abrupt, with non-specific symptoms such as fever, headache, chills, and myalgias. Gastrointestinal symptoms are particularly common in children. Rash occurs in 20–54% of patients near the end of the first week of illness. It typically begins as a maculopapular eruption on the trunk and spreads peripherally. The rash does not typically involve the face, palms of the hands, or soles of the feet. Symptoms of severe CNS disease such as seizures, stupor, and ataxia are infrequent, found in <5% of patients. However, cases of subacute aseptic meningitis or meningoencephalitis and CNS hemorrhage have been reported in patients with murine typhus without rash or other systemic findings. These cases suggest that neurological involvement in murine typhus is more common than previously described and that murine typhus should be included in the diagnosis of subacute meningitis and meningoencephalitis, especially if an appropriate epidemiological history is present.

Scrub typhus

Scrub typhus is extremely common in Asia and specifically in Southeast Asia. It is transmitted by the trombiculid mite larva. Scrub typhus may begin insidiously with headache, anorexia, and malaise, or start abruptly with chills and fever after a 10-day incubation period. Macular or maculopapular rash is infrequent. More than 50% of patients have an eschar at the inoculation site. The eschar may develop before the onset of systemic symptoms, and can occur in multiple locations. Generalized lymphadenopathy occurs in the majority of patients. Periorbital edema, edema of

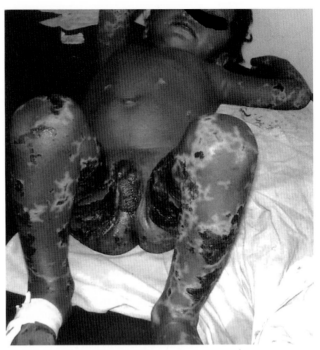

Figure 77.2 Extensive gangrene in a child with Rickettsial vasculitis. For color details, please refer to the color plates section.

dorsum of hand or foot, or generalized edema, polyserositis, and hepatosplenomegaly are sometimes seen. The neurological signs are similar in many respects to other rickettsial diseases in that the headache is nearly always present. Meningismus or meningitis has been found in 5.7–13.5% of patients. However, in a series of 25 patients who underwent lumbar puncture in the absence of overt signs, 48% had reactive spinal fluid showing a mild mononuclear pleocytosis. Scrub typhus should be considered one of the causes of aseptic meningitis in areas of endemy. A small proportion of patients develop tremors, delirium, altered mental status, and coma. Acute hearing loss occurred in 6 out of 72 patients in Thailand.

Complications

Disseminated intravascular coagulation, non-cardiogenic pulmonary edema, gangrene of digits and earlobe, and hemophagocytic syndrome are some of the dreaded complications seen in rickettsial diseases (Figure 77.2).

Scoring system for diagnosis

The Rathi, Goodman, and Aghai (RGA) scoring system (Table 77.2) uses clinical, laboratory, and epidemiological features to diagnose spotted fever group rickettsias in resource-poor settings. On receiver operating characteristic (ROC) curve analysis, the cut-off score with the highest accuracy was found to be 14, with a sensitivity and specificity of 96.15% and 98.84%, and a positive predictive value (PPV) and negative predictive value (NPV) of 98.0% and 97.7%, respectively. When applied to patients presenting with fever of unknown source, a clinical score of 14 or more on the RGA scoring system has sensitivity and specificity similar to the detection of specific IgM antibody by enzyme-linked immunosorbent assay (ELISA).

Table 77.2 RGA scoring system to diagnose spotted fever rickettsioses (total score = 35). Source: Rathi 2011. Reproduced with permission.

Clinical feature	Score	Laboratory feature	Score
Living in rural area	1	Hemoglobin <9gm/dL	1
Pets in household	1	Platelets <1,500,000/dL	1
Tick exposure	2	CRP ≥50mg/dL	2
Tick bite	3	Serum albumin <3gm/dL	1
Non-exudative conjunctival congestion	2	Urine albumin >2+	1
Maculopapular rash	1	SGPT >100 U/L	2
Purpura	2	Serum Na <130meq/L	2
Palpable purpura/ecchymosis/necrotic rash	3		
Rash appearing 48–96 hrs after fever	2		
Pedal edema	2		
Rash on palms/soles	3		
Hepatomegaly	2		
Lymphadenopathy	1		
TOTAL	**25**	**TOTAL**	**10**

Investigations

Culturing remains extremely difficult for these organisms, and diagnosis mainly relies on serology, PCR, and immunological detection. The reference technique for serology is microimmunofluorescence (MIF). Many cross-reactions are observed, and determination of the precise infecting species may be difficult. Testing of several antigens on the same slide to compare reactivity may help in discriminating among cross-reacting agents. Western blot may be more specific in early sera and cross-absorption may help to discriminate SFG rickettsiae.

PCR is an appropriate tool for the diagnosis of rickettsioses and can be used on samples of blood, skin, and arthropods. Skin biopsy of the inoculation eschar is the best clinical sample for the SFG rickettsiae, preferably before antibiotic therapy. Molecular amplification with PCR from eschar biopsy or ethylenediamine tetraacetic acid (EDTA) blood or from ticks targets different genes (17-kd protein, citrate synthase, *ompA*, *ompB*, "gene D") and allows the detection and identification of the causal agent with certitude. Biopsies can also be used for immunochemistry. Blood sample is the best clinical sample for PCR in scrub typhus. Immunological detection using specific antibodies or monoclonal antibodies allows detection in blood and other tissues.

Treatment

Early empirical antibiotic therapy should be prescribed in any suspected rickettsioses before confirmation of the diagnosis. Early treatment may prevent many but not all cases in which CNS complications occur. Other variables such as age and G6PD deficiency may be important factors in the risk of neurological complications. The most useful treatment in children and in adults is doxycycline. The length of treatment is unknown, but it should be continued orally for at least 3 days post fever. In children, the risk of dental staining by doxycycline is negligible when a single, relatively short (5–10 days) course of treatment is administered. It can be prescribed in a shorter course (1 day) for typhus, scrub typhus, and MSF. Doxycycline should not be given to pregnant women; therefore chloramphenicol should be used. Typhus group rickettsias are also susceptible to erythromycin. Sulfonamides are contraindicated in rickettsial diseases, as they increase morbidity and mortality, either by delaying institution of appropriate antibiotics or directly stimulating the growth of organisms.

Further reading

Drevets DA, Leenen PJ, Greenfield RA. Invasion of the central nervous system by intracellular bacteria. *Clin Microbiol Rev* 2004;17(2):323–346.

Marrie TJ, Raoult D. Rickettsial infections of the central nervous system. *Semin Neurol* 1992;12(3):213–224.

Parola P, Paddock C, Raoult, D. Tick-borne rickettsioses around the world: Emerging diseases challenging old concepts. *Clin Microbiol Rev* 2005;18(4):719–756.

Rathi N, Rathi A. Rickettsial diseases in central India: Proposed clinical scoring system for early detection of spotted fever. *Ind Ped* 2011;48(11):867–872.

PART 9   Prion Diseases and Neurovirology

78   Prion diseases

Ellen Gelpi[1] and Herbert Budka[2]

[1] Neurological Tissue Bank, Biobank-Hospital Clinic-IDIBAPS, Barcelona, Spain
[2] Institute of Neuropathology, University Hospital Zurich, Switzerland

Transmissible spongiform encephalopathies (TSEs) or prion diseases are irreversible diseases of the central nervous system (CNS), invariably leading to death. These diseases are thought to be caused by a misfolded host prion protein that is expressed predominantly in the brain, but also in other tissues. Different forms of human diseases have been described: *sporadic* (arising spontaneously with no obvious origin), including sporadic Creutzfeldt–Jakob disease (CJD), sporadic fatal insomnia (sFI), and variably protease-sensitive prionopathy (VPSPr); *genetic* (mutations or insertions in the prion protein gene on chromosome 20), including genetic (familial) CJD, fatal familial insomnia (FFI), and Gerstmann–Sträussler–Scheinker disease (GSS); and *acquired* (transmitted from contact with external prions), including variant CJD (contact with bovine spongiform encephalopathy [BSE] prions), iatrogenic CJD (inadvertent transmission by invasive medical procedures), and kuru (transmission by ritualistic cannibalism). Animal TSEs comprise scrapie affecting sheep and goats, chronic wasting disease affecting North American cervids, transmissible mink encephalopathy, feline spongiform encephalopathy, and bovine spongiform encephalopathy (BSE). This chapter deals only with human disease.

Epidemiology

Creutzfeldt–Jakob disease (CJD) is rare, with a worldwide incidence of about 1–2 cases per million per year. Sporadic CJD is the most frequent form, occurring spontaneously with an average age of onset between 60 and 70 years. There is a familial/genetic basis to 5–15% of CJD cases, inherited as an autosomal dominant trait. More than 400 cases of iatrogenic CJD have been reported. The most important sources of iatrogenic transmission have been human dura mater grafts and cadaveric human growth hormone (hGH). The duration of hGH treatment ranged between 1 and 13 years (median 6.4 years), with symptoms appearing 11–15 years later. The long incubation period could be explained by low titers of infectivity after dilutions, admixture from different donors, and the peripheral route of administration. Cadaveric human hormone preparations were used until the mid-1980s, when synthetic recombinant hormones were produced, which have been used since. Cases of iatrogenic CJD after transplantation of lyophilized dura mater obtained from commercial dura mater grafts (produced before 1987) have most frequently been reported in Japan. The incubation period varies between 1.5 and 23 years. Single cases were reported after neurosurgery and corneal grafting.

Kuru was recognized in the late 1950s in the Fore linguistic group in Papua New Guinea to be due to ritualistic cannibalism. It affected mostly adult women and children over 4 years of age, since in the cannibalistic feasts, women and children ate the less desirable tissues, including CNS tissue.

In 1996, variant CJD was identified in the United Kingdom. A causal link between variant CJD and BSE was first hypothesized, and there is now overwhelming epidemiological and experimental evidence that prions causing BSE and variant CJD are the same. The most plausible route of exposure is via BSE-contaminated food. Contamination of the human food chain most likely resulted from CNS tissue in mechanically recovered meat used to manufacture processed products. The incubation period might be about 10 years, but a period of several decades cannot be excluded. Variant CJD mostly affects individuals under 40 years of age. As of September 2014, 229 cases had been reported, mostly in the United Kingdom (177) and France (27), and a few cases in Spain (5), Ireland (4), the United States (4), the Netherlands (3), Portugal (2), Italy (2), Canada (2), Saudi Arabia (1), Taiwan (1), and Japan (1).

There is one important polymorphism at codon 129 of the prion protein gene *PRNP* that encodes either methionine (M) or valine (V). MM homozygosity there represents a risk factor for iatrogenic and variant CJD, and influences the clinical and neuropathological phenotype of sporadic and genetic TSEs. In the normal population, MV heterozygotes represent 50%, MMs 39%, and VVs 11%, in contrast to sporadic CJD, where MM homozygotes represent around 70%. To date, all manifest variant CJD cases are MM homozygotes, although asymptomatic MV infection carriers have been observed. Additionally, the phenotype of certain genetic TSEs is strongly influenced by codon 129, such as in the D178N mutation: when the mutated allele encodes methionine in codon 129, FFI is observed, whereas a CJD phenotype predominates when the mutated allele encodes valine.

The combination of this polymorphism with the prion protein type (type 1 and type 2; see "Pathophysiology") is the basis of the molecular and phenotypic classification of sporadic CJD into six main subtypes (MM1, MV1, MM2, MV2, VV1, and VV2).

Pathophysiology

The term "prion" designates a "proteinaceous infectious particle." The *protein-only* hypothesis supposes that the infectious agent (prion) causing TSEs represents a conformational change of the normal host-encoded cellular prion protein, PrP^c, present in all cells of the body but predominantly expressed in the brain on the surface of neurons. The disease-associated, newly formed PrP^{sc} (sc derives from scrapie) is enriched in beta sheets and may interact with PrP^c and cause the latter to adopt the beta sheet conformation of PrP^{sc}, initiating a self-perpetuating process that results in increasing PrP^{sc} concentrations. PrP^{sc} is not degraded by common enzymatic activity and accumulates around neurons and axons. It is suggested that the loss of function of PrP^c combined with the accumulation of PrP^{sc} in the brain induces neurodegeneration. Some mutations and insertions in the *PRNP* gene apparently favor spontaneous conversion of PrP^c to PrP^{sc}, which could account for genetic forms of human prion diseases.

Western blot isoform patterns of protease-resistant PrP (PrP^{res}) are classified on the basis of electrophoretic mobility of the non-glycosylated protein band as type 1 (21 kDa) or type 2 (19 kDa) and by differences in the glycoform ratio after proteinase K digestion. Recently, two disease forms (variably protease-sensitive sporadic prionopathy [VPSPr] and rapidly progressive dementia with thalamic degeneration) have shown significant PrP^{sc} sensitivity to proteinase kinase digestion in conventional Western blot studies and have led to the recognition of protease-sensitive PrP^{sc} or senPrP^{sc}. This PrP form is distinguishable from PrP^c by its conformational state and seeding capacity or infectivity. In VPSPr, it is accompanied by some PrP^{res}, while in rapidly progressive dementia with thalamic degeneration there is a complete absence of PrP^{res}.

Transmission of prions can occur within the same species or between species. Infection by the oral route, as in kuru and variant CJD, requires that prions enter the body via the digestive tract, after which PrP^{sc} can be found in Peyer's patches and the enteric nervous system. It has been suggested that myeloid dendritic cells mediate transport within the lymphoreticular system, and that follicular dendritic cells replicate prions locally. Neuroinvasion is thought to occur through the peripheral nervous system via the autonomic splanchnic nerves that enter the spinal cord, or via the vagus nerve to the brain.

The infectivity of different tissues can be demonstrated by bioassays. Experimental data reveal the highest transmission rates to non-human primates for iatrogenic CJD (100%), kuru (95%), and sporadic CJD (90%), with considerably lower rates for most familial forms of disease (68%).

Clinical features

Sporadic Creutzfeldt–Jakob disease

The most frequent initial symptoms of sporadic CJD are cognitive decline, cerebellar symptoms, ataxia, behavioral change, dizziness, and visual complaints (especially cortical blindness). Later, a combination of various neurological symptoms, including movement disorders and pyramidal signs, accompany dementia, indicating a rapidly progressive global encephalopathy. Myoclonus and, in the terminal phase, akinetic mutism are usually prominent. Disease leads invariably to death, generally due to respiratory or systemic infection in the terminal stage, after less than 2 years, on average within 6 months. The six molecular subtypes of sporadic CJD show variability in age, clinical signs at onset, and duration of illness.

Genetic transmissible spongiform encephalopathies

Genetic or familial CJD is similar to sporadic CJD in clinical parameters and laboratory variables, but might have earlier onset and longer duration of disease. In familial fatal insomnia (FFI), the age of onset is younger, mainly 25–60 years, and the duration can range from 6 months to 3 years. The main clinical manifestations of FFI are alterations of circadian rhythm and autonomic disturbances with insomnia and autonomic dysregulation, but myoclonus and dementia are also prominent. The principal clinical features of Gerstmann–Sträussler–Scheinker are cerebellar and spinal, followed later by cognitive decline.

Iatrogenic Creutzfeldt–Jakob disease

The clinical presentation of iatrogenic CJD seems to depend on the site of inoculation, with dementia predominating after neurosurgery, and cerebellar symptoms after peripheral transmission (e.g., growth hormone). In dural grafts, the location of the graft does not appear to influence the clinical manifestation of disease, which is mostly cerebellar and myoclonic.

Kuru

Kuru is characterized by intense tremor and instability in gait, bulbar signs such as dysarthria and dysphagia, and, less prominently, cognitive decline.

Variant Creutzfeldt–Jakob disease

Variant CJD differs from classical sporadic CJD in that psychiatric and sensory symptoms are the most frequent initial clinical features. Because no neurological alterations may be detected at early stages of the disease, patients are often referred to a psychiatrist. Duration of disease is also longer than in sporadic CJD, with a median of 14 months (6–38 months). Later, dementia and myoclonus are frequent, but choreiform movements, pyramidal signs, cerebellar symptoms and rigidity, and vertical gaze weakness also develop.

Investigations

There is no test to definitely diagnose prion disease *in vivo*, although promising results are being obtained by some new methods, including real-time quaking-induced conversion for PrP^{sc} on cerebrospinal fluid (CSF) or olfactory mucosal cells obtained by nasal brushing.

Current clinical criteria (Table 78.1) cover suspected cases with high sensitivity (97%) and moderate specificity (65%). Additional techniques such as electroencephalography (EEG), immunoblot detection of 14-3-3 protein in CSF, and magnetic resonance (MR) neuroimaging improve diagnosis. Differential diagnoses include Alzheimer's disease, diffuse Lewy body disease, vascular dementia, inflammatory encephalopathies in younger people, Hashimoto encephalopathy, or paraneoplastic syndromes.

Electrophysiological studies

In sporadic CJD, the electroencephalogram (EEG) shows periodic sharp-wave complexes (PSWC), some with triphasic morphology, with a duration of 100–600 ms and an intercomplex interval of 500–2000 ms. Note that other disorders such as hepatic encephalopathy, hypoglycemia, SIADH (syndrome of inappropriate ADH secretion), brain abscesses, and drugs (lithium, baclofen) may cause similar EEG alterations. Accordingly, EEG has a sensitivity of 66%

Table 78.1 Clinical diagnostic criteria for surveillance. Source: WHO 2010. Reproduced with permission of WHO.

Sporadic CJD
Definite:
 Neuropathological/immunohistochemical confirmation
Probable:
 Rapidly progressive dementia and at least two of the following:
 – Myoclonus
 – Visual/cerebellar problems
 – Pyramidal or extrapyramidal features
 – Akinetic mutism
 And typical EEG and/or positive 14-3-3 (disease duration <2 years) and/or high signal abnormalities in caudate/putamen on MRI scans
Possible:
 • Like probable, but disease duration <2 years, and EEG and/or 14-3-3-negative or not performed.

Variant CJD
I (A) Progressive neuropsychiatric disorder
 (B) Duration of illness >6 months
 (C) Routine investigations suggesting no alternative diagnosis
 (D) No history of potential iatrogenic exposure
 (E) No evidence of familial TSE
II (A) Early psychiatric symptoms*
 (B) Persistent painful sensory symptoms**
 (C) Ataxia
 (D) Myoclonus, chorea or dystonia
 (E) Dementia
III (A) EEG does not show typical appearance of sporadic CJD*** or no EEG performed
 (B) Bilateral pulvinar high signal on MRI scan
IV (A) Positive tonsil biopsy§
Definite: IA **and** neuropathological confirmation of variant CJD****
Probable: I and 4/5 of II **and** IIIA **and** IIIB, or I and IVA

*Depression, anxiety, apathy, withdrawal, delusions. ** Both frank pain and/or dysesthesia. ***Generalized triphasic periodic complexes at approx. 1/sec. §Tonsil biopsy is not recommended routinely or in cases with EEG appearances typical of sporadic CJD, but may be useful in suspected cases in which clinical features are compatible with variant CJD and MRI does not show bilateral pulvinar high signal. ****Spongiform change and extensive PrP deposition with florid plaques throughout the cerebrum and cerebellum.

and a specificity of 74%, and PSWC can be observed during progression of the disease, but may disappear at terminal stages. In variant CJD, PSWC have been only observed in single cases at late disease stage.

Cerebrospinal fluid

The detection by immunoblotting of 14-3-3, a neuronal protein that is increased in CSF after tissue damage, has the greatest sensitivity (94%) and specificity (84%) to diagnose sporadic CJD. Nevertheless, the protein is not diagnostic for CJD, since it may be present in conditions with neuronal destruction such as stroke, encephalitis, or tumor. False negatives have been reported, especially at the onset of clinical symptoms or even as the disease progresses. In genetic forms and in variant CJD, 14-3-3 is not a useful marker. Other proteins that have been studied are tau, beta-amyloid, neuron-specific enolase, and S100 protein, which have lower sensitivity and specificity and are not the first choice, even though tau shows a multifold increase in patients with sporadic CJD beyond the range seen in Alzheimer's disease or other dementing disorders.

Neuroimaging

Brain MRI may demonstrate bilateral areas of increased signal intensity in the caudate nuclei and putamina on long repetition time images in sporadic CJD and bilateral increased signal in pulvinar in variant CJD ("hockey-stick" sign). In fluid-attenuated inversion recovery images and diffusion-weighted MRI, ribbon-like high-signal intensity changes in cerebral cortex can be found. Due to high sensitivity and specificity, MRI alterations are considered supportive of a clinical diagnosis and are now included in the updated World Health Organization (WHO) diagnostic criteria (Table 78.1). False-positive MRI findings may be associated with inflammatory conditions that are treatable, such as viral encephalitis.

Genetic analysis

Genetic analysis is recommended in all suspected cases when possible, since an abnormality is suggested by a family history in only half of genetic cases. Furthermore, knowledge of the codon 129 polymorphism is important to predict the clinical course and to interpret the result of additional investigations such as EEG and presence of 14-3-3 protein.

Brain biopsy

Brain biopsy has a role in suspected CJD only when treatable alternative diagnoses are under consideration. Because of local variability in the distribution of typical histological changes and PrP^{sc} deposits, the chance of false-negative results of brain biopsy must be considered. In addition to its presence in CNS tissue and retina, PrP^{sc} in variant CJD may also be present in the thymus, lymph nodes, tonsils, spleen, liver, adrenal gland, colon, ileum, jejunum, and rectum. Tonsillar biopsy has been advocated as a potentially relevant examination in the diagnosis of variant CJD and is currently included in clinical diagnostic criteria for variant CJD (Table 78.1).

Postmortem investigations

Every suspected case of any form of CJD should be confirmed by neuropathology after death of the patient whenever possible. To ensure adequate safety precautions for the postmortem examination, the pathology laboratory should be notified of the suspected diagnosis. Classical histopathological features (Figure 78.1a–c) include spongiform change, neuronal loss, astrogliosis, and microglial activation. Amyloid plaques are rarely seen in sporadic CJD, whereas variant CJD shows abundant amyloid plaques, many of which are surrounded by vacuoles ("florid plaques"). In GSS, multicentric amyloid plaques predominate (Figure 78.1d), while FFI is characterized by severe gliosis of the thalamus and olivary nuclei without prominent spongiform change. Immunohistochemistry or Western blot for the detection of PrP^{sc} is needed for definitive neuropathological diagnosis in cases with non-classic histopathology (Figure 78.1e–h).

Treatment

There is no effective treatment of prion diseases.

Preventive measures

An important characteristic of prions is their extreme resistance to conventional sterilization procedures such as heat, irradiation (UV and ionic), and chemicals (alcohol, formaldehyde, ethylene oxide, and others). To avoid and prevent transmission to others, surgical instruments must undergo special decontamination procedures or be disposed of after potential contact with prions. Proven inactivating methods include treatment with sodium hydroxide or bleach and

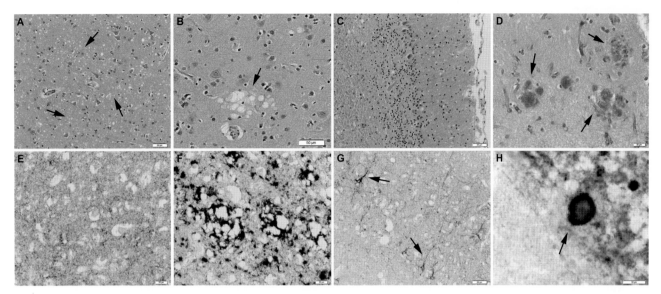

Figure 78.1 (A) Classic histopathology of sporadic CJD is characterized by small vacuoles (arrows) in the neuropil of gray matter (spongiform change) associated with neuronal loss and reactive astrogliosis and microglial proliferation (hematoxylin and eosin stain). (B) In some sporadic CJD subtypes (e.g., MM2C and focally in about one-third of MM/MV1 cases), clusters of large confluent vacuoles are seen (arrow). (C) The cerebellum is severely affected in the ataxic VV2 subtype and shows prominent depletion of granular cells, segmental reduction of Purkinje cells with some axonal swelling (torpedoes), and mild narrowing of the molecular layer with moderate spongiform change of the neuropil. (D) In GSS, large multicentric PAS-positive PrP^{sc} amyloid plaques (arrows) are detected throughout the brain (PAS staining). (E–H) Different PrP^{sc} immunoreactivity patterns in sporadic CJD: classic synaptic type as seen in MM/MV1 (E), patchy-perivacuolar accumulations usually detected in MM2C (F), perineuronal deposits as seen in VV2 (G, arrow), and unicentric, kuru-type PrP^{sc} amyloid plaques in the granule cell layer of the cerebellum as detected in MV2K patients (H, arrow). For color details, please refer to the color plates section.

subsequent autoclaving at 134 °C. Conventional care of patients in hospital or at home is not associated with transmission risk.

Blood elements might also be a vehicle of prions in variant CJD (not in sporadic CJD), with five cases of transfusion-associated variant CJD reported to date. Because the incubation period of variant CJD can be several years, asymptomatic carriers (including MV/VV subjects) might be blood donors, with implications for transfusion services and blood products.

Further reading

Brown P, Gibbs CJ, Jr, Rodgers Johnson P, *et al.* Human spongiform encephalopathy: The National Institutes of Health series of 300 cases of experimentally transmitted disease. *Ann Neurol* 1994;35:513–529.
Budka H. Neuropathology of prion diseases. *Br Med Bull* 2003;66:121–130.
McCutcheon S, Alejo Blanco AR, Houston EF, *et al.* All clinically-relevant blood components transmit prion disease following a single blood transfusion: A sheep model of vCJD. *PLoS One* 2011;6:e23169.
Parchi P, Giese A, Capellari S, *et al.* Classification of sporadic Creutzfeldt–Jakob disease based on molecular and phenotypic analysis of 300 subjects. *Ann Neurol* 1999;46:224–233.
Trevitt CR, Collinge J. A systematic review of prion therapeutics in experimental models. *Brain* 2006;129(9):2241–2265.
Will RG, Ironside JW, Zeidler M, *et al.* A new variant of Creutzfeldt–Jakob disease in the UK. *Lancet* 1996;347:921–925.
World Health Organization (WHO). Guidelines on tissue infectivity distribution in transmissible spongiform encephalopathies. 2006, and updated in 2010. http://www.who.int/bloodproducts/tablestissueinfectivity.pdf?ua=1 (accessed November 2015).
Zerr I, Kallenberg K, Summers, DM, *et al.* Updated clinical diagnostic criteria for sporadic Creutzfeldt–Jakob disease. *Brain* 2009;132:2659–2668.
Zerr I, Pocchiari M, Collins S, *et al.* Analysis of EEG and CSF 14-3-3 proteins as aids to the diagnosis of Creutzfeldt-Jakob disease. *Neurology* 2000;55:811–815.
Zou WQ, Puoti G, Xiao X, *et al.* 2010. Variably protease-sensitive prionopathy: A new sporadic disease of the prion protein. *Ann Neurol* 2010;68:162–172.
For the current epidemiology of vCJD and BSE, see http://www.cdc.gov/prions/vcjd/index.html (accessed November 2015).

79 Acute, recurrent and chronic viral meningitis

Larry E. Davis

Neurology Service, New Mexico VA Health Care System, and Department of Neurology, University of New Mexico School of Medicine, Albuquerque, NM, USA

Viral meningitis is the most common infection of the central nervous system (CNS). The illness occurs worldwide, with the highest incidence in children and young adults. Viral meningitis now outnumbers bacterial meningitis by more than 25:1 in many countries. This is particularly true for countries offering the *Haemophilus influenzae* type b conjugate vaccine to infants and *Streptococcus pneumoniae* vaccines to both children and adults, which has dramatically reduced the incidence of bacterial meningitis.

The term meningitis refers to inflammation of the meninges. Aseptic meningitis is a broad term that includes most meningeal mononuclear cell inflammatory processes not due to pyogenic bacteria, tuberculosis, or fungi. The US Centers for Disease Control and Prevention define aseptic meningitis as a clinically compatible illness diagnosed by a physician, with no laboratory evidence of bacterial or fungal meningitis. The syndrome has multiple etiologies, but viruses cause most cases. Recurrent meningitis refers to meningitis that recurs. Between episodes, the patient is asymptomatic and the cerebrospinal fluid (CSF) is normal. Chronic meningitis refers to the persistence of clinical meningitis symptoms and CSF inflammatory cells for 3–4 weeks. Meningoencephalitis is a term used when an infectious agent infects both the meninges and brain parenchyma, with the patient developing symptoms and signs of both meningitis and encephalitis.

Epidemiology

Viral meningitis occurs worldwide and reports of aseptic meningitis regularly appear from all regions. When a viral etiology is determined, most are enteroviruses. Often the same enterovirus serotype circulates simultaneously around the world. Herpes simplex type 2 is the second most common cause of viral meningitis.

The true incidence of viral meningitis is unknown, as it is not a reportable disease in most countries. In the United States, estimates of the number of aseptic meningitis cases per year range up to 150,000. Generally, the incidence of adult viral meningitis worldwide ranges between 10 and 20 per 100,000 population per year. However, one report from Finland found the annual incidence of viral infections of the meninges and/or brain of children to be about 700 per 100,000.

Most viral meningitis is caused by enteroviruses, herpes simplex 2 virus, arboviruses, and mumps virus. Mumps meningitis now occurs almost exclusively in countries not routinely administering the mumps vaccine. Herpes simplex 2 (HSV-2) meningitis occurs mainly in young sexually active adults. Most viral meningitis occurs in the summer in temperate climates when enteroviruses prevail. Table 79.1 lists many of the viruses that cause meningitis.

Table 79.1 Causes of viral meningitis.

Common viruses	Comments
Enteroviruses	Accounts for over 50% of all meningitis cases in every country. A few strains, HEV-68, -70, and -71, also occasionally cause acute flaccid paralysis or brainstem encephalitis.
Herpes simplex, types 2 and rarely 1	Develops mainly in young sexually active adults who acquire genital herpes.
Arboviruses (West Nile virus, Western equine, Eastern equine, St. Louis, California, Powassan, Japanese B, Jamestown Canyon, Toscana, tick-borne encephalitis, and many others)	Incidence is seasonal when the vector is prevalent in the community. Types of arbovirus infection vary by country. These viruses primarily cause encephalitis rather than meningitis.
Mumps	Very common in children from countries that do not routinely administer childhood mumps vaccine, but sporadic cases occur from vaccination failures or waning immunity to mumps virus in developed countries.
Less common causes	
Varicella zoster virus	Can occur in immunocompetent and immunosuppressed patients with or without a rash. Frequency is increasing due to better identification owing to more use of cerebrospinal fluid polymerase chain reaction (CSF PCR) assays and antibody assays.
Lymphocytic choriomeningitis virus	Can occur from exposure to infected wild or pet rodents.
Human immunodeficiency virus	Patients are symptomatic mainly during the primary infection, but CSF viral persistence occurs.
Human T-cell lymphotropic virus, type 1	Low-grade lymphocytic meningitis with slowly progressive myelopathy.
Poliovirus	Sporadic or clusters of cases occur in developing countries that lack strong poliovirus immunization programs. Meningitis without paralysis occurs in about 4% of primary infections.
Uncommon causes	
Parvovirus B19	Identified so far only in children or with immunosuppression.

International Neurology, Second edition. Edited by Robert P. Lisak, Daniel D. Truong, William M. Carroll and Roongroj Bhidayasiri
© 2016 John Wiley & Sons, Ltd. Published 2016 by John Wiley & Sons, Ltd.

Adenovirus	Occurs rarely in immunosuppressed individuals.
Reovirus	Mainly occurs in infants.
Rhinovirus	Rare even in children.
Cytomegalovirus	Mainly in immunosuppressed individuals, especially those with AIDS.
Human herpesvirus 6	Rare in infants.
Epstein–Barr virus	Mainly in immunosuppressed individuals.
Parainfluenza and Influenza virus	Rare even in epidemics. Most patients with influenza and meningismus have normal CSF.
Rubeola virus (measles)	Occurs mainly as a meningoencephalitis or postviral encephalitis and occurs in countries without active childhood immunization programs.
Rotavirus	Mainly seen in young children.
Live virus vaccines (mumps, measles, rubella, poliovirus)	Very uncommon.

Pathophysiology

Viral meningitis begins with a primary focus of infection associated with the virus's route of entry: gastrointestinal (GI) tract for enteroviruses, respiratory tract for mumps, subcutaneous tissue following mosquito or tick bite for arboviruses, and genital skin infection for HSV-2 virus.

Spread to distant areas from the primary site occurs by lymphatic spread of progeny virions from the respiratory tract, GI tract, or subcutaneous tissue to blood, producing a viremia or by infection of adjacent peripheral nerves in skin, such as in HSV-2 virus infection. Viremia is the most common route by which the virus reaches the meninges. For a viremia to cause meningitis, several important host barriers must be overcome. The reticuloendothelial system (RES) efficiently filters viruses circulating in blood.

Humoral and cellular immune responses effectively terminate viremia. Antibody production, usually of IgM antibody, begins days after the primary infection. Immunosuppression may hamper the humoral immune response.

The final obstacle to the virus reaching the CNS is the blood–brain barrier. This is a complex barrier between cerebral endothelial cells that prevents infectious agents and many circulating molecules from entering the brain. The actual mechanism of meningitic virus entering the CSF is poorly understood. Thus, most viral infections are asymptomatic or cause minimal illness due to infection of other organs.

Eradication of a viral infection within the meninges depends primarily on the host's immune system, particularly since antiviral drugs are available for only a few neurotropic viruses. Unfortunately, viral clearance of a CNS infection is less efficient than for infections elsewhere in the body, since the brain and meninges have limited host defenses. For example, antibody titers in CSF are markedly lower than in serum; few lymphocytes are in normal CSF; and the brain lacks a lymphatic system. Nevertheless, during active viral infection, immune monocytes invade the meninges, gamma interferon and other cytokines are released by CNS monocytes, and neutralizing antibody enters the CSF, normally to destroy the virus. Because the virus is located only in the meninges in viral meningitis, clearance of the CNS virus usually occurs within 1–2 weeks and seldom causes neurological sequelae.

Enterovirus infections cause up to 80% of viral meningitis. Enteroviruses, now classified as human enterovirus species A, B, C, and D, are a family of over 77 serotypes. These virions are small (30 nm diameter) and survive readily in water and sewerage. Enteroviruses are shed in the stool for weeks and transmission is usually person to person via fecal contamination, such as using the toilet and not washing the hands afterwards.

Clinical features

Acute viral meningitis

Most cases of viral meningitis have a mild prodrome consisting of gastrointestinal symptoms, pharyngitis, herpangina, conjunctivitis, or rash on the hand, foot, or mouth that begins a few days before the typical meningitis headache. Patients with herpes simplex meningitis may have genital vesicles 1–7 days earlier, but in many instances there are no genital lesions. Although parotitis is the classic sign of mumps several days before meningitis, up to half of patients develop meningitis before parotid gland swelling. Patients with mumps meningitis may also develop abdominal pain due to pancreatitis with an elevated serum amylase level, or mumps oophoritis in women and testicular pain in men.

There is often a seasonal distribution to viral meningitis depending on the etiology. Meningitis due to enteroviruses (Coxsackie and ECHO) is common in summer. Arthropod-borne viruses cause aseptic meningitis as well as encephalitis in late summer and fall. In winter, when mice carrying lymphocytic choriomeningitis (LCM) virus seek warmth and invade homes, humans develop acute LCM; also in winter, mumps is common. Both type-2 herpes simplex virus and varicella zoster virus (VZV) can cause aseptic meningitis at any time of year.

The signs and symptoms of meningitis usually have an abrupt and explosive onset, often becoming intense within a few hours. The classic triad for viral meningitis is fever (which is seldom high), severe diffuse headache (which is often pounding), and stiff neck of varying severity. Table 79.2 lists the frequency of symptoms and signs of viral meningitis. Patients with aseptic meningitis have a relative preservation of their mental status. However, due to the headache they seldom concentrate well or perform difficult mental tasks, but are generally not disoriented, confused, or hallucinating. If the mental status is markedly depressed, the diagnosis of meningoencephalitis should be considered. Although nuchal rigidity has been considered typical for viral meningitis, it is present only in about half of patients. The presence of papilledema, focal neurological deficit, or coma suggests that the patient may have brain parenchymal involvement. Of note is that occasional patients with acute enterovirus D68, 70, or 71 infections can develop an acute flaccid paralysis and brainstem encephalitis.

Viral meningitis can develop in anyone. However, children less than 5 years old have the highest incidence. Immunocompromised individuals who are immunocompromised from disease or medications that suppress the immune system are also at greater than normal risk. Examples would be chemotherapeutic agents, specific drugs aimed at suppressing the immune system such as monoclonal antibodies, patients with recent organ or bone marrow transplants, and those with human immunodeficiency virus (HIV)/acquired immunodeficiency syndrome (AIDS). Infants less than 2 years of age often present with non-specific signs such as fever, anorexia, lethargy, and irritability. Nuchal rigidity is found in only one-fourth of infant cases. Signs of an upper respiratory or gastrointestinal infection and rash may also be present.

Table 79.2 Signs and symptoms of acute viral meningitis.

Common findings	%
Fever	85
Headache	85
Stiff neck	60
Anorexia, nausea, vomiting	75
Photophobia	20
Irritability	40
Relative preservation of mental status	75
Less common findings Stupor	5
Seizures	5
Rare findings Focal neurological signs	2
Papilledema	<1
Babinski sign	<1
Coma	<1

In addition to viruses, drugs can induce aseptic meningitis. The most common ones are non-steroidal anti-inflammatory drugs (e.g., ibuprofen), antimicrobial drugs such as those containing sulfa, monoclonal antibodies, vaccines, and intravenous immunoglobulins. See Table 79.3 for many non-viral causes of aseptic meningitis.

Table 79.3 Non-viral causes of aseptic meningitis.

Other infectious agents

Bacteria: Borrelia Burgdorferi (Lyme disease), *Treponema pallidum* (syphilis), *Leptospira sp.*, *Brucella sp.*, *Bartonella sp.* (cat-scratch fever), agents of bacterial endocarditis, *Mycoplasma pneumonia*
Rickettsia: *Rickettsia rickettsii* (Rocky Mountain spotted fever), *Rickettsia prowazekii* (typhus), *Rickettsia conorii*, *Orientia tsutsugamushi*, *Ehrlichia chaffeensis*, *Anaplasma sp.* (human granulocytic ehrlichiosis), *Babesia sp.*
Protozoa and helminths: Taenia solium (cysticercosis), *Toxoplasma gondii*, *Trichinella spiralis* (trichinosis), *Chlamydia trachomatis*, *Strongyloides stercoralis* (eosinophilic meningitis or hyperinfection syndrome), *Angiostrongylus cantonensis* and *Baylisacaris procyonis* (eosinophilic meningitis), *Naegleria fowleri* (amoebic meningitis)

Parameningeal conditions
Sinusitis, epidural or subdural empyema, mastoiditis, cranial osteomyelitis, infection or inflammation related to ventricular shunts, deep brain stimulator leads, posterior fossa surgery, brain abscess, venous sinus thrombosis, subarachnoid hemorrhage

Drugs
Trimethoprim-sulfamethoxazole, ibuprofen, sulindac, tolmetin, naproxen, rofecoxib, diclofenac, ketoprofen, azathioprine, sulfasalazine, ciprofloxacin, amoxicillin, metronidazole, cephalosporins, pyrazinamide, isoniazid, carbamazepine, lamotrigine, ranitidine, phenazopyridine, chemical meningitis from drugs, air, or radiographic agents instilled in cerebrospinal fluid, chymopapain infections into spinal area, and intrathecal drug injections

Biological products
Monoclonal antibodies such as cetuximab, adalimumab, infliximab, ipilimumab, efalizumab, muromonab-CD3, and intravenous gammaglobulin

Systemic or immunologically mediated diseases
Sarcoidosis, systemic lupus erythematosus, rheumatoid arthritis, polyarteritis nodosa, granulomatous arteritis, mixed connective tissue disease, Sjögren's syndrome, lymphomatoid granulomatosis, Wegener's granulomatosis, Behçet's disease, Kawasaki disease, Vogt-Koyanagi-Harada syndrome, familial Mediterranean fever, status epilepticus, postinfectious syndromes

Neoplastic diseases
Leukemia, leptomeningeal carcinoma, lymphoma, craniopharyngioma, teratoma, astrocytoma, medulloblastoma, dermoid and epidermoid cysts

Recurrent viral meningitis

Recurrent viral meningitis is uncommon. More than 90% of cases are caused by herpes simplex virus (95% of those by HSV-2 and 5% by HSV-1). HSV-2 infections are common worldwide. In Sweden the seroprevalence in childbearing women is around 25%, and in the United States about 45 million adults are infected. Most patients are older children and adults, with a slight female predominance. A prodrome of low back and buttock pain, often radicular, may develop, followed by fever, nausea, headache, photophobia, and meningismus lasting 2–7 days. Spontaneous recovery is typical over several weeks. Some, but not all, patients develop genital vesicles. The total number of episodes ranges from 3–9, with the time to recurrence varying from weeks to months or years. Over time, recurrences become less common. The syndrome originally called Mollaret's meningitis appears to be mainly due to recurrent HSV meningitis.

About 5% of patients with recurrent meningitis lack evidence of HSV infection in the CSF. Rare cases have been associated with recurrent enterovirus infections, often of different serotypes. Importantly, recurrent aseptic meningitis may be due to repeated exposures to drugs or biological products that trigger aseptic meningitis, intracranial and intraspinal tumors and cysts that periodically leak antigenic material into the CSF, and systemic connective tissue diseases (see Table 79.3). Despite the presence of many thousands of cells in CSF, predominantly neutrophils, and of hypoglycorrhachia, the CSF in chemical aseptic meningitis is sterile. The specific irritating substance in the cyst fluid is unknown. Aseptic meningitis occurs not only with dermoid cysts, but also with craniopharyngiomas, and even in patients with glioblastoma multiforme.

Chronic viral meningitis

Persistence of viruses in the CNS is extremely rare in otherwise healthy individuals. When it happens, the viral persistence has been mainly due to adaptation of the virus to evade the host immune response or when the host immune response is deficient. HIV is the most common persistent meningeal virus; its persistence is the result of the virus evading and impairing the host immune response. Viral persistence develops early during the primary infection, with viral invasion of the brain and meninges. From that point, the CSF contains HIV in varying titer, usually accompanied by a low-grade lymphocytic pleocytosis. HIV may cause symptomatic meningitis during the primary infection, but seldom causes chronic meningeal symptoms. However, HIV may progress to a progressive HIV encephalopathy.

Viral and other infectious agents can persist in meninges when the host immune system is impaired, such as in AIDS or other immunosuppressive illnesses. Chronic viral infections of the meninges of immunosuppressed patients are recognized for several viruses, including cytomegalovirus, enteroviruses, poliovirus, West Nile, Epstein–Barr, herpes simplex, and varicella zoster. The best-recognized viral chronic meningitis occurs in patients with agammaglobulinemia who develop persistent enterovirus meningitis.

Differential diagnosis

The differential diagnosis of acute aseptic meningitis is broad, but the majority are due to viruses (Table 79.1). In addition, there are other causes that include bacteria, Rickettsia, protozoa, helminths, parameningeal conditions, drugs, biological products, systemic or immunologically mediated diseases, and neoplasms, as listed in Table 79.3. The cause of recurrent viral meningitis is mainly HSV-2, but a variety of different non-viral causes can produce recurrences (Table 79.3).

The causes of chronic meningitis are broad and rarely include viruses. More common causes include other infectious agents (bacteria, fungi, parasites), vasculitis, connective tissue diseases, sarcoidosis, chronic administration of drugs producing idiosyncratic meningitis, chemical meningitis from antigen leakage of CNS tumors into the CSF, and leptomeningeal cancer metastases (Table 79.3).

Investigations

In the workup of a patient, the first step is to utilize the history and neurological exam to establish a high suspicion of meningitis and to help distinguish meningitis from other CNS problems. The key to proving that the patient has meningitis is to perform a lumbar puncture and examine the CSF. The presence of CSF white blood cell pleocytosis establishes the diagnosis of meningitis. The opening CSF pressure should be obtained. From 10–20 ml of CSF should be collected in several sterile tubes. Important tests to be ordered include CSF cell count with differential white cell count, glucose level, protein level, Gram stain of spun CSF sediment, and tests to determine the etiology that include bacterial culture, relevant CSF polymerase chain reaction (PCR) assays, and possibly viral culture. Other CSF cultures such as for fungi and tuberculosis may be indicated.

Analysis of the CSF usually allows a distinction between bacterial and aseptic meningitis. Table 79.4 lists CSF findings supportive of viral and bacterial meningitis. In viral meningitis, the lumbar CSF opening pressure with the patient lying horizontal is at the upper limits of normal or slightly elevated, but not dramatically elevated. The CSF of most viral meningitides contains a predominance of mononuclear cells, with a mean of 60–150 cells/mm^3 and total CSF white blood cells ranging from 10–600/mm^3. Occasionally, if the CSF is examined in the first 12–24 hours of the viral meningitis, a transient predominance of neutrophils can be seen that converts to a lymphocytic predominance the following day.

A simultaneous serum glucose is helpful in determining whether the CSF glucose is depressed. CSF/serum glucose ratios below 50% are usually considered abnormal, as is a CSF glucose level below 40 mg/dL. Although viral meningitis usually has a normal glucose level, a few viruses, including varicella zoster, mumps, and lymphocytic choriomeningitis virus, may produce mildly depressed CSF glucose levels, typically from 30–40 mg/dL. In patients with CSF glucose levels less than 25 mg/dL, bacterial, fungal, or tuberculous meningitis should be considered. CSF protein levels are usually at the upper limit of normal or elevated as high as 100 mg/dL, but not highly elevated. CSF oligoclonal bands are unusual in the acute CSF sample.

In general, the fever in viral meningitis is mild, while it may be quite high in bacterial meningitis. Likewise, the peripheral white blood cell count in viral meningitis is often normal or slightly elevated, while in bacterial meningitis it may be quite elevated.

Once the CSF points to aseptic meningitis, the final diagnostic step is to identify the viral etiology. In general, the yield of virus isolation from CSF is below 50% and rapidly declines to less than 10% over several days. Viruses that are most commonly isolated from CSF in tissue culture or by animal inoculation include enterovirus, mumps, and lymphocytic choriomeningitis and the first episode of HSV-2. It is also possible to isolate the virus from other body sites that can include throat, nasopharynx, stool, and skin lesions. These sites may yield the virus when the CSF culture is negative. Unfortunately, virus isolation from non-CNS sites does not automatically mean that virus was the cause of the viral meningitis. False-positive isolations are particularly common for enteroviruses that often cause asymptomatic gastrointestinal infections in the summer, or for herpes simplex virus that often produces a silent salivary viral reactivation with any acute febrile illness.

Because of the difficulty in isolating virus from CSF, PCR assays have become popular. Viral PCR assays are rapid (often less than 1 day), less expensive than virus culture, have over 80–95% sensitivity and specificity depending on the virus, and can detect viral nucleic acid up to 1–2 weeks after disease onset. CSF PCR assays for enterovirus, herpes simplex, HIV, mumps, and varicella zoster viruses are readily available in many hospital laboratories.

A newly available advanced technology is "multiplex" reverse transcription (RT) PCR assays to identify common viruses and bacteria simultaneously in CSF in a reaction mixture to detect their nucleic acid. Commercial multiplex RT PCR assays report that analysis of a single CSF sample can detect nine different RNA and DNA neurotropic viruses, plus often common bacteria that cause meningitis. However, clinical judgment must be used in interpreting the results of these CSF assays, since occasionally dual viral infections are found and patients not suspected of a meningeal infection have had positive PCR assays.

A third method for establishing the etiology of viral meningitis is by demonstration of specific intrathecal antibody synthesis. Identification of specific IgM antibody in CSF is a common method to diagnosis West Nile virus neuroinvasive disease. CNS infection with varicella zoster virus can also be diagnosed by demonstration of varicella zoster antibody in CSF.

In patients with viral meningitis, the cranial CT or MRI scan with gadolinium is generally normal. However, in chronic viral meningitis or meningoencephalitis, the MRI may show focal brain or spinal cord abnormalities such as is seen in varicella zoster meningomyelitis. Electroencephalography is usually normal in aseptic meningitis, but occasionally shows transient diffuse abnormalities that normalize by 1 week.

Treatment

Typically, patients with aseptic meningitis are hospitalized, and given antinausea medication, intravenous fluids for dehydration, and age-appropriate medications for fever and headache. The majority of patients receive broad spectrum antibiotics until the CSF

Table 79.4 Distinguishing cerebrospinal fluid (CSF) features between viral and bacterial meningitis.

CSF feature	Viral meningitis*	Bacterial meningitis*
White blood cells	40 to <500 cells/mm^3	500 to >1000 cell/mm^3
White blood cell differential	Predominantly mononuclear	Predominantly neutrophils
Protein	Normal to mildly elevated	Elevated
Glucose	Normal to minimally depressed	Depressed
Lactate	Normal	Elevated
Gram stain of sediment	Negative	Positive
Bacterial culture	Negative	Positive

*These CSF features are usually present, but all the features will not necessarily be present in every patient.

bacterial cultures return, and also get acyclovir for possible atypical herpes simplex encephalitis until the CSF HSV PCR assay returns. The hospital duration ranges from 3–15 days.

Until recently, there has been little emphasis on establishing the specific etiology of the aseptic meningitis, because seldom did a specific viral diagnosis affect treatment options. The increasing availability of enterovirus and HSV PCR assays in children and adults with aseptic meningitis has shown that early use of this CSF PCR test can significantly shorten the duration of hospitalization by several days, reduce the need for neuroimaging and electroencephalography, and reduce total hospital costs by up to 50%.

Under ideal circumstances, a patient with enterovirus meningitis could be discharged after 24 hours if the following circumstances pertain:

- The patient's history, examination, and CSF findings, including a negative CSF Gram stain, are consistent with an aseptic meningitis and the patient is not immunosuppressed.
- CSF enterovirus PCR assay is positive (possibly because enterovirus PCR assay results usually are available within 1 day) and the HSV PCR assay is negative.
- The patient is improved symptomatically at 24 hours with respect to rehydration, nausea, and vomiting.
- CSF bacterial cultures are negative at 24 hours (most patients with acute bacterial meningitis have positive CSF bacterial cultures by 24–36 hours). It is extremely rare to have a CSF co-infection of both a virus and bacteria.
- There is a responsible caregiver who can monitor the patient and return them to the hospital if there is deterioration.

Currently there is no antiviral drug approved by the US Food and Drug Administration for treatment of enteroviral meningitis. If the CSF HSV PCR assay is positive and the patient does not have encephalitis, the patient often can be discharged early with pain medication. Use of antiviral drugs will depend on the severity of the meningitis. If the patient has recurrent mild HSV meningitis, the individual often can be discharged from the emergency room if the CSF HSV PCR assay is positive. Acute management of HSV meningitis is similar to that of enterovirus meningitis. However, patients are often also treated with anti-HSV drugs. Unfortunately, there have been no controlled studies to demonstrate that these anti-HSV drugs given intravenously or orally significantly shorten the duration of the headache and meningism. For patients hospitalized with severe HSV meningitis, treatment often consists of intravenous acyclovir, 10 mg/kg every 8 hours for several days. For treatment of subsequent episodes of recurrent meningitis, the patient may be given prescriptions for valacyclovir, 1 g 3 times per day for 1 week.

Currently use of anti-HSV drugs is neither thought to prevent future attacks nor to cure the sacral ganglia viral latency. Although daily prophylactic treatment with an anti-HSV drug reduces recurrent genital herpes simplex episodes, it is unclear whether it prevents recurrent HSV meningitis.

Management of mumps meningitis often depends on the severity of the parotitis or orchitis, but it also is symptomatic since there are no proven antiviral drugs for mumps.

Recovery and prognosis

Over 95% of patients with viral meningitis make a complete recovery. In one study of adults, 43% were symptom free at hospital discharge and over 50% were symptom free by 3 months. Mild cognitive deficits were reported in 7%, mainly in concentration, but studies examining cognition 1–2 years after acute aseptic meningitis found that the large majority of patients were normal. In very young infants, viral meningitis may cause more long-lasting nonspecific cognitive problems. Patients with enterovirus meningitis rarely have subsequent episodes of viral meningitis from the same virus serotype.

Recurrent episodes of HSV-2 meningitis usually decrease in frequency over several years. Full recovery is common after each episode. For individuals with persistent viral meningitis, such as chronic enterovirus meningitis in patients with agammaglobulinemia, the prognosis is poorer.

Further reading

Davis LE. Subacute and chronic meningitis. *Continuum* 2006;12:27–57.

DeBiasi RL, Tyler KL. Recurrent aseptic meningitis. In: Davis LE, Kennedy PGE (eds.). *Infectious Diseases of the Nervous System*. Oxford: Butterworth-Heimann; 2000: 445–479.

Hviid A, Rubin S, Muhlemann K. *Mumps. Lancet* 2008;371:932–944.

Jubelt B, Lipton H. Enterovirus/Picornavirus infections. In: Tselis AC, Booss J (eds.). *Handbook of Clinical Neurology*, Vol. 123 (3rd series). Amsterdam: Elsevier; 2014:379–416.

Leveque N, Van Haecke A, Renois F, *et al.* Rapid virological diagnosis of central nervous system infections by use of a multiplex reverse transcription-PCR DNA microarray. *J Clin Microbiol* 2011;49:3874–3879.

Mohseni MM, Wilde JA. Viral meningitis: Which patients can be discharged from the emergency department? *J Emerg Med* 2012;43:1181–1187.

Nowak DA, Boehmer R, Fuchs H-H. A retrospective clinical, laboratory and outcome analysis in 43 cases of acute aseptic meningitis. *Eur J Neurol* 2003;10:271–280.

Shaiabi M, Whiteley RJ. Recurrent benign lymphocytic meningitis. *Clin Infect Dis* 2006;43:1194–1197.

Steiner I, Benninger F. Update on herpes virus infections of the nervous system. *Curr Neurol Neurosci Rep* 2013;13:414–418.

80 Acute viral encephalitis

Heng Thay Chong[1] and Chong Tin Tan[2]

[1] Department of Neurology, Western Health, Melbourne, VIC, Australia
[2] Division of Neurology, University of Malaya, Kuala Lumpur, Malaysia

Overview of acute encephalitis

Encephalitis indicates inflammation of brain parenchyma. Often, there is concomitant meningitis. Viruses are the most common cause of encephalitis.

Epidemiology

The incidence of viral encephalitis is estimated to be 1–7.4/100,000 persons yearly, but may be as high as 16.7/100,000 in children under 2 years of age. This is in contrast to bacterial meningitis, which affects 36.3/100,000 persons yearly.

There are many viral causes of encephalitis (Table 80.1). The most important agents are the herpesviruses (see Chapter 81) and arbovirus-

Table 80.1 Viruses that affect the central nervous system.

Primary human viruses	
Herpesviruses	Herpes simplex type 1 & 2, varicella zoster, Epstein–Barr virus, cytomegalovirus, human herpes virus 6
Enteroviruses	Poliovirus 1–3, coxsackievirus A1–22, 24, B1–6, echovirus 1–7, 9, 11–27, 29–33, enterovirus 68–71
Other	Mumps, measles, rubella, human immunodeficiency virus, human T-cell lymphoma virus, adenovirus, parvovirus B19, JC virus, human metapneumovirus
Zoonotic viruses	
Arenavirus	Lymphocytic choriomeningitis virus, Lassa virus, Junin virus, Machupo virus, Guanarito virus, Sabia virus
Filovirus	Marburg virus, Ebola virus
Paramyxovirus	Nipah virus, Hendra virus
Rhabdovirus	Rabies virus, Mokola virus, Lyssavirus
Herpesvirus	B virus (Herpes simiae or Cercopithecine herpesvirus 1)
Arthropod viruses	
Flaviviridae	Mosquito-borne: St. Louis encephalitis virus, Japanese encephalitis virus, Murray Valley encephalitis virus, Kunjin virus, West Nile virus, Ilheus virus, Rocio virus
	Tick-borne: Far Eastern, Siberian, and Western European tick-borne encephalitis viruses, Negishi virus, Louping ill virus, Langat virus, Powassan virus, Omsk hemorrhagic fever virus, Kyasanur forest disease virus, Kadam virus and Royal farm virus (subtypes Karshi virus, Gadgets Gulley virus, and Alkhumra virus)
Bunyaviridae	California encephalitis virus, LaCrosse encephalitis virus, Jamestown Canyon virus, Snowshoe hare virus, Tahyna virus, Inkoo virus, Rift Valley virus, Toscana virus
Togaviridae (alphaviruses)	Eastern equine virus, Western equine virus, Venezuelan equine virus
Reoviridae (Orbivirus)	Colorado tick fever virus

es (arthropod-borne viruses). Japanese viral encephalitis is the most common encephalitis worldwide, while West Nile viral encephalitis is more widespread, occurring in Europe, Russia, Africa, the Middle East, India, Indonesia, and, recently, North America. In Eastern Europe, tick-borne encephalitis is highly prevalent. Rabies virus infection is endemic in Latin America, Asia, and Africa (see Figure 80.1).

Rabies, an exception to the generally limited zoonotic viruses, is carried worldwide by dogs and other wildlife, while the similar bat lyssavirus is found only in Australia. Zoonotic viruses are viruses carried by animals, and those affecting humans are primarily carried by rodents, primates, horses, bats, pigs, birds, dogs, and other small mammals, which also serve as reservoirs and amplifying hosts. Domesticated animals such as horses, pigs, buffalo, sheep, cattle, and camels serve as reservoirs for some of these viruses – such as Japanese encephalitis, West Nile, alphaviruses, and the Henipah (Hendra and Nipah virus) viruses. Most arboviruses are transmitted by mosquitoes and ticks.

Pathophysiology

Most encephalitic viruses are introduced through skin, respiratory, or gastrointestinal mucosal via insect bites, respiratory droplets, or contaminated food. Many of these viruses first replicate in the peripheral tissues, causing prodromal symptoms, before accessing the central nervous system (CNS) through hematogenous spread. Some viruses traverse the blood–brain barrier by replicating in the cerebrovascular endothelial cells and then infecting leukocytes that enter the CNS, whereas others may cross directly into cerebrospinal fluid (CSF) through the porous capillaries of the choroidal plexus. Other viruses, such as herpes simplex, varicella zoster, and rabies viruses, enter nerve terminals in end organs and utilize neuronal transport to infect neuronal cell bodies. The Henipah viruses cause both vasculitis with resultant thrombosis and infarct, as well as neuronal infection. Once inside the CNS, most viruses target the neurons; and some viruses have predilection for neurons in specific locations, such as the herpes simplex virus, which prefers the hippocampal neurons, Japanese encephalitis virus those in basal ganglia, and poliovirus the motor neurons in spinal cord and brainstem. These viruses travel within the neurons using the neuronal microtubule system and spread from neurons to neurons via synapses. Viral infection and replication, as well as the inflammatory response by activated astrocytes, microglial cells, monocytes, and lymphocytes, cause neuronal death. Gliosis ensues if the patient survives.

International Neurology, Second edition. Edited by Robert P. Lisak, Daniel D. Truong, William M. Carroll and Roongroj Bhidayasiri
© 2016 John Wiley & Sons, Ltd. Published 2016 by John Wiley & Sons, Ltd.

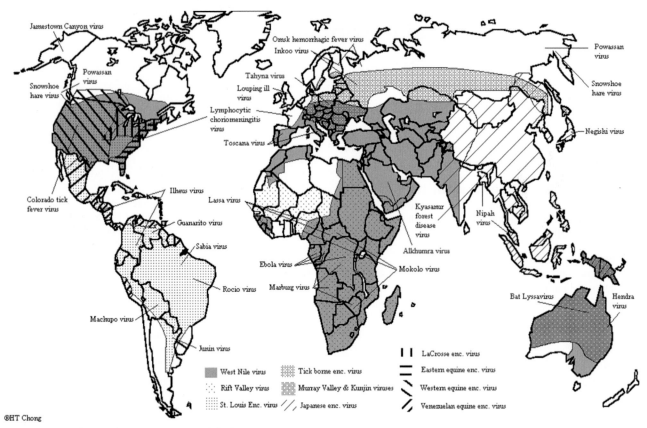

®HT Chong

Figure 80.1 Distribution of viruses causing encephalitides.

Viral elimination in infected but surviving cells involves immune mediated cytolysis, but because neurons are irreplaceable and neuronal death leads to loss of function, infected neurons are often spared cytolysis. A non-cytolytic mechanism does not eliminate viral RNA from neurons, therefore long-term immunological suppression by antibodies is required to prevent viral reactivation and progression of infection. When the immune system is compromised, viral reactivation and reinfection occur, such as in varicella zoster infection. Other viruses may target the glial cells, such as human immunodeficiency virus (HIV) and JC virus, and cause encephalopathy and demyelination, respectively.

Clinical features

Patients with acute encephalitis present with fever, headache, seizures, respiratory and abdominal symptoms, such as abdominal pain, nausea, vomiting, and diarrhea. Neurological examination shows impaired consciousness, confusion, and focal neurological deficits.

Investigations

Laboratory abnormalities are often non-specific. A complete blood count may show lymphocytosis. The clotting profile may be abnormal in patients with viruses that cause hemorrhagic complications, such as some arenaviruses and flaviviruses (see Table 80.2).

Electroencephalogram (EEG) often shows non-specific slow waves, although periodic lateralized epileptiform discharges are seen in herpes simplex encephalitis and severe Nipah encephalitis. Imaging studies are also non-specific, showing gray- and sometimes

Table 80.2 Laboratory investigations.

Investigation	Differential diagnoses and complications
Blood tests	Serum electrolytes, glucose level, renal function, liver function, arterial blood gases, thyroid function, peripheral blood picture, creatinine kinase, autoimmune markers, thick and thin film for malaria parasite; blood culture; serology for bacterial, treponemal, and rickettsial infection
Chest X-ray	Pneumonia or pneumonitis (atypical pneumonia, Nipah encephalitis), orthostatic or aspiration pneumonia (complication), pulmonary tuberculosis, pulmonary aspergillosis, disseminated candidiasis or cryptococcomas
EEG	Non-convulsive status epilepticus, triphasic waves (hepatic and metabolic encephalopathy), periodic lateralized epileptiform discharges, and focal slow waves
Brain CT scan	Brain abscess, subdural hematoma, vasculitic stroke
Brain MRI	Hyperintense signal in gray or white matter, diencephalon, brainstem, and cerebellum; tuberculoma, cryptococcomas, toxoplasma encephalitis, vasculitic stroke, and venogram (for sagittal sinus thrombosis)
Lumbar puncture	Opening pressure, cell count, and biochemical analysis; Gram stain and Ziehl–Nielsen stain; serology for bacterial, treponemal, and viral infection, cryptococcal antigen, bacterial and mycobacterial culture; PCR for tuberculosis, enterovirus, herpes simplex virus, cytomegalovirus, and other viruses; viral culture; quantitation of herpes simplex virus DNA copies for prognostication
Brain biopsy	Necrosis, hemorrhage, intraneuronal or intranuclear inclusion body, Negri body, vasculitic changes, fluorescence in situ hybridization.

white-matter involvement. CSF examination typically shows high opening pressure, lymphocytosis and increased protein levels; glucose levels are often normal.

Specific etiological diagnosis is based on serological studies, viral culture, and polymerase chain reaction (PCR) to detect specific viral genomes in CSF (Table 80.3). Differential diagnoses of viral encephalitis include other CNS infections, autoimmune and metabolic diseases (Table 80.4). In up to 75% of patients, specific viral studies such as serology, PCR, and viral culture are negative. Acute disseminated encephalomyelitis and autoimmune encephalitis are particularly difficult to distinguish from viral encephalitis, although magnetic resonance imaging (MRI) in acute disseminated encephalomyelitis often shows multifocal asymmetric white-matter lesions and less prominent gray-matter involvement. Auto-antibodies, such as anti-NMDAR, anti-VGKC, anti-neuronal, and anti-TPO antibodies, are generally helpful in the diagnosis of autoimmune encephalopathy.

Table 80.3 Specific clinical features of viruses causing encephalitis.

Clinical features	Suggestive virus
Children	Japanese encephalitis virus, Venezuelean equine virus, LaCrosse virus, enterovirus, adenovirus, Tahyna virus and human metapneumovirus; poor outcome in Japanese encephalitis, Western and Eastern equine encephalitis
Elderly	West Nile virus, alphaviruses; worse outcome in St. Louis, West Nile, Eastern equine, and Nipah encephalitis
Immunosuppressed host	Cytomegalovirus, JC virus (progressive multifocal leucoencephalopathy), measles virus (measles inclusion body encephalitis), recurrent enterovirus infection
Chronic or recurrent encephalitis	Measles virus (measles inclusion body encephalitis and subacute sclerosing panencephalitis), Nipah virus, Hendra virus, enterovirus in patients with immunoglobulin deficiency
Biphasic fever	Tick-borne encephalitis virus, Kyasanur forest disease virus
Parkinsonism	Japanese encephalitis virus, West Nile virus, tick-borne encephalitis virus, Western equine virus
Cerebellar involvement	Varicella zoster virus, Junin virus
Brainstem involvement	West Nile virus, tick-borne encephalitis virus, St. Louis virus, enterovirus 71, Nipah virus, Hendra virus
Spinal cord involvement	Japanese encephalitis virus, West Nile virus, rabies virus (paralytic rabies), tick-borne encephalitis virus, cytomegalovirus, human T-cell lymphoma virus type 1, human immunodeficiency virus
Autonomic involvement	Herpes simplex virus, Nipah virus, and rabies virus (furious rabies)
Meningeal involvement	Enterovirus, Epstein–Barr virus, West Nile virus, parvovirus B9, lymphocytic choriomeningitis virus, Toscana virus, Colorado tick fever virus
Coexisting retinitis	Cytomegalovirus
Myoclonus, opsoclonus	Nipah virus, Japanese encephalitis virus, rabies virus, St. Louis encephalitis virus
Urinary symptoms	St. Louis encephalitis virus
Respiratory and/ or abdominal involvement	LaCrosse virus, Nipah virus, Venezuelan equine virus, Guanarito virus, human metapneumovirus
Bleeding diasthesis	Kyasanur forest disease virus, arenavirus (Lassa, Junin, Machupo, Guanarito, and Sabia viruses), filovirus (Marburg and Ebola viruses)

Table 80.4 Differential diagnoses of viral encephalitis. Source: Kennedy 2002. Reproduced with permission of Springer.

Infective causes	
Bacterial	Abscess, actinomycoses, *Bartonella henselae*, *Borrelia burgdorferi*, brucella, legionella, leptospira, *Listeria monocytogenes*, *Mycobacterium tuberculosis*, *Mycoplasma pneumoniae*, nocardia, *Salmonella typhi*, *Treponema pallidum*, *Tropheryma whippeli* (Whipple disease)
Rickettsial	Ehrlichiosis, Q fever, Rocky Mountain spotted fever, typhus
Fungal	Aspergillosis, blastomycosis, candidiasis, coccidioidomycosis, cryptococcosis, histoplasmosis
Parasitic	Malaria, *Nagleria fowleri*, toxoplasmosis, trypanosomiasis, schistosomiasis
Non-infective causes	
Autoimmune diseases	Acute demyelinating encephalomyelitis, Bickerstaff encephalitis, vasculitides involving the central nervous system, autoimmune encephalopathy, Rasmussen syndrome, system lupus erythematosus
Metabolic diseases	Mitochondrial disease, thyrotoxic storm, neuroleptic malignant syndrome, thrombotic thrombocytopenic purpura, severe systemic sepsis, hepatic encephalopathy, uremia, diabetic complications (hypoglycemia, hyperglycemia hyperosmolar syndrome, diabetic ketoacidosis), nutritional deficiency (e.g., Wernicke's encephalopathy)
Other systemic diseases	Hypoxic encephalopathy, malignant hypertension, non-convulsive status epilepticus, sagittal sinus thrombosis, poisoning

Treatment

Treatment of viral encephalitis is broadly divided into supportive care and treatment of complications, specific antiviral therapy, and rehabilitation. The patient's vital signs and state of consciousness should be closely monitored, which is often best done in an intensive care unit. If consciousness is impaired, as indicated by a low or rapidly deteriorating Glasgow Coma Scale score, or if the patient is in status epilepticus, intubation and mechanical ventilation should be applied to provide airway protection and prevent aspiration pneumonia. Intravenous hydration and nasogastric tube feeding are necessary, with meticulous attention to fluid, electrolyte, and acid-base balance. Ripple mattress, coma nursing, regular positional change to prevent pressure sores, chest physiotherapy to prevent orthostatic pneumonia, and deep vein thrombosis prophylaxis are essential. Urinary catheters, if used, must be changed regularly and aseptically. Seizures must be rapidly controlled. Specific antiviral therapy is only available in a few instances (Table 80.5).

Generally, the outcome of viral encephalitis is relatively good. The overall mortality in children is only 4.5%, and only 8.1% develop neurological sequelae. Japanese encephalitis, Nipah encephalitis, and Eastern equine encephalitis have higher mortality rates of 5–30%, 30–40%, and 30–80%, respectively. Viral encephalitis may be complicated by cerebral salt-losing syndrome, syndrome of inappropriate antidiuretic hormone secretion (SIADH), and venous thrombosis.

Table 80.5 Specific treatment for viral infections of the central nervous system

Virus	Therapy
Herpes simplex virus	Acyclovir 10 mg/kg, 3 times daily IV for 10–14 days, or valacyclovir/famciclovir
Cytomegalovirus	Ganciclovir 5 mg/kg, 2 times daily IV with/without foscarnet 60 mg/kg, 3 times daily IV, valganciclovir, cidofovir
Herpes zoster virus	Acyclovir 800 mg, 5 times daily IV for 7–10 days, or famciclovir 500 mg, 3 times daily for 7 days, or valacyclovir 1 g, 3 times daily IV for 7 days
Enterovirus	Pleconaril 5 mg/kg, 3 times daily IV for 10 days, or IV Ig for patients with Ig deficiency
Nipah virus	Ribavirin 2 g day 1, 1.2 g 3 times daily from days 2–4, 1.2 g 2 times daily from days 5–6, 0.6 g 2 times daily for another 1–4 days orally
JC virus in HIV infection	Highly active antiretroviral agent therapy

Rabies and bat lyssavirus

Pre-exposure vaccination

– Human diploid cell or purified chick embryo cell vaccine on days 0, 7, and 28 in the deltoid; boost 1 year later and then every 2–5 years depending on exposure.

Post-exposure prophylaxis

– Swab all wounds for bacterial culture, thoroughly cleanse with soap and water, and irrigate with a virucidal agent such as povidone–iodine solution; give tetanus toxoid and antibiotics for Gram negatives and anaerobes.
– If not previously vaccinated, administer human rabies Ig 20 IU/kg. If possible, infiltrate the full dose around and into the wounds; if not, administer remaining volume IM at sites distant from vaccine administration. Human diploid cell or purified chick embryo cell vaccine 1 mL IM in deltoid (or lateral thigh in small children) on days 0, 3, 7, and 14. If immunosuppressed, administer an extra dose on day 28. Do not administer into gluteal region.
– If previously vaccinated with tissue culture rabies vaccine or if vaccinated with older vaccine and has documented adequate antibodies response, *do not* use human rabies Ig. Administer human diploid cell or purified chick embryo cell vaccine 1 mL IM in deltoid (or lateral thigh in small children) on day 0 and in contralateral deltoid on day 3. Do not administer into gluteal region.

Specific viral encephalitides: Rabies

Rabies virus is a RNA virus of the genus *Lyssavirus*, of the family *Rhabdoviridae*. Infection is almost universally fatal and it is the commonest fatal CNS infection. Except for Australia, the Antarctic, and a few island states, the virus has a worldwide distribution.

Epidemiology

Rabies remains an important worldwide health problem, with more than 35,000 reported human infections yearly; an estimated 25,000 of these occur in India alone. The incidence is less than 0.1–1.0 case/100,000 persons in most countries, but it is as high as 3 cases/100,000 persons in South Asia, probably because of the large number of stray dogs in the country. The primary dog variant of rabies virus was eliminated in North America through extensive mass vaccination and stray control programs. Recent phylogenetic analysis and epizootiological data show no evidence of enzootic dog rabies in the United States for the last 13 years. The virus, however, persists in wild carnivores, which causes occasional outbreaks in domestic dogs in the past. A related virus, bat lyssavirus, is found in Australia. In the developing world, rabies-infected dogs are the primary vector and are responsible for 90% of human infections, while in developed countries, rabies is more often caused by infected bats and small terrestrial mammals.

Pathophysiology

At the site of inoculation, the rabies virus infects muscle fibers and, by binding to the nicotinic acetylcholine receptor at the neuromuscular junction, gains entry into neurons. The virus then spreads retrogradely along the peripheral nerves to the CNS via fast axonal transport. After establishing infection in the CNS, the virus spreads along the sensory nerves to various parts of the body such as the skin, visceral organs, muscle spindles, and salivary glands.

Rabies causes an acute non-suppurative meningoencephalomyelitis. Autopsy specimens show perineural and perivascular mononuclear cell infiltrates, neuronophagia, ganglion cell degeneration, and glial nodules distributed widely in the brain, brainstem, spinal cord, and peripheral nerves. Intracytoplasmic inclusion bodies (Negri bodies) contain viral ribonucleoprotein and are found in 80% of human patients, particularly in the pyramidal cells of Ammon's horn in the hippocampus, in Purkinje cells in the cerebellum, and in the medulla.

Clinical features

Rabies infection can be divided into four clinical stages: namely, incubation, prodrome, neurological manifestations, and death. Incubation can range from 5 days to 12 months, but usually lasts between 3 and 8 weeks. Facial inoculation, multiple severe bites, transmission by corneal transplantation, and accidental inoculation are associated with a shorter incubation period. The prodromal symptoms, usually lasting a few days, consist of fever, flu-like symptoms, and in one-third of patients, localized pruritus, pain, or paraesthesiae at the site of the bite. After the prodromal period, about two-thirds of patients develop periodic spasms, autonomic dysfunction, hydrophobia, and aerophobia ("furious" rabies), whereas the other one-third develop ascending lower motor neuron weakness without phobia or spasms ("paralytic" rabies). Without intensive care, death, often preceded by coma, occurs within 1–2 weeks.

Furious rabies

Furious rabies is characterized by hydrophobia, aerophobia, and episodic generalized arousal interrupted by periodic spasm involving the diaphragm and other respiratory muscles. This is followed by generalized spasm and opisthotonos, with episodic generalized arousal associated with hyperesthesiae, hallucination, and agitated confusion. Between these episodes, the patient is alert, lucid, and rational. Other findings include rhisus sardonicus, meningism, cranial nerve palsy, upper motor neuron weakness, muscle fasciculations, and abnormal involuntary movement. Patients with furious rabies often progress to coma, flaccid paralysis, and then death within 1 week.

Dumb rabies

Patients with paralytic rabies develop paralysis, paraesthesiae, pain, and muscle fasciculations, starting in the inoculated limb and gradually ascending to other parts of the body, causing quadriplegia, sphincteric disturbance, bulbar and respiratory muscle palsy. Hydrophobia and aerophobia are usually absent and the patient may survive for several weeks even without intensive treatment. Similar to furious rabies, death is preceded by coma. Rabies with atypical clinical features are increasingly seen, including tetanus-like trismus, transverse myelitis, myoclonus, hemichorea, and Horner's syndrome, especially in infection from bats.

Investigations

During the prodromal phase, MRI shows T2 hyperintensities in the brachial plexus, nerve roots, and spinal cord in both furious and paralytic ("dumb") rabies. This is followed by T2 hyperintensities in the midline structures of the brain, such as the brainstem, thalamus, hypothalamus, basal ganglia, and limbic structure, with minimal or no gadolinium enhancement in the non-comatose phase. When the patient becomes comatose, the blood–brain barrier breaks down and enhancement is seen in these midline structures, especially the brainstem. Confirmatory tests include serum-neutralizing antibodies, nuchal skin biopsy, corneal impression smears, and brain biopsy. Recent advances in diagnostics include the use of PCR to detect the virus in saliva, skin, and CSF. PCR assay is nearly 100% sensitive if three serial saliva samples or three different samples (such as saliva, CSF, urine, or hair follicles) are analyzed simultaneously.

Treatment

Table 80.5 summarizes pre-exposure vaccination and treatment of rabid animal bites. Wound cleansing is the most effective means of rabies prevention. Modern tissue culture vaccine (human diploid cell vaccine or purified chick embryo cell vaccine) may cause mild local symptoms in approximately 15% of patients if given intramuscularly (IM) or in 35% if given intradermally. Transient constitutional symptoms such as fever, headache, or flu-like symptoms occur in approximately 7% of patients and 10% may suffer from mild immune complex disease 3–13 days after booster injections. Human rabies immunoglobulin (Ig) is administered to patients without prior vaccination up to 7 days post exposure; given after this point, Ig administration could suppress antibody production from vaccination and is therefore not recommended. Supportive treatments include benzodiazepines, ketamine, barbiturates, and morphine. Coma induction is no longer recommended. Nimodipine to relieve vasospasm should be used with caution, since it may cause hypotension and shock.

Japanese encephalitis

Epidemiology

Japanese encephalitis virus, a flavivirus, is transmitted by the *Culex tritaeniorhynchus* mosquito between birds and pigs, both of which develop high viremia and are important in maintaining, amplifying, and transmitting the disease. Humans do not develop significant viremia and are thus dead-end hosts, but can become infected when living close to the enzootic cycle of the virus in rural areas. Japanese encephalitis has spread from East and Southeast Asia to Russia, the Guam islands, India, and the northern tip of Australia. Today, it is the most common cause of arboviral encephalitis, with an annual incidence of 1.8/100,000 in adults and 5.4/100,000 in children. It causes some 67,900 infections and at least 15,000 deaths annually, accounting for more infections and death than all other arboviruses combined. Half of the infections occur in China. In endemic areas, it is a disease of children and young adults, with 75% of infections worldwide occurring in children aged 0–14 years, although non-immune adults, who are more likely to develop symptomatic infection, are also affected during outbreaks. In northern Asia, epidemics occur during the summer months; in the south, the disease is endemic, with outbreaks occurring in the monsoon months.

Pathophysiology

After the bite of an infected mosquito, the virus multiplies in skin and lymph nodes, followed by transient viremia. The mechanism of entry into the CNS is unclear, but passive transfer through endothelial cells is thought to be important. In the brain, the virus causes diffuse encephalitis, seen macroscopically in autopsy specimen as focal petechiae or hemorrhage involving gray matter. The thalamus, basal ganglia, and midbrain are severely affected. Microscopically, there is perivascular cuffing, mononuclear cell infiltration, and phagocytosis of dead cells. Immunologically, the patient mounts a rapid and effective IgM response within days, which limits viral replication and may facilitate lysis of infected cells. Cytotoxic T-cells are believed to be important in the clearance of the virus.

Clinical features

Only 1 in 25 to 1 in 1000 patients infected with Japanese encephalitis virus becomes symptomatic. Naïve adults are more likely to be symptomatic than local populations in endemic areas, for reasons that may be related to the age of patients when first exposed, different genetic susceptibilities, partial protection from previous infections of other flaviviruses, or reporting bias. Symptoms range from mild, non-specific, flu-like illness to fatal meningoencephalitis. Severity depends on the route of viral entry, the size and virulence of the inoculum, and host factors such as age, prior immunity, genetic factors, and general health.

After a variable incubation period of 2–14 days and non-specific viral prodromal symptoms, patients present with headaches, abdominal pain, nausea, vomiting, fever, and lethargy, followed by meningism such as neck stiffness and photophobia. Seizure occurs in 50–85% of children and 10% of adults, including convulsive and non-convulsive status epilepticus, and carries a poorer prognosis.

On examination, mask-like facies, tremor, generalized hypertonia, and cogwheel rigidity are seen in 70–80% of adults and 20–40% of children. Titubation, pill-rolling tremor, choreoathetosis, orofacial dyskinesia, and upper motor facial nerve palsy are seen in about 10% of patients, presumably due to the involvement of the thalamus and basal ganglia. Opisthotonus, opsoclonus, myoclonus, changes in respiratory pattern, decerebrate or decorticate posturing, and pupillary and vestibulo-ocular reflex abnormalities indicate brainstem involvement and may herald a poorer prognosis. Mortality is 5–30%, particularly in younger children, and nearly one-third of survivors have serious neurological sequelae. Some patients present with flaccid paralysis of one or more limbs, probably due to anterior horn cell damage, and one-third of these eventually develop encephalitis.

Investigations

Routine blood tests may show peripheral leukocytosis and hyponatremia due to SIADH. EEG shows diffuse slowing, alpha-, theta-, or delta-coma, burst suppression, or epileptiform activity. Brain MRI shows more extensive involvement of the cerebral hemispheres, thalamus, basal ganglia, cerebellum, brainstem, and spinal cord. Single-photon emission tomography shows hyperperfusion in the thalamus and putamen.

Definitive diagnosis is made with IgM and IgG enzyme-linked immunosorbent assays (ELISAs), which have more than 95% sensitivity and specificity if tested in CSF after 4 days and in serum after 7 days of symptom onset. Previous infection by or vaccination against another flavivirus could cause cross-reactivity. PCR can detect small amounts of viral RNA though it should not be used to exclude the diagnosis.

Treatment

Prevention of Japanese encephalitis includes mosquito control programs and prevention of mosquito bites. For individuals 1–17 years of age, inactivated mouse brain–derived vaccine is given in three doses (days 0, 7, and 30). Up to 20% of vaccine recipients report local side effects, such as swelling, tenderness, and redness, while 10% report mild systemic side effects of fever, chills, malaise, and headache. The risk of severe neurological side effects, such as encephalitis or encephalopathy, seizure, and peripheral neuropathy, is only 0.1–0.23 cases/100,000 recipients. Recently, up to 1/100 recipients in Europe, North America, and Australia reported a new pattern of side effects consisting of pruritus, urticaria, and facial angioedema. Production of this vaccine has ceased and the remaining stock in the United States is reserved for children. A live attenuated vaccine (SA 14-14-2, produced by Chengdu Institute of Biological Products, Chengdu, China) with proven effectiveness of 88–96% is given in only 2 doses at short intervals of 1–2.5 months. It causes infrequent (0.2–6%) mild side effects and virtually no neurotoxicity. Although it has been shown to be effective and safe in children, it is only available in some Asian countries. Another purified formalin-inactivated whole virus vaccine (IXIARO/JESPECT IC51, produced by Intercell, Vienna, Austria) has a high seroconversion rate of 83% in 1 year when given in 2 doses of 6 μg with a 28-day interval. The vaccine is available worldwide, but is only approved by the US Food and Drug Administration (FDA) for persons 17 years or older. A fourth vaccine based on a chimeric virus (IMOJEV/ChimeriVax-JE, produced by Acambis/Sanofi-Aventis, Paris, France) elicits protective neutralizing antibodies in 96–99% of subjects 1 month after a single dose. It has been tested and approved for individuals ≥1 year of age in some countries (Australia, Malaysia, and Thailand), although a booster dose after 1–2 years is necessary for those ≤18 years of age. There have been no safety concerns, but the efficacy beyond 5 years is unknown. Travelers who visit endemic areas during rainy seasons, or who stay near pig farms, or in rural or agricultural areas or for long durations (≥30 days), need to be vaccinated.

There is no definitive antiviral agent for Japanese encephalitis, although various compounds, such as isoquinoline and α-interferon, have been tried. Treatment is therefore mainly supportive and symptomatic.

West Nile encephalitis

Epidemiology

Birds are natural reservoirs of West Nile virus, a flavivirus transmitted by the *Culex* mosquito from birds to humans and animals such as horses, domestic animals, and other mammals, which are dead-end hosts. The virus is widely distributed across Africa, the Middle East, India, Southern Europe, Russia, and North America. In the Nile Delta, about 40% of humans have antibodies against it. Although it is asymptomatic in endemic populations, outbreaks have occurred in South Africa, Europe, and Russia. Phylogenetic studies reveal at least five lineages of the virus, with lineage 1 clade 1a found in North America, Europe, the Middle East, and Africa, generally causing more severe human neurological disease and being responsible for almost all recent outbreaks. Lineage 2 (endemic in sub-Saharan Africa and Madagascar, with occasional outbreaks in Europe) and lineage 1 clade 1b (also known as Kunjin virus, found in Australia) generally cause milder disease. Lineage 1 clade 1c is found only in India. Lineage 3 contains of a single isolate from

mosquitoes in Austria in 1997, and lineage 4 has been found circulating in Russia since 1988. Little is known about lineage 5.

Pathophysiology

West Nile virus causes encephalomyelitis and leptomeningitis. Histologically, microglial nodules with neuronal loss are seen in the gray and white matter of the cerebrum, hippocampus, thalamus, medulla, and, possibly, anterior horn cells. There is perivascular infiltration by mononuclear cells and focal inflammation of cranial nerves and leptomeninges. Immunohistochemical staining shows viral antigens in neuronal cytoplasm and processes associated with glial nodules.

Clinical features

In endemic areas, over 80% of infection is asymptomatic, and most symptomatic infections are mild, self-limiting febrile illnesses. About 1–5% of symptomatic patients, usually the elderly, suffer from neurological disease. Generally, symptomatic patients present 3–15 days after incubation with flu-like illness (i.e., headache, myalgia, nausea, vomiting, and chills). Half of patients have a non-pruritic roseolar or maculopapular rash that generally lasts no more than a week. Some patients suffer from severe fatigue during recovery. CNS involvement includes aseptic meningitis, encephalitis, optic neuritis, and myelitis with anterior horn cell involvement causing flaccid paresis.

Severe neurological involvement is seen in non-endemic areas. In these patients, 30% develop meningitis while 60%, particularly those ≥50 years of age, develop encephalitis. In those with encephalitis, common symptoms include fever, headache, nausea, vomiting, chills and rigors, myalgia, backache, and weakness. Common signs are confusion, drowsiness, tremor, neck stiffness, myoclonus, ataxia, parkinsonism such as rigidity, bradykinesia, and postural instability, cranial nerve palsies such as dysphagia and absent corneal and gag reflexes, and brainstem dysfunction such as nystagmus and apnoeic episodes. Some patients develop an asymmetric flaccid paralysis with areflexia and bladder dysfunction due to anterior horn cell involvement.

The overall mortality from West Nile infection is 3–16%, but twice as high in those hospitalized. Patients ≥68 years of age and those with flaccid paralysis fare the worst.

Investigations

In patients with encephalitis or meningitis, mild peripheral blood leukocytosis is common. MRI shows bilateral, focal T2 hyperintense lesions in the thalamus, basal ganglia, pons, and sometimes spinal cord in severely ill patients, and evidence of meningitis. EEG shows diffuse, irregular slow waves with sharp waves or seizure activity. Electromyography may show axonal neuropathy, probably reflecting anterior horn cell involvement, although a demyelinating neuropathy is also seen in some patients. Depending on when the sample is obtained, CSF shows polymorphonuclear or lymphocytic pleocytosis.

Infection is diagnosed with a rising convalescent titer in serum or in CSF 8–21 days after symptom onset, or with detection of IgM using ELISA. Because West Nile virus cross-reacts with antibodies directed against other flaviviruses, the presence of specific IgM should be confirmed via plaque reduction assay to detect neutralizing antibodies. Viral isolation using the Vero cell line is less sensitive, but very specific. Other tests include virus gene sequencing and PCR. Viral load can be quantified with real-time PCR if CSF samples are obtained early in infection.

Treatment

Apart from supportive management, there is no specific treatment for West Nile encephalitis.

Tick-borne encephalitis

Epidemiology

Tick-borne encephalitis is the most common encephalitis in Europe, where there are three subtypes of the virus species: Far Eastern (formerly designated Russian spring and summer), Siberian (formerly West Siberian), and Western European (formerly Central European).

The virus is transmitted by *Ixodes* and *Haemaphysalis* ticks. *Ixodes* ticks are found in Europe, the Baltic States, Central Asia, and North Africa. Small mammals such as rodents and wolves act as major reservoirs and amplifying hosts, while insectivores such as moles, hedgehogs, and shrews serve as additional reservoirs. Humans are dead-end hosts. Worldwide, 10,000–20,000 clinical cases are reported annually, particularly in Central and Eastern Europe, where the viruses account for 29–54% of encephalitis with a diagnosis. The risk is highest among farmers, hunters, forest workers, and, in Russia, the unemployed. In more affluent countries, infection is contracted during outdoor leisure activities where men are at higher risk of infection. The incidence is as high as 80 cases/100,000 persons yearly in parts of Finland, but generally ranges from 10–30 cases/100,000 persons yearly. Seroprevalence varies from 1% (France) to 32.4% (Lithuania). The virus has been shown to be transmitted by goat milk in Slovakia. Encephalitis caused by the Far Eastern subtype is also found in the Jilin and Yunan provinces in China, and in Hokkaido, Japan.

Pathophysiology

Tick-borne encephalitis virus is found in tick saliva and is introduced into the skin via tick bites. The virus first infects the Langerhans cells before invading the lymphoid and reticuloendothelial system, where it spreads hematogenously to other organs, including the CNS, probably by infecting and seeding through capillary endothelial cells. Once inside the CNS, it causes widespread inflammation in the leptomeninges, cortical gray matter, brainstem, cerebellum, and spinal cord. Histologically, neuronal degeneration, necrosis, and neuronophagia are observed, with prominent perivascular inflammatory cell infiltration.

Clinical features

Serological surveys suggest that 70–95% of human infection is subclinical. Symptomatic patients have a biphasic illness. After a median incubation period of 8 days (range 4–28 days), the patient complains of fever, myalgia, nausea, fatigue, and headache. This viremic phase usually lasts for 4–18 days. After an interval of 8–133 days, 74–87% of patients present with CNS infection. Because the virus invades the CNS widely, tick-borne encephalitis can present in many clinical forms; 45–56% of patients have encephalitis, while others have meningitis, radiculitis, or myelitis ("poliomyelitic" form). Encephalitic patients present with fever, headache, ataxia, meningism, dyskinesia, confusion, altered consciousness, tremor, cranial nerve palsies, and, rarely, seizure. Ataxia is typical, and when cranial nerves are involved, motor nerves are affected. Approximately half have meningitis, presenting with fever, headache, nausea, vomiting, vertigo, and meningeal irritation; 11–15% of patients have radiculitis

or polyradiculoneuritis. Patients with myelitis present with lower motor neuron weakness of the neck and upper limbs, sparing the lower limbs. The paresis is occasionally preceded by severe pain. Autonomic dysfunction with heart rate abnormality has been reported. Diffuse involvement of the CNS causing meningoencephalomyelitis is the most severe form of the disease.

Central brainstem involvement and diffuse cerebral edema are common causes of death, usually within 5–10 days from onset. Mortality is ≤1% in many European countries, but is reportedly higher in Siberia (6–8%) and the Far East (20–40%). This could be due either to more virulent strains of virus in these regions or bias in case ascertainment and hospitalization. Mortality is higher among adults than children. Up to 10% of patients suffer from permanent spinal paralysis and as many as 26–46% have long-term disabilities. Mortality is higher in older patients, those with reduced consciousness, ataxia, abnormal MRI, pleocytosis of more than 300 cells/μL in CSF, and impairment of the blood–brain barrier.

Laboratory features

Thrombocytopenia, leukopenia, and elevated liver enzymes are seen in 10–20% of patients in the viremic phase. In the meningoencephalitic phase, white cell counts and inflammatory markers are elevated in the majority and CSF analysis is similar to that of other viral encephalitides, although the serum:CSF albumin ratio often shows serious blood–brain barrier damage. Computed tomography (CT) scan is often normal, while MRI shows T2 hyperintensity in the thalamus, putamen, pallidum, caudate nucleus, brainstem, and cerebellum. Because most patients present during the second phase of the illness when the antibody titer is high, viral isolation and PCR are not useful. ELISA of specific IgM is the main diagnostic method. However, antibodies to other flaviviruses cross-react in this assay, so that neutralizing tests may be necessary in patients previously exposed to other flaviviruses or to vaccination. In those with incomplete vaccination, demonstration of intrathecal synthesis of specific antibodies is necessary for diagnosis. Almost all patients have specific antibodies in the CSF 2 weeks after the onset of symptoms.

Management

There is no specific treatment for tick-borne encephalitis, and management is largely supportive. Two similar vaccines with a protection rate of 95–98% are available and given IM in three doses (the second dose in 2–12 weeks, the third dose in 5–12 months), preferably during winter, with subsequent booster doses every 3–5 years, depending on exposure risk.

St. Louis encephalitis

Epidemiology

St. Louis encephalitis virus, a flavivirus, is the second most common cause of viral encephalitis in the United States. Although it occurs primarily in the Ohio–Mississippi Valley, human infection has been documented throughout the United States and the virus has been isolated from southern Canada to Argentina. It is carried by the *Culex* mosquito and amplified by passage between mosquitoes and birds. The virus spills out of the zoonotic cycle when there are sufficient infected mosquitoes, causing waves of epidemic outbreaks in humans approximately every 10 years. Sentinel cases often occur in the elderly due to the increased risk of clinical encephalitis and mortality.

Pathology

St. Louis virus causes meningoencephalitis with leptomeningeal infiltration by lymphocytes, macrophages, polymorphonuclear leukocytes, and plasma cells, particularly around the brainstem, cerebellum, and in the Virchow–Robin spaces. Neuronal death and neuronophagia occur in the brain parenchyma, where cellular nodules composed of monocytes, lymphocytes, and microglial cells are seen. Gray matter, the substantia nigra, and thalamic nuclei are the most severely affected, although the cerebellum, pontine tegmentum, medulla, striatum, and spinal cord are variably affected as well.

Clinical features

The number of people infected by St. Louis virus who actually develop clinical disease ranges widely (1:800 to 1:100,000). Of those with clinically apparent illness, 40% of young adults and children suffer only from mild aseptic meningitis, while 90% of the elderly develop encephalitis. The onset of encephalitis can be abrupt or slow and is usually marked by fever, headache, dizziness, nausea, and malaise. Other clinical features include meningism, confusion, disorientation, tremor, unsteady gait, and apathy. Although the pathogenesis of urinary tract involvement is unknown, 25% of patients have urinary frequency, urgency, incontinence, or retention. Cranial nerve palsies are seen in 20% of patients. SIADH is occasionally seen. The disease progresses for up to a week before resolution, although 30–50% of patients exhibit prolonged asthenia, irritability, tremor, insomnia, depression, poor memory, headache, and, in more severe cases, gait and speech disturbances. Mortality is 5–20%, but as high as 70% in those ≥75 years old.

Investigation

Imaging studies are usually unhelpful and diagnosis is made using serological tests.

Treatment

There is no specific antiviral agent; management, therefore, is largely supportive.

LaCrosse encephalitis

Epidemiology

The commonest type of arboviral encephalitis in the United States is caused by the California serogroup of viruses, which are bunyaviruses. Of the 15 viruses in this group, nearly all infection is caused by LaCrosse virus. The virus is transmitted by the *Aedes triseriatus* mosquito, with chipmunks and squirrels serving as reservoirs and amplifying hosts. Humans are incidental dead-end hosts. The incidence of LaCrosse encephalitis has been stable over the years at 70–100 cases/year, with sharp peaks in the summer months. More than 90% of cases occur in the central eastern states of Minnesota, Wisconsin, Iowa, Illinois, Indiana, and Ohio, and ≥90% occur in those under 15 years of age. Males are twice as likely to contract the infection, probably reflecting differences in outdoor activity involvement. In endemic areas, 12.5–18% of residents are seropositive.

Pathophysiology

LaCrosse virus causes an encephalitic process similar to that of other viruses, with neuronal and glial damage, perivascular cuffing around capillaries and venules, and, in fatal cases, cerebral edema. However, it has a predilection for the cortical gray matter of the frontal, temporal, and parietal lobes as well as the basal ganglia, midbrain, and pons.

Clinical features

The ratio of persons with clinical versus subclinical infection is not clear, but may be as low as 1:1000. It mainly affects children, and the median age of patients is 7 years. Fever is almost universal. About 75% of patients have headache and 50% have meningism; other features include seizure, altered state of consciousness, focal neurological deficits, abdominal pain, cough, and sore throat; 12% progress to coma. The outcome is generally good, with mortality rate of approximately 0.5% and an estimated 2% experiencing neurological sequelae other than seizures, although 75% of children have abnormal EEG findings 3–4 years after infection. About 6–20% of patients develop remote symptomatic epilepsy.

Investigations

Diagnosis is made with virus-specific IgM ELISA or a four-fold IgG rise in convalescent serum detected by complement fixation, hemagglutination inhibition, or immunofluorescence. Serology is specific and sensitive.

Treatment

Treatment is supportive, since there is no specific antiviral agent. Salicylates should be avoided because the disease affects mainly children, who are at risk of Reye's syndrome.

Alphaviruses

The alphaviruses belong to the Togaviridae family. Three of the viruses in this family are of human significance: the Western, Venezuelan, and Eastern equine encephalitis viruses, which are all transmitted by mosquitoes and found in North and Central America.

Western equine virus

The Western equine virus is mainly transmitted by the *Culex tarsalis* mosquito. Birds are the main reservoirs; however, in late summer, mosquitoes switch their feeding pattern from birds to mammals, causing outbreaks in horses, mules, and humans. Fewer than 5 cases have been reported annually since the last outbreaks in the Red River Valley in 1975 and Colorado in 1988.

Postmortem findings of the brain of a patient with Western equine encephalitis showed edema and multiple necrotic foci, with or without cellular infiltrate, especially in the striatum, globus pallidus, substantia nigra, cerebral cortex, thalamus, pons, and, occasionally, spinal cord.

The ratio of clinical to subclinical infection ranges from 1:100 cases to 1:2000 cases, with an incubation period of 5–10 days. The virus causes a spectrum of clinical manifestations, from mild fever to aseptic meningitis to encephalitis. Infants are more susceptible to CNS disease and neurological sequelae. In encephalitic patients, onset is sudden, heralded by fever, chills, headache, nausea, vomiting, and, uncommonly, respiratory symptoms. Within days, patients develop lethargy, drowsiness, meningism, photophobia, vertigo, conscious state impairment, and, in severe cases, coma. In infants younger than 1 year old, irritability, focal or generalized seizure, tremor, upper or lower motor neuron weakness, rigidity, and dyskinesia are common. Recovery usually begins after 10 days, and adults often recover fully. Mortality is only 3–5%, which usually occurs within 1 week. However, 56% of infants ≤1 month, 16% of infants between 1 and 2 months, and 11% of infants between 2 and 3 months of age develop seizures and permanent and severe cognitive or motor impairment.

Venezuelan equine virus

Venezuelan equine virus consists of at least six subtypes, with types 1AB and 1C causing periodic but unpredictable outbreaks in Central and South America; the remaining serotypes are mainly enzootic and do not cause human infection. Rodents are the main reservoir, equines the main secondary amplifying host, and *Culex* mosquitoes the main vector. In epidemic outbreaks, *Ochlerotatus* and *Psorophora* species of mosquitoes are common vectors as well. Humans are infected when living in areas close to animals, such as in agricultural areas.

In human autopsy specimens, virus-induced meningoencephalitis with intense necrotizing vasculitis and cerebritis with macroscopic congestion and hemorrhage are seen. The same is observed in the gastrointestinal and respiratory tracts.

The incubation period is 2–5 days, with most infections being clinically apparent, although often misdiagnosed as dengue fever or other arboviral infection. Clinical manifestations start abruptly with fever, chills, occipital or retro-orbital headache, malaise, and myalgia of the back and thighs. Other symptoms include tachycardia, nausea, vomiting, and diarrhea. Neurological involvement is evidenced by photophobia, seizure, drowsiness, and confusion. In most patients, the illness subsides after 4–6 days, followed by a few weeks of asthenia. In some patients, however, the infection may be biphasic and recur 4–8 days after the initial onset. A small proportion of patients become comatose, although mortality is ≤1%.

Eastern equine virus

Eastern equine virus is the most lethal arboviral encephalitis in the United States. The chief vector is *Culiseta melanura*, a fastidious mosquito that is strictly ornithophilic and breeds only in a specific microenvironment of peat soil and dark, organic-rich water. Human infection only occurs when other, less fastidious mosquitoes venture into this environment. The virus is found in the Atlantic and Gulf Coast regions of the United States, and in Wisconsin, Michigan, and Indiana. In the last 10 years, the virus has spread northward to southeastern Canada. A different strain of Eastern equine virus is found in Central and South America, although human infection is very rare outside the United States.

Eastern equine virus infection occurs in small outbreaks with high fatalities, causing either systemic or CNS infection. In the CNS, it causes an encephalomyelitis with neuronal death and vasculitic lesions in the frontal cortex, basal ganglia, and brainstem. Autonomic dysfunction may be severe and can lead to fatal heart failure and pulmonary edema.

Nearly all human infection is symptomatic. Adults and older children may suffer only from systemic infection, although this can be followed by encephalitis. Young children are more susceptible to encephalitis and serious neurological sequelae. Systemic infection is characterized by abrupt onset of high fever, malaise, arthralgia, and myalgias, which usually last 1–2 weeks. In those with encephalitis, onset is abrupt with high fever, headache, confusion, restlessness, drowsiness, nausea, vomiting, anorexia, diarrhea, seizure, and rapid progression to coma. Children may present with periorbital, facial, or generalized edema, tremor, muscle twitching, and meningism.

Mortality, which occurs 2–10 days after the onset of symptoms, is approximately 30%, although it can be as high as 80%, especially in the extremes of age. Serious neurological sequelae, which include severe intellectual impairment, personality changes, spastic paralysis, cranial nerve palsies, and epilepsy, occur in 70% of children. Long-term outcome is dismal, with only 10% surviving beyond 9 years and 3% having no neurological sequelae.

Investigations

Diagnosis of alphaviral infection is made serologically. For example, diagnosis of Venezuelan equine virus infection is made by ELISA, hemagglutination inhibition, neutralizing tests, or detection of viral antigen using indirect fluorescent antibody tests.

Treatment

There is no specific antiviral therapy and treatment is supportive. There are, however, effective equine vaccines.

Other encephalitides

Dengue virus

Dengue virus is a flavivirus transmitted by *Aedes* mosquitoes and primarily infects humans and primates. The virus is endemic in the tropics and subtropics, especially in crowded, large metropolises, causing acute febrile illness with rash and severe myalgia and, in more severe cases, hemorrhage and hemorrhagic shock. Neurological manifestations are seen in 0.5–5.4% of infections of all severity and are more common in children. Dengue encephalitis is distinguished from dengue encephalopathy caused by systemic organ failure, shock, metabolic disturbances, cerebral edema, or hemorrhage. Dengue encephalitis does not produce distinctive histopathological features. Encephalitic patients present with headache, dizziness, drowsiness, confusion, and seizure, including generalized status epilepticus and status epilepticus partialis continua. Brain MRI and EEG findings are non-specific. Since patients with dengue encephalopathy display similar clinical features, diagnosis of encephalitis is made by CSF PCR or NS1 antigen detection or finding of dengue-specific IgM. The sensitivity of these techniques is low. Treatment is supportive, and consists of intravenous fluid and blood product replacement, as well as management of complications, such as electrolyte imbalance, bleeding, and liver and renal failure.

Nipah virus

The Nipah virus is a paramyxovirus found in bats. After causing an outbreak in Malaysia in 1999, it continues to cause sporadic outbreaks in Bangladesh and the neighboring state of West Bengal in India. It is transmitted to and amplified in pigs through bat excretion, and then to humans. Human-to-human transmission was rare in the initial outbreak, but was the dominant mode of transmission in some of the Bangladeshi outbreaks.

Acute Nipah infection is characterized by systemic vasculitis with endothelial cell damage and necrosis, as well as syncytial giant cell formation, which causes extensive thrombosis and parenchymal necrosis, particularly in the CNS and lungs. The virus then invades neurons, forming viral cytoplasmic and, less commonly, nuclear inclusion bodies, leading to diffuse encephalitis with focal neuronophagia, microglial nodule formation, and perivascular cuffing.

Following an incubation period of approximately 9 days (range 2–45 days), the patient presents with fever, headache, chills, myalgia, giddiness, drowsiness, seizures, confusion, and respiratory and abdominal symptoms. Severe hypertension, tachycardia, hyperthermia, segmental myoclonus, and focal neurological deficits are prominent features. Late onset and relapse encephalitis are seen in up to 10% of patients up to 53 months after the initial infection.

Mortality is approximately 40%. Poor prognostic factors include brainstem involvement, past history of diabetes mellitus, and presence of the virus in CSF. Ribavirin was shown in an open-label, historical control trial to reduce mortality by about 36%, although supportive management is equally important. The Hendra virus vaccine under development may protect against Nipah virus.

Enterovirus and EV71

The enteroviruses are the most common cause of aseptic meningitis worldwide, and 3% of infected patients develop encephalitis. Enteroviruses are transmitted via fecal–oral route, and humans are the only significant host. Among the many serotypes, certain ones predominate in a particular geographic locality; each serotype causes cyclic outbreaks when there are sufficient non-immunized individuals present, usually young children. Enteroviral infection of the CNS is usually mild and self-limiting, with the exception of enterovirus 71, which causes fatal outbreaks among young children in Bulgaria and the Asia-Pacific region. Enterovirus 71 infection manifests as the childhood exanthema known as hand–foot–mouth disease and is clinically indistinguishable from that caused by Coxsackie virus. In the CNS, the virus infects anterior horn cells, causing neuronal death and acute flaccid paralysis. Elsewhere, the virus causes meningitis, cerebellitis, and postinfectious neurological syndromes. The most severe form is brainstem encephalitis. Patients with brainstem encephalitis, usually young children under the age of 5 years, present with fever, myoclonus, ataxia, nystagmus, and cranial nerve palsies. Although most recover, 10–20% manifest neurological sequelae. Children with severe disease develop rapidly progressive neurogenic pulmonary edema, with mortality ≥80%. Treatment is largely supportive, although agents such as pleconaril and intravenous Ig have been tried.

Rift Valley encephalitis

Rift Valley virus, a zoonotic virus first discovered in the 1930s in Kenya, is a phlebovirus in the Bunyaviridae family. The vector is the *Aedes* mosquito; buffaloes, cattle, sheep, and goats serve as reservoirs and amplifying hosts. It causes major and recurring outbreaks of animal and human disease in sub-Saharan Africa and has recently spread to northern Africa, the Sinai and Arabian peninsulas. The virus is transmitted by both mosquito bites and contact with infected animal carcasses, abortion tissue and blood products.

In most patients, infection presents with fever, nausea, vomiting, abdominal and respiratory symptoms. Less than 5% of patients develop meningoencephalitis, often late in the illness, with confusion, meningism, hyperreflexia, and depressed conscious state. Less than 8% of patients develop severe disease, characterized by hemorrhage, hepatitis, renal failure, retinitis, and encephalitis. Mortality is 0.5–1.0%, but as high as 29–34% in patients with severe disease. Laboratory investigation shows elevated liver enzymes, hepatic and renal failure, and prolonged prothrombin and partial thromboplastin times. Treatment is supportive since there is no specific antiviral agent.

Powassan and deer tick virus encephalitis

Powassan and deer tick viruses belong to the tick-borne encephalitis serogroup of flaviviruses. The two are closely related and indistinguishable serologically. They are found in the northern United States, Canada, and the Primorski region of Russia. Powassan virus is transmitted by *Ixodes cookei* and deer tick virus *Ixodes scapularis*. The viruses are also isolated from *Dermacentor andersoni*, *Ixodes marxi*, and *Ixodes spinipalpis*. *Ix. cookei* infests groundhogs and skunks, *Ix. Scapularis*, white-footed mice, and *Ix. Marxi*, squirrels.

Pathologically, these viruses cause widespread inflammation with perivascular and focal parenchymal lymphocytic infiltration with associated necrosis, especially in the cortical gray matter, and to a lesser degree the cerebellum, brainstem, and spinal cord, followed by gliosis. Meningeal infiltration occurs in some patients.

The viruses cause 1–2 cases of infection yearly in North America, although the actual incidence is probably higher due to underreporting, asymptomatic infections, and cross-reactivity of serology test with other flaviviruses. After an incubation period of 8–34 days, patients present with prodrome of fever, headache, lethargy, weakness, and, occasionally, maculopapular rash. This is followed by aseptic meningitis, meningoencephalitis, or encephalitis. Patients with encephalitis suffer from drowsiness, confusion, seizure, ataxia, tremor, ocular symptoms, dysarthria, and respiratory failure. MRI shows T2 hyperintensities in the temporal lobes, basal ganglia, caudate nuclei, and, occasionally, in brainstem and cerebellum. CSF shows non-specific pleocytosis and elevated protein.

Diagnosis is based on serum or CSF serology test, confirmed by detection of virus-specific IgM, and rising plaque reduction neutralizing test titer in paired serum or by PCR. Mortality is 10%, with half of survivors suffering long-term sequelae. Treatment is supportive and there is no effective vaccine.

Australian encephalitis: Murray Valley encephalitis and Kunjin encephalitis

Both Murray Valley encephalitis and Kunjin encephalitis are caused by closely related mosquito-borne flaviviruses endemic in Australia and Papua New Guinea. The primary vectors of both are *Culex* and *Aedes* mosquitoes. Water birds appear to be the major hosts. Murray Valley encephalitis can also be transmitted by *Anopheles* mosquitoes and, based on serological findings, other domestic and wild animals have also been implicated as hosts. Outbreaks follow periods of heavy rain and flooding.

Clinical Murray Valley encephalitis occurs in 1/1000 infections, while Kunjin virus infection is less common. The two are indistinguishable clinically. Patients with Kunjin virus infection present with mild fever, headache, photophobia, rash, arthralgia, myalgias, lymphadenopathy, and, less often, encephalitis, exhibiting cranial nerve palsies, dyskinesia, tremor, parkinsonism, and flaccid paralysis due to anterior horn cell involvement; seizure may occur in children. Murray Valley encephalitis is more severe, with mortality in 20–30%, usually due to neurogenic respiratory failure, and severe neurological sequelae in 20% of survivors.

Brain CT scan in Murray Valley encephalitis shows hypodensity in the thalami, while brain MRI shows bilateral thalamic T2 hyperintensity and T1 hypointensity. Diagnoses of both encephalitides are made by ELISA and treatment is supportive.

Hendra virus

Hendra virus is a paramyxovirus closely related to the Nipah virus. It causes infrequent small outbreaks among horses and humans in Queensland and northern New South Wales in Australia. Like the Nipah virus, its natural reservoir is the *Pteropus* fruit bat, and the virus is transmitted to humans through the respiratory secretion of sick horses. Hendra virus causes widespread vasculitis in the brain, lung, heart, and kidney. Small necrotic and vacuolar plaques, and parenchymal inflammation, are seen in the brain, together with mild meningitis.

Human infection occurs 5–21 days after contact and presents as flu-like symptoms of fever, headaches, lethargy, myalgia, nausea, and vomiting, followed by drowsiness, confusion, ataxia, ptosis, cranial nerve palsy, and seizures. Blood tests show thrombocytopenia and elevated liver enzymes, and CSF shows pleocytosis and raised protein. MRI shows multifocal T2 hyperintensities scattered in gray and white matter, brainstem, and cerebellum. EEG shows diffuse slow waves with periodic sharp waves and epileptiform discharges in more severe infection. Mortality is ≥50%, with a single case report of recurrent infection after 13 months.

Diagnosis is made by serology tests and treatment is supportive. Ribavirin was used based on the similarity between Hendra and Nipah virus, but the efficacy is unproven. A vaccine is under development.

Further reading

Carod-Atal FJ, Wichmann O, Farrar J, *et al*. Neurological complications of dengue virus infection. *Lancet Neurol* 2013;12:906–919.

Chong HT, Tan CT. Central nervous system infections. In: Feigin VL, Bennett DA (eds.). *Handbook of Clinical Neuroepidemiology*. Hauppauge, NY: Nova Science; 2007:339–389.

Griffin DE. Viral encephalomyelitis. *PLoS Pathogens* 2011;7(3):e1002004.

Haglund M, Günther G. Tick-borne encephalitis – pathogenesis, clinical course and long-term follow-up. *Vaccine* 2003;21(Suppl 1):S11–S18.

Hemachudha T, Ugolini G, Wacharapluesadee S, *et al*. Human rabies: Neuropathogenesis, diagnosis and management. *Lancet Neurol* 2013;12:498–513.

Kennedy PGE. Viral encephalitis. *J Neurol* 2005;252:268–272.

Rossi SL, Ross TM, Evans JD. West Nile virus. *Clin Lab Med* 2010;30:47–65.

Solomon T. Exotic and emerging viral encephalitides. *Curr Opin Neurol* 2003;16:411–418.

Solomon T, Michael BD, Smith PE, *et al*. Management of suspected viral encephalitis in adults – Association of British Neurologist and British Infection Association National Guidelines. *J Infection* 2012;64:347–373.

81 Neurological complications of human herpesvirus infections

Don Gilden[1,2] and Maria A. Nagel[1]

[1] Department of Neurology, University of Colorado School of Medicine, Aurora, CO, USA

[2] Department of Microbiology and Immunology, University of Colorado School of Medicine, Aurora, CO, USA

The clinical features and imaging abnormalities produced by infection of the nervous system by the various human herpesviruses are different. Many human herpesvirus infections can be treated. This chapter focuses on the neurological complications of the human herpesviruses, optimal virological tests to identify the etiological agent, and state-of-the-art treatment for these disorders.

Herpes simplex virus (HSV-1) encephalitis

Clinical features
Both HSV-1 and HSV-2 cause encephalitis. HSV-1 encephalitis is much more common than HSV-2 encephalitis, which occurs primarily, but not exclusively, in newborns. Unlike most viral encephalitides, HSV-1 encephalitis is focal. Thus, the clinical features reflect the combination of virus replication in the medial temporal lobe and orbital surface of the frontal lobe, along with inflammation and brain swelling. Fever, headache, lethargy, irritability, and confusion are typical. Seizures (major motor, complex partial, focal, and even absence attacks) are common. When the dominant temporal lobe is involved, aphasia develops along with focal motor or sensory deficits. Progressive hemorrhagic necrosis and temporal lobe edema may lead to uncal herniation, commonly characterized by tachycardia, hyperventilation, flexor (and later extensor) posturing, and a dilated pupil, usually on the side of the herniated temporal lobe.

Because HSV-1 becomes latent and periodically reactivates to produce recurrent skin sores (herpes labialis), the misconception exists that HSV encephalitis is protracted or chronic. Although survivors of HSV encephalitis may have a permanent seizure disorder, mental changes, aphasia, or motor deficit, the neurological disease is acute, as in other viral encephalitides. While HSV-1 infects approximately 70% of individuals, HSV-1 encephalitis is rare. Defects in the Toll-like receptor-3/interferon (IFN) and IFN-responsive pathways, which normally confer immunity to HSV-1 central nervous system (CNS) infection, may predispose to HSV-1 encephalitis.

Investigations

Imaging studies
Computed tomography (CT) shows hypodense lesions involving the medial temporal regions. An important diagnostic clue is a sharp transition from the hypodense temporal lesion to the normal basal ganglia. Edema and mass effect occur in 80% of cases, and contrast enhancement appears in more than 50% of cases. Magnetic resonance imaging (MRI) reveals a decrease in T_1 (the spin-lattice/longitudinal relaxation time) and an increase in T_2 (the spin-spin/transverse relaxation time) signal (Figure 81.1). The signal abnormality includes a larger area of brain than is usually seen with CT. Unlike CT, MRI of the temporal lobes is not subject to artifact from the petrous and sphenoid bones, which may obscure the temporal fossa. In addition, MRI may visualize temporal lobe inflammation days before CT.

Cerebrospinal fluid
The cerebrospinal fluid (CSF) is usually abnormal in HSV encephalitis. The CSF opening pressure is often elevated and may be very high if there is brain swelling and impending temporal lobe herniation. CSF examination is usually performed in the first few days of illness, before significant brain swelling develops, decreasing the potential

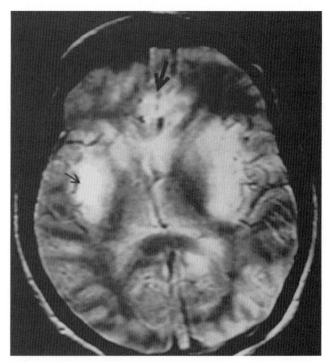

Figure 81.1 HSV-1 encephalitis. T2-weighted brain MRI shows bilateral involvement of temporal lobes and the cingulate gyrus.

International Neurology, Second edition. Edited by Robert P. Lisak, Daniel D. Truong, William M. Carroll and Roongroj Bhidayasiri
© 2016 John Wiley & Sons, Ltd. Published 2016 by John Wiley & Sons, Ltd.

for herniation after lumbar puncture. Mononuclear CSF pleocytosis is found in more than 90% of patients. Red blood cells (RBCs) and a xanthochromic CSF are often seen, reflecting the hemorrhagic nature of brain lesions. Instead of attributing the presence of RBCs in CSF to a traumatic tap, the astute clinician may use this finding to support the presumptive diagnosis of HSV encephalitis. CSF protein is usually elevated, and rarely hypoglycorrhachia occurs. Polymerase chain reaction (PCR) amplification of HSV-1 DNA in CSF is both sensitive and specific and has become the gold standard for diagnosis in suspected cases of HSV encephalitis. Nonetheless, clinicians should note that PCR may be negative for HSV DNA in the first few days. Increased anti-HSV antibody titers are not usually detected until 2 weeks or more after the onset of disease, such that their practical value lies more in retrospective analysis than in identifying acute encephalitis. Although HSV can be isolated from cerebral biopsy or autopsy material, isolation of HSV from CSF during acute disease is rare.

Electroencephalography

The electroencephalogram (EEG) is usually abnormal and often exhibits features highly suggestive of HSV encephalitis. In early disease, background disorganization with generalized or focal slowing occurs, predominantly over the involved temporal region. Within days, widespread, periodic, stereotypical sharp-wave and slow-wave complexes develop, usually at regular intervals of 2–3 seconds. Bilateral periodic complexes appear if both sides of the brain are involved. Although these features can be seen in other CNS disorders (e.g., tumor, abscess, syphilis, infarct, and anoxia), their presence in the clinical setting of fever and rapidly progressive neurological disease is presumptive evidence of HSV encephalitis.

Differential diagnosis

Other viral and bacterial infections, cerebral abscess, tumor, and stroke can mimic the clinical features of HSV encephalitis. A focal area of decreased density and increased vascularity that extends into subcortical areas is consistent with cerebritis, which heralds frank abscess formation and helps distinguish evolving abscess from HSV encephalitis. Ring-enhancing lesions characteristic of cerebral abscess or tumor are not seen in the first few days of HSV encephalitis. Glioma and infarct are not likely to be associated with fever, and brain imaging reveals lesions that are not restricted to the medial temporal lobe.

Treatment

Patients should be treated with intravenous (IV) acyclovir, 15–30 mg/kg/day in three divided doses for at least 10 days. Early use of acyclovir has reduced mortality to slightly lower than 30%, which ranged previously from 60–70%. Early treatment (before coma ensues) is associated with a more favorable outcome. Acyclovir is generally safe, with only mild hematological, hepatic, and renal function abnormalities reported.

Cerebral edema may be the most frequent cause of death resulting from HSV encephalitis. Thus, the benefits of a short course of steroids to control cerebral edema and impending herniation outweigh the small risk of potentiating HSV infection. Dexamethasone is administered IV at an initial dose of 10 mg and then 4–8 mg every 4–5 hours for the next 3 days. Incipient herniation may be managed with osmotic diuretics. Mannitol is given in repeated doses of 0.25–2.0 g/kg. Serum osmolality should be monitored closely and kept below 310 mOsm/L. The effectiveness of mannitol decreases

with repeated use, and rebound increases in intracranial pressure may occur. Treatment involves reducing the total fluid intake to between one-half and two-thirds of that required for maintenance and elevating the patient's head to 30°. Edema is treated by intubation and hyperventilation to bring the partial pressure of carbon dioxide to 25 mmol/L, reducing intracranial pressure by constricting the intracranial vasculature. After 24 hours, hyperventilation is less effective.

Anticonvulsants are used to treat seizures. For initial seizures, diazepam may be administered IV in doses of 2 mg/min for a maximum total dose of 15–20 mg; alternatively, lorazepam may be administered IV in doses of 2 mg/min for a maximum total dose of 5–10 mg. These treatments are followed by fosphenytoin administered in a loading dose of 20 mg/kg at 150 mg/min. Blood pressure and electrocardiographic monitoring should be employed during treatment with fosphenytoin. Maintenance doses of phenytoin average 300–400 mg/day. Anticonvulsants should be continued for several months after acute illness. There are no controlled studies on prophylactic use of steroids or anticonvulsants in HSV encephalitis.

While relapse after acyclovir therapy is uncommon, the CSF of some patients with relapsing HSV encephalitis contains N-methyl-D-aspartate receptor (NMDAR) antibodies. Antibody synthesis begins 1–4 weeks after HSV encephalitis. NMDAR-related symptoms are potentially responsive to immunotherapy.

HSV-2 infection

Clinical presentations

Primary HSV-2 infection may be asymptomatic or produce genital herpes. HSV-2 becomes latent in sacral ganglia. The neurological complications of HSV-2 reactivation are more protean than for HSV-1. Rarely does HSV-2 cause encephalitis. More commonly, HSV-2 reactivation leads to meningitis or radiculopathy, either of which may be recurrent.

Encephalitis

HSV-2 encephalitis occurs most often in newborns and immunocompromised adults, and infection is more diffuse than the focal medial-temporal and orbital-frontal lesions produced by HSV-1. Nevertheless, seizures, alterations in state of consciousness, and focal neurological deficits, all common clinical features of HSV-1 encephalitis, also characterize HSV-2 encephalitis. Treatment is with IV acyclovir, 15–30 mg/kg, 3 times daily for 10–14 days. Acquired immune deficiency syndrome (AIDS) patients may require long-term oral antiviral maintenance to prevent further virus reactivation.

Aseptic meningitis

Aseptic meningitis is the main neurological complication of HSV-2 infection. In the United States, HSV-2 accounts for 5% of all aseptic meningitis. Unlike viral meningitides that have a seasonal association, HSV-2 meningitis occurs any time of year. Typical symptoms and signs are headache, fever, and stiff neck. A marked CSF lymphocytic pleocytosis is common. Because HSV-2 causes genital infection, meningitis may be preceded by genital or pelvic pain. The astute clinician who suspects HSV-2 meningitis will ask about recent symptoms of pelvic inflammatory disease or penile lesions. The workup for suspected HSV-2 meningitis should include a careful search for vesicular lesions over the external genitalia and a pelvic examination for vaginal or cervical lesions. The cause of aseptic meningitis in one patient with recurrent dermatomal skin lesions was shown to be HSV-2.

PCR has also revealed that the primary agent causing benign recurrent lymphocytic meningitis is HSV-2, less often HSV-1. Brain imaging is normal in HSV-2 meningitis. A suspected diagnosis of HSV-2 meningitis is supported by a history of previous episodes of meningitis, recurrent skin lesions, genital herpes, and intermittent radicular symptoms; careful examination of the entire skin may reveal active patchy HSV-2 lesions (see later). HSV-2 meningitis is self-limited; although antiviral therapy is given, patients historically recover completely without treatment.

Radiculopathy

HSV-2 produces recurrent radicular pain. Pain may be accompanied by genital herpes, patchy vesicular skin lesions, and/or meningitis, which may also recur. Thus, clues to the diagnosis of HSV-2 infection are (1) a history of recurrent meningitis; (2) a history of genital herpes; (3) recurrent patchy zosteriform skin lesions with neuropathy (e.g., sciatica); and (4) recurrent patchy skin eruptions with no history of neuropathy or genital herpes, but with meningitis. Figure 81.2 shows patchy lesions produced by HSV-2, which differ from dermatomal distribution lesions produced by varicella zoster virus.

Zosteriform eruptions with radicular pain are often characterized by a prodrome of diffuse neuralgia, often with malaise and fever, followed within a few days by vesicular eruption. Lesions occur on the face in one or more areas served by the trigeminal nerve, as well as on the trunk, extremities, and genitalia. Reports of recurrent sciatica associated with HSV are particularly interesting, because they identify a form of sciatica that can be treated with antiviral agents. A first episode may be confused with herpes zoster, but recurrent episodes of dermatomal neuralgic pain and zosteriform eruptions are usually caused by HSV-2.

Although HSV neuropathy is well documented as a clinical entity, more information is needed to know the exact type of HSV responsible for each disease. Clinicians attribute herpetic lesions above the neck to HSV-1 reactivation, while lesions below the waist are thought to indicate HSV-2 reactivation. Future DNA analysis of herpes isolates by PCR with primers specific for HSV-1 or HSV-2 will determine the relative contribution of each virus to HSV neuropathy.

Most clinical reports of HSV neuropathy were made before the development of antiviral agents against human herpesviruses. Historically, patients with recurrent HSV-2 meningitis recovered spontaneously. Today, patients with HSV-2 meningitis are routinely treated with antiviral agents, although it is not known how long patients should be treated, whether intravenous antiviral therapy is superior to oral antiviral agents, or even if antiviral treatment is beneficial. Nevertheless, antiviral treatment is likely to reduce the number of days that patients have pain and rash; thus, patients are usually treated with oral valacyclovir (1 g, 3 times daily) or famciclovir (500 mg, 3 times daily) for 7–10 days. Neither HSV-1 nor HSV-2 is eradicated by antiviral therapy. Rather, resolution of acute disease is followed by a return of herpes to the latent state, with the potential for reactivation.

Varicella zoster virus

Clinical presentations

Varicella zoster virus (VZV) causes varicella (chickenpox), after which the virus becomes latent in ganglionic neurons along the entire neuraxis. As cell-mediated immunity to VZV declines with aging, as well as in immunocompromised individuals and AIDS patients, the virus reactivates to cause herpes zoster. Zoster is frequently complicated by chronic pain (postherpetic neuralgia, PHN) and multiple neurological and ocular disorders.

Zoster

Herpes zoster is characterized by pain and rash (a vesicular eruption on an erythematous base) in one or several dermatomes. Rash and pain usually develop within a few days of each other, although pain may precede rash by 7 to more than 100 days. Any dermatome may be involved. The trunk from T3 to L2 is the most heavily involved area, followed by the face and extremities.

Pathologically, zoster is characterized by inflammation and hemorrhagic necrosis with associated neuritis, localized leptomeningitis, unilateral segmental poliomyelitis, and degeneration of related motor and sensory roots. Demyelination is seen in areas

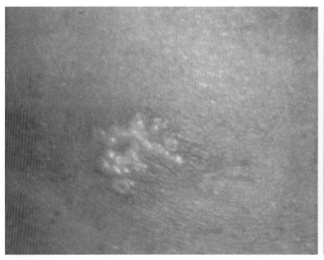
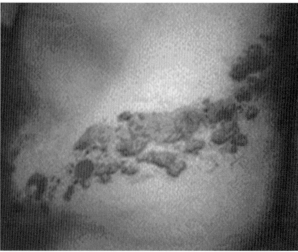

Figure 81.2 HSV-2 skin lesions. HSV-2 causes patchy lesions (left), which differ from the dermatomal lesions caused by varicella zoster virus (right).

with mononuclear cell (MNC) infiltration and microglial proliferation. Intranuclear inclusions, viral antigen, and herpesvirus particles are present in acutely infected ganglia.

Antiviral drugs (e.g., valacyclovir, 1 g, 3 times daily for 7–10 days) speed healing of rash and shorten the duration of acute pain. In immunocompromised patients, IV acyclovir (5–10 mg/kg, 3 times daily for 5–7 days) is recommended. Because zoster pain may be accompanied by an inflammatory response, a short course of oral prednisone (1 mg/kg for 5–7 days) may help.

Postherpetic neuralgia
PHN is operationally defined as pain that persists for at least 3 months (sometimes years) after zoster. PHN occurs in approximately 40% of patients more than 60 years of age. The cause and pathogenesis of PHN are unknown. Analysis of ganglia from a case of PHN of 2.5 months' duration revealed diffuse and focal infiltration by chronic inflammatory cells, an observation confirmed by prominent collections of lymphocytes found in ganglia from another patient with PHN of 2 years' duration. At autopsy from a case of severe thoracic PHN for 5 years, the most striking pathological finding was atrophy of the dorsal horn over five segments, with only one ganglion affected by fibrosis and cellular loss and with involvement only of the nerve roots at that level. Further studies in three PHN cases revealed not only dorsal root atrophy and ganglionic changes, but also marked inflammation in the dorsal horn and loss of axons and myelin in the sensory root and peripheral nerve. The inflammatory response in ganglia of these subjects raises the possibility of prolonged viral infection. Further evidence that PHN may be produced by low-level ganglionitis comes from the detection of VZV DNA and proteins in blood mononuclear cells (MNCs) of patients with PHN (presumably acquired by MNCs trafficking through productively infected ganglia) and from the favorable response of some PHN patients to antiviral treatment. PHN is difficult to manage. No universally accepted treatment exists. Many patients benefit from combinations of gabapentin, pregabalin, tricyclic antidepressants, topical lidocaine, and opiates.

Zoster paresis
Zoster paresis (weakness) is manifest by arm weakness or diaphragmatic paralysis after cervical distribution zoster, leg weakness after lumbar or sacral distribution zoster, and by urinary retention after sacral distribution zoster. MRI of patients with zoster paresis reveals involvement not only of the posterior horn and posterior roots, but also of the anterior roots and anterior horn at the spinal level corresponding to the patient's clinical deficit. Rarely, clinical deficit in cervical zoster paresis extends to the brachial plexus, confirmed by both electrodiagnostic testing and MRI. Functional recovery occurs in 55–67% of cases.

Cranial nerve involvement
Optic neuritis, sometimes bilateral, may develop after zoster. Third nerve palsies are more common than the sixth; least affected is the fourth. Combinations of third, fourth, and sixth nerve palsies are not unusual. Zoster affects the head in approximately 19% of cases, with nearly all rashes (97%) in the trigeminal distribution, most often ophthalmic. Maxillary-distribution zoster may be accompanied by alveolar bone necrosis and tooth loss. Weakness of facial muscles is usually associated with lesions in the ear (Ramsay Hunt syndrome; geniculate zoster) or on the anterior two-thirds of the tongue. Deficits commonly involve the eighth nerve. Although the

mechanism by which cranial nerves are involved in zoster is not clear, many cases occur days to weeks after zoster. One possible explanation for VZV-induced late-onset cranial neuropathy is microinfarction. VZV particles could spread along trigeminal (and other ganglionic) afferent fibers to small vessels supplying cranial nerves. The blood supply of cranial nerves comes from the carotid circulation and may receive input from trigeminal afferent fibers, as has been demonstrated for larger extracranial and intracranial blood vessels. Multiple cases of trigeminal and geniculate zoster, as well as polyneuritis cranialis due to VZV, occur in the absence of rash.

Meningoencephalitis
VZV can cause acute meningoencephalitis, with or without rash. Many cases of VZV encephalitis are actually VZV vasculopathy. In some cases of meningoencephalitis, cerebellitis (gait ataxia and tremor) predominates and CSF glucose is low. Acute VZV cerebellitis without rash has also been documented virologically; in one instance, the primary clue leading to virological tests for VZV in CSF was the patient's early age of chickenpox. Interestingly, 44% of 174 patients with acute CNS disease caused by VZV had no rash.

Myelopathy
VZV myelopathy presents in various ways. One form is a self-limiting, monophasic spastic paraparesis, with or without sensory features and sphincter problems. This so-called postinfectious myelitis usually occurs in immunocompetent patients days to weeks after acute varicella or zoster. Its pathogenesis is unknown. The CSF usually contains a mild mononuclear pleocytosis, with normal or slightly elevated protein. Steroids are used to treat these patients, although some improve spontaneously. Rarely, VZV myelitis recurs, even in immunocompetent patients. VZV myelopathy may also present as an insidious, progressive, and sometimes fatal myelitis, mostly in immunocompromised individuals. AIDS has commonly and increasingly become associated with VZV myelitis. MRI reveals longitudinal serpiginous enhancing lesions. Diagnosis is confirmed by the presence of VZV DNA or anti-VZV IgG or both in CSF. In fatal cases, pathological and virological analyses of the spinal cord reveal frank invasion of VZV in the parenchyma and adjacent nerve roots. Not surprisingly, some patients respond favorably to antiviral therapy. Importantly, VZV myelitis may develop without rash. Early diagnosis and aggressive treatment with IV acyclovir have been helpful, even in immunocompromised patients. The benefit of steroids in addition to antiviral agents is unknown. VZV also produces spinal cord infarction as identified by diffusion-weighted MRI and confirmed virologically.

Vasculopathy
VZV vasculopathy due to productive virus infection of cerebral arteries occurs after varicella or zoster and is often chronic and protracted, producing waxing and waning neurological symptoms and signs. Clinical features include headache, fever, mental status changes, and/or focal deficit. Brain MRI is abnormal in virtually all patients and usually reveals ischemic and/or hemorrhagic infarcts, unifocal or multifocal, more deep-seated than cortical lesions, particularly at gray–white matter junctions (Figure 81.3), a clue to diagnosis. Cerebral angiography may show focal arterial stenosis and beading or occlusion, involving large or small arteries but more commonly both, and also aneurysm or hemorrhage. The CSF often contains a mononuclear pleocytosis and, not uncommonly, red blood cells. Oligoclonal bands representing IgG antibody directed

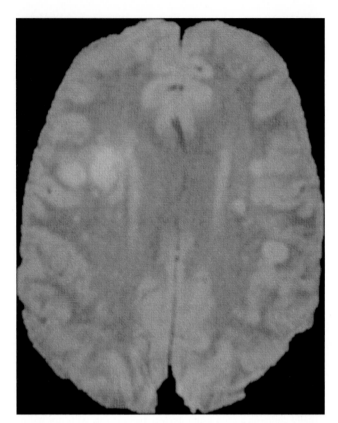

Figure 81.3 Varicella zoster virus vasculopathy. Proton-density brain MRI shows multiple areas of infarction in both hemispheres, particularly involving white matter and extending to gray–white matter junctions.

against VZV are often found. Importantly, more than one-third of patients with virologically verified VZV vasculopathy do not have a CSF pleocytosis or history of zoster rash.

Furthermore, the CSF does not always contain PCR-amplifiable VZV DNA, but does contain anti-VZV IgG (30% vs. 93% in 30 virologically verified cases), indicating that detection of anti-VZV antibody in CSF is the most sensitive test to diagnose VZV vasculopathy. Rarely is anti-VZV IgM antibody found in serum or CSF, but when present, it provides strong virological evidence of active VZV infection. In immunocompetent or immunocompromised patients experiencing a transient ischemic attack or stroke with a history of recent zoster or varicella rash, the clinician should test for both VZV DNA and anti-VZV antibodies in CSF. Because not all patients with VZV vasculopathy have a history of zoster or varicella rash, the CSF of all patients with CNS angiitis of unknown etiology should be analyzed for VZV DNA and anti-VZV antibody. When the diagnosis of VZV vasculopathy is being considered and CSF virological studies are underway, patients should be treated with IV acyclovir, 10–15 mg/kg, 3 times daily for at least 14 days. Because there is often an inflammatory response in cerebral arteries, oral prednisone, 1 mg/kg daily for 5 days (no taper needed), may help, although it remains unclear whether steroids confer additional benefit. Finally, steroid treatment after antiviral medication has been discontinued can potentiate virus infection.

Ocular disorders

VZV produces multiple ocular disorders, including acute retinal necrosis (ARN) and progressive outer retinal necrosis (PORN).

ARN develops in both immunocompetent and immunocompromised hosts. Patients present with periorbital pain and floaters, with hazy vision and loss of peripheral vision. Treatment is typically IV acyclovir, steroids, and aspirin followed by oral acyclovir. Intravitreal injections of foscarnet and oral acyclovir are used in early, milder cases.

PORN presents with sudden painless loss of vision, floaters, and constricted visual fields with resultant retinal detachment. Multifocal, discrete opacified lesions begin in the outer retinal layers peripherally and/or the posterior pole; only late in disease are inner retinal layers involved. Diffuse retinal hemorrhages and whitening with macular involvement bilaterally are characteristic findings. Although PORN can be caused by HSV and cytomegalovirus, most cases are produced by VZV, primarily in immunosuppressed individuals. PORN may be preceded by retrobulbar optic neuritis and aseptic meningitis, central retinal artery occlusion, or ophthalmic-distribution zoster, and may coexist with multifocal vasculopathy or myelitis. Treatment with IV acyclovir has given poor or inconsistent results, and even when acyclovir helped, VZV retinopathy recurred when drug was tapered or stopped. PORN patients treated with ganciclovir alone or in combination with foscarnet had a better final visual acuity than those treated with acyclovir or foscarnet. The best treatment for PORN in AIDS patients may be prevention with highly active retroviral therapy (HAART), which appears to decrease its incidence.

As with VZV neurological disease, ocular disorders caused by VZV can also occur in the absence of rash. Multiple cases of PORN, as well as a case of severe unremitting eye pain without rash, were proven to be caused by VZV based on detection of VZV DNA in nasal and conjunctival samples. In addition, third cranial nerve palsies, retinal periphlebitis, uveitis, iridocyclitis, and disciform keratitis that occurred without rash were confirmed virologically to be caused by VZV.

Zoster sine herpete

Zoster sine herpete is defined as chronic radicular pain without rash and is virologically confirmed by detection of VZV DNA in CSF. Electromyography (EMG) of paraspinal muscles may demonstrate fibrillation potentials restricted to chronically painful thoracic root segments. CSF without amplifiable VZV DNA may contain anti-VZV IgG, with reduced serum/CSF ratios indicative of intrathecal synthesis. Persistent radicular pain without rash can be also be caused by chronic active VZV ganglionitis.

Detection of VZV DNA or anti-VZV antibody in patients with meningoencephalitis, vasculopathy, myelitis, cerebellar ataxia, and polyneuritis cranialis, all in the absence of rash, has broadened the spectrum of zoster sine herpete, which is more appropriately termed "VZV reactivation without rash."

Investigations

Diagnosis of VZV-induced neurological disease is straightforward when the characteristic dermatomal distribution rash of zoster is present. When zoster rash is absent in a patient with neurological disease that might be caused by VZV (e.g., chronic radicular pain, meningoencephalitis with our without cerebellitis, vasculopathy, myelitis, or retinal necrosis), examination of CSF for VZV DNA or anti-VZV antibody is essential. The presence of amplifiable VZV DNA in CSF in patients with any of the above disorders confirms the diagnosis of VZV-induced disease. Importantly, many cases of VZV vasculopathy and myelitis are protracted, and the best virological test to confirm

VZV causality is detection of anti-VZV IgG and/or anti-VZV IgM in CSF or anti-VZV IgM in serum. Practically, the CSF most often contains only anti-VZV IgG and rarely anti-VZV IgM antibody. The detection of anti-VZV IgG antibody in CSF with intrathecal synthesis is superior to detection of VZV DNA in CSF to diagnose VZV vasculopathy. It is also critical to establish the diagnosis of recurrent VZV myelopathy, VZV brainstem encephalitis, and zoster sine herpete.

Cytomegalovirus

Clinical presentations

Cytomegalovirus (CMV) infects approximately 70% of individuals in the United States by the age of 40. After primary infection, CMV becomes latent in lymphoid tissue, specifically in cells of the myeloid lineage. When acquired *in utero*, CMV can cause cytomegalic inclusion body disease in newborns with serious neurological complications, including microcephaly, deafness, and blindness. In immunocompetent adults, infection is usually asymptomatic. Virtually all other neurological complications of CMV infection are in immunocompromised individuals, particularly those with AIDS. The most common disorder is retinitis with and without neurological complications.

Guillain–Barré syndrome

CMV is one of the infectious agents associated with Guillain–Barré syndrome (GBS). Serological studies reveal recent CMV infection in 13% of GBS patients. While the pathogenesis of CMV-associated GBS is unknown, CMV-infected fibroblasts express gangliosidelike epitopes, and anti-ganglioside 2 (GM2) antibodies have been detected in 22–67% of CMV-infected patients, supporting the notion of molecular mimicry between GM2 and CMV antigens in these patients. Likewise, in the axonal form of GBS associated with *Campylobacter jejuni* infection, anti-ganglioside antibodies crossreact with lipooligosaccharides in the outer membrane of *C. jejuni*.

Polyradiculopathy

A serious neurological complication is CMV polyradiculopathy, which presents with subacute leg weakness, paraesthesia, and urinary retention. Untreated patients develop ascending paralysis and die within weeks. In 103 cases of AIDS-related CMV polyradiculopathy, lumbar pain was present in 36%, paraesthesias in 79%, weakness and hyporeflexia in 100%, sensory loss in 80%, urinary retention in 94%, and fecal incontinence in 67%. Either MNCs or neutrophils may predominate in CSF, the latter perhaps reflecting chronic active disease. Hypoglycorrhachia is common. Positive PCR for CMV DNA in CSF clinches the diagnosis. MRI with gadolinium may be normal or reveal meningeal enhancement, and EMG reveals denervation in all cases. Untreated patients die within 8 weeks of symptom onset. Ganciclovir and foscarnet monotherapy increase survival time by only 3–4 months. Pathological changes include necrosis with inflammatory infiltrates and focal vasculitis of nerve roots.

Ventriculoencephalitis

AIDS patients may develop ventriculoencephalitis due to CMV infection of ependymal cells lining the ventricular system. Clinical features include confusion and gait disturbances, often with cranial nerve palsies, hyperreflexia, and abnormal serum electrolytes. Ventriculitis often coexists with CMV retinitis. Brain imaging reveals ventriculomegaly with periventricular enhancement. Pathological examination shows CMV inclusion-bearing cells and necrotizing periventriculitis with involvement of the meninges and adjacent cranial nerve roots.

Encephalitis

Diffuse CMV encephalitis occurs mostly in human immunodeficiency virus (HIV) infected individuals. A MEDLINE search revealed 676 cases of pathologically verified CMV encephalitis (microglia nodules and cytomegalic inclusion bodies), 85% of whom were HIV+, 12% were otherwise immunosuppressed, and only 3% were immunocompetent. Neurological features include headache, confusion, seizures, and cranial nerve palsies. Progressive cognitive changes are often misdiagnosed as HIV dementia. CSF is normal or contains a mononuclear pleocytosis. PCR is often positive for CMV DNA.

Cases of transverse myelitis and myeloradiculitis have also been reported. Rarely does CMV cause a multifocal neuropathy affecting the radial, ulnar, peroneal, or cranial nerves.

Treatment

CNS infection is treated with IV ganciclovir, 5 mg/kg every 12 hours for 14–21 days followed by maintenance with 5 mg/kg daily. In HIV-infected patients with CD4+ counts <100 cells/mm3, additional therapy consists of IV foscarnet, 60 mg/kg every 8 hours for 14–21 days followed by 90–120 mg/kg daily. Serial CSF PCR for CMV DNA can be used to monitor response to therapy. Long-term maintenance is often required in severely immunosuppressed patients. Despite treatment, prognosis is poor. Polyradiculoneuropathy often recurs when antiviral therapy is discontinued.

Epstein–Barr virus

Clinical features

Epstein–Barr virus (EBV) is highly prevalent in all human populations. Primary infection is usually asymptomatic, but also causes infectious mononucleosis. In most humans, primary infection occurs in childhood or adolescence. By 30 years of age, more than 90% of adults have antibody to EBV. The exact incidence of neurological complications due to EBV is unknown, but has been estimated to occur in 1–5% of individuals with infectious mononucleosis. EBV mononucleosis may be followed by recurrent meningitis.

EBV becomes latent in B lymphocytes. Reactivation causes a wide range of disorders of the CNS and peripheral nervous system. The most common presentation is meningoencephalitis. Other protean neurological manifestations of EBV include optic neuritis, myelitis, radiculopathy, and plexopathy. EBV causes cranial neuropathies with ophthalmoplegia, including acute autonomic neuropathy. In a fascinating case of acute demyelinating disease after EBV infection, a patient presented with behavioral abnormalities, visual illusions, and a seizure. Chronic active EBV infection has been associated with calcification in the basal ganglia. A study of four patients with myeloradiculitis, encephalomyeloradiculitis, meningomyeloradiculitis, and meningoencephalomyeloradiculitis revealed CSF pleocytosis, predominantly mononuclear, with elevated protein and normal glucose.

Investigations

MRI of the brain, spinal cord, or nerve roots may show enhancement or be normal. No distinct imaging features are diagnostic of

EBV infection. EBV DNA and anti-EBV IgM and IgG antibodies may be present in the CSF with a reduced serum-to-CSF ratio of EBV antibody compared to ratios for total IgG or albumin, consistent with intrathecal synthesis of anti-EBV antibody. It should be noted that in many CNS inflammatory and infectious disorders, the CSF contains a large mononuclear pleocytosis in which EBV DNA can be amplified from latently infected B-cells. Thus, before attributing neurological disease to EBV infection, the CSF should also be shown to contain anti-EBV antibody. The mechanism by which EBV causes neurological disease is unknown, and there is no specific treatment. Aside from neurological complications, EBV is also detected in CNS lymphoma seen in organ transplant recipients and AIDS patients.

Human herpesvirus-6 (HHV-6) encephalitis

Clinical features
HHV-6 was initially isolated in patients with lymphoproliferative disorders in 1986. There are two variants, HHV-6A and HHV-6B. HHV-6B causes roseola, characterized by high fever in infants followed by a macular rash over the trunk, face, and legs that develops with defervescence. Seizures are common after HHV-6 infection. After primary infection, virus becomes latent in T-cells. HHV-6 rarely reactivates in AIDS or other immunosuppressed patients, particularly bone marrow or solid organ transplant recipients, or in immunocompetent individuals.

HHV-6 encephalitis is characterized by the subacute onset of seizures, memory loss, insomnia, and agitation. Focal neurological deficits are less frequent.

Investigations
MRI is either normal or shows increased signal and mild swelling of the medial temporal lobe, distinct from the markedly increased signal and massive edema seen in HSV-1 encephalitis. Unlike other herpesvirus CNS infections, a CSF pleocytosis is often absent, particularly in immunocompromised individuals. Diagnosis is confirmed by detection of HHV-6 DNA in CSF.

Treatment
Disease is often fatal. There are several reports of successful treatment with ganciclovir and foscarnet, but no clinical trial data exist.

Acknowledgments
This work was supported by Public Health Service grants AG006127, AG032958 (DG), and NS 067070 (MAN) from the National Institutes of Health. We thank Marina Hoffman for editorial review and Cathy Allen for manuscript preparation.

Further reading
Armangue T, Leypoldt F, Malaga I, *et al*. Herpes simplex virus encephalitis is a trigger of brain autoimmunity. *Ann Neurol* 2014;75:317–323.

Nagel MA, Gilden D. The challenging patient with varicella zoster virus disease. *Neurol Clin Pract* 2013;3:109–117.

Nagel MA, Cohrs RJ, Gilden D. Varicella zoster virus infections. In: Jackson AC (ed.). *Viral Infections of the Human Nervous System*, Basel: Springer; 2013:87–114.

Nagel MA, Khmeleva N, Boyer PJ, *et al*. Varicella zoster virus in the temporal artery of a patient with giant cell arteritis. *J Neurol Sci* 2013;335:229–230.

Zhang SY, Abel L, Casanova JL. Mendelian predisposition to herpes simplex encephalitis. *Handbook Clin Neurol* 2013;112;1091–1097.

82 Chronic viral diseases of the central nervous system

Maria A. Nagel[1] and Don Gilden[1,2]
[1] Department of Neurology, University of Colorado School of Medicine, Aurora, CO, USA
[2] Department of Microbiology and Immunology, University of Colorado School of Medicine, Aurora, CO, USA

Subacute sclerosing panencephalitis (SSPE) is a chronic fatal encephalitis characterized by progressive mental and motor deterioration due to measles virus infection of the central nervous system (CNS). The first indication that SSPE was caused by a virus came in 1933–34 from J.R. Dawson's examination of the brains of two children who died after progressive involuntary jerking of the limbs and mental deterioration. He found encephalitic changes with intracellular eosinophilic inclusion bodies in numerous cortical neurons suggestive of viral infection. Subsequent pathological examination of brains from children with similar clinical features revealed inflammation and nodular sclerosis in white and gray matter, demyelination with glial proliferation, and intraneuronal inclusion bodies. In 1965, electron microscopy identified paramyxovirus nucleocapsids in SSPE brain, and in 1967, high titers of anti-measles virus antibodies in blood and cerebrospinal fluid (CSF) of SSPE patients were found. In 1969, measles virus was isolated from SSPE brain.

Epidemiology

Since the advent of measles vaccination in 1969, the incidence of both measles and SSPE has decreased dramatically. Nevertheless, vaccine delivery is difficult in many areas. Worldwide, there are 20 million cases of measles annually; there were approximately 585 cases in the United States in 2014 (http://www.cdc.gov/measles/cases-outbreaks.html). Since 4–11 cases of SSPE are expected for every 100,000 cases of measles, 800–2200 cases of SSPE are predicted worldwide yearly. In children younger than 5 years, the incidence of SSPE is higher (18/100,000), and in the Middle East the incidence is 360/100,000 for individuals infected with measles before 1 year of age. SSPE is more prevalent in boys than girls. The average time from measles to onset of SSPE is 6–10 years, but ranges from 1–24 years.

Pathophysiology

Pathological findings in SSPE brain include diffuse encephalitis of both gray and white matter and cerebral and brainstem structures. Perivascular cuffing of mononuclear cells and proliferation of both macroglia and microglia are also present. Demyelination and astrocyte proliferation are pronounced in white matter. Neuronal loss is severe. Cowdry type A inclusion bodies are present in neurons, astrocytes, and oligodendrocytes. Electron microscopy reveals paramyxovirus nucleocapsids. Some measles virus isolates from SSPE brain have mutations in the matrix (M) protein gene.

A recent report described a 52-year-old man who was treated for hepatitis C with interferon and ribavirin and developed chronic focal encephalitis attributed to measles virus, based on elevated titers of measles virus antibody in serum and CSF and detection of measles virus RNA in the brain biopsy. The patient responded favorably to steroid therapy. While different than SSPE, the focal nature of the chronic disease and steroid responsiveness expand the spectrum of chronic encephalitis produced by measles virus.

Clinical features

SSPE begins in childhood or adolescence. Mental and behavioral regression is the most frequent initial manifestation, along with apathy, irritability, and sometimes psychosis. School performance deteriorates due to poor memory and intellectual decline. Focal neurological signs subsequently develop, including dysphasia and hemiparesis, as well as athetoid and myoclonic movements. Visual abnormalities are common – bilateral and homonymous if visual pathways or the striate cortex are involved, or monocular if the macula is involved. Myoclonic seizures are most frequent, but generalized and partial complex seizures are also common. Myoclonus frequently heralds the late stages of SSPE in which the patient becomes increasingly demented and stuporous as decorticate rigidity develops. Pain, headache, and fever do not occur. Table 82.1 lists the clinical stages of SSPE.

Table 82.1 Clinical staging of subacute sclerosing panencephalitis.

Stage	Clinical features
I	Personality changes accompanied by deterioration in school performance and behavioral abnormalities
II	Axial (especially characteristic rapid neck flexion) myoclonus, causing frequent falls
III	Generalized rigidity with extrapyramidal features and progressive unresponsiveness
IV	Impaired state of consciousness progressing to akinetic mutism with severe autonomic failure

Investigations

Serology and cerebrospinal fluid analysis

Definitive diagnosis based on clinical presentation and demonstration of high titers of measles virus antibody in serum and CSF obviates brain biopsy. In SSPE, antibody titers to measles virus in serum can be >10 times higher than during convalescent measles infection or after vaccination. Antibody titers to measles virus in CSF are also elevated, but are much higher in serum (serum:CSF ratios range from 5:1 to 80:1). CSF opening pressure is normal and CSF is clear. A moderate pleocytosis (5–20 mononuclear cells/mm^3) is usually present. CSF glucose is normal, and CSF protein is normal or mildly elevated; if >90 mg/100 mL, disorders other than SSPE should be considered. CSF IgG, expressed as percent of total protein, is markedly increased (normal <13%). Bands of oligoclonal IgG are present, nearly all of which are directed against measles virus antigen.

Magnetic resonance imaging

High signal intensity lesions on T2-weighted images involving periventricular and subcortical white matter is the most common finding. Lesions typically start in cortex-subcortical white matter and progress, with periventricular and other white matter involvement, along with diffuse cerebral atrophy (Figure 82.1). Pial and parenchymal contrast enhancement is common. Brainstem and basal ganglionic lesions are rare. The extent and location of

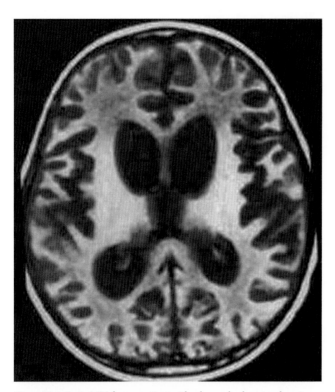

Figure 82.1 Brain MRI from a patient with advanced subacute sclerosing panencephalitis. T$_1$-weighted axial image shows diffuse, symmetric involvement of periventricular and subcortical white matter in the frontal and parietal regions bilaterally. Signal intensity increased on proton density and T$_2$-weighted images (not shown), and decreased on T$_1$. Enlarged ventricles and cortical sulci indicate cerebral atrophy.

periventricular white matter lesions and cerebral atrophy do not correlate with clinical findings.

Electroencephalography

Electroencephalography (EEG) may be helpful in diagnosis, depending on the stage of disease. Early on, the EEG may be normal or show moderate non-specific generalized slowing. As disease progresses, periodic stereotyped high-voltage discharges appear, usually during sleep, without myoclonic jerks. Later, these discharges are seen during wakefulness associated with myoclonic jerks. The discharge pattern consists of bilateral, synchronous symmetric bursts at amplitudes of 200–500 uV and with polyphasic, monomorphic rhythmic delta waves every 4–10 seconds. In advanced disease, this pattern is replaced with disorganized slow delta waves, and voltage gradually declines, possibly becoming almost isoelectric by stage IV (coma).

Prognosis and treatment

SSPE is fatal within 2–3 years after onset in 95% of cases. Treatment is supportive. Several patients treated with interferon-α and ribavirin, which are broad antiviral agents active against both RNA and DNA viruses, as well as isoprinosine, which disrupts viral replication and may have immune modulatory effects, showed only a 35% benefit at best, defined as slower disease progression, prolonged survival, or clinical improvement. Recently, progressive mental deterioration and loss of motor function were stopped in a 15-year-old girl with early SSPE treated with oral isoprinosine (100 mg/kg/day), intraventricular interferon-α, and intraventricular ribavirin; 3 years later, she was alive and able to have special assistance schooling, at which time[18] fludeoxyglucose-positron emission tomography showed that cortical glucose metabolism was preserved rather than decreased as in untreated SSPE patients.

Other viruses that cause chronic progressive panencephalitis

Other viruses that can cause chronic progressive panencephalitis are rubella virus, tick-borne encephalitis virus (TBEV, a flavivirus), and HIV. Progressive rubella panencephalitis is a rare CNS disorder that develops about a decade after congenital rubella infection. Fewer than 20 cases have been described. The clinical features are similar to those of SSPE, including progressive mental and motor deterioration, ataxia, chorea, and myoclonic seizures. CSF reveals a mild mononuclear pleocytosis with elevated protein and IgG levels. High titers of antibody to rubella are present in serum and CSF, distinguishing this disorder from SSPE.

A chronic progressive form of tick-borne encephalitis has been reported in Siberia and far-eastern Russia (Russian spring–summer encephalitis) after infection with the Siberian TBEV subtype; only two cases of infection with the European subtype have been reported. Approximately 1.7% of patients with acute encephalitis develop chronic progressive disease. Clinical features and survival rates are diverse. Patients may present with epilepsia partialis continua, progressive neuritis, lateral sclerosis, parkinsonian-like disease, and progressive muscle atrophy. Mental deterioration also leads to dementia and death. Chapter 85 is devoted to HIV encephalitis.

Conclusion

While measles vaccination has significantly reduced the incidence of SSPE, the disease still occurs in several regions, particularly India, the Middle East, and the Philippines, where vaccination coverage is poor and measles is still widespread.

Acknowledgments

This work was supported by Public Health Service grants AG006127, AG032958, (DG), and NS 094758 (MAN) from the National Institutes of Health. We thank Marina Hoffman for editorial review and Cathy Allen for manuscript preparation.

Further reading

Anlar B, Saatci I, Kose G, Yalaz K. MRI findings in subacute sclerosing panencephalitis. *Neurology* 1996;47:1278–1283.

Dawson JR. Cellular inclusions in cerebral lesions of epidemic encephalitis. *Arch Neurol Psychiatry* 1934;31:685–700.

Poponnikova TV. The clinical picture of chronic tick-borne encephalitis in children. *Int J Med Microbiol* 2008;298 (Suppl 1):351–355.

Steiner I, Livneh V, Hoffmann C, *et al*. Steroid-responsive, progressive, focal measles virus brain infection. *Ann Neurol* 2014;75:967–970.

83 Progressive multifocal leukoencephalopathy

Salim Chahin,[1] Thomas Weber,[2] and Joseph R. Berger[1]

[1] Multiple Sclerosis Division of the Department of Neurology, Perelman School of Medicine, University of Pennsylvania, PA, USA

[2] Department of Neurology, Marienkrankenhaus Hamburg, Hamburg, Germany

Progressive multifocal leukoencephalopathy (PML) is a rare, often fatal opportunistic infection of the central nervous system (CNS) that is caused by JC virus (JCV). The landscape of PML has changed over the years. First described as a distinct entity by Aström, Mancall, and Richardson in 1958 in patients with an underlying B-cell lymphoproliferative disorder, it became a well-recognized and common neurological complication of human immunodeficiency virus (HIV)/acquired immune deficiency syndrome (AIDS). The incidence of AIDS-associated PML decreased following the introduction of highly active antiretroviral therapy (HAART). In 2005, PML was recognized as a complication of natalizumab and has also been associated with other immunosuppressive drugs.

Epidemiology

Urine–oral and respiratory transmission has been suggested as the primary mechanism of viral spread; however, the precise mode of contagion remains unknown. No clinical disease is associated with primary infection.

Approximately 10% of children 1–5 years of age have antibodies to JCV. By age 10, 40–60% of the population is antibody positive, and 50–60% of individuals 50–60 years of age are seropositive. Although exposure to JCV is common, PML is rare. A significant underlying abnormality in cell-mediated immunity is seen in all patients with PML.

PML and HIV/AIDS

Until 1984, PML was seen most often in patients with an underlying lymphoproliferative disorder; however, it was observed with other conditions including myeloproliferative diseases, carcinoma, granulomatous disease, and inflammatory or connective tissue diseases, especially system lupus erythematosus (SLE).

The first description of AIDS-associated PML was in 1982. HIV/AIDS rapidly became the most common underlying disorder predisposing to PML. The prevalence of AIDS-related PML before the introduction of antiretrovirals was ~5%, higher than with any other immunosuppressive disorder. Quickly, the demographics of PML reflected those of AIDS: PML became more common in men between the ages of 20 and 50 years, whereas prior to that PML had been chiefly a disease of the elderly with equal gender distribution. After HAART, both the incidence and mortality rate of PML declined, but PML remains a significant complication of AIDS.

PML in other populations

The 2010s saw the recognition of PML as a complication of treatment with immunomodulatory and immunosuppressive agents. This was brought to light by the report of cases of PML in patients using natalizumab for the treatment of multiple sclerosis (MS) or Crohn's disease (two diseases not known to predispose to PML) and focused attention on a direct role for these agents in the pathogenesis of the disease. Because not all agents carry the same PML risk, a classification scheme was proposed in which there are three distinct classes that differ by frequency of PML, time between treatment initiation and PML, and the nature of underlying illness.

Class I agents include natalizumab and efalizumab; the latter was withdrawn from the market in 2009. These agents are associated with a latency of several months to years from starting drug to the onset of PML. Natalizumab is a monoclonal antibody targeting $\alpha4\beta1$ and $\alpha4\beta7$ integrin, thus preventing lymphocyte trafficking through brain and gut endothelium, respectively, and approved for the treatment of MS and Crohn's disease. Risk factors for natalizumab-associated PML include JCV seropositivity, duration of treatment, and immunosuppressive therapy before starting natalizumab. The risk of PML ranges from <1/1000 for patients with no risk factors to around 13/1000 for patients with all three risk factors. The level of anti-JCV antibodies (measured as an index in the serum) may help further stratify the risk of PML: patients who were anti-JCV antibody positive with no prior immunosuppressant use with an index from ≤0.9 to ≤1.5 had a significantly lower risk of PML compared to patients with an index >1.5.

Class II agents have a much lower risk of PML. Most cases occur in patients with predisposing illnesses or on other immunosuppressants. The development of PML with these agents is stochastic with no evidence for latency. The drug most commonly associated with PML among class II agents is rituximab, a monoclonal antibody targeting CD 20+ T-cells. To date, rituximab-associated PML has almost exclusively been described in the setting of lymphoproliferative and connective tissue disorders. Other class II agents include mycophenolate mofetil, brentuximab vedotin, and belimumab. Like rituximab, all cases of PML associated with these agents had an underlying illness known to predispose to PML or were on other immunosuppressants. Furthermore, the risk of PML developing appears to be orders of magnitude below the risk observed with class I agents.

Class III agents, rarely associated with PML, are similar to class II agents. They are used to treat conditions that predispose to PML

International Neurology, Second edition. Edited by Robert P. Lisak, Daniel D. Truong, William M. Carroll and Roongroj Bhidayasiri
© 2016 John Wiley & Sons, Ltd. Published 2016 by John Wiley & Sons, Ltd.

or in conjunction with other agents that increase the risk of PML. PML in patients taking the class III agent alemtuzumab occurred on a background of immunosuppression or malignancy and no cases have developed in MS patients. The risk of PML with other class III agents (e.g., TNF-alpha inhibitors adalimumab, etanercept, and infliximab) is small and confounded by use of other immunosuppressive agents. At least two cases of PML have occurred in patients taking dimethylfumarate, a fumaric acid agent, and others have been described in association with fumaric acid ester use. Fingolimod, an agent that impedes the egress of effector memory T-cells from lymph nodes, has also been associated with two cases of PML, although both remain to be published and details from the first reported case suggest that neuromyelitis optica spectrum disorder may have been responsible for the clinical and radiographic findings rather than PML. At least 11 PML cases occurred in patients as they ceased natalizumab and switched to fingolimod.

Geographic differences

Curiously, the epidemiology of PML has some geographic differences. PML is rare in Africa and Asia, possibly explained by underdiagnosis, differences in medical care, or death of PML patients from other AIDS-related complications. It is also possible that less virulent strains of JCV are more common in those areas and that the predominant HIV strains predispose to a lower PML risk in parts of Africa and Asia. The incidence of non-HIV PML in these regions follows the incidence of the predisposing disorders and is likely affected by differences in treatment patterns with immunosuppressive agents and underdiagnosis.

Pathophysiology

JCV belongs to the genus Polyomavirus, in the family Papovavirus. The virus has a double-stranded DNA genome that encodes several regulatory, non-structural proteins, three structural capsid proteins, and a non-coding control region. Mutations result in different tissue tropism and clinical expression. For example, mutations in the non-coding control region distinguish viruses capable of replicating effectively in glial tissues from those replicating chiefly in renal tissues, and mutations in the capsid protein genes have been implicated in a cerebellar syndrome caused by JCV.

The virus uses a sialic acid receptor that is facilitated by a serotonin receptor 5-HT2a (5-HT2AR, a potential treatment target) for binding, although other, as yet unidentified receptors may also be important for cell binding and entry. After binding, the virus enters the cell and is transported to the endoplasmic reticulum through caveosomes, and from there it enters the nucleus.

Pathogenesis

Several lines of evidence suggest that PML results from reactivation of a latent infection and not as a primary infection. The evidence most supportive of this is the observation that virtually all individuals developing natalizumab-associated PML were JCV antibody testing six or more months before the PML.

Acute infection with JCV appears to be subclinical, as no clinically distinct disorder has been observed at primary infection. The primary site of JCV infection remains uncertain, although tonsillar stromal cells have been suggested. From there, the virus likely propagates to hematopoietic precursor cells and genitourinary tract tissues, where it remains latent.

Active infection is characterized by JCV infection of oligodendrocytes and astrocytes with a characteristic histopathological triad of demyelination, abnormal oligodendroglial nuclei, and giant astrocytes (Figure 83.1).

Clinical features

The onset of PML symptoms is usually subacute and insidious. PML heralds AIDS in 1% of all HIV-infected persons and can therefore lead to diagnostic difficulty in an individual with unsuspected HIV infection. Similarly, diagnostic confusion can occur in MS because of potential clinical and radiographic overlap between the two diseases. The most common symptoms of PML are weakness (hemiparesis), cognitive abnormalities, gait disorders, headaches, visual impairment (visual field loss), and sensory loss. Seizures are seen in 5–10% of patients. Subtle differences in PML symptoms can occur depending on the underlying illness; for example, in natalizumab-associated PML cognitive impairment is the most frequent symptom, followed by motor abnormalities, language disorders, and visual impairment.

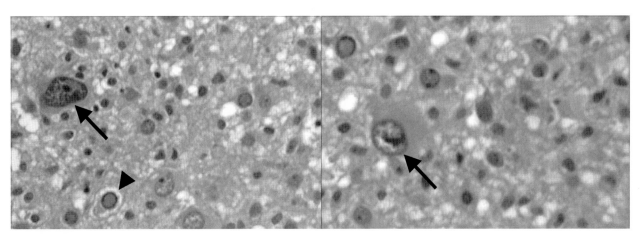

Figure 83.1 Pathology of progressive multifocal leukoencephalopathy – haematoxylin and eosin (H&E) staining of a typical PML lesion showing the bizarre astrocytes (arrows) and the enlarged oligodendrocyte nuclei (arrowhead).

PML–immune reconstitution inflammatory syndrome

The immune reconstitution inflammatory syndrome (IRIS) is the paradoxical worsening of symptoms of an opportunistic infection concomitant with recovery of a suppressed immune system. PML-IRIS can be fatal if untreated. It is most commonly seen in HIV-associated disease after initiation of HAART, and is characterized by new or increased deficits, increase in number and size of lesions, as well as contrast enhancement and edema on magnetic resonance imaging (MRI). IRIS is also common with natalizumab-associated PML following removal of the monoclonal antibody by plasma exchange. At the height of PML-IRIS, there is prominent inflammation (particularly CD8+ T-cells), B-cells, plasma cells, and monocytes. MS lesions can flare up after natalizumab is withdrawn, further complicating the clinical state.

Prognosis

The survival of HIV-associated PML changed from less than 10% in the pre-HAART era to 50% after the introduction of effective antiretroviral agents. Factors associated with prolonged survival in HIV-associated PML include PML as the presenting manifestation of AIDS, higher CD4 lymphocyte count, presence of perivascular inflammatory infiltrates in PML lesions, and contrast enhancement. Survival with natalizumab-associated PML is ~80%. Factors associated with survival include early diagnosis, prompt removal of natalizumab by plasma exchange, treatment of IRIS, and lower disability before PML.

Other forms of infection

Granule cell neuronopathy (GCN-PML) is characterized by cerebellar atrophy with lytic infection of cerebellar granule cells. Another form of PML is typified by cortical lesions with lytic infection of pyramidal neurons and cortical astrocytes by JCV.

Investigations

Imaging

Radiographic imaging strongly supports the diagnosis of PML. Brain computed tomography (CT) reveals hypodense white-matter lesions without mass effect and infrequent contrast enhancement. Brain MRI is more sensitive and shows T2 hyperintense and T1 hypointense lesions. Contrast enhancement is recognized, but uncommon, and is often seen in IRIS. The lesions of PML are usually multifocal, but can be monofocal and often have a distinctive "ground glass" appearance on T2-weighted images. The frontal and parieto-occipital regions are the most commonly affected, but involvement of the basal ganglia, external capsule, cerebellum, and brainstem has also been reported.

Laboratory studies

Detection of JCV by polymerase chain reaction (PCR) in cerebrospinal fluid (CSF) helps to confirm PML in the appropriate clinical setting and MRI findings. JCV PCR is highly sensitive and specific. Frequently, the CSF JCV DNA copy count is low, particularly with natalizumab-associated PML where as many as two-thirds of patients have <500 copies of JCV DNA per μL. Ultrasensitive PCR is mandatory and multiple CSF collections may be required. CSF cell count in PML is usually <20 cells/mm3 and more than half of PML cases have a mildly elevated CSF protein. In HIV-infected individuals, the peripheral lymphocyte counts generally reveal a profound CD4 lymphopenia with <200 cells/mm3.

Histopathology

The cardinal feature of PML pathology is microscopic or macroscopic demyelination, ranging in size from 1 mm to several centimeters. The histopathological hallmarks of PML are a triad of multifocal demyelination; hyperchromatic, enlarged oligodendroglial nuclei; and enlarged bizarre astrocytes with lobulated hyperchromatic nuclei (Figure 83.1). Electron microscopic or immunohistochemistry examination reveals papova virions in oligodendrocytes. Although the gold standard for diagnosis of PML is demonstration of the histopathological triad, the diagnosis is more often established when patients present with a compatible clinical picture, a typical brain MRI, and PCR-amplified JCV DNA in CSF.

Treatment

Most reports of effective treatment of PML remain anecdotal. Nucleoside analogs (such as cytarabine) have demonstrated some efficacy against the virus *in vitro*, but have failed in clinical trials. Interferons do not improve survival. Topoisomerase inhibitors prevent JCV replication *in vitro*, but are toxic and have not been shown to be clinically efficacious. Cidofovir has demonstrated selective antipolyomavirus activity, but a clinical trial failed to show any benefit. The use of mefloquine, an antimalaria agent, in PML was advocated based on laboratory studies, but also lacked clinical efficacy in a study that was terminated prematurely. The observation that the JCV binding is dependent on the serotonin receptor 5HT2a has led to the anecdotal use of serotonin receptor antagonists (risperidone, ziprasdisone, and mirtazapine) as a potential therapeutic modality, but their effectiveness remains questionable and is unsupported by any well-controlled clinical trials.

Treatment of PML-IRIS includes high-dose steroids. Although not without potential risks, steroids seem to improve survival. The CCR5 blocker maraviroc has also been proposed as a potential therapy for PML-IRIS.

Prevention (risk-mitigation strategies)

With the observation that certain drugs may predispose to PML, risk mitigation strategies have been proposed (Table 83.1). Risk mitigation has been employed regularly in patients treated with natalizumab where three factors have been identified as substantially increasing the risk of PML: (1) longer treatment durations (>24 months); (2) JCV antibody positivity, particularly JCV antibody indices <1.5; and (3) prior use of an immunosuppressive agent. Monitoring patients with serial MRIs and for JCV antibody seropositivity has been widely implemented, but there have been no controlled trials demonstrating that this strategy decreases the risk of PML and, to date, the number of patients developing PML while being treated with natalizumab has not seemed to be decreasing. Nonetheless, the strategy appears prudent. Whether a similar strategy is of value in patients being treated with other agents that increase the risk of PML is uncertain. In light of the significantly lower risk of PML with drugs other than natalizumab, such a strategy cannot be recommended at this time.

Table 83.1 Medications previously reported with progressive multifocal leukoencephalopathy.

Treatment	Drug(s)	
Oral glucocorticoids	All	
Alkylating agents	• Cyclophosphamide (Cytoxan®) • Camustine (BiCNU®)	• Dacarbazine (DTIC-Dome®)
Purine analogs	• Fludarabine (Fludara®) • Cladribine (Leustat®)	• Azathioprine (Imuran®) • Nelarabine (Arranon®)
Antimetabolite	• Methotrexate (Trexall®)	
Monoclonal antibodies	• Rituximab (Rituxan®) • Infliximab (Remicade®) • Natalizumab (Tysabri®) • Basiliximab (Simutect®) • Belimumab (Benlysta®)	• Daclizumab (Zenapax®) • Muromonab-cd3 (Orthoclone OKT3®) • Efalizumab (Raptiva®) • Alemtuzumab (Campath®, Lemtrada®)
Fusion proteins	• Etanercept (Enbrel®) • Belatacept (Nulojix®)	• Brentuximab vedotin (Adcetris®)
Immunosuppressants	• Cydosporin • Cyclosporine (Sandimmune®) • Tacrolimus (Prograf®)	• Sirolimus (Rapamune®) • Mycophenolate (CellCept®)
Immunomodulatory agents	• Dimethyl fumarate (Tecfidera®) • Fingolimod (Gilenya®)	

Further reading

Berger JR, Khalili K. The pathogenesis of progressive multifocal leukoencephalopathy. *Discov Med* 2011;12(67):495–503.

Chahin S, Berger JR. A risk classification for immunosuppressive treatment-associated progressive multifocal leukoencephalopathy. *J Neurovirol* 2015;21(6):623–631.

Clifford DB, De Luca A, Simpson DM, *et al.* Natalizumab-associated progressive multifocal leukoencephalopathy in patients with multiple sclerosis: Lessons from 28 cases. *Lancet Neurol* 2010;9(4):438–446.

Plavina T, Subramanyam M, Bloomgren G, *et al.* Anti-JC virus antibody levels in serum or plasma further define risk of natalizumab-associated progressive multifocal leukoencephalopathy. *Ann Neurol* 2014;76(6):802–812.

Shankar SK, Satishchandra P, Mahadevan A, *et al.* Low prevalence of progressive multifocal leukoencephalopathy in India and Africa: Is there a biological explanation? *J Neurovirol* 2003;9(Suppl 1):59–67.

84 Biology of HIV and overview of AIDS

Alexandros C. Tselis

Department of Neurology, Wayne State University School of Medicine, Detroit, MI, USA

The human immunodeficiency virus (HIV) is a highly neurotropic virus and a common cause of viral encephalitis worldwide. This chapter discusses the biology of HIV and clinical features of early and late disease.

Although there are two different types of HIV (HIV-1 and HIV-2), HIV-1 produces the most disease and will be referred to as HIV throughout the chapter.

History and overview

Disease due to HIV infection first manifested itself in the United States in June of 1981, when the Centers for Disease Control and Prevention reported five cases of young gay men in Los Angeles with pneumocystis carinii pneumonia (PCP), mucosal candidiasis, and cytomegalovirus (CMV) infection. The following month, similar clusters of patients were reported with Kaposi's sarcoma in New York. Each of these infections is generally only seen in patients with profound suppression of cell-mediated immunity; not surprisingly, in the initial cases later identified as HIV/AIDS (acquired immune deficiency syndrome), there was profound CD4+ lymphopenia.

As the number of cases increased and clinical experience with the disease accumulated, it was noted that the disease was not always transmitted sexually (with multiple sexual partners a strong risk factor), but also by blood transfusions, and sharing of needles between intravenous drug users. HIV was isolated from the lymph node of a patient with lymphadenopathy in 1983. It was only the second retrovirus shown to cause human disease (human T-lymphotropic virus-1 [HTLV-1] was the first). The development of methods for isolation and propagation of HIV was important for the production of test kits that allowed for detection of the virus before the AIDS clinical manifestations were present, and for screening antiviral drugs.

In 1987, zidovudine, the first antiretroviral drug, was approved for clinical use by the US Food and Drug Administration (FDA), and the first Western blot test kit was approved for diagnosis of HIV infection. The first protease inhibitor, saquinavir, was approved in 1995 and the first non-nucleoside reverse transcriptase inhibitor, nevirapine, in 1996. The FDA approved HIV viral load as a valid and reliable method to monitor patients in 1996. By 1997, combination antiretroviral therapy (cART) was the standard of care. The combination of antiretroviral drugs with different mechanisms of action reduced the generation of resistance mutations in the virus, thus sustaining antiviral efficacy. This resulted in a dramatic decrease in AIDS and death from AIDS and its complications.

Viral molecular epidemiology

There are three groups of HIV: M (or Main), O (Outlier), and N (non-M and non-O) groups. M consists of nine subgroups or clades: A, B, C, D, F, G, H, J, and K. These clades, or subtypes, differ with respect to efficiency of viral replication, ability to infect certain types of cells, vulnerability to drug resistance, and certain types of clinical manifestations, including those affecting neurocognitive function. Each clade differs from the others by >20% in the ENV (viral glycoproteins/viral envelope) region of the genome (see later) and by >15% in the GAG region, which encodes capsid proteins. The O and N groups appear to affect only a minority of patients. There is a geographic distribution of local clade prevalence; for example, clade B is found in North America and Europe, while clades A, C, D, and H are found in Africa, and clades J and K in Zaire and Cameroon, respectively. Some viral isolates have sequences from different clades in their genomes. These arose as recombinants from simultaneous infection of one individual by viruses from two or more clades, and are now known as circulating recombinant forms (CRFs).

Antigens for most commercially available enzyme-linked immunosorbent assay (ELISA) tests are based on clade B viruses from North America and Europe, which have been used most in clinical trials. Viruses from different clades respond differently to antiretroviral drugs. HIV-1 group O and HIV-2 viruses are often resistant to non-nucleotide reverse transcriptase inhibitors (NNRTIs), and HIV-1 clade G appears to be less susceptible to protease inhibitor drugs *in vitro*.

Viral structure

The HIV virion consists of two identical (diploid) single-strand 9 kb RNA molecules enclosed within a capsid surrounded by a viral envelope. The virus transcribes its RNA into DNA by reverse transcriptase (RT) and inserts DNA into the genome of the infected cell by an integrase (IN).

The viral genome consists of the typical retroviral LTR-GAG-POL-ENV-LTR structure that incorporates the regulatory long terminal repeat (LTR) and the genes for structural (GAG, or group-specific antigen), polymerase (POL), and envelope (ENV) proteins along with accessory genes (tat, vpr, vpu, nef), as shown in Figure 84.1. The viral genome is translated as a polyprotein, which is then cleaved into functional component proteins by the viral-encoded protease (PR) segment of the polyprotein. GAG encodes for the structural proteins, which includes the matrix (MA), capsid protein (CA), p7, and the nucleocapsid protein (NC). POL encodes three proteins: PR, RT, and an IN. Finally, ENV encodes for the

International Neurology, Second edition. Edited by Robert P. Lisak, Daniel D. Truong, William M. Carroll and Roongroj Bhidayasiri

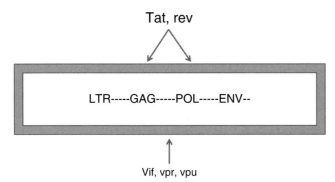

Figure 84.1 The HIV genome.

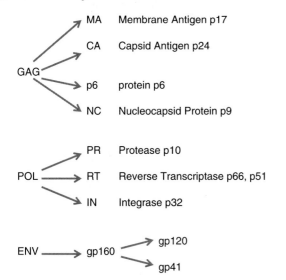

Figure 84.2 HIV proteins.

envelope glycoprotein gp160, which is cleaved into two viral surface proteins, gp120 and gp41. Gp120 attaches the virus to the cell, and gp41 induces fusion between the viral envelope and the cell membrane (Figure 84.2).

Pathogenesis

HIV infects many cell types, but CD4+ T-lymphocytes and macrophages are most prominently affected. To achieve infection, the HIV envelope glycoprotein gp120 attaches to a CD4+ molecule as well as to one of two possible co-receptors, CXCR4 or CCR5. CD4 is expressed on lymphocytes and macrophages and is considered the main viral receptor. CXCR4 co-receptors, expressed on T-cells, select for infection by so-called X4 viruses, while CCR5 co-receptors are expressed on macrophages and select for R5 viruses. The precise tropism by the virus is in part determined by sequences in gp120 that bind either to CXCR4, resulting in a T-lymphotropic (T-tropic) virus or to CCR5, resulting in a macrophage-tropic (or M-tropic) virus. T-tropic strains replicate to high titer in MT-2 cells, causing them to produce syncytia (syncytium inducing or SI) and cell death. M-tropic strains replicate to low titer in MT-2 cells, do not produce syncytia, and have low pathogenicity.

Once the virus penetrates the cell, subsequent events depend on the viral strain and type of cell infected. HIV RNA, bound to viral

proteins including RT, is released into the cell cytoplasm. If the cell is permissive, RT reverse transcribes the viral RNA into a complementary DNA copy, cDNA, which is then converted into double-stranded DNA (dsDNA). The ds cDNA, along with viral proteins MA, vpr, and IN, forms the preintegration complex, which is then directed into the nucleus of the cell, where ds cDNA is inserted into the host cell's genomic DNA. At that point, infection may become latent or productive, transcribing incorporated cDNA into viral RNA and producing virions.

The process of infection described provides a number of therapeutic targets. These include drugs that act as reverse transcriptase inhibitors (RTI), which are nucleoside analogs (nRTI) and non-nucleoside analogs (nnRTI), protease inhibitors (PI), fusion inhibitors (FI), integrase inhibitors, and CCR5 co-receptor blockers (see Table 84.1).

Table 84.1 Antiretroviral medications used in the treatment of HIV infections.

Nucleoside analog reverse transcriptase inhibitors (NRTI)
Zidovudine (ZDV)
Didanosine (ddI)
Zalcitabine (ddC)
Emtricitabine (FTC)
Lamivudine (3TC)
Stavudine (d4T)
Abacavir (ABC)
Tenofovir (TDF)
Non-nucleoside analog reverse transcriptase inhibitors (N-NRTI)
Delavirdine (DLV)
Efavirenz (EFV)
Etravirine (ETR)
Nevirapine (NVP)
Rilpivirine (RPV)
Protease inhibitors (PI)
Atazanavir (ATV)
Darunavir (DRV)
Fosamprenavir (FPV)
Indinavir (IDV)
Nelfinavir (NFV)
Ritonavir (RTV)
Saquinavir (SQV)
Tipranavir (TOV)
Fusion inhibitors (FI)
Enfuvirtide (T20)
Entry inhibitors CCR5 blockers (EI)
Maraviroc (MVC)
Integrase inhibitors (II)
Dolutegravir (DTG)
Raltegravir (RAL)

Course of infection and clinical features

Clinical HIV infection is classified into several stages depending on viral load, clinical characteristics, and CD4+ count. Acute retroviral infection is defined as the first few weeks of HIV infection before HIV antibodies appear. Early HIV infection is defined as the first few months after the development of HIV antibodies. This is followed by a clinically latent state, in which there are no signs or symptoms of disease. Advanced HIV infection, or AIDS, is defined by several criteria, including a low CD4+ cell count (<200 cells/μL), the presence of any one of several opportunistic infections, and certain HIV-specific syndromes, such as HIV dementia, HIV-associated neuropathy, and HIV-associated vacuolar myelopathy.

Acute HIV infection

Acute HIV infection may be entirely asymptomatic, but is often characterized by an acute illness, with fever, sore throat, fatigue, weight loss, macular rash, lymphadenopathy, and myalgia. Some findings on physical examination include oral ulceration, exudative pharyngitis, thrush, genital or rectal ulceration, and adenopathy. Acute retroviral syndrome can resemble other acute systemic infectious diseases such as infectious mononucleosis, secondary syphilis, hepatitis A or B, measles, and toxoplasmosis, and may be accompanied by aseptic meningitis.

In acute infection, blood-borne dissemination results in viral deposition in various organs and can manifest as organ-specific syndromes. These may be the result of cytopathic effects or an immunopathology.

HIV can be isolated from the cerebrospinal fluid (CSF) early in the course of infection. Occasionally, acute retroviral syndrome can involve the central nervous system (CNS). HIV syndromes in the CNS include encephalitis and acute myelopathy. In the peripheral nervous system (PNS), Bell's palsy, acute brachial plexopathy, and inflammatory demyelinating polyneuropathy can occur. Sensory ganglionitis, cranial nerve palsies, progressive myopathy, and acute rhabdomyolysis have also been reported. The pathogenesis of these syndromes is unclear and may not involve direct infection of neural cells; instead, these syndromes may reflect the effects of generalized immune activation. The outcome of these illnesses is unpredictable, but often quite good.

Early HIV

Early HIV disease has little neurological manifestation, except for the lingering effects of facial palsy, plexopathy, or chronic inflammatory demyelinating polyneuropathy.

Advanced HIV/AIDS

Advanced HIV/AIDS is dominated by opportunistic infections and the secondary effects of HIV infection. Many patients are asymptomatic for a considerable time, and develop systemic opportunistic infections. These include oral thrush, Kaposi's sarcoma, PCP, cytomegalovirus (CMV) retinitis, esophagitis, or colitis, as well as some neoplasms. Neurological opportunistic infections include cryptococcal meningitis, progressive multifocal leukoencephalopathy (PML), CMV encephalitis, retinitis, or radiculomyelitis, and primary CNS lymphoma (actually an opportunistic neoplasm driven by Epstein–Barr virus).

Neurological sequelae of HIV infection

HIV can affect the nervous system independently of opportunistic infections. Three clinical entities have been identified. These are HIV dementia, HIV-associated painful polyneuropathy, and HIV myelopathy.

HIV dementia consists of a variably but subacutely progressive difficulty with memory, mood, fine motor skills, steadiness of gait, and ability to organize. These can be mild enough not to interfere even with very demanding tasks or severe enough that the patients cannot live independently. Brain MRI shows atrophy and diffusely abnormal signal in the white matter. Histopathology shows perivascular infiltrates, microglial nodules, myelin pallor, and the characteristic multinuclear giant cells. It is of note that HIV does not infect neurons or oligodendrocytes, but abortively infects astrocytes and productively infects microglia and giant cells. This suggests that damage to neurons in a "bystander" fashion rather than directly lysing the cells.

The polyneuropathy consists of loss of elementary sensations (especially sharp–dull) in a glove-and-stocking distribution and selectively involves small fibers more than large fibers. A clinically identical condition is seen in patients who took the antiretrovirals didanosine, zalcitabine, or stavudine (all of which are no longer being used). The condition can be quite uncomfortable and can have a major impact on quality of life. There is no specific treatment for HIV polyneuropathy.

HIV myelopathy is characterized by a slowly progressive spastic paraparesis, usually late in the course of diseases where competing diseases make the diagnosis difficult. The diagnosis is made by neurological examination, which shows lower-extremity weakness and hyperreflexia with no sensory level, an MRI that now shows abnormal signal in the cord, and possibly mild atrophy and an otherwise negative workup for myelopathy. There is a vacuolar degeneration in the long tracts of the cord, similar to what is seen in vitamin B_{12} deficiency. There is no specific treatment.

Viral dynamics

On initial infection, particularly with M-tropic strains, only part of the viral inoculum replicates to high initial titer. The virus crosses the mucosal barrier (in the genitals or rectum) and encounters Langerhans cells, which express both CD4+ and CCR5 molecules, probably favoring transmission of the M-tropic part of the inoculum. The Langerhans cells migrate to local draining lymph nodes, become activated dendritic cells, and infect CD4+ lymphocytes. Virus becomes detectable in local lymph nodes within a few days. This is followed by a burst of viremia and systemic dissemination. The blood viral load is initially high (between 10,000 and 80,000 HIV RNA copies/mL), but as cell-mediated immunity is activated, drops to a steady level or "set point." A high set point is predictive of a more rapid progression to AIDS. In one study of HIV+ patients followed for 2 years, the initial median viral set point in those who developed AIDS was 80,000 RNA copies/mL plasma compared with 40,000 HIV RNA copies/mL plasma in those who did not. Initially, the number of CD4+ T-cells drops, while the number of CD8+ T-cells increases, resulting in an inverted CD4:CD8 ratio. As the set point is approached (in 20–120 days), the CD4+ count recovers. In the untreated host, the CD4+ count then decreases slowly and symptomatic AIDS occurs in about 10 years.

After the set point is achieved and antiretroviral medication is initiated, measurements of viral load reveal the dynamics of viral generation. Cells productively infected with virus have an average lifespan of approximately 2 days. Plasma viral load has a half-life of about 6 hours; decay of plasma virus is faster than that of peripheral blood mononuclear cell-associated virus. The viral generation time, from release of a virion to release of "daughter" virions after infection of a new cell, is approximately 2.6 days. It is estimated that 10 billion virions are produced every 24 hours.

In the original burst of viremia, HIV is deposited in various tissues and establishes infection in each of them, particularly in the CNS. Usually, the initial virus is of R5 M-tropic phenotype. The different tissue compartments (plasma, brain parenchyma, CSF, gut mucosa, testicles, lymph nodes, etc.) can be relatively isolated from one another and virus evolves in each compartment independently from the others. Thus, early on HIV isolates from blood and CSF may have the same initial phenotype, but late in the course of infection the phenotypes can differ. A large reservoir of CD4+ T-cells in mucosa of the gastrointestinal tract is rapidly eliminated during acute infection. Studies of diarrhea in HIV patients showed loss of mucosal CD4+ T-cells along with villus atrophy and resultant malabsorption. If no other cause is discovered, this disease process is known as HIV enteropathy. There is a preferential loss of Th17 cells in the mucosa. Th17 cells elaborate IL-17, which helps protects the gastrointestinal tract from bacterial and fungal infection. Loss of Th17 cells allows microbes access to the systemic circulation (microbial translocation). Bacterial lipopolysaccharides (LPS) help activate systemic inflammation with an increase in activated CD8+ T-cells and interferon α (IFNα). HIV+ patients are at greater risk of morbidity and mortality if they have a generally hyperinflammatory state, as determined by increased IL-6, C-reactive protein, and d-dimer at baseline at the beginning of HIV enteropathy.

Treatment and management

Appropriate therapy depends on the stage of HIV disease and comorbidities such as diabetes or hepatitis B and hepatitis C infection. Hepatitis C co-infection results in a poorer prognosis for both HIV and hepatitis C, and hepatitis C has its own effects on both the central and peripheral nervous systems. US National Institutes of Health (NIH) guidelines for evaluation and treatment of HIV in adults and adolescents are periodically updated and should be consulted on an NIH web page (http://aidsinfo.nih.gov/contentfiles/lvguidelines/AdultandAdolescentGL.pdf). NIH also publishes guidelines for the management of HIV/AIDS in children.

First, antiretroviral drugs are given to suppress viral production. Second, opportunistic infections such as cryptococcal meningitis or PCP are treated with appropriate antimicrobials. Third, active concurrent infections such as hepatitis B and hepatitis C are suppressed with appropriate antivirals. Finally, other comorbidities such as diabetes and dyslipidemias need to be dealt with, since the symptoms and complications of these diseases are amplified in patients who also have chronic HIV infection.

Antiretroviral therapy (ART) reduces the viral burden and slows the progression of disease. Therapy consists of a combination of drugs (cART) with different mechanisms of action. Therapy is also designed to reduce the risk of virus transmission *in utero* and through sexual activity. There are a number of considerations in choosing a cART regimen and advice from an infectious disease expert is needed. An extensive number of baseline studies are also required. CD4 counts and viral load are measured at baseline, along with routine labs, and resistance genotypic assays.

The CD4 count and viral load are measured again every 3–6 months or when changing therapies or a clinical event such as unexpected opportunistic infection occurs. The aim of antiretroviral therapy is to reduce viral loads to undetectable levels (most assays have a sensitivity of <20/mL copies HIV RNA).

The success of cART in suppressing viral load and restoring immune function has led to unanticipated complications. One is the so-called immune reconstitution inflammatory syndrome (IRIS), which occurs in the context of decreasing HIV viral load and increasing CD4+ T-cell counts. IRIS often affects areas that were previously affected by an opportunistic infection, and may be confused with a relapse of a previously resolved disease. An important clue to the presence of IRIS is that of occurrence during immune reconstitution, with increased CD4 counts and decreasing viral load. Other atypical features can suggest IRIS. An edematous ring-enhancing white-matter brain lesion may arise in an area of apparently inactive PML. Another example would be a decreased cryptococcal antigen in a patient with what appears to be a clinically relapsed cryptococcal meningitis. Other infections commonly showing reactivation include cytomegalovirus, cryptococcosis, mycobacterium tuberculosis, and PML. IRIS due to HIV itself has also been reported. Occasionally IRIS can become severe or even life-threatening. While there is no data to guide clinical management, most clinicians treat with high-dose corticosteroids.

Conclusion

HIV disease is an important pathogen that has affected many millions, and has taught us much about the different ways in which the nervous system can be affected. This includes the effects of HIV by itself, through opportunistic infections and neurotoxicity. The success of the fight against HIV is due to a multidisciplinary approach. The ultimate success would be an effective vaccine.

Further reading

Chun TW, Fauci AS. HIV reservoirs: Pathogenesis and obstacles to viral eradication and cure. *AIDS* 2012;26:1261–1268.

Cornblath D, McArthur J, Kennedy P, Witte A, Griffin J. Inflammatory demyelinating neuropathies associated with human T-cell lymphotropic virus type III infection. *Ann Neurol* 1987;21:32–40.

Davis L, Hjelle B, Miller V, *et al.* Early brain invasion in iatrogenic human immunodeficiency virus infection. *Neurology* 1992;42:1736–1739.

Douek D, Picker L, Koup R. T cell dynamics in HIV-1 infection. *Ann Rev Immunol* 2003;21:265–304.

Haseltine W. Molecular biology of the human immunodeficiency virus type1. *FASEB J* 1991;5:2349–2360.

Hollander H, Levy J. Neurologic abnormalities and recovery of human immunodeficiency virus from cerebrospinal fluid. *Ann Intern Med* 1987;106:692–695.

Kassutto S, Rosenberg S. Primary HIV type 1 infection. *Clin Infect Dis* 2004; 38: 1447–1453.

Martin-Blondel G, Delobel P, Blancher A, *et al.* Pathogenesis of the immune reconstitution syndrome affecting the central nervous system in patients infected with HIV. *Brain* 2011;134:928–946.

Panel on Antiretroviral Guidelines for Adults and Adolescents. Guidelines for the use of antiretroviral agents in HIV-1-infected adults and adolescents. Washington, DC: Department of Health and Human Services. http://aidsinfo.nih.gov/contentfiles/lvguidelines/AdultandAdolescentGL.pdf (accessed November 2015).

Parry G. Peripheral neuropathies associated with human immunodeficiency virus infection. *Ann Neurol* 1988;23:S49–S53.

Peeters M, Toure-Kaane T, Nkengasong J. Genetic diversity of HIV in Africa: Impact on diagnosis, treatment, vaccine development and trials. *AIDS* 2003;17:2547–2560.

Schacker T, Collier A, Hughes J, Shea T, Corey L. Clinical and epidemiological features of primary HIV infection. *Ann Intern Med* 1986;125:257–264.

Simpson D, Bender A. Human immunodeficiency virus-associated myopathy: Analysis of 11 patients. *Ann Neurol* 1982;4:79–84.

85 HIV encephalitis and myelopathy

Girish Modi, Kapila Hari, and Andre Mochan
Department of Neurology, University of the Witwatersrand, Johannesburg, South Africa

HIV-associated cognitive impairment

Cognitive impairment in the human immunodeficiency virus (HIV) is caused either by the virus itself, by HIV-related opportunistic disease, or from unrelated neuropathology. HIV-related opportunistic disease is typically associated with immunosuppression and includes infections (cryptococcosis, toxoplasmosis, varicella zoster virus infection, progressive multifocal leukoencephalopathy [PML]), and neoplasms (lymphoma). Unrelated neurodegenerative disorders like Alzheimer's dementia or cerebrovascular disease can contribute to cognitive impairment in aging patients with chronic HIV infection. Neurocognitive illness caused by the virus itself ranges from clinically asymptomatic through moderate disease to severe disease, where significant loss of cognition and activities of daily living occurs.

The focus of this section is the spectrum of primary HIV-related neurocognitive illness.

Terminology

During the early stages of the HIV epidemic the entity of subacute encephalitis was recognized in HIV-infected patients with features of dementia. The neuropathological hallmark was the presence of multinucleated giant cells on autopsy and the absence of other potential pathogens. The term AIDS dementia complex (ADC) was coined later and described the clinical features and neuropathology of this primary HIV infection of the brain. ADC was soon recognized as a spectrum of cognitive deficiency ranging from mild (neuropsychologically impaired, NPI), to moderate (minor cognitive motor disorder, MCMD), to severe (HIV-associated dementia, HAD). The currently advocated terminology for HIV-associated neurocognitive disorders (HAND) is in the Frascati criteria. These are based on and include neuropsychological testing and assessment of functional status. The neuropsychological component of the evaluation requires assessment of the following ability domains: verbal/language; attention/working memory; abstraction/executive; memory (learning, recall); speed of information processing; and sensory-perceptual and motor skills. Functional status is based on activities of daily living and may rely on self-reporting, and require corroboration or long-term follow-up. Three categories are described based on the severity of the impairment.

- Asymptomatic neurocognitive impairment (ANI): neurocognitive test performance 1 standard deviation (SD) below an appropriate normative mean in at least two cognitive domains, but no decline in functional status.
- Mild neurocognitive disorder (MND): neurocognitive test performance 1 SD below mean in at least two cognitive domains and mild impairment in activities of daily living.
- HIV-associated dementia (HAD): severe cognitive impairment in two or more domains by 2 SD below mean combined with notable impairment in activities of daily living.

The Frascati criteria rely on neuropsychological testing and are not applicable at the bedside. The diagnosis of HIV-associated neurocognitive disorder requires that other causes of dementia be excluded and the possibilities of psychiatric illness and drug abuse be considered.

Epidemiology

The introduction of highly active antiretroviral therapy (HAART) during the mid-1990s delineated two distinct phases in the epidemiology of HIV-related neurocognitive disorders. The pre-HAART era was characterized by a high prevalence of HAD. Pre-HAART data from the San Diego HIV Neurobehavioral Research Center (HNRC) cohort on subjects enrolled between 1988 and 1995 show cognitive impairment rates of 25% in patients in stage Centers for Disease Control (CDC)-A, 42% in CDC-B, and 52% of patients in CDC-C. Similarly, data from Baltimore and Los Angeles in the Multicenter AIDS Cohort Study (MACS), a longitudinal study following 7000 homo-/bisexual men, described the incidence of acquired immunodeficiency syndrome (AIDS) dementia in a cohort of 492 patients; 64 patients (15%) developed severe dementia between initial recruitment and death. Other large longitudinal cohort studies, including EuroSIDA (a prospective observational cohort study started in 1994 of more than 16,000 patients followed in 31 European countries plus Israel and Argentina) and the National Australian AIDS Registry, concur in the observation that neurocognitive impairment was common and overt dementia was more prevalent in patients with advanced disease and low CD4 counts. A meta-analysis of 12 studies involving approximately 1200 patients from sub-Saharan Africa found neurocognitive impairment in 42% pre-HAART.

The use of potent HAART regimes has strikingly reduced the number of patients developing frank dementia. The CNS HIV Anti-Retroviral Therapy Effects Research (CHARTER) study, a large multicenter study based in the United States, estimates the prevalence of HAD at less than 5%. The EuroSIDA cohort showed that HAART was associated with a 41% reduction in the risk of HAD. The milder subtypes of HAND, however, continue to be reported in patients despite sustained virological control. In the CHARTER study, mild neurocognitive impairment (NCI) was detected in 45% of patients, ANI in 33%, and MND in 12%. About half of HAART-treated patients remain with the milder forms of NCI.

International Neurology, Second edition. Edited by Robert P. Lisak, Daniel D. Truong, William M. Carroll and Roongroj Bhidayasiri
© 2016 John Wiley & Sons, Ltd. Published 2016 by John Wiley & Sons, Ltd.

Several reasons for this apparent treatment failure have been postulated:

- The "legacy effect" of HIV infection: permanent damage predating initiation of HAART.
- Ongoing central nervous system (CNS) disease activity resulting from lack of viral suppression due to poor CNS penetration effectiveness (CPE) of antiretrovirals (ARVs).
- Potential neurotoxicity of HAART.
- Confounding comorbidities like psychiatric illness, substance abuse, and cerebrovascular disease.
- Aging.

The current epidemiological pattern dominated by milder forms of HAND largely pertains to developed countries. Globally, the overwhelming majority of HIV patients are to be found in developing countries with sub-Saharan Africa bearing the brunt of the disease burden. The World Health Organization in 2013 estimated that globally there were 31.8 million adults living with HIV, and 21.8 million were resident in sub-Saharan Africa. The number of new adult HIV infections worldwide was estimated to be 1.9 million and of this, 1.3 million were in the sub-Saharan region. HAART availability in these regions has lagged behind, but a meta-analysis of nine studies post HAART, involving over 1300 patients, showed that NCI occurred in 30% of patients on therapy. Increasing access to antiretroviral therapy will have the same effects as seen in developed regions of the world, with a considerable decrease in the disease burden of HAD and an increase in milder HAND subtypes.

The role, if any, of clade subtypes on the development of HAND has not been resolved. Clade D may be the most neurovirulent subtype, followed by B, C, and A. The subtypes have possibly an effect on the severity of NCI in a specific patient population rather than determining whether it occurs or not.

Pathophysiology

HIV invades the brain during viremia after primary infection. Infected monocytes and lymphocytes cross the blood–brain barrier and establish reservoirs in the brain. Chronic productive infection of resident macrophages and microglial cells ensues. Restricted, nonproductive infection of astrocytes contributes to neuronal dysfunction. Oligodendrocytes and neurons are not infected by the virus.

Within the brain, HIV segregates selectively, with the highest levels found in the basal ganglia, subcortical (especially frontal) white-matter regions, and frontal cortex. This regional distribution is unexplained, but may be related to viral entry via cerebrospinal fluid (CSF), to patterns of monocyte trafficking within the brain, or to relative differences in the selective vulnerability of particular neuronal populations or brain regions. Neuropathological features include white-matter pallor, microglial nodules, multinucleated giant cells, and gliosis, a constellation termed HIV encephalitis (HIVE). Damage to synaptic and dendritic structures dominates over neuronal loss. The extent of histopathological involvement and severity of clinical dementia correlate poorly, indicating that biochemical and immunological factors determined by host–virus interactions rather than structural damage are responsible for neuropathogenesis. Neurotoxicity occurs directly from viral proteins (gp120, gp41, tat, nef, and vpr) or indirectly from macrophage factors (quinolinic acid, prostaglandins, leucotrienes, arachidonic acid, nitric oxide, superoxide anions), cytokines, and chemokines (TNF-α, IL-1, 6, -10, interferons, macrophage inflammatory proteins [MIP], regulated on activation normal T-cell expressed and secreted [RANTES], and platelet activating factor). Blood–brain barrier disruption may additionally promote access of neurotoxins from the systemic infection to the extracellular central nervous system (CNS) compartment. Excitotoxicity via activation of N-methyl-D-aspartate (NMDA) receptors may be the final common pathway of neuronal dysfunction.

Clinical features

Asymptomatic neurocognitive impairment is, by definition, an asymptomatic condition with a normal clinical neurological examination. The diagnosis requires formal neuropsychological testing revealing decreased performance in two or more domains. Cognitive domains initially affected include verbal and visual memory (retrieval rather than recognition), complex sequencing, mental flexibility, and visual construction.

Patients with mild neurocognitive disorder may complain of mild neurocognitive impairment and minor functional impairment in daily living. These patients usually are unable to complete complex tasks both at work and at home, but may continue to work, albeit at a decreased level of efficiency. This presents clinically with impaired short-term memory, poor concentration and attention, and executive dysfunction with mental slowing and impaired judgment. Mild early motor symptoms become noticeable and consist of psychomotor slowing, leading to difficulties with fine finger movements and balance problems. Patients report deterioration of handwriting and a tendency to drop things. Subtle gait difficulties are present at this stage, resembling impaired postural reflexes as seen in patients with extrapyramidal disease. At this stage of illness, neurological examination is normal except for mild slowing of repetitive movements (e.g., finger tapping), subtle saccadic and smooth pursuit eye-movement abnormalities, and increased deep tendon reflexes.

Patients with HIV-associated dementia have definitive features of neurological dysfunction. Cognitive fallout involves multiple domains. Behavioral abnormalities include apathy, inertia, loss of libido, irritability, blunting of emotional responses, and waning interest in work and hobbies, ultimately leading to social withdrawal. As disease progresses, spasticity (especially of lower limbs), clonus, frontal release signs, tremor, and ataxia develop. Seizures and myoclonus can occur in late disease. In advanced dementia, signs of co-occurring myelopathy and/or peripheral neuropathy may contribute to abnormal motor findings.

Focal neurological signs such as hemiplegia, hemianopia, and hemisensory impairment are absent; in fact, their presence suggests other pathologies. In late- or end-stage disease, dementia becomes global, with mutism, abulia, and incontinence. This advanced clinical picture is uncommon in regions where HAART usage is widespread, but continues to occur in patients with treatment failure, non-adherence, and limited access to antiretroviral therapy.

HAART has had an overall beneficial effect on the neurocognitive performance of patients living with HIV, but the prevalence of cognitive disorders has not decreased. There has been a shift toward milder forms of the disease, with ANI being reported in up to 60% of patients. Early detection of ANI is significant, as the CHARTER Group has shown that it confers an increased risk for development of symptomatic HAND.

Investigations

Screening tests

Neuropsychological testing can be used for screening purposes in high-risk asymptomatic or early symptomatic patients and for follow-up evaluation in patients with established cognitive impairment. They are also needed for classification purposes and categorization into ANI, MND, and HAD. Appropriate normative standards are not available for large parts of the developing world. The HIV Dementia Scale (HDS) is a useful bedside tool. The revised cut-off score of 14 out of a possible 16 points is sufficiently sensitive and specific.

Blood tests

Laboratory tests cannot reliably establish the diagnosis of HIV-associated cognitive impairment. In the pre-HAART era, current CD4 count and viral load indicated the risk of developing NCI. In the HAART era, the nadir CD4 count is relevant as a risk marker.

CSF analysis

CSF is usually normal or shows non-specific abnormalities, with a lymphocytic pleocytosis and/or mildly elevated protein (aseptic meningitis syndrome). HAART results in CSF viral suppression in most patients. HIV CSF escape denotes virus undetectable in the blood, but present in the CSF. This phenomenon occurs in less than 10% of patients, but the relevance to HAND is unclear.

Neuroimaging

Structural imaging with computed tomography (CT) or magnetic resonance imaging (MRI) is integral to diagnostic evaluation. Age-inappropriate cerebral atrophy with corresponding ventricular enlargement is a typical finding. Increasing ventricular size consistent with subcortical tissue loss mirrors progressive clinical deterioration. On T2-weighted MRI sequences, this appears as patchy confluent high-intensity white-matter signal changes sparing subcortical U fibers (Figure 85.1).

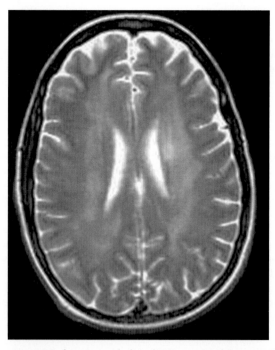

Figure 85.1 MRI of a patient with clinical HIV=associated dementia. T2-weighted image showing confluent white-matter hyperintensities, sparing the subcortical U fibers. The cortical sulci are prominent, consistent with cerebral atrophy. Source: Sakaie 1999. Reproduced with permission of The American Association for the Advancement of Science.

Magnetic resonance spectroscopy (MRS) can document abnormal metabolite levels suggestive of HAND in frontal white matter and the basal ganglia.

Diffusion tensor imaging (DTI) could prove to be a useful modality in early detection of white-matter abnormalities, gauging the extent of disease and monitoring response to therapy.

Functional MRI (fMRI) provides dynamic information on blood-flow abnormalities seen in asymptomatic patients and in mild NCI.

Therapy

The management of HAND requires suppression of the virus and treatment of associated psychiatric, neurological, and neuropsychological dysfunction. HAART has led to a decreased frequency of HIV dementia and improved cognitive performance in some patients with established deficits, and may delay or prevent the onset of symptoms in others. Despite this, there are no specific consensus treatment guidelines on when to initiate antiretrovirals (ARVs) and which drug combination to use. Current evidence supports commencement of HAART at the earliest stage of neurocognitive impairment irrespective of immunological suppression, because the severity of impairment at initiation correlates strongly with persistent neuropsychological deficits, the so-called legacy effect. Studies, including the CHARTER cohort, have identified a low nadir CD4 cell count as a strong predictor of cognitive impairment. Conversely, HIV-positive individuals who never had low CD4 counts are unlikely to develop NCI. These findings support initiation of treatment at CD4 cell counts above the currently recommended level of 500 cells/μL.

The role of brain penetration of antiretroviral drugs is contentious. CNS penetration effectiveness (CPE) assigns a number to each antiretroviral drug based on chemical parameters, CSF concentration, and resulting CSF viral load reduction. The cytopathic effect score of a particular HAART combination is simply determined by adding the respective numbers. Higher CPE scores correlate with better CSF viral load suppression, but not necessarily with better neuropsychological performance. A high CPE regime is currently recommended for patients with HAND.

HIV-associated myelopathies

Myelopathies in HIV/AIDS are uncommon and occur mainly with advanced disease. HIV-related spinal cord syndromes can be caused by the virus itself, as in HIV myelitis and vacuolar myelopathy (VM), or can be secondary to infectious or neoplastic opportunistic disease, vascular disease, or metabolic derangement. Infectious aetiologies include CMV, HSV-1 and 2, varicella zoster virus (VZV), human T-lymphotrophic virus-1 (HTLV-1), JC virus, tuberculosis (TB), syphilis, *Nocardia*, *Cryptococcus*, *Aspergillus*, and *Toxoplasma gondii*. Neoplastic causes are primary CNS lymphoma (PCNSL), metastatic lymphoma, astrocytoma, and plasmacytoma. Necrotizing vasculitis and disseminated intravascular coagulation (DIC) are some of the described vascular causes.

This section will concentrate on VM, the commonest primary HIV myelopathy that typically occurs with immunosuppression.

Epidemiology

The early data on vacuolar myelopathy (VM) is predominantly based on two large autopsy series by Petito *et al.* (1985) and Dal Pan *et al.* (1994). Petito documented the clinical and neuropathological features in 89 patients who died of AIDS. Of these, 20 patients

(22%) had the pathological diagnosis of VM, but only half had clinical features consistent with myelopathy. Dal Pan in his series of 215 consecutive AIDS autopsies found VM in 47%; 56 patients with pathologically diagnosed VM had clinical evaluations, but only 15 (27%) had symptoms and signs of myelopathy. These and other studies showed that clinical myelopathy is uncommon, even though frequently described at autopsy.

VM, the most common spinal cord disease in HIV/AIDS, is symptomatic in 5–10% of AIDS patients. VM is less commonly reported in developing regions. In a clinical study of 506 HIV-positive inpatients from South Africa, we diagnosed VM in 9 patients (2%). The frequency in a Brazilian study of 653 inpatients was less than 1%. In these regions infectious aetiologies predominate and in our study of 50 HIV-positive myelopathy patients, 56% had a presumed infectious cause.

The influence of HAART on the occurrence of VM is poorly documented. HAART is readily available in the developed world and patients with advanced disease are uncommon, which may account for the dearth of recent literature on VM.

Pathophysiology

The pathological feature of VM is patchy vacuolation of white matter, occurring mainly in the thoracic region and predominantly affecting the lateral and dorsal columns (Figure 85.2). Axonal damage is secondary. There is no significant inflammatory infiltrate. The exact pathogenesis of VM is unknown. HIV-infected macrophages, microglia, and astrocytes secrete immunoactive substances that are myelin toxic. These include TNF-α, IL-1, and IL-6. TNF-α mediates oligodendrocyte and myelin injury through the generation of reactive oxygen species. Oxidative damage to oligodendrocyte membranes causes increased consumption of antioxidants (e.g., glutathione) and methyl groups, which are essential for myelin maintenance. S-adenosylmethionine (SAM), the universal methyl group donor, is deficient in HIV patients with VM and in vitamin B_{12} deficiency, accounting for the striking pathological similarities (i.e., the vacuolar change). It is likely that cytokines released by HIV-infected macrophages lead, via SAM depletion, to a metabolic disorder that causes white-matter vacuolization in VM. Co-occurrence of

SAM depletion and macrophage activation in immunosuppressed HIV-negative individuals (e.g., those with hematological malignancies or in organ transplant recipients) can produce a clinically and pathologically identical myelopathy.

Clinical features

VM presents as a spastic-ataxic dorsolateral thoracic spinal cord syndrome evolving over weeks to months. Upper limbs are spared. Motor features include symmetric lower limb weakness with hyperreflexia, spasticity, and extensor plantar responses. Sensory findings are less prominent, although loss of vibration and position sense result in sensory ataxia. A distinct sensory level is unusual and suggests other etiologies. Neurogenic bladder disturbance and erectile dysfunction may be present.

VM and distal sensory polyneuropathy frequently occur in the same patient. This combination can lead to a mixed clinical picture where lower limb hyperreflexia and extensor plantar responses are seen in conjunction with absent ankle jerks.

Investigations

The diagnosis of VM is by exclusion. Serum vitamin B_{12} and copper levels should be normal, and syphilis and HTLV-1 serology should be negative.

The CSF may be normal or show a slightly elevated protein with mild lymphocytic pleocytosis, a well-recognized non-specific finding in asymptomatic HIV-positive individuals. CSF analysis is important to exclude the infectious etiologies listed earlier.

MRI is usually normal, but there may be atrophy of the thoracic cord and non-specific tract hyperintensities on T2 images. These lesions typically do not enhance.

Somatosensory evoked potentials may demonstrate prolonged central conduction time, indicative of spinal cord involvement.

Treatment

There is no specific therapy for VM. Neither HAART nor vitamin B_{12} supplementation has provided consistent improvement or delayed progression. The effect of high-dose supplemental methionine was evaluated in a placebo-controlled phase 2 trial on 56 patients. There was a modest, but not significant improvement in central conduction time, but no benefit clinically. Intravenous immunoglobulin was used in a pilot trial of 17 patients with VM, which showed improved strength only but no effect on overall disability.

Supportive therapy remains the mainstay in the management of VM. Symptomatic treatment of spasticity, urinary urgency, and erectile dysfunction is warranted.

Further reading

Antinori A, Arendt G, Becker JT, *et al*. Updated research nosology for HIV – associated neurocognitive disorders. *Neurology* 2007;69:1789–1799.

Berger JR, Levy RM. *AIDS and the Nervous System*, 2nd ed. Philadelphia, PA: Lippincott-Raven; 1997.

Brew JB, Chan P. Update on HIV dementia and HIV-associated neurocognitive disorders. *Curr Neurol Neurosci Rep* 2014;14:468.

Clifford DB, Ances BM. HIV-associated neurocognitive disorder. *Lancet Infect Dis* 2013;13:976–986.

Dal Pan GJ, Glass DG, McArthur JC. Clinicopathologic correlations of HIV-1-associated vacuolar myelopathy: An autopsy-based case-control study. *Neurology* 1994;44:2159–2164.

Heaton RK, Franklin DR, Ellis RJ, *et al*. HIV-associated neurocognitive disorders before and during the era of combination antiretroviral therapy: Differences in rates, nature, and predictors. *J Neurovirol* 2011;17:3–16.

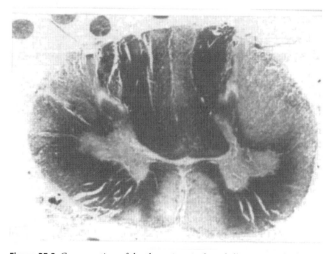

Figure 85.2 Cross-section of the thoracic spinal cord showing marked confluent vacuolation in the posterior and lateral columns and mild vacuolation in the anterior columns of a case with vacuolar myelopathy. Source: Tan 1995. reproduced with permission of OUP.

McArthur JC, Brew BJ, Nath A. Neurological complications of HIV infection. *Lancet Neurol* 2005;4:543–555.

Modi G, Hari K, Modi M, Mochan A. The frequency and profile of neurology in black South African HIV infected (clade C) patients – a hospital-based prospective audit. *J Neurol Sci* 2007;254:60–64.

Modi G, Ranchhod J, Hari K, Mochan A, Modi M. Non-traumatic myelopathy at the Chris Hani Baragwanath Hospital, South Africa – the influence of HIV. *Q J Med* 2011;104:697–703.

Mothobi NZ, Brew BJ. Neurocognitive dysfunction in the highly active antiretroviral therapy era. *Curr Opin Infect Dis* 2012;25:4–9.

Sakaie KE, Gonzalez RG. Imaging of neuroaids. *NeuroAids* 1999;2(7). http://aidscience.org/neuroaids/zones/articles/1999/08/Imaging/index.asp (accessed November 2015).

Tan SV, Guiloff RJ, Scaravilli F. AIDS-associated vacuolar myelopathy: A morphometric study. *Brain* 1995;118:1247–1261. doi:10.1093/brain/118.5.1247

86 Neuromuscular complications of HIV

David M. Simpson[1] and Kara Stavros[2]

[1] Department of Neurology, Icahn School of Medicine at Mount Sinai, New York, USA
[2] Warren Alpert School of Medicine at Brown University, Rhode Island Hospital, Providence, RI, USA

Many different types of peripheral neuropathy and myopathy are associated with human immunodeficiency virus (HIV) infection. These disorders may result from the virus itself, through indirect, immune-mediated mechanisms, or may be the result of antiretroviral medications. The types of neuropathy and myopathy as well as the clinical presentations and sometimes treatments of these disorders can differ in the HIV population compared to non-immunosuppressed individuals. Additionally, opportunistic infections can produce neuropathic and myopathic symptoms. A further challenge is that many HIV patients may present with multiple overlapping central and peripheral neurological disorders, resulting in a complex clinical picture. This chapter reviews the common peripheral neuropathies and myopathies that occur in the HIV population and their treatments (Table 86.1).

Epidemiology

Many studies have investigated risk factors for the development of HIV distal sensory polyneuropathy (DSP), the most common type of neuropathy seen in this population. Incidence of HIV DSP varies depending on the cohort studied, but estimates range from about one-third to one-half of HIV patients in the United States. Before highly active antiretroviral therapy (HAART), risk factors included low CD4 count, elevated plasma viral load, and the use of neurotoxic antiretroviral medications, in particular the dideoxynucleoside reverse transcriptase inhibitors also known as the "d-drugs." Studies performed after the widespread use of HAART identified risk factors such as older age and greater height, which suggests that HIV neuropathy is a length-dependent process. These more recent studies did not confer an additional risk of DSP with low CD4 count or elevated viral load. Study of the genetics of the risk of developing HIV DSP has revealed that certain mitochondrial DNA haplogroups are associated with a lower risk of sensory neuropathy.

Risk factors for neuropathy in association with HIV have been studied in other parts of the world. Studies done in South Africa, Nigeria, and Australia have found a similar prevalence of neuropathy in HIV patients. A cross-sectional study of eight Asia Pacific countries found a comparatively lower prevalence of neuropathy at a rate of about 20%. Risk factors identified in these studies also include greater height and age, as well as exposure to stavudine.

Pathophysiology

Neurotoxicity in DSP occurs by various indirect immunomodulatory mechanisms as a result of HIV infection, including the release of inflammatory cytokines, chemokines, glutamates, and viral proteins, such as the envelope protein gp120. Antiretroviral-induced DSP is thought to occur via mitochondrial dysfunction through inhibition of polymerase gamma. In fact, d-drugs impair mitochondrial DNA to varying degrees, with stavudine being particularly potent. HIV myopathy is also suspected to be due, at least in some cases, to mitochondrial dysfunction. Furthermore, some opportunistic infections have been associated with HIV myopathy, including toxoplasmosis, cryptococcus, and mycoplasma avium intracellulare.

Clinical features

When symptomatic, patients with HIV DSP typically report numbness, burning pain, or paresthesias in the extremities, predominantly distal, occurring in a length-dependent manner. Examination reveals diminished sensation in a stocking-glove pattern, reduced or absent ankle jerks, and sensory ataxia. Clinical presentations of other HIV neuropathies – inflammatory demyelinating polyneuropathies (IDP), polyradiculopathy, or mononeuritis multiplex – are similar to presentations in non-HIV patients and are described later.

HIV-associated myopathy presents with myalgia and progressive, symmetric weakness of the proximal muscles. Patients report difficulty rising from a seated position or trouble climbing stairs. Examination reveals weakness, greater proximally, typically with preservation of sensation and normal reflexes unless there is concomitant neuropathy. If there is an opportunistic infection underlying the myopathy, such as toxoplasmosis, then there may be additional clinical signs and symptoms resulting from a focal central nervous system lesion.

HIV-associated neuropathy and myopathy produced by either virus or antiretroviral medications are clinically indistinguishable. To determine whether symptoms are medication induced, it is necessary to stop the potentially offending drug and observe the patient for improvement; however, it may take months to see any change. Furthermore, symptoms may worsen before they improve, a phenomenon known as "coasting." This poses a significant challenge to the physician, who may need to weigh the risk of discontinuing an effective HIV medication against that of producing a side effect such as DSP.

Myopathies

Several myopathies are associated with HIV. These include inflammatory myopathies, such as polymyositis and inclusion body myositis (IBM), as well as nemaline rod myopathy and antiretroviral

International Neurology, Second edition. Edited by Robert P. Lisak, Daniel D. Truong, William M. Carroll and Roongroj Bhidayasiri
© 2016 John Wiley & Sons, Ltd. Published 2016 by John Wiley & Sons, Ltd.

Table 86.1 Summary of selected HIV-associated neuropathies and myopathies.

Diagnosis	Clinical features	Diagnostic workup	Treatment
DSP	• Length-dependent sensorimotor disturbances including numbness, pain, paresthesias	• Serum B$_{12}$, TSH, SPEP, A1c, HCV, RPR, metabolic panel • EMG/NCS • Skin biopsy	• Numerous options have been tested with mostly negative results (see text).
IDP	• Acute ascending weakness, paresthesias, autonomic dysfunction • May be cranial nerve or respiratory involvement • May occur at the time of seroconversion • Chronic forms are also possible	• HIV testing in patients without a known history • Lumbar puncture, albumino-cytological dissociation may be disrupted in HIV • EMG/NCS	• IVIG • Plasma exchange • Caution with steroids for CIDP
Mononeuritis multiplex	• Multiple mononeuropathies, variable clinical presentation	• Vasculitis and neoplastic workup • Lumbar puncture for CMV PCR • EMG/NCS • Nerve and/or muscle biopsy	• IVIG • Ganciclovir/foscarnet for underlying CMV • Caution with steroids or immune-modulating therapy
Polyradiculopathy	• Lower back pain radiating to the legs, urinary incontinence, leg weakness, saddle anesthesia • May extend to include arm weakness or cranial nerve involvement	• Lumbar puncture with CMV PCR • EMG/NCS • MRI of lumbar spine	• Ganciclovir/foscarnet
Inflammatory myopathies	• Progressive symmetric proximal muscle weakness in polymyositis • Weakness of finger flexors and knee extensors in IBM • Myalgia • Difficulty climbing stairs or rising form a squatting position	• CK level • EMG/NCS • Muscle biopsy	• Caution with steroids or immune-modulating therapy • IVIG • Discontinue toxic ARV

ARV = antiretroviral; CIDP = chronic inflammatory demyelinating polyneuropathy; CK = creatine kinase; CMV = cytomegalovirus; DSP = distal symmetric polyneuropathy; EMG = electromyography; HCV = hepatitis C virus; IBM = inclusion body myositis; IDP = inflammatory demyelinating polyneuropathy; IVIG = intravenous immunoglobin; MRI = magnetic resonance imaging; NCS = nerve conduction study; PCR = polymerase chain reaction; RPR = rapid plasma reagin; SPEP = serum protein electrophoresis; TSH = thyroid-stimulating hormone

or opportunistic infection-associated myopathies. There have also been reports of acute rhabdomyolysis in HIV, and there may be muscle involvement in the AIDS wasting syndrome.

The most common myopathy in HIV is polymyositis. The presentation is similar to that seen in HIV-negative cases: slowly progressive proximal muscle weakness that may be associated with myalgia. There may be elevated serum creatine kinase (CK) level, myopathic findings on EMG (including small, polyphasic motor unit potentials with early recruitment), and inflammatory cell infiltrates on muscle biopsy. Similarly, IBM also presents as it does in non-HIV patients; typically slowly progressive asymmetric weakness with predilection for the finger flexors and knee extensors, elevated CK levels, and myopathic electromyography (EMG). Muscle biopsy reveals intracellular vacuoles and inclusion bodies. Polymyositis typically responds to steroids or other immunosuppressive treatments, while IBM does not. In HIV patients, these agents should be used with caution to avoid opportunistic infection; concurrent use of prophylaxis against pneumocystis pneumonia may be considered. Intravenous immunoglobin (IVIG) is an alternative to immunosuppressive treatment, although controlled studies are lacking.

Antiretroviral-associated myopathies may result from exposure to zidovudine (AZT) or stavudine. There is also an HIV-associated diffuse infiltrative lymphocytosis syndrome (DILS). This is a CD8 hyperlymphomatosis with visceral organ infiltration and peripheral nerve involvement that may present with myopathy or peripheral neuropathy.

Neuropathies

HIV-DSP

A history and examination suggestive of DSP (see earlier) should prompt an investigation to rule out chronic alcoholism, hypothyroidism, hepatitis C, diabetes mellitus, paraproteinemia, vitamin B$_{12}$ deficiency, or other causes of peripheral neuropathy. Further workup may include EMG, which can show reduced or absent sensory and motor potentials affected in a length-dependent manner and active or chronic denervation patterns. Electrodiagnostic studies may be normal if predominantly small fibers are affected, and in that case skin biopsy may aid in diagnosis by showing a reduction in the intraepidermal nerve fiber density.

Among symptomatic treatments, only the 8% transdermal capsaicin patch and an alternative treatment, smoked cannabis, have proven efficacy. Other symptomatic agents, even those that have been shown to be efficacious in the treatment of non-HIV-associated neuropathic pain, are not proven in HIV DSP. These include topical lidocaine, gabapentin, lamotrigine, pregabalin, amitriptyline, duloxetine, peptide T, and mexiletine. Neuroregenerative treatments, such as acetyl L-carnitine, prosaptide, and recombinant human nerve growth factor, have been tested without positive results or clinical applicability. Given the dearth of effective pharmacological therapies for DSP, non-pharmacological therapies such as acupuncture and hypnosis have also been investigated. Physicians often employ rational polypharmacy to treat patients using a combination of medications and non-pharmacological treatments to control symptoms.

Inflammatory demyelinating polyneuropathies (IDP)

Acute inflammatory demyelinating polyradiculoneuropathy (AIDP) may occur at the time of HIV seroconversion. In such cases, the presenting symptoms are similar to those of a non-HIV patient presenting with AIDP; typically progressive, ascending weakness associated with paresthesias, autonomic dysfunction, occasional cranial nerve involvement, and potential respiratory dysfunction. Examination reveals symmetric weakness and areflexia. An important difference in the cerebrospinal fluid (CSF) of these patients is that there may be modest pleocytosis not seen in typical AIDP. Electrophysiology may yield evidence of demyelination with slowed conduction velocities, conduction block, or prolonged distal latencies; there may also be absent or prolonged late responses. Spinal neuroimaging can show enhancement of the nerve roots.

Treatment is the same as for non-HIV patients, IVIG or plasma exchange. It is important that in an otherwise healthy patient presenting with AIDP, HIV testing should be considered as part of the patient's workup, given that AIDP may be the first presentation of acute HIV infection.

Chronic inflammatory demyelinating polyradiculoneuropaty (CIDP) is more common than AIDP in HIV patients. These patients present with relapsing or progressive motor and sensory symptoms. CSF may contain a pleocytosis and electrophysiology may show demyelinating features described earlier. Treatment is with IVIG or steroids, which should be used cautiously to avoid opportunistic infections.

Polyradiculopathy

Most polyradiculopathy in HIV patients is produced by cytomegalovirus (CMV). Patients present with progressive weakness, sensory loss, pain, and urinary dysfunction resembling a cauda equina syndrome, including the typical saddle distribution of pain and sensory loss. The virus may infect the cauda equina leading to inflammation of the lumbosacral nerve roots; in some cases the arms and cranial nerves may be affected.

Workup includes neuroimaging to rule out a structural lesion. Imaging may show meningeal enhancement of the cauda equina. CSF should be examined by polymerase chain reaction (PCR) for amplifiable CMV DNA. The CSF contains a pleocytosis in which neutrophils or lymphocytes predominate, with low glucose and elevated protein. Electrophysiology may show evidence of axonal injury and denervation. Despite treatment with ganciclovir, often combined with foscarnet, the prognosis is poor.

Mononeuropathy multiplex

The presentation of mononeuritis multiplex is variable, with occurrence of multiple mononeuropathies, typically described as painful "stepwise" deficits. This presentation is similar in patients with and without HIV. The etiology may be vasculitic and diagnostic workup includes cryoglobulins, antineutrophil cytoplasmic antibodies (ANCA), rheumatoid factor, antinuclear antibodies (ANA), and neoplastic workup. Additionally, HIV mononeuritis multiplex may be associated with CMV polyradiculopathy. Electromyogram and nerve conduction studies (EMG/NCS) may show evidence of axonal injury and denervation. Nerve biopsy may reveal vasculitic neuropathy, including necrotizing vasculitis. IVIG is considered safe treatment; steroids or immunomodulating therapy should again be considered with caution to avoid opportunistic infection. In the case of concomitant CMV, treatment with ganciclovir and/ or foscarnet should be initiated. One Japanese case study reported mononeuritis multiplex as a manifestation of acute HIV infection.

Conclusion

In summary, numerous neuropathies and myopathies can affect HIV patients. The clinician must be aware of the increased risk for neuropathy and myopathy in this population, and the ways in which the clinical presentation can differ from non-HIV patients. Treatment can be challenging in these patients. Few agents have proven efficacy for symptomatic treatment in DSP. The best approach is to work closely with patients' primary care and infectious disease specialists to determine the best antiretroviral regimen with the least possible neurotoxic side effects, or, in the case of some myopathies and neuropathies, to weigh the risks versus benefits of steroid treatment.

Further reading

Cherry CL, Skolasky L, Lal L, et al. Antiretroviral use and other risks for HIV-associated neuropathies in an international cohort. *Neurology* 2006;66:867–873.

Morgello S, Estanislao L, Simpson D, et al. HIV associated distal sensory polyneuropathy in the era of highly active anti-retroviral therapy: The Manhattan HIV Brain Bank. *Arch Neurol* 2004;61:546–551.

Phillips TJC, Cherry C, Cox S, Marshall SJ, Rice AS. Pharmacological treatment of painful HIV-associated sensory neuropathy: A systematic review and meta-analysis of randomized controlled trials. *PLoS One* 2010;5(12):e14433.

Simpson DM, Kitch D, Evans SR, et al. HIV neuropathy natural history cohort study: Assessment measures and risk factors. *Neurology* 2006;66(11):1679–1687.

Wright E, Brew B, Arayawichanont A, et al. Neurologic disorders are prevalent in HIV-positive outpatients in the Asia-Pacific region. *Neurology* 2008;71:50–56.

Opportunistic infections in HIV-positive subjects and AIDS patients

Bruce J. Brew and Aoife Laffan

Departments of Neurology and HIV Medicine, St Vincent's Hospital, Sydney, Australia

Opportunistic infections result from the reactivation of latent infection and occur in the setting of advanced human immunodeficiency virus (HIV) disease with CD4 cell counts usually below 200 cells/µL. Occasionally, the CD4 cell count may be higher, as in progressive multifocal leukoencephalopathy. Sometimes these infections occur even when the CD4 cell count is rising and the HIV viral load is dropping, typically with the recent introduction of highly active antiretroviral therapy (HAART) as part of the "immune reconstitution syndrome." Several infections may occur simultaneously in the same patient. For example, up to one-third of patients with cryptococcal meningitis in developing countries also have tuberculous meningitis. The best clinical approach to these conditions rests on neurological evaluation to decide whether the disease is diffuse or focal. This chapter focuses on infections that are common and some of these infections, such as varicella zoster virus and neurosyphilis, are discussed in further detail in this textbook and in other more specialized texts.

HIV-associated lymphoma can either be a primary central nervous system lymphoma (PCNSL) or secondary metastases from systemic lymphoma. These conditions differ in terms of epidemiology, pathophysiology, clinical features, and treatment, and are therefore discussed separately.

Opportunistic infections: Diffuse complications

Cryptococcal meningitis

Cryptococcal meningitis is a relatively frequent complication of advanced HIV disease. It is certainly treatable, if not curable, in most patients. Clinical vigilance is paramount, since headache may be the only presenting feature.

Epidemiology

Cryptococcal meningitis is a feature of advanced HIV disease (CD4 cell counts <100 cells/µL). It has a variable prevalence dependent on geography (2% in Northern Europe to 20–30% in parts of Africa and Southeast Asia in advanced disease patients), whether fluconazole is being taken for prophylaxis or treatment against candidiasis and whether HAART is being administered. Patients with HIV-associated cryptococcal infections account for up to 90% of all cases.

Pathophysiology

More than 50 species of Cryptococcus exist, but almost all cases of human disease are related to *Cryptococcus neoformans* and less commonly *Cryptococcus gatii*. Transmission is primarily via the respiratory route, with deposition of yeast spores into the pulmonary alveoli followed by phagocytosis by alveolar macrophages. *Cryptococcal neoformans* pulmonary disease can be asymptomatic and therefore meningitis may be the presenting feature.

Clinical features

Headache, personality change, and confusion develop over days to weeks. Fever and neck stiffness are less common. Drowsiness, nausea, and vomiting can indicate raised intracranial pressure, which occurs in 20% of cases. Less common presentations include cranial neuropathies, choreoathetoid movements, ataxia, seizures, and transient ischemic-like episodes.

Investigations

Virtually all patients will test positive for cryptococcal antigen in the blood. Further evaluation with computed tomography (CT) or magnetic resonance imaging (MRI) brain scanning followed by cerebrospinal fluid (CSF) analysis should be performed. Imaging will define the presence of any associated mass lesions compatible with cryptococcomas and give a baseline evaluation of the size of the ventricles that may or may not preclude CSF sampling.

In 75% of patients, CSF analysis shows a mononuclear pleocytosis (usually <20 cells/mm^3), elevated protein, and, less frequently, low glucose. A raised opening pressure is common. CSF cryptococcal antigen is almost always positive. Fungal cultures should be performed on CSF to determine the sensitivities to various antifungal agents.

The most important prognostic factor is a CSF opening pressure ≥25 cm H_2O, which indicates a poor outcome. Other poor prognostic factors include a depressed level of consciousness, hyponatremia, markedly depressed CSF glucose, CSF white cell count <20/mm^3, and CSF cryptococcal antigen titer >1024.

Treatment

Antifungal therapy should start as soon as the diagnosis is confirmed, or even before confirmation in very ill patients. To prevent an immune restoration exacerbation of cryptococcal disease, HAART is usually commenced within 1 month of antifungal therapy. If the patient is already on HAART, it should be continued.

Antifungal therapy usually consists of amphotericin B with 5-flucytosine. Fluconazole is less often used as the initial treatment in light of increasing data pointing to the superiority of amphotericin B, particularly if the patient is obtunded.

International Neurology, Second edition. Edited by Robert P. Lisak, Daniel D. Truong, William M. Carroll and Roongroj Bhidayasiri

Treatment regimens consist of amphotericin B at 0.7–1 mg/kg/day for 2 weeks, with 2 weeks of 5-flucytosine at 100 mg/kg/day in four divided doses. Unfortunately, 5-flucytosine is not widely available in developing countries, and mortality rates from cryptococcal meningitis are higher without it. Most clinicians advise amphotericin B and 5-flucytosine followed by fluconazole at 400 mg daily for at least 8–10 weeks. If fluconazole is used as initial treatment, it should be administered as a loading dose intravenously followed by at least 400 mg/day. A progress CSF analysis is often recommended after initial treatment at the 10–12-week mark.

If the patient responds, a maintenance dose of 200 mg daily of fluconazole is recommended. Raised intracranial pressure should be treated aggressively with acetazolamide, frequent lumbar punctures, possibly mannitol, and, in difficult patients, by a lumbar drain or ventriculostomy. Maintenance therapy can be discontinued if the HIV viral load becomes undetectable and CD4 cell counts are consistently above 200/μL for several months.

Tuberculous meningitis

Tuberculous meningitis (TBM) is a significant cause of a non-focal deficit in Africa and parts of Asia and may even be more common than cryptococcal meningitis. The disorder is treatable in most patients as long as diagnosis is made early. In general, HIV-related TBM is associated with a higher burden of TB than in non-HIV-infected patients.

Epidemiology

TBM can occur in up to 10% of HIV-infected patients, especially in the developing world and the intravenous drug use population. Most TBM patients have a CD4 cell count <200 and virtually all have a CD4 cell count <400 cells/μL.

Pathophysiology

TBM manifests in two stages. First, TB droplets infect the alveolar macrophages, causing a localized infection or primary complex that accumulates in the lung and spreads to the surrounding lymph nodes. In those who develop central nervous system TB, bacilli seed the meninges and/or brain parenchyma, forming small subpial or subependymal caseous lesions, also known as Rich foci. The second stage involves an increase in Rich foci size leading to rupture into the subarachnoid space, causing meningitis. Tuberculous exudate triggers a hypersensitivity reaction that precipitates marked inflammatory changes, particularly at the base of the brain.

Clinical features

Fever (83–89%), headache (59–83%), and altered mental status (43–71%) are the most common symptoms. A productive cough occurs in about 20% of cases. Meningeal signs occur in 65% and cranial nerve deficits or hemiparesis in 19%. Approximately half of patients have no preceding symptoms related to TB.

Investigations

Imaging often reveals meningeal enhancement and hydrocephalus. Focal brain lesions are seen less often. CSF analysis is usually abnormal, with a lymphocytic pleocytosis (occasionally a neutrophil predominance) of approximately 200 cells/μL. Up to 16% have an acellular CSF, 43% a normal protein, and 14% a normal glucose.

Elevated CSF concentrations of adenosine deaminase may be useful as an adjunct to diagnosis, although this is non-specific. Direct smears of CSF are positive for TB in approximately 25%, while polymerase chain reaction (PCR) is positive in about 80%. Approximately half of TBM patients have an abnormal chest X-ray, showing pulmonary infiltrates and cavitating lesions.

Treatment

Combination therapy, probably initially with corticosteroids, is required for the treatment of TBM. The only difference in HIV-related TBM treatment is the higher rate of adverse drug reactions, especially with rifampin: the dose should be halved when used in combination with protease inhibitors. Isoniazid (with pyridoxine 50–100 mg/day) and pyrazinamide should be components of the drug regimen, since they are bactericidal and cross the blood–brain barrier. Additional drugs should include rifampin rather than ethambutol because the former is bactericidal.

Patients who are not on HAART at the time of diagnosis should be commenced on this in conjunction with their antituberculosis regimen. The exact timing of HAART initiation is challenging, since if given too early, the risk of drug interactions, toxicity, reduced tolerability, and immune reconstitution is higher, whereas morbidity and mortality are increased when HAART is given too late. Usually, HAART is started within a few weeks of antituberculous drugs.

Three drugs should be given for at least 2 months and then two drugs for 4 months. Shortly after initiation of therapy, deterioration may occur because of hydrocephalus, immune reconstitution inflammatory syndrome, or arteritis-related infarcts. Response should be assessed at 2 months with repeat CSF analysis. Continuation of therapy for at least 9 months may be necessary.

Cytomegalovirus encephalitis

Cytomegalovirus (CMV) encephalitis is an uncommon complication of advanced HIV disease, typically with CD4 counts <50/μL. Nonetheless, it is treatable if diagnosed early.

Epidemiology

CMV encephalitis occurs in at least 6% of patients with advanced HIV disease who are not on HAART; it is much reduced in HAART-treated patients. The mean CD4 cell count is 13 cells/μL, with almost all having a count <50 cells/μL. Without treatment, the mean time to death is 8.5 weeks.

Pathophysiology

CMV is a member of the herpesvirus family. CMV encephalitis is the consequence of reactivation of a previously latent infection, usually in some other part of the body with secondary seeding to the brain. Very uncommonly it is a consequence of reactivation of latent infection in the brain.

Clinical features

Most commonly, patients experience confusion (70–90%), apathy (60%), headache (30–50%), fever (16%), incoordination (10%), and sometimes seizures developing over an average of 3.5 weeks. Approximately one-quarter will have brainstem involvement, with vertical or horizontal gaze-evoked nystagmus, internuclear ophthalmoplegia, and cranial neuropathies. There is often evidence of

CMV infection elsewhere, usually in the retina. CMV encephalitis can arise in patients who are on maintenance therapy for CMV elsewhere (e.g., patients with colitis). There is a strong association between CMV retinitis and encephalitis.

Investigations

Brain imaging often shows periventricular ependymal or meningeal enhancement. Mass lesions are rare. CSF shows a polymorphonuclear pleocytosis (25%), low glucose (33%), and elevated protein (83%). CSF PCR for CMV DNA is positive in more than 90% of cases, sensitivity and specificity values are approximately 80%, while the positive and negative predictive values are 86–92% and 95–98%, respectively.

Treatment

While randomized clinical trial data are lacking, most clinicians treat with both ganciclovir and foscarnet for approximately 3 weeks followed by half the dose as maintenance therapy, until there is a sustained increase in CD4 cell count above 100 cells/μL. Response rates vary, with about half of patients improving and the other half stabilizing or deteriorating. HAART should be commenced usually 1 month after anti-CMV treatment to minimize immune reconstitution inflammatory syndrome.

Opportunistic infections: Focal complications

Toxoplasmosis

Cerebral toxoplasmosis is one of the most common causes of a focal brain lesion in patients not on HAART, even in the developing world where tuberculosis can have a similar presentation. Indeed, a good practical guide is that all focal brain lesions in patients with advanced HIV disease reflect cerebral toxoplasmosis until proven otherwise.

Epidemiology

The seroprevalence of past toxoplasmosis infection varies from up to 80% in parts of Europe to 30% in North America. Most patients with toxoplasmosis have a CD4 count <100 cells/μL.

Pathophysiology

Toxoplasma gondii is an intracellular parasite that exists in three forms: (1) tachyzoite (the replicating organism that causes disease); (2) bradyzoite (the non-replicating organism responsible for latent disease); and (3) oocyst. Eating undercooked red meat, which contains the bradyzoite, increases the risk of contracting toxoplasmosis, as does eating food contaminated by cat feces containing the oocysts.

Clinical features

Headache (up to 60%) and a focal deficit (hemiparesis or visual field deficits) occur, usually with fevers (up to 70%), occasionally confusion (up to 40%) and seizures (25%). Less common are movement disorders and brainstem deficits. Systemic manifestations such as retinitis and pneumonitis are very uncommon.

Investigations

Evidence of seropositivity to *Toxoplasma* is critical to establishing the possibility of cerebral toxoplasmosis, but up to 16% of patients may be seronegative; that is, there may be loss of previous antibody responses with advanced immunodeficiency. Brain imaging, especially with MRI, is useful: a single lesion or a periventricular lesion(s) favors cerebral lymphoma over toxoplasmosis, while lesions involving the deeper parts of the brain, especially the basal ganglia, favor toxoplasmosis. Thallium brain single photon emission computed tomography (SPECT) scanning can be helpful in distinguishing between toxoplasmosis and cerebral lymphoma (as discussed later). CSF PCR for *Toxoplasma gondii* is positive in approximately 60% of patients.

Treatment

Pyrimethamine (75–100 mg/day), folinic acid (10–15 mg/day), and sulfadiazine (6–8 g/day) are recommended; clindamycin can be used (2400–4800 mg/day) in the sulfa-allergic patient. In countries where sulphadiazine is not available, cotrimoxazole may be effective. Approximately 30% of cases will require alternate therapy (azithromycin, clarithromycin, atovaquone, doxycycline, or dapsone). Patients may deteriorate in the first few days because of hemorrhage or edema. The latter can be treated in the short term with mannitol; corticosteroids should be avoided because of their confounding effect if the diagnosis is lymphoma rather than toxoplasmosis. Clinical and radiological responses occur after about 10 days, and by 6 weeks 30% will have complete resolution. Persistent lesion enhancement on brain imaging is an indication for continuation of treatment. Maintenance therapy (half the initial doses) can be instituted when there is no lesion enhancement. HAART should commence approximately 1 month after the start of antitoxoplasmosis therapy.

Tuberculosis

As mentioned, TB involvement of the central nervous system (CNS) occurs at an earlier stage of HIV disease than other infections. Indeed, one report has recorded a median CD4 cell count of 326 cells/μL in patients with TB and HIV disease.

Clinical features

There are two forms of focal tuberculous brain involvement, tuberculoma (tuberculous granuloma) and tuberculous abscess, although the clinical features of headache, focal deficits, and seizures are the same. Tuberculous abscess is more often associated with fever, while tuberculomas are often multiple, and very occasionally associated with tuberculous meningitis. Approximately half of patients will have respiratory disease.

Pathophysiology

As with TB meningitis, the initial respiratory infection via bacilli droplet inhalation is the same. Tuberculomas, however, are a collection of caseous granulomatous foci within the brain tissue as opposed to the meninges, and can grow to considerable sizes even in the absence of TB meningitis. Clinically silent lesions are often found in the setting of meningitis. In the immune compromised host, tuberculomas can progress to abscess formation.

Investigations

A positive Mantoux test can be helpful, but a negative result may occur in up to 66% of patients with a CD4 cell count <200 cells/μL. Interpretation of a negative Mantoux test may be assisted by assessing the presence of cutaneous anergy. Interferon-γ release assays can also be useful, with a negative result making TB unlikely but not excluding it, while a positive result indicates latent or active TB. Importantly, these assays are not affected by previous BCG (Bacillus Calmette–Guérin) vaccination. BCG vaccines are manufactured from attenuated live bovine tuberculosis that is no longer virulent to the human host. Chest X-rays, sputum smears, blood cultures, and PCR for TB from blood may be helpful. Tuberculomas on CT brain scan are solid enhancing or ring enhancing, possibly with calcification and mild to minimal mass effect. MRI shows nodular rim-enhancing lesions that are hypointense, isodense, or hyperintense on T2-weighted images. Tuberculous abscesses on CT scanning are hypodense lesions with significant mass effect and peripheral enhancement, while MRI additionally shows lesions with central hyperintensity on T2 images.

Treatment

Tuberculoma or TB abscess treatment follows the guidelines provided for TB meningitis. Indeed, the diagnosis of parenchymal TB is often made when imaging is performed for suspected TB meningitis, and therefore treatment is as already outlined. In cases of obstructive hydrocephalus, ventricular drains or shunts may be required. In contrast to other CNS mass lesions, conservative medical management is preferred, reserving surgery for significant clinical deterioration.

Progressive multifocal leukoencephalopathy

Progressive multifocal leukoencephalopathy (PML) is a subacute demyelinating disease of the CNS, resulting from productive infection of oligodendrocytes and astrocytes by the JC virus, named after John Cunningham, the first patient with this infection. PML is now a relatively common neurological complication of HIV disease. Because HAART can stabilize and occasionally improve the clinical deficit, it is important for neurologists to be familiar with the disease.

Epidemiology

Up to 4% of patients with advanced HIV infection develop PML, and this figure has not significantly changed with the introduction of HAART. The mean CD4 cell count in several studies has ranged from 30–104 cells/μL, but some have a CD4 cell count >200 cells/μL. Approximately one-third of patients have a plasma HIV viral load below detection. Untreated, the average survival is between 3 and 4 months. Patients with a CD4 cell count >50 cells/μL have a better prognosis, as do patients <45 years of age. Approximately 10% of patients experience spontaneous remission and prolonged survival beyond 1 year, while about 5% will live beyond 1 year, with a mean survival time of 42 months.

Pathophysiology

The JC virus is a member of the polyoma group of viruses. It is a double-stranded DNA virus encapsulated in an icosahedral protein. It remains latent in cells of the reticuloendothelial system (particularly bone marrow and kidney, but probably not brain) until reactivated, usually in the context of immunodeficiency. Most clinicians believe that JC virus is transported into the brain by infected B-cells. Neurovirologically, the virus may productively infect oligodendrocytes and B-cells, but probably not cells of the monocytic lineage.

Clinical features

Hemiparesis, speech disturbances, cognitive dysfunction, headache, and ataxia are the most common presenting symptoms, usually developing over several weeks in the absence of fever. In 60% of patients, there is a single clinical localization.

Investigations

Seropositivity in normal adults is approximately 50% with the two-step enzyme-linked immunosorbent assay (ELISA), which minimizes false positives from cross-reactivity with other polyoma viruses. PCR amplification of JC DNA as well as RNA in peripheral blood mononuclear cells, plasma, and urine is not helpful, since periods of asymptomatic viremia occur in normal individuals. CT of the brain is either normal or shows an area of hypodensity without mass effect that rarely enhances. Cranial MRI reveals single or multiple areas of T2 high-signal intensity, largely in the white matter. Mild contrast enhancement may occur in 15% of cases. CSF cell count and glucose are usually normal, but CSF protein is mildly to moderately elevated in about 50% of cases.

CSF PCR for JC virus DNA has sensitivity and specificity rates of approximately 65% and 92%, respectively. The most definitive test is brain biopsy.

Treatment

Most patients on HAART improve significantly, with a median survival of 46.4 weeks versus 11 weeks for those not receiving HAART. Protease inhibitor–containing HAART regimens may be preferable. Some patients worsen significantly during the first few weeks of HAART, probably due to immune reconstitution inflammatory syndrome. Cytarabine or cytosine arabinoside (ara-C) has a limited role. A randomized clinical trial did not show benefit, although there are criticisms of the study design. Cidofovir, interferon-α, and topotecan have proven to be largely ineffective.

HIV-associated lymphoma

HIV-associated lymphoma may involve the nervous system, either as primary central nervous system lymphoma (PCNSL) or systemic lymphoma with neurological metastases. These conditions differ in terms of epidemiology, pathophysiology, clinical features, and treatment, and are therefore discussed separately.

Primary central nervous system lymphoma

Epidemiology

In the pre-HAART era, PCNSL occurred in 6–18% of advanced disease patients; HAART has halved this figure. PCNSL is distinctly uncommon in children. In HAART-naïve patients not taking cotrimoxazole, PCNSL is the second most common cause of a mass lesion after toxoplasmosis; the effect of HAART is unknown. The median CD4 cell count is <50/μL in all series (even in the HAART era), although occasional cases may occur, even in the normal range. HAART has improved the median survival from 32 to 48 days and the 12-month survival from 4% to 12%.

Pathophysiology

PCNSL is a diffuse large cell non-Hodgkin's lymphoma of B-cell origin arising in the central nervous system. It is almost always secondary to Epstein–Barr virus (EBV) infection. Immune deficiency leads to unchecked reactivation of EBV infection, promoting B-cell proliferation with consequent gene arrangements and development of PCNSL.

Clinical features

Usually patients present with confusion (51%), focal deficits (30–60%), headache (30–40%), seizures (22%), and fever. Ocular involvement (vitreous, uvea, or retina) is rare.

Investigations

Brain imaging with CT scan or MRI often shows a single enhancing lesion with edema, usually in the frontal lobe, periventricular region, or, less often, the basal ganglia. Posterior fossa involvement is found in less than 10%. Magnetic resonance spectroscopy may show changes in phosphorylethanolamine, consistent with the diagnosis. Thallium SPECT imaging has some diagnostic utility. Patients with lesions ≥2 cm in dimension have increased thallium uptake, which has 100% sensitivity and 89% specificity.

Provided that a lumbar puncture can be safely performed, PCR for EBV has a sensitivity of 83–100% and specificity of 94–100%. However, there is some concern that these figures are less favorable in patients who develop PCNSL while taking HAART. CSF cytology can be positive in up to 30% of patients.

Brain biopsy can be useful. A false-negative rate of 5–33% has been reported, with a morbidity and mortality of up to 11% and 8%, respectively. The use of corticosteroid therapy should be avoided if possible before a formal diagnosis, since necrosis of lesions can occur prior to brain biopsy. Sampling errors can also occur, making diagnosis difficult.

Treatment

No consensus on treatment of PCNSL exists. Treatment can be considered when diagnosis is definitive or when there has been failure to respond to a trial of antitoxoplasmosis therapy. While there is no curative therapy, treatment can certainly increase life span and quality in appropriate patients. Good prognostic factors are the completion of radiotherapy, especially at least 30y, administration of HAART, few or no previous AIDS-defining illnesses, and absence of non-focal neurological symptoms such as confusion.

Treatment usually consists of high-dose methotrexate in addition to corticosteroids and HAART. In some patients, induction therapy with high-dose methotrexate, temozolomide, and rituximab, as used for non-HIV primary CNS lymphoma, may result in a complete response and reduce the need for radiotherapy. Radiotherapy can be considered, but may not prolong survival by any meaningful degree. It may be useful in palliation.

Because PCNSL is multicentric, there is no value in surgical removal of identifiable tumors. The HAART-related improvement in immune function decreases the risk of death from an opportunistic infection and possibly curtails PCNSL progression, at least in some patients.

Metastatic lymphoma

Epidemiology

Systemic lymphoma occurs in approximately 5–10% of advanced HIV disease patients, although this estimate may change as patients live longer on HAART, given that there is evidence suggesting that the risk of developing lymphoma is related in part to the duration of HIV disease. Data thus far have shown that HAART has not led to a decrease in the incidence of lymphoma, contrary to its effects on PCNSL incidence.

The CNS is involved by systemic lymphoma in approximately 20% of patients and usually takes the form of leptomeningeal disease. The median CD4 cell count for systemic non-Hodgkin's lymphoma is just below 200 cells/μL.

Pathophysiology

Systemic lymphoma with CNS metastases is almost always of the non-Hodgkin's type. However, unlike PCNSL, it is related to EBV infection in only half of patients.

Clinical features

Brain metastases lead to confusion, focal deficits, and sometimes seizures. Leptomeningeal involvement occurs in up to 10% of cases, causing a compressive spinal cord syndrome or multilevel deficits with the characteristic finding of scattered absent deep-tendon reflexes.

Investigations

In patients with brain metastases, brain imaging with CT or MRI shows multiple enhancing lesions. In leptomeningeal disease, CSF cytology is frequently positive.

Treatment

Intrathecal chemotherapy, usually with methotrexate or cytarabine, should be given in addition to systemic chemotherapy. While there is some controversy as to whether HAART should be given at the same time due to additive myelotoxicity, most specialists do recommend concomitant HAART. Caution must be taken when both HAART and chemotherapy are administered due to (1) the additive myelotoxicity when zidovudine is a component of HAART; (2) the additive risk of neuropathy when stavudine or didanosine is a component of HAART and when vinca alkaloids are given as part of chemotherapy; and (3) the compromise of chemotherapy efficacy when protease inhibitors are part of HAART because of their effects on the cytochrome P450 system.

Radiotherapy for localized disease with chemotherapy has some efficacy. The precise chemotherapy regimens have varied (e.g., cytoxan, adriamycin, and methotrexate; cyclophosphamide, doxorubicin, vincristine, and prednisone; CCNU, etoposide, cyclophosphamide, and procarbazine; cyclophosphamide, doxorubicin, and etoposide). Granulocyte-macrophage colony-stimulating factor (GM-CSF) is used for chemotherapy-induced neutropenia. Leptomeningeal disease is treated with intrathecal methotrexate. Appropriate opportunistic infection prophylaxis should be added to treatment plans.

Further reading

Brew BJ. Chapters 7–11. In: Brew BJ. *HIV Neurology*. New York: Oxford University Press; 2001:91–123.

Day JN, Chau TT, Lalloo DG. Combination antifungal therapy for cryptococcal meningitis. *N Engl J Med* 2013;368:2522–2523.

Dedicoat M, Livesley N. Management of toxoplasmic encephalitis in HIV-infected adults (with an emphasis on resource-poor settings). *Cochrane Database Syst Rev* 2006;19:CD005420.

Gerstner E, Batchelor T. Primary CNS lymphoma. *Exp Rev Anticancer Ther* 2007;7:689–700.

Gupta NK, Hwang J, Rubenstein JL. High-dose methotrexate is effective, safe, and leads to durable responses in patients with AIDS-related primary central nervous system lymphoma treated during the era of combined anti-retroviral therapy (abstract 1792). *Blood* 2013.

Naidoo K, Baxter C, Abdool Karim SS. When to start antiretroviral therapy during tuberculosis treatment? *Curr Opin Infect Dis* 2013;26:35–42.

Offiah CE, Turnbull IW. The imaging appearances of intracranial CNS infections in adult HIV and AIDS patients. *Clin Radiol* 2006;61:393–401.

Quinn D, Newell M, De Graaff B, *et al.* Human immunodeficiency virus related primary central nervous system lymphoma: Factors influencing survival in 111 cases. *Cancer* 2004;100:2627–2636.

Rubenstein JL, Hsi ED, Johnson JL, *et al.* Intensive chemotherapy and immunotherapy in patients with newly diagnosed primary CNS lymphoma: CALGB 50202 (Alliance 50202). *J Clin Oncol* 2013;31:3061.

Thwaites GE, Duc Bang N, Huy Dung N, *et al.* The influence of HIV infection on clinical presentation, response to treatment, and outcome in adults with tuberculous meningitis. *J Infect Dis* 2005;192:2134–2141.

88 Neurological complications of human T-cell lymphotropic virus type-1 infection

Abelardo Q. C. Araujo[1,2], Marco A. Lima[1,2], and Marcus Tulius Silva[1]

[1] Laboratory for Clinical Research in Neuroinfections, National Institute of Infectious Diseases (INI), Oswaldo Cruz Foundation (FIOCRUZ), Brazilian Ministry of Health, Rio de Janeiro, Brazil

[2] Federal University of Rio de Janeiro, Rio de Janeiro, Brazil

The human T-cell lymphotropic virus type 1 (HTLV-1) is a member of the Retroviridae family, the Orthoretrovirinae subfamily, and the delta-retrovirus genus, and was the first human retrovirus to be discovered. HTLV-1 preferentially infects CD4+ lymphoid cells *in vivo* to cause various diseases, including adult T-cell leukemia/lymphoma (ATLL) and HTLV-1-associated myelopathy/tropical spastic paraparesis (HAM/TSP). ATLL is due to a neoplastic clonal growth of HTLV-1-infected CD4+ T-cells and is characterized by unique clinical features, including hypercalcemia and severe organ infiltration by leukemic cells. HAM/TSP is an immune-mediated disease of the central nervous system (CNS), but the precise mechanism by which disease develops remains a matter of debate.

Epidemiology

HTLV-1 is endemic largely in the southwestern part of Japan, sub-Saharan Africa, South America, and the Caribbean, with some foci in the Middle East and the southeast region of Oceania (Australia and Melanesia). The virus can be transmitted through breastfeeding, sexual intercourse, and contact with contaminated cellular blood products. The prevalence of HTLV-1 increases gradually with age, especially among women. The total number of HTLV-1 carriers is currently estimated to vary from 5–20 million individuals worldwide.

Unlike HIV-1 infection, which causes AIDS in most patients, only 2–3% of HTLV-1-infected individuals develop ATLL and another 0.25–3.8% develop HAM/TSP, with most infected individuals becoming lifelong asymptomatic carriers. Both host and virological factors play a role in the neurological outcome after infection.

Pathophysiology

To date, the best predictor of becoming ill from HTLV-1 is a high proviral load (PVL); that is, a high percentage of peripheral blood mononuclear cells (PBMCs) carrying the provirus. Japanese studies report a median PVL more than 10 times higher in HAM/TSP patients than in asymptomatic carriers, consistent with studies from the Caribbean, South America, and the Middle East. Genetic factors such as the human leukocyte antigen (HLA) genotype appear to be related to the high PVL in HAM/TSP patients and their relatives. In chronic HTLV-1 infection, 90–95% of the PVL is carried by CD4+ T-cells and 5–10% by CD8+ T-cells.

HAM/TSP is characterized by an overstimulation of the immunological compartment, including increased expression of inflammatory cytokines and chemokines, and an increase in the number of highly activated circulating CD8+ T-cells directed against the Tax_{11-19} viral epitope in both peripheral blood (PB) and cerebrospinal fluid (CSF).

The mechanism(s) by which HTLV-1 induces HAM/TSP remains unknown, but is currently thought to rest in "bystander damage," whereby interferon (IFN)-γ-secreting HTLV-1-infected CD4+ T-cells and their recognition by virus-specific CD8+ cytotoxic T-lymphocytes in the CNS induce microglia to secrete cytokines, for example tumor necrosis factor-α, which may be toxic for myelin. Both anatomically determined hemodynamic conditions and adhesion molecule-mediated interactions between circulating infected T-cells and endothelial cells may contribute to the localization of the main lesions. After induction of HTLV-1 antigens on the surface of infected T-cells in the CNS, expansion of the responses of immunocompetent T-cells to viral proteins may result in CNS tissue damage mediated by the released cytokines. More recently, a model has been proposed in which HTLV-1-infected cells in the CNS produce IFN-γ to induce secretion of the chemokine CXCL10 by astrocytes, in turn recruiting additional infected cells via the chemokine receptor CXCR3 and thus constituting a T-helper type 1–centric continuous positive feedback loop that results in chronic inflammation of the spinal cord.

In necropsy cases of HAM/TSP in Japan, the spinal cord shows symmetric atrophy, especially of the thoracic cord, in proportion to the severity of neurological deficit. Infiltration of mononuclear cells and degeneration of both myelin and axons are the essential microscopy findings of cases with a relatively short clinical course of disease. Inflammatory lesions extend throughout the entire spinal cord, but are most severe in the middle–lower thoracic region. Similar but milder lesions are seen scattered in the brain. In patients with a more prolonged clinical history, the spinal cord shows a monotonous degeneration and gliosis, with a few inflammatory cells in perivascular areas. Fibrous thickening of the vessel walls and pia mater are frequently noted. Degeneration of the spinal cord white matter is symmetric and diffuse, but more severe at the anterolateral column and inner portion of the posterior column, where inflammatory lesions are accentuated in the active–chronic phase. There are no focal demyelinating plaques. HTLV-1 proviral DNA is detectable by polymerase chain reaction (PCR) analysis of DNA extracted from affected spinal cords in HAM/TSP, although levels

International Neurology, Second edition. Edited by Robert P. Lisak, Daniel D. Truong, William M. Carroll and Roongroj Bhidayasiri

tend to decrease with disease progression in parallel with a decrease in CD4+ T-cell numbers. Together, these findings suggest a preceding inflammatory process in such areas, although investigators outside of Japan speculate that the neuraxis is affected in a more systemic axial fashion as seen in neurodegenerative diseases, and that lesions do not seem to be secondary to vascular or inflammatory abnormalities.

Pathological examination of patients with other neurological manifestations of HTLV-1 infection show various degrees of inflammatory changes with necrotic and degenerating muscle fibers and focal invasion of HTLV-1-infected CD4+ cells, mainly in HTLV-1-associated myositis; anterior horn cell loss with surrounding infiltration of CD8+ lymphocytes, gliosis, axonal, and myelin loss of the pyramidal tracts in all spinal cord levels and thickened and infiltrated leptomeninges in those ALS-like cases; and both demyelination/remyelination and axonal degeneration/regeneration or, less often, inflammatory infiltrates in the peripheral nerves in those patients with polyneuropathy.

Clinical features

The neurological features of HTLV-1 infection are varied, and consist of a mixture of central, peripheral, and autonomic nervous system involvement.

HTLV-1-associated neurological complex

HAM/TSP is a neurological condition defined clinically and serologically according to guidelines proposed by a World Health Organization (WHO) panel of experts in 1988. Although still largely used, these guidelines have important shortcomings, including frequent use of vague terminology and criteria that encompass many syndromes. Table 88.1 lists new diagnostic guidelines to classify HAM/TSP disease according to different levels of ascertainment.

HAM/TSP is a slowly progressive disease, with some large prospective studies showing that patients progressed from disease onset to wheelchair confinement over a median of 21 years.

Although HAM/TSP is only one of the HTLV-1-associated neurological diseases, other neurological syndromes are found in HTLV-1-positive individuals without myelopathy, suggesting that the neurological spectrum of HTLV-1 disease is broader than previously thought.

HTLV-1-associated polymyositis (HAPm)

Most HAPm cases described are associated with HAM/TSP. HAPm is an important diagnosis to consider if patients with HAM/TSP develop a new pattern of muscular weakness (more proximal), myalgias, and increased serum creatine kinase levels. Compared to idiopathic polymyositis, HAPm follows a more protracted course and is particularly resistant to steroids.

HTLV-1-associated polyneuropathy (HAPn)

Peripheral neuropathies have been consistently found in association with HAM/TSP. The clinical picture is of paresthesiae, burning sensations, and abnormal superficial sensation distally in a sock-and-glove distribution, generally associated with abolished ankle jerks. Although in most cases peripheral nerve involvement is associated with HAM/TSP, HAPn cases can also be found in isolation, manifesting as a predominantly sensory axonal polyneuropathy with no spinal cord involvement.

HTLV-1-associated dysautonomia (HAD)

Autonomic disturbances are always associated with HAM/TSP and so far have never been described in isolation. HAD is characterized by impaired cardiovascular and sweat control, and clearly indicates a major dysfunction of the sympathetic nervous system. Postural hypotension is a common feature of HAM/TSP and should always be investigated and treated symptomatically. Dysautonomia may be more frequent than previously suggested, and in some cases may be severe enough to warrant specific treatment.

Amyotrophic lateral sclerosis-like syndrome associated with HTLV-1 (ALS-HTLV)

ALS-HTLV pictures have been occasionally described as a sole manifestation of HTLV-1 infection. The main difference between these patients and typical HTLV-1-negative ALS cases is the longer evolution and slower progression in HTLV-1-infected individuals.

Chronic diffuse encephalomyelopathy

Diffuse brain white-matter magnetic resonance imaging (MRI) abnormalities, reflecting a chronic perivascular inflammation with progressive gliosis, can explain the mild cognitive disturbance reported in some HTLV-1-infected individuals, with psychomotor slowing and deficits in verbal and visual memory, attention, and visuomotor abilities.

Table 88.1 Diagnostic guidelines for HAM/TSP according to levels of assessment.

Definite
1. Non-remitting progressive spastic paraparesis with impaired gait perceptible by the patient. Sensory symptoms or signs may be present, but remain subtle and without a clear-cut sensory level. Urinary and anal sphincter signs or symptoms may be present.
2. Presence of HTLV-1 antibodies in serum and cerebrospinal fluid (CSF) confirmed by Western blot and/or a positive polymerase chain reaction (PCR) for HTLV-1 in blood and/or CSF.
3. Exclusion of other disorders that can resemble HAM/TSP.

Probable
1. Monosymptomatic presentation. Spasticity or hyperreflexia in the lower limbs or isolated Babinski sign with or without subtle sensory signs or symptoms, or neurogenic bladder only confirmed by urodynamic tests.
2. Presence of HTLV-1 antibodies in serum and/or CSF confirmed by Western blot and/or a positive PCR for HTLV-1 in blood and/or CSF.
3. Exclusion of other disorders that can resemble HAM/TSP.

Possible
1. Complete or incomplete clinical presentation.
2. Presence of HTLV-1 antibodies in serum and/or CSF confirmed by Western blot and/or a positive PCR for HTLV-1 in blood and/or CSF.
3. Disorders that can resemble HAM/TSP have not been excluded.

Investigations

A variety of systemic laboratory abnormalities can be found in patients with HAM/TSP, such as the presence of "flower cells" (atypical lymphocytes with petal-shaped nuclei, typical of ATLL), hypergammaglobulinemia, an increased proportion of CD4+ to CD8+ cells, the presence of autoantibodies, and false-positive serological tests, such as Venereal Disease Research Laboratory (VDRL) and Lyme serology. A higher PVL in the blood appears to distinguish HAM/TSP from asymptomatic carriers as well as from individuals with more rapid disease progression. PVL values vary widely among individuals, but are relatively constant within individuals.

The CSF may be normal or may reveal a small/moderate mononuclear pleocytosis along with a modestly elevated protein content. Oligoclonal IgG bands, increased levels of cytokines (neopterin, TNF-α, IL-6 and IL-γ), and increased intrathecal antibody synthesis specific for HTLV-1 antigens have also been described. Some authors have advocated the use of PVL measurement in the CSF as a diagnostic aid in defining HAM/TSP. Indeed, the percentage of HTLV-1-infected cells in the CSF cells and the CSF/PBMC HTLV-1 PVL ratio are always >10% and >1, respectively, in patients with HAM/TSP, in contrast to <10% and <1, respectively, in asymptomatic carriers.

Cerebral white-matter lesions and spinal cord abnormalities are frequently observed in HAM/TSP. Early in the course of the myelopathy, spinal cord edema might be found, reflecting an active inflammatory process. As disease progresses, the spinal cord becomes progressively atrophic.

Differential diagnosis

HAM/TSP can be occasionally mistaken for other neurological conditions such as the "progressive" spinal form of multiple sclerosis, the vacuolar myelopathy of AIDS, sporadic cases of familial spastic paraparesis, primary lateral sclerosis, some slowly progressive spinal cord compressions, vitamin B_{12} or copper deficiency, idiopathic transverse myelitis, Lyme disease, and neurosyphilis. Most of these conditions can be ruled out by an initial screening with a brain and spinal MRI, CSF examination, and specific blood tests.

Treatment

HAM/TSP is a highly incapacitating myelopathy, but clinical trials of specific drugs to treat it are lacking. Oral or intravenous corticosteroids are still the mainstay of HAM/TSP treatment, particularly in the initial phase of the disease when inflammation is more prominent than demyelination and gliosis. Motor disability, pain, and urinary dysfunction may be ameliorated with steroids, but improvement is usually not sustained.

Since HAM/TSP is associated with a high HTLV-1 PVL, reducing this load could treat or even prevent disease. However, despite *in vitro* evidence that certain nucleoside/nucleotide analog reverse transcriptase inhibitors (NRTIs) are active against HTLV-1, *in vivo* results have been disappointing, with no clinical improvement or reduction of the PVL. Valproic acid arose as a potential treatment for HAM/TSP based on evidence that this drug can activate viral gene expression and expose virus-infected cells to the immune system, leading to a reduction of the PVL. However, the drug was ineffective in improving motor and other disabilities. Other drugs such as IFN-α, cyclosporin A, methotrexate, pentoxifylline, azathioprine, and danazol may be tried if steroids fail or cannot be tolerated, but their use should be balanced in terms of their risk–benefit profile. More recently, small open trials of prosultiamine, a vitamin B_1 derivative known to induce apoptosis in HTLV-1-infected cells, and of pentosan polysulfate sodium, a heparinoid with hemorheological properties, have provided evidence of some clinical improvement in HAM/TSP. Confirmation of these results awaits larger, double blind studies.

Symptomatic treatment using drugs and physical therapy to alleviate pain (which strongly correlates with a low quality of life of these individuals) and spasticity and to improve bladder control are the current mainstay in the treatment of HAM/TSP.

Further reading

Araujo AQ. Update on neurological manifestations of HTLV-1 infection. *Curr Infect Dis Rep* 2015;17:459.

Araujo AQ, Silva MT. The HTLV-1 neurological complex. *Lancet Neurol* 2006;5: 1068–1076.

Araujo A, Lima MA, Silva MT. Human T-lymphotropic virus 1 neurologic disease. *Curr Treat Options Neurol* 2008;10:193–200.

Cartier LM, Cea JG, Vergara C, Araya F, Born P. Clinical and neuropathological study of six patients with spastic paraparesis associated with HTLV-I: An axomyelinic degeneration of the central nervous system. *J Neuropathol Exp Neurol* 1997;56: 403–413.

Izumo S. Neuropathology of HTLV-1-associated myelopathy (HAM/TSP). *Neuropathology* 2010;30:480–485.

PART 10   Demyelinating Disorders

89   Multiple sclerosis

Robert P. Lisak[1] and Jun-Ichi Kira[2]
[1] Wayne State University School of Medicine and Detroit Medical Center, Detroit, MI, USA
[2] Department of Neurology, Kysuhu University, Fukuoka, Japan

Multiple sclerosis (MS) is the most common cause of neurological disability among young adults in the temperate regions of the Western hemisphere, Europe, and Australia/New Zealand. There has been an increase in our understanding of the pathogenesis of MS, although the etiology is unknown. More remarkable has been the emergence of disease modifying treatments (DMTs) that have been shown to have a positive effect on the course of the disease. Imaging studies have been critical in allowing earlier diagnosis as well as to understand the evolution of the disease from its earliest presentation.

Epidemiology

MS is not evenly distributed geographically, but increases, in general, as one moves north or south from the equator. In countries with long north/south dimensions, the same pattern is observed, although Japan is an exception to this; here the incidence and prevalence are much lower than other highly industrialized countries at the same latitude. Prevalence worldwide varies, with highs of 30–150/100,000, a mid-range of 5–30/100,000, and lows of fewer than 30/100,000, to virtually no disease. Migration studies support the concept that for MS it is important where one is born and raised for the first 10–15 years of life. Increased risk of developing MS by being born and raised in regions of high prevalence accompanies the migrant to low prevalence regions and vice versa. Ashkenazi Jews, however, who have a high prevalence, and their offspring who are born in Israel, a region where Sephardic Jews and Arabs have a relatively low prevalence, retain the high risk even though they were predicted to acquire the low prevalence. Some of these differences are becoming less striking, particularly for certain populations such as white females in the United States, and are non-existent for other populations such as black men. The incidence of MS is increasing, and cannot be solely attributed to better and more widely available diagnostic techniques or newer diagnostic criteria.

There are clearly racial/ethnic differences that likely represent genetic factors rather than being solely related to environmental factors; genetic/environmental interactions are likely involved. Prevalence in Asia is much lower than in Western countries and frequently has a different clinical presentation. However, probably due to rapid "westernization," the prevalence of MS in Japan rose from 1.4/100,000 to 7.7/100,000 over 30 years. Potential environmental factors postulated to contribute to the higher incidence and prevalence of MS in certain geographic regions include genetic/ethnic differences, amount of sunlight, infectious agents (particularly viral), products of industry in the environment, smoking, obesity, and dietary differences. In the case of viruses, infection with common viruses at a later age, perhaps because of better hygiene, is a popular theory, as is infection with a particular virus in a susceptible population. Differences in the immune system in individuals living in temperate climates, where the predominant intracellular infectious agents are viruses requiring a Th1- and/or a Th17-weighted response, as opposed to tropical climates, where parasitic diseases elicit Th2-weighted responses, have been suggested to contribute to the geographic distribution of MS. This theory is in part based on the current evidence for Th1/Th17-initiated responses in MS.

In countries with highly heterogenous ethnic/racial populations such as the United States, the disease is seen more frequently in Caucasians when compared with African Americans, although MS is much more common than previously believed in that population. MS is virtually unknown in black Africans in Africa, perhaps representing environmental and genetic factors, and rare in individuals of Oriental origin in both countries of origin and living in countries such as the United States. The relapsing–remitting presentation of the disease (relapsing–remitting MS, RRMS) is more common in women than men (approximately 2:1), which is driving the increase of MS. Patients with progressive disease without remissions from the onset (primary progressive MS, PPMS) seem to be equally represented (1:1) and are usually older at onset. Onset is most frequently between 20 and 40 years of age, but there is increasing recognition of clinical onset in teenage and prepubertal children as well as patients >40 years old (see Chapter 90). There is an increased familial incidence of MS, with 1–5% incidence in first-degree relatives. Concordance in siblings is 1–2%, dizygotic twins 2–5%, and monozygotic twins about 30–40%.

MS is not an inherited disease in the sense of a mutation in a single gene. It is more likely the effect of modest changes in multiple genes and their protein products that are not pathogenic on their own, or of interactions between genes and environmental factors.

International Neurology, Second edition. Edited by Robert P. Lisak, Daniel D. Truong, William M. Carroll and Roongroj Bhidayasiri
© 2016 John Wiley & Sons, Ltd. Published 2016 by John Wiley & Sons, Ltd.

In addition there is evidence that there are genes involved in resistance to MS and others that may determine the severity or course of the disease. Recent results of genome-wide association studies (GWAS) suggest that as many as 160 genes, most related to the immune system, may be involved in disease pathogenesis. Epigenetic factors, microRNAs, the gut microbiome, relative insufficiency of vitamin D, perhaps other factors related to sunlight that we cannot readily measure, smoking tobacco, childhood obesity (see Chapter 90), and viral infections, particularly Epstein–Barr virus, seem to affect susceptibility and severity. High sodium intake has been postulated as another factor.

Pathophysiology

Pathology

MS has been considered a multifocal inflammatory disease of central nervous system (CNS) white-matter myelin with late secondary axonal/neuronal damage. Modern immunopathological studies show that there is damage to axons in the white matter early in the course of the disease, as well as early damage in cortical and deep gray matter, changes that were actually shown in some of the very earliest pathological studies. Neuroimaging has also been instructive to understanding the pathology and clinical course. Two distinct processes have been postulated in the pathogenesis of CNS lesions, inflammation and (neuronal) degeneration. This is an oversimplification, partly dependent on a definition of inflammation as gadolinium-enhancing lesions on magnetic resonance imaging (MRI). Newer techniques including tractography, double inversion recovery-related techniques for cortical pathology, ultra-high-strength magnets to demonstrate venocentric lesions, various approaches to quantitate atrophy, magnetization transfer resonance for myelin, as well as the use of spectroscopy to provide *in vivo* studies of biochemical changes, are contributing to increased understanding of changes in the CNS during the evolution of disease. Nevertheless, the relative emphasis on inflammation and degeneration mirrors the clinical features of relapsing and progressive clinical courses.

The hallmark lesions in the white matter of RRMS patients are the perivascular (postcapillary/perivenular) inflammatory lesions consisting of T- and B-lymphocytes, monocytes/macrophages, and plasma cells. Demyelination, often in a vesicular pattern with myelin phagocytosis by macrophages, is characteristic. Microglial activation and reactive astrocytes are seen. These are acute lesions, thought to evolve into chronic active lesions with inflammatory cells at the edge of the lesion. Further evolution results in areas of demyelination with few infiltrating inflammatory cells: chronic inactive lesions. Collectively these lesions constitute the plaques, which are frequently confluent and often macroscopic (Figure 89.1).

Some acute lesions resemble delayed hypersensitivity reactions (type I). In biopsy and early autopsy material, the most common lesions (type II) are similar to the type I lesions, but with deposition of immunoglobulin and activated complement. They likely represent a combination of delayed hypersensitivity and antibody-mediated immune reaction. Increase in IgG is found in the CNS in patients with MS and some of this IgG is specific for several myelin antigens. Type I and II lesions contain oligodendrocytes (OL) and oligodendrocyte precursors (OPC). There is some remyelination and those lesions with significant remyelination are termed shadow plaques, but if insufficient or subjected to repeated attacks or other factors, eventually remyelination fails.

Two less common types of acute lesions have been identified. Type III is characterized by OL death probably by apoptosis, with characteristics suggestive of a dying-back oligodendrogliopathy and uneven demyelination. There are similarities to hypoxic lesions of myelin. Type IV lesions, quite rare, show an even pattern of demyelination and OL appear as if they are undergoing cytotoxic death, perhaps via toxin or infection. Modest numbers of inflammatory cells are found in type III and IV lesions. It has been proposed that all acute lesions in individual patients are of one type throughout the relapsing course of their disease. Other researchers posit that individuals may have different types of lesions in different sites and at different times in their disease course, and further that one type of lesion may evolve into another.

Additionally, immunohistological and proton magnetic resonance spectroscopic (MRS) studies of so-called normal-appearing white matter (NAWM) reveal abnormalities that apparently precede the classic pathological changes described earlier, before focal abnormalities can be seen on standard diagnostic MRI. Clusters of apoptotic OL occur in NAWM with activated microglia in the absence of other inflammatory changes, suggesting that inflammatory lesions in white matter are reactive, a consequence of primary changes in OL in patients with the appropriate genetic makeup. The rediscovery of axonal pathology including axonal spheroids (due to axonal transection) in early inflammatory lesions, as well as changes in N-acetyl aspartate (NAA) by MRS in lesions, are responsible for a change in paradigm, MS being viewed as a neurodegenerative disease. Early inflammation, later diffuse infiltration of inflammatory cells, and ongoing microglial activation contribute to the "neurodegenerative" component of MS. White-matter inflammation likely leads to dysfunction and damage to axons and neurons upstream early in the disease. Much of the permanent disability in MS is due to loss of axons and neurons, which may also be a result of direct damage to these cells. In patients with SPMS and PPMS, conventionally viewed as non-inflammatory because of lack of gadolinium enhancement of focal lesions, there is diffuse inflammation in the brain (SPMS and PPMS), including lymphocytes and marked activation of microglia and germinal follicle-like lesions in the meninges (SPMS). Diffuse meningeal inflammation also occurs in PPMS and in patients with very early RRMS, and is associated with highly characteristic and specific subpial cortical lesions devoid of inflammation and lymphocytic infiltration.

Gray matter is involved, starting in the earliest stages of the disease. Pathological findings in cortical gray matter include (1) inflammatory lesions with demyelination that also involve adjacent juxtacortical white matter (leukocortical; type I lesions); (2) demyelination surrounding small venules with minimal inflammation (intracortical; type II); and (3) most commonly, demyelination and axonal/neuronal damage in layers I–IV, sometimes extending to the deepest layers, in the absence of any infiltrating inflammatory cells, immunoglobulin deposition, or evidence of complement activation (subpial; type III). A striking correlation is seen between the amount of cortical gray matter pathology and the intensity of the overlying meningeal inflammation, suggesting that one or more toxic factors diffuse from the meninges and contribute to the cortical pathology. Axonal pathology in underlying white matter and a "dying back" of neurons in the cortical gray matter may also be involved in producing cortical pathology. Inflammation in deep gray matter, including thalamus and basal ganglia, is intermediate in intensity between white matter and cortical gray matter.

Some writers hold that one-third of Asian MS patients who clinically have predominantly optic nerve and spinal cord clinical

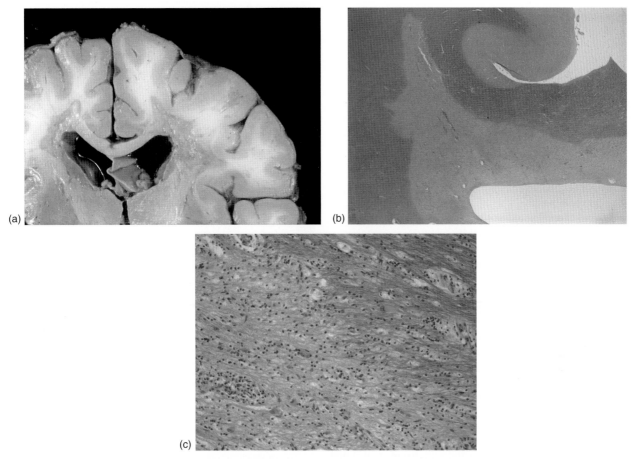

Figure 89.1 (a) Whole brain gross demonstration of several large plaques, including those in periventricular regions. (b) Large periventricular plaque (hematoxylin & eosin [H&E] and luxol fast blue [LFB]; low power). (c) Perivascular lesions within plaque (high power). Source: Reproduced with permission of Dr. William Kupsky. For color details, please refer to the color plates section.

manifestations (optic spinal MS phenotype, OSMS) are without antibodies to aquaporin 4 (AQP4), and that at least 50–60% of these patients actually have neuromyelitis optica (NMO) with AQP4 autoantibodies (see Chapter 91). Yet a substantial and increasing number of Japanese patients appear to have MS by the usual clinical and imaging criteria. In OSMS, MS lesions severely affect both the optic nerve and the spinal cord and are frequently necrotic (see also Chapter 91). Tissue destruction is most prominent at the optic chiasm and from the lower cervical to the thoracic spinal cord. Not only demyelination but also axonal degeneration, cavity formation, and in some cases microhemorrhage are seen in the lesions. Vessel wall thickening and capillary proliferation are also common. Many lipid-laden macrophages are present; however, the degree of perivascular inflammatory cell cuffing is variable. Thus, there is pronounced infiltration of lymphocytes together with neutrophils and eosinophils in some and virtually no inflammatory cells in others. It remains to be elucidated whether the wide range of variability in inflammatory cell infiltrates reflects distinctions of immune mechanisms operative for lesion development. The deposition of IgM and complement components, as well as the preferential loss of GFAP and AQP4 in astrocytes in excess of myelin basic protein loss in myelin in perivascular lesions, has been described in autopsied Asian cases with an optic spinal phenotype, supporting the predominant involvement of humoral immunity in such cases and leading some researchers to view these as part of the NMO spectrum disorder

(NMOSD), even in the absence of demonstrable AQP4 serum antibodies, affecting many Asian populations and not confined to Japan (see Chapter 91).

Pathogenesis and etiology

MS is widely viewed as an autoimmune disease, and while the immune system is clearly involved in the pathogenesis, the evidence for true autoimmunity is indirect. The current concept of the pathogenesis of RRMS is that CD4+ Th1 and/or Th17 cells, capable of recognizing a component of CNS myelin, become activated, perhaps in response to an infectious agent by molecular mimicry and through sequential/orchestrated pathways, and that cytokines and chemokines affecting adhesion molecules and their ligands enter the CNS through an altered blood–brain barrier, the meninges, and/or choroid plexus. On recognizing their cognate antigen presented by antigen-presenting cells (APC), it is likely that microglia, cytokines, and chemokines recruit additional inflammatory cells. These additional CD4 and CD8 cells, monocytes/macrophages, dendritic cells, B-cells, and plasma cells also contribute to lesion formation. Plasma cells are maturational products of B-cells. B-cells, monocytes/macrophages, and dendritic cells, as well as microglia, are APC, can interact with T-cells, and further contribute to lesion formation. These cells and their products, such as tumor necrosis factor-α and lymphotoxin, directly and indirectly, by generating toxic products such as nitric oxide, peroxynitrite, and free radicals/reactive oxygen species, mediate damage to myelin, OL, and axons, all amplified by age-related Fe++ deposition. In type II lesions antibodies directed at one or more components of myelin bind to myelin and cause damage by deposition and activation of complement cascade.

Th17 cells producing IL-17 and other cytokines are also important in lesion formation. CD8+ T-cells may cause damage to axons, and excitatory neurotransmitters may also damage OL, axons, and neurons. Cytokines and chemokines may alter the function of OL, astrocytes, and neurons/axons. Demyelinated axons upregulate sodium channel numbers, which then spread along the bare internode and in the short run may allow demyelinated axons to resume impulse transmission. Continued excess activation of channels may eventually lead to axonal damage via loss of normal mitochondrial metabolism and failure of normal ion exchange, leading to relative hypoxia and consequent influx of calcium. "Proinflammatory" cytokines may contribute to this process, as many cytokines are capable of up-regulating genes for proteins associated with hypoxia. Deposition of increased amounts of iron in a toxic valence in cells that are not generally rich in iron likely contribute to pathology and degeneration.

The steps leading to these changes are not fully understood. Downregulatory cytokines are important in limiting lesion activity. Astrocyte hypertrophy and hyperplasia (gliosis) lead to scarring, and are thought eventually to limit remyelination, the restoration of faithful impulse transmission, and functional recovery. Decreased levels of growth factors and mistiming of up- and downregulation of factors involved in different stages of myelination/remyelination may also limit remyelination, along with the inability of OL to re-myelinate damaged axons. However, astrocytes are capable of protecting cells of the oligodendrocyte lineage and neurons from toxic molecules, including excess glutamate. The pathogenic mechanisms mediated by the inflammatory cells and activated microglial nodules in SPMS and PPMS are not known, but are likely to contribute to axonal loss. Microglia may also be important in regeneration and protection by phagocytizing myelin debris and secreting downregulatory cytokines.

Clinical presentation

Symptoms, signs, and course

Symptoms and signs of MS involve dissemination in space in the CNS, and in RRMS dissemination in time. Symptoms and signs can be variable, although there are some that are more common, particularly early in the course of the disease (Table 89.1). Many patients present with subacute, occasionally acute, onset of a single symptom representing a single lesion (monosymptomatic); others less commonly have polysymptomatic onset. Subtle signs of other lesions may be apparent in monosymptomatic-onset patients. Clinically isolated syndrome (CIS) is a commonly used, imperfect term for the presentation of a first demyelinating event or attack (relapse) of MS occurring in a patient of appropriate age, with all other possible etiologies being excluded. The chances of a patient going on to a diagnosis of MS are often predictable from the MRI and cerebrospinal fluid (CSF) findings with this first episode. More recently, individuals who have MRI scans done for unrelated symptoms, such as headaches or head injuries, are found to have changes suggestive of MS. The term of radiologically isolated syndrome (RIS) has been used and longitudinal studies show that some of these individuals develop additional lesions and others also eventually manifest clinical symptoms and signs of MS.

Table 89.1 Symptoms in multiple sclerosis.

Blurred vision or loss of vision
Diplopia
Loss of balance and/or clumsiness of limbs
Weakness of limbs
Paresthesias with/without decreased sensation
Lhermitte's symptom or phenomenon
Band-like (cuirass) sensation around chest or abdomen
Fatigue
Bladder dysfunction
Bowel dysfunction
Sexual dysfunction
Pain of various types including trigeminal neuralgia
Stiffness/spasms
Vertigo
Dysarthria
Dysphagia
Cognitive complaints
Depression
Seizures
Pseudobulbar behavior (pseudobulbar affect, PBA)
Paroxysmal episodes
Trigeminal neuralgia

The most common symptoms at onset are paresthesias and/or decreased sensation, weakness, abnormal gait and/or limb ataxia, decreased vision (optic neuritis), and diplopia. Vertigo or sphincter dysfunction can be experienced early in disease, and sphincter and sexual dysfunction are very common as progressive disability accumulates. Fatigue is common, causing major difficulties in work and daily living. Cognitive problems are also common and can be detected in up to 30–50% of patients; severe dementia is rare. Disorders in mood including depression are frequent and inappropriate euphoria and inappropriate crying and/or laughter (pseudobulbar affect/behavior) are seen. Seizures occur, usually later in the course, but are uncommon. Signs on neurological examination confirm the multifocal and diffuse nature of the disease, especially over time (Table 89.2).

In Asian patients with OSMS, selective and severe involvement of the optic nerves and spinal cord is characteristic, as is seen in NMOSD (see Chapter 91). Compared to patients with the conventional form of MS (CMS), these patients are often older, have a greater female preponderance, greater disability, poorer recovery from attacks/relapses, and are less likely to enter a progressive course. OSMS patients show a higher frequency of longitudinally extensive spinal cord lesions (LESCLs) than CMS patients (Figure 89.2).

In typical Western MS patients, less than 3% have such LESCLs. By contrast, in Asians, LESCLs are seen in more than half of OSMS patients, while about one-quarter of CMS patients also have these lesions. LESCLs in OSMS patients are present from the lower cervical to thoracic cord, whereas they are preferentially found in the cervical cord in CMS patients. Not unexpectedly given their definitions, cranial MRI shows a significantly lower frequency of brain lesions fulfilling Barkhof criteria in OSMS than in CMS patients.

Table 89.2 Common neurological signs in multiple sclerosis.

Abnormal reflexes (hyperreflexia, Babinski, hyporeflexia*, absent superficial abdominal and cremasteric reflexes)
Weakness
Spasticity
Impairment of vibratory sensibility
Decrease in proprioception/position sense
Impairment of sense of pain, light, touch, and/or temperature
Ataxia of gait and/or trunk
Limb ataxia with/without tremor
Abnormalities of eye movement including internuclear ophthalmoplegia, nystagmus
Decrease in visual acuity, visual fields, and color vision
Pallor of the optic disc
Afferent pupillary defect
Dysarthria (cerebellar, spastic [pseudobulbar and/or bulbar])
Decrease in facial sensation
Facial weakness
Abnormalities of mood (signs of depression)
Cognitive dysfunction

* Patients with marked segmental sensory deficits, lower motor neuron weakness, or marked increase in tone may manifest hypo- or even arreflexia in some regions.

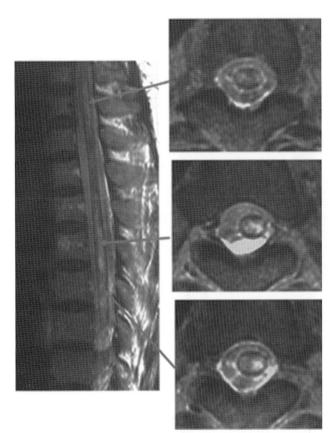

Figure 89.2 MRI of cervical spinal cord in a Japanese patient with ocular spinal MS (OSMS); T2-weighted image.

These findings, even in the absence of AQP4 antibodies, as noted in the pathology section (and in Chapter 91), have led to the suggestion that OSMS patients are part of the NMOSD.

Untreated MS patients have a 10–12-year decrease in life expectancy. Somewhere between 50% and 80% of patients in the era preceding the introduction of DMTs developed a progressive course and significant disability. It is still not definitively proven that DMTs prevent or even delay the onset of SPMS, as long-term placebo-controlled studies are not possible. Some series report that 10–30% of patients have benign disease at 10 and 20 years of disease; the percentage at 30 or more years is likely to be no more than 5–10%.

Investigations

Diagnosis of MS is still based on dissemination of lesions in the CNS in time and space, with no alternative diagnosis by a physician experienced in the diagnosis of MS. Currently criteria employ MRI (T2/FLAIR/proton-weighted density and double inversion recovery [DIR] sequences for white- and gray-matter lesions; Figure 89.3), CSF oligoclonal bands, and visual evoked responses (VEP), which added to the clinical history and neurological examination allow for an earlier diagnosis. One can make the diagnosis in some patients with classic presentations with a single MRI scan if there are non-gadolinium-enhancing lesions as well as gadolinium-enhancing lesion(s) that are not responsible for the clinical episode, which together satisfy dissemination in space. CSF analysis may still be important, particularly in patients with atypical features. Other laboratory tests and imaging studies help eliminate other diagnostic possibilities.

Diagnosis is not difficult when there are clear-cut relapses of typical symptoms with objective evidence of dissemination of lesions in time and limited to the CNS by neurological examination, such as visual loss, dyschromatopsia, disc pallor, an afferent pupillary defect, internuclear ophthalmoplegia and other brainstem findings, paraparesis with or without spasticity, ataxia of gait and/or limbs, and sensory deficits. PPMS can still pose problems in diagnosis, as can atypical presentations of RRMS. The differential diagnosis varies with the clinical presentation depending on the part of the nervous system implicated, as well as whether the onset and course are acute, subacute, or progressive. In non-Western regions of the world, NMOSD is the principal alternative diagnosis (see Chapter 91). With an acute/subacute onset the differential also includes vascular diseases, certain infectious processes, and immunologically mediated diseases, including vasculitides, subacute onset from tumors, certain subacute infections, other immunologically mediated diseases, as well as combined systems degeneration, deficiency states, and paraneoplastic syndromes, and a progressive pattern from tumors, lymphomas, inherited disorders, spinal cord compression, and HTLV-1-associated myelopathy. Imaging, CSF, and laboratory testing should be rational, based on the symptoms, signs, and onset/course of the disease.

In CSF oligoclonal bands (OCB) and an increase in the IgG index are found significantly less frequently in OSMS than CMS or Western MS patients (about 25% versus 60% respectively in Japan and 80–90% in MS in Western countries, depending in part on the technique employed), while marked pleocytosis (50 cells/μL) and neutrophils and eospinophils are encountered significantly more commonly in OSMS than CMS (in Asian countries where the terms are used) or MS patients in Western countries. AQP4 antibodies

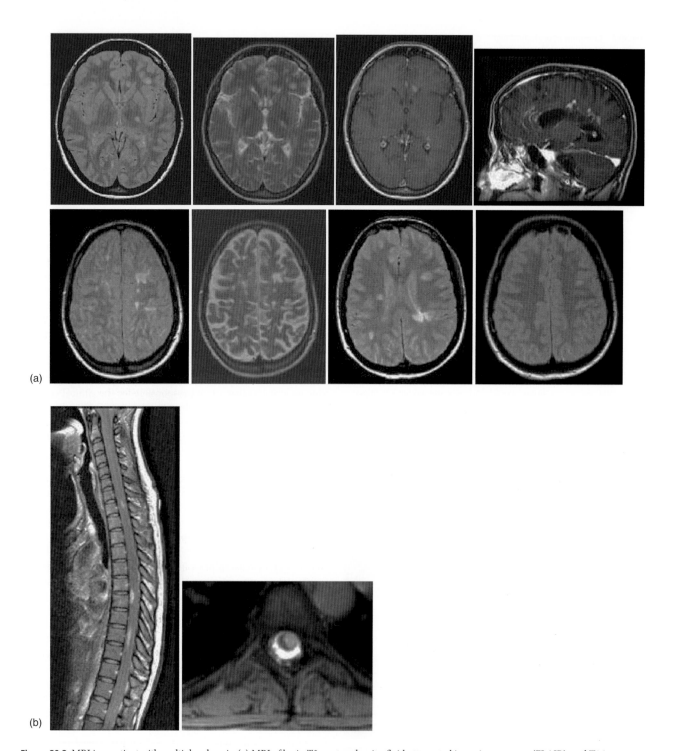

Figure 89.3 MRI in a patient with multiple sclerosis. (a) MRI of brain T2, proton density, fluid-attenuated inversion recovery (FLAIR), and T1 images demonstrating typical lesions including gadolinium enhancement on T1 sequences. (b) MRI of cervical and thoracic spine demonstrating three separate lesions on sagittal sequences and one of the lesions in a typical peripheral or excentric location on axial sequence. Source: Reproduced with permission of Dr. Omar Khan.

(NMO-IgG) are found in 50–60% of patients having OSMS with LESCLs (in Japanese patients, 30% of OSMS with and without LESCLs, and about 15% of all Japanese MS cases). In Japan both AQP4 antibody-positive MS and AQP4 antibody-negative OSMS patients with LESCLs demonstrate higher frequencies of severe optic neuritis and acute transverse myelitis than AQP4 antibody-

negative CMS patients. With spinal cord MRI, LESCLs in AQP4 antibody-positive MS patients predominantly involve the central gray matter of the thoracic cord, while those in AQP4 antibody-negative OSMS patients extend from the cervical through the thoracic spinal cord and may show a pattern of entire cord involvement. However, even in AQP4 antibody-positive MS patients, ovoid lesions in the periventricular white matter of the cerebrum and short lesions in the peripheral white matter of the spinal cord frequently coexist with LESCLs. Thus, there are overlap and transition among AQP4 antibody-positive MS patients who fulfill the definite NMO criteria, AQP4 antibody-negative OSMS patients, and anti-AQP4 antibody-negative CMS patients. AQP4 antibodies occur in up to 75% of patients with classic NMO (see Chapter 91).

Treatment

Treatment of MS is required to encompass five areas: (1) maintenance of general health; (2) symptomatic therapy; (3) treatment of relapses; (4) disease modifying therapy (at this time treatments are primarily immunomodulatory and/or immunosuppressive); and (5) prevention of progressive disability.

Maintenance of general health and prevention or lowering the risk of MS

Besides screening for and preventing comorbid conditions, there are other considerations. One is discontinuation of smoking tobacco, smoking not only being a risk factor for many diseases and for MS itself, but also a factor in MS progression. Childhood/adolescent obesity is a risk factor, as are low levels of vitamin D_3 and low levels of exposure to UVB. Supplementation of vitamin D in the form of vitamin D_3 has become popular, because lower levels of vitamin D are a risk factor for the development of MS and lower levels of vitamin D in patients with established MS (25 hydroxy vitamin D) are associated with increased relapses. Because of the known effects of vitamin D on the immune system and some of the epidemiology of MS (distance from the equator), some studies suggest an additional benefit of vitamin D_3 supplementation when added to DMT and the apparent safety of supplementation of vitamin D_3 in individuals who are not hypercalcemic. Whether supplementation inhibits the disease process is not clear, nor is the dose of vitamin D_3 or desirable serum level. Supplementation with other vitamins, in the absence of demonstrated deficiencies, is of dubious value.

Treatment of symptoms

Treatment involves the use of medications as well as non-pharmacological physical treatments, generally related to the nature of the symptom and the lesions responsible for those symptoms, with some modification based on the disease. Not all symptoms need to be treated and one must balance therapeutic effects with side effects and tolerability. In earlier stages of the disease these symptoms are not as problematic as in patients with longer-standing disease, particularly in progressive phases. Close communication between physicians and other health professionals with patients and families in helping patients deal with this chronic disorder is important.

Spasticity is best treated by a combination of physical therapy and medication. Occupational therapy is often helpful for problems with hands. Some degree of spasticity is frequently useful for patients in helping with ambulation; in some it is critical for the ability to transfer. Baclofen is useful, safe, and well tolerated. Doses are best titrated, ranging from 5 mg twice or three times a day to 160–200 mg/day, the higher doses generally reserved for non-ambulatory or limited ambulatory patients; intrathecal infusions by programmable pump may be required. Limiting side effects include an increase in weakness, sleepiness, and fatigue. Other medications include tinazidine, as a solitary agent or in combination with baclofen, the drugs acting on different channels/receptors within the CNS. It is

necessary to build this agent up very gradually, since sleepiness, fatigue, lightheaded sensation, and hypotension are not uncommon. Benzodiazepines can be helpful, particularly as a night-time dose; side effects can limit use. Dantrolene may prove effective, but weakness and significant hepatic damage can occur with chronic use. Repeated local injections of botulinum toxin can provide help for months, but eventually need to be repeated. Casting by physiatrists and other combined treatments may be required for deforming spasticity. Paroxysmal hypertonia, including "spasms," can sometimes be effectively treated with anticonvulsant drugs such as carbemazapine.

4-aminopyridine has been used off label for years to improve motor function. A sustained release form has been approved, taken as 10 mg twice a day. There are beneficial effects on speed of ambulation, endurance, and power in approximately one-third of patients and in other motor functions. Whether there are other benefits has been difficult to demonstrate on standard neurological examination. The drug is contraindicated in patients who have had or have seizures or abnormal renal function.

Fatigue is a frequent and often disabling symptom in MS. Patients experience several types, including fatigue due to effort (work- and exercise-induced worsening, which improves with rest), fatigue due to depression (often present early in the day, even on wakening), fatigue due to difficulties with sleep (nocturia, sleep apnea, severe paroxysmal spasms, etc.), and the classic sense of fatigue that is often overwhelming and triggered by very little if any effort. Treatment for the latter includes energy conservation, naps, or other periods of rest. Amantadine (100 mg once or twice a day) and modafinil (100–400 mg/day) can be helpful.

Bladder dysfunction is common, interfering with daily activities, and can lead to complications including urinary tract infections, skin breakdown and infection, nephrolithiasis, and rarely renal failure. Three basic patterns of dysfunction exist; urodynamics may sometimes be needed to plan therapy. Patients have difficulty in retaining urine, with urgency, frequency, incontinence, and at times nocturia. Others have difficulty voiding, with hesitancy, double voiding, and at times overflow incontinence. Most have a combination of problems because of detrusor sphincter dysynergy. Urinary retention (>100–150 ml post-voiding residual) should be avoided and requires intervention. Anticholinergic drugs, including long-acting and skin patch formulations, or tricyclic antidepressants, can prove useful if there is not excessive urinary retention. With significant retention and recurrent infections or ureteral reflux, intermittent catheterization is preferable to indwelling urethral or suprapubic catheters. In some, suprapubic catheters, ileal conduits, and electrical stimulation of S1/2 territory will be useful. Intravesical botulinum toxin is proving very useful in appropriate patients. Bowel dysfunction can result in mixed symptoms, such as urgency, constipation, obstipation, and/or incontinence. The latter is hardest to manage. A bowel training program and working with patients on both bladder and bowel management permit patients to manage their lives better.

Sexual dysfunction is common, underappreciated, and affects women as well as men. Treatment with phosphodiesterase type 5 inhibitors, intrapenile suppositories, or injections of prostaglandin alone or in combination with other drugs is helpful for some men. Counseling of couples is very important.

Pain is common in patients with MS, being characteristic of the hidden effects of MS, and treatment depends on the type of pain. Abnormal gait or posture may lead to accentuated musculoskeletal pain and degenerative spine disease. Spasticity including spasms can be painful and treatment should be directed at the spasticity/spasms. Neurogenic pain, paroxysmal tonic spasms, segmental pruritus, and band-like sensations may require a combined approach. If simple analgesics do not suffice, anticonvulsant drugs such as gabapentin, pregabalin, carbamazepine, phenytoin, and topiramate can help control pain. Trigeminal neuralgia can be treated in the same manner. There is seldom any reason to treat Lhermitte's phenomenon. Anticonvulsants cannot restore sensory function like "numbness" and the use for this purpose is futile. Cannabinoids have been suggested as providing some beneficial effect on pain and nausea.

Depression can usually be satisfactorily treated with antidepressant medications and counseling. Mood swings and inappropriate euphoria are harder to treat. A combination of dextromethorphan with a very small amount of quinidine sulfate has been shown to be effective for pseudobulbar affect. Off-label uses of other psychoactive drugs alone or in combination may be partially effective. Cognitive problems are difficult to treat and there is little evidence that inhibitors of CNS acetylcholinesterase or of CNS excitotoxicity are particularly effective in most individuals. Tremor and ataxia are difficult to treat. Agents used for essential tremor have limited efficacy, but botulinus toxin and lead weights are worth consideration. Rarely, patients may benefit from deep brain stimulation.

Exercise including pool therapy, yoga, and aerobic exercise as tolerated are helpful for improvement in mood, reduction of fatigue, improved ambulation and sitting, and reduction of certain types of pain. In severely disabled patients nutrition, regular stretching, and prevention of pressure sores and contractures are important components of comprehensive multidisciplinary care. Avoiding malnutrition and aspiration may occasionally require enteral feeding devices.

Treatment of relapses

Many relapses need not be treated. Preventing relapses is an important goal, but there is little evidence that treating relapses affects long-term prognosis. Relapses that cause a significant adverse effect on a patient's activities of daily living or ability to work are treated with corticosteroids (CS), generally intravenous methylprednisolone (MP) at a total of 1 g/day for 2–5 days. Oral CS in similar doses may be equally effective. While various post-intravenous methylprednisolone (IVMP) oral CS tapering schedules are employed, there are no large controlled prospective randomized studies indicating that they have any effect on degree of recovery from the relapse or the onset of the next relapse. The use of adrenocorticotropic hormone (ACTH), a melanocortin, may be equally effective, but its use has been limited by current costs. Plasma exchange may be useful for CS refractory relapses. There are no randomized controlled studies to support the use of intravenous IgG in patients with poor recovery from a relapse after treatment with CS.

Disease modifying therapies

The development of agents that modify the course of MS has changed the face of the disease's management. In many countries there are currently seven unique classes of approved available therapies for RRMS, more properly relapsing forms of MS: the interferons (IFN)-βs, glatiramer acetate (GA), natalizumab, fingolimod, terifIouramide, dimethyl fumarate, and alemtuzumab. In some countries there are two formulations of recombinant IFN-β: IFN-β1b (non-glycosylated and differing in two amino acids from human IFN-β1a), administered subcutaneously (SC) every other day; and IFN-β1a (glycosylated), given either SC three times a week or intramuscularly once a week. Pegylated IFNb-1a given every two weeks or even once per month is now available.

Evidence suggests that dose and particularly frequency of administration matter; two head-to-head studies favored high-dose/high-frequency regimes over weekly injections. In addition, neutralizing antibodies (NAbs) occur commonly in patients treated with the subcutaneous non-pegylated IFN-β medications and persistent high titers of NAbs reduce the therapeutic effect. Controversy exists over the best way to measure NAbs and availability, and the cost of testing in some countries limits the widespread routine use of NAbs. Patients receiving IFN-β1 therapy require monitoring of blood counts and liver function tests (LFTs). Significant long-term adverse effects have not been seen in patients receiving these medications when properly monitored. There are significant side effects involving tolerability, including injection site reactions and flu-like symptoms, but these can generally be managed. IFNs have multiple mechanisms of action, with inhibition of breakdown of the blood–brain barrier being important.

Glatiramer acetate (GA) is a preparation of random polymers of four basic amino acids, which inhibits the development of experimental autoimmune encephalomyelitis (EAE). Not an interferon, GA seems to have several mechanisms of action that differ from the interferons. Administered at 20 mg SC daily or 40 mg SC three times a week, there do not seem to be any NAbs. GA does not affect either bone marrow elements or LFTs and it is very well tolerated, with manageable local injection site reactions. Some patients develop occasional self-limited immediate post-injection systemic reactions and others chronic lipoatrophy. Large, randomized, prospective, double blind, head-to-head studies comparing GA with subcutaneous frequently injected IFN in RRMS show GA to be as effective and more effective than weekly IFN β1a. GA has several mechanisms of action, with induction of a Th1 to Th2 shift and upregulation of the function of T regulatory (Treg) cells seeming to be most important.

Natalizumab is a partially humanized monoclonal antibody directed against the α4 integrin peptide of VLA4, a ligand for vascular adhesion molecule (VCAM). The interaction of VLA4 and VCAM is required for the entry of pro-inflammatory CD4 T-cells into the CNS through the altered blood–brain barrier. Blocking the entry of inflammatory cells is likely the primary mechanism of action of this agent. Natalizumab administered intravenously every 28 days markedly reduces both relapse rate and gadolinium enhancement on MRI compared to placebo. The comparative efficacy of natalizumab with other treatments for RRMS is uncertain, since no head-to-head study has been performed, but clinical experience suggests that it can be highly effective in patients when other agents fail. Side effects including a slight increase in serious infections compared to placebo were acceptable, and there were occasional infusion reactions. Progressive multifocal leukoencephalopathy (PML) in MS patients treated with natalizumab has now been reported in hundreds of patients not on any concomitant DMT. Natalizumab has usually been reserved for relapsing forms of MS or patients with explosive disease with high-risk factors for poor prognosis, although the trials did not test only this population. The availability of a sensitive and specific antibody (Ab) assay to detect patients who carry the causative JC virus (see Chapter 46) and more recently a quantitative index (titer) has lead to more wide use of natalizumab earlier in the course of the disease. Known risk factors for development of PML

Table 89.3 Risk for progressive multifocal leukoencephalopathy (PML).

Months	JCV Ab+, no IS	JCV Ab+, prior IS
1–24	1/429	1/526
25–48	1/189	1/89
49–72	1/164	insufficient data

Risk for JCV Ab- patients is estimated at 0.1/1000 based on approximate 3% false negative for the JCV Ab test.
IS = immunsuppressive therapy

include the presence of a carrier state for the JC virus, duration of therapy, and/or number of infusions and prior chemotherapy for any indication. Others may yet emerge (Table 89.3).

Diagnosis of PML requires demonstration of JC virus in CSF or brain. A program of very close monitoring for patients treated with natalizumab is required, including testing for JCV Ab at least twice per year. In patients without chemotherapy with low-index JCV antibodies, recent data suggest it may be possible to continue patients on treatment with natalizumab. Patients discontinuing natalizumab not only may have a return to relapses (8–12 weeks) but sometimes a rebound phenomenon, and rarely, particularly in patients who have had plasma exchange to rapidly clear natalizumab, in patients suspected of PML, this can lead to immune reconstitution inflammatory syndrome (IRIS); see Chapter 84. Given the early return of relapses and rebound phenomenon, there is no reason for a prolonged washout period after discontinuing natalizumab before beginning another DMT. There have now been cases of PML reported in patients treated with fingolimod (see later) not previously exposed to natalizumab, as well as several cases of PML reported with dimethyl fumarate (see later) and a related medication used for psoriasis, in patients who have not been previously treated with natalizumab or immunosuppressive agents. It is too soon to know how frequently this will occur and what are the risk factors, although severe and prolonged lymphopenia may well be important with the fumarate agents.

Fingolimod, an oral agent, binds to several sphingosine-1 phosphate receptors (S1PR) leading to internalization of the receptor, functionally reducing available S1PR. The lack of available S1PR leads to trapping of lymphocytes in secondary lymphoid organs, as S1PR are required for lymphocytes to exit secondary lymphoid structures. Fingolimod enters the CNS, where it may have additional effects. In addition to reduction of relapse rate and disability, MRI data demonstrate some reduction in atrophy. Widespread expression of S1PRs explains many of the side effects, including bradycardia with initiation of therapy, increase in infections, particularly lower pulmonary, lymphopenia (a result of therapeutic effect), increase in blood pressure, and macular edema, a rare event early in the course of treatment and of most concern in patients who have had uveitis or have diabetes. There has been concern for more severe herpes infections, particularly herpes zoster (varicella zoster virus, VZV), and patients should be tested for evidence of VZV immunity. There have been several cases of posterior reversible encephalopathy syndrome (PRES) in patients treated with fingolimod (see Chapter 16). There are absolute and relative cardiac and concomitant medication contraindications to the use of fingolimod. Monitoring liver function tests is also required.

Terifluoramide, an oral agent, is an inhibitor of pyrimidine metabolism, resulting in inhibition of activated lymphocytes. Reduc-

tion of relapse rate, MRI activity, and a beneficial effect on disability and disease progression have been demonstrated. Terifluoramide is well tolerated, but monitoring of blood count and liver function tests is required. Temporary thinning of hair is seen along with a slight increase in infections. However, terifluoramide has an "X" rating from the US Food and Drug Administration (FDA) for pregnancy, with GA having a "B" rating and the other agents, to date, a "C" rating. The pregnancy issue is compounded by enterohepatic recirculation requiring 6–8 months to clear, although this can be shortened to approximately 2 months by the use of cholystiramine or activated charcoal. Terifluoramide has also been detected in sperm, raising concern about use for men planning on becoming a father.

Dimethylfumarate (DMF), an oral agent taken twice per day, results in reduction of relapse rate and MRI activity. It is thought to work by activation of the anti-inflammatory stress protein HO and cytoprotection by upregulation of Nrf2 inducing an antioxidant effect. DMF does enter the nervous system, but the active compound is likely monomethylfumarate (MMF), since oral DMF is rapidly metabolized to MMF. The drug has a very short serum half-life. The agent is relatively safe, with a minor increase in infections and uncommon reduction of blood count and liver function test abnormalities. DMF has two tolerability side effects that can be troublesome. Approximately 40% of patients develop significant gastrointestinal symptoms, including abdominal pain and diarrhea, usually clearing after one month. The other is flushing sensation in approximately 40% of patients, which may continue past one month. There are now well-documented cases of PML in patients who have received DMF or related MMF who have had no exposure to natalizumab or chemotherapy.

Alamtuzumab, a monoclonal antibody directed at CD52, a molecule on the surface of many inflammatory cells, results in long-term reduction in circulating lymphocytes and monocytes, with reduction of T-cells lasting for a year or longer. Despite this, the incidence of serious infections was only modestly increased compared to placebo or interferon. Since the infusions are given over 5 days once per year, discontinuing the agent to allow return of mononuclear blood cells is not an option. A major concern is the increase in autoimmune diseases, primarily Grave's disease, but also immune thrombocytopenia, Goodpasture's syndrome, and glomerulonephritis. In addition to infusion reactions, alamtuzumab also carries a "black box" warning for possible neoplasia. Phase II studies demonstrated striking effects on relapse rates, disability, and lack of MRI activity, including for up to 5 years after the end of infusions (two sets of infusions a year apart). Phase III studies were also positive, but the effects and the superiority to INFβ 1a three times weekly for all metrics was not nearly as striking. At this time alamtuzumab is approved in many but not all countries. The relative efficacy of alamuzumab when compared to other DMTs, other than IFN β1a 44 µg three times a week, is at this time unknown.

RRMS patients who are rapidly progressing with frequent relapses may be considered for immunosuppressant medications such as cyclophosphamide or mitoxantrone to induce remission, followed by other treatments, but there are no large randomized studies to support this approach routinely. In the future it is likely that a number of other medications will be available for this situation. IFN-β 1b was approved for SPMS and mitoxantrone is approved for treatment of SPMS, but two of the side effects, congestive heart failure and leukemia, have greatly reduced its use in MS.

Treatment of clinically isolated syndrome

Treatment of patients with clinically isolated syndrome (CIS) with several DMTs delays the onset of the defining second relapse and/or MRI-defining lesion to meet the criteria of MS. This is not surprising; CIS with defined MRI criteria and other disorders ruled out usually is the first clinical episode of MS. Combining the findings with CIS and RRMS, early treatment seems to be beneficial, but whether this should include all such patients in the absence of a helpful biomarker remains controversial. Severity of persisting deficit from the first attack, lesion load or volume, evidence of atrophy or non-gadolinium-enhancing T1 hypointensities on initial or repeat MRI in 3–6 months have all been suggested as guidelines to treat CIS patients with DMTs. The latest guidelines for diagnosis of MS, which allow a single MRI scan meeting certain criteria, will reduce the number of patients with the "diagnosis" of CIS. Patients with MRI done for other indications with findings typical of MS, such as RIS, may go on to have MS, but treatment at that stage is currently controversial.

Treatment of SPMS, PPMS, and PRMS

SPMS treatment remains a major challenge. Although IFN-β1b is an approved treatment for SPMS, it seems clear that this should be reserved for patients with superimposed relapses or gadolinium-enhancing lesions. There might be a subset of mitoxantrone-responsive SPMS patients, but the drug has significant side effects (cardiac, increased susceptibility to infection, and leukemia) and tolerability issues and is used infrequently at this time. There is little to recommend methotrexate or azathioprine and there are no large controlled studies of other agents. As noted, short-term use of cyclophosphamide in patients with rapidly progressing SPMS, particularly with gadolinium-enhancing lesions, may be helpful. Autologous stem cell, embryonic, and mesenchymal stem cell therapy should be considered experimental. At this time no treatments have been approved to slow progression of PPMS. Patients with progressive onset but with one or more clear-cut relapses (PRMS) are often treated as SPMS, since there are no studies on patients with this relatively uncommon pattern of disease and the recent suggested classification eliminates this as a separate MS disease pattern. Rituximab may prove effective in patients with SPMS or PPMS with superimposed exacerbations or gadolinium-enhancing lesions.

Overview of treatment of relapsing forms of MS

It is fashionable to provide a flow diagram for a suggested sequence for treatment of patients with a certain disease. It should be based on class I evidence and such evidence does not exist, because of the paucity of head-to-head studies of the currently approved agents and the tremendous heterogeneity of RRMS. Suggested sequences do not take into account the multiple factors independent of MS that influence the choice of agents at initiation of treatment, or when it is thought that a switch in agents is indicated. Even the decision of if and when to switch agents is more art than science, and again other factors influence this decision. The choice should be what is best for the individual patient, not tiering based on costs

of drug, on lowest-cost deals between individual payers and individual pharmaceutical companies, or marketing to physicians or to patients. Based on approval by regulatory agencies, all of the currently approved agents for relapsing forms of MS should be allowed to be used to initiate therapy, and choices for switching should also be independent of costs. The guiding principle accepted by most clinicians worldwide is to treat all disease activity as aggressively as possible, which has led to the conceptual goal of no evidence of disease activity (NEDA).

Treatment pipeline

At the time of writing, multiple agents are being studied for use in MS. Some are modifications of current agents. Others are monoclonal antibodies directed against cytokines or surface molecules on particular subsets of cells, including agents that eliminate B-cells, as well as one directed against interleukin-2 receptor alpha, among others. There continue to be studies of different types of stem cells or precursor cells in patients with severe disease. There are ongoing studies of therapies approved for relapsing forms of MS, or variations of those agents, in patients with progressive forms of the disease. Finally, there are studies underway looking at agents that might provide direct neuroprotection and/or remyelination in patients with MS.

Further reading

Borghi M, Cavallo M, Carletto S, et al. Presence and significant determinants of cognitive impairment in a large sample of patients with multiple sclerosis. *PLos One* 2013;8:e69820.

Coles A. Multiple sclerosis, *Pract Neurology* 2009;9:118–126.

Granberg T, Martola J, Kristoffersen-Wiberg M, et al. Radiologically isolated syndrome-incidental magnetic resonance imaging findings suggestive of multiple sclerosis: A systematic review. *Mult Scler* 2013;19:271–280.

Kira J. Multiple sclerosis in the Japanese population. *Lancet Neurol* 2003;2:117–127.

Kira J. Genetic and environmental backgrounds responsible for the change in the phenotype of MS in Japanese subjects. *Mult Scler Relat Disord* 2012;1:188–195.

Lassmann H. Mechanisms of white matter damage in multiple sclerosis. *Glia* 2014;62:1816–1830.

Lassmann H. Multiple sclerosis: Lessons from molecular neuropathology. *Exp Neurol* 2014;2622PA:2–7.

Lisak RP, Hohlfeld R. Repair and retention of neuronal structures in multiple sclerosis: Identifying markers, metrics and correlates of treatment success. *Neurology* 2007;68(Suppl 3):S1–S96.

Lublin FD, Reingold SC, Cohen JA, et al. Defining the clinical course of multiple sclerosis: The 2013 revisions. *Neurology* 2014;83:278–286.

Lucchinetti C, Bruck W, Parisi J, et al. Heterogeneity of multiple sclerosis lesions: Implications for the pathogenesis of demyelination. *Ann Neurol* 2000;47(6):707–717.

Matsuoka T, Matsushita T, Kawano Y, et al. Heterogeneity of aquaporin-4 autoimmunity and spinal cord lesions in multiple sclerosis in Japanese. *Brain* 2007;130:1206–1223.

Miller DH, Weinshenker BG, Filippi M, et al. The differential diagnosis of suspected multiple sclerosis: A consensus approach. *Mult Scler* 2008;14:1157–1174.

Misu T, Fujihara K, Kakita A, et al. Loss of aquaporin 4 in lesions of neuromyelitis optica: Distinction from multiple sclerosis. *Brain* 2007;130:1224–1234.

Multiple Sclerosis Coalition. *The use of disease-modifying therapies in multiple sclerosis: Principles and current evidence.* Hackensack, NJ: Consortium of Multiple Sclerosis Centers; 2014. www.mscare.org/CMSC-DMT (accessed November 2015).

Polman CH, Reingold SC, Banwell B, et al. Diagnostic criteria for multiple sclerosis: 2010 revisions to the McDonald criteria. *Ann Neurol* 2011;69:292–302.

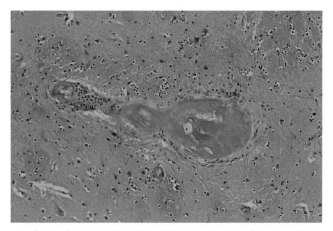

Figure 4.1 Lipohyalin mural change in a caudate nucleus arteriole, with possible microaneurysm formation. (Hematoxylin and eosin stain x200.)

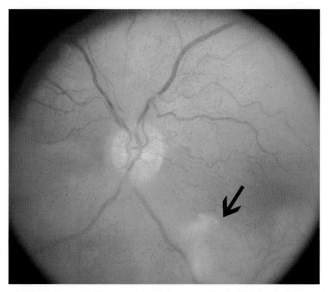

Figure 24.1 Top panel: fundus photograph of a patient with Susac syndrome showing multiple BRAOs, the largest of which is identified by the black arrow.

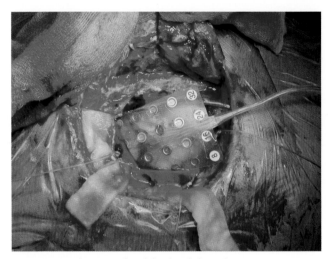

Figure 37.1 Implantation of a subdural grid electrode.

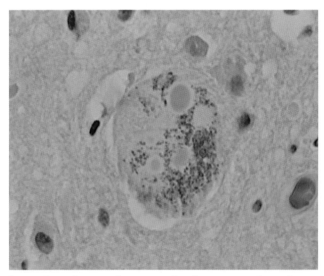

Figure 40.1 Multiple Lewy bodies in the cytoplasm of pigmented neurons in the substantia nigra. Original magnification 400X.

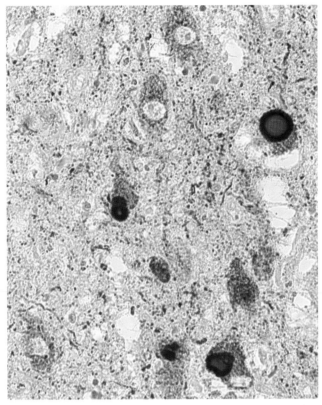

Figure 40.2 Lewy bodies in the cytoplasm of pigmented neurons in the substantia nigra positive in an immunohistochemical reaction using a monoclonal antibody against α-synuclein. Original magnification 400X.

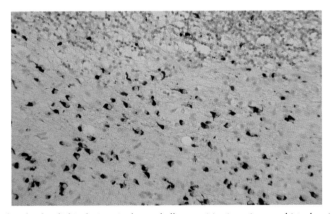

Figure 40.3 Numerous Papp–Lantos oligodendroglial inclusions in the cerebellum positive in an immunohistochemical reaction using a monoclonal antibody against α-synuclein. Original magnification 400X.

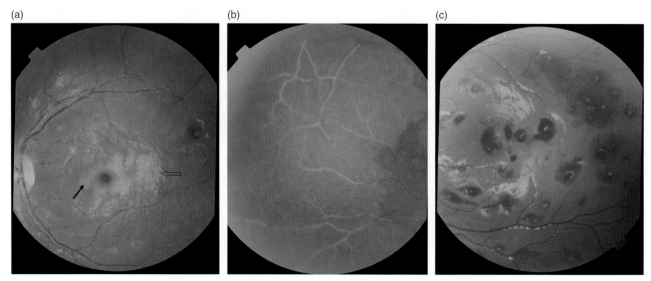

Figure 71.2 a Severe macula whitening (solid arrow) completely surrounding the foveola of a child with cerebral malaria. Papilledema is present as well as a white-centered hemorrhage temporal to the macula and cotton-wool spots above superior temporal arcade. The open arrow indicates glare. Figure 71.2b. White retinal vessels in an area of confluent peripheral retinal whitening. Figure 71.2c. Large number of retinal hemorrhages in a child with cerebral malaria.

Source: Beare 2006. Reproduced with permission of *American Journal of Tropical Medicine and Hygiene*.

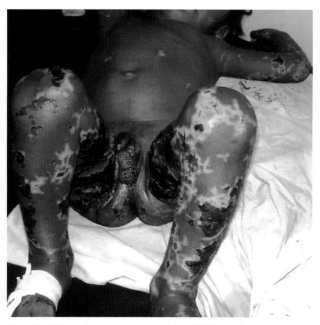

Figure 77.2 Extensive gangrene in a child with Rickettsial vasculitis.

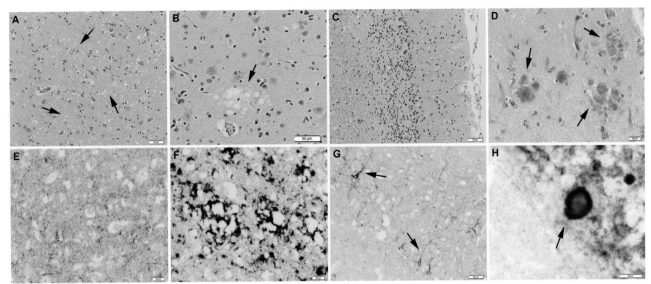

Figure 78.1 (A) Classic histopathology of sporadic CJD is characterized by small vacuoles (arrows) in the neuropil of gray matter (spongiform change) associated with neuronal loss and reactive astrogliosis and microglial proliferation (hematoxylin and eosin stain). (B) In some sporadic CJD subtypes (e.g., MM2C and focally in about one-third of MM/MV1 cases), clusters of large confluent vacuoles are seen (arrow). (C) The cerebellum is severely affected in the ataxic VV2 subtype and shows prominent depletion of granular cells, segmental reduction of Purkinje cells with some axonal swelling (torpedoes), and mild narrowing of the molecular layer with moderate spongiform change of the neuropil. (D) In GSS, large multicentric PAS-positive PrPsc amyloid plaques (arrows) are detected throughout the brain (PAS staining). (E–H) Different PrPsc immunoreactivity patterns in sporadic CJD: classic synaptic type as seen in MM/MV1 (E), patchy-perivacuolar accumulations usually detected in MM2C (F), perineuronal deposits as seen in VV2 (G, arrow), and unicentric, kuru-type PrPsc amyloid plaques in the granule cell layer of the cerebellum as detected in MV2K patients (H, arrow).

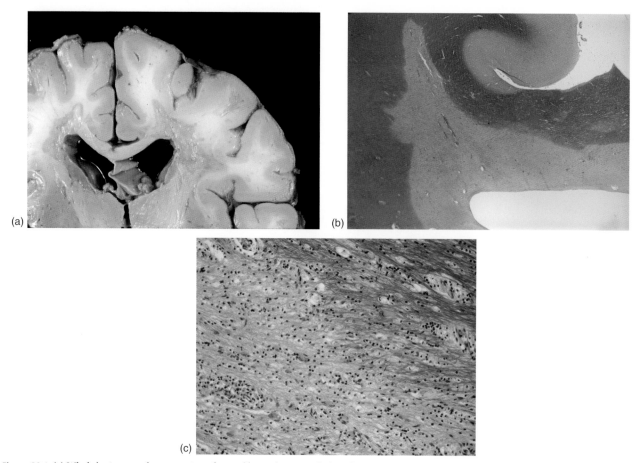

Figure 89.1 (a) Whole brain gross demonstration of several large plaques, including those in periventricular regions. (b) Large periventricular plaque (hematoxylin & eosin [H&E] and luxol fast blue [LFB]; low power). (c) Perivascular lesions within plaque (high power). Source: Reproduced with permission of Dr. William Kupsky.

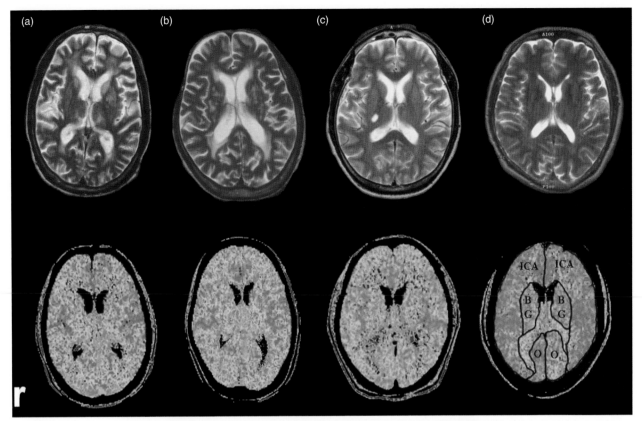

Figure 96.2 Brain MRI changes in carbon disulfide (CS_2) intoxication.(A) (Top) Brain MRI findings on T2 weighted images in three patients with CS_2 intoxication (a–c) and a normal control (d) showing multiple high signal intensity lesions in the subcortical white matter and basal ganglia.(B) (Bottom) Brain CT perfusion scan with a regional mean transit time (MTT) map in three patients with CS2 intoxication (a–c) and a normal control (d) showing a statistically significant prolongation of MTT in the brain parenchymal area and the basal ganglia. (BG = basal ganglia; ICA = internal carotid artery; O = occipital area)

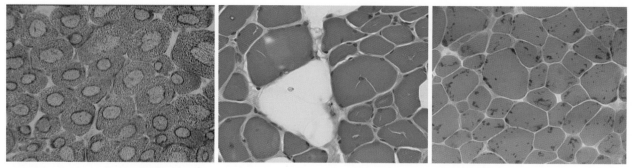

Figure 117.1 The characteristic histological features of congenital myopathies: central core disease (left, NADH-Tr, × 400), centronuclear myopathy (middle, H&E, × 400), and nemaline myopathy (right, Gomori trichrome, × 200).

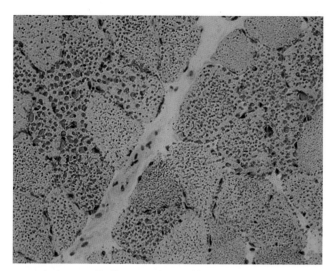

Figure 165.1 Pathological lipid storage in muscle. Intermyofibrillar accumulation of fatty acids as seen in lipid storage diseases, mitochondrial myopathies, and fatty acid oxidation disorders (Oil Red O staining).

90 Multiple sclerosis in children

Sarah E. Hopkins[1], Yael Hacohen[2], Sona Narula[1], and Brenda L. Banwell[1]

[1] Children's Hospital of Philadelphia, Division of Neurology, University of Pennsylvania, Philadelphia, PA, USA
[2] Nuffield Department of Clinical Neurosciences, John Radcliffe Hospital, Oxford, UK

Multiple sclerosis (MS) is an inflammatory demyelinating disease of the central nervous system (CNS) that is typically seen in young adults, with onset between the ages of 20 and 40 years. Up to 5% of all patients, however, experience their first clinical symptom in childhood. Among pediatric patients, MS is most common in adolescents, and less common in children younger than 10 years of age. Children are more likely than adults to have monophasic demyelination, and younger patients are more likely to have atypical presentations of MS. As such, differentiating patients with monophasic demyelination from those who will go on to have a confirmed diagnosis of MS is an important area of focus. The differential diagnosis of demyelinating disease in children is extensive and includes infectious disease, malignancies, metabolic, and other autoimmune conditions.

There are limited data regarding the effectiveness of treatments for pediatric MS, although treatments approved for adults have been utilized with some success in children. Formal pediatric trials are planned. Further studies of the pathophysiology and course of pediatric-onset MS are important, as pediatric patients are closer to the time of any environmental exposures or triggers and present unique opportunities for investigation.

Epidemiology

Adult-onset MS is more common in women. In prepubertal children, the male-to-female ratio is about equal. However, the numbers then shift with the hormonal changes of puberty, so that MS is more commonly diagnosed in female adolescents and adults. MS predominantly affects Caucasians, although there is greater racial and ethnic variability in children than in adults.

Genetic risk factors for MS remain an important area of study. As in adults, children with HLA-DRB1*15 alleles are more likely than those without to develop MS. Additionally, there is also evidence that 57 genes associated with immune modulation identified as increasing risk for adult MS also increase risk for pediatric MS, even controlling for the risk conferred by the HLA-DRB1*15 alleles. These genes do not appear to increase risk for monophasic demyelination.

MS is more common in those residing further from the equator, and children who move to a new area before their 15th birthday take on an MS risk profile closer to that of their new region. Suboptimal vitamin D status and obesity have also been implicated as contributors to multiple sclerosis risk. Additionally, lower vitamin D levels are associated with increase in subsequent relapse rate and new T2 lesions or contrast-enhancing lesions on brain magnetic resonance imaging (MRI). Passive smoking appears to raise the risk of pediatric-onset MS as much as two-fold.

Viral exposures play an important role in the risk for developing MS in children. Children with MS are more likely than other children to have had remote exposure to Epstein–Barr Virus (EBV). By contrast, a remote cytomegalovirus (CMV) infection is independently associated with a lower risk of MS or CIS (clinically isolated syndrome), even in models including EBV status. The interplay of environmental and genetic risk factors is complex; large-scale studies are needed to investigate further these factors and their relationships.

Pathophysiology

The contributions of genetic, environmental, and infectious risk factors to the development of pediatric MS have already been discussed. It is unclear whether there are major differences in the pathophysiology of pediatric and adult MS. Our knowledge is limited by the fact that biopsy specimens are rare in children with multiple sclerosis, and generally limited to patients with tumefactive disease. As in adult MS, active demyelinating lesions are accompanied by mononuclear cell infiltrates and macrophages in a perivascular distribution. One recent case series suggests that there may be more axonal damage in children with MS than in adults. Pediatric MS patients have a sizable burden of T1 lesions and demonstrate early brain atrophy, suggesting that the destructive aspects of MS are evident even in the youngest patients.

Clinical features

In children the first presentation of an acquired demyelinating syndrome (ADS) is more likely to be monophasic than in adults, with 15–46% being diagnosed with MS within the first 5 years of presentation. Pediatric MS is nearly always relapsing–remitting. Cognition is impaired in up to 35% of cases, but this is also seen in patients following CIS – albeit at lower frequencies – consistent with the observation that cognitive impairment in children with multiple sclerosis progresses over time, or limits expected cognitive gains. Fatigue and depression are far more common in children with ADS than in controls, with difficulties with emotional and executive function frequently reported in children with MS.

The International Pediatric MS Study Group published consensus criteria for the diagnosis of pediatric MS and other acquired demyelinating disorders of the CNS in 2007, in hopes of improving

International Neurology, Second edition. Edited by Robert P. Lisak, Daniel D. Truong, William M. Carroll and Roongroj Bhidayasiri
© 2016 John Wiley & Sons, Ltd. Published 2016 by John Wiley & Sons, Ltd.

consistency and facilitating the collaborative research required to study these relatively rare disorders. These criteria were revised in 2013. According to the 2013 criteria, the diagnosis of pediatric MS can be made by any one of the following: (1) two or more clinical CNS events without encephalopathy, separated by more than 30 days and involving more than one area of the CNS; (2) one episode of inflammatory demyelination typical of MS associated with MRI findings that meet the 2010 Revised McDonald criteria for dissemination in space, and a follow-up MRI that shows at least one new lesion demonstrating dissemination in time; (3) one episode of ADEM (acute disseminated encephalomyelitis) followed at least 3 months later by an non-encephalopathic clinical event with new MRI lesions that meet 2010 Revised McDonald criteria; or (4) a first event in a patient older than 12 that is not consistent with ADEM when the 2010 Revised McDonald criteria for dissemination in space and time are met. The 2010 Revised McDonald criteria are more difficult to apply to children under 12 years of age, as many younger children will not have a second demyelinating attack. In a study estimating the positive predictive value of these criteria for pediatric MS, the positive predictive value was only 55% for younger children who were not encephalopathic at the time of presentation.

Less than 1% of pediatric patients have prepubertal onset of MS. Children less than 12 years of age are more likely to present with a polysymptomatic initial episode, with encephalopathy, and with motor and brainstem findings. Additionally, in younger children the final diagnosis is often less clear at the onset. Documenting past clinical attacks may be more difficult in younger children who are less able to describe clinical symptoms. A thorough ophthalmological examination, including optical coherence tomography (OCT) and possibly visual evoked potentials, may help to elucidate evidence of past optic neuritis.

Investigations

MRI

As already mentioned, many children, particularly adolescents, will present with MRI findings similar to those in adults, and the 2010 Revised McDonald criteria have been found to be 100% sensitive and 86% specific for MS in children older than 11 years of age, with a positive predictive value of 76%. Findings include the typical ovoid lesions that are hyperintense on T2 and FLAIR (fluid attenuated inversion recovery), with enhancement of areas of active inflammation and dark areas on T1 imaging indicating areas of myelin injury.

Pediatric patients tend to have a higher volume of brain lesions earlier in the disease when compared to adult patients, with a higher infratentorial burden of both T1- and T2-weighted lesions. Studies of diffusion tensor imaging (DTI) in pediatric MS have shown reduced fractional anisotropy in normal-appearing white matter, suggesting that the integrity of myelin may be disrupted in spite of the fact that there may be a lower burden of supratentorial T1 lesions in children with MS compared to adults, which could suggest some ability for lesional repair. Figure 90.1 demonstrates findings more consistent with pediatric than adult MS.

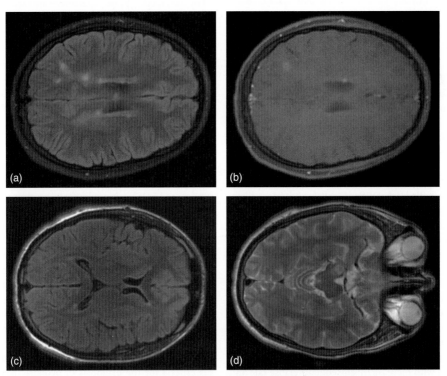

Figure 90.1 Imaging findings typical of pediatric multiple sclerosis. (a) Axial T2/fluid attenuation inversion recovery image demonstrating typical ovoid lesion in the periventricular white matter orientation perpendicular to the ventricles. (b) T1 post-contrast images demonstrating enhancement of the right periventricular and parietal lesions demonstrated in (a). (c and d) Axial T2/fluid attenuation inversion recovery images demonstrating involvement of the corpus callosum (c) and a large right medullary lesion (d).

Laboratory tests

Evidence of inflammation in the cerebrospinal fluid (CSF) demonstrated by the presence of oligoclonal bands has long been recognized as a key diagnostic feature of MS in adults. Children may not have oligoclonal banding at the time of first presentation and this tends to be detected less often in younger children. Repeat sampling of CSF may reveal oligoclonal banding later in the disease course when initial testing is negative, with one recent study demonstrating oligoclonal bands in CSF in 91% of children under the age of 11 and 85% of children aged 14–16 years with subsequent attacks. In addition to these differences, younger patients may be less likely to have an elevated immunoglobin G (IgG) index but more likely to have higher white blood cell counts in the CSF, with a higher number of neutrophils than their adult counterparts.

Differential diagnosis

The differential diagnosis of pediatric MS is most complex at the time of presentation and often becomes clearer over time. Diagnoses that should be considered when a patient presents with neurological symptoms and imaging findings concerning for multiple sclerosis include ADEM, encephalitis (including Lyme disease), vasculitis, malignancy (such as lymphoma), and metabolic causes of leukodystrophy. History and physical examination are key. For instance, patients with metabolic leukodystrophies are more likely to have a baseline history of developmental delay with regression, seizures, or other neurological issues. Mitochondrial disease should be considered in patients with vision loss unresponsive to steroids. Some malignancies, including CNS lymphoma, may have imaging characteristics similar to pediatric MS and could present with remittance of disease when treated with steroids. Tumefactive demyelination may be distinguished from tumor by the presence of multiple lesions, absence of cortical involvement, and decrease in lesion size or detection of new lesions on serial imaging.

Features that should raise questions about a diagnosis of pediatric-onset multiple sclerosis include a progressive course, seizures, and peripheral nerve involvement. Basic recommendations for workup of the initial presentation of demyelinating disease are included in the chapter on ADEM (Chapter 92).

Treatment

The basic treatment of pediatric MS parallels that of adult patients. Clinical trials of disease-modifying treatments in children with MS are just now getting underway. At this time clinical decisions in pediatric MS are based on data from observational studies in children and clinical trials performed in adults.

Acute treatment

Acute treatment of exacerbations is with high-dose intravenous corticosteroids (generally 20–30 mg/kg methylprednisolone daily for 3–5 days), sometimes followed by an oral taper at the discretion of the provider. In cases resistant to corticosteroid treatment, intravenous immunoglobulin (IVIG) may be considered, with plasma exchange an option for treatment of fulminant demyelination unresponsive to other treatments.

Disease-modifying therapies

Injectable therapies, specifically interferon beta and glatiramer acetate, are the current mainstays and first-line therapies for the treatment of pediatric MS. Both have a favorable safety profile. While transaminase elevation can occur with interferon beta, this is rare and may be mitigated by slow dose escalation or reduction in dose. Medication may rarely need to be discontinued because of side effects.

Fortunately, there are many new medications that have recently received approval for use in adult MS, including fingolimod, teriflunomide, and dimethyl fumarate. Unfortunately, there are limited data regarding the safety and efficacy of these medications in children. There are plans, however, to proceed with clinical trials of these medications in children to obtain high-quality data regarding their efficacy and safety prior to widespread use. Second-line therapies sometimes must be considered when there is progression of disease in spite of interferon beta and glatiramer acetate. Natalizumab is the most widely used. The major risk of natalizumab is progressive multifocal leukoencephalopathy, and this risk is minimal in patients who test negative for anti-JC virus antibodies prior to treatment and who remain unexposed during treatment. For those who have been exposed, the risk can be stratified by considering duration of treatment and past immunosuppressant use. Table 90.1 illustrates dosing, administration considerations, and side effects of commonly used disease-modifying therapies in pediatric multiple sclerosis.

Table 90.1 Commonly used disease-modifying therapies in pediatric multiple sclerosis. Oral therapies are currently under investigation in pediatric trials.

Medication (brand name) website	Frequency	Preparation and administration	Adverse effects	Recommended laboratory monitoring
Interferon beta-1a (Avonex) www.avonex.com	30 µg weekly, titration kit available	Intramuscular, autoinjector available	Flu-like symptoms, injection site reaction, leukopenia, transaminase elevation	Monthly complete blood count (CBC) and liver functions for the first 6 months, then every 6 months thereafter, periodic thyroid studies
Interferon beta-1a (Rebif) www.rebif.com	22 or 44 µg three days a week, titration pack available	Subcutaneous, autoinjector available	Flu-like symptoms, injection site reaction, leukopenia, transaminase elevation	Monthly CBC and liver functions for the first 6 months, then every 6 months thereafter, periodic thyroid studies
Interferon beta-1b (Betaseron/ Extavia) www.betaseron.com www.extavia.com	0.25 mg every other day, titration pack available for Betaseron	Subcutaneous, autoinjector available, must be reconstituted prior to use	Flu-like symptoms, injection site reaction, leukopenia, transaminase elevation	Monthly CBC and liver functions for the first 6 months, then every 6 months thereafter, periodic thyroid studies

(Continued)

Medication (brand name) website	Frequency	Preparation and administration	Adverse effects	Recommended laboratory monitoring
Glatiramer acetate (Copaxone) www.copaxone.com	20 mg every day or 40 mg three times weekly	Subcutaneous, autoinjector available	Injection site reactions, potential systemic reaction with flushing and chest pain	None
Second-line therapies				
Natalizumab (Tysabri) www.tysabri.com	300 mg, every 4 weeks	Intravenous infusion over an hour	Infections, including progressive multifocal leukoencephalopathy (PML) and leukopenia	Anti-JCV antibodies prior to and periodically through treatment (every 3 months), periodic CBCs, baseline and periodic MRI brain (at 3 months, 6 months, and then every 6–12 months). MRIs should be done more frequently when PML risk is high (positive JC virus antibody and duration of treatment is greater than 2 years)

Multidisciplinary team approach

A team approach is integral to the care of children with MS. Given the cognitive changes noted in many pediatric MS patients, baseline cognitive testing is essential so that academic performance can be optimized and changes can be monitored over time. Ophthalmology involvement is essential to detect changes that may be associated with optic neuritis. Early involvement of physical and occupational therapists can help to limit issues with mobility and coordination, and help to anticipate equipment needs.

Future directions

Diagnostic criteria of multiple sclerosis in children are now well established, with approximately 3000 pediatric MS patients currently identified worldwide. Accurate estimates of prevalent pediatric MS patients remains challenging, as most pediatric-onset MS patients are diagnosed between 12 and 15 years of age, and are thus "pediatric" for only a few years. The next 5–10 years will witness the first clinical trials in pediatric MS. Such trials will be challenged by the rarity of pediatric MS and by the need for multinational collaboration.

Further reading

Chabas D, Ness J, Belman A, *et al.* Younger children with MS have a distinct CSF inflammatory profile at disease onset. *Neurology* 2010;74(5):399–405.

Charvet LE, O'Donnell E, Belman A, *et al.* Longitudinal evaluation of cognitive functioning in pediatric multiple sclerosis: Report from the US Pediatric Multiple Sclerosis Network. *Mult Scler* 2014;20(11):1502–1510.

Harding KE, Liang K, Cossburn MD, *et al.* Long-term outcome of paediatric-onset multiple sclerosis: A population-based study. *J Neurol Neurosurg Psychiatry* 2013;84(2):141–147.

Huppke B, Ellenberger D, Rosewich H, *et al.* Clinical presentation of pediatric multiple sclerosis before puberty. *Eu J Neurol* 2014;21:441–446.

Krupp, LB, Tardieu M, Amato M, *et al.* International Pediatric Multiple Sclerosis Study Group criteria for pediatric multiple sclerosis and immune-mediated central nervous system demyelinating disorders: Revisions to the 2007 definitions. *Mult Scler* 2013;19(10):1261–1267.

Pfeifenbring S, Bunyan R, Metz I, *et al.* Extensive acute axonal damage in pediatric multiple sclerosis lesions. *Ann Neurol* 2015;77(4):655–667. doi:10.1002/ana.24364

Sadaka Y, Verhey LH, Shroff MM. 2010 McDonald criteria for diagnosing pediatric multiple sclerosis. *Ann Neurol* 2012;72(2):211–223.

Van Pelt ED, Mescheriakova JY, Makhani N, *et al.* Risk genes associated with pediatric-onset MS but not with monophasic acquired CNS demyelination. *Neurology* 2013;81(23):1996–2001.

Waldman A, Ghezzi A, Bar-Or A, *et al.* Multiple sclerosis in children: An update on clinical diagnosis, therapeutic strategies, and research. *Lancet Neurol* 2014;13:936–948.

Waubant E, Mowry EM, Krupp L, *et al.* Common viruses associated with lower pediatric multiple sclerosis risk. *Neurology* 2013;76(23):1989–1995.

91 Neuromyelitis optica spectrum disorders

William M. Carroll

Western Australian Neuromuscular Research Institute, University of Western Australia, Sir Charles Gairdner Hospital, Perth, WA, Australia

Neuromyelitis optica spectrum disorder (NMOSD) is arguably one of the most rapidly expanding neurological topics today. From its eponymous origins with Eugene Devic and his student Fernand Gault in 1894 through to late in the twentieth century, neuromyelitis optica (NMO) or Devic's disease was little known outside of neurology circles. It is now acknowledged to have had original descriptions dating back as far as 1844 and more recently it has been an important catalyst in our understanding of central nervous system (CNS) inflammation. All of the early historical descriptions are but the central characteristics of what is now regarded as a humorally immune-mediated astrocytopathy, both pathogenetically and therapeutically distinct from multiple sclerosis (MS). With the more recently added refinement of testing for neuromyelitis optica immune globulin (NMO-Ig), which targets aquaporin-4 (AQP4), the antigenic epitope of the principal water channel of the CNS, the spectrum of disease has broadened to encompass a range of other manifestations within and outside of the CNS, but which can later manifest as myelitis and optic neuritis, the essential elements of the originally described neuromyelitis optica.

The descriptions from 1894 highlighted a monophasic, often catastrophic illness, rendering the patient paralyzed and blind. Nowadays, it is recognized that relapsing forms are more common, often causing diagnostic difficulty in distinguishing it from MS, particularly the so-called opticospinal (OSMS) phenotype that occurs relatively more commonly in Asia. Additional typical features have also emerged such as area postrema syndromes of intractable singultus (hiccup) and/or vomiting. The development and subsequent refinement of an NMO-Ig antibody assay originally developed in 2004 have greatly increased diagnostic certainty, the recognition of a broad range of diverse manifestations, and more timely therapeutic intervention.

NMOSD is now recognized worldwide to occur with a prevalence ranging from 0.52–4.4 cases per 100,000, with the higher prevalence being found in areas where typical oligodendrocyte-targeted MS is relatively less frequent, such as Asia, South America, and Africa.

Current status

NMOSD is recognized and treated as distinct from other inflammatory diseases of the CNS, especially MS, and its status is evolving. While seropositivity for NMO-Ig is proving most helpful for diagnosis, the exact relationship between seronegativity for NMO-Ig and NMOSD is less clear. Patients in the seronegative group include a high percentage of males with typical clinical features, a smaller percentage of pediatric cases, and those with monophasic neuromyelitis optica. Some of these have been shown to have anti-MOG (myelin oligodendrocyte glycoprotein) antibody disease and it may be that there are other pathogenic antibodies yet to be identified.

For the present, cases with similar clinical features (see later) are separated into AQP4- seropositive and AQP4-seronegative groups, and some of the latter are divided further into anti-MOG-seropositive cases. There is ongoing discussion based on the need for scientifically rigorous clinical trials and early treatment to help refine the current terminology with findings that can be used to argue either for or against NMOSDs, NMOSD, NMO, aquaporin antibody-associated disease, or aquaporin astrocytopathy, a discussion that is beyond the scope of this chapter.

The most recent iteration of the terminology followed an extensive literature review and the deliberation and consensus of international experts regarding the essential clinical, imaging, and serological features required to support a diagnosis of NMOSD, recognizing the likelihood of future changes that will accompany the acquisition of new information.

Pathology and pathophysiology

NMO pathology is centered on the optic nerve and spinal cord, typically longitudinally extensive in both structures, and involves the central areas of the spinal cord, the juxta-ependymal areas, including gray matter, from the corpus callosum and diencephalon to the medulla. Indeed, up to 60% of patients with NMO will have brain lesions, ranging from those with typical appearances in regions of high AQP4 content through reversible fluffy lesions to relatively non-specific lesions.

There are two main forms of NMO lesion, one typically more destructive and one relatively reversible. The first is characterized by non-selective necrosis of white and gray matter, perivascular demyelination with oligodendrocyte depletion, and dramatic astrocyte loss. The prominent perivascular inflammation includes T and B lymphocytes, neutrophils, eosinophils, and plasma cells. The second comprises myelin change without demyelination, but with axonal sparing, associated microglia and astrocyte reactivity, and an inflammatory infiltrate that is more granulocytic. The later stages of the destructive lesions are characterized by cavitation, atrophy, and gliosis with thickening and hyalinization of vascular walls and limited remyelination.

Immunopathologically there are also distinctive features. IgG and IgM deposits with complement activation products (C_9neo) in a rosette or rim vasculocentric pattern with associated eosinophilic

International Neurology, Second edition. Edited by Robert P. Lisak, Daniel D. Truong, William M. Carroll and Roongroj Bhidayasiri
© 2016 John Wiley & Sons, Ltd. Published 2016 by John Wiley & Sons, Ltd.

and neutrophilic infiltration are considered unique to NMO. Both eosinophils and neutrophils are emerging as key drivers of the tissue-destruction type of NMO lesion. AQP4-reactive T-cells are now thought to contribute to neutrophil recruitment, possibly via IL17, and it is likely that the T-cell infiltrates contain such cells. B-cells are found in the infiltrate and are increased in the cerebrospinal fluid (CSF) in addition to plasma cells, among which CD19+ B-cells are prominent.

Immunohistochemical studies, largely from Japan, have confirmed the AQP4 targeting of the injury. Heavily localized in astrocyte foot processes at sites adjoining CSF, perivascular spaces, and brain parenchyma, AQP4 is lost in acute lesions in a pattern matching, or exceeding, that of GFAP (glial fibrillary acid phosphorylase, an astrocyte cell marker) and resembling the vasculocentric rosette and rim deposits of immunoglobulin and complement activation products. In the brain, lesions compatible with NMO occur in those regions where AQP4 is strongly located in the brainstem and cerebral hemispheres. In the area postrema, the tissue comprises decompacted or loose-looking parenchyma, vascularly rich without endothelial tight junctions and with thin ependyma, suggesting a readily permeable blood–brain barrier. NMO lesions of the area postrema comprise decompacted tissue, thickening of capillary walls, absence of axonal and myelin injury, but with a marked loss of AQP4 staining associated with complement deposition and perivascular lymphocyte infiltration. In the cerebral cortex, lesions occur rarely despite heavy AQP4 expression, but when they do, both AQP4 and GFAP staining are absent in cortical layer I.

Aside from the standard histological changes in NMO lesions and the central role of the targeted AQP4, animal models and *in vitro* studies have provided the framework for the understanding of the NMO lesion pathogenesis. These studies have shown immunoglobulin binding to AQP4-expressing membranes, followed by complement activation and downregulation of AQP4, leading to cell lysis. Other observations indicate that NMO-IgG binding to AQP4 on astrocytes, even in the absence of complement, potentially injures oligodendrocytes through increased calcium ion permeability via glutamate receptors. The effects of NMO-IgG binding to AQP4 appear to be isoform specific. The M23 isoform seems to accentuate the injury through formations of orthogonal arrays of protein (OAP), which increase complement activation, whereas the M1 isoform does not. Whether there is a direct effect of altering AQP4 channel function, which then results in cellular edema, remains contentious, although strongly suspected. In any event, it appears most likely that the AQP4-NMO-IgG is pathogenic and central to the pathological changes so far identified.

Clinical, imaging, and laboratory features

The core clinical features of NMOSD are myelitis, which is typically longitudinally extensive on magnetic resonance imaging (MRI), involving three or more vertebral segments and located centrally in the axial plane of the cord; and optic neuritis, to which is now added area postrema syndromes of intractable nausea and vomiting or hiccups. In addition, a number of other clinical syndromes have broadened the clinical spectrum and are now accepted as part of the disorder. These include the first attack of longitudinally extensive transverse myelitis (LETM), recurrent or bilateral optic neuritis, cerebral and diencephalic syndromes, those associated with other autoimmune conditions like systemic lupus erythematosus (SLE), Sjögren's syndrome (SS), and myasthenia gravis, and importantly many of those previously considered to have what is called "Asian

MS" with a typical opticospinal phenotype. Most cases recognized nowadays follow a relapsing course, often with a severe persisting deficit, as distinct from the originally described phenotype of essentially monophasic optic neuritis and myelitis. The clinical characteristics of the myelitis are that it is often in the thoracic and cervical regions of the spinal cord, it is frequently severe, and it is usually symmetric in the lower limb deficit. Similarly, there are features of the optic neuritis that are typical, such as persistent severe loss of vision, simultaneous or bilateral and closely sequential involvement, chiasmal lesions on MRI, or an altitudinal hemianopia not due to ischemic optic neuropathy. In area postrema, syndromes of intractable nausea and vomiting or hiccups have a linear T2 signal hyperintensity in the ventral medulla; such episodes are experienced by almost half of those with relapsing forms of NMOSD. Diencephalic syndromes of hypersomnia are associated with bilateral hypothalamic lesions and encephalopathies, including posterior reversible encephalopathy syndrome (PRES), and can have large, fluffy T2 lesions with "cloud-like" gadolinium enhancement. A clinical diagnosis requires at least two attacks, although the interval between the first and the subsequent events can be highly variable in individual cases. Given the severity of the attack-related disability, early diagnosis and initiation of treatment to prevent further attacks are urgent.

There are other clinical features that also are important to note. Typically the age of the patient at the time of their first attack is older than in those with MS. Women are more frequently affected than men, particularly with the relapsing form, and progression of disability is rare if it occurs at all. The question of cognitive involvement is not settled, and in the absence of much cortical disease on MRI, the pathogenesis of such an effect is yet to be determined. As with MS, pregnancy affords protection from attacks, and among the pediatric population the diagnosis is essentially the same as in adults, but can be more difficult. A subgroup of NMOSD is also being defined among those who are AQP4 seronegative; about a quarter of these will have anti-MOG (short-length) antibody detectable in their serum. These cases have a different phenotype in that they are more often male, older, and have monophasic illness, and so resemble more the original description of Devic; in other cases lesions may be confined to the optic nerve or spinal cord, frequently in the lower thoracolumbar region or the conus medullaris. These cases are often associated with less severe disability. No doubt further subgroups will be identified over time.

It is now well recognized that there are certain typical MRI brain lesions and patterns that signal a high likelihood of NMOSD. On the other hand, in some cases lesions considered typical of MS can also occur, which may confound the use of MRI to distinguish NMOSD from MS. Indeed, up to 13% of NMOSD cases can have MRI appearances that fulfill the Barkhof MS MRI criteria. Typical brain MRI appearances include involvement of the corpus callosum, which may comprise longitudinal lesions, fluffy and edematous or heterogeneous lesions in the acute phase or that extend confluently into the hemispheres, extensive periependymal disease, including that of the area postrema, tumefactive-like hemisphere lesions, and long corticospinal pathway lesions. Gadolinium enhancement patterns differ from those of MS, showing a patchy so-called cloud-like appearance rather than the peripheral open ring characteristic of MS. Some typical MRI lesions of MS are rare in NMOSD, such as cortical lesions, inferior temporal periventricular lesions, and so-called Dawson's fingers. On 7T MRI images, the central venule-associated lesion pattern described in MS is rarely seen in NMOSD. Over time as many as one-quarter of brain lesions will disappear. More than half will shrink, more than half become less intense on T2 or FLAIR (fluid attenuation inversion recovery) images, up to half will show focal T1 hypointensity, and almost one-fifth will develop cystic change.

The CSF findings in initial attacks of NMO may inform the likely diagnosis. About half will have pleocytosis, at times with up to 50 lymphocytes. In one study, the acute attack median was 19 cells/μl with a range of 6–380/μl and frequently included neutrophils, eosinophils, activated lymphocytes, and/or plasma cells. Less than a quarter will have oligoclonal bands. GFAP will be elevated in the CSF in acute attacks, often markedly.

In terms of diagnosis, the refinement of testing for NMO-Ig directed to AQP4 since the original description has improved the accuracy of the early diagnosis of NMOSD, and also has led to a broadening of the clinical spectrum of manifestations of NMOSD. Indeed, the clinical features are now recognized to extend beyond the CNS and to include elevated serum creatine kinase, generalized pruritus, and endocrinopathies. Among patients with these less well-recognized clinical manifestations, many will at some time experience typical myelitis and optic neuritis. Serological testing has clearly identified area postrema syndromes as a frequent manifestation of NMOSD. At present it is recommended that AQP4 serology testing be performed by a recognized laboratory with a validated technique; in cases where there is any doubt of the diagnosis, the testing should be repeated, preferably by another laboratory. The value of CSF testing for AQP4 antibody is not yet certain, but it may help in some cases. It is believed that AQP4 antibody is passively transferred from serum to CSF in the acute phase.

Finally, electrophysiological testing for subclinical visual or spinal pathway involvement is not helpful given the risk of spurious or anomalous results and the much less likely occurrence of subclinical lesions in NMOSD.

Serological testing

Since the presence of NMO-Ig was first described, there have been progressive advances in the specificity and sensitivity of the techniques employed to measure it, and also in the knowledge of this unique biomarker. The antibody is IgG class I. It is directed to the AQP4 water channel, the main water channel in the CNS, which is concentrated on astrocyte foot processes and belongs to a class of membrane water channels that facilitate the passive osmotic transport of water across cell membranes. It is richly concentrated near the blood–brain barrier and the ependymal CSF surfaces of the brain and spinal cord, in the area postrema where the blood–brain barrier is relatively deficient, and in the cerebellum. It is also found in the renal collecting duct epithelium, lung, and skeletal muscle. It exists in one of two isoforms, M1 and M23. The latter are conformationally clumped in so-called orthogonal arrays of particles, leading to more accessible binding by the anti-AQP4 antibody, and they are therefore the preferred target for the detection of this antibody. There have been a number of excellent comparative studies of the different techniques used to measure anti-AQP4 antibody. At present, cell-based assay systems using microscopy or flow cytometry detection are preferred over enzyme-linked immunosorbent, fluorescence immuno-precipitation, and radioimmunoprecipitation techniques.

The AQP4-IgG antibody is diagnostic and predictive of the risk of relapse in patients who have had a first attack. In a comprehensive review of AQP4 antibody serological testing, Waters *et al.* described the specificity and sensitivity of six different assays from a total of 37 studies and found the 9 cell-based assays to have the

highest mean specificity (99.8%) and mean sensitivity (76.7%). In a smaller single study of 146 serum samples from 35 NMO and 45 MS patients that compared the six different techniques from three centers, all were 100% specific, but those based on live transfected cells expressing M23–AQP4 were the most sensitive at 68.6–71.4%. These findings suggest that this form of cell-based assay is likely to be the most useful.

In practice, it is also important to note that females have a much higher rate of seropositivity than males (in some series up to ten-fold), relapsing disease is more frequently seropositive than monophasic disease, and levels of seropositivity can vary with time – often decreasing with treatment – and do not predict the time of an attack.

Diagnosis

Since the publication of the original diagnostic criteria for NMO in 1999, there was a revision in 2006 and a 2015 revision has been published (Table 91.1). The latest criteria were developed by a group of experts convened as an international panel for NMO diagnosis to incorporate into the updated guidelines the widening spectrum of the disorder, enhanced understanding of the pathogenesis, course, and treatment, the relationship with OSMS, and especially the central role of serological testing for the AQP4 antibody. Consequently, the new criteria offer a simpler diagnosis for patients who have clinical features of NMOSD and who are AQP4 seropositive. For those who are AQP4 seronegative, or who are unable to be tested serologically, the clinical criteria and imaging features are more exacting, given the importance of accurate diagnosis.

Table 91.1. NMOSD diagnostic criteria. Source: Wingerchuk 2015. Reproduced with permission of Wolters Kluwer.

1.0 AQP4-IgG seropositive NMOSD
1. At least 1 core clinical characteristic (see below)
2. Positive test for AQP4-IgG
3. No better explanation for the clinical syndrome

1.1 AQP4-IgG seronegative (or serostatus unknown) NMOSD
1. At least 2 core clinical characteristics which satisfy all of the following:
   a. At least 1 core clinical characteristic must be optic neuritis, acute myelitis with LETM, or area postrema syndrome
   b. Dissemination in space
   c. Fulfillment of additional MRI requirements, as below
2. Negative test(s) for AQP4-IgG using best available assay, or testing unavailable
3. No better explanation for the clinical syndrome

1.2 Core clinical characteristics
1. Optic neuritis
2. Acute myelitis
3. Area postrema syndrome (an episode of otherwise unexplained hiccups or nausea and vomiting)
4. Acute brain stem syndrome
5. Symptomatic narcolepsy or acute diencephalic clinical syndrome with NMOSD-typical diencephalic MRI lesion(s)
6. Symptomatic cerebral syndrome with NMOSD-typical brain lesion(s)

1.3 Additional MRI requirements for AQP4-IgG seronegative (or serostatus unknown) NMOSD
1. Acute optic neuritis: requires brain MRI showing a) normal findings or only nonspecific white matter lesions; or b) Optic nerve MRI with T2-hyperintense lesion or T1-weighted gadolinium-enhancing lesion extending over >1/2 optic nerve length or involving optic chiasm
2. Acute myelitis: requires associated intramedullary MRI lesion extending over ≥3 contiguous segments (LETM) or ≥3 contiguous segments of focal spinal cord atrophy in patients with prior history compatible with acute myelitis
3. Area postrema syndrome: requires associated dorsal medulla/area postrema lesion(s)
4. Acute brain stem syndrome: requires associated peri-ependymal brain stem lesion(s)

Seropositive NMOSD

For cases in whom a diagnosis of NMOSD is suspected and who are seropositive (1), the following additional criteria are required: (2) at least one core clinical characteristic of optic neuritis, acute myelitis, area postrema syndrome, acute diencephalic syndrome, or symptomatic cerebral syndrome with typical NMOSD brain lesions (Figure 91.1), and (3) no better explanation.

Seronegative NMOSD or of unknown serostatus

Of cases in whom the serostatus is unknown or negative, diagnosis requires at least two of the core clinical characteristics for seropositive NMOSD and additional MRI specificity.

Optic neuritis

A diagnosis of optic neuritis requires a normal brain MRI or non-specific white-matter lesions or optic nerve gadolinium on T1- or

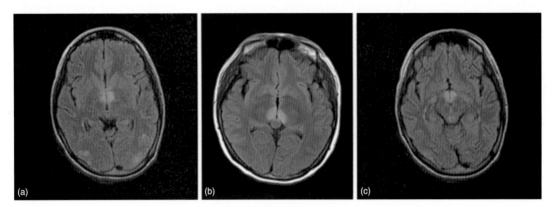

Figure 91.1 MRI lesions characteristic of NMOSD. Source: Kim 2015. Reproduced with permission of Wolters Kluwer.
A. Diencephalic lesions surrounding (a) the third ventricles and cerebral aqueduct, (b) which include thalamus, hypothalamus, and (c) anterior border of the midbrain.

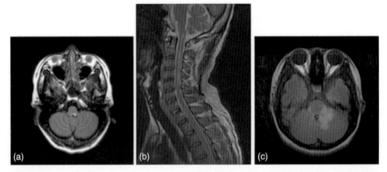

B. (a) Dorsal brainstem lesion adjacent to the fourth ventricle; (b) linear medullary lesion that is contiguous with cervical cord lesion; (c) edematous and extensive dorsal brainstem lesion involving the cerebellar peduncle.

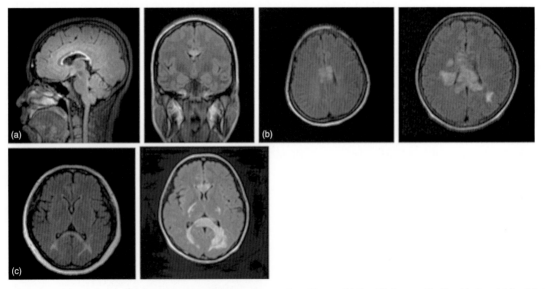

C. (a) Callosal lesion immediately next to the lateral ventricle, following the ependymal lining; (b) "marbled pattern" callosal lesion; (c) "arch bridge pattern" callosal lesion.

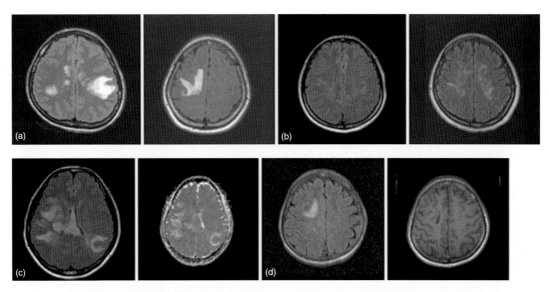

D. (a) Tumefactive hemispheric white-matter lesions; (b) a long spindle-like or radial-shape lesion following white-matter tracts; (c) extensive and confluent hemispheric lesions showing increased diffusivity on apparent diffusion coefficient maps suggesting vasogenic edema; (d) hemispheric lesions in the chronic phase showing cystic-like cavitary changes.

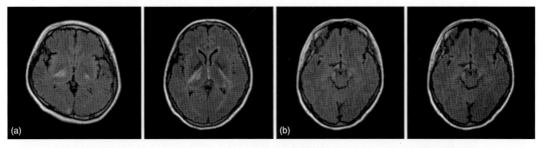

E. (a) Corticospinal tracts lesions involving the posterior limb of the internal capsule and (b) cerebral peduncle of the midbrain; (c) longitudinally extensive lesion following the pyramidal tract.

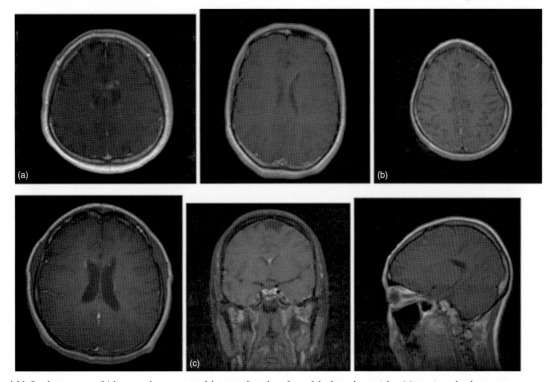

F. (a) "Cloud-like" enhancement; (b) linear enhancement of the ependymal surface of the lateral ventricles; (c) meningeal enhancement.

T2-weighted images showing lesions extending for more than half the length of the optic nerve or involving the chiasm (Figure 91.2).

Myelitis

For myelitis, MRI must show an intramedullary lesion extending over >3 contiguous vertebral segments (LETM), or atrophy of >3 vertebral segments in those with a prior history of myelitis (Figure 91.3).

Area postrema syndromes

Area postrema syndromes have a longitudinal central dorsal medulla MRI lesion.

Acute brainstem or diencephalic syndromes

These are accompanied by periependymal brain MRI lesions.

In the same way that there are specific MRI features to be satisfied to support the diagnosis of NMOSD, so too are there imaging and clinical features that should signal the need for caution in establishing

a diagnosis of NMOSD. For example, in brain MRI, typical MS lesions with an elongated morphology perpendicular to the ventricular surfaces, inferior temporal lateral ventricular lesions, juxtacortical and cortical lesions, and persistence of gadolinium enhancement should all herald caution, as should those in the spinal cord that are <3 contiguous vertebral segments, peripherally located on axial images, asymptomatic, show persistent gadolinium enhancement of >3 months, are localized to specific tracts, or comprise diffuse indistinct lesions.

Treatment

The established dominant role for humoral immunity in NMOSD signals that the treatment of NMOSD will be different from that of MS. Furthermore, a number of treatments useful for MS may exacerbate NMOSD. Consequently, the need for a quite separate therapeutic approach is absolute. Given the severity of many NMO

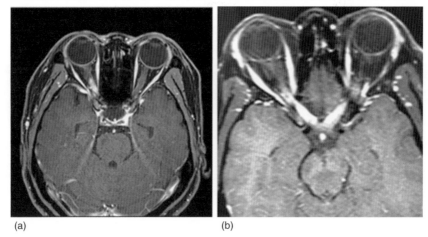

(a) (b)

Figure 91.2 Optic nerve MRI lesions characteristic of NMOSD.(a) Dense gadolinium-enhancing lesion at posterior part of right optic nerve. (b) Extensive gadolinium-enhancing lesion at bilateral posterior part of optic nerve/chiasm. Source: Kim 2015. Reproduced with permission of Wolters Kluwer.

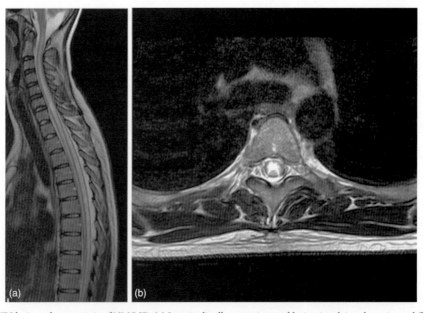

Figure 91.3 Spinal cord MRI lesions characteristic of NMOSD. (a) Longitudinally extensive cord lesion involving thoracic cord.(b) Exclusive involvement of gray matter (H-shaped cord lesion). Source: Kim 2015. Reproduced with permission of Wolters Kluwer.

attacks and the resulting disability, early and accurate diagnosis is critical until a treatment that is safe for both MS and NMO is developed.

For acute attacks, high-dose methylprednisolone can be given, preferably in tandem with, or prior to, plasma exchange. Although there is no class I level of evidence, most clinicians use 1 g/day of intravenous or oral methylprednisolone for 3–5 days. Plasma exchange regimens can incorporate 5 exchanges each of approximately 1.5 L over 7–10 days, or a total exchange of 1.1 times the plasma volume in 7 equal treatments over 10–14 days. Subsequent to the acute treatment, and especially if there is a high titer of AQP4-NMO-IgG indicating a likely future relapse, treatment with one of several immunosuppressant agents or B-cell-targeted monoclonal antibody immunotherapy should be commenced. In the absence of class I level evidence, agents such as azathioprine, given at 2–3 mg/kg per day, or mycophenolate mofetil at 1 g twice per day, with or without oral prednisolone at about 20 mg per day, seem to be effective treatments. Rituximab, a chimeric monoclonal antibody targeting CD20+ memory and naïve B-cells, has proven efficacious in a small trial and is a preferred treatment in those countries where it can be afforded, or if immunosuppressant agents fail. It can be given as a single dose, repeated when the B-cells are replenished to about 2% of the lymphocyte population, or more frequently at lower doses titrated against the B-cell population.

A range of other therapeutic approaches are being developed or evaluated in clinical trials that show promise. These include (1) anti-CD19+ monoclonal antibodies, which also target plasmablasts and plasma cells that actively secrete the AQP4-NMO-IgG antibody; (2) monoclonal antibodies to IL6 (e.g., tocilizumab) or IL17 (e.g., secukinumab) cytokines, which are involved in driving the production of pathogenic antibody and granulocyte lesion infiltration, respectively; (3) novel approaches to limit neutrophil elastase elaboration with sivelestat, and eosinophil stabilization with antihistamines like cetirizine and ketotifen that may offer assistance both acutely and prophylactically; (4) blockade of AQP4 antibodies to AQP4 with agents such as modified non-pathogenic AQP4 monoclonal antibody (aquaporumab), which competitively outbinds the pathogenic AQP4 antibody and also shows no undesirable effect on the water channel; (5) other novel therapies to interfere with the Fc effector region of AQP4-NMO-IgG or the formation of OAP by the M23 isoform, both of which may limit the extent of immune-dependent cytotoxicity; and (6) repurposing of cladribine, given its likely effectiveness in both MS and NMO, permitting earlier prophylaxis in cases of suspected NMO that are AQP4 seronegative.

Further reading

Jarius S, Wildemann B. The history of neuromyelitis optica. *J Neuroinflamm* 2013;10:8.

Kim HJ, Paul F, Lana-Peixoto MA, et al. MRI characteristics of neuromyelitis optica spectrum disorder: An international update. *Neurology* 2015;84:1165–1173. doi:10.1212/WNL.0000000000001367

Kitley J, Waters P, Woodhall M, et al. Neuromyelitis optica spectrum disorders with aquaporin-4 and myelin-oligodendrocyte glycoprotein antibodies: A comparative study. *JAMA Neurol* 2014;71:276–283. doi:10.1001/jamaneurol.2013.5857

Kowarik MC, Soltys J, Bennett JL. The treatment of neuromyelitis optica. *J Neuro Ophthalmol* 2014;34:70–82.

Lucchinetti CF, Guo Y, Popescu BF, et al. The pathology of an autoimmune astrocytopathy: Lessons learned from neuromyelitis optica. *Brain Pathol* 2014;24:83–97.

Waters PJ, Pittock SJ, Bennett JL, et al. Evaluation of aquaporin-4 antibody assays. *Clin Exper Neuroimmunol* 2014;5:290–303.

Wingerchuk D, Banwell B, Bennett JL, et al. International Consensus Diagnostic Criteria for NMO spectrum disorders. *Neurology* 2015;85(2):177–189.

92 Acute disseminated encephalomyelitis

Sona Narula[1], Sarah E. Hopkins[1], Yael Hacohen[2], Brenda L. Banwell[1]

[1] Children's Hospital of Philadelphia, Division of Neurology, University of Pennsylvania, Philadelphia, PA, USA
[2] Nuffield Department of Clinical Neurosciences, John Radcliffe Hospital, Oxford, UK

Acute disseminated encephalomyelitis (ADEM) is considered to be a monophasic fulminant inflammatory demyelinating syndrome, more common in children, manifesting with encephalopathy and polyfocal neurological deficits. ADEM is thought to occur as a consequence of mistaken immunological targeting of central nervous system (CNS) antigens following infectious exposures and, rarely, vaccinations. ADEM occurs in approximately 1/1000 children following acute infection with measles, which remains a major health issue in countries that do not have a universal vaccination program. Post-vaccination ADEM is most clearly associated with exposure to vaccines that utilize neural tissue cultures as part of their production. However, this is now quite rare, as these vaccines have been replaced by recombinant protein vaccines.

Current therapeutic strategies for ADEM include corticosteroids, intravenous immunoglobulin (IVIG), and plasma exchange, with the choice of therapy dictated by the clinical severity of the presentation. Up to 18% of children and 40% of adults with ADEM may experience at least one subsequent demyelinating event, and most patients with recurrent disease will ultimately be diagnosed with multiple sclerosis (MS; see Chapters 89 and 90). Clinical, laboratory, and magnetic resonance imaging (MRI) features that reliably predict MS risk at the time of an acute ADEM presentation are currently lacking.

Clinical features

ADEM is characterized by encephalopathy (manifesting as behavioral change, irritability, or altered consciousness) that cannot be explained by fever or illness, and polyfocal neurological deficits. Neurological symptoms are heterogeneous and may include visual loss due to unilateral or bilateral optic neuritis; limb weakness and/or sensory dysfunction due to spinal cord involvement or cerebral lesions; ataxia, dysarthria, tremor, or nystagmus; or cranial nerve abnormalities and possibly respiratory depression resulting from brainstem involvement. Although less common, seizures and meningismus also occur with ADEM.

Systemic symptoms such as fever, headache, and fatigue often precede the development of neurological deficits in ADEM. Once neurological symptoms begin, the course is rapidly progressive and patients typically develop maximal symptoms within 3–5 days. Symptoms of ADEM may occur spontaneously without antecedent illness, or more typically occur within a few days to weeks of an infectious illness of presumed viral etiology. By definition, the clinical symptoms of ADEM can fluctuate and evolve over a period of 3 months.

The International Pediatric Multiple Sclerosis Study Group (IPMSSG) has published and recently updated consensus definitions for ADEM, MS, and other acquired demyelinating syndromes (Table 92.1). While the definition of ADEM was created based on the typical presentation seen in children, there are no accepted diagnostic criteria for ADEM in adults, and in a study looking at a cohort of 40 adult patients with ADEM, encephalopathy was not part of the inclusion criteria.

Laboratory findings in ADEM

A mild to moderate lymphocytic pleocytosis (cell count $>10/\mu L$) and/or elevated cerebrospinal fluid (CSF) protein is found in the majority of cases of ADEM. CSF oligoclonal bands (OCBs) have been reported to be acutely present in up to 19% of patients with ADEM. OCBs are more likely to be detected in patients with an initial demyelinating event who are ultimately confirmed to have MS. The methodology for CSF OCB evaluation is critical.

MRI features of ADEM

MRI features of ADEM most commonly include large multifocal, bilateral, asymmetric, T2-hyperintense lesions scattered diffusely in the CNS white matter, and areas of increased signal in the deep gray matter. Spinal cord lesions are present in up to 28% of patients with ADEM, and can be longitudinally extensive. Although radiological findings are typically present at the time of clinical symptoms, they can sometimes lag behind by 5–7 days.

Despite the fact that ADEM is a fulminant and acute process, it is rare for all radiological lesions to enhance with gadolinium, and some patients have no enhancing lesions. Meningeal enhancement is also uncommon in ADEM, as is the presence of lesions with complete ring enhancement.

The presence of T1 hypointense white-matter lesions is uncommon in ADEM and can be more suggestive of a chronic process such as MS. Typical MRI features of ADEM and MS are contrasted in Table 92.2 and shown in Figure 92.1. MRI features at presentation, however, cannot be used to reliably distinguish ADEM from the first attack of MS. The onset of MS in very young children may demonstrate MRI features typical of ADEM at the first demyelinating attack, but then evolve over time into a pattern more consistent with MS. Serial imaging with MRI is important when trying to differentiate an episode of ADEM from an initial attack of a chronic demyelinating disease, as lesions in ADEM should at least partially

International Neurology, Second edition. Edited by Robert P. Lisak, Daniel D. Truong, William M. Carroll and Roongroj Bhidayasiri
© 2016 John Wiley & Sons, Ltd. Published 2016 by John Wiley & Sons, Ltd.

Table 92.1. Summary of the proposed definitions for acquired demyelinating syndromes.

Diagnosis	Definition	Key clinical features	Key MRI features	Specific exclusions
Monophasic ADEM	• A first clinical attack with a presumed inflammatory demyelinating cause, with acute or subacute onset that affects multifocal areas of the CNS	• Polyfocal neurological symptoms • Encephalopathy*	• Bilateral, asymmetric, large T2 hyperintense lesions in white matter and/or deep gray nuclei • Chronic T1 hypointense lesions are rare	• Acute CNS infection • Prior events consistent with demyelination
Multiphasic ADEM	• ADEM followed by a new clinical attack also meeting criteria for ADEM, characterized either by new symptoms/areas of CNS involvement or by re-emergence of initial clinical symptoms • Attack occurs at least 3 months after initial ADEM episode	• Polyfocal neurological symptoms • Encephalopathy*	• MRI can show new lesions, although this is not a requirement • Original lesions may have enlarged or resolved	• Attack occurs within 3 months of first clinical episode (considered a part of the initial ADEM illness)
Clinically isolated syndrome	• An initial CNS inflammatory demyelinating event that does not meet criteria for ADEM, MS, or NMOSD	• Heterogeneous; either monofocal or polyfocal symptoms can occur • Symptoms must last at least 24 hours	• Heterogeneous – common sites of involvement include the optic nerve, spinal cord, and brainstem	• Encephalopathy (unless there is prominent brainstem involvement) • Diagnosis of MS is met based on MRI features
Multiple sclerosis	• Clinical or radiographic evidence of lesion dissemination in both time and space	• Relapsing disease course • Monofocal or polyfocal features	• New lesions on repeat imaging are common	• Children with a first demyelinating event consistent with ADEM must have one non-ADEM-like event that is (1) non-encephalopathic, (2) occurs at least three months after the initial CNS event, and (3) is associated with new MRI findings consistent with dissemination in space
Neuromyelitis optica spectrum disorder	• Must have ON and TM • Spinal cord lesion extending over three cord segments or anti-aquaporin-4 antibody positive	• Monophasic (i.e., single ON and TM episode) • Relapsing NMOSD (recurrent ON and TM episodes)	• Longitudinally extensive spinal cord lesions • Increased T2 signal, swelling, or Gd enhancement of optic nerves • Brain lesions tend to be in hypothalamic region, midbrain, or in a pattern not otherwise consistent with MS	• Clinical features more consistent with MS

ADEM = acute disseminated encephalomyelitis; CNS = central nervous system; Gd = gadolinium; IgG = immunoglobulin; MRI = magnetic resonance imaging; MS = multiple sclerosis; NMOSD = neuromyelitis optica spectrum disorder; ON = optic neuritis; TM = transverse myelitis.
* Encephalopathy is defined by (1) behavioral change (confusion, excessive irritability) or (2) alteration in consciousness (lethargy, coma).

Table 92.2. Demographic, clinical, and radiological features of acute disseminated encephalomyelitis (ADEM) and multiple sclerosis (MS).

	ADEM	MS
Demographics	More common in children, slight male predominance in a few pediatric cohorts	More common in adolescents and adults, female predominance
Course	Typically monophasic	Relapsing or progressive
Presence of cerebrospinal fluid (CSF) oligoclonal bands	Rare (0–19%) and likely transient	Common (>95% when evaluated by an experienced laboratory) and persistent
Brain MRI	Lesions are large, confluent, multifocal, with ill-defined borders Lesions in gray-matter nuclei are often visible T1 hypointense lesions are rarely noted	Lesions have well-defined margins Corpus callosum, subcortical, and periventricular white matter are often involved T1 hypointense lesions are commonly present at onset
Follow-up MRI	Complete or partial resolution of lesions without accrual of new lesions	New lesions appear
Prognosis	Good, with minimal if any residual dysfunction	Risk of accrual of physical and cognitive disability over time

resolve on follow-up scans and new clinically silent lesions should not appear.

Novel myelin imaging techniques, such as measurement of myelin water fraction, could be helpful in further characterizing lesions in ADEM and may provide insight as to whether changes seen represent loss of myelin integrity versus just inflammation and edema. Having the ability to measure the extent of myelin damage *in vivo* would be helpful in terms of predicting prognosis and further understanding the pathophysiology of this syndrome.

Differential diagnosis

The differential diagnosis of acute neurological illness in a previously well child or adult is broad. The key disorders that require exclusion include (1) active, viral, or bacterial infection; (2) systemic or isolated CNS inflammatory disorders, including vasculitis; (3) disseminated CNS malignancy (such as lymphoma, leukemia, or metastatic disease); (4) macrophage activation syndromes; (5) metabolic or mitochondrial disease; (6) acute necrotizing encephalitis (associated with the RANBP2 mutation); and (7) in all patients one must consider whether the acute demyelinating event is the first manifestation of MS. The key clinical features and specific investigations appropriate for the exclusion of these disorders are listed in Table 92.3.

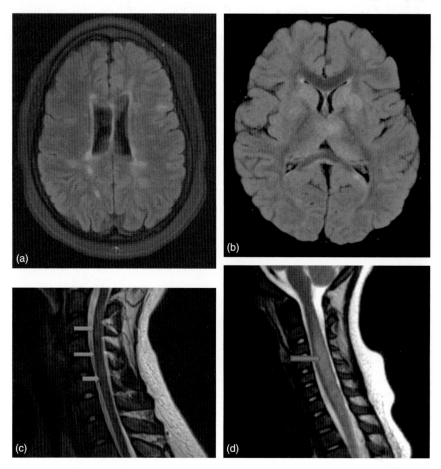

Figure 92.1 Typical MRI images of acute disseminated encephalomyelitis (ADEM) and multiple sclerosis (MS). The figure contrasts the typical MRI features of MS and ADEM.

(a) Axial fluid-attenuated inversion recovery (FLAIR) image: the typical MRI appearance of MS is characterized by multifocal ovoid lesions with a predilection for the periventricular and subcortical white matter.

(b) Axial FLAIR image: brain MRI lesions in ADEM tend to be large, with ill-defined borders. Involvement of the deep gray nuclei is commonly seen.

(c) Sagittal T2 image: spinal MRI in a patient with MS that demonstrates small, focal spinal lesions.

(d) Sagittal T2 image: spinal MRI in a patient with ADEM that demonstrates a longitudinally extensive lesion spanning multiple cord segments.

Treatment

To date, there have been no formal treatment trials for ADEM and standard of care is based on observational data and expert consensus. Treatment of acute ADEM typically consists of high-dose intravenous (IV) corticosteroids (CS) with the additional use of IVIg in CS-resistant or life-threatening cases. Although evidence-based treatment guidelines are lacking, proposed treatment protocols typically begin with IV CS (20–30mg/kg/day for 3–5 days). If there are ongoing symptoms or deficits, oral prednisone can subsequently be administered (initial dose of 1 mg/ kg/day), and tapered over 2 weeks. Case series–level evidence exists for the use of IVIg (2g/kg divided over 2–5 days) for patients who do not respond to CS therapy, and level II evidence exists for the use of plasma exchange (PE; 5–7 exchanges every other day) in acute, life-threatening demyelination.

Prognosis

The outcome of ADEM is generally favorable, and over 85% of patients will recover with little or no sequelae. The average time to full recovery ranges from 1–6 months, although patients often experience immediate improvement of symptoms after beginning treatment with corticosteroids. Minor cognitive deficits occur in a small number of children with ADEM.

Although ADEM is typically a monophasic illness, this can only be confirmed after long-term observation. Rare patients experience more than one ADEM attack (termed multiphasic ADEM). As already stated, an ADEM-like episode can also be the first attack of MS, in which case the subsequent relapses do not meet ADEM criteria. According to IPMSSG consensus, a patient meets criteria for MS after an initial event consistent with ADEM if the second clinical event is non-encephalopathic, occurs 3 or more months after the incident neurological event, and is associated with revised radiological criteria for dissemination in space.

The reported percentage of patients with an ultimate diagnosis of MS varies in different cohorts based on the inclusion criteria and definition of ADEM used. For example, while one prospective study reported that 18% of its ADEM cohort eventually had a confirmed diagnosis of MS, a national prospective study of patients with initial acute demyelinating syndromes and strict definitions for ADEM

Table 92.3. Differential diagnosis of a patient with acute disseminated encephalomyelitis (ADEM).

Disorder	Key clinical clues	Investigations
Central nervous system (CNS) infection	• Persistent fever • Systemic evidence of infection • Predominantly gray-matter involvement • Endemic or environmental exposures	• Blood and cerebrospinal fluid (CSF) cell counts and cultures • Polymerase chain reaction (PCR) testing for infection • Tuberculosis testing • Fungal culture
Systemic inflammatory disorders, vasculitis, and sarcoidosis	• Persistent and prominent headache • Systemic evidence of vasculitis • *Note: clinical, laboratory, and radiographic evidence of systemic disease may be absent in CNS vasculitis	• Erythrocyte sedimentation rate (ESR), C-reactive protein (CRP), antinuclear antibody (ANA), dsDNA • Angiotensin-converting enzyme (ACE) level • Antiphospholipid and anticardiolipin antibodies • Chest X-ray • MR angiography of head • Cerebral angiography • Brain biopsy
Malignancy	• History of prior malignancy • Pre-existing systemic symptoms (weight loss, night sweats, fever)	• Blood smear • CSF cytology • Brain biopsy
Macrophage activation syndromes	• History of similarly affected sibling • Systemic signs of liver, skin, renal, or bone marrow involvement • Persistent fever	• Ferritin level • Triglycerides • Soluble IL-2 receptor level • Blood, CSF, and bone marrow evaluation for hemophagocytosis • Perforin expression in lymphocytes
Metabolic or mitochondrial disease	• Symptomatic worsening with fever • Pre-existing progressive neurological deterioration, developmental delay, or cognitive dysfunction	• Lactate/pyruvate (serum, CSF) • MR spectroscopy • Consider plasma amino acids, urine organic acids, ammonia, acylcarnitine profile
Multiple sclerosis	• History of prior transient neurological deficits or symptoms • Fatigue • Recurrent disease • Family history of MS	• CSF oligoclonal bands • Rigorous and longitudinal observation • Serial MRI scans

reported that only 4 of 77 patients (5%) diagnosed with ADEM were subsequently diagnosed with MS.

Rarely, an ADEM-like attack may be the first presentation of neuromyelitis optica spectrum disorder (NMOSD; see Chapter 91). Anti-aquaporin-4 antibody testing should be done in cases characterized by longitudinally extensive spinal cord lesions, or if there is brainstem, optic nerve, or hypothalamic involvement.

Pathobiology

Pathological studies of ADEM are restricted to biopsies of tumefactive lesions and autopsy studies of extremely fulminant disease. Pathological features that appear to distinguish ADEM from typical MS include that (1) all lesions appear to be of similar age; (2) inflammatory cells (T-cells and macrophages) in ADEM tend to congregate in a sleeve-like pattern around CNS venules; and (3) inflammatory cells may invade vessel walls. Acute hemorrhagic leukoencephalitis (AHLE), a severe form of ADEM, is characterized by necrotizing angiitis of the venules and capillaries with ball and ring hemorrhage, myelin edema, and demyelination.

The role of myelin-specific autoantibodies in the pathogenesis of ADEM is an area of active research and studies are ongoing to try to determine serological biomarkers for ADEM and other demyelinating syndromes. Antibodies to myelin oligodendrocyte glycoprotein (MOG) have been reported in up to 40% of children with ADEM, and also in other acquired demyelinating syndromes. Although these antibodies are associated with both monophasic and relapsing presentations, they have been shown to correlate with active disease, with normalization in patients with ADEM, and with

persistent levels in patients with MS. Nevertheless, their relevance in disease pathogenesis remains controversial.

In summary, prototypical ADEM is an acute, monophasic inflammatory demyelinating illness of the CNS. Prognosis is typically excellent and with rare reports of persistent sequelae. At the current time, diagnosis can only be fully confirmed as monophasic after prolonged observation. Biomarkers that reliably distinguish ADEM from an ADEM-like first MS attack will be of clinical importance.

Further reading

Banwell B, Bar-Or A, Arnold DL, *et al.* Clinical, environmental, and genetic determinants of multiple sclerosis in children with acute demyelination: A prospective national cohort study. *Lancet Neurol* 2011;10(5):436–445.

Hynson JL, Kornberg AJ, Coleman LT, *et al.* Clinical and neuroradiologic features of acute disseminated encephalomyelitis in children. *Neurology* 2001;56(10):1308–1312.

Krupp LB, Tardieu M, Amato MP, *et al.*; International Pediatric Multiple Sclerosis Study Group. International Pediatric Multiple Sclerosis Study Group criteria for pediatric multiple sclerosis and immune-mediated central nervous system demyelinating disorders: Revision to the 2007 definitions. *Mult Scler* 2013;19(10):1261–1267.

Mikaeloff Y, Caridade G, Husson B, *et al.*; Neuropediatric KIDSEP Study Group of the French Neuropediatric Society. Acute disseminated encephalomyelitis cohort study: Prognostic factors for relapse. *Eur J Paediatr Neurol* 2007;11(2):90–95.

Polman CH, Reingold SC, Banwell B, *et al.* Diagnostic criteria for multiple sclerosis: 2010 revisions to the McDonald Criteria. *Ann Neurol* 2011;69(2):292–302.

Tenembaum S, Chamoles N, Fejerman N. Acute disseminated encephalomyelitis: A long-term follow up study of 84 pediatric patients. *Neurology* 2002;59(8):1224–1231.

Tenembaum S, Chitnis T, Ness J, Hahn JS; International Pediatric MS Study Group. Acute disseminated encephalomyelitis. *Neurology* 2007;68(16 Suppl 2):S23–S36.

Verhey LH, Branson HM, Shroff MM, *et al.*; Canadian Pediatric Demyelinating Disease Network. MRI parameters for prediction of multiple sclerosis diagnosis in children with acute CNS demyelination: A prospective national cohort study. *Lancet Neurol* 2011;10(12):1065–1073.

93 Isolated inflammatory demyelinating syndromes

Ernest Willoughby

Department of Neurology, Auckland City Hospital, Auckland, New Zealand

This chapter describes disorders characterized by focal, acute or subacute, non-infective areas of inflammation of the central nervous system (CNS), defined by the site affected; that is, optic nerve (optic neuritis), spinal cord (myelitis), brainstem, or cerebral hemisphere. Usually only one area is affected clinically, but isolated inflammatory demyelinating syndromes (IIDS) may be clinically multifocal, and an isolated focal clinical syndrome may be accompanied by asymptomatic lesions in other areas on magnetic resonance (MR) scan. An alternative, less precise term is "clinically isolated syndrome" (CIS), used most commonly in situations where the features of the attack and the MR changes suggest that it represents the first clinical attack of multiple sclerosis (MS; see Chapter 90).

Of particular significance is the likelihood that these syndromes may be the first clinical manifestation of a chronic relapsing inflammatory disease of the CNS, especially multiple sclerosis (MS) or neuromyelitis optica (NMO). In the case of MS, that is usually indicated by the presence of asymptomatic, previously established lesions in the CNS on MR scan, or oligoclonal immunoglobin G (IgG) bands in the cerebrospinal fluid (CSF). NMO may be suggested by the severe nature of the attack and the MR appearances, particularly in the spinal cord or brainstem (see Chapter 91). The differential diagnosis of IIDS is extensive and varies in different parts of the world.

The focal inflammation may follow vaccination or a systemic viral infection, which may also precede the related disorder, acute disseminated encephalomyelitis (ADEM), where there are widespread, multifocal inflammatory CNS lesions with more diffuse clinical features, including encephalopathy. In that disorder, the inflammation is isolated with respect to time but not to area of involvement in the CNS. ADEM is covered in Chapter 92.

Note that IIDS as outlined here do not include low-grade chronic inflammatory disorders affecting the CNS such as neurosarcoidosis, which progress over months to years, although those may also selectively affect the spinal cord or brain (see Chapter 26).

Features common to all isolated inflammatory demyelinating syndromes

Epidemiology
IIDS occur in all parts of the world and affect all racial groups, but there is considerable variation in the frequency of the syndromes in different parts of the world. The typical syndromes are most common in Western Europe and North America and in other temperate areas where the population is of predominantly European origin and where the prevalence of MS is high, reflecting the fact that the single most common cause of IIDS is a first clinical attack of MS. In Asia, Africa, and the Middle East, where the prevalence of MS is much lower, IIDS are less frequent and often represent the first clinical attack of NMO, which is more common in populations of Asian origin and probably also in Polynesians. In all regions, IIDS may also be a manifestation of a systemic connective tissue disorder such as systemic lupus erythematosus (SLE), Sjögren's syndrome, or Behçet disease.

In general, optic neuritis and myelitis are substantially more common in all areas than syndromes affecting the brainstem or cerebral hemispheres, and are the characteristic syndromes seen as a manifestation of NMO. Women are affected about twice as often as men, with a peak age of onset of 20–35.

Pathophysiology
The inflammatory pathology of IIDS has been studied mainly in large cerebral lesions after biopsy. It is probably much the same at different sites, with infiltration of lymphocytes and macrophages with myelin breakdown and variable amounts of axonal damage. There is controversy about the extent of oligodendrocyte loss as a common early feature. Subsequent healing is characterized by remyelination with gliosis. It is now well established that the pathological process in NMO is related to aquaporin-4 antibody-mediated damage to astrocytes, where there is also involvement of small vessels with necrosis, and relatively little selective demyelination, as is the case with the inflammation in MS.

Clinical features
Symptoms occur relatively suddenly and characteristically worsen over several days, or may take 2–3 weeks to reach a plateau. Even without treatment, there is then gradual improvement over several weeks or months. Resolution may be complete or there may be residual neurological deficit. Overall, a rough guide is that one-third of attacks resolve completely, one-third recover with mild residual symptoms, and one-third leave significant residual disability.

Clinical manifestations are due primarily to involvement of major white-matter tracts in the affected area. The severity varies considerably with respect to the peak symptoms, their duration, and the amount of residual disability. The degree of recovery relates in large measure to the extent of initial axonal damage.

Pain may be a prominent symptom. It is related mainly to involvement of sensory pathways in the affected area.

Except for general fatigue, there is usually no associated systemic upset such as fever, unless that is a manifestation of a preceding viral infection that may trigger an IIDS. There may be features of an underlying systemic connective disorder.

Investigations

MR scanning of the affected area is the key diagnostic investigation in distinguishing IIDS from other pathological processes producing similar symptoms (see Figure 93.1). In addition, by demonstrating white-matter scars resulting from previous, asymptomatic patches of CNS inflammation in other areas, particularly in the brain, MR also has a role in determining the likelihood of further attacks (i.e., whether the IIDS is the first clinical manifestation of an already established, but previously asymptomatic, chronic relapsing process, or is potentially an isolated event).

CSF may show a mild lymphocytic pleocytosis and raised protein, and the presence on electrophoresis of oligoclonal IgG bands substantially increases the chances of further attacks in the future, indicating MS in particular. Serum antibodies to aquaporin-4 are a highly specific marker for NMO and other autoantibodies may indicate an underlying systemic connective tissue disorder.

Treatment

The main consideration is the use of high-dose corticosteroids, typically methylprednisolone 0.5–1 g daily, intravenously (IV) or orally, for 3–5 days, at times followed by a tailing course of oral steroids for 2–3 weeks. There is no established consensus on the most appropriate regimen. Steroids relieve acute symptoms, especially pain, and produce more rapid improvement, but evidence is lacking that the treatment reduces the amount of long-term residual disability. For severe attacks with limited improvement on steroids, plasmapheresis has been shown to be of benefit and IVIg may possibly have a place.

After recovery from an IIDS, if there is evidence that the episode represents the first manifestation of MS or NMO, or is associated with a systemic connective tissue disorder, the main issue is consideration of ongoing immunomodulatory or immunosuppressive treatment to reduce the chances of future attacks. That is a complex decision, dependent on the likely nature of the underlying disease process and the availability of a number of costly treatments. There are indications that immunomodulatory therapy that is effective for MS may cause worsening in NMO, and access to long-term treatment varies considerably in different parts of the world.

The clinical syndromes

Optic neuritis

Clinical features

Optic neuritis usually affects one eye, but may be bilateral. Impairment of vision is most marked centrally, with early reduction of color vision and worsening typically over several days. Pain in the eye is usual and aggravated by eye movement, a feature that helps distinguish optic neuritis from other causes of acute visual impairment. Severity of visual impairment is very variable. A common and characteristic feature during the acute phase and also after recovery is temporary aggravation of visual impairment by exercise or exposure to heat (Uhthoff's phenomenon). Swelling of the optic disc is seen in only about one-third of cases, because, most often the inflammatory process (retrobulbar neuritis) does not extend anteriorly to involve the optic nerve head. Characteristically, even when visual impairment is mild there is reduced pupillary constriction to light, demonstrated most sensitively by alternately shining a light in each eye (relative afferent pupil defect). After several weeks, even with good return of vision, pallor of the optic disc (optic atrophy) due to loss of optic nerve axons commonly develops.

Differential diagnosis

This includes other disorders affecting the optic nerve, especially anterior ischemic optic neuropathy (usually painless and more abrupt in onset, often with altitudinal visual field defects), Leber's hereditary optic neuropathy (painless and progressive over weeks or months), and orbital idiopathic or tuberculous granulomatous disease or tumors. Chronic raised intracranial pressure or severe hypertension with papilledema may present with acute impairment of vision in one eye, as may disease of the eye itself, especially neuroretinitis (most commonly due to cat-scratch disease), other retinal disorders, anterior uveitis, ocular larva migrans, toxoplasmosis, and acute glaucoma. In tropical countries, Eale's disease, an idiopathic retinal vasculopathy (especially in India and the Middle East), and onchocerciasis also need consideration. In temperate areas in Europe and North America, Lyme disease should be considered, and in all areas, neurosyphilis. Occasionally, recurrent episodes of optic neuritis occur without other evidence of CNS inflammation (chronic recurring idiopathic optic neuropathy or CRION). The disorder overlaps with aquaporin-4 antibody-negative NMO spectrum disorder, where attacks are confined to the optic nerves.

(Transverse) myelitis

Clinical features

Depending on the site of the main inflammatory focus (cervical or thoracic), there is paraparesis or quadriparesis of variable degree, often asymmetric, with sensory impairment below the level of the lesion, plus bladder and bowel dysfunction. The term transverse myelitis relates to that clinical pattern, with discrete demarcation of sensory change at a particular segmental level. A characteristic feature of cervical myelitis is Lhermitte's symptom, where there is shock-like discomfort down the spine on neck flexion. However, that is not specific for inflammatory cord lesions and also occurs with cord injury and myelopathy due to vitamin B$_{12}$ deficiency. Relatively mild disease with involvement of only part of the spinal cord cross-section is particularly likely to be a feature of a first MS attack. Pain in the spine may be marked and the distal sensory impairment may also be painful. If weakness is severe and develops rapidly, tone may be flaccid rather than spastic, and tendon reflexes absent in the early stages. The extent of recovery is very variable.

Differential diagnosis

The first step is to distinguish myelitis from other causes of acute weakness, especially polyneuropathy. MR scanning usually will distinguish myelitis from tumors, abscesses, and vascular malformations involving the spinal cord. However, at times it may be difficult to distinguish acute inflammation from cord ischemia, which is much less common. The inflammation in IIDS may be localized, as in MS, to fewer than three spinal segments, with peripheral asymmetric cord involvement on axial sections on MR, or be more extensive over several spinal segments with central cord involvement with diffuse cord swelling and patchy areas of enhancement

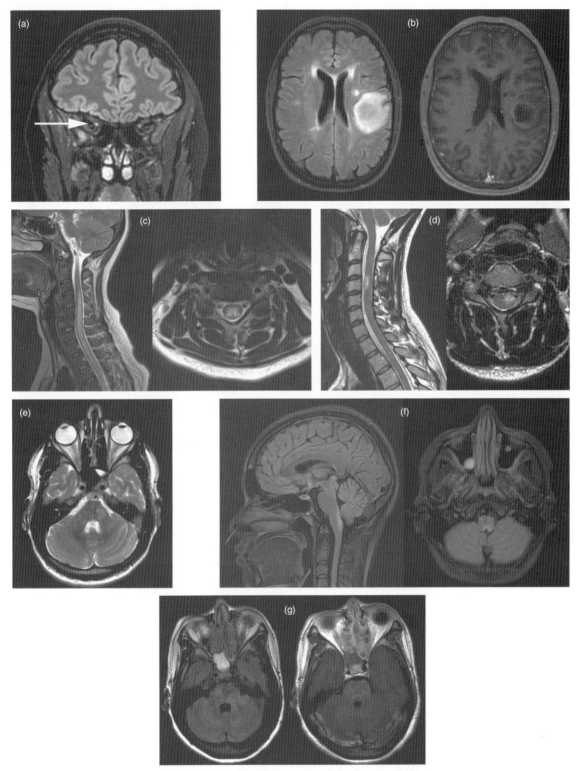

Figure 93.1 MR scans.

(a) Right optic neuritis (hyperintensity of optic nerve – arrow). Coronal T2 FLAIR.
(b) Left cerebral lesion (incomplete ring enhancement). Axial T2 FLAIR and T1 with gadolinium.
(c) Cervical myelitis – neuromyelitis optica (long central lesion). Sagittal and axial T2.
(d) Cervical myelitis – multiple sclerosis (short eccentric lesion). Sagittal and axial T2.
(e) Brainstem inflammation – multiple sclerosis (patchy pontine lesions). Axial T2.
(f) Brainstem inflammation – neuromyelitis optica (dorsal medullary lesion). Sagittal and axial T2 FLAIR.
(g) Brainstem inflammation – CLIPPERS ("pepperpot" multifocal enhancement + incidental sinus inflammatory disease). Axial T2 FLAIR and T1 with gadolinium.

with gadolinium, as in NMO, where CSF neutrophils are more commonly seen. CSF and blood tests will also help distinguish infections of the cord, especially with herpes zoster and West Nile viruses, neurosyphilis and tuberculosis, and, in sub-Saharan Africa and South America, schistosomiasis. Unusual causes to be considered in particular circumstances are nitrous oxide toxicity (usually after recreational inhalation), ischemic myelopathy due to cocaine abuse, myelopathy of uncertain mechanism in heroin addicts, surfer's myelopathy, probably of ischemic origin in novice surfers and reported most often in Hawaii, and atopic myelitis associated with systemic allergic reactions, described mainly in Asia. An unusual form of focal myelitis that may be subacute in onset, but is followed by gradual progressive worsening over months or years, has been termed solitary sclerosis.

Brainstem inflammatory lesions

Clinical features
Motor and sensory dysfunction in the limbs may be similar to that seen in cervical myelitis, with the additional features of cranial nerve lesions, particularly diplopia and impairment of eye movements and/or cerebellar dysfunction. Lesions due to NMO characteristically affect the dorsal medulla and are associated with nausea and hiccups, while MS and Behçet disease produce more irregularly sited lesions in the pons and midbrain. A particular form of brainstem inflammation of uncertain cause with characteristic multifocal small areas of contrast enhancement on MR scan has been named CLIPPERS (chronic lymphocytic inflammation with pontocerebellar perivascular enhancement responsive to steroids).

Differential diagnosis
Tumors, vascular malformations, and infective processes such as listeriosis affecting the brainstem are usually distinguishable by MR scan and CSF, but at times brain biopsy may be needed to confirm the diagnosis.

Cerebral hemisphere inflammatory lesions

Clinical features
The most common are hemiparesis, hemisensory symptoms, dysphasia, or homonymous visual field defects. Headache is not consistently present and seizures may occur.

Differential diagnosis
Symptomatic lesions are usually large, characteristically with incomplete peripheral ring enhancement with contrast on CT or MR scan. Baló's concentric sclerosis is an unusual type of cerebral inflammation with concentric rings of demyelination that may be more common in Asia (see Chapter 95). The lesions may be multifocal and there is overlap with MS. A feature that helps distinguish these types of idiopathic inflammation from tumors and abscesses on MR scan is a relative lack of mass effect for the size of the lesion. Where there is doubt, brain biopsy should be definitive.

Further reading

Miller D, Barkhof F, Montalban X, Thompson A, Filippi M. Clinically isolated syndromes suggestive of multiple sclerosis. Part 1: Natural history, pathogenesis, diagnosis and prognosis. *Lancet Neurol* 2005;4:281–288.

Miller D, Barkhof F, Montalban X, Thompson A, Filippi M. Clinically isolated syndromes suggestive of multiple sclerosis. Part 2: Non-conventional MRI, recovery processes and management. *Lancet Neurol* 2005;4:341–348.

Pelayo R, Tintore M, Rovira A, *et al.* Polyregional and hemispheric syndromes: A study of these uncommon first attacks in a CIS cohort. *Mult Scler* 2007;13:731–736.

Toosy AT, Mason DF, Miller DH. Optic neuritis. *Lancet Neurol* 2014;13(1):83–99.

West TW, Hess C, Cree BA. Acute transverse myelitis: Demyelinating, inflammatory, and infectious myelopathies. *Seminars in Neurol* 2012;32(2):97–113.

94 Osmotic demyelination syndromes

Ovidiu-Alexandru Bajenaru

Faculty of Medicine, University of Medicine and Pharmacy "Carol Davila," and Department of Neurology, University Emergency Hospital, Bucharest, Romania

Osmotic demyelination syndrome (ODS) is a clinicopathological entity first described by Adams *et al.* in 1959 in chronic alcoholic patients, as central pontine myelinolysis, and defined pathologically as a symmetric area of myelin disruption in the center of the basis pontis. During the following years patients were described with similar lesions, preferentially in the basis pontis but also with extrapontine myelinolysis or only in other brain areas without pons injury. The cause most often identified for this condition is the rapid medical correction of chronic hyponatremia, but during the last few years more cases have been reported with ODS determined by other metabolic conditions, not necessarily accompanied by hyponatremia.

Epidemiology

Osmotic demyelination syndrome is not a common medical condition. There are no epidemiological data concerning it. Initial descriptions of ODS were based on autopsy findings, so it has been considered as a medical entity with a high mortality. As imaging techniques have improved, diagnosis and supportive care have also advanced, and two types of consequences have emerged: the number of survivors with or without neurological sequelae reported is greater than initially expected, but also new difficulties in differentiating ODS from other pathological entities have appeared.

Pathophysiology

ODS seems to be most often a consequence of a hyperosmotically induced demyelination process, resulting from rapid intracellular/extracellular to intravascular water shifts producing relative glial dehydration and myelin degradation and/or oligodendroglial apoptosis. When chronic hyponatremia is rapidly corrected, reaccumulation of brain organic osmolytes is delayed and brain cell shrinkage occurs, finally leading to ODS. To date, experimental models demonstrate brain demyelination when sodium is rapidly corrected and usually not with slow correction. However, these models do not take into account the underlying disorders that may be present in human patients. Myelinolysis has also been reported when sodium correction occurs at recommended rates. The nature and degree of insult required to trigger osmotic injury remain unclear, as long as patients with normonatremia (alcoholic cirrhosis and intravenous fluid resuscitation, therapy with interferon alpha) and also with hypernatremic states (hyperosmolar diabetic coma, hypernatremia after peritoneal lavage with saline solution), hypokalemia, hypophosphatemia, or hyperammonemia have also been reported to develop ODS (see later).

Histological characteristics of ODS include symmetric, midline demyelinating lesions in the pons and/or extrapontine areas (mostly in the bundles of myelinated fibers in the gray matter and in the white matter surrounded by massive gray matter, including the cerebellar and neocortical white/gray matter junctional areas, thalamus and striatum, and even hippocampus), loss of oligodendrocytes, reactive glial cell infiltration, and relative preservation of axonal fibers. More recently, lesions in the spinal cord have also been described.

Proposed hypotheses concerning the developmental mechanism of ODS also include osmotic injury to the endothelium resulting in myelinotoxic factors, or vasogenic edema and brain dehydration resulting in separation of the axon from its myelin sheath with resultant injury of oligodendrocytes, particularly at interfaces of gray and white matter; more recent studies imply other mechanisms such as decreased concentration of Na^+,K^+-ATPase in endothelial cell membrane in hyponatremia complicated by hypokalemia, and particular vulnerability of oligodendrocytes to apoptosis. A detrimental role of secondary inflammation, microglial activation, and finally demyelination has also been proposed. Massive accumulation of microglia that express proinflammatory cytokines and complement activation in the demyelinative lesions, following blood–brain barrier disruption, have been noticed in animal models. The role of microglia in ODS is time dependent and its detrimental activity manifests during the early phase after rapid correction of osmolarity, while astrocytes play a protective role in the late phase. Based on this observation, therapeutic modulation of excessive proinflammatory responses in microglia during the early phase of the disorder might represent a therapeutic target for ODS.

Clinical features

As chronic hyponatremia is the most frequent condition associated with ODS, the first step in the diagnosis is the recognition of the predisposing risk factors for these electrolyte derangements. As we have mentioned, the first patients described with ODS were chronic alcoholic patients; the association with alcoholism continues to be particularly frequent (in up to 40% of cases), probably because alcohol itself interferes with sodium/water regulation by suppression of antidiuretic hormone (ADH), and also because these patients often have inadequate nutrition or have profound hyponatremia caused by the combined effects of potomania associated with multiple drugs (such as thiazide diuretics and serotonin reuptake inhibitors) and hypovolemia. ODS has also been reported in patients with alcohol withdrawal without hyponatremia. Other reported risk factors associated with ODS are hyperosmolar hyperglycemia (even though

International Neurology, Second edition. Edited by Robert P. Lisak, Daniel D. Truong, William M. Carroll and Roongroj Bhidayasiri
© 2016 John Wiley & Sons, Ltd. Published 2016 by John Wiley & Sons, Ltd.

ODS is rare in diabetes mellitus, despite the frequent electrolyte derangements), liver disease and liver transplantation, sepsis, acute necrotic-hemorrhagic pancreatitis, correction of hypophosphatemia related to refeeding syndrome in the context of mental anorexia or other pathology in children, correction of hyperammonemia in a case of ornithine transcarbamylase deficiency, severe hypokalemia with metabolic acidosis as in type 1 renal tubular acidosis, gastroenteritis with repeated vomiting, adrenal insufficiency, the syndrome of inappropriate secretion of ADH (and the etiological conditions generating this syndrome), postpartum pituitary hemorrhage, surgery for sellar and suprasellar tumors inducing different pathophysiological mechanisms (diabetes insipidus, inappropriate secretion of ADH, central adrenal insufficiency), dehydration and electrolyte disturbance due to hyperemesis gravidarum, amyotrophic lateral sclerosis, use of antineoplastic agents such as cyclophosphamide, or drugs such as angiotensin-converting enzyme inhibitors and thiazide diuretics. Anorexia nervosa represents a particular condition in which serum electrolyte abnormalities are attributable to malnutrition, excessive water intake, or laxative and/or diuretic misuse followed by medical rapid correction. Although hemodialysis has been reported as a risk factor for ODS, the frequency of this association is much less than one would expect, probably because urea is acting in renal failure as an "ineffective solute" that contributes to measured osmolarity, but does not contribute to hypertonicity because it easily crosses cell membranes, thus protecting from the rapid shifts in sodium content. Also, in some cases complicated by neurological disturbances suspected to be due to ODS, the magnetic resonance imaging (MRI) examination noted on apparent diffusion coefficient (ADC) map changes, suggestive for interstitial brain edema (increased ADC) associated with first hemodialysis. It is important to mention that the clinical manifestations of ODS usually develop after a delay of some days (on average 4–6 days) after changes in sodium levels.

The classic presentation of ODS is related to its most frequent topographic location of lesions in the CNS: the central pons. The most suggestive clinical manifestations are dysphagia, dysarthria, ophthalmoplegia, and focal or generalized weakness, progressing to quadriplegia and neurocognitive changes. Less frequently, the central pons involvement generates a clinical picture of "locked-in" syndrome.

Extrapontine demyelinating lesions (usually but not always associated with central pontine involvement) have been described as having clinical manifestations in about 10% of cases, including ataxia, parkinsonism, athetosis, dystonia, secondary tics associated with ODS, confusion, behavioral or personality changes, hallucinations, seizures, catatonia, and akinetic mutism, depending on the areas involved. Extrapyramidal symptoms are sometimes masked by pyramidal tract lesions and brainstem dysfunction. Symptoms may progress over days, and in severe cases may lead to coma or death or survival in a prolonged vegetative state, sometimes accompanied by attacks of myoclonus. Movement disorders and cognitive problems resulting from ODS affecting the basal ganglia may occur early in the course of the illness, or may present as delayed manifestations after the patient survives the acute phase.

In contrast to the classic view concerning the prognosis of ODS, the possibilities offered by modern imaging techniques have shown that there are also patients with a favorable evolution, with clinical improvement during the months after the acute stage of the disease, and also in many cases accompanied by remission of the lesions detected by MRI. There are more cases reported with movement disorders sequelae after ODS, as parkinsonism, dystonia, or myoclonus associated or not with cognitive disorders. Of particular interest is the observation that the parkinsonism after ODS is usually dopa responsive.

Investigations

Modern non-invasive imaging techniques, in particular MRI, supersede the auditory evoked potentials that were used before the implementation of computed tomography (CT) in clinical practice. Today, brain MRI is the imaging technique of choice, because it has a net superiority over CT for the demonstration of lesions in central pons, but especially of the extrapontine osmotic demyelinating lesions. These are hyperintense on T2- and hypointense on T1-weighted images. It is important to note that the appearance of MRI lesions can be significantly delayed, which implies in some cases the necessity to repeat the investigation after 10–14 days. Bilateral signal changes in the MRI may be seen in other conditions too: perinatal hypoxic-ischemic injury, carbon monoxide poisoning, and metabolic disorders. Patchy multifocal signal change may also be seen in acute demyelinating encephalomyelitis, Creutzfeldt–Jakob disease and other encephalitis, small vessel disease, inflammatory microangiopathies, and mitochondrial diseases. Diffusion-weighted imaging (DWI) might have the capability of detecting the lesions not detected on T2. DWI could in some cases differentiate between demyelinating lesions and vasogenic edema; in other conditions such as ODS and posterior reversible encephalopathy syndrome, DWI could only differentiate in correlation with the clinical etiopathogenic context.

Treatment

As ODS usually develops after aggressive treatment of hyponatremia by any method, including water restriction, treatment should be extremely cautious, especially when hyponatremia has lasted for more than 48 hours. There is no consensus about the optimal treatment of symptomatic hyponatremia, but a 5% increase in serum sodium concentration, not exceeding 12 mmol/L per day, could be recommended as a guiding target on an individual basis. New data suggest that reintroduction of hyponatremia in those patients who have undergone inadvertent rapid correction of the serum sodium and corticosteroids could be beneficial in prevention of ODS. Reinduction of hyponatremia seems to be effective in treating ODS if started immediately after diagnosis.

Concerning the treatment of ODS, there are no clinical trials. Currently, there is no standard therapy other than supportive therapy. Supportive treatment is all that can be recommended with certainty. Other therapy includes steroids, plasma exchange, IVIg, and thyrotropin-releasing factor, but these therapies have not been shown to be particularly effective. Combined saline solution and desmopressin might be a reasonable strategy for correcting severe hyponatremia, but studies comparing this regimen with other therapeutic strategies are needed. In a recent experimental rat model of ODS, treatment with minocycline significantly decreased brain demyelination, alleviated neurological manifestations, and reduced mortality associated with rapid correction of hyponatremia.

Further reading

de Souza A. Movement disorders and the osmotic demyelination syndrome. *Parkinsonism Relat Disord* 2013;19(8):709–716.

Huq S, Wong M, Chan H, Crimmins D. Osmotic demyelination syndromes: Central and extrapontine myelinolysis. *J Clin Neurosci* 2007;14(7):684–688.

King JD, Rosner MH. Osmotic demyelination syndrome. *Am J Med Sci* 2010; 339(6):561–567.

Martin RJ. Central pontine and extrapontine myelinolysis: The osmotic demyelination syndromes. *J Neurol Neurosurg Psychiatry* 2004;75(Suppl 3):22–28.

Ruiz-Sandoval JL, Chiquete E, Alvarez-Palazuelos LE, Andrade-Ramos MA, Rodríguez-Rubio LR. Atypical forms of the osmotic demyelination syndrome. *Acta Neurol Belg* 2013;113(1):19–23.

95 Concentric sclerosis (Baló's disease)

Takeshi Tabira

Department of Diagnosis, Prevention and Treatment of Dementia, Juntendo University, Tokyo, Japan

Concentric sclerosis is a demyelinating disease of the central nervous system (CNS), which is characterized by the annual ring-like alternating pattern of demyelinating and myelin-preserved regions. The first case showing such lesions was reported by Otto Marburg in 1906 as "akute multiple Sklerose." Twenty years later, a similar case was reported by Joseph Baló as "encephalitis periaxialis concentrica." Because of the pathological characteristics, it is now widely accepted as concentric sclerosis or Baló's concentric sclerosis (disease). Although it is a rare condition worldwide, increased prevalence was observed several decades ago in the Philippines.

Epidemiology

Concentric sclerosis abruptly disappeared from the Philippines in the late 1990s. In previously pathologically verified cases, the age of onset was 19–49 years (mean 32.5 years) and the male-to-female ratio was 1:1.8. The prevalence of the disease did not vary seasonally or geographically and no environmental factors have been associated with its development.

Pathophysiology

Seventeen autopsy cases were collected in the Philippines from 1981–99. All cases showed the typical concentric pattern of demyelination (Figure 95.1). Histological studies demonstrate both demyelination and some axonal damage. Perivascular cuffs were seen in active demyelinating areas in one study and inflammatory cells including CD4, CD8, T-cells, and macropaghes are also observed. It has been suggested by some researchers that there are similarities between lesions observed in Baló's concentric sclerosis and the type III lesions characteristic of relapsing–remitting multiple sclerosis (RRMS).

Clinical features

Prodromal symptoms and signs such as fever and headache were present in 8 of 14 patients with documents 4–30 days prior to onset of the disease. Reticence (muteness), urinary incontinence, and pyramidal signs were present in all patients. Generalized seizure was observed in 4 out of 16 cases. All cases except for one showed acute onset of the disease and died during the acute stage without showing any remission. One case showed a relapse 4 years after the first attack, and died on the 28th day of the second attack. Ten patients died of secondary infections such as pneumonia and sepsis. It is

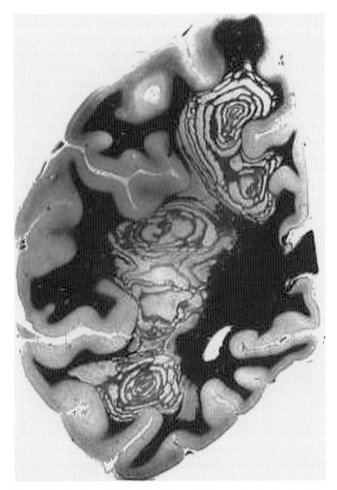

Figure 95.1 Section of brain stained for myelin demonstrating the typical pattern of demyelination in Baló's concentric sclerosis.

interesting to note that four cases died of brain herniation. Duration of the illness was 5 days to 8 months (mean 2.38 months), except for the one case that relapsed. There are some atypical presentations, but the clinical course, although not the pathology, is similar to what is now often called Marburg's variant of MS, a rapidly progressive "acute MS." The relationship between Baló's disease, particularly as described in the Philippines, Marburg's acute MS, and Baló-like lesions in more typical MS is not clear.

International Neurology, Second edition. Edited by Robert P. Lisak, Daniel D. Truong, William M. Carroll and Roongroj Bhidayasiri
© 2016 John Wiley & Sons, Ltd. Published 2016 by John Wiley & Sons, Ltd.

Investigations

Laboratory findings
Cerebrospinal fluid (CSF) findings were subtle. White blood cells (WBCs) were increased in 5 out of 15 cases, and the highest count was 59/mm^3. Total protein was also mildly elevated (44–100 mg/dL) in 5 of the 15 cases. WBCs in the peripheral blood were elevated in 10 of the 15 cases, but this was thought to be due to secondary infections.

Imaging
MRI scans can be suggestive of concentric sclerosis with large lesions that enhance in layers and are inhomogenous on T2-weighted images. Although such lesions are highly suggestive of this disease, other conditions such as infections or tumors must be ruled out.

Treatment
There have been no large series and no controlled clinical trials. Treatment with corticosteroids has been reported to have some effect in case reports/small series.

Further reading
Baló J. Encephalitis periaxialis concentrica. *Acta Neurol Psychiat* 1928;19:242–264.

Kuroiwa Y. Concentric sclerosis. In: Koetsier JC (ed.). *Demyelinating Diseases*. Amsterdam: Elsevier; 1985:409–417.

Marburg O. Die sogenannte "akute multiple sklerose" (encephalomyelitis periaxialis scleroticans). *J Psychiatr Neurol* 1906;27:217–312.

Matsouka T, Suzuki SO, Iwaki T, *et al*. Aquaporin-4 astrocytopathy in Baló's disease. *Acta Neuropathol* 2010;120:651–660.

Stadelmann C, Ludwin S, Tabira T, *et al*. Tissue preconditioning may explain concentric lesions in Baló's type of multiple sclerosis. *Brain* 2005;128:979–987.

PART 11   Specific Toxicities and Deficiencies

96   Neurotoxicology

Chin-Chang Huang and Nai-Shin Chu
Department of Neurology, Chang Gung University College of Medicine and Chang Gung Memorial Hospital, Taipei, Taiwan

Neurotoxicity deals with the adverse effects on the structure and/or function of the nervous system that are caused by exposure to chemical, biological, or physical agents. These neurotoxic effects are manifest at many levels of neuronal organization, leading to a disorder or disease.

Hundreds of agents are recognized as having neurotoxic potential in humans. These agents may have direct or indirect effects on the nervous system. The nervous system is particularly vulnerable because it has a complex structure and function, it has a prolonged period of development, and even after maturation it is very active and has a high metabolic demand. Therefore, the nervous system's vulnerability to toxic agents depends heavily on its developmental state and the postdevelopmental functional specialization.

According to Schaumburg, there are five well-recognized sources of postnatal human neurotoxic disorders: (1) pharmaceutical agents; (2) biological neurotoxic agents; (3) environmental chemical exposure; (4) occupational chemical exposure; and (5) self-administration of harmful agents. Therefore, many disorders are not necessarily caused by occupational or environmental exposure, but are patient initiated. Clinicians should be aware of these possibilities when dealing with neurotoxic diseases.

The chapter is divided into 12 sections: heavy metal intoxication, organic solvents or compounds, gases, pesticides, defoliant agents, animal toxins, plant toxins, bacterial toxins, illicit drugs, specific drugs, hypervitaminosis, and regionally specific toxicities.

Heavy metal intoxication

Arsenic

Exposure to potentially toxic levels of arsenic may occur from drinking contaminated groundwater, working in mining and ore-smelting plants, accidental ingestion of pesticides, and, infamously, intentional poisonings. Most cases of acute arsenic poisoning are due to accidental ingestion of pesticides or insecticides, or by inhalation in occupational settings.

Both neuropathy and encephalopathy are common manifestations of acute arsenic exposure. Clinical features may include nausea, vomiting, bloody diarrhea, dizziness, diffuse muscle weakness, numbness, and paresthesia of the distal extremities. Respiratory symptoms can be seen in cases of inhalation exposure. Hypotension, cardiac arrhythmias, myoglobulinuria, and acute renal failure are not infrequent. In severe cases, seizures, coma, and death may follow.

Chronic encephalopathy is more common after exposure to organic arsenic than to inorganic arsenic. The symptoms may include confusion, irritability, paranoid delusions, and auditory or visual hallucinations.

The neuropathy is a painful, axonal, length-dependent, sensory polyneuropathy affecting all extremities. Symptoms usually begin 2–3 weeks after initial exposure and start with pain in the distal lower extremities, eventually involving the distal upper extremities. Subsequently, generalized muscle weakness and muscle wasting develop.

Systemic abnormalities that may provide important clues to the diagnosis include weight loss, severe hyperkeratosis, alopecia, and white horizontal lines on the nails (Mees' lines). Diagnosis can be confirmed by detecting elevated arsenic levels in the blood, urine, hair, or nail clippings.

Standard treatment consists of cessation of continued arsenic exposure and removal of arsenic by use of sulfur chelators, including dimercaptosuccinic acid or D-penicillamine.

Lead

Due to its extensive commercial use, lead has historically been one of the most common sources of heavy metal intoxication. Lead toxicity may occur from occupational exposure – that is, metal soldering, ore smelting, battery manufacturing, or industrial painting – or from non-occupational exposure, including accidental ingestion of lead paint by children, or exposure to contaminated water and foods. Children are at particular risk from oral ingestion of paint chips or contaminated soil.

Characteristic systemic features of lead poisoning are abdominal pain, constipation, and a microcytic, hypochromic anemia. In general, peripheral neuropathy is commonly seen in adults, whereas acute lead encephalopathy is most common in children.

The peripheral neuropathy of lead toxicity is a motor-predominant neuropathy affecting the upper limbs more than the lower limbs, presenting as a symmetric or asymmetric wrist drop. The weakness may also involve other muscle groups of the distal upper extremities. Involvement of lower extremities, including isolated foot drop, also may occur.

International Neurology, Second edition. Edited by Robert P. Lisak, Daniel D. Truong, William M. Carroll and Roongroj Bhidayasiri
© 2016 John Wiley & Sons, Ltd. Published 2016 by John Wiley & Sons, Ltd.

Electrophysiological studies reveal a wide range of abnormalities, from mild motor conduction slowing to denervation, indicating axonal involvement. Nerve biopsy reveals increased paranodal demyelination and internodal remyelination in mild-to-moderate neuropathies, and axonal degeneration in advanced neuropathies.

Symptoms of acute lead encephalopathy include lethargy, irritability, confusion, ataxia, and impaired motor functions. Chronic low-level lead exposure also causes encephalopathy. The symptoms are similar to those of acute lead toxicity, but the onset is insidious. The long-term effects of chronic low-level lead exposure have especially devastating effects on the still-developing nervous system of young children. Occasionally a subgingival "lead" line may be seen and a dense "lead line" in the metaphysical plate appears in long bone X-ray, particularly in children.

Laboratory diagnostic indicators of lead toxicity include elevated blood lead level, decreased blood delta-aminolevulinic acid (ALA-D), and basophilic stippling on blood smear.

Treatment requires eliminating continued exposure and initiating therapy to enhance excretion with chelating agents, such as ethylenediaminetetraacetic acid (EDTA), D-penicillamine, and British antilewisite.

Manganese

Manganese was initially used by the Egyptians and Romans in the manufacture of glass and ceramic. Today, it is widely employed in industry, primarily in the manufacture of steel and alloys. Several hundred cases of manganese poisoning have been reported, not only from mining regions of Chile, Egypt, Cuba, Morocco, India, and China, but also from industrial countries processing this metal for metal alloys, dry-cell batteries, paints, varnish, enamel, colored glass, and an antiknock agent in lead-free gasoline. Rarely, central nervous system (CNS) manganism occurs in agricultural workers who have chronic exposure to fungicide containing manganese.

The history of manganese neurotoxicity dates back to 1837, when Couper of Glasgow first reported a peculiar neurological syndrome somewhat similar to Parkinson's disease in five men working in a manganese ore-crushing plant in France. This report of "manganese crusher's disease" appeared only 20 years after Parkinson's essay on the shaking palsy in 1817.

Chronic manganese toxicity causes an extrapyramidal syndrome with features resembling those found in Parkinson's disease, Wilson's disease, and postencephalitic parkinsonism.

The clinical course of manganism can be divided into three phases: an initial phase of subjective symptoms, with or without a psychotic episode, lasting for a few months; an intermediate phase of evolving neurological symptoms, again for a few months; and an established phase with persisting neurological deficits. The onset is usually insidious and progressive. In general, miners have more severe neurological deficits than victims of other types of exposure.

The initial symptoms are usually subjective and non-specific, and may include fatigue, restlessness, headache, poor memory, reduced concentration, apathy, insomnia, diminished libido, somnolence, lumbago, muscle aches and cramps, and a generalized slowing of movement. Usually seen in miners, an episode of psychomotor excitement can be among the presenting symptoms, which include nervousness, irritability, nightmare, emotional lability, aggressive and destructive behavior, and bizarre compulsive acts. It has been referred to as *locura manganica* or "manganese madness."

In the intermediate phase, speech becomes monotonous, low in volume, halting, and sometimes stuttering; the face is expressionless with dazed appearance and intermittent grimace; handwriting can become tremulous, micrographic, and cramped; movements are generally slow and clumsy; gait is most impaired, body turn tends to be "*en bloc*," and walking backward is particularly difficult.

In the established phase, there is aggravation of neurological deficits and walking difficulty becomes more pronounced. A peculiar wide-based slapping gait and dystonic posturing of the foot with sustained plantar flexion may be seen and is termed "cock-walk" or "peacock gait" (Figure 96.1).

Inability to walk backward because of severe retropulsion is generally the most striking feature. Tremor is not a common finding, but when it does occur, it is usually postural rather than resting, and of low amplitude. Dystonic features are common, and tend to involve the face and foot.

Neurological deficits tend to become established 1–2 years after onset of the disease. Thereafter, neurological deficits may remain stable or improve following cessation of exposure, or continue to progress, even after elimination of the source of exposure. In our

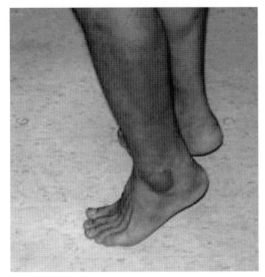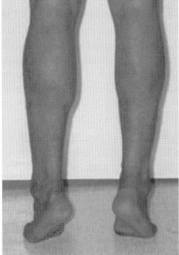

Figure 96.1 "Cock walk" posture and foot dystonia. Note that the patient walks on the metatarsopharyngeal joints.

long-term, 20-year follow-up study, neurological symptoms continued to progress in the first 10 years and then stabilized in the second 10 years.

Manganese concentrations in the blood, urine, scalp hair, and pubic hair are usually high, ranging from 3–300 times higher as compared with non-exposed normal controls in a few weeks to months, but may return to normal 1–3 years later.

Neuropathological studies, although few, have consistently shown that the hallmark is degeneration of the basal ganglia, principally confined to the medial segment of the globus pallidus and the pars reticulata of the substantia nigra. The putamen and the caudate nuclei are often affected, but to a lesser degree.

Because manganese has a paramagnetic quality and causes a shortening of the proton T1 relaxation time, signal intensities are increased symmetrically in the globus pallidus (GP) and midbrain, particularly the substantia nigra pars reticularis (SNr) on T1-weighted brain magnetic resonance imaging (MRI) in patients with manganism and in non-human primates with experimental manganese poisoning. Signals on the brain MRI are commonly increased, with a frequency of 41.6% in exposed workers. In addition, the hyperintensity lesions may resolve 6 months to 1 year after cessation of exposure. Many workers who do not have any clinical symptoms may have hyperintensities in the brain MRI. Therefore, increased signal intensities on T1-weighted images may reflect exposure to or accumulation of manganese, but not necessarily manganism.

Our positron emission tomography (PET) studies, employing 6-fluorodopa to investigate the integrity of the dopaminergic nigrostraital pathways and D2 receptor ligand raclopride to investigate dopaminergic postsynaptic function, show generally normal or slightly impaired dopaminergic function. Our recent study on dopamine transporter binding using 99mTc-TRODAT-1 single photon emission computed tomography (SPECT) also reveals only a slight decrease of the uptake in the putamen in patients with manganism when compared to normal subjects, indicating that presynaptic dopaminergic terminals are not the main target of chronic manganese intoxication.

Experimental studies with rhesus monkeys were conducted by injecting intravenous (IV) manganese chloride at weekly intervals for 2–3 months. These monkeys developed a parkinsonian syndrome characterized by bradykinesia, rigidity, and facial dystonia, but no tremors. They did not respond to levodopa. Autopsy demonstrated that the gliosis was confined to the GP and the SNr. Mineral deposits in the perivascular region were found in the GP and SNr. The mineral deposits were composed of iron and aluminum. These studies demonstrated that manganese primarily damaged the GP and SNr, and relatively spared the nigrostriatal dopaminergic system.

Although levodopa has been shown to be effective in some reports, others have failed to detect a meaningful improvement.

Mercury

Neurological damage may occur in adults and children after poisoning with mercury compounds due to occupational exposure to fungicides containing organic mercury, ingestion of grain treated with these fungicides, or consumption of fish and shellfish contaminated by industrial wastes containing organic mercury (Minamata disease). Rarely, poisoning may result from inhalation of elementary mercury vapor in factories reprocessing mercury batteries or in glass blowers.

Mercury exists in elemental, organic, and inorganic forms. It is the only metal that is in a liquid state in its elemental form. The inorganic form may be classified in accordance with the oxidative state of the metal, whereas the organic form may covalently bind to an organic (carbon-containing) moiety, either as arylmercury or alkylmercury. The arylmercury is readily degraded into inorganic mercury ions in the biological system, whereas the alkylmercury is relatively stable and resists biodegradation.

Various forms of mercury are found in household items, manufacturing products, and water supplies. Among them, elementary mercury vapor and alkylmercury compounds are considered to be most neurotoxic.

Elemental mercury

Metallic mercury vaporizes readily even at room temperature. When inhaled, mercury vapor is efficiently absorbed through the alveolar membrane and has high affinity for the CNS, especially the gray matter of the occipital cortex, cerebellum, and various nuclei of the brainstem.

Prolonged exposure to mercury vapor, generally due to occupational exposure, produces "battery refiner's disease" in workers reprocessing mercury batteries. This consists of a fairly well-defined neuropsychiatric syndrome usually called erethism, including fatigue, tremor, poor memory, cognitive impairment, social withdrawal, excitability, personality change, and emotional lability. In more severe cases, a fine trembling tremor appears in the fingers, tongue, eyelids, and lips. In addition, there is a progressive and incapacitating movement disorder consisting of titubation, truncal ataxia, generalized tremor, and multifocal myoclonus. The visual field may be constricted. The combination of increased excitability, tremor, and gingivitis has been thought of as the classic triad of chronic mercury exposure.

Inorganic mercury salts

Human mercurous mercury poisoning is mainly due to the use of calomel in children's teething powder in the early twentieth century. Because of the redness of the hands and feet, it is referred to as "pink disease." Symptoms include acrodynia, photophobia, profuse sweating, anorexia, and insomnia. However, the primary target for mercuric salts is the kidney.

Neurotoxicity from mercury salts is usually not prominent, although prolonged exposure to mercuric oxide and mercuric nitrate may result in "mad hatter syndrome," which historically affected workers in the felt hat industry. This syndrome is similar to that observed in mercury vapor poisoning.

Inorganic mercury intoxication also can induce peripheral neuropathy. Electrophysiological studies revealed axonal polyneuropathy involving both motor and sensory fibers. Sural nerve biopsy demonstrates axonal degeneration with demyelination and a predominant loss of large myelinated fibers.

Organomercury compounds

The most neurotoxic of the mercury compounds are methylmercury and ethylmercury, and the most notorious poisoning was the massive outbreak of methylmercury intoxication in Japan in the 1950s. This is called "Minamata disease" because it occurred in Minamata Bay, Kumamoto, due to industrial dumping of mercury-containing waste into the water supply. After entering the water, mercury was methylated by micro-organisms and in turn ingested by aquatic species – that is, fish and shellfish – which were finally consumed by humans.

Outbreaks have occurred also following the use of methyl mercury as a fungicide in 1940 by Hunter and Russels, and in Pakistan and Iraq, because intoxication occurs if treated seed for planting is eaten instead by humans.

Neurological manifestations of methylmercury toxicity are paresthesia, tremor, ataxia, spasticity, visual and hearing loss, and encephalopathy. Visual field loss usually affects the periphery and central vision is spared. Funnel vision is more common than tunnel vision. Other features are ataxia, chorea, athetosis, ballismus-like movements, and coarse tremor. Cognitive and memory deficits may be present. In severe cases, coma and death may occur.

The pathological hallmark of mercury poisoning is severe damage affecting the visual cortex and the granule cell layer of the cerebellum. In the cerebral cortex, degeneration and loss of neurons with gliosis are found particularly in the precentral and postcentral gyri. Damage to the basal ganglia, especially the putamen, is frequent and usually moderate to severe, but may be minimal.

Organic solvents or compounds

Acrylamide

Acrylamide, a water-soluble vinyl monomer, is an important industrial compound and has been widely used in chemical industries, including polyacrylamides such as flocculants for waste-water treatment, cosmetics, soil stabilization, adhesives and grouts, and polyacrylamide gels in molecular laboratories.

Acrylamide monomer can be absorbed via inhalation, ingestion, and skin exposures, and is toxic to the peripheral nervous system (PNS) and CNS, while the acrylamide polymer is not. Numbness, muscle weakness in the distal limbs, and diffuse hyporeflexia or areflexia are experienced in the initial stage of acute intoxication. Action or intention tremor and a wide-based gait are common early signs. Excessive sweating, peeling skin, and contact dermatitis are frequently found.

Motor nerve conduction studies are characterized by mild abnormalities with reduced motor conduction velocities, while sensory nerve conduction studies are almost abnormal, particularly in the sensory nerve action potentials. The reduction of amplitudes is the most common early abnormality. Recent quantitative electrophysiological field studies indicate that significant differences in the vibratory thresholds of index fingers and great toes are noted between acrylamide-exposed workers and healthy controls.

Previously, distal axonopathy has been considered in acrylamide intoxication based on the observation that there is distal swelling and degeneration of large myelinated axons in both PNS and CNS. The fundamental axonal change is an accumulation of 10 nm neurofilaments. In recent animal studies, acrylamide-intoxicated rats showed ataxia, hindlimb weakness, foot splay, and autonomic dysfunction. In the peripheral nerves, axonal degeneration is an epiphenomenon related to long-term low-dose intoxication. With exposure to a higher dose of acrylamide for a shorter duration, nerve terminal dysfunction and degeneration are noted in electrophysiological, neurochemical, and morphological studies. In particular, recent animal studies have shown that nerve terminals are the primary site of intoxication in both the CNS and PNS, and that acrylamide produces a terminal neuropathy, not an axonopathy. In immunohistochemical studies of human skin biopsies, acrylamide also induces degeneration of small-diameter sensory nerves, with epidermal nerve swelling in the early stage and a progressive loss of epidermal nerves in the late stage.

In addition, acrylamide disrupts presynaptic function via decreased release of neurotransmitters. Evidence also suggests that acrylamide may cause changes in thiol groups of proteins that are critically involved in the synaptic vesicle-membrane fusion and recycling.

Carbon disulfide

Carbon disulfide (CS_2) is a colorless liquid organic solvent at room temperature and is used in the production of viscose rayon fibers and cellophane films. Acute exposure to large amounts of CS_2 may cause narcosis, psychosis with delirium, seizure, mental impairment, and even death. In chronic exposure or repeated low-dose exposure to CS_2, there may be polyneuropathy, parkinsonism, intention tremor, and neuropsychological symptoms, such as sleep disturbance, depression, decreased concentration, and impotence.

Peripheral neuropathy induced by CS_2 includes distal muscle weakness, paresthesia, a glove-and-stocking-like sensory impairment, and decreased or absent tendon reflexes. Electrophysiological studies show a reduction of compound muscle action potentials, prolonged distal latencies, and slowed nerve conduction velocities. The pathological studies on sural nerve biopsy reveal a decrease of fiber density, relative loss of large myelinated fibers, and degeneration of both axon and myelin. In animal studies, multiple axonal swelling with secondary demyelination develops in the node of Ranvier region. Electron microscopic examination reveals an accumulation of neurofilaments that is very similar to that with n-hexane, methyl n-butyl ketone, or acrylamide intoxication.

After exposure to moderate amounts of CS_2 for a few months, symptoms of manic-depressive psychosis, hallucination, and suicidal behavior may appear. Subsequently depressive mood is accompanied by tremor, incoordination, ataxia, and memory impairment. Following long-term exposure, there may be pyramidal tract symptoms and parkinsonism, with cogwheel rigidity, bradykinesia, and loss of balance.

Long-term exposure to CS_2 may lead to an increase in mortality due to coronary artery diseases, bradycardia, tachycardia, and/or other arrhythmias. Laboratory studies reveal an increase in β-lipoprotein, total cholesterol, triglyceride, and low density β-lipoprotein cholesterol. In addition, cerebral vascular diseases with multiple infarctions and reduced regional blood flow in the brain are observed (Figure 96.2). Long-term exposure to CS_2 may also impair the vision, including optic neuropathy, absent pupillary and corneal reflexes, retinal hemorrhage, and other retinal changes. A small vessel vasculopathy may be responsible.

The carbamide 2-mercapto-2-thiazolinone-5, 2-thiothiazolidine-4-carboxylic acid (TTCA) is the most important metabolite in CS_2 intoxication. TTCA in the urine has been generally used as a biomarker of exposure. The level of urinary TTCA can reflect the previous day's exposure.

The natural course of illness in patients with CS_2 exposure has been rarely studied. In a few long-term follow-up studies, persistent damage to the peripheral nerves was noted even after CS_2 exposure had ceased for 3 years. Exposure to CS_2 may induce parkinsonian features that may be confused with idiopathic Parkinson's disease. However, dopamine transporter studies with ^{99m}Tc-TRDAT-1 brain SPECT show normal uptake in CS_2-parkinsonism patients. In addition, the CS_2-induced parkinsonism and cerebellar damage cannot be recovered even with levadopa treatment.

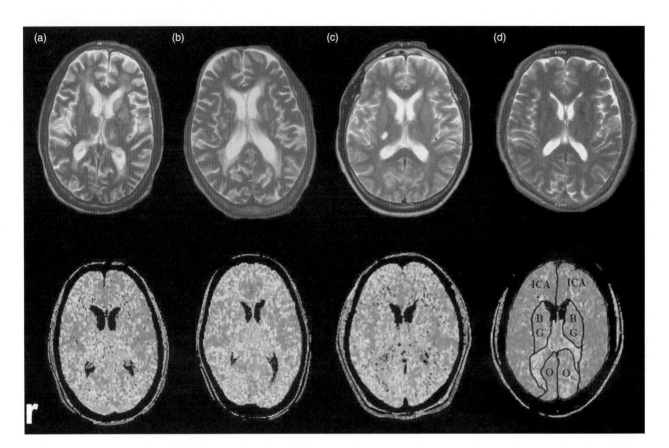

Figure 96.2 Brain MRI changes in carbon disulfide (CS_2) intoxication. (A) (Top) Brain MRI findings on T2 weighted images in three patients with CS_2 intoxication (a–c) and a normal control (d) showing multiple high signal intensity lesions in the subcortical white matter and basal ganglia. (B) (Bottom) Brain CT perfusion scan with a regional mean transit time (MTT) map in three patients with CS2 intoxication (a–c) and a normal control (d) showing a statistically significant prolongation of MTT in the brain parenchymal area and the basal ganglia. (BG = basal ganglia; ICA = internal carotid artery; O = occipital area). For color details, please refer to the color plates section.

N-hexane and methyl-n-butyl ketone

N-hexane is an aliphatic hexacarbon and an organic solvent. It has been widely used in many industrial processes, particularly in the production of glues, paints, adhesives, coating products, laminating plastics, press proofing, cleaning agents, shoes, leather, furniture, and vulcanizing procedures.

Exposure to n-hexane may cause a subacute onset and progressive course of axonal polyneuropathy in humans, involving both motor and sensory fibers in the distal extremities. N-hexane is also present in certain glues and cements. Therefore n-hexane-induced polyneuropathy also has been found in those who sniff glue for recreation. Common symptoms include distal numbness, muscle weakness, and muscle wasting in the intrinsic muscles of the hand and foot. A loss of pin-prick, temperature, touch, vibratory, and position sensations is usually accompanied by diminished ankle jerks. In severely intoxicated patients, weight loss, anorexia, abdominal pain, and muscle cramps are also found. Some glue sniffers with high and prolonged exposure may develop dysarthria, swallowing difficulty, blurred vision, and autonomic disturbances. Hyperhidrosis or anhidrosis, blue discoloration, impotence, and reduced temperature of the distal limbs have been reported in patients with moderate or severe glue sniffing.

In patients with severe n-hexane intoxication, nerve action potentials usually cannot be elicited, particularly in the distal peroneal nerves. In other nerves, there are prolonged distal latencies, reduced amplitudes of compound muscle action potentials and sensory nerve action potentials, and profound slowing of nerve conduction velocities. Focal conduction block with temporal dispersion may occur in some cases, indicating a demyelinating nature. There are frequent fibrillation potentials and positive sharp waves with reduced recruitment pattern. Somatosensory, brainstem auditory, and pattern-reversal visual-evoked potentials also demonstrate abnormalities in the central pathways as well as the PNS.

Nerve biopsies and postmortem pathological studies reveal giant axons with segmental demyelination in the paranodal region. In giant axons, 10 nm neurofilaments accumulate in the distal nerve fibers and spinal cord. The histograms of the sural nerve biopsy confirm a predominant loss of large myelinated fibers. In experimental studies, degeneration of myelinated fibers may also occur in the spinal cord, medulla, inferior cerebellar peduncles, and cerebellar vermis.

The neurotoxic property of n-hexane and the related substance methyl n-butyl ketone is attributable to the common gamma-diketone metabolite 2, 5-hexanedione (2, 5-HD). This is a potent neurotoxin. However, other gamma-diketones including 3, 6-octanedione can also cause neuropathy. In addition, detection of 2, 5-hexanedione in the urine has been proved to be a biological marker.

A continuous progression of the neurological features is noted one to a few months after cessation of the toxic exposure. Prognosis is generally favorable if exposure to n-hexane ceases. Patients with mild or moderate polyneuropathy usually recover completely within 1–2 years. Severely affected patients also improve but sometimes have neurological sequelae, such as mild weakness, leg spasticity, and hyperreflexia 2–3 years later.

Toluene

Toluene is a major component of glue vapor. The acute CNS effects of toluene intoxication include headache, nausea, vomiting, confusion, euphoria, hallucination, ataxia, and conscious disturbance. Chronic exposure to toluene may also induce mainly CNS manifestations such as permanent encephalopathy with cognitive disturbance, cerebellar dysfunction, optic neuropathy, and neurosensory-type hearing loss. Cerebellar dysfunction is characterized by nystagmus, unsteady gait, ataxia, and intention tremor in both hands. Behavioral toxicology study reveals that toluene can induce hyperactivity, ataxia, addiction, insomnia, and memory impairments.

In addition to the CNS manifestation, chronic progressive polyneuropathy is also common in glue sniffers. Patients may develop muscle wasting, distal numbness, and hyporeflexia or areflexia. Although polyneuropathy resulting from glue sniffing is well recognized, the glue may contain other substances such as n-hexane, methyl-n-butyl ketone, benzene, and acetone. In a few reports, toluene was reported as the sole agent to induce peripheral neuropathy.

Brain MRI shows diffuse cerebral, cerebellar, and brainstem atrophy, loss of differentiation between the gray and white matters, and increased periventricular white-matter lesions. Among the persistent neurological deficits attributed to toluene, cerebellar dysfunction is the commonest. Toluene appears to have only a low toxicity to the peripheral nerves.

Thallium

Thallium salts have been used for the treatment of many diseases, including tuberculosis, gonorrhea, syphilis, and scalp fungal infection. Recently, thallium has been utilized in the manufacturing of optical lenses, semiconductors, scintillation counters, imitation jewelry, and chemical catalysts.

Thallium toxicity generally occurs after ingestion of thallium-containing chemicals, rat poison, or contaminated foods. An outbreak of thallium poisoning was reported in California in 1932 and attributed to the use of a rodenticide for control of a ground squirrel infestation. Thallium poisoning became rare after thallium was banned from use in pesticides in the 1970s. Currently, thallium toxicity is seen only in unintentional ingestion, usually linked to intentional poisoning.

The clinical manifestations of acute thallium poisoning consist of the characteristic dermatological findings of alopecia, hyperkeratosis, and Mees' lines on the nails, as well as neurological symptoms including dysesthesia, painful neuropathy, muscle weakness, cranial nerve palsies, ataxia, tremor, convulsions, coma, and death.

Painful neuropathy is usually severe and excruciating, and is often the most prominent symptom of thallium poisoning. A debilitating encephalopathy may also occur and its symptoms may include hallucinations, paranoia, and cognitive impairment. The term "encephalopathia thallica" implies a variety of conditions, from giddiness, lack of drive, and memory impairment to a decline in intelligence and irreversible dementia. It should be pointed out that neuropathic and systemic symptoms of thallium toxicity are strikingly similar to those of arsenic poisoning. Quantitative sensory tests reveal an impairment of pin-prick, temperature, and touch sensations. Cutaneous nerve biopsy confirmed a loss of epidermal nerves, indicating an involvement of the small sensory nerves.

Electrodiagnostic and sural nerve biopsy findings are consistent with an axonal degeneration primarily of the distal nerves, involving both large and small myelinated fibers, and even unmyelinated fibers, particularly in the lower extremities.

The concentrations of thallium in the blood, urine, hair and stool may return to normal 3 months later after treatment with Prussian blue. A recent study with brain fluorodeoxyglucose positron emission tomography (^{18}FDG PET) disclosed a decreased uptake of glucose metabolism in the cingulate gyrus, bilateral frontal, and parietal lobes.

There is no specific therapy for neuropathy and encephalopathy, but gastric lavage, activated charcoal, hemoperfusion, and Prussian blue may assist in blocking further absorption and facilitating elimination.

Gases

Carbon monoxide

Carbon monoxide (CO) is a worldwide environmental toxin and a leading cause of deliberate or accidental poisoning. Acute CO intoxication may induce hypoxic encephalopathy with variable degrees of brain damage, ranging from confusion to deep coma. Although approximately one-third of patients succumb during the acute intoxication, most of the remaining patients can recover completely from the first episode. However, 0.2–40% of the survivors develop delayed encephalopathy within 2–6 weeks after pseudorecovery.

The common clinical features of CO toxicity include cognitive changes, sphincter incontinence, akinetic mutism, parkinsonism, and dystonia. Most patients have a prominent improvement after conservative treatment, particularly in sphincter incontinence and akinetic mutism, although some sequelae such as dystonia and cognitive impairment persist. The common neuroimaging changes are hyperintensity lesions in the basal ganglia, particularly in the globus pallidus and subcortical white matter (Figure 96.3). A steady improvement is also noted in the basal ganglia and subcortical white matter in serial brain MR images.

The neuropathological changes in acute CO intoxication include necrosis, ischemia, and demyelination in the globus pallidus and cerebral white matter, spongy changes in the cerebral cortex, and necrosis in the hippocampus. In delayed encephalopathy, the characteristic findings are small necrotic foci and demyelinating changes in the cerebral white matter and globus pallidus. Demyelination with relative preservation of axons is prominent in the frontal lobes. The pathogenesis of the predominant involvement of the globus pallidus remains unclear, but ischemic changes may precede irreversible changes in some patients with CO intoxication.

Recovery from acute CO intoxication usually depends on the CO concentration, duration of hypoxia, and individual variation, while the prognosis of delayed CO encephalopathy is relatively good. Immediate oxygen (O_2) administration is adequate in most patients, but occasional hyperbaric oxygen therapy may be helpful. For long-term sequelae of CO intoxication only symptomatic therapy is available.

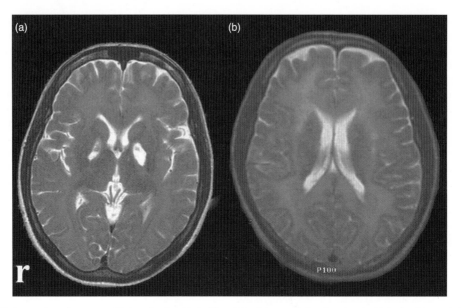

Figure 96.3 Brain MRI changes in carbon monoxide intoxication. Brain T2-weighted image studies showing the high signal intensity lesions in the bilateral basal ganglia (a) and subcortical white matter in the bilateral frontal and occipital areas (b). On image, make A read (a) and B read (b).

Hydrogen sulfide

Hydrogen sulfide (H_2S) is a noxious and toxic gas that first causes an olfactory paralysis after a short exposure to a relatively low concentration. The sudden loss of smell is thought to be responsible for unawareness of continuous exposure, which results in fatalities. The toxicity of hydrogen sulfide is thought to be mainly due to the reversible inactivation of mitochondrial cytochrome oxidase, which in turn disrupts the electron transport chain, with resultant inhibition of aerobic metabolism. Nitrites, the antidotes for cyanide poisoning, produce methemoglobin that can inactivate sulfide by competitive binding of the toxic hydrosulfide anion, and thus in turn presumably reactivate and protect cytochrome oxidase.

Hydrogen sulfide intoxication has occurred in some industrial environments, such as in the refinement and manufacturing of heavy water and the production of coal gas. It may also occur in manure storage places, in deep mines, in sewers, and even in hospital settings. Physically, the classic signs and symptoms of acute H_2S intoxication include loss of consciousness, cyanosis, repetitive tonic convulsions, conjunctivitis, respiratory depression, and circulatory collapse. The treatment of H_2S intoxication includes amyl nitrile inhalation and intravenous administration of sodium nitrile and sodium thiosulfate in addition to oxygen supply.

Nitrous oxide

Nitrous oxide (N_2O) is a stable gas commonly used as laughing gas or happy toxic gas, which has been noted to interfere with inactivation of vitamin B_{12}, a coenzyme for methionine synthase activity. It has remained one of the most commonly used anesthetics in dental applications and is also used in some non-medical areas, including the semiconductor industry, car racing, and food processing. Excessive occupational exposure to the gas in dentists has been known to cause bone marrow changes. Agranulocytosis and subacute combined degeneration developed after repeated exposure.

Nitrous oxide is administered by inhalation, absorbed by diffusion through the lungs, and illuminated via respiration. Victims exposed to high doses of N_2O may experience severe hypotension, loss of consciousness, or death. N_2O may be abused as a euphoriant among young people and can cause a toxic myeloneuropathy. The initial symptom is numbness commonly found in the distal hands and legs and combined with weakness, tightness of fingers, and gait disturbance. Neurological examinations reveal impairment of the vibration and position sensations in the fingers and toes, and decreased tendon reflexes. Romberg's sign and Lhermite's sign may also occur. In severe cases, spasticity in the legs, severe loss of vibration, position, and pin-prick sensations, and Babinski sign are found. An encephalopathy including altered consciousness, mood changes, poor concentration, memory difficulty, and intellectual decline may accompany myeloneuropathy. The clinical features may improve following cessation of exposure. Laboratory studies show megaloblastic anemia, decreased vitamin B_{12} level, and increased homocysteine level. Nerve conduction and electromyographic studies are consistent with a distal axonal motor and sensory polyneuropathy. Somatosensory evoked potential study reveals a prolongation of latency or even absence of cortical potentials following tibial and median nerve stimulation.

Withdrawal of nitrous oxide is the most important treatment in patients with N_2O poisoning. Patients may also respond to vitamin B_{12} therapy and methionine supplementation. The toxic mechanism is that N_2O may inhibit the methionine synthetase, an enzyme involved in the synthesis of methionine and tetrahydrofolate from the substrates homocysteine and methyl tetrahydrofolate.

Pesticides

Organophosphates

Organophosphates have been used in several major industries as pesticides, helminthicides, petroleum additives, modifiers of plastics, and in chemical warfare. Organophosphates can be easily absorbed through pulmonary alveoli, skin, eyes, and the gastrointestinal tract following intentional (suicidal) ingestion, accidental exposure, or homicide attempts. Most organophosphates can cause an acute cholinergic crisis via inhibition of acetylcholinesterase and then an intermediate syndrome due to blockade of neuromuscular junctions. Occasionally a delayed peripheral neuropathy may occur 2–3 weeks after exposure.

Acute effects of organophosphates are caused by slowly reversible or irreversible binding to acetylcholinesterase, leading to increased bronchial secretion, sweating, abdominal pain, and diarrhea. CNS effects include convulsions, confusion, irritability, and anxiety. Overactivity at the nicotinic receptors may produce fasciculation and muscle weakness.

The intermediate syndrome usually develops within 24–96 hours after poisoning and affects the bulbar and ocular muscles, neck flexors, proximal limb muscles, and respiratory muscles. Electromyographic studies show fade on titanic stimulation, absence of fade on low-frequency stimulation, and absence of post-titanic facilitation, indicating a postsynaptic defect. The neuromuscular function defect has been the predominant cause of the paralytic symptoms. Atropine therapy has no effect on the intermediate syndrome.

Some organophosphates can produce delayed axonopathy with muscle cramps, muscle weakness, paresthesia, and decreased or absent tendon reflexes following single exposure. The pathogenic mechanisms are inhibition and aging of the enzyme-neuropathy target esterase. The delayed neuropathy involves motor and sensory function and even myelopathy. Recovery is sometimes incomplete, with residual muscle weakness and spasticity.

Triorthocresyl phosphate (TOCP) is a lipid-soluble, oily substance and its intoxication has been found in axonal neuropathy epidemics after drinking the adulterated Jamaica ginger extract known as "Jake." Severe damage to the PNS and spinal cord has resulted in permanent "Jake leg paralysis" in the United States.

Electrophysiological studies vary during the course of exposure in the acute, intermediate, and delayed syndromes. In acute intoxication and the intermediate syndrome, an atypical decremental response to repetitive nerve stimulation can be observed. In the delayed neuropathy, nerve conduction studies show reduced sensory and motor responses, with signs of denervation.

The drug of choice in the treatment of acute muscarinic effects is atropine. Phosphorylated cholinesterase can be treated with oxime compounds such as pyrine-2-aldoxime methylchloride (2-PAM pralidoxime).

Organic tin

Triphenyl tin acetate (TPTA) is commonly used in the manufacture of plastic products and in farming due to its characteristic heat stability and bactericidal properties. It has been used to kill golden apple snails (*Pomacea canaliculata*), which have become a major pest to aquatic crops and have caused serious economic and agricultural damage. However, TPTA is toxic to the CNS as it causes interstitial edema in the subcortical white matter, and may cause pathological changes in cerebellar Purkinje's cells or limbic system structures. Attempted suicide with molluscidal agent is the main cause of intoxication. Cognitive impairments including acalculia and ataxia disorientation have been documented. In addition, delayed sensorimotor polyneuropathy has been noted, which was reversible during the follow-up period.

Defoliant toxins

2, 4-Dichlorophenoxyacetic acid

2, 4-Dichlorophenoxyacetic acid (2, 4-D) was developed during World War II and is a common systemic herbicide used for the control of broadleaf weeds. The powerful defoliant and herbicide "Agent Orange," used extensively throughout the Vietnam War, contained 2, 4-D contaminated with a form of dioxin 2, 7-dichlorodibenzo-p-dioxin (DCDO), which is toxic to the liver and a possible carcinogen. Although the chlorophenoxy herbicides may act as plant growth hormones, they have no hormonal action in humans. However, 2, 4-D may cause myopathy, myonecrosis, myoglobinuria, and possible myotonia. Several cases of distal symmetric motor-predominant polyneuropathy were reported. In addition, an epidemiological study of workers employed in the manufacture of phenoxy herbicides revealed mild abnormalities in a nerve conduction velocity study attributed to peripheral neuropathy. However, there are no reports of nerve biopsies, or long-term follow-up studies, in 2, 4-D–induced peripheral neuropathy.

Animal toxins

Marine toxins including ciguatoxin, saxitoxin, and tetrodotoxin

Ciguatoxin

Ciguatoxin is a heat-stable, lipid-soluble compound elaborated by the photosynthetic dinoflagellates *Gambierdiscus toxiques*. The toxin can accumulate in the flesh of certain marine fish such as grouper or snapper. The toxin can cause neurological, gastrointestinal, cardiac, and autonomic dysfunction known as ciguatera, which is the most common food-borne illness in some areas. Ciguatoxin is usually characterized by neurological dysfunction including paresthesia in the four limbs and perioral region within 6–12 hours and gastrointestinal symptoms. "Dry-ice" phenomenon is highly characteristic of ciguatera, in which cold is misperceived as hot. Generalized weakness, sensory impairment, and gait disturbance may persist for months. Cardiovascular instability associated with hypotension and bradycardia occurs less frequently. Neurological dysfunction is the most common cause of morbidity, including weakness, pain, and sensory dysfunction. Occasionally, cerebellar dysfunction, myopathy, retrobulbar pain, and urinary frequency can occur. No specific antidote exists, and treatment is usually symptomatic. Atropine may combat bradycardia and hypotension. Amitriptyline can ameliorate paresthesia and pain. Intravenous mannitol within 2 days of ingestion can decrease the acute morbidity of ciguatera due to a reduction in intracellular edema.

Puffer fish

The puffer fish, or fugu in Japanese, has become well known in tales of fatal poisoning after ingestion of improperly prepared fugu, which is an expensive Japanese delicacy. There are 100–200 cases of puffer fish poisoning each year in Japan. The poisoning comes from tetrodotoxin, which is highly concentrated in the viscera (particularly the liver and ovaries) of the tetrodontiform fishes, including puffer fish (*Fugu poecilonotus*) and porcupine fish (*Diodon hystrix*).

Tetrodotoxin is an exceptionally potent voltage-gated sodium channel blocker, and the organs that contain sodium channels are affected. They include the brain, peripheral nerves, and skeletal muscle. Cardiac muscle and its sodium channels are less sensitive to tetrodotoxin than are those of nerves.

Tetrodotoxin poisoning causes a rapidly progressive sensorimotor polyneuropathy that may affect bulbar and respiratory muscles. Numbness of the tongue and lips develops within minutes after ingestion. Limb weakness develops soon after and may result in flaccid quadriparesis. Symptoms of the autonomic nervous system are frequent, including vomiting, profuse salivation, excessive sweating, hypotension, bradycardia, and hypothermia.

Tetrodotoxin intoxication can be divided into four stages based on clinical signs: (1) numbness of the tongue and lips, and often of fingers; (2) rapidly progressing numbness and limb paralysis; (3) motor incoordination and paralysis; and (4) progressively deteriorating consciousness and respiratory paralysis, which may result in death.

Sodium channel blockade underlies the pathophysiology of tetrodotoxin poisoning, which impairs the propagation of the nerve action potentials. Electrophysiological studies reveal reduced amplitudes of compound muscle action potentials and sensory nerve action potentials, slowing of sensorimotor conduction velocity without conduction block or temporal dispersion, and prolongation of distal and proximal (F-wave) motor latencies. Wave forms of compound muscle and sensory nerve action potentials appear normal. These abnormalities can be explained by the fact that, in mammalian myelinated fibers, most of the sodium channels are located at the node of Ranvier, with few in the internodal axonal membrane. The nerve conduction abnormalities may rapidly improve in parallel with clinical recovery and a decrease in the urinary excretion of tetrodotoxin.

Treatment of puffer fish poisoning is supportive. No chemical antidotes are known and patients must be ventilated until the tetrodotoxin level is sufficiently reduced. Recovery may be dramatic.

Saxitoxin: Paralytic shellfish

Saxitoxin (STX) is a heat-stable neurotoxin, produced by marine dinoflagellates binding to voltage-sensitive sodium channels. The organisms that produce these molecules are thought to be responsible for "red tides." A connection between red tides and poisonous shellfish was proposed. It was suspected that dinoflagellates, on which the mussels are feeding, might be poisonous. The dinoflagellate was identified as *Gonyaulax catanella*. The major neurotoxin found in extracts of *G. catanella* was named saxitoxin.

Initial symptoms of STX poisoning are characterized by a tingling and burning sensation of the lips, gums, tongue, and face and then the sensation spreading to the neck, arm, fingertips, legs, and toes. Subsequently the tingling sensation turns to numbness. Weakness and muscle paralysis develop in the following 6–12 hours and diarrhea is an associated symptom.

Death may occur due to paralysis of the respiratory muscles. Treatment of paralytic shellfish poisoning is mainly symptomatic. No specific antidote is noted, but emetics may be helpful to remove the poison from the stomach in the early stage.

Plant toxins

Datura

Datura or jimson weed plants, including *Datura stramorium*, *Datura alba*, and *Datura suaveolens*, grow in the wild throughout the world, particularly in tropical and subtropical areas.

Datura stramorium comprises several kinds of alkaloids, including atropine, hyoscyamine (daturine), and scopolamine. Scopolamine and atropine, which are structurally similar to the neurotransmitter acetylcholine, may interfere with the transmission of nerve impulses in the parasympathetic nervous system. Hyoscyamine has atropine-like effects more potent than natural atropine.

Ingestion of *D. stramorium* can cause acute anticholinergic syndrome, with dryness of the mouth, pupillary dilation, blurred vision, facial flushing, palpitation, hypertension, disorientation, and even coma. This poisoning is usually caused by medication to relieve asthma, hallucinogens, or ingestion of contaminated grains. The onset of symptoms usually develops within 30 minutes to 2 hours after ingestion of *Datura*.

The severity of *Datura* poisoning appears to be related to the dosages of atropine and scopolamine and the pattern of onset. In cases of severe intoxication, patients may progress to convulsions, respiratory depression, stupor, coma, or even death. Recently, the incidence of this poisoning seems to have increased in Asian countries because the plants have been used for loss of vitality or in herbal drugs used as remedies. Most of the abnormalities are reversible. The treatment of acute *Datura* poisoning includes gastric lavage and administration of activated charcoal. In severely intoxicated patients with seizures, uncontrolled hypertension, hallucinations, arrhythmia, or coma, physostigmine salicylate is indicated.

Mushrooms

Exposure to poisonous mushrooms usually occurs by accidental ingestion or in the setting of intended recreational use. Mushrooms that predominantly affect the nervous system produce an immediate response. Poisonous mushrooms belong to the genus *Amanita*, including *A. muscaria*, *A. regalis*, and *A. panthirina*, and the genus *Psilocybe*.

The CNS toxicity of *A. muscaria* is due to ibotenic acid and its derivative, muscimol. Ibotenic acid has structural and functional similarities to the excitatory neurotransmitter glutamate. It is estimated to be approximately eight times more active than glutamate and equivalent to N-methyl-D-aspartate (NMDA) in provoking the activity of cat spinal interneurons and Renshaw cells. In human experiments, both *Amanita* and muscimol poisonings produce ataxia, myoclonic jerks, somnolence, and euphoria. The effects of muscimol cannot be distinguished from those of ibotenic acid.

The CNS symptoms often include alterations in mental state, visual changes, hallucinations, agitation, and ataxia. In severe cases, seizures and psychosis may occur. Muscle fasciculations and anticholinergic symptoms such as flushing, mydriasis, and urinary retention are commonly seen.

Psilocybe mushrooms contain psilocybin and its more potent metabolite psilocin. These indole alkylamines are structurally similar to serotonin and interact with CNS receptors to produce a lysergic acid diethylamide (LSD)-like syndrome, including visual illusions, vivid hallucinations, euphoria, and restless behavior. Anxiety, drowsiness, and dysphonia are common. Flushing, hypertension, tachycardia, and hyperthermia also occur frequently.

The acute neurotoxicity of mushrooms typically resolves completely without intervention and without chronic sequelae.

Podophyllotoxin (Bajiaolian)

Podophyllum, or a herbal medicine referred to as Bajiaolian in Chinese, is the dried resin from the roots and rhizomes of *Podophyllum pelatum*. It has been applied as a cathartic, helminthic ointment for a variety of tumors and anogenital condylomata. Podophyllotoxin is thought to be the major ingredient of podophyllum. The toxin may affect the nervous system, bone marrow, liver, kidneys, and gastrointestinal system. The clinical features of podophyllotoxin poisoning include diarrhea, nausea, vomiting, tachycardia, oliguria, paralytic ileus, and nervous system symptoms. The CNS toxicity includes an acute confusional state: hallucination, convulsion, coma, and even death. The PNS toxicity consists of autonomic and sensorimotor polyneuropathy. In most patients, sensory ataxia with a prominent loss of vibration and position sensations is noted.

The mechanism of cytotoxicity induced by podophyllotoxin is similar to that of colchicine: arrest of cellular mitosis in metaphase through the inhibition of microtubule formation and increased assembly of neurofilaments. Experimental animal studies reveal a disturbance of axonal transport, with extensive disintegration of Nissl bodies in the ganglion neurons. Human sural nerve pathology shows a decrease in the number of large myelinated fibers, axonal degeneration, and disruption of myelin. On ultrastructural examination, atrophic axons with disorganized neurofilaments are very similar to those of vincristine-induced axonal-type polyneuropathy. There is improvement in motor weakness in 1-year follow-up; however, impairment of position and vibration sensations may still be present in the legs, consistent with the changes in nerve conduction studies.

Bacterial toxins

Botulinum toxin

Botulinum toxin is the most potent biological neurotoxin, and can cause a neuromuscular transmission disorder called botulism. Botulism is a specific intoxication caused by a heat-labile, highly potent toxin produced by clostridium botulinum and frequently found in poorly preserved food products. Botulism was first described in 1897 by van Ermengem in Belgium. At least seven distinct botulinum neurotoxins (types A–G) were found. Food-borne botulism is caused by ingestion of food that contains botulinum toxin. The neurotoxin can bind rapidly to acetylcholine receptors at the neuromuscular junction, autonomic ganglia, and postganglionic parasympathetic endings.

In food-borne botulism, abdominal distention, nausea, vomiting, and diarrhea have been noted several hours after ingestion and then followed by constipation. Neurological symptoms include diplopia, blurred vision, dysarthria, dysphagia, and dizziness. Autonomic dysfunction includes dilated or unreactive pupils, dryness of eyes, postural hypotension, and urinary retention. The pattern of muscle weakness is usually symmetric limb weakness, and respiratory muscle weakness.

Treatment of botulism is mainly supportive. Antitoxin should be given as early as possible by intravenous or intramuscular administration. The antitoxin can only neutralize the circulating botulinum neurotoxin. Nasogastric suctioning and enemas may help remove toxin in food-borne cases. In wound botulism, infected wounds should be debrided. In some patients with other infections, other antibiotics should be given, but aminoglycoside should be avoided because it may impair the presynaptic neuromuscular transmission function.

Tetanus

Tetanus (lock jaw) remains a considerable health problem in many parts of the world. It is an infection with *Clostridium tetani* that causes localized or generalized spasm of muscles due to the toxin produced by the causative organism. The organism is present in the excreta of humans and most animals, and in putrefying liquids and dirt. It is especially prevalent in fertilized or contaminated soil. The organism gains entrance to the human body through puncture wounds, compound fractures, or cut wounds.

Tetanus toxin blocks the inhibitory interneurons that synapse with motor neurons, and also blocks the inhibition by the intermediolateral cells in the spinal cord.

The incubation period is usually between 5 and 10 days. Symptoms may be localized or generalized. Localized tetanus develops when the toxin spreads through the nerve. The symptoms are muscular spasms and contractions that are confined to the wounded limb or region. However, localized tetanus is relatively rare.

Generalized tetanus is usually ushered in by stiffness of the jaw (trismus), which is followed by stiffness of the neck, irritability, and restlessness. As the disease progresses, muscle stiffness and rigidity become generalized. The spasm of the back muscles may become so severe that the patient assumes the posture of opisthotonus. Rigidity of the facial muscles may give the characteristic facial expression of the so-called risus sandonicus. In addition, there are paroxysmal tonic muscle spasms, or generalized convulsions that may occur spontaneously, or may be precipitated by an external stimulus, such as a sudden noise or a touch. Spasm of the pharyngeal muscles may cause dysphasia, and spasm of the glottis or respiratory muscles may produce cyanosis and asphyxia.

Basic management consists of tetanus toxoid (500–3000 U), human tetanus immunoglobulin, sedation, and debridement of the wound. Penicillin G is the most effective antibiotic for inhibiting further growth of the organism. Sedatives, muscular relaxants, and anticonvulsants are given to combat generalized spasms and convulsions. Intrathecal baclofen or intravenous dantrolene may be tried. Artificial ventilation may be required.

Illicit drugs

1-Methyl-4-phenyl-1,2,3,6-tetrahydropyridine

The neurotoxin 1-methyl-4-phenyl-1,2,3,6-tetrahydropyridine (MPTP) was first identified as a contaminant of synthetic illicit drugs that can cause parkinsonian manifestation in drug addicts in 1979. The affected victims may develop rapid onset and progression of major parkinsonian features including tremor, rigidity, bradykinesia, and postural instability, in addition to other features such as masked face, micrographia, and seborrhea. The clinical features are very similar to idiopathic Parkinson's disease (IPD). MPTP patients also respond to levodopa treatment and develop the typical side effects of "peak-dose dysknesia" and "weaning off" phenomena as do IPD patients. PET scans using ^{18}F-fluorodopa as the tracer showed a marked reduction of uptake in the nigrostriatal radioactivity in MPTP-exposed subjects compared with IPD patients.

MPTP can be distributed throughout the body tissues and crosses the blood–brain barrier. It may convert to the neurotoxic substance 1-methyl-4-phenylpyridium (MPP$^+$), which exerts its toxic effect in the nigrostriatal dopaminergic neurons. MPP$^+$ molecules can bind with high affinity to neuromelanin and could selectively damage the neuromelanin-containing neurons of the substantia nigra. MPTP-affected patients also show a significant motor improvement after implantation of bilateral fetal dopamine-rich neuronal tissues. The positive effect supports the view that the clinical effects of MPTP result from selective damage of the nigrostriatal dopaminergic neurons.

Specific drugs

Disulfiram

Disulfiram (tetraethylthiuramdisulfide) has been used in the treatment of chronic alcoholism. Neuropathies and encephalopathies are associated with chronic disulfiram intoxication. The neuropathy is characterized by symmetric distal axonopathy. A tingling sensation starts in the face, followed by unsteady gait, decreased pin-prick, temperature, position sense, and absent reflexes, which are noted in most patients several months after a standard therapeutic dose (250–500 mg daily). Parkinsonian symptoms after acute or chronic disulfiram intoxication are usually transient. Persistent extrapyramidal syndrome after acute intoxication is exceedingly rare. Of four reported cases, two had akinetic symptoms while the remaining two had akinetic plus dystonic symptoms. Although dystonia was not the dominant feature, it progressed slowly over months or years. Computed tomography (CT) scans of two patients disclosed bilateral pallidal lesions. Autopsy study of another revealed bilateral cystic destruction of the outer segment of the globus pallidus, slight gliosis and demyelination of the putamen, and normal appearance of the caudate.

The neurotoxicity of disulfiram remains unclear. Disulfiram and its metabolites may interfere with enzyme systems, including cellular oxidation. If combined with alcohol, the reaction may cause irreversible inhibition of acetaldehyde dehydrogenase and subsequent accumulation of acetaldehyde, with resultant hypotension and possible hypoperfusion of the basal ganglia. Disulfiram may be metabolized to CS$_2$ to cause further damage to the basal ganglia and other CNS regions.

Cyanide

Cyanide intoxication is a histological hypoxia due to inhibition of neuronal cytochrome oxidase and other oxidative enzymes. Cyanide ion is the common toxic agent among cyanide compounds, including potassium cyanide, nitroprusside, and laetrile. Because cyanide is a potent and rapidly acting toxin, the mortality rate is extremely high and death usually occurs in seconds or minutes. The CNS is highly susceptible to this toxin, and rapid death is attributed to failure of the medullary respiratory center.

The first clinicopathological study of parkinsonism as a result of cyanide intoxication was reported in an 18-year-old man. Neurological examination 4 months later revealed marked generalized

rigidity and bradykinesia, slight tremor of the tongue and eyelids, intermittent resting and postural tremors in the arms, and postural instability with prominent propulsion and retropulsion. The patient died 1 year later after another suicide attempt. Autopsy study revealed spongy degeneration of the striatum including the putamen and globus pallidus, complete loss of neurons and marked gliosis in the zona reticularis of the substantia nigra, and some nerve cell loss and astrocytic proliferation in the subthalamic nuclei. There was segmental atrophy of cerebellar folia with complete loss of Purkinje's cells and partial loss of granule cells. In contrast to experimental findings, central demyelination was not found. Most of the neocortex, the hippocampus, the zona compacts of the substantia nigra, and the brainstem exhibited normal or nearly normal cytoarchitecture.

Hexachlorophene

Hexachlorophene is a poorly soluble white powder synthesized from 3,4,5-trichlorophenol; the preparations may contain minute amounts of the toxic compound 2,3,7,8-tetrachlorodebezo-p-dioxin. Hexachlorophene was used as an antimicrobial agent at high concentrations (3% solution) and as a cosmetic preservative at lower concentrations (<1%).

In human studies, toxicity may develop after topical application of hexachlorophene, particularly in an event in France in 1972 that accidentally contained hexachlorophene at a concentration of 6.3%. Patients may exhibit increased intracranial pressure, seizures, paresis, and mental state alteration. The lesions are primarily in the reticular formation and in the myelinated long tracts of the brainstem. Personally we have experienced a young child who accidentally ingested 30 ml hexachlorophene solution and then developed dilated pupils, optic atrophy, transient weakness in bilateral legs, and urinary incontinence. Although his leg weakness improved bilaterally, blurred vision and optic atrophy persisted.

Hexachlorophene can bind to myelin and lead to an increased water content of the brain, diffuse white-matter edema, and vacuolar degeneration of myelin.

The specific toxic mechanism of hexachlorophene-induced myelin degeneration is unknown, but biochemical effects of hexachlorophene include mitochondrial dysfunction, the uncoupling of oxidative phosphorylation, and the inhibition of protein and lipid synthesis in nerves.

Methanol

Acute methanol intoxication was common in the past. The early phase of CNS depression is similar to that caused by other aliphatic alcohols. It is metabolized to formaldehyde in the liver by alcohol dehydrogenase and catalase. Formaldehyde is in turn metabolized to formic acid by liver and red blood cell aldehyde dehydrogenase. Formic acid with or without acidosis is thought to be responsible for pathogenesis of CNS lesions.

Acute methanol intoxication can induce CNS depression after an asymptomatic latent period of 12–24 hours. Gastrointestinal disturbances include nausea, vomiting, and occasional diarrhea. Early visual symptoms are common, such as photophobia. Cloudy or diminished vision, especially loss of light perception, and even complete blindness occurs within hours or gradually over several days. Visual field defects are common. Other symptoms include headache, dizziness, amnesia, muscle weakness, somnolence, delirium, seizures, rigidity, opisotonus, and then coma.

The major finding in methanol intoxication is severe metabolic acidosis with a profound decrease in serum bicarbonate levels, an elevation of lactate and pyruvate concentrations, and reduced blood pH. If the patient survives the acute intoxication, neurological sequelae are usually confined to the ocular and extrapyramidal systems. Blindness is associated with optic atrophy. The prognosis is usually poor if the acidosis is not corrected rapidly. Extrapyramidal findings such as rigidity, akinesia, and dystonia may occur associated with spasticity, hyperreflexia, clonus, and extensor plantar responses. Putaminal necrosis can be found by CT and MRI. Rigor and akinesia may improve spontaneously after the acute event. Levadopa has no therapeutic effect. The amount of ethanol ingested with methanol, and the folate and vitamin B_{12} concentrations of the victim, may influence the outcome.

Treatment of the acute intoxication includes gastric lavage with 3% sodium bicarbonate, and correction of the severe metabolic acidosis with intravenous bicarbonate to maintain a blood pH >7.35. Intravenous administration of ethanol to retard the metabolism of methanol and hemodialysis to remove methanol and formic acid from body fluids are helpful in the treatment of acute methanol intoxication.

Hypervitaminosis

Vitamin A
Vitamin A (retinol), a family of lipophilic compounds, is essential for phototransduction, embryogenesis, and growth. Vitamin A is transported from the gut to the liver and stored in the liver. It may bind to specific intracellular receptor proteins. The targets of hypervitaminosis A toxicity include the brain, liver, bone, and blood vessels. Hypervitaminosis A may induce pseudotumor cerebri, a condition of increased intracranial pressure, and hepatomegaly, abnormal liver function, cortical thickening, and periosteal reaction of the bone, particularly in children, as well as ossification of ligaments. In addition, the increased triglyceride level and decreased high-density lipoproteins are also suggested to be a potential risk factor for cardiovascular diseases.

Short-term toxic effects after a large dose of vitamin A include headache, papilledema, visual disturbance, drowsiness, irritability, muscle weakness, and hemorrhages in mucosa.

Frequent skin changes include hair loss, dry skin, yellowish skin, and mouth blisters. Ocular changes may be present, including conjunctivitis, photodermatitis, corneal opacity, and decreased night vision.

The treatment is mainly based on cessation of the excessive intake. Therapy may include acetazolamide or corticosteroids for pseudotumor cerebri, and improvement may start several days to weeks later.

Regional-specific toxins

Polychlorinated biphenyls
Polychlorinated biphenyls (PCBs) and the products of polychlorinated dibenzofurans (PCDFs) are toxic chemicals that have been widely used in the past. They contain approximately 209 congeners in active ingredients with variable toxicity to humans, most through contaminated food or environmental exposure. PCBs have been used as capacity insulators, in adhesion, and in electronics since the 1950s. Because thousands of tons of PCBs have been dispersed into the environment, leading to serious contamination and slow breakdown, the use of these chemicals was abandoned in the United States in 1977.

There have been two notorious outbreaks of PCB intoxication: "Yusho" in Japan in 1968 and "Yu-Cheng" in Taiwan in 1979. The victims who consumed the contaminated rice oil developed chloracne, arthritis, headache, and general fatigue. In addition, hypothyroidism, menstrual abnormalities, reproductive disorders, and even slow cognitive development in the patients' descendants have been noted.

In about half of patients, there are neurological manifestations such as headache, dizziness, memory impairment, mental dullness, paresthesia or pain in the extremities, and hearing difficulty. Sensory symptoms are more prominent than motor symptoms. Nerve conduction velocity (NCV) tests show abnormalities of sensory or motor nerves in about half of patients. In the CNS, acute PCB poisoning may induce irreversible neurobehavioral changes and persistent depression in adults, while chronic exposure to PCBs may produce sequential memory and learning deficits.

In long-term follow-up studies, sensory disturbance is usually more prominent than motor disturbance in PCB-intoxicated victims. However, the PNS abnormalities are not well correlated with the concentrations of PCBs/PCDFs in the blood.

In experimental studies, PCBs are profoundly neurotoxic to the dopaminergic system, causing neurobehavioral abnormalities and movement disorders in rats.

Dimethylamine-borane
Dimethylamine-borane (DMAB) is a new synthetic agent used in the manufacturing of thin metal film, floppy discs, power transistors, and high-temperature printed circuit boards. The toxicity of DMAB was first reported in humans. In 2005, a 40-year-old man working in a semiconductor plant developed acute confusion and general weakness in four extremities following exposure to this new toxic chemical, which was then unfamiliar to the public. This was the first episode of human DMAB poisoning. Acute polyneuropathy with bilateral weakness in both legs, hyporefexia in both knee jerks and ankle jerks, and sensory impairment was noted 2 weeks later. Following exposure, the patient also developed mild Parkinsonism and cognitive deficits. A brain F-[18] FDG-PET scan also showed a relatively decreased cerebral metabolism at the anterior cingulate gyrus and bilateral frontal lobes. The polyneuropathy presented more motor symptoms, generally in the lower extremities. Sural nerve biopsy study revealed axonal degeneration, and loss of free nerve ending was noted in the skin biopsy staining with PGP 9.5.

Tetramethylammonium hydroxide
Tetramethylammonium hydroxide (TMA) is an etchant or developer used in the photoelectric or semiconductor industries. TMA intoxication from dermal exposure may be fatal and is becoming a serious concern in Taiwan. The structure of TMA ion is similar to the cationic portion of acetylcholine. TMA may stimulate the muscarinic or nicotinic autonomic ganglion and lead to depolarization blockade. The neurological manifestations of TMA intoxication include paralysis of respiratory muscles due to a ganglionic block-

ing effect. Cholinergic symptoms by accumulation of acetylcholine were first reported in Taiwanese patients.

Conclusions

Neurotoxicity due to occupational or environmental exposure is not only an individual illness, but also a public health matter. It is therefore important for clinicians to understand these neurotoxic diseases. Furthermore, many neurotoxic diseases are preventable.

In dealing with neurotoxic diseases, it is important to employ a multidisciplinary approach that may include neurobiological, neurophysiological, neuropathological, neurobehavioral, neuroimaging, neurogenetic, and public health specialties. Through such an approach, a better understanding of the neurotoxic disease may be achieved, and hopefully better treatment may be realized.

Further reading

Chang CC, Chang WN, Lui CC, *et al.* Clinical significance of the pallidoreticular pathway in patients with carbon monoxide intoxication. *Brain* 2011;134:3632-3646.

Chang LW, Dyer RS (eds.). *Handbook of Neurotoxicology.* New York: Marcel Dekker; 1995.

Chen RC, Tang SY, Miyata H, *et al.* Polychlorinated biphenyl poisoning: Correlation of sensory and motor nerve conduction, neurologic symptoms, and blood levels of polychlorinated biphenyls, quaterphenyls, and dibenzofurans. *Environ Res* 1985;37:340–348.

Huang CC. Carbon disulfide neurotoxicity: Taiwan experience. *Acta Neurologica Taiwanica* 2004;13;3-9.

Huang CC, Chu NS, Lu CS, *et al.* The natural history of neurological manganism over 18 years. *Parkinsonism Relat Disord* 2007;13:143–145.

Kuo HC, Huang CC, Tsai YT, *et al.* Acute painful neuropathy in thallium poisoning. *Neurology* 2005;65:302–304.

Kutsuma M (ed.). *Minamata Disease.* Study Group of Minamata Disease. Japan: Kumamoto University; 1968.

Liu CH, Huang CY, Huang CC. Occupational neurotoxic disease in Taiwan. *Saf Health Work* 2012;3:257–267.

Oda K, Araki, Totoki T, *et al.* Nerve conduction study of human tetrodotoxication. *Neurology* 1989;39:743–745.

Senenayake N, Karalliedde L. Neurotoxic effects of organophosphorus insecticides: An intermediate syndrome. *N Engl J Med* 1987;316:761–763.

Shih RD. Mushroom poisoning. In: ViccellioP (ed.). *Emergency Toxicology,* 2nd ed. Philadelphia, PA: Lippincott-Raven; 1998:1081–1086.

Spencer PS, Schaumburg HH, Ludolph AC (eds.).*Experimental and Clinical Neurotoxicology,* 2nd ed. New York: Oxford University Press; 2000.

97 Alcohol-related neurological disorders

Yuri Alekseenko
Department of Neurology and Neurosurgery, Vitebsk State Medical University, Vitebsk, Republic of Belarus

Alcohol-related neurological disorders cover a wide variety of conditions that affect the brain and peripheral nervous system. There are various neurological and psychoneurological conditions that are associated with long-term alcohol misuse and related vitamin deficiencies.

Based on the temporal relationship between alcohol abuse and onset of neurological symptoms, all these conditions may be subdivided into three main categories: acute intoxication, withdrawal syndrome, and a varied group of acute or subacute disorders secondary to chronic alcohol abuse. The best evidence indicates that between 0.5% and 1.5% of the adult population in different countries will have neurological disorders as a consequence of excessive alcohol misuse. The prevalence may rise to as much as 30% in heavy and long-term drinking categories of patients. In primary and secondary medical care, alcohol-related neurological disorders are usually underdiagnosed. In addition, the frequency of alcohol misuse is often underestimated in women and elderly populations. At the same time there is clear evidence that 75% of people with alcohol-related neurological disorders do improve with appropriate care.

Pharmacological aspects

Alcohol can influence various structures of the nervous system and cause some potentially dangerous conditions. Development of alcohol-related disorders of the nervous system depends on the extent and duration of alcohol abuse, nutrition and metabolic activity, and a variety of individual factors. Alcohol is toxic to the central and peripheral nervous system in a dose-dependent manner. Metabolism of ethanol is carried out in the liver by several enzymes, including alcohol dehydrogenase, aldehyde dehydrogenase, microsomal ethanol-oxidizing system, and peroxisomal catalase. Non-habituated patients metabolize ethanol at 13–25 mg/dL/h. In alcoholic persons, this rate increases to 30–50 mg/dL/h. Metabolism rates vary greatly between individuals. Clinical presentation of alcohol intoxication depends on blood concentrations and tolerance to ethanol. Acetaldehyde is a highly toxic metabolite of ethanol and probably the major factor of alcohol-related damage of the nervous system. Chronic alcohol consumption is usually accompanied by malnutrition and vitamin deficiency, particularly of thiamine. On the other hand, alcohol may itself be one of the most important causes of malnutrition, vitamin deficiency, and metabolic and electrolyte disorders.

Alcohol affects several neurotransmitter systems within the brain: glutamate, gamma-amino-butyric acid (GABA), dopamine, serotonin, and opioid systems. Alcohol produces opioid-related analgesia, pleasure, and stress-reducing effects. At the same time, alcohol increases dopamine neurotransmission, which mediates the pleasurable effects of alcohol via the mesolimbic dopamine system. Serotonin may also be linked to the pleasurable effects of alcohol, so different brain serotonin levels may provide for anxious and aggressive behavior in alcohol misusers. The interaction between alcohol and the GABA-benzodiazepine receptors is probably the major pathogenic mechanism responsible for alcohol dependency and withdrawal syndrome. Alcohol may interact with neurological and psychiatric medications, with some undesirable effects and life-threatening complications.

Acute alcohol intoxication

Acute alcohol intoxication is a transient exogenous condition resulting from acute intake of a sufficiently large amount of alcohol. The clinical manifestations of acute alcohol intoxication depend on its amount, but do not directly reflect the blood alcohol concentration. The subject's weight, individual metabolic rate, pre-existing somatic and neurological disorders, and some other additional intrinsic and environmental factors contribute to the clinical effects of ethanol intoxication.

There are three levels of severity of acute alcohol intoxication. Mild alcohol intoxication (blood alcohol concentration <1.5‰) is usually characterized by reduction of psychomotor capacities, loss of inhibitions, increased sociability and volubility, reduced control, and positional nystagmus. Moderate alcohol intoxication (blood alcohol concentration 1.5–2.5‰) is typically manifested by euphoria or aggressive irritability, reduced self-criticism, daze, behavior strongly dependent on external cues, and primitive explosive reactions. Severe alcohol intoxication (blood alcohol concentration greater than 2.5‰) is usually associated with disturbance of consciousness, disorientation, anxiety, and agitation. Ataxia, dizziness, dysarthria, and nystagmus develop as a result of alcohol-induced dysfunction of the vestibulocerebellar system. At high concentrations, alcohol can cause severe autonomic dysfunction, coma, and death from respiratory depression and cardiovascular collapse. Concomitant traumatic brain injury, intoxication with psychotropic drugs, and metabolic coma should be excluded in patients with severe alcohol intoxication and progressive disorders of consciousness.

International Neurology, Second edition. Edited by Robert P. Lisak, Daniel D. Truong, William M. Carroll and Roongroj Bhidayasiri
© 2016 John Wiley & Sons, Ltd. Published 2016 by John Wiley & Sons, Ltd.

Pathological intoxication may be observed in some special circumstances in predisposed subjects, for instance in patients with brain injury and other neurological disorders. In such cases even a small amount of alcohol may cause a state of agitation or drowsiness with disorientation, illusions, anxiety, fury, and violent behavior, with complete amnesia for these events.

The symptomatic treatment of severe alcohol intoxication should be provided according to standard protocols that are suitable for intoxications. In some cases haloperidol may be effective in the treatment of agitation with a low risk of cardiovascular side effects. Special therapy for patients with mild or moderate alcohol intoxication is usually not necessary.

Alcohol withdrawal

Alcohol withdrawal syndrome occurs in alcohol-dependent individuals after cessation or sufficient reduction of their heavy and prolonged alcohol consumption. Approximately 50% of subjects with alcohol dependence experience clinically relevant symptoms of withdrawal. Severe consequences of alcohol withdrawal, especially seizures or delirium tremens, occur in less than 5% of alcohol-dependent individuals.

Patients with alcohol withdrawal demonstrate a spectrum of different signs and symptoms, ranging from mild sleep disturbance to alcoholic delirium. The severity of this withdrawal syndrome relates to a number of factors, but most importantly to the abruptness of withdrawal, amount of alcohol intake, and the contribution of residual effects of previous drinking. Alcohol withdrawal usually starts 8–12 hours after cessation or sufficient reduction of chronic alcohol consumption. The main symptom of all varieties of alcohol withdrawal is a 6–8 Hz tremor of the hands, which may also extend to the tongue and the eyelids. Alcohol withdrawal may cause insomnia, anxiety, hyperkinesias, nausea, vomiting, and signs of vegetative hyperactivity such as tachycardia, hypertension, hyperhidrosis, and mild hyperpyrexia. Some patients may complain of dryness of the mouth and headache.

Alcoholic delirium develops in more serious cases and is clearly differentiated from uncomplicated alcohol withdrawal by disturbed orientation and clouded consciousness with agitation. These patients experience frightening visual or auditory hallucinations that last usually 5–6 days. Visual hallucinations typically consist of scenes with small moving animals or objects.

Seizures may occur; they are usually brief, generalized, and tonic–clonic in nature without an aura. They occur in a cluster of 1–3 seizures with a short postictal period. Partial seizures are not uncommon. In 30–50% of patients, the seizures progress to alcoholic delirium. Most seizures terminate spontaneously or are easily controlled with benzodiazepines. The peak incidence for seizures is around 36 hours (usually occurring between 12 and 48 hours) and for delirium around 72 hours. Alcoholic delirium is a self-limited disorder that resolves spontaneously. At the same time it is always a life-threatening condition because of severe autonomic dysregulation (i.e., hyperthermia, respiratory disturbances, cardiac arrhythmias) and uncontrolled seizures.

Medical treatment of alcoholic delirium consists of the administration of benzodiazepines (diazepam or chlordiazepoxide) or clomethiazole to reduce agitation and the incidence of seizures. Alternatively, gamma-hydroxy-butyric-acid may be used. Beta blockers (such as atenolol) reduce tremor and autonomic dysfunction. Neuroleptic drugs may be useful as an adjunctive therapy, but may

provoke seizures. In addition, parenteral thiamine should be recommended. Any associated infection, dehydration, hypoglycemia, or electrolyte disturbances should be treated.

Alcohol-related dementia

Alcohol may have a direct neurotoxic effect on cortical neurons. Chronic alcohol consumption causes cerebral atrophy, particularly of the frontal lobes, with the involvement of both white and gray matter, and ventricular dilatation, which are confirmed by computed tomography (CT) of the brain. Neuropathological studies show reduced numbers of neurons within the superior frontal cortex in alcoholic patients with dementia. Neuropsychological investigations demonstrate that alcohol-related dementia involves generalized cognitive abnormalities and predominantly affects visuospatial and problem-solving abilities, whereas the Wernicke–Korsakoff syndrome is distinguished by selective amnesia. At the same time diffuse brain damage, predominantly subcortical in alcoholic patients, may be caused by concomitant thiamine deficiency leading to Wernicke–Korsakoff syndrome. In general, cognitive impairment is quite common in alcoholics and usually reflects varying combinations of acute and chronic brain damage, including alcohol intoxication, vitamin deficiency, metabolic disorders, cerebrovascular diseases, and previous traumatic brain injuries. In some cases, cognitive impairment in alcoholic patients without any history of apparent head injury may be due to subdural hematoma.

Some investigations have demonstrated that radiological signs of cerebral atrophy are at least partially reversible after the cessation of alcohol consumption. The reduction of cerebral atrophy seems to be accompanied by an improvement in cognitive function and takes some weeks to months. However, the extent of this improvement as well as its underlying mechanisms are still a matter of discussion. It is unclear what level of drinking may pose a risk for the development of brain damage or, in fact, whether lower levels of alcohol may protect against other forms of dementia.

Alcoholic cerebellar degeneration

Mild clinical signs of cerebellar dysfunction may be found in about one-third of all chronic alcoholics. This alcohol-related cerebellar degeneration affects men more often than women and peaks in the fifth decade of life. The structural substrate of the disease is a degeneration of the anterior and middle parts of the cerebellum vermis. Purkinje cells of the cerebellar cortex are more severely affected than other cerebellar neurons. Cerebellar degeneration not only seems to result from the direct toxic effects of alcohol or its metabolites, but also reflects some other factors, such as thiamine deficiency in Wernicke's encephalopathy. The clinical picture is characterized by a severe ataxia of stance and gait. Coordination of hands is only mildly disturbed. Dysarthria and oculomotor abnormalities are unusual. In many patients peripheral neuropathy of alcoholic or thiamine deficiency origin usually contributes to the ataxia. Although generally of gradual onset, alcoholic cerebellar degeneration may evolve to become relatively acute over the course of several weeks. The incidence of cerebellar ataxia does not quite correlate with the extent of lifetime alcohol consumption or the degree of cerebellar atrophy on CT of the brain. It remains unclear why thiamine deficiency may cause Wernicke's encephalopathy in some patients but selective lesions of separate cerebellar regions in others. Cessation of alcohol consumption and administration of thiamine and other B vitamins should be recommended to all patients. If alcohol consumption is ceased, a further progression of the disease can be avoided, and in some cases a certain improvement may be observed.

Marchiafava–Bignami disease

Marchiafava–Bignami disease is characterized by symmetric demyelination and necrosis of the central parts of the corpus callosum and occasionally of the anterior and posterior commissures. It is usually observed in alcoholic patients after excessive and long-term (greater than 20 years) consumption of alcohol. The exact mechanisms of this disease remain poorly understood. The onset of the disease is usually acute. Disturbances of consciousness, seizures, gait apraxia, spasticity, signs of pyramidal tract involvement, dysarthria, and dementia are the most typical clinical features. The clinical presentation of this disorder is quite variable. The damage of the corpus callosum and adjacent cerebral white matter can be detected by magnetic resonance imaging (MRI) or high-resolution CT scanning. Modern imaging techniques (MRI, CT scan) allow differentiation of various alcohol-related conditions, including central pontine myelinolysis and Wernicke's encephalopathy, during the patient's life. The disease is usually progressive and in most cases patients die after only a few days to a few months, or survive for many years with severe dementia. No specific proven treatment measures are known that reliably influence the outcome of the disease. However, high-dose intravenous corticosteroid treatment may be considered as an option in rapidly progressive cases as well as thiamine, folate, and other B vitamins (especially B_{12}).

Alcoholic amblyopia

Alcoholic amblyopia (or tobacco-alcohol amblyopia) is a selective optic neuropathy that may be observed in some alcoholic patients. Alcoholic optic neuropathy seems to be associated with any deficiency of the B vitamins, as well as with exposure to cyanides, methanol, or combinations of these factors. The substrate of this optic neuropathy is symmetric, bilateral papillomacular demyelination, which starts in the retrobulbar region and develops retinofugally. Blurred vision or loss of vision is the main complaint of patients. These symptoms appear gradually within several days or weeks. Examination usually reveals symmetric central scotomas and pallor of the temporal parts of the optic disk. Without appropriate treatment, alcoholic optic neuropathy can lead to irreversible optic nerve atrophy. Therapy includes the administration of B vitamins and a well-balanced diet and should be started as soon as possible. If the symptoms persist for more than a couple of weeks after the beginning of the therapy, the prognosis with regard to a full functional recovery remains doubtful.

Alcoholic myopathy

There are three clinical manifestations of acute and chronic alcohol-related damage of muscles that may be observed in patients with alcohol abuse: rhabdomyolysis, hypokalemic alcohol myopathy, and chronic alcohol myopathy. Alcohol is probably the most frequent cause of acute rhabdomyolysis of non-traumatic origin. Seizures, vascular occlusion, physical exercise, prolonged muscle compression, drugs, toxins, infections, and extremes of temperature are less frequent, but can also be responsible. Episodes of acute muscle weakness due to rhabdomyolysis usually follow bouts of

excessive alcohol consumption and are associated with myoglobinuria. At the same time, such an apparently slight muscle injury is often asymptomatic, with only elevation of muscle enzymes in the serum. The most typical clinical manifestations are pain, swelling, weakness of affected muscles, and dark urine. The muscle lesion(s) can lead to hyperkalemia and increased serum myoglobin and creatine kinase levels. Renal failure is a common complication of acute rhabdomyolysis. The possibility of rhabdomyolysis should be considered in any intoxicated patient with muscle tenderness and acute muscle paralysis. There is no specific therapy, but common measures of intensive therapy usually include water and electrolyte balance correction, enforced diuresis, and hemodialysis.

Hypokalemic myopathy in alcoholic patients usually develops because of frequent vomiting and increased loss of potassium through the gastrointestinal tract, whereas renal excretion of potassium is not changed. Painless muscle weakness, mainly affecting the proximal parts of the limbs, and decreased serum potassium level are the most typical clinical features. Significant increases in serum levels of liver and muscle enzymes may be found. The therapy consists mainly of slow intravenous infusion of potassium chloride or potassium lactate. Monitoring of the electrocardiogram is necessary. The muscle weakness usually improves within 7–14 days.

Chronic alcoholic myopathy is probably one of the most prevalent skeletal muscle disorders and occurs in approximately 50–70% of alcohol misusers. This myopathy occurs independently of peripheral neuropathy, malnutrition, and secondary liver disease. Chronic alcoholic myopathy is characterized by selective atrophy of type II muscle fibers and the entire muscle mass may be reduced by up to 30%. Alcohol and acetaldehyde are potent inhibitors of muscle protein synthesis, and both contractile and non-contractile proteins are usually affected by acute and chronic alcohol exposure. Some possible mechanisms include free radical effects, and calcium and immunological disturbances may play a role. The extent of the myopathy significantly correlates with the overall amount of the patient's alcohol consumption during his or her lifetime. Malnutrition or electrolyte disturbances are not thought to be important contributing factors. The main clinical features are painless atrophy and paresis of the proximal limb muscles. The pelvic girdle musculature is usually affected much more than the shoulder girdle. An associated cardiomyopathy is common. In addition, alcoholic myopathy may be accompanied by alcoholic polyneuropathy, which usually involves the more distal parts of the limbs. The serum creatine phosphokinase level may be elevated in one-third of patients. Electromyography and histological examination show non-specific myopathic features, which may be demonstrated in a sufficient number of all alcohol misusers with minimal or even absent clinical symptoms. Abstention from alcohol is considered to be the most important treatment measure. A well-balanced diet and physiotherapy should be recommended in addition. In general, alcoholic myopathy has a more favorable prognosis in comparison with alcoholic polyneuropathy.

Alcoholic polyneuropathy

The clinical presentation of alcohol-related polyneuropathy was first described more than 200 years ago. Meanwhile, the precise mechanisms of pathogenesis of alcoholic neuropathy remain unclear. Polyneuropathy may be found in 10–50% of alcoholic patients, according to different diagnostic criteria and patient selection. Alcohol appears to exert a toxic effect on the peripheral nervous system in a time- and dose-dependent manner, so polyneuropathy is usually associated with frequent, heavy, and continuous alcohol consumption.

Direct neurotoxic effects of ethanol or its metabolites can cause alcoholic polyneuropathy. Acetaldehyde is one possible mediator of these effects among the ethanol metabolites. At the same time, nutritional and vitamin deficiencies including thiamine, other B-complex vitamins, and folic acid are quite common in alcoholic patients with polyneuropathy. However, it is always difficult to separate alcohol effects from nutritional and vitamin deficiencies, especially thiamine. Although clinicopathological features of the pure form of alcoholic polyneuropathy are uniform, they show extensive variations when thiamine deficiency is present. Hereditary polymorphism of aldehyde dehydrogenase-2 can explain the association of acetaldehyde accumulation due to enzyme inactivity with alcoholic polyneuropathy in some selected patients. It has also been suggested that alcohol-induced neuropathy may be in part associated with increased oxidative stress leading to free radical damage to nerves.

Alcoholic polyneuropathy is predominantly axonal, with the involvement of both afferent and efferent fibers. Clinical manifestations of alcoholic polyneuropathy can be summarized as slowly progressive (over months) abnormalities in sensory, motor, and autonomic functions. In general, symptoms are not quite specific and often indistinguishable from those in other forms of sensorimotor axonal neuropathy. The legs are usually affected earlier than the arms and more severely; so are the distal parts of the extremities in contrast to the proximal ones. Sensory symptoms include early numbness, hyperalgesia, paresthesias, dysesthesias, and allodynia of the feet and legs, especially at night. The character of the pain may be variable: dull and constant or sharp. Sometimes patients complain of cramping sensations in the muscles of the feet and calves, as well as sensation of heat and burning. When the symptoms extend above the ankle level, the fingertips often get similarly involved, giving rise to the well-known stocking-and-glove pattern of sensory disturbances. When the proprioception fibers become involved, sensory ataxia occurs, contributing to gait difficulty, independent of possible concomitant alcoholic cerebellar ataxia. Motor manifestations usually include distal weakness and muscle wasting. Frequent falls and gait unsteadiness are common. These are secondary, mainly due to ataxia that is caused by cerebellar degeneration, sensory ataxia, or distal muscle weakness. Cranial nerve involvement is not common and is usually confined to the oculomotor and lower cranial nerves. Symptoms such as dysphagia and dysphonia may appear secondary due to degeneration of the vagus nerve.

Autonomic disturbances are quite relevant clinical features. Excessive sweating of the soles and palmar surfaces of the feet, palms, and fingers is a common manifestation of alcoholic polyneuropathy. There are some signs of parasympathetic dysfunction including depressed heart rate responses, abnormal pupillary reactions, erectile dysfunction, and sleep apnea. Sympathetic dysfunction is quite rare, but it can lead to orthostatic hypotension and hypothermia. There are some visible trophic abnormalities such as thinning of the skin and alteration of nails, but trophic ulcers occur rarely.

Examination usually reveals distal sensory abnormalities, pain in muscles and superficial nerves, loss of tendon reflexes in the legs and less frequently in the arms, distal weakness, muscle atrophy, sweating of the feet and palms, sometimes ataxia and gait disorders.

Occasionally subjective complaints predominate over the mild sensory and motor disturbances.

Clinical features of alcoholic polyneuropathy without thiamine deficiency are characterized by slowly progressive, sensory-dominant symptoms. Superficial sensation is predominantly impaired and painful symptoms are the major complaint. Pathological features are characterized by small-fiber-predominant axonal degeneration. In contrast, the clinicopathological features of alcoholic polyneuropathy with concomitant thiamine deficiency are variable, constituting a spectrum ranging from a picture of a pure form of alcoholic polyneuropathy to a presentation of non-alcoholic thiamine-deficiency polyneuropathy.

The natural course of alcoholic polyneuropathy is quite variable. Manifestations of polyneuropathy may not be apparent clinically, in spite of continued alcohol consumption. In most cases, well-known clinical symptoms steadily increase over the course of several weeks or months. Sometimes alcoholic polyneuropathy may present as acute- or subacute-onset sensorimotor polyneuropathy, clinically mimicking Guillaine–Barré syndrome. Alcoholics with generalized axonal polyneuropathy are prone to pressure palsies at multiple sites. The prognosis of alcoholic polyneuropathy is generally good in the case of a complete abstention from alcohol. Patients with mild to moderate polyneuropathy can significantly improve, but the improvement is usually incomplete in those with severe disorders. The recovery is presumed to be due to regeneration and collateral sprouting of damaged axons. The prognosis does not depend on age. At the same time, some findings suggest that the evidence of vagal neuropathy in long-term alcoholics is associated with a significantly higher mortality rate than in the general population. Deaths due to cardiovascular disease are a major factor.

The diagnosis is based on an accurate history of prolonged and excessive alcohol intake, clinical signs and symptoms, and electrophysiological testing. Electromyography examination of the distal muscles of the lower extremities shows active denervation as well as chronic changes in the form of reinnervation patterns. Nerve conduction tests may be abnormal even before the emergence of clinical symptoms. Sural nerve biopsy often shows evidence of generalized distal axonal loss affecting both large and small fibers, with secondary segmental demyelination but without distinctive pathological features. Thiamine levels are not consistently reduced, but the thiamine-mediated enzyme transketolase is often abnormal. In all alcoholic patients with sensorimotor polyneuropathy, other causes of neuropathy (e.g., malignancy, diabetes, and nerve trauma) should be routinely excluded. In cases of acute or subacute manifestation of alcohol-related polyneuropathy, Guillain–Barré syndrome may be considered, although biopsy and electrodiagnostic studies usually reveal an axonal neuropathy, with normal cerebrospinal fluid (CSF) parameters. Patients have an increased risk of compression neuropathy, and the interpretation of electrodiagnostic findings can be confusing because of superimposed mononeuropathies.

The treatment program usually includes alcohol abstinence, a nutritionally balanced diet supplemented by all the B vitamins, physical therapy, and rehabilitation. Benfotiamine 320 mg/day for 4 weeks followed by 120 mg/day for at least 4 more weeks may be recommended. However, in the setting of ongoing alcohol consumption, vitamin supplementation alone is not sufficient for improvement in most patients. Painful dysesthesias can be treated using gabapentin or amitriptyline.

Fetal alcohol syndrome

Maternal alcohol consumption during pregnancy can cause serious birth defects, of which fetal alcohol syndrome is the most devastating. Recognized by characteristic craniofacial abnormalities (smooth philtrum, thin vermillion, and small palpebral fissures) and growth retardation (intrauterine growth restriction and failure to have catch-up growth), this condition produces severe alcohol-induced damage in the developing brain and leads to cognitive impairment, learning disabilities, and behavioral abnormalities.

Ethanol and its metabolite acetaldehyde can alter fetal development by disrupting cellular differentiation and growth, disrupting DNA and protein synthesis, and inhibiting cell migration. Both ethanol and acetaldehyde modify the intermediary metabolism of carbohydrates, proteins, and fats. They also decrease the transfer of amino acids, glucose, folic acid, zinc, and other nutrients across the placental barrier, indirectly affecting fetal growth due to intrauterine nutrient deprivation.

The principal structural and functional neurological features of children with fetal alcohol syndrome include microcephaly, delayed or deficient myelination, agenesis or hypoplasia of the corpus callosum, intellectual impairment (mild to moderate mental retardation), cognitive impairment, developmental delay, irritability in infancy, hyperactivity in childhood or attention deficit/hyperactivity disorder, ataxia, and seizures.

Neuroimaging studies reveal that in addition to the overall reduction of brain size, prominent brain shape abnormalities with narrowing in the parietal region and reduced brain growth in portions of the frontal lobe are present. Volumetric and tissue density findings demonstrate disproportionate reductions in the parietal lobe, cerebellar vermis, corpus callosum, and the caudate nucleus, suggesting that certain areas of the brain may be especially vulnerable to prenatal alcohol exposure.

In the absence of sensitive and specific biomarkers of exposure and given the common reluctance or inability of women to disclose the quantity and frequency of their alcohol consumption accurately, validating maternal reports of alcohol use is usually difficult. The risk of alcohol-related effects increases according to maternal alcohol consumption in a dose-dependent fashion. Furthermore, heavy episodic or binge drinking is the riskiest pattern of consumption. No level of alcohol consumption in pregnancy is known to be safe. So far as alcohol primarily affects brain development, drinking in all three trimesters poses a risk. As a consequence, pregnant women can reduce their risk of alcohol-related birth outcomes by reducing the dose or by discontinuing the consumption of alcohol as soon as possible, or better, before the pregnancy.

Further reading

Koike H, Sobue G. Alcoholic neuropathy. *Curr Opin Neurol* 2006;19:481–486.

McIntosh C, Chick J. Alcohol and the nervous system. *J Neurol Neurosurg Psychiatry* 2004;75;16–21.

Welch K. Neurological complications of alcohol and misuse of drugs. *Pract Neurol* 2011;11:206–219.

98 Vitamin deficiencies

Jacques Serratrice[1] and Volodymyr Golyk[2]

[1] Internal Medicine Department, Hôpitaux Universitaires de Genève, Geneva, Swizerland
[2] Neurology and Border States Department, Ukrainian State Institute of Medical and Social Problems of Disability, Dnipropetrovsk, Ukraine

Although diseases resulting from vitamin deficiencies have been historically known for millennia, such disorders were generally attributed to toxic or infectious causes until the "vitamin doctrine" was developed in the early twentieth century. Recently, however, as more and more health enthusiasts have integrated complicated vitamin regimens into their preventive efforts, physicians are increasingly encountering patients with syndromes associated with vitamin neurotoxicity from overdose.

The first recognized vitamin toxicity was related to the fat-soluble vitamins (A, D, E, and K), but water-soluble vitamins can also be harmful when they are ingested in large quantities. Both vitamin deficiencies and vitamin toxicity can affect the central and peripheral nervous systems in several ways. Formerly, knowledge about beriberi was responsible for the discovery of thiamine and for the concept of vitamin B_1 deficiency. Even now there is still a significant incidence of beriberi in specific populations in developing countries (up to 6.5% affected). Moreover, in these countries alcoholism is a major contributor to nutritional disorders as well as avitaminosis. At least some drugs utilized in the treatment of tuberculosis or hypertension are able to interfere with the enzymatic function of vitamin B_6. Recent studies have discovered not only dietary, absorption, and depletion factors responsible for vitamin deficiency syndrome, but some genetic abnormalities with certain predispositions.

In this chapter, after a brief review of physiology, we will describe the most relevant neurological manifestations of vitamin deficiency or overload. Clinical manifestations of vitamin deficiencies are summarized in Table 98.1.

Table 98.1. Clinical manifestations of vitamin deficiencies.

Water-soluble vitamin deficiencies
Thiamine (B_1)
– Gayet–Wernicke encephalopathy (acute ataxia, encephalopathy/alterations in level of consciousness and oculomotor disturbances)
– Korsakoff's (amnesic) syndrome
– Polyneuropathy (neuropathic beriberi)
– Cerebellar degeneration
– Central pontine myelinolysis (progressive gait disturbance, hallucinations, paraparesis, dysphagia, locked-in-like syndrome)
Nicotinic acid/niacin
– Pellagra (dermatitis, diarrhea, and dementia)
– Encephalopathy in alcoholic patients
– Hartnup's disease (dermatitis), intermittent cerebellar ataxia, and psychosis-like symptoms (only under certain conditions)
Cobalamin (B_{12})
– Pernicious anemia, dementia, subacute combined degeneration, optic nerve atrophy
Pyridoxine (B_6)
– Microcytic anemia, neuropathy, dizziness, drowsiness, lethargy, anorexia
Pantothenic acid (B_5)
– Fatigue, headache, and weakness
– Gastrointestinal disturbances, sleep disturbances, personality and emotional disorders
Ascorbic acid (C)
– Scurvy (fatigue, depression, widespread abnormalities in connective tissues and bleeding into body cavities)
Fat-soluble vitamin deficiencies
Retinol (A)
– Night blindness and corneal ulceration
Alpha-tocopherol (E)
– AVED (ataxia with vitamin E deficiency)
– Loss of tendon reflexes, ophthalmoparesis, proximal muscle weakness, elevated creatine kinase
Vitamin D
– Childhood muscle hypotonia, skull deformation
Vitamin K
– Bleeding

Group B vitamins

The most important nutrients for the nervous system are vitamins, and more specifically members of the vitamin B group.

Thiamine

Dietary thiamine (B_1) is absorbed as either thiamine or thiamine monophosphate in the small intestine. It is then taken up by specific transporters into the cell and converted to the active form (co-factor), thiamine pyrophosphate (TPP), by thiamine pyrophosphokinase (TPK) in the cytosol. From there it can be transported into mitochondria. In humans there are two isoforms of thiamine transporters in the plasma membrane encoded by *SLC19A2* and *SLC19A3*. TPP is either bound to the cytosolic thiamine-dependent enzyme transketolase from the pentose phosphate cycle, or transported into mitochondria by means of the mitochondrial thiamine pyrophosphate carrier encoded by *SLC25A19*. In the mitochondria, TPP is involved in three distinct ketoacid dehydrogenases: pyruvate dehydrogenase (PDH), which converts pyruvate to acetyl coenzyme A; α-ketoglutarate dehydrogenase, which catalyzes the conversion of α-ketoglutarate to succinate in the Krebs cycle; and branched-chain α-keto acid dehydrogenase. Thiamine regulates the expression of genes that code for enzymes using thiamine as a co-factor. TPP deficiency reduces the mRNA levels of transketolase and PDH, followed by elevated levels of serum pyruvate and

International Neurology, Second edition. Edited by Robert P. Lisak, Daniel D. Truong, William M. Carroll and Roongroj Bhidayasiri
© 2016 John Wiley & Sons, Ltd. Published 2016 by John Wiley & Sons, Ltd.

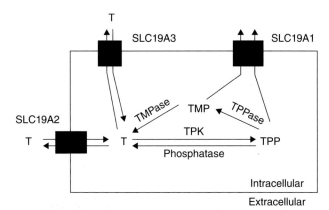

Figure 98.1 A model of the transcellular fluxes of thiamine, its phosphorylated metabolites and folates mediated by the reduced folate carrier (*SLC19A1*) and the thiamine transporters *SLC19A2* and *SLC19A3*. Source: Zhao 2013. Reproduced with permission of Elsevier.

occasionally lactate, reduced red blood cell (RBC) transketolase activity, and a corresponding increase in transketolase activity in response to added TPP (TPP effect; Figure 98.1).

Several syndromes of both genetic and somatic origin have been identified that feature different types of thiamine metabolism protein deficiency. Thiamine transporter-2 (hTHTR-2) deficiency is a rare inherited childhood-onset autosomal recessive disease caused by mutations in the *SLC19A3* gene, followed by decreased intracellular thiamine uptake in the context of normal extracellular thiamine levels. Other conditions affecting thiamine transporter proteins include different types of cancer. *SLC19A3* RNA levels have been reported to be downregulated by breast, lung, and gastric cancer cell lines. It is important to note that normal levels of circulating thiamine diphosphate or transketolase activity in red blood cells do not guarantee normal thiamine diphosphate or thiamine triphosphate levels in the brain, because of possible neuronal transport problems. Furthermore, the activity levels of any enzyme involved in thiamine metabolism are not necessarily connected to the activity levels of other enzymes; that is, just because one enzyme is acting normally does not mean that all the others are as well.

Alimentary sources most abundant with thiamine are yeast, pork, legumes, cereal grains, and rice. The recommended daily allowance of thiamine is 0.5 mg/1000 kcal. The total body store is 30–100 mg, and it is present in heart, skeletal muscle, liver, kidneys, and brain. Because there is a limited quantity of thiamine stored, the supply must be constantly replenished. The half-life of thiamine is approximately 2 weeks, and patients may suffer severe neurological complications and even death after 6 weeks of total thiamine depletion. Patients at high risk for thiamine deficiency include adults who derive most of their carbohydrates from milled rice, alcoholics, and infants who are breastfed by malnourished mothers. Other potentially thiamine-deficient states include anorexia nervosa, post-gastric or jejunoileal bypass, intractable vomiting following gastric stapling for morbid obesity, prolonged total parenteral nutrition, hyperemesis gravidarum, and severe malabsorption. Thiamine deficiency is also found in those who are prisoners of war or those who engage in a hunger strike. Thiamine deficiency has also been reported after long-standing peritoneal dialysis and hemodialysis.

Nicotinic acid/niacin

Vitamin B_3 is also known as nicotinic acid or niacin. Originally referred to as nicotinic acid, its name was changed to niacin in order to prevent confusion with the tobacco derivative, nicotine. Niacin includes both nicotinic acid and nicotinamide, which form the metabolically active nicotinamide adenine dinucleotide (NAD), and NAD phosphate (NADP), an end-product of tryptophan metabolism. More than 200 enzymes are dependent on NAD and NADP to carry out oxidation and reduction reactions, and these enzymes are involved in the synthesis and breakdown of all carbohydrates, lipids, and amino acids.

Recent studies have identified several major biochemical metabolic pathways that are disturbed in niacin deficiency, which include N-methyl-D-aspartate (NMDA) receptor stimulation and release of neurotoxic intermediate metabolites, breakdown of DNA repair processes and genomic integrity, abnormal cell respiration and ATP synthesis, and others. Genetic disorders caused by mutations in the gene *SLC6A19* encoding the angiotensin I type receptor transporter (B^0AT1) in kidneys and small intestine lead to defects of tryptophan absorption and niacin deficiency. Although niacin is endogenously produced in humans, exogenous intake is required in order to prevent deficiency. Niacin is found in meats, liver, fish, legumes, peanuts, enriched bread, coffee, and tea.

Cobalamin

Cobalamin (B_{12}) is absorbed in the small intestine, where the vitamin B_{12}+intrinsic factor (B_{12}–IF) complex binds to a specific receptor (cubam) and is adsorbed via an endocytotic process. Mutations in the genes coding different subunits of the receptor as well as gastric achlorhydria lead to a vitamin B_{12} malabsorption syndrome. This is accompanied by proteinuria, because cubam also mediates the tubular reabsorption of protein from the primary urine. Achlorhydria, lack of IF, and dysfunction of the cubam receptor all predispose to vitamin B_{12} deficiency. The transport of vitamin B_{12} in the blood, as well as its tissue and hepatic uptake, require the presence of transporter proteins known as transcobalamins (TCBs). TCB types I (TCB I) and III (TCB III) ensure the binding of 80% of circulating vitamin B_{12}; however, TCB type II (TCB II) plays the predominant role in the key processes of tissue and hepatic uptake of vitamin B_{12}.

Methylcobalamin is a co-factor of methionine synthase, a cytosolic enzyme that catalyzes the conversion of homocysteine and methyltetrahydrofolate to produce methionine and tetrahydrofolate. Methionine is further metabolized to S-adenosylmethionine, which is necessary for the methylation of myelin sheath phospholipids and proteins. Tetrahydrofolate is the required precursor for purine and pyrimidine synthesis. In the mitochondria, adenosylcobalamin catalyzes the conversion of L-methylmalonyl-CoA to succinyl-CoA. Vitamin B_{12} deficiency affects the neurological and hematological systems by impairing the function of these two enzyme systems.

The total body store of cobalamin is 2000–5000 µg, half of which is stored in the liver. Liver storage of vitamin B_{12} is mediated by endothelial cells, hepatocytes being naturally devoid of TCB II receptors. The enterohepatic cycle (5–7 mg daily) and proximal tubular reabsorption of vitamin B_{12} help maintain physiological reserves of cobalamin at significant levels; 2–5 years elapse before a patient develops cobalamin deficiency from malabsorption, and as long as 10–20 years are needed to induce a dietary deficiency from a strict vegetarian diet. The recommended daily allowance is 6 µg/day, and the average diet provides 20 µg/day.

Hypercobalaminemia, or high serum vitamin B_{12}, is defined by a level >950 pg/mL (701 pmol/L), which corresponds by biological standards to the upper limit of biological normality (ULN), in the absence of any sign and/or clinical anomaly. The high prevalence of hypercobalaminemia was exemplified in a 2009 retrospective study of 3072 hospitalized patients conducted by Deneuville and colleagues, which found high levels of vitamin B_{12} in 12% of cases, in contrast to B_{12} deficiency, which was observed in 10% of cases.

A high plasma level of vitamin B_{12} may be an indicator of a functional deficit with clinical consequences similar to those of vitamin B_{12} deficiency. Indeed, an increase in the binding of vitamin B_{12} to transporter proteins, secondary to an elevation in their plasma levels (especially for TCB I and III, which are by far the majority), leads to a potential decline in its attachment to TCB II and therefore alters its delivery to the cells. Thus, a functional deficit in vitamin B_{12} with an increase in homocysteine and/or methylmalonic acid levels can occur, even though the initial anomaly in this instance is not a deficiency in vitamin B_{12}. Aside from this mechanism, functional deficiency may also be caused by the failure of a damaged liver to take up cobalamin from the serum and/or by leakage of total vitamin B_{12} from the liver tissue into the plasma.

Pyridoxine

Pyridoxal phosphate is the active biochemical form of pyridoxine (B_6). It is a co-enzyme of amino acid metabolism, particularly tryptophan and methionine. By inhibiting methionine metabolism, excessive S-adenosylmethionine accumulates, which inhibits nerve lipid and myelin synthesis. Because tryptophan is required in the production of niacin, pyridoxine deficiency can produce a secondary niacin deficiency indistinguishable from primary pellagra. Pyridoxine is also involved in lipid and neurotransmitter synthesis. Dopamine, serotonin, epinephrine, norepinephrine, and gamma-aminobutyric acid (GABA) all require pyridoxine for their production.

The recommended daily allowance of pyridoxine is 2 mg. Pyridoxine is found most abundantly in enriched breads, cereals and grains, chicken, orange and tomato juice, bananas, and avocados. Patients at risk for pyridoxine deficiency include those with general malnutrition, prisoners of war, refugees, alcoholics, infants of vitamin B_6-deficient mothers, and patients using isoniazid and hydralazine. Pyridoxine is unique in that both the deficient and toxic states can cause peripheral neuropathy.

Pantothenic acid

Pantothenic acid (vitamin B_5) is part of co-enzyme A, an essential element of carbohydrate and fatty acid synthesis and degradation. Dietary reference intake is 5 mg/day of pantothenic acid for males and females 14 years of age and older, 6 mg/day during pregnancy, and 7 mg/day during lactation. Because of its ubiquity, no single neurological syndrome is known to be caused by pantothenate deficiency.

Vitamin B deficiency syndromes

Thiamine deficiency

Gayet–Wernicke encephalopathy

Gayet–Wernicke encephalopathy (GWE) is a medically emergent condition characterized by abrupt onset of ataxia, changes of consciousness, and abnormal eye movements. Morphologically the disorder typically presents as polioencephalitis hemorrhage with pathological changes primarily affecting the gray matter around the third and the fourth ventricles and aqueduct of Sylvius, as well as mammillary bodies, with petechial hemorrhages and associated with variable degrees of necrosis, vascular proliferation, and astroglial and microglial proliferation. Magnetic resonance imaging (MRI) abnormalities are characterized by high signal intensity on T2-weighted sequences and breakdown of the blood–brain barrier evident on contrast-enhanced images. Besides the more frequently reported structures involved in GWE, there are many other typically less affected areas, such as the caudate nucleus, perirolandic cortex, and posterior putamina, which can show abnormal signal intensity on MRI and help toward confirming this diagnosis. Cranial nerve nuclei such as hypoglossal, medial vestibular, facial, and abducens nuclei may also be involved.

Postmortem prevalence rates of GWE with Korsakoff's syndrome (see later) range from 1–2% in the general population and 12–14% in the alcoholic population. All these lesions are due to vitamin B_1 deficiency, related either to inadequate dietary intake, alcoholism-associated neurotoxicity, damage to apoenzymes, and/or increased metabolic demands, impaired absorption of thiamine due to active transport, liver damage, and/or reduced thiamine phosphorylation, and reduction in the rate of conversion to the active metabolite. One or more of these factors may be implicated. Other factors affecting the availability of thiamine to enter the brain are genetic predisposition; thiamine transport problems in the gastrointestinal tract, blood–brain barrier, or neurons; increased demand for thiamine due to alcohol withdrawal, delirium tremens, or NMDA receptor hyperactivation; organ damage (especially liver damage and reduced thiamine phosphorylation); deficiencies of other nutrients such as B_{12} or folate; predisposing diseases (e.g., those requiring hemodialysis); and inadequate treatment.

The onset of GWE is usually abrupt, with mental status changes that may include a global confusional state, memory loss, and agitation. Rarely, patients develop stupor and coma. Ocular abnormalities include nystagmus, lateral rectus palsies, conjugate gaze palsy, ptosis, retinal hemorrhages, pupillary abnormalities, and scotomas. Ataxia may be severe, preventing an affected patient from standing without assistance. Finger-to-nose and heel-to-shin tests are often normal when the patient is tested in the bed. Truncal ataxia frequently becomes obvious only on standing or sitting, reflecting midline degeneration of the superior division of the vermis. Polyneuropathy is present in over 80% of patients with GWE. It presents with slowly progressive muscular weakness, sensory impairment, and hyporeflexia, accompanied by burning feet and lancinating pains. Calf tenderness is a prominent feature. Bilateral foot drop and even wrist drop may occur. Patients may also develop an autonomic neuropathy with orthostatic hypotension. The classic clinical triad of ataxia, changes of consciousness, and oculomotor abnormalities is present in only a minority of patients. Clinical presentation is usually subtle, especially in non-alcoholic patients and in those with deep coma whose neurological evaluation is limited. Pyruvic acid is elevated. Some individuals are at increased risk because of a genetic predisposition, which means that their thiamine requirements are increased and higher blood concentrations are required for thiamine to enter the brain cells. Patients with thiamine deficiency may become acutely symptomatic when challenged with large doses of carbohydrate.

GWE is reversible if treated with a timely and adequate dose of parenteral thiamine. If it is undiagnosed or inadequately treated, it is likely to proceed to the chronic state, Korsakoff's syndrome (KS). In cases when GWE results from thiamine deficiency alone (e.g., due to alimentary deprivation or hyperemesis of different origin), low-dose oral/subcutaneous thiamine treatment is usually successful in preventing progression to KS. When GWE occurs in individuals with an alcohol problem the situation is more complicated, because alcohol is thought to compromise thiamine transport systems and to interfere with thiamine utilization. Changes to thiamine transport and utilization mean that higher doses of thiamine are required to treat the condition successfully in alcohol misusers, and that the thiamine must be given parenterally. Immediate thiamine replacement is required with 500 mg intravenously (IV) three times daily for 2–3 consecutive days, followed by 250 mg daily IV for the next 3–5 days and 100 mg orally three times daily for the rest of the hospital stay and during outpatient treatment. This should be accompanied by magnesium and fluid replacement, according to separate guidelines from the Royal College of Physicians (2001), British Association for Psychopharmacology (2004), European Federation of Neurological Societies (2010), and National Institute for Health and Care Excellence (2011).

Korsakoff's syndrome

KS is an amnesic syndrome linked to thiamine deficiency in a chronic alcoholic patient, either spontaneously or after a GWE. The salient features include anterograde amnesia (impaired ability to acquire new information) and retrograde amnesia (impaired ability to recall events that has been well established before the onset of the syndrome). Immediate memory (digit repetition) and remote memory (early life events) are relatively unaffected. Confabulation (momentary and fantastic memory) is not constant and often is associated with false recognition. A collateral history from family or friends should be taken to determine the premorbid functioning state of the patient, alcohol use history and complications, and the observed decline in functioning. Physical examination may uncover peripheral neuropathy and cerebellar ataxia. Assessment of cognitive function should not be carried out until at least 4 weeks post alcohol withdrawal.

Pathologically, there are symmetric lesions in both mammillary bodies with necrosis, neuronal loss, and hemorrhages, and in the bilateral medial thalami.

A clear difference is present between GWE-KS due to dietary restrictions alone and that due to thiamine deficiency and alcohol misuse. The evidence rests on the fact that KS rarely supervenes in the former situation, but frequently occurs in alcoholic patients. The best treatment for KS is timely recognition of GWE and appropriate intervention and prevention. Unfortunately, complete recovery occurs in only 20% of patients.

Polyneuropathy (neuropathic beriberi)

The main pathological change in polyneuropathy is axonal degeneration with destruction of both axon and myelin sheath. The most pronounced changes are observed in the distal part of the largest myelinated fibers. The nerve roots can be affected. Anterior horn and dorsal root ganglion cells undergo chromatolysis, indicating axonal damage.

Clinically there are three forms of beriberi: dry beriberi, wet beriberi, and infantile beriberi. Dry beriberi is characterized by a sensorimotor, painful, distal, axonal peripheral neuropathy. Wet beriberi is associated with high-output heart failure with peripheral neuropathy. The terms wet and dry beriberi have been used to describe the presence or absence of edema in neuropathic beriberi.

The dry form of neuropathy is characterized by symmetric impairment and hyporeflexia, most marked in the distal segments of the limbs. Pain is common in the initial period. Dysesthesias are prominent with a dull, constant ache in the feet and legs, or lightning pains. Cramps, band-like feelings, coldness of the feet, and burning in the soles are also common, and are worsened by contact with bedclothes or the ground (burning feet). The signs are those of sensory-motor neuropathy, initially with distal weakness and predominant cutaneous sensory loss. Nerve conduction study and electromyography generally reveal a moderate decrease of motor and sensorimotor nerve velocity. Sensory action potentials are markedly reduced.

The wet form manifestations include severe leg edema, heart murmur, accentuated secondary pulmonary sounds, and cardiac enlargement, together with a severe neuropathy, predominantly affecting distal motor function. The majority of patients with the wet form cannot stand or walk. Serum level and urinary excretion of thiamine are reduced, while lactate in serum is increased. Good recovery is achieved by thiamine treatment.

Cerebellar degeneration

Thiamine deficiency probably plays a part in cerebellar degeneration, particularly in alcoholics. More frequent in men, this disorder is characterized by gait instability and ataxia. The full clinical spectrum of cerebellar syndrome evolves gradually. MRI shows cortical cerebellar atrophy. The pathological changes consist of degeneration of the cerebellar cortex, particularly of the Purkinje cells. The syndrome is caused by nutritional deficiency rather than the toxic effects of alcohol. Cerebellar ataxia improves with thiamine therapy.

Central pontine myelinolysis

Central pontine myelinolysis is related to a profound electrolytic disturbance, associated with hypoxia and vitamin B_1 deficiency, also called osmotic demyelinization syndrome. The nature of the lesions is essentially demyelination involving the basis pontis. Most patients who develop this syndrome have chronic medical illnesses that are treated by hemodialysis. Central pontine myelinolysis is induced by a rapid correction of hyponatremia, causing the extracellular fluid to be relatively hypertonic, with secondary damage to the pontine and extrapontine cells of the brain. Primary clinical manifestations consist of progressive gait disturbance, postural instability, hallucinations, and mild cognitive dysfunction, progressing to paraparesis or quadriparesis, dysphagia, dysarthria, diplopia, and loss of consciousness (locked-in-like syndrome) over a period of several days. CT and MRI of the brain show a central pontine hypodensity (see also chapter 94 and 97).

A slow correction of hyponatremia prevents the syndrome. It is suggested that hyponatremia should be corrected at a rate of no more than 8–10 mmol/L of sodium per day to prevent central pontine myelinolysis. Therefore, hemodialysis correction of hyponatremia should also be done carefully, adapting the sodium level of the dialysate to the patient's serum level with subsequent vitamin B_1 supplementation.

Nicotinic acid/niacin deficiency

Pellagra

Pellagra, or rough skin, continues to occur in parts of Africa and Asia, especially in populations dependent on corn as the principal source of carbohydrate. In developed countries niacin deficiency is seen in alcoholics and patients taking isoniazid. There is a single case report of a patient developing nicotinic acid deficiency after valproic acid and phenobarbital therapy. Pregnant women are protected from niacin deficiency owing to their enhanced ability to convert tryptophan to niacin endogenously, particularly during the third trimester. In human pellagra, neuropathological abnormalities consistently observed are chromatolysis in motor neurons (Betz cells in the motor cortex, brainstem nuclei, anterior horn cells of the spinal cord), characterized by cytoplasmic swelling, disappearance of Nissl granules, and displacement of flattened nucleus to the periphery of the cell body.

Pellagra affects the skin, the gastrointestinal system, and the central nervous system. Hence the classic triad of the "three Ds": dermatitis, diarrhea, and dementia. In industrialized countries, particularly among alcoholics, niacin deficiency may present only with encephalopathy. Patients may have altered sensorium, diffuse rigidity of the limbs, and grasping and sucking reflexes. Dementia and confusion are the most consistent findings, followed by diarrhea (50%) and dermatitis (about 30%). The initial symptoms can be insomnia, fatigue, nervousness, irritability, and depression. The detailed neurological examination may disclose psychomotor slowing, apathy, and memory impairment. Sometimes, an acute confusional psychosis dominates the clinical picture. Spinal cord and peripheral nerve defects have also been reported. Peripheral neuropathy is frequent and may be indistinguishable from the neuropathic beriberi. Spinal cord involvement is different from spinal spastic syndrome (frequent in prisoner-of-war camps) or from tropical spastic paraparesis (caused by human T-lymphotropic virus [HTLV] infection or a toxic effect of cassava ingestion). Coexisting deficiencies of thiamine and pyridoxine are common, especially in alcoholics. Whenever pellagra is suspected, treatment with oral nicotinamide 100 mg three times daily for 3–4 weeks prior to laboratory confirmation is recommended as an inexpensive, safe, and potentially life-saving intervention.

Hartnup's disease

Hartnup's disease is an autosomal recessive defect in tryptophan absorption in the gastrointestinal system and kidney. It is caused by mutations in the gene *SLC6A19* encoding the B^{0}AT1 transporter. Even though B^{0}AT1 is the major neutral amino acid transporter in the kidney and small intestine, patients develop normally and may present symptoms, other than aminoaciduria, resembling pellagra (including light-sensitive dermatitis), intermittent cerebellar ataxia, and psychosis-like symptoms only under certain conditions (infections, malnutrition, etc.). The aminoaciduria is attributed to the defective transporter in the kidney, but the impact of the transport defect on intestinal absorption and its connection to pellagra or neurological manifestations is still unclear. Hartnup's disease is also responsive to niacin administration.

Carcinoid syndrome

Carcinoid syndrome can produce niacin deficiency. Because all tryptophan is diverted to the production of serotonin in this disorder, none is available for the production of nicotinic acid, thereby predisposing to deficiency in the absence of supplementation.

Supraphysiological doses of niacin (1.5–3 g daily) have been used successfully in the treatment of hypercholesterolemia, further reducing the mortality caused by coronary artery disease. Side effects of high-dose niacin include flushing, hyperuricemia, hyperglycemia, and elevations in liver enzymes.

In the evaluation of potential niacin deficiency, nicotinic acid metabolites can be identified in the urine; however, clinical suspicion and general availability of niacin make this measurement impractical and unnecessary. The administration of 40–250 mg of niacin daily is usually adequate to reverse most of the symptoms and signs of niacin deficiency. With proper therapy, the prognosis for the resolution of neurological symptoms is excellent.

Nicotinic acid deficiency encephalopathy in alcoholic patients

In 1940, Jolliffe *et al.* described a syndrome characterized by clouding of consciousness, cogwheel rigidity, and grasping reflexes. Those patients were treated with nicotinic acid and recovered rapidly. Although endemic niacin deficiency has essentially been eradicated in most Western countries, alcohol withdrawal delirium may in many cases account for pellagra. There are several case reports of patients who misuse alcohol presenting with laryngitis and psychosis due to nicotinic acid deficiency. Recent investigations have shown that pellagra should be considered in the differential diagnosis for all patients with chronic alcohol dependence and others at risk of malnutrition, such as the homeless and those positive for human immunodeficiency virus (HIV).

Chronic niacin deficiency

Chronic niacin deficiency is a dramatic example of how nutritional deficiency can affect mental function in childhood.

Cobalamin deficiency

Cobalamin (vitamin B$_{12}$) deficiency causes a wide range of hematological, gastrointestinal, psychiatric, and neurological disorders. Hematological presentations of cobalamin deficiency – pernicious anemia or autoimmune parietal cell dysfunction – range from the incidental increase of mean corpuscular volume and neutrophil hypersegmentation to symptoms of severe anemia such as angor, dyspnea on exertion, and fatigue, or symptoms related to congestive heart failure, such as ankle edema, orthopnea, and nocturia. Neuropsychiatric symptoms may precede hematological signs and are represented by myelopathy, neuropathy, dementia, and less often optic nerve atrophy. The spinal cord manifestation is called subacute combined degeneration (SCD), to designate the spinal cord lesion in pernicious anemia and to distinguish it from other forms of so-called combined system disease, in which the posterior and lateral columns are affected.

The mean age of diagnosis of pernicious anemia is 60 years, with the female-to-male ratio approximately 1.5:1. In white populations, the incidence of the disease increases with age, peaking after 65 years of age. In Hispanic and African populations, there is an overall younger age distribution, especially among women. When using radioassay-derived serum cobalamin levels below 200 pg/mL or elevated levels of homocysteine and methylmalonic acid as diagnostic criteria, the prevalence of vitamin B$_{12}$ deficiency from all causes ranges from 7–16%.

The brain, spinal cord, optic nerves, and peripheral nerves may also be involved in pernicious anemia. The spinal cord is usually affected first and often exclusively. SCD occurs in the majority of patients with pernicious anemia. The initial symptoms are usually generalized weakness and paresthesias, described as tingling, pins and needles, or other vague sensations. They are localized to the distal parts of all four limbs in a symmetric pattern; occasionally the lower extremities are involved before the upper ones. As the illness progresses, the gait becomes unsteady. Then, the legs are weak and spastic. If the disease remains untreated, an ataxic paraplegia with variable degrees of spasticity and contracture may develop.

The paresthesias and ataxia are due to lesions in the posterior columns, and these may also account for the loss of tendon reflexes. Weakness, spasticity, increased reflexes, and Babinski signs depend on the involvement of corticospinal tracts. Involvement of the spinothalamic tract explains the finding of a sensory level on the trunk. The distal and symmetric impairment of superficial sensation and the loss of tendon reflexes that occur in some cases are due to the involvement of peripheral nerves.

When only paresthesias are present, there may be no objective signs. The examination may disclose the impairment of the posterior and lateral columns of the spinal cord, predominantly of the former. Loss of vibration sense is by far the most consistent sign; it is more pronounced in the legs than in the arms, and frequently it extends over the trunk. Position sense is usually impaired as well. The motor signs include weakness, spasticity, and changes in tendon reflexes, and clonus associated with extensor plantar responses. These signs are usually limited to the legs. The patellar and Achilles reflexes can be diminished, increased, or even absent. With treatment, the reflexes may return to normal or become hyperactive. The gait at first is predominantly ataxic, but later is ataxic and spastic. Sensory disturbances are of spinal or peripheral distribution.

Psychiatric disturbances are frequent and range from irritability, apathy, somnolence, paranoia, and emotional lability to a marked confusional, depressive psychosis, or intellectual deterioration.

Visual impairment may be the sole manifestation in pernicious anemia; examination discloses symmetric centrocecal scotoma and optic atrophy in the most advanced cases. The cerebrospinal fluid (CSF) is usually normal.

In clinical practice, normal concentrations of serum B_{12} do not exclude the diagnosis of B_{12} deficiency. The analysis of serum metabolite concentrations, such as methylmalonic acid (MMA) and homocysteine, can reveal patients with borderline B_{12} concentrations (<300 pg/mL). MMA or homocysteine concentration can be corrected after treatment for B_{12} deficiency unless renal failure or other causes of increased metabolites coexist. Screening for vitamin B_{12} deficiency should start from clinical awareness of the population at risk, including elderly persons, vegans, alcoholics, malnourished persons, and patients with gastrointestinal diseases, neuropsychiatric symptoms, or autoimmune diseases. Common laboratory findings suggestive of cobalamin deficiency include macrocytosis with or without anemia and hypersegmented neutrophils. Special attention should also be given to patients on medications such as proton pump inhibitors, H2-receptor antagonists, metformin, colchicine, cholestyramine, and patients chronically on anticonvulsants or antibiotics. An adequate cobalamin supply is suggested by serum B_{12} concentrations above 350 pg/mL. Assessment of MMA in patients whose serum cobalamin concentrations are below 350 pg/mL is strongly recommended.

The most consistent MRI finding in SCD is a symmetric abnormally increased T2 signal intensity, commonly confined to posterior or posterior and lateral columns in the cervical and thoracic spinal cord (Figure 98.2). In acute and severe cases, the spinal cord might also present as swollen. Involvement of anterior columns has occasionally been reported. T2 hyperintensity of spinal cord columns has been related to demyelination. Intramyelin edema in the white matter of the spinal cord is the histopathological hallmark in experimental models of SCD. Sometimes, enhancement is noted after the administration of gadolinium, due to the disruption of the blood–brain barrier. Spinal MR imaging assists in early diagnosis and treatment of the disease; follow-up MR imaging findings correlate with clinical outcome after treatment with vitamin B_{12} supplementation. The abnormal MR signals on the spinal cord might either disappear on follow-up after months, or sometimes they might persist, especially in cases diagnosed and treated at an advanced stage. Nerve conduction velocity is reduced. Reduction of sensory action potentials is usual. The pathophysiology of nervous alteration is not known.

Diagnosis is based on assays of cobalamin serum concentration, megaloblastic and macrocytic anemia, and antibodies to IF, parietal cells, and immunoglobin G (IgG). Treatment is aimed at the underlying disorder and may include rectifying dietary imbalance, supplementation of pancreatic enzymes, administration of antibiotics, taenicides, corticosteroids, intestinal motility-decreasing drugs, and bile salt-sequestering agents, as well as cobalamin (parenteral) substitution therapy with cobalamin 2000 µg intramuscularly per day during the first 2 weeks, and 100 µg intramuscularly every month thereafter. Some reports have found that oral supplementation is effective.

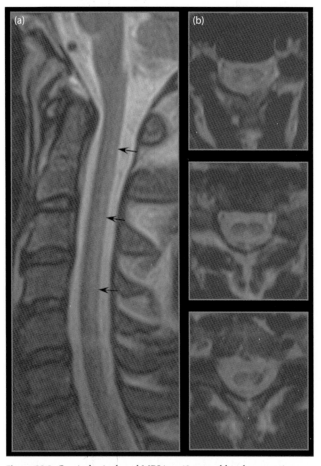

Figure 98.2 Cervical spinal cord MRI in a 49-year-old male presenting with subacute combined degeneration due to a deficit of B_{12}. (a) The midsagittal T2-weighted image shows linear hyperintensity in the posterior portion of the cervical tract of the spinal cord (black arrows). (b) Axial T2-weighted images reveal the selective involvement of the posterior columns. Source: Briani 2013. Reproduced with permission of MDPI.com.

Pyridoxine deficiency

Antagonists of pyridoxine (vitamin B_6) are used in patients with tuberculosis and in those with hypertension. Hydrazines and isoniazid (INH) produce pyridoxal hydrazones, biologically inactive compounds that are excreted, suggesting a carbonyl-trapping effect, which also may occur with other compounds such as furadantine. Excretion of xanthurenic acid is increased under these conditions. Pyridoxine deficiency affects the blood, skin, and nervous system. The skin changes are indistinguishable from pellagra, probably due to the close interaction of niacin and pyridoxine. Pyridoxine improves the microcytic anemia of alcoholics as well as the anemia associated with pyridoxine-responsive seizures in infants. Pyridoxine deficiency neuropathy in humans has been produced in long-term experiments with the antagonist desoxypyridoxine, and it also occurs during concomitant treatment with antagonist drugs. The characteristic peripheral nerve involvement usually affects distal symmetric sensory nerves with "burning feet" sensations. Pain can be so severe that it interferes with sleep. Weakness generally occurs later, with initial motor disturbances usually consisting of moderate weakness of toe and foot. The nerve lesions are primarily axonal. The pathogenesis of hydralazine neuropathy and clinical manifestations are similar to those of INH neuropathy. Favorable response to vitamin B_6 administration is observed.

CNS involvement is manifested by dizziness, drowsiness, lethargy, anorexia, vomiting, or psychotic episodes occasionally resembling Korsakoff's syndrome. In children, hyperexcitability is common, generally culminating in seizures. Pyridoxine dependency is a rare disease, inherited as an autosomal recessive trait. It is characterized by early-onset seizures, sometimes even *in utero*, failure to thrive, hypertonia-hyperkinesia, irritability, tremulous movements ("jitter-baby"), exaggerated auditory startle (hyperacusis), and later, if untreated, psychomotor retardation. Excretion of pyridoxine and its catabolic end product, 4-pyridoxic acid, is decreased. The specific laboratory abnormality is an increased excretion of xanthurenic acid in response to a tryptophan load. Neuropathologically, brain weight is below normal, with a decreased amount of central white matter in the cerebral hemispheres and a depletion of neurons in the thalamic nuclei and cerebellum, with gliosis. The administration of 50–100 mg of vitamin B_6 ablates the seizure, and daily doses of 40 mg permit normal development. Excess pyridoxine also results in a peripheral neuropathy.

Pyridoxine overload also results in a peripheral neuropathy. Megadoses of pyridoxine, generally in excess of 2 g/day, produce a sensory neuropathy, but this has also been reported to occur with long-term use of as little as 200 mg/day. Symptoms of paresthesias, ataxia, and burning feet occur 1 month to 3 years after starting pyridoxine. Sural nerve biopsies show reduced myelin fiber density and myelin debris, suggesting axonal degeneration. After stopping pyridoxine, all patients improve, but the condition resolves entirely in only a few.

Pantothenic acid deficiency

Deficiency of pantothenic acid (vitamin B_5) may possibly induce a sensory polyneuropathy characterized by numbness and tingling of hands and feet. However, there is no firm evidence that lesions of peripheral nerves are caused by pantothenic acid deficiency alone. The triad of fatigue (including apathy and malaise), headache, and weakness has been the most consistent finding. Other common effects include gastrointestinal disturbances (nausea, abdominal cramps, occasional vomiting, increased flatulence, and epigastric burning sensations); sleep disturbances; and personality changes and emotional disorders. A less frequent occurrence is signs of cardiovascular instability (tachycardia and lability of arterial blood pressure, with a tendency to orthostatic hypotension). Paresthesias, burning sensations of the hands and feet, and muscle cramps and weakness have occurred in several patients. Impaired motor coordination also occurs in some patients, and may be accompanied by a peculiar gait. In some clinical trials, infections were common among people with pantothenic acid deficiencies, whereas in other trials they were not. Administration of pantothenic acid may reverse the painful dysesthesias of the "burning feet" syndrome. Experimentally, neuropathy with degeneration of large-diameter fibers in nerves and dorsal roots is noted.

Other vitamins

Vitamin E

Alpha-tocopherol is the most active form of vitamin E in humans. Tocopherol is absorbed and incorporated into chylomicrons in the small intestine and carried in portal blood to the liver. In the liver, alpha-tocopherol transfer protein (α-TTP) binds and recycles vitamin E for incorporation into low-density lipoproteins and very low-density lipoproteins. Once delivered to cells, alpha-tocopherol serves as an antioxidant, preventing free radical peroxidation and injury to cell membranes. It is stored in adipose tissue, liver, and muscle. Deficiency can occur at any stage of tocopherol metabolism: reduced intake, fat malabsorption, inhibition of enterohepatic circulation, mutation of α-TPP, and abetalipoproteinemia.

Vitamin E is a fat-soluble vitamin found in abundance in vegetable oils and wheat germ. The recommended daily allowance is 10 mg for men and 8 mg for women. Patients at risk for the development of vitamin E deficiency include those who have hypobetalipoproteinemia or abetalipoproteinemia (Bassen–Kornzweig syndrome), other disorders of the pancreas and liver, such as cystic fibrosis and primary biliary atresia, familial vitamin E deficiency due to a defect in α-TTP, and other malabsorptive states that result in cholestasis, such as Crohn's disease, ulcerative colitis, and celiac disease. Pregnancy increases maternal vitamin E serum concentrations, but premature infants often have low levels of vitamin E due to a lack of adipose tissue as well as difficulty in transplacental migration of the vitamin. The majority of patients who have vitamin E deficiency are those with severe malabsorptive states present since birth or rare familial vitamin E deficiency due to transfer protein abnormalities. Vitamin E deficiency leads to axonal membrane injury, with resultant axonal degeneration of peripheral nerve, dorsal root ganglia, and posterior columns.

Vitamin C

The pharmacokinetic profile of vitamin C (ascorbic and dehydroascorbic acid) – that is, absorption, distribution, metabolism, and elimination – is quite complex and involves several different active and passive transport mechanisms as well as intracellular reduction, which permits the recycling of vitamin C within specific tissues. The tight regulation of vitamin C homeostasis is primarily controlled by four regulatory systems: intestinal uptake (bioavailability); tissue accumulation and distribution; rate of utilization and recycling; and renal excretion and reabsorption. Most mammals synthesize vitamin C in the liver by enzymatic conversion of glucose; however, a few species, including humans, guinea pigs, and bats, lack a functional L-gulono-lactone oxidase enzyme catalyzing the final step in the biosynthesis and, therefore, rely completely on a dietary supply of vitamin C.

After ingestion, vitamin C is absorbed from the intestinal lumen and released into the bloodstream. In the gastrointestinal tract, the ionized form of vitamin C, ascorbate (ASC), and its oxidized counterpart, dehydroascorbic acid (DHA), are absorbed through different transporter systems, with an increased affinity for ASC compared to DHA. Following uptake across the intestinal epithelium, vitamin C is released into the bloodstream as ASC (>95% of vitamin C in human plasma is in the form of ASC). Here, ASC is easily oxidized and the produced DHA is rapidly taken up through glucose transporters (GLUT1) transporters on the erythrocytes.

Within the body, the brain has a uniquely high vitamin C level and is able to maintain a superior concentration relative to most other organs during periods of vitamin C deficiency, placing the brain as an organ of particular interest when assessing the effects of vitamin C deficiency. The entry of ASC into the brain is hampered by the blood–brain barrier, which is impermeable to ASC and lacks the expression of sodium-dependent vitamin C transporters (SVCT2). Instead, ASC is thought to enter the cerebrospinal fluid of the brain through SVCT2 transporters in the choroid plexus. DHA, on the other hand, readily crosses the blood–brain barrier due to the expression of GLUT1. The DHA now present in the extracellular space can then be transported to the bloodstream by GLUT1 in the blood–brain barrier, or taken up by astrocytes expressing GLUT1, recycled back to ASC, and, concomitantly, released to the extracellular space by a yet undisclosed mechanism or possibly by diffusion.

Ascorbic acid readily oxidizes to dehydroascorbic acid in aqueous solution. Because the latter can be reduced *in vivo*, it possesses vitamin C activity. Therefore, total vitamin C is measured as the sum of ascorbic and dehydroascorbic acid concentrations. Because of its antioxidant properties, it serves primarily as a biological antioxidant in aqueous environments. Biosyntheses of collagen, carnitine, bile acids, and norepinephrine, as well as proper functioning of the hepatic mixed-function oxygenase system, depend on this property. Vitamin C in foodstuffs increases the intestinal absorption of non-heme iron. Overt deficiency is uncommon in developed countries. Tobacco smoking lowers plasma and leukocyte vitamin C levels.

Recent data from a dose-response analysis demonstrated that an increase in vitamin C intake of 100 mg/day was marginally associated with a reduced risk of stroke. There was an association between vitamin C intake and risk of stroke, with the greatest risk reduction observed at an intake of 200 mg/day, and it remained protective until an intake of 550 mg/day.

Vitamin A

Vitamin A, derived from β-carotene, is necessary for normal vision and reproduction. Deficiency leads to night blindness and corneal ulceration. Hypervitaminosis in pregnant mothers may lead to birth defects and learning disabilities.

Vitamin D

Vitamin D is necessary for calcium absorption in the gut. Deficiency leads to osteomalacia, hypocalcemia, and hypophosphatemia, contributing to muscle weakness.

Other vitamin deficiencies

Vitamin E deficiency

Vitamin E deficiency could account for some ataxia, loss of tendon reflexes, ophthalmoparesis, and proximal muscle weakness with a high level of creatine kinase. However, the primary characteristic syndrome is AVED (ataxia with vitamin E deficiency), which differs from Freidreich's ataxia in three principal ways: the frequency of head titubation, decreased visual acuity, and retinitis pigmentosa. Mutation 744 del A of the *aTTP* gene is present.

Another rare autosomal recessive disorder related to vitamin E deficiency is Bassen–Kornzweig syndrome, which results from malabsorption of vitamin E owing to the carrier lipoprotein not being synthesized in the liver. It is characterized by a near absence of β-lipoprotein and a low level of cholesterol in the serum, retinal degeneration, and acanthocytosis, a thorny appearance of the red cells, and a chronic, progressive deficit, usually beginning in childhood, steatorrhea, and retarded growth. The first neurological sign is hyporeflexia or absence of tendon reflexes in the second year of life. Later, a loss of position sense is found in the legs. Cerebellar ataxia of gait, trunk and extremities, titubation, dysarthria, muscle weakness, ophthalmoparesis, Babinski's sign, and loss of pain and temperature are other neurological abnormalities. Learning disabilities occurs. Progression occurs over a few years and many patients are no longer able to stand and walk by the time of adolescence. Retinal pigmentation is observed.

Neuropathological findings consist of demyelination of peripheral nerves and degeneration of nerve cells in the spinal gray matter and cerebellar cortex. Diagnosis is confirmed by the finding of acanthocytes, low serum cholesterol, and β (low-density) lipoproteins.

Vitamin A deficiency

Vitamin A deficiency is very uncommon except in developing countries among children, in which it manifests as xerophthalmia inducing blindness. Avitaminose A is the main cause of blindness in the world. Electroretinogram and electronystagmogram are useful tests. Vitamin A deficiency is sometimes induced by antiepileptic drugs (e.g., dihydantoin). Hypervitaminosis may also cause neurological symptoms, for example pseudotumor cerebri (increased intracranial pressure and visual disturbances with normal brain imaging), ataxia, and bone and muscle pain. Chronic toxicity may occur with a habitual daily intake of >10,000 µg.

Vitamin C deficiency

The classic vitamin C deficiency syndrome is scurvy, characterized by fatigue, depression, and widespread abnormalities in connective tissues, such as inflamed gingiva, petechiae, perifollicular hemorrhages, impaired wound healing, coiled hairs, hyperkeratosis, and bleeding into body cavities. In infants, defects in ossification and bone growth may occur. In some adults living on canned foods (due to the thermolability of vitamin C), asthenia, myalgias, and hemorrhages could appear. Ascorbic acid level is low in leucocytes and in plasma.

Vitamin D deficiency

Vitamin D deficiency gives a few neurological signs that generally occur in childhood, including muscle hypotonia and skull deformation. Adult patients often complain of pronounced fatigue with bone pain. The reason muscle weakness occurs in such patients is unclear, and the phenomenon is explained only in part by low serum calcium.

Vitamin K deficiency

The term vitamin K actually denotes a group of lipophilic, hydrophobic vitamins that belong to the class of 2-methyl-1,4-naphthoquinone derivatives. The naturally occurring compounds are vitamin K1 (phylloquinone, phytomenadione, or phytonadione) and vitamin K2 (menaquinone or menatetrenone). The former compound is the primary source of vitamin K in humans. It is acquired through the diet and is prevalent in leafy green vegetables such as spinach, Swiss chard, Brassica (e.g., cabbage, kale, cauliflower, turnip, and Brussels sprouts), some fruits such as avocado, banana, and kiwi, as well as in some vegetable oils, especially soybean oil. Interestingly, cooking does not remove significant amounts of vitamin K from these foods. Many bacteria that colonize the human intestine (especially Bacteroides) synthesize vitamin K2 or menaquinone, which is used as a redox reagent in electron transport and oxidative phosphorylation. There is, however, an ongoing debate about whether bacterial synthesis of vitamin K in the intestine provides a significant supply of this vitamin in humans. The colon contains a large reservoir of bacterial vitamin K2 (~2 mg), but it is now undeniable that this pool represents only about 10% of normal human requirements and is, therefore, insufficient to satisfy these requirements. Furthermore, there is some evidence of poor bioavailability of this intestinal source of vitamin K. Bile salts are necessary for effective absorption of vitamin K, but are not present in the colon, and the intestinal synthesis of vitamin K is not sufficient to compensate for deficiency due to biliary obstruction. Moreover, intestinal menaquinones are enveloped within the bacterial membranes and are, therefore, poorly available for intestinal adsorption. Taken together, these data argue against the concept of the colon as a significant source of vitamin K for human use, so that patients at risk of deficiency remain those who cannot absorb vitamin K from the small intestine. Fasting vitamin K1 reference values in healthy adults range from 0.15–1.0 µg/L (median 0.5 µg/L). The thresholds of adequate vitamin K intake were set as 2 µg/day for infants in the first 6 months of life and 2.5 µg/day for infants aged 7–12 months. After this age, the adequate intake progressively increases from 30 µg/day in children aged 1–3 years, up to 75 µg/day in adolescents (up to 18 years old).

Vitamin K is essential for the function of several proteins involved in blood coagulation (prothrombin, also known as factor II, factors VII, IX, and X, protein C, protein S, and protein Z), bone metabolism (osteocalcin, periostin, and matrix Gla protein), as well as vascular biology, cell growth, and apoptosis (growth-arrest-specific gene 6 protein). A poor vitamin K status is, therefore, currently regarded as a risk factor not only for bleeding, but also for increased postmenopausal bone loss and arterial calcification, especially in diabetics and in patients with chronic renal disease.

Dietary deficiency of vitamin K is extremely rare in adults, and when it does occur, it is usually associated with profoundly inadequate dietary intake, intestinal disorders (e.g., regional enteritis, cystic fibrosis, intestinal resection), malabsorption, and, to a lesser extent, decreased production by normal flora (e.g., during the use of a broad spectrum antibiotic) and renal failure.

Vitamin K deficiency is, however, much more frequent in neonates, due to both endogenous and exogenous deficiency. The former case, which is probably less clinically significant, has been attributed to insufficient intestinal colonization by bacteria, whereas the latter case arises from poor placental transport of the vitamin and its low concentration in breast milk. The main exogenous source of vitamin K in neonates, which is almost exclusively milk, cannot adequately compensate for deficient endogenous production, since human breast milk contains between 1 and 4 µg/L of vitamin K1 (and a much lower concentration of vitamin K2).

Vitamin K deficiency-related bleeding (VKDB) is defined as a bleeding disorder in which the coagulation is rapidly corrected by vitamin K supplementation. The diagnosis is suggested by an international normalized ratio of 4 or a prothrombin time of 4 times the control value in the presence of a normal platelet count and normal fibrinogen level. Confirmation of the diagnosis requires measurement of the specific vitamin K-dependent factors (II, VII, IX, X), whose levels are rapidly corrected by the parenteral administration of 1 mg vitamin K1. VKDB is usually classified by etiology (idiopathic and secondary) and by age of onset (early, classical, and late).

Early VKDB presents within 24 hours of birth and is almost exclusively seen in infants of mothers taking drugs that inhibit vitamin K: anticonvulsants (carbamazepine, phenytoin, and barbiturates), antituberculosis drugs (isoniazid, rifampicin), some antibiotics (cephalosporins), and vitamin K antagonists (coumarin, warfarin). The clinical presentation is often severe, with cephalic hematoma and intracranial and intra-abdominal hemorrhages. The incidence of early VKDB in neonates of mothers taking these drugs without vitamin K supplementation varies from 6–12%. Classical VKDB occurs between 24 hours and 7 days of life and is associated with delayed or insufficient feeding. The clinical presentation is often mild, with bruises, gastrointestinal blood loss, or bleeding from the umbilicus and puncture sites. Blood loss can, however, be significant, and intracranial hemorrhage, although rare, has been described. Estimates of the frequency vary from 0.25–1.5% in older reviews and 0–0.44% in more recent reviews. Late VKDB is associated with exclusive breastfeeding. It occurs between the ages of 2 weeks and 12 weeks. The clinical presentation is severe, with a mortality rate of 20% and intracranial hemorrhage occurring in 50%. Persistent neurological damage is frequent in survivors. In fully breastfed infants who did not receive vitamin K at birth, the incidence is between 1/15,000 and 1/20,000. Babies with cholestasis or malabsorption syndromes are at particular risk.

Conclusion

Adequate dietary intake of micronutrients is not necessarily achieved even in resource-rich areas of the world wherein overeating is a public health concern. Disorders due to vitamin deficiencies are still observable in different parts of the world, both highly and less developed. Neurologists must be aware of such possible reasons for neurological symptoms and be able to diagnose and adequately treat them.

Further reading

Briani C, Dalla Torre C, Citton V, *et al.* Cobalamin deficiency: Clinical picture and radiological findings. *Nutrients* 2013;5(11):4521–4539.

Chawla J, Kvarnberg D. Hydrosoluble vitamins. *Handb Clin Neurol* 2014;120:891–914.

de Souza A. Movement disorders and the osmotic demyelination syndrome. *Parkinsonism Relat Disord* 2013;19(8):709–716.

Galvin R, Bråthen G, Ivashynka A, *et al.* EFNS guidelines for diagnosis, therapy and prevention of Wernicke encephalopathy. *Eur J Neurol* 2010;17(12):1408–1418.

Kumar N. Neurologic presentations of nutritional deficiencies. *Neurol Clin* 2010; 28(1):107–170.

Lindblad M, Tveden-Nyborg P, Lykkesfeldt J. Regulation of vitamin C homeostasis during deficiency. *Nutrients* 2013;5(8):2860–2879.

López M, Olivares JM, Berrios GE. Pellagra encephalopathy in the context of alcoholism: Review and case report. *Alcohol Alcohol* 2014;49(1):38–41.

Pfeiffer RF. Neurologic manifestations of malabsorption syndromes. *Handb Clin Neurol* 2014;120:621–632.

Shearer MJ, Fu X, Booth SL. Vitamin K nutrition, metabolism and requirements: Current concepts and future research. *Adv Nutr* 2012;3:182–195.

Thomson AD, Guerrini I, Marshall EJ. The evolution and treatment of Korsakoff's syndrome: Out of sight, out of mind? *Neuropsychol Rev* 2012;22(2):81–92.

Zhao R, Goldman ID. Folate and thiamine transporters mediated by facilitative carriers (SLC19A1-3 and SLC46A1) and folate receptors. Mol Aspects Med 2013;34(0): 10.1016/j.mam.2012.07.006.

99 Starvation, Strachan's syndrome, and postgastroplasty syndrome

Ivan G. Milanov and Vesselina T. Grozeva

Neurology Department, Medical University, and Movement Disorders Clinic, St. Naum University Hospital for Active Treatment in Neurology and Psychiatry, Sofia, Bulgaria

Starvation

Starvation, where the intake of food (calories, vitamins, and minerals) is insufficient and below the minimum dietary requirement, is the most extreme form of malnutrition. Malnutrition contributes to more than one-third of all childhood deaths. Interestingly, epidemiological studies have suggested that individuals who were prenatally exposed to famine had less DNA methylation, pointing out that early life environmental conditions can cause epigenetic changes in humans that persist throughout life.

Malnutrition during development has been linked to poor cognitive function and greater susceptibility to neuropsychiatric disorders. Neurological deficits in adults may be classified as primary and secondary. The primary deficits arise from inadequate food intake in restrictive diets (e.g., veganism), food avoidance (anorexia nervosa, hunger strike), and incarceration (prison camp). The secondary deficits are due to other diseases/conditions that have led to low food ingestion, inadequate nutrient absorption, or nutrient losses. Secondary causes can include parasitism, infectious diseases, especially severe chronic infections associated with chronic diarrhea, critical illness, cachexia, and specific medical conditions with inability to digest and assimilate required nutrients (e.g., pernicious anemia, celiac disease, malignancy), or bariatric/weight-loss surgery. Specific neurological conditions are associated with vitamin and micronutrient deficiencies of vitamins A, B_1, B_6, B_{12}, and E, folic acid, iodine, and non-metal (iodine, selenium) and metal ions (zinc, iron, copper, magnesium).

The effects of malnutrition can be mild, moderate, or severe. The clinical forms of severe protein–energy malnutrition are marasmus and kwashiorkor. Kwashiorkor arises predominantly from protein deficiency, while marasmus is mainly associated with a severe energy-deficient state. Marasmic kwashiorkor is a combination of chronic deficiency and chronic or acute protein deficit. These conditions lead to shrinkage of vital organs (lungs, heart, ovaries, or testes) and reduction of their functional capacity. Clinically, patients present with chronic diarrhea, anemia, reduction in muscle mass, weakness, low body temperature, decreased ability to digest (lack of digestive acid production), irritability, immune deficiency, and edema associated with deficiency of glutathione, an important cellular antioxidant. In adults, anemia is the first sign of malnutrition, followed by edema of extremities and loss of resistance to infections. Specific symptoms of nutrient deficiencies may appear subsequently.

Clinical features

Reduced nerve conduction velocity is evident in the upper and/or lower extremities of children with kwashiorkor and marasmus. Deficiency of thiamine and riboflavin following severe protein deprivation causes peripheral sensory and sensorimotor axonal neuropathy. Other neurological signs of malnutrition in children include learning deficits, behavioral problems, and poor manual dexterity, motor weakness with muscle atrophy, hypotonia, and hyporeflexia. Nerve biopsies show retarded segmental myelination with abnormal motor nerve conduction. Nutritional deficiency can cause optic neuropathy, which is usually bilateral, painless, chronic, insidious, slowly progressive, and responsive to vitamin therapy. Peripheral neuropathy with increased risk of focal compression neuropathies is present in malnourished patients with anorexia nervosa.

Studies involving prisoners who underwent a hunger strike showed electrophysiological changes of prolonged distal motor latencies of the tibial nerve and prolonged latencies of visual evoked potentials. Many developed Wernicke–Korsakoff syndrome, with altered consciousness, amnesia, gaze-evoked horizontal nystagmus, and truncal ataxia. Physiological responses included a lower body temperature, respiration, and heart rate. Many of the participants developed anemia, fatigue, apathy, extreme weakness, lower-extremity edema, irritability, severe emotional distress, depression, hysteria, and hypochondriasis.

A form of cachexia, with severe malnutrition, loss of body weight, muscle atrophy, fatigue, and weakness, can be associated with certain chronic inflammatory diseases, including acquired immune deficiency syndrome (AIDS), tuberculosis, and cancer.

Treatment

Treatment consists of a well-balanced diet consisting of all essential nutritional supplements. The condition of severe malnutrition requires parenteral feeding of a carefully selected diet.

Strachan's syndrome

In the nineteenth century, Dr. Henry Strachan first described a neuropathy with an undefined cause affecting some sugar cane workers in Jamaica. The constellation of symptoms differed from beriberi and pellagra. The condition was characterized by a combination of visual deficits (amblyopia), sensorineural deafness, painful sensorimotor polyneuropathy with ataxia, and lesions of the skin and mucous membranes (orogenital dermatitis). Additional symptoms

International Neurology, Second edition. Edited by Robert P. Lisak, Daniel D. Truong, William M. Carroll and Roongroj Bhidayasiri
© 2016 John Wiley & Sons, Ltd. Published 2016 by John Wiley & Sons, Ltd.

were found in individuals liberated from prison camps following World War II, including vertigo, confusion, spastic leg weakness, and myasthenic bulbar weakness.

In a series of autopsies carried out by Fisher, the most prominent pathological finding was demyelination of the posterior columns of the cervical and thoracic spinal cord. In 1955, Fisher named the syndrome after Henry Strachan, since the so-called Jamaican neuritis was similar to that seen in Canadian prisoners of war in Japanese concentration camps during World War II.

Later, from 1991–93, an epidemic of a similar syndrome appeared in Cuba due to food shortages on the island. The Cuban Ministry of Health reported 50,862 cases of neuropathy. The syndrome manifested with retrobulbar optic neuropathy (decreased vision, bilateral and symmetric central or cecocentral scotoma, and loss of color vision), sensory (distal axonopathy lesion affecting predominantly large myelinated axons) and dysautonomic peripheral neuropathy, dorsolateral myeloneuropathy (dorsal column and pyramidal involvement of the lower limbs with spastic bladder), sensorineural deafness (selective high frequency, 4–8 kHz, hearing loss), dysphonia and dysphagia, spastic paraparesis, and mixed presentations. The endemic ceased after B-group vitamins and folate supplements were given to the population. The primary cause for the epidemic appeared to be deficiency of the micronutrients thiamine, cobalamine, folate, and sulfur amino acids. Most patients improved significantly after treatment and less than 0.1% of them continued to have sequelae. Increased risk for developing the syndrome was observed among smokers due to their exposure to cyanide, heavy drinkers, and those with a low protein diet, weight loss, and excessive sugar consumption. Scott also reported optic nerve degeneration among workers in a Jamaican sugar cane (a cyanogenic plant) plantation in 1918.

Subsequently, many cases of Strachan's syndrome were described in prisoners in Singapore and concentration camps in Germany, and in people from Thailand and Senegal. Multiple variants with different names were observed: Madrid syndrome, paresthesia-causalgia syndrome, syndrome of the burning feet, Cuban epidemic optic and peripheral neuropathy, tropical ataxic neuropathy, "camper foot," and others. Some conditions like tropical ataxic neuropathy and tropical spastic paraparesis caused by viral human T-lymphotropic virus (HTLV-1) infection may occasionally have a peripheral manifestation of Strachan's syndrome, although they are characterized by spasticity and other signs of corticospinal involvement.

Pathophysiology

The pathogenesis of Strachan's syndrome is unknown. The condition was suspected to be caused by a toxin (e.g., arsenic, cyanide) or malnutrition. Riboflavin deficiency was also hypothesized as a possible cause. It is now accepted that the main etiology of Strachan's syndrome is deficiency of the microelement vitamins such as A, D, E, thiamine, cobalamine, folic acid, and sulphur-containing amino acids. Deficiency of microelements can be due to malnutrition and tropical enteropathy caused by remitting infections, impairing the mucous of small intestines, accompanied by a syndrome of malabsorption. Mitochondrial deletion is another proposed pathogenic mechanism. All result in damage to the most sensitive neurons of the dorsal root ganglia and bipolar neurons of the retina.

Histopathology shows axonal loss of myelinated and non-myelinated nerve fibers. Demyelination and axonal loss are present in the dorsal columns of the cervical and thoracic spinal cord. Papillomacular bundle fibers are lost in the optic nerve.

Clinical features

Progressive sensorial deficits including pain, numbness, dysesthesia with burning feet sensation, loss of vibration and position, and a slightly impaired temperature sensation appear in the lower limbs and are more pronounced distally. The gait may be disturbed. Only the upper or only the lower limbs may be affected symmetrically. Tendon reflexes in the lower limbs may be absent, but the muscle tone and strength are preserved. Muscle weakness involves predominantly the proximal muscles of the lower limbs. Muscular hypotrophy and cramps may also appear. Spastic paraparesis may be observed, although spasticity is not that prominent. Cerebellar symptoms of tremor and dysmetria are pronounced in 20% of patients. Impotence, constipation, and urinary incontinence may develop. The disease progresses slowly over the course of several years. The optic neuritis and hearing loss are more often seen in patients from Jamaica (15%) in comparison to other parts of the world.

Ophthalmic disturbances such as amblyopia are more typical for the Cuban form of the syndrome. Other ophthalmic findings included central or centrocecal visual scotoma, diminished visual acuity, paleness of the pupil of the optic nerve, and progress to total blindness. Laryngeal symptoms are less often seen in patients with sensorineural deafness, vertigo, glossitis, stomatitis, gingivitis, and dermal desquamation. Dermatitis affects the mucocutaneous junctions of the mouth and eye angle, preputium, anus, and vulva.

Investigations

Nerve conduction studies show chronic axonal injury in the limbs. Nerve biopsy reveals axonal degeneration of large myelinated fibers.

Differential diagnosis

Strachan's syndrome must be differentiated from beriberi, vitamin B_{12} deficiency, pellagra, tropical spastic paraparesis, Leber's optic neuropathy, and toxic/nutritional optic neuropathy (Table 99.1).

Treatment

Treatment includes administration of vitamin B complex and folic acid.

Postgastroplasty syndrome

Neurological complications such as sensorimotor painful polyneuropathy may appear in up to 62% of patients who have undergone a gastrectomy (Roux-en-Y, jejunal pouch interposition, Billroth I, and Billroth II method) due to peptic ulcer, carcinoma, stomach bypass (jejunoileal bypass), or restriction operations (bariatric/weight-loss surgery), or in patients who suffer from malnutrition due to inappropriate diet, alcoholism, or malabsorption syndrome.

Nowadays open or laparoscopic bariatric surgery offers the most effective treatment for obesity – a growing epidemic. As obesity significantly increases the risk of developing metabolic and cardiovascular disorders and reduces life expectancy, the number of bariatric procedures is increasing. The most commonly performed bariatric surgeries are Roux-en-Y gastric bypass, which involves the creation of a small gastric pouch and intestinal rerouting; sleeve gastrectomy, in which 75% of the stomach is removed; and adjustable gastric banding, the placement of a silicone ring around the stomach that limits the amount of food that can be consumed. Regardless of the surgical method used, bariatric procedure outcome is rapid weight loss, with physiological effects that resemble those of a starvation diet.

Table 99.1. Differential diagnosis of Strachan's syndrome.

	Etiology	Clinical characteristics	Treatment
Strachan's syndrome	Vitamin deficiency Cyanide-containing foods (cassava/manioc) Apricot kernels	Amblyopia Sensorineural deafness Painful sensorimotor polyneuropathy with ataxia Orogenital dermatitis	Vitamin B, folic acid, riboflavin supplement Well-balanced diet
Beriberi	Vitamin B_1 (thiamine)	"Dry" beriberi – peripheral nervous system involvement "Wet" beriberi – cardiovascular and other systems Wernicke–Korsakoff syndrome	Vitamin B1 supplement Well-balanced diet
Pellagra	Vitamin B_3 (nicotinamide, niacin) deficiency	Dermatitis, diarrhea, hematopoiesis, peripheral neuropathy, and dementia Acute cases: spasticity, psychoneurosis (stupor and mania, delirium, and paranoia) Mild cases: weakness, tremor, anxiety, depression, irritability, confusion, fear, dizziness, and poor memory	Vitamin B3 supplement Well-balanced diet
Vitamin B_{12} (cobalamin) deficiency	Gastritis pernicious anemia Bariatric and gastric surgeries Crohn's disease Alcoholism Grave's disease Lupus erythematosus Vegan diet	Progressive hematological, psychiatric, and neurological disease Sensory nerve abnormalities Cranial (including optic) nerve and cerebellar abnormalities	Vitamin B_{12} supplement
Tropical spastic paraparesis/Konzo	HTLV-1 Cyanide-containing foods	Spastic paraparesis Sphincter dysfunction Sensory impairment	Corticosteroids Interferons Plasmapheresis Myorelaxants
Leber's optic neuropathy	Mitochondrial genetic defect	Severe optic atrophy with permanent decrease of visual acuity	Medications are going through trials
Toxic/nutritional optic neuropathy	Toxic (heavy metals, fumes, solvents) Drug-induced (ethambutol, isoniazid, amiodarone) Nutritional (tobacco, alcohol, thiamine, vitamin B12 deficiency)	Bilateral optic neuropathy Dimness of vision Color vision anomaly (dyschromatopsia)	Balanced diet Vitamin B_{12} Hydroxycobalamin

Recent studies show that maternal obesity and overeating during pregnancy are potential risk factors for obesity, type II diabetes, and cardiovascular disease in the offspring. Genetic expression related to disease risk may be modified by the environment. The term "epigenetic changes" describes DNA methylation and alterations to histone proteins that alter the likelihood that certain genes will get transcribed. Epigenetic changes usually occur during prenatal development or the early postnatal period. Proper maternal intake of folate, methionine, and vitamin B_{12} is very important during pregnancy, as it affects DNA methylation. Nutritional signals reaching the developing hypothalamic neurons during pregnancy are hypothesized to influence their sensitivity to respond to similar signals postnatally. Infant nutrition in the neonatal period may also affect future risk for obesity and its complications. Despite the known positive effects, weight-reduction surgery may lead to serious neurological complications, such as peripheral neuropathy, burning feet syndrome, meralgia paresthetica, posterolateral myelopathy, myotonic syndrome, Wernicke–Korsakoff encephalopathy, optic neuropathy, and lumbosacral plexopathy.

Pathophysiology

Neurological complications associated with postgastroplasty syndrome arise mostly as a result of the acquired deficiency of thiamine (vitamin B_1) and cyanocobalamin (vitamin B_{12}). The nervous system may be affected in 31% of patients through similar mechanisms to those in pernicious anemia.

The pathogenesis may be explained by the aberrant absorption and subsequent deficiency of cyanocobalamin, thiamine, pyridoxine, panthenol, niacin, vitamin A, and copper. There may also be a role for decreased gastric juice secretion, inadequate production of intrinsic factor, and minimal food intake, together with reduced exposure of ingested food in the duodenum. Some unknown inflammatory factors may also contribute. Iron deficiency is present in 50% of patients, most probably due to aberrant calcium absorption, deficiency of vitamin D, and secondary hyperparathyroidism. The most critical deficiencies after bariatric procedures appear to be those of albumin, vitamins B_1, B_{12}, and D, iron, and zinc. Drugs such as antidepressants, antimicrobials, and metformin, which is prescribed to bariatric patients, may also affect bioavailability and absorption. Histopathological studies of peripheral nerves in these patients confirmed the presence of severe axonal neuropathy.

Cinical features

The disease begins with remitting vomiting and rapid severe weight loss. A mixture of symptoms appear, resulting from inadequate supplementation of key nutrients. Neurological complications can involve any part of the nervous system: the brain, spinal cord, nerves leaving the spinal cord, or the peripheral nerves. Often more than one part of the nervous system is involved.

Peripheral neuropathies are the most frequent complication after gastrectomy. They present as sensorimotor polyneuropathy – predominantly sensitive – with insidious onset (acute or subacute) and chronic evolution; mononeuropathy, which can develop at any time postoperatively; or radiculoplexopathy, which is always acute or subacute in onset. Impairment of the peripheral nervous system may start abruptly, as in acute inflammatory demyelinating polyneuropathy, or subacutely, as in distal sensorimotor polyneuropathy. Distal symmetric sensory and motor disturbances appear. The first symptoms are numbness, burning sensation of pain, and paresthesias in the feet, followed by subacute development of sensorimotor neuropathy. Some patients present with distal motor weakness of the hands and feet, and "drop foot." Muscle weakness can be considerable and it can seriously disturb walking. In some patients muscle atrophy may be present relatively early in the clinical course. Cramps and involvement of cranial (double vision, difficulty to swallow) and trunk nerves may occur.

Mononeuropathies may affect the great occipital nerve, the median nerve (i.e., carpal tunnel syndrome), the radial nerve (sensitive neuropathy of the superficial radial nerve), the ulnar nerve, the lateral femoral cutaneus nerve, the sciatic nerve, and the fibular nerve. Carpal tunnel syndrome and paresthetic meralgia (neuropathy of the lateral femoral cutaneous nerve) are most frequent.

Rarely, neuropathies involve the nerve radices and plexi (brachial plexus/Parsonage–Turner syndrome). Radiculoplexoneuropathies may affect cervical and lumbosacral regions. Initially, symptoms are asymmetric and include severe burning, sharp pain, shocks, or allodynia and numbness, followed by muscle weakness of the involved limb.

Autonomic symptoms such as constipation, fainting, syncope, hypotension, impotency, and urinary urgency or incontinence may develop.

Neurological complications of bariatric surgery also may include myelopathy, myotonia, Wernicke–Korsakoff encephalopathy (confusion, memory complaints, and coordination difficulty), and optic neuropathy.

A Brazilian study group described demyelination of the central nervous system, clinically manifested as multiple sclerosis, with findings fulfilling the magnetic resonance imaging (MRI) criteria for diagnosis, in several patients with bariatric surgeries. They also observed some cases with rapidly progressing tetraparesia and electrophysiological signs of motor neuron disease. Whether nutritional deficiencies might be responsible for these central nervous system manifestations remains unknown.

Neurological complications after bariatric surgery primarily include Guillian–Barré syndrome (GBS), occurring as a result of inflammation. Classic symptoms after surgery are protracted nausea, vomiting, and lower extremity weakness. Generalized weakness can progress over days to weeks. GBS can present also with cranial nerve deficits and respiratory compromise. Symptoms of confusion, inappropriate behavior, profound weakness, and paraplegia may appear.

Investigations

Nerve conduction studies show a slight decrease of conduction velocity (up to 20%) of sensory and motor fibers and decreased amplitude of compound muscle action potentials (CMAPs) and sensory nerve action potentials (SNAPs), which are most evident in the lower limbs. Distal latency (DL) can be mildly prolonged in

some patients. The electromyography (EMG) findings are consistent with an axonal sensorimotor polyneuropathy. The needle EMG is usually normal.

Treatment

Preoperative evaluation of nutritional parameters is recommended. Levels of vitamins, calcium, alkaline phosphatase, and iron, together with lipid profile, should be controlled before and after the surgical intervention. Treatment includes avoiding or reducing severe and rapid weight loss and administering nutritional, vitamin, and mineral supplements. Some cases need complete parenteral feeding and reconstruction of the bypass.

Thiamine deficiency in bariatric patients should be treated with thiamine, other B-complex vitamins, and magnesium. Early symptoms of neuropathy can be resolved by oral thiamine doses of 20–30 mg/day until symptoms disappear. Patients with protracted vomiting and advanced neuropathy are to take intravenous or intramuscular thiamine in 50–100 mg/day doses. Those with Wernicke–Korsakoff encephalopathy require ≥100 mg intravenous thiamine for several days or longer, followed by intramuscular thiamine or high oral doses, until symptoms have resolved or improved, which may take months or sometimes years. Lifelong thiamine treatment is required to prevent reoccurrence of neuropathy.

Vitamin B_6 1.6 mg/day is recommended in the early postoperative period. Supplementation with 350–500 μg/day may prevent postoperative vitamin B_{12} deficiency.

Folate does not affect myelin, so neurological complications are rare in cases of folate deficiency, as compared to vitamin B_{12} deficiency. Patients with folate deficiency often present with forgetfulness, irritability, hostility, and paranoid behaviors. Folate deficiency requires a daily folate intake of 1000 mg. Folate supplementation >1000 mg/day is not recommended because of the potential for masking vitamin B_{12} deficiency.

Iron deficiency is corrected with 50–100 mg elemental iron daily.

Deficiency of vitamins A, E, and K, as well as zinc, has also been noted after bariatric procedures. The recommended dosages after surgery are 50,000 IU for vitamin A (every 2 weeks) and 500 mg daily for vitamin E.

Symptoms of myelopathy (i.e., ataxia, paresthesia) appear when copper is deficient. Copper deficiency can cause a demyelinating neuropathy. Copper should be administered as a dose of 2 mg/day to resolve the deficiency.

Life-long use of multivitamins and minerals such as zinc, vitamin D, and calcium is recommended. The required vitamin A daily intake is 10,000 IU. A daily dose of 300 μg vitamin K is sufficient after bariatric procedures.

The tricyclic antidepressants amitriptyline and nortriptyline and the anticonvulsants gabapentin and carbamazepine are the drugs of choice for neuropathic pain secondary to polyneuropathies. Physical therapy also has an important role in patient rehabilitation.

Prognosis

Treatment is effective only if started on time. If treatment is delayed after the onset of complications, neuropathy symptoms may persist. Neuropathies may add to the potential cases of serious and often permanent neurological complications of bariatric surgery. Some patients have a complete resolution of neurological symptoms, but others – those with a longer time between the development of symptoms and beginning treatment – usually have persistent distal sensitive and/or motor deficits. Neurological complications are among the most feared, due to the potential for irreversibility.

Further reading

Allied Health Sciences Section Ad Hoc Nutrition Committee; Aills L, Blankenship J, Buffington C, *et al.* ASMBS Allied Health nutritional guidelines for the surgical weight loss patient. *Surg Obes Relat Dis* 2008;∫(5 Suppl):S73–S108.

Chin RL, Langsdorf J, Feuer N, Carey B. Nutritional and alcoholic neuropathies. In: DonofrioPD (ed.). *Textbook of Peripheral Neuropathy*. New York: Demos Medical Publishing; 2012: 69–85.

Fragoso YD, Alves-Leon SV, Anacleto Ade C, *et al.* Neurological complications following bariatric surgery. *Arq Neuropsiquiatr* 2012;70(9):700–703.

Guénard F, Tchernof A, Deshaies Y, *et al.* Methylation and expression of immune and inflammatory genes in the offspring of bariatric bypass surgery patients. *J Obes* 2013;492170.

Heijmans BT, Tobi EW, Stein AD. Persistent epigenetic differences associated with prenatal exposure to famine in humans. *Proc Natl Acad Sci USA* 2008;105(44): 17046–17049.

Kumar N. Obesity surgery: A word of neurologic caution. *Neurology* 2007;68(21): E36–E38.

Menezes MS, Harada KO, Alvarez G. Painful peripheral polyneuropathy after bariatric surgery. Case reports. *Rev Bras Anestesiol* 2008;58(3):252–259.

Spencer PS, Palmer VS. Interrelationships of undernutrition and neurotoxicity: Food for thought and research attention. *Neurotoxicology* 2012;33(3):605–616.

PART 12 Peripheral Neuropathies

100 Peripheral neuropathies overview

Friedhelm Sandbrink

Department of Neurology, Veterans Affairs Medical Center, and Georgetown University, Washington, DC, USA

Peripheral neuropathies are disorders affecting the peripheral nervous system. While the term is often used rather imprecisely to imply a polyneuropathy, it refers to any disorder of the peripheral nerves, including focal neuropathies and radiculopathies. Polyneuropathy describes a disorder affecting numerous peripheral nerves simultaneously and usually fairly symmetrically. Mononeuropathy indicates involvement of a single nerve, usually due to trauma, compression (entrapment), vasculitis, or tumor infiltration. Often, the term *focal neuropathy* is used to describe a localized nerve lesion. Mononeuropathy multiplex or multifocal mononeuropathy signifies simultaneous or sequential damage to multiple non-contiguous nerves, due to vasculitis or other systemic disease. If inflammatory, the term *mononeuritis multiplex* may be used. In advanced stages, the deficits may become confluent and resemble polyneuropathy. In a broad sense, multiple focal mononeuropathies from several distinct nerve compressions or hereditary neuropathy with liability to pressure palsies (HNPP) may also present as mononeuropathy multiplex. Neuronopathies are diseases of nerve cell bodies, including motor neuron diseases such as spinal muscular atrophies or sensory ganglionopathies.

Epidemiology

Polyneuropathies are among the most common neurological disorders. Population-based estimates indicate a prevalence of 2–7% overall, and an estimated annual incidence of 25–200/100,000 persons per year. They are more common in the elderly, with an estimated prevalence of 5–10%. In Western countries, the most common causes are diabetes mellitus and alcoholism. In other countries infectious etiologies are prominent, especially leprosy.

In Italy, a study of people 55 years and older documented a probable diagnosis of polyneuropathy in 4% and possible diagnosis in 7%. The most common risk factor was diabetes, present in 44% of patients diagnosed with probable polyneuropathy. The prevalence of polyneuropathy among patients with no risk factors was 1.6%, for patients with one risk factor 11.8%, and for patients with two risk factors 17.3%. The prevalence of polyneuropathy was highest in diabetics (18.3%), followed by patients with a diagnosis of alcoholism (12.5%), non-alcoholic liver disease (10.9%), and tumor (7.1%).

Table 100.1 includes some of the many causes of polyneuropathy. Even after diagnostic workup, the etiology remains unknown in one-third of patients.

Table 100.1. Causes of polyneuropathy.

Hereditary
– Hereditary motor and sensory neuropathies
– Hereditary sensory and autonomic neuropathies
– Refsum disease
– Familial amyloidosis
– Friedreich ataxia
– Metachromatic leukodystrophy
– Krabbe disease
– Abetalipoproteinemia
– Tangier disease
– Fabry's disease
– Porphyrias

Acquired
Immune-mediated

– Guillain–Barré syndrome
– Chronic inflammatory demyelinating polyneuropathy
– Multifocal motor neuropathy
– Vasculitis

Neoplastic and paraproteinemic

– Paraproteinemias
– Amyloidosis
– Paraneoplastic
– Tumor infiltration/compression

Metabolic

– Diabetes
– Vitamin B_1, B_6, and B_{12} deficiency
– Copper deficiency/zinc excess
– Hypothyroidism
– Uremia
– Liver disease

Infective and granulomatous

– HIV-related
– Leprosy
– Lyme
– Syphilis
– Diphtheria
– Sarcoidosis
– Sepsis/multiorgan failure

Drug-induced and toxic

– Alcohol
– Drugs, including chemotherapeutic agents, antiviral medication, antibiotics fluroquinolone, phenytoin, pyridoxine (vitamin B_6)
– Toxins, including heavy metals, solvents, pesticides

Pathophysiology and clinical features

Most polyneuropathies fit the typical pattern of symmetric sensory predominant symptoms with distal onset, consistent with "length-dependent" or "dying-back" *axonal polyneuropathy*. The primary insult to neuron or axon, often toxic or metabolic, causes degeneration in the distal parts of the nerve, most removed from the trophic influence of the nerve cell body. Failure to maintain the axonal transport results in *Wallerian-type degeneration* distally with centripetal progression. Clinically, sensory symptoms begin in the toes and feet with numbness and paresthesias, often described as tingling, pins-and-needles sensation, or stabbing or burning pain. Neuropathic pain from small fiber involvement is suggested by the perception of pain to a non-noxious tactile stimulation (allodynia) or increased pain response to noxious stimulation (hyperalgesia). The report of pain more bothersome at rest, such as during the night, usually suggests neuropathic origin. When the sensory deficit reaches to below knee level, the hands become affected and stocking-and-glove sensory deficit develops. Patients with advanced sensory neuropathy may show hypesthesia over the anterior chest and abdomen, typically when the sensory level in the legs reaches the mid-thigh. In general, sensory complaints predominate and motor deficits occur late in the course and are typically limited to the distal muscles. Patients may have weakness of toe/foot extensor muscles followed by interossei hand muscles, and atrophy of intrinsic foot and hand muscles.

In a patient with this typical pattern who has a history or laboratory documentation of diabetes mellitus, alcohol abuse, B_{12} deficiency, uremia, or preceding exposure to a known neurotoxin or drug, further diagnostic workup is unlikely to change the diagnosis. Patients without an obvious cause or any patient with an atypical clinical presentation should undergo further testing, including electrophysiological testing.

Any atypical clinical presentation of a polyneuropathy, other than the sensory predominant fiber-length-dependent pattern described earlier, requires a thorough workup that is based on the clinical features, with usually a shorter list of diagnostic considerations (see Figure 100.1). All patients with early-onset or predominant weakness, or an asymmetric or anatomically restricted pattern of deficits, or an acute or relapsing time course should undergo EMG/NCS testing to delineate the underlying pathophysiology as well as targeted laboratory testing.

The clinical features of *myelinopathies* include proximal muscle weakness, the pattern of disproportionately mild muscle atrophy despite marked weakness, early loss of deep tendon reflexes, tremor, and enlarged nerves. A *hereditary* polyneuropathy usually has a chronic indolent course over years, and patients often have few or no complaints of paresthesias despite sensory deficit on examination.

Patients with small fiber neuropathy have impairment of pain and temperature modalities and autonomic dysfunction. Autonomic symptoms include postural hypotension and syncope, heat intolerance due to impaired sweating, or coldness of the extremities. Bladder or bowel dysfunction is common, and erectile dysfunction occurs early in men. Gastroparesis may result in anorexia, nausea, or vomiting. Small fiber involvement is common in amyloidosis, diabetes mellitus, human immunodeficiency virus (HIV)/acquired immune deficiency syndrome (AIDS), leprosy, Sjögren's syndrome, and in the inherited hereditary sensory and autonomic neuropathies, Fabry's disease, and Tangier disorder. Autonomic deficits often occur also in uremia, porphyria, paraneoplastic neuropathies, and variants of Guillain–Barré syndrome.

The differential diagnosis of painful polyneuropathies includes the small fiber neuropathies, and also vasculitis, alcohol and other toxins (arsenic, thallium), porphyria, Guillain–Barré syndrome, entrapment neuropathies, plexopathy from neuralgic amyotrophy or diabetic lumbosacral radiculoplexopathy, and radiculopathies.

Investigations

The electrophysiological findings in axonal neuropathy include nerve conduction studies (NCS) characterized by reduced amplitudes of nerve action potentials with normal or only minor slowing of conduction velocities, affecting sensory more than motor fibers, in legs more than arms. The needle electromyography (EMG) documents acute denervation in distal muscles, usually accompanied by chronic de- and reinnervation changes of the motor unit action potentials (MUAPs).

The NCS/EMG in hereditary demyelinating polyneuropathies shows uniform slowing of conduction velocities. The neurophysiology finding of segmental demyelination is typical for *acquired* immune-mediated myelinopathies. NCS show marked slowing of conduction velocity (less than 70% of lower normal limit), severely prolonged distal latencies, and in particular conduction block or temporal dispersion. Conduction block is responsible for weakness and sensory loss.

Electrodiagnostic evaluation with routine NCS and EMG assesses *large myelinated* nerve. Routine nerve conduction studies do not assess small fiber nerve function and thus may be normal in selective (isolated) small fiber neuropathies.

The electrodiagnostic assessment of *small fiber and autonomic nerve function* relies on quantitative sensory testing of cold and heat pain thresholds, testing of sudomotor (sweating) function including the quantitative sudomotor axon reflex test (QSART), and cardiovascular/cardiac autonomic testing (heart rate response to tilt table/orthostasis, heart rate variability with respiration, and blood pressure/heart rate change to Valsalva maneuver).

Laboratory testing in patients with undiagnosed polyneuropathy routinely includes full blood count, glucose (hemoglobin A1c, fasting glucose, oral glucose tolerance test), creatinine, erythrocyte sedimentation rate, liver function tests, vitamin B_{12}, serum protein and immune electrophoresis, and thyroid function, and commonly also HIV antibody, rapid plasma reagin (RPR)/Venereal Disease Research Laboratory (VDRL). Further testing is done based on the clinical presentation and electrophysiological findings.

Cerebrospinal fluid (CSF) analysis in acquired demyelinating polyneuropathies typically shows markedly increased protein in the setting of normal or only mildly increased cell count. CSF protein to a lesser degree is also elevated in diabetes and some inherited demyelinating neuropathies. CSF pleocytosis occurs in HIV/AIDS or Lyme disease. Paraneoplastic neuropathies may result in increased CSF protein and cell count. Abnormal cytology may be noted in meningeal carcinomatosis or lymphomatosis.

A nerve biopsy is most useful in patients with suspected vasculitis and amyloidosis, and may be needed in sarcoid, leprosy, or neoplastic infiltration. It may be helpful in acquired or hereditary demyelinating disorders, but is usually not required for diagnosis, except of polyglycosan body neuropathy. Skin biopsy has become a commonly used tool to document loss of

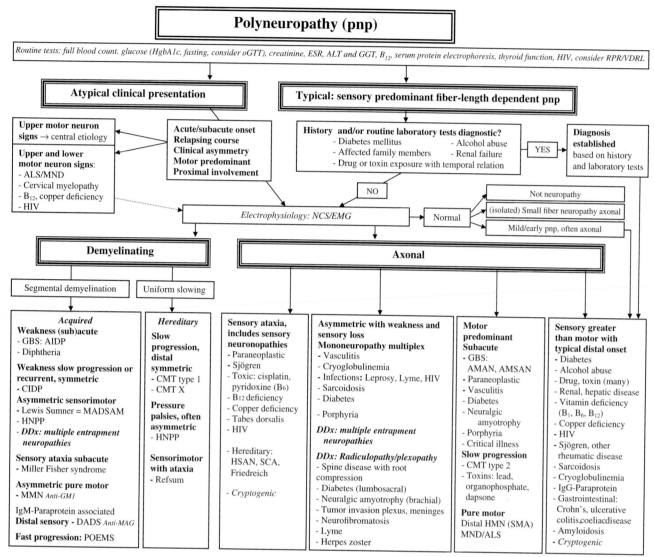

Figure 100.1 Diagnostic considerations in patients with polyneuropathy depending on clinical and electrophysiological pattern.
AIDP = acute inflammatory demyelinating polyneuropathy; ALS = amyotrophic lateral sclerosis; ALT = alanine aminotransferase; AMAN = acute motor axonal neuropathy; AMSAN = acute motor sensory axonal neuropathy; CIDP = chronic inflammatory demyelinating polyneuropathy; CMT = Charcot–Marie–Tooth; DADS = distal acquired demyelinating sensory neuropathy; DDx = differential diagnosis; EMG = electromyography; ESR = erythrocyte sedimentation rate; GBS = Guillain–Barré syndrome; GGT - gamma glutamyl transferase; HIV = human immunodeficiency virus; HMN = hereditary motor neuropathy; HNPP = hereditary neuropathy with liability to pressure palsies; HSAN = hereditary sensory and autonomic neuropathy; MADSAM = multifocal acquired demyelinating sensory and motor neuropathy; MAG = myelin-associated glycoprotein; MMN = multifocal motor neuropathy; MND = motor neuron disease; NCS = nerve conduction studies; oGTT = oral glucose tolerance test; POEMS = peripheral neuropathy, organomegaly, endocrinopathy, M-component and skin changes; RPR = rapid plasma reagin; SCA = spinocerebellar ataxia; SMA = spinal muscular atrophy; VDRL = Venereal Disease Research Laboratory

intraepidermal nerve fibers in small fiber neuropathies, when routine NCS are normal.

Treatment

Medical treatment of neuropathic pain is often difficult. Ideally, therapy is directed at the underlying cause, and if available, this is described in subsequent sections. There are several sets of recommendations for the symptomatic treatment of neuropathic pain, including one by the International Association for the Study of Pain (IASP), two European, one Canadian, and one Latin American

guideline. Simple analgesics including acetaminophen (paracetamol) and non-steroidal anti-inflammatory drugs (NSAIDs) are usually not effective. Treatment relies primarily on selected antidepressants and anticonvulsants and topical agents. The antidepressant and anticonvulsant medications usually require gradual titration, with benefit expected after several weeks (to months) of therapy.

Tricyclic antidepressants and serotonin-norepinephrine reuptake inhibitors are the antidepressants with documented benefit as adjuvant analgesics. Tricyclic medication may relieve burning and dysesthetic pain, and improve sleep. The more selective secondary amine tricyclic antidepressants (nortriptyline, desipramine) are often recommended over amitriptyline due to fewer side effects, with overall similar efficacy. Treatment is initiated with 10–25 mg at bedtime and gradually increased as tolerated. Side effects including sedation, dry mouth, and constipation are common and frequently dose limiting. Particular caution is advised in the elderly and any patient with cardiac arrhythmias. Serotonin-norepinephrine reuptake inhibitors are often better tolerated than the tricyclic antidepressants, especially in full antidepressant dosage. Duloxetine is initiated at 30 mg/day (elderly 20 mg) and increased to 60 mg/day, sometimes higher; if venlafaxine is used, a gradual increase to a higher dosage (150–225 mg/day) is usually required for analgesic benefit.

Anticonvulsant medications for pain are primarily the calcium channel alpha 2-delta ligands (gabapentinoids). Gabapentin and pregabalin have overall similar indications and side effects. Gabapentin is initiated with 100–300 mg three times a day (usually in gradually increasing steps) and then further increased as tolerated and needed to 600–900 mg three times a day. Pregabalin is easier to titrate and is begun with 150 mg divided in two or three daily doses, and increased to a target dosage of 300 mg/day. The usual side effects are sedation/drowsiness, peripheral edema, and over time weight gain. If it is too sedating, a single daily dosage at bedtime may improve tolerability and also improve sleep. The use of other anticonvulsants including carbamazepine and other sodium channel blocking agents may be considered as second-line agents.

Combination therapy of two medications with different mechanisms of action may result in greater pain reduction, but is often associated with greater side effects. The topical agents include lidocaine and capsaicin (both are formulated as cream/ointment and in patch form).

Opioid treatment is controversial and usually not recommended for chronic (long-term) therapy in neuropathic pain. Opioids may be considered for acute or episodic exacerbation of severe pain, and when prompt pain relief is required until the slower-acting adjuvant

analgesics become effective. If opioid medication is used, then tramadol (an opioid agonist and serotonin-norepinephrine reuptake inhibitor) is often preferred due to a more favorable risk/benefit ratio than others. Tramadol has limitations due to dosage limitation (maximal dosage is 100 mg every 6 hours), drug–drug interactions (in particular with antidepressants), and side effects including nausea (which may be avoided by initiating at a low dose of 25–50 mg twice a day as needed). While there are randomized studies documenting the efficacy of opioid therapy for painful neuropathy, treatment of neuropathic pain usually requires higher dosages than for nociceptive pain, and over time the risks likely outweigh the benefits for most patients. Situations when opioids may be justified include acute, cancer-related, or episodic exacerbation of severe pain, when prompt pain relief is required, and until the slower-acting adjuvant pain medication becomes effective.

Treatment of severe chronic pain should include non-pharmacological strategies in accordance with the biopsychosocial model of chronic pain, including behavioral pain therapy, physical therapy and other rehabilitation modalities, and integrative approaches.

Further reading

Attal N, Cruccu G, Baron R, *et al*. EFNS guidelines on the pharmacological treatment of neuropathic pain: 2010 revision. *Eur J Neurol* 2010;17:1113–e88.

Beghi E, Monticelli ML. Chronic symmetric symptomatic polyneuropathy in the elderly: A field screening investigation of risk factors for polyneuropathy in two Italian communities. Italian General Practitioner Study Group (IGPST). *J Clin Epidemiol* 1998;51:697–702.

Mygland A. Approach to the patient with chronic polyneuropathy. *Acta Neurol Scand* 2007;115 (Suppl 187):15–21.

O'Connor AB, Dworkin RH. Treatment of neuropathic pain: An overview of recent guidelines. *Am J Med* 2009;122(10 Suppl):S22–S32.

Vrancken AF, Kalmijn S, Buskens E, *et al*. Feasibility and cost efficiency of a diagnostic guideline for chronic polyneuropathy: A prospective implementation study. *J Neurol Neurosurg Psychiatry* 2006;77:397–401.

101 Hereditary neuropathies

Liying Cui and Mingsheng Liu

Department of Neurology, Peking Union Medical College Hospital, Beijing, China

The classification of hereditary neuropathies has been a source of confusion, as both clinical and genetic schemes are used. Based on clinical patterns, hereditary neuropathies are generally subdivided into three categories, reflecting the selective or predominant involvement of the motor or sensory peripheral nervous system. The most common group is hereditary motor and sensory neuropathy (HMSN). HMSN was first described by Charcot and Marie in France and Tooth in England in 1886 and is also called Charcot–Marie–Tooth (CMT) disease. In HMSN (CMT), both the motor and sensory nerves are affected. The second group is hereditary sensory and autonomic neuropathy (HSAN), in which sensory dysfunction prevails and the autonomic nervous system is also involved to varying degrees. The third group is distal hereditary motor neuropathy (distal HMN), in which only the peripheral motor nervous system is affected. Each of these subtypes will be described in detail in this chapter.

Hereditary motor and sensory neuropathy

HMSN or CMT neuropathy refers to a heterogenous group of inherited peripheral neuropathies that affect motor and sensory nerves. More than 50 distinct genetic causes have been identified, yet these mutations account for only half of patients with the CMT phenotype. Table 101.1 provides a framework for HMSN based on clinical and genetic information.

Clinically, HMSN with autosomal dominant inheritance is subdivided on the basis of nerve conduction velocity into two types: HMSN I (or CMT1), with severely slowed conduction velocities (demyelinating), and HMSN II (or CMT2), with normal or near normal conduction velocities (axonal). HMSN III (or CMT3) is the clinical category for hypertrophic neuropathy with onset during infancy, also called Dejerine–Sottas disease. CMTX is X-linked and most patients have intermediately slowed nerve conduction velocities.

Epidemiology

HMSN as a group represents the most common form of inherited peripheral neuropathy and is one of the most common inherited neurological diseases. The frequency of the disease cannot be stated with precision because of its clinical heterogeneity, but the usually quoted prevalence is about 40/100,000 of the population. According to recent studies, a molecular diagnosis may be established in one-half to two-thirds of patients with a clinical diagnosis of HMSN.

Pathophysiology

Inheritance of HMSN is most often autosomal dominant, with almost complete penetrance. In the Western hemisphere, X-linked dominance is the second most common inheritance pattern. Autosomal recessive forms are more commonly seen in countries with ethnically homogenous populations and higher rates of consanguineous marriages. Some cases, probably a small number, arise as *de novo* mutations.

The common types of HMSN that are connected to chromosomes 1 or 17 cannot be easily distinguished from one another on clinical grounds, but they have distinctive electromyographic (EMG) features. Of CMT1 cases, 70% result from duplication of the gene for a peripheral myelin protein (*PMP22*) on chromosome 17 p11 (type CMT1A). Other studies of the *PMP22* and *P0* (another myelin protein) gene expression in CMT1 and CMT3 cases (Dejerine–Sottas disease) have yielded discordant results because mutations on different loci, including one on chromosome 1, lead to different presentations. Hereditary neuropathy with pressure palsies (HNPP) also displays an aberration on chromosome 17, but in the form of a deletion rather than a duplication of the *PMP22* gene. The identification of many new genes associated with CMT demonstrates the role of axonal transport and abnormal protein trafficking in the etiology of various forms of CMT. Axonal signaling and the molecular architecture of both Schwann cells and neurons are of considerable importance in the pathogenesis of CMT.

Nerve biopsies in CMT1 demonstrate reduced numbers of myelinated nerve fibers. Myelinated fiber histograms demonstrate a unimodal distribution with a broad middle peak and deficiency of both large and small myelinated fibers. Striking Schwann cell proliferation forming "onion bulbs" is a typical feature. The fascicular area is expanded because of endoneurial fibrosis. Teased nerve fibers show paranodal segmental demyelination and internodal remyelination.

In CMT2, the pathology demonstrates a decreased number of large-diameter myelinated nerve fibers with greater loss at more distal sites. In plastic-embedded sections, features include loss of myelinated nerve fibers, axonal atrophy as demonstrated by an increase in the axon-caliber myelin thickness ratio, and small clusters of thinly myelinated, regenerating axons. Occasional onion bulbs may also be encountered. Nerve fiber teasing shows myelin wrinkling, Wallerian-like degeneration, and remyelination. Remyelination can be distinguished from a primary demyelination by its increased number of consecutive short internodal segments.

In Dejerine–Sottas disease (CMT3), nerve biopsy shows a marked reduction of myelinated nerve fibers. Thinly myelinated fibers are prominent. Onion bulb formation is usually more severe

---

International Neurology, Second edition. Edited by Robert P. Lisak, Daniel D. Truong, William M. Carroll and Roongroj Bhidayasiri

Table 101.1 Hereditary sensorimotor neuropathies.

Disorder	Locus/gene	Inheritance	Protein/function of gene
CMT1A	17p11.2/Pmp22 (duplication)	AD	PMP22, myelination cell growth
HNPP	17p11.2/Pmp22 (deletion)	AD	PMP22, myelination cell growth
CMT1B	1q22-23/MPZ (P0)	AD	MPZ, adhesion
CMT1C	16p13.1-p12.3/LITAF (SIMPLE)	AD	SIMPLE, stimulator of inflammatory mediators
CMT1D	10q21.1-q22.1/EGR2	AD	Early growth response protein 2, PNS P myelin development and maintenance
CMT1E	8q21/NEFL	AD	Neurofilament organization, axonal transport
CMT2A1	1p36/KIF1B	AD	Kinesin-like protein KIF1B
CMT2A2	1p36/MFN2	AD	Motor protein, transport mitochondria
CMT2B CMT2B1 CMT2B2	3q21/RAB7 1q21/LMNA MED25	AD AR AR	Ras-related protein Rab-7, regulator of vesicular transport and membrane trafficking Structural protein of the nuclear lamina, transcription Chromatin modification
CMT2C	12q23-24/TRPV4	AD	Cation channel transient receptor potential vanilloid 4
CMT2D	7p15/GARS	AD	Protein synthetase
CMT2E	8p21/NEFL	AD	Neurofilament triplet L protein, axonal transport
CMT2F	7q11-21/HSPB1 (HSP27)	AD	Regulates and maintains cytoskeleton
CMT2G CMT2H/K	12q12-q13.3 8q21.1/GDAP1	AD AR	N/A Transcriptional regulation; maintains mitochondrial networks
CMT2I/J	1q22/MPZ	AD	Compact myelin protein, adhesion
CMT2k	GDAP1	AD	Expressed in neurons, maintains mitochondrial networks
CMT2L	12q24/HSPB8 (HSP28)	AD	Mutation promotes intracellular aggregation
CMT2N	AARS	AD	Attaches amino acids to their cognate tRNA molecules for protein synthesis
CMT2O	DYNC1H1	AD	Role in retrograde axonal transport in neurons
CMT2P	LRSAM1	AD	Membrane vesicle fusion during viral maturation
CMT3	PMP22, MPZ, PRXEGR2, FIG4	AR	N/A
CMT4A	8q13-q21/GDAP1	AR	Ganglioside-induced differentiation-associated protein 1
CMT4B1	11q22/MTMR2	AR	Myotubularin-related protein 2, maintains mitochondrial networks
CMT4B2 CMT4B3	11p15/SBF2/MTMR13 22q13.33/SBF2/MTMR	AR AR	SET binding factor 2, control of myelination SET binding factor 2, control of myelination
CMT4C	5q32/ SH3TC2(KIAA1985)	AR	SH3TC2 associated control of myelination
CMT4D	8q24.3/NDRG1	AR	NDRG1 protein, required for myelination and integrity of node of Ranvier
CMT4E	10q21.1-q22.1/EGR2	AR	Early growth response protein 2, role in differentiation, protein shutting
CMT4F	19q13.1-q13.2/PRX	AR	Periaxin, PNS myelin development and maintenance
CMT4G	10q23.2/unknown	AR	Maintenance of peripheral nerve myelin
CMT4H	12q11-q13/FGD4	AR	N/A
CMT4J	6q21/FIG4	AR	N/A
CMTX1	Xq13.1/GJB1(Cx32)	X-linked D	Gap junction beta-1 protein (connexin 32) in non-compact myelin
CMTX2	Xp22.2	X-linked R	N/A
CMTX3	Xq26.3-q27.3	X-linked R	N/A
CMTX4	AIFM1	X-linked R	N/A
CMTX5 CMTX6	Xp22.2, Xp22.3/PRPS1 Xp22.11/PDK3	X-linked R X-linked D	N/A N/A
DI-CMTA	Unknown	AD	N/A
DI-CMTB	DNM2	AD	Vesicular traffic, endocytosis protein synthesis
DI-CMTC	YARS encoding tyrosyl-Trna synthetase	AD	N/A
DI-CMTD	MPZ	AD	N/A
RI-CMTA	GDAP1	AR	Transcriptional regulation
RI-CMTB	KARS Encoding lysyl-Trna synthetase	AR	Role in translation, involved in a signaling pathway leading to gene activation

than in CMT1. Teased nerve fiber preparations demonstrate segmental demyelination or uniform, thinly myelinated fibers, giving the appearance of hypomyelination. The unmyelinated fiber population remains relatively spared.

In HNPP, the number of myelinated nerve fibers is variable. In many cases there is only a slight reduction, while others show an obvious loss. The diagnostic finding on nerve biopsy is the presence of sausage-shaped structures composing redundant loops of myelin folded over and back on themselves. In plasticized sections, the nerve fibers may appear hypermyelinated when the redundant loops adhere to the contour of the axon. In teased nerve fiber preparation, the thickened or swollen areas appear globular or sausage-like, and in longitudinal section these thickened areas appeared as focal enlargements. Electron microscopy of the large thickened fibers shows increased numbers of myelin lamellae and some demyelinated fibers, but the axons and Schwann cell are normal (Figure 101.1).

Clinical features

CMT1

CMT1 is the most common subtype of HMSN. It is autosomal dominant with onset in the first or second decade of life. About 20% of cases have no family history and represent new mutations. There are four genetic variants of this condition: 70% of individuals have CMT1A, 20% CMT1B, and 10% CMT1C or CMT1D. These genetic variants cannot be distinguished by clinical or electrophysiological studies, although some evidence suggests that CMT1B may be slightly more severe than the other variants.

The clinical presentation of CMT1 includes complete symmetry, and slow progression over decades. Difficulty running, frequent weakness and ankle sprains, or stumbling and slapping of the feet

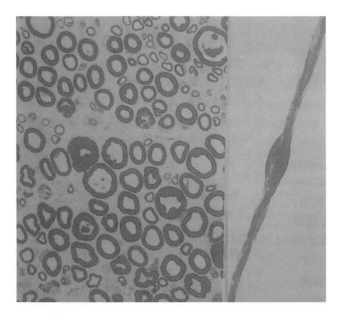

Figure 101.1 Sural nerve biopsy from patient with hereditary neuropathy with liability to pressure palsies shows abnormally thickened myelin (tomacula). Many fibers have abnormally thin myelin. Teased nerve fiber preparations show regions of myelin thickening (tomaculi) that appear sausage-like (×400). Source: Chen Lin 1997. Reproduced with permission of the Chinese Medical Association.

are noted by the parents of young children. Adult patients have difficulty dating the onset of symptoms. With milder forms, they may not even be aware of having a neuropathy, and examination of family members may identify patients without symptoms. Distal muscle weakness and atrophy begin in the feet and legs and later involve the hands. The majority of patients have pes cavus and hammer toes. Sometimes it is these skeletal abnormalities that bring the patient to medical attention. In severe cases, clawing of the fingers may be seen. An early age of onset of motor impairment is predictive of a more severe course. Most patients have no sensory complaints despite clear sensory involvement on clinical examination. Vibratory sensation is usually diminished, with preserved joint position sense. Muscle stretch reflexes are absent, especially in lower limbs. The feet may become cold, swollen, and blue, secondary to muscle inactivity. There is usually no disturbance of autonomic function.

CMT2

CMT2 is less common than CMT1. Genetic linkage has been established for six types of CMT2, all autosomal dominant. Clinically, CMT2A shows a striking resemblance to CMT1, except that the onset is often slightly later than CMT1, sometimes in the second decade or even after. Families with CMT2B have been reported to have mutilating neuropathic ulcers. CMT2C may have vocal cord paralysis and respiratory muscle weakness. In severe cases, symptoms begin in infancy. The majority of patients have a more insidious onset. CMT2D more severely affects distal upper limbs than the legs. The distinguishing feature is onset of disease with hand weakness and atrophy, and there is preferential loss of muscle stretch reflexes and sensory loss in the upper extremities.

X-linked CMT neuropathy

The most common form of X-linked CMT neuropathy (CMTX) is CMTX1 (sometimes also called CMT1X). It is caused by genetic defects on the proximal long arm of the X chromosome (Xq13.1), the locus of the gap junction beta-1 (*GJB1*) gene encoding the connexin 32 (Cx32) protein, which is expressed by myelinating Schwann cells and is necessary for the formation of gap junctions. More than 150 different mutations of the Cx32 gene have been identified. CMTX is more commonly diagnosed nowadays and represents the second most common form of CMT, representing at least 10–15% of all HMSN. Clinical findings are similar to CMT1. Females carrying the Cx32 mutation may be asymptomatic or only mildly affected. In males, onset occurs late in childhood or in adolescence. The patient shows symmetric distal muscle weakness and atrophy. Pes cavus and hammer toes are common. A cane or a wheelchair may be required in the fifth or sixth decade because of a significant gait disturbance. Sensory complaint is usually minimal. Muscle stretch reflexes are lost in most patients. In comparison to CMT1, peripheral nerves are often not palpably enlarged in CMTX. A "split hand syndrome" may be observed in CMTX1, with greater atrophy of the thenar muscle group than the interossei muscles in the hands. The disease has an expanded clinical spectrum, including transient central nervous system dysfunction, mental retardation, and hearing loss.

Dejerine–Sottas disease (CMT3)

The clinical classification of Dejerine–Sottas disease or HMSN III refers to a more severe demyelinating form of HMSN with onset in early childhood and autosomal recessive inheritance. In recent classifications, Dejerine–Sottas disease as CMT3 identifies all the severe sensory and motor neuropathies with early onset, including autosomal recessive or dominant forms. The genes known to cause CMT3 include *PMP22*, *P0*, and *EGR2*. Clinical onset is at birth or early childhood. Pain and paresthesia in the feet occur early, followed by symmetric weakness and wasting distally. Delayed motor milestones lead to inability to walk. Talipes equinovarus postures with claw feet and later claw hands are common. All sensory modalities are impaired distally, and the tendon reflexes are absent. Miotic, unreactive pupils, nystagmus, and kyphoscoliosis have been observed. The enlarged nerves are not tender.

Hereditary neuropathy with pressure palsies

HNPP (also termed tomaculous neuropathy) is autosomal dominant, with onset in the second or third decade typically as multiple mononeuropathy. It is caused by a deletion of the *PMP22* gene from one chromosome, so that the PMP22 protein is predicted to be at half normal level. In contrast, in the previously described CMT1A the gene is duplicated, resulting in overexpression. Patients usually present with recurrent transient focal motor and sensory neuropathies caused by traction or compression. Weakness and sensory loss occur in the anatomic distribution of a specific peripheral nerve. The focal neuropathies and plexopathies are generally not painful. Focal nerve lesions are often provoked by only slight or brief compression. The most commonly affected are the ulnar nerve (elbow), peroneal nerve (fibula head), median nerve (wrist), and radial nerve (spiral groove of the humerus). In addition to recurrent focal neuropathies, most individuals with HNPP have a mild, slowly progressive, demyelinating sensorimotor neuropathy.

Investigations

The contribution of electrophysiology to our understanding and diagnosis of inherited neuropathy cannot be overemphasized. In both CMT1 and CMT2, the compound muscle action potentials (CMAPs) and sensory nerve action potentials (SNAPs) are reduced in amplitude, and severe sensory nerve conduction abnormalities are present despite the lack of subjective sensory complaints. The electrophysiological differentiating criterion is the degree of slowing of conduction velocity. Most CMT patients can be classified as either CMT1 (demyelinating) or CMT2 (axonal) using the median nerve conduction velocity cut-off value of 38 m/s. Some CMT families, however, are difficult to classify according to this criterion, leading to the concept of intermediate CMT with nerve conduction velocity between 35 and 45 m/s, or a broad range of conduction velocities for different members of the same family.

In CMT1 there is severe and uniform slowing of nerve conduction velocity without conduction block, with lower limbs more affected than arms. Most patients have conduction velocities between 15 and 30 m/s. Longitudinal studies in CMT1 have shown no significant changes in nerve conduction velocity over decades, but CMAP amplitudes and muscle strength decrease over time. CMT1, CMT3, and CMT4 are considered demyelinating. In contrast, CMT2 is axonal: motor nerve conduction velocities are normal or mildly slow and CMAP amplitudes are greatly reduced. SNAPs are also significantly reduced or absent, more severely in lower limbs. CMAP and SNAP amplitudes are more severely reduced in CMT2 than in CMT1, but dispersion is more severe in CMT1. Conventional electromyogram (EMG) studies show neurogenic changes, including increased duration and amplitude of motor unit potentials

and decreased recruitment patterns, more severe in distal lower limb muscles.

CMTX is a heterogenous group defined by inheritance pattern and includes demyelinating and axonal forms. CMTX1, X4, X5, and X6 are demyelinating neuropathies. In CMTX1, the conduction velocities are often in the intermediate range and slowing of conduction velocities may be asymmetric.

The cerebrospinal fluid (CSF) in CMT1 and CMT2 is usually normal. Some patients may have mildly elevated CSF protein up to 80 mg/dL, rarely higher in CMT1.

Genetic tests for the most common types (CMT1A, CMT1B, CMT2, and CMTX) are available, and it is now possible to identify many more cases, including sporadic ones. It is seldom necessary to resort to nerve biopsy for diagnosis; occasionally biopsy is necessary for patients with negative genetic testing to exclude chronic inflammatory demyelinating polyneuropathy.

In CMT3, unlike other forms of CMT, the CSF protein is usually elevated and spinal nerve roots are enlarged. Nerve conduction velocities are markedly reduced, even when there is little or no functional impairment.

In HNPP, electrophysiological studies show focal slowing of conduction velocities and a loss of amplitude at sites of entrapment affecting the motor and sensory nerves. HNPP patients have some slowing of conduction velocities of distal motor and sensory nerve, favoring a more generalized demyelinating neuropathy. CSF protein may be elevated. Nerve biopsies document localized nerve sheath thickening with duplication of the myelin lamellae.

Hereditary sensory and autonomic neuropathy

The HSANs are a clinically and genetically heterogeneous group with five different clinical subtypes. With the exception of the autosomal dominant HSANI, the other four types are autosomal recessive. Molecular genetic research has shown that at least eight loci and six genes are associated with HSANs. Because HSAN is rare, incidence and prevalence data are not available.

Clinical features

HSANI

HSANI, the most common form of HSNA, is linked to chromosome 9q22. Onset of this autosomal dominant peripheral neuropathy occurs between the second and fourth decades as a slowly progressive but marked sensory impairment, with variable motor and minimal autonomic involvement. Patients come to clinical attention for foot ulcers or spontaneous pain. Usual sites of ulceration are the first metatarsal head or the tips of the toes. The neuropathic ulcers may lead to recurrent cellulitis, deep fistulas, and ultimately osteomyelitis. Some patients have repeated stress fractures, with resorption of bone resulting in foot deformities. Severe burning or lancinating pain is another main symptom, which may recur in bouts of variable frequency and intensity. Shooting pains may be experienced in various parts of the body, including the hands, shoulders, back, and legs. Impaired sensation in the lower limbs causes foot deformities and ulcerations, and some patients have Charcot joints. The sensory deficit is symmetric and more severely affects the lower limbs. Sensory loss for pain and temperature predominates. Some patients showed hyperhidrosis and anhidrosis at different stages, caused by denervation to the sweat glands. Muscle stretch reflexes are usually depressed or absent at the ankle and preserved at other joints. Distal muscle weakness is not a prominent symptom.

HSANII

HSANII is a rare autosomal recessive form. Patients present in early childhood with distal stocking-and-glove numbness in upper and lower limbs. Later, the sensory loss affects all modalities, with impairment of pain, temperature, and touch sensations, and may extend to the trunk. Tendon reflexes are often absent. The patients usually have digital ulcers and recurrent fractures. Muscle weakness is usually absent or mild. Autonomic dysfunction is minimal. In most cases, the neurological deficits are not or are only slowly progressive.

HSANIII

HSANIII (also called infantile dysautonomia or Riley–Day syndrome) is autosomal recessive. It affects the development and survival of sensory and autonomic neurons, and is a catastrophic illness starting at birth. Patients demonstrate swallowing problems, episodes of vomiting, and intermittent, unexplained fever. Absent lacrimation, profuse seating, and labile blood pressure are common. On physical examination, the absence of fungiform papillae of the tongue is particularly important. Muscle stretch reflexes are usually absent. Muscle strength is normal. There is decreased nociception and temperature sensation over the entire body, whereas touch, vibration, and position sensation are retained. Many patients die in early childhood from recurrent pneumonia.

HSANIV

HSANIV represents a congenital variant of autosomal recessive HSAN and is characterized by disease onset at birth. It is also known as congenital insensitivity to pain and anhidrosis. Autonomic disturbances are a predominant feature. Sweating is markedly decreased or absent, leading to episodic fever and recurrent hyperpyrexia. Absent pain sensation promotes repeated traumatic and thermal injuries and severe mutilations of the hands and feet. The patients always show multiple sites of trauma, and the tip of the tongue, parts of the lips, and the distal ends of the fingers may be missing. Joint deformities and entrapment neuropathies may be apparent. Hyperactivity and emotional lability are common, and children often show mild mental retardation. On examination there is widespread anhidrosis, decreased pinprick and temperature sensation, with normal touch, vibration, and proprioception. Muscle strength and deep tendon reflexes are preserved. Patients may die from hyperpyrexia within the first years of life.

HSANV

HSANV, the least common HSAN, begins in infancy. Impaired nociception and temperature sensation lead to acral ulcers, painless fractures, and neurogenic arthropathies. Other sensory modalities are preserved, and autonomic function is normal except for decreased sweating in some patients. Muscle strength and tendon reflexes are normal. There is no mental retardation.

Investigations

Motor conduction velocity is normal or only mildly reduced in HSANs. EMG may reveal large motor unit potentials in the distal limb muscles. SNAPs are reduced in amplitude or absent in HSANI,

II, or III, and normal in HSANIV and V. Sympathetic skin response is absent.

Distal hereditary motor neuropathy

The distal HMNs are often included in the inherited neuropathies and comprise about 10% of all inherited motor neuropathies. They are neuronopathies and are usually termed spinal muscular atrophies (SMAs). Chapter 108 is devoted to their discussion. Patients usually present with weakness and atrophy in the distal muscles. Sensory abnormalities are usually absent, although older patients may have mild decreases in vibration sensation. Distal HMNs had been tentatively classified into many subtypes on the basis of mode of inheritance. Thirteen subtypes are autosomal dominant, four subtypes are autosomal recessive, and one subtype is X-linked. Detailed features and genetic changes are presented in Table 101.2. The electrodiagnostic examination of the SMAs reveals normal or near-normal SNAPs. Motor conduction velocities are normal or minimally slow, despite clinical evidence of weakness and atrophy and EMG evidence of denervation–reinnervation. Fasciculations may be encountered, but are not nearly as prominent as in amyotrophic lateral sclerosis.

Table 101.2 Clinical and genetic features of distal hereditary motor neuropathy subtypes

Subtypes	Locus/gene	Clinical features
Autosomal dominant	7q34-q36	Distal motor involvement; pyramidal tract involvement
	HSPB8(HSP22)	Distal motor involvement; adult or juvenile onset
	HSPB1(HSP27)	Distal motor involvement; fat atrophy in lower limbs; adult or juvenile onset
	BSCL2	Distal motor involvement;; adult onset; upper limbs predominance; pyramidal tract involvement
	GARS	Distal motor involvement
	TRPV4	Distal motor involvement; vocal cord paresis
	DYNC1H1	Distal motor involvement
	HSPB3	Distal motor involvement
	DCTN1	Distal motor involvement; vocal cord paresis
	SLC5A7	Distal motor involvement; upper limbs predominance; vocal cord paresis
	SETX	Distal motor involvement; pyramidal tract involvement
	4q34-q35	Distal motor involvement; pyramidal tract involvement
	REEP1	Distal motor involvement
Autosomal recessive	GARS	Distal motor involvement; upper limbs predominance
	11q13	Distal motor involvement; diaphragmatic paresis
	9p21.1-p12	Distal motor involvement; pyramidal tract involvement
	IGHMPB2	Distal motor involvement; respiratory distress type 1
X-linked X	ATP7A	Distal motor involvement

Other hereditary neuropathies

Refsum's disease

Refsum's disease (sometimes termed HMSNIV) is an autosomal recessive disorder (chromosome 10) resulting in accumulation of phytanic acid. Peripheral neuropathy is usually present by age 20 years. Other features include retinitis pigmentosa (night blindness), ichthyosis, and cerebellar ataxia. Muscle weakness and atrophy begin in the legs distally and later become generalized, accompanied by areflexia and large fiber sensory impairment. Pes cavus and over-riding toes (due to short fourth metatarsals) are diagnostic clues. CSF protein is elevated. Motor conduction velocities are markedly slowed, with either uniform or non-uniform changes. SNAPs are decreased or absent. Refsum's disease is treated by elimination of phytanic acid from the diet, and plasmapheresis may be helpful to reduce body stores of phytanic acid.

Familial amyloid polyneuropathy

Familial amyloid polyneuropathy (FAP) often presents as small fiber neuropathy, but large fiber function and motor fibers are usually affected in advanced disease. Decreased pain and temperature sensation are accompanied by stabbing, lancinating pains in the feet, and autonomic dysfunction (e.g., impaired sweating, postural hypotension, constipation or diarrhea, etc.). Nerve entrapment such as carpal tunnel syndrome may occur from amyloid deposition. Several subtypes have been described, with types I and II linked to the transthyretin (TTR) gene on chromosome 18q11.

Friedreich's ataxia

Friedreich's ataxia (see Chapter 55) manifests as childhood-onset ataxia and sensory more than motor polyneuropathy. The disorder is autosomal recessive and is caused by triplet repeat expansion in a non-coding region of the frataxin gene on chromosome 9q. Features include ataxic gait, clumsiness, and other features of cerebellar ataxia, reduced or absent deep tendon reflexes, distal weakness and atrophy, scoliosis, and electrocardiogram (ECG) abnormalities.

Hereditary disorders of lipid metabolism

In hereditary disorders of lipid metabolism, dysmyelination usually affects central and peripheral myelin, and central manifestations often overshadow the peripheral neuropathy. Polyneuropathy occurs in children with metachromatic leukodystrophy and Krabbe's disease (globoid cell leukodystrophy), both of which are autosomal recessive. Adrenoleukodystrophy or adrenomyeloneuropathy is X-linked dominant; abetalipoproteinemia and Tangier disease are autosomal recessive.

Fabry's disease

Fabry's disease (see Chapter 131) is caused by X-linked deficiency of alpha-galactosidase. Affected boys or young men complain of burning or stabbing pain in hands and feet, especially with heat exposure or fever. Angiokeratomas (reddish purple skin lesions) are typical. Premature arteriosclerosis causes renal disease and early strokes. Routine nerve conduction studies are normal in this small fiber neuropathy. Enzyme replacement therapy is available.

Porphyrias

The porphyrias (see Chapter 170) are inherited disorders of heme synthesis. Three autosomal dominant forms cause peripheral neuropathy. Most common is acute intermittent porphyria; the others are variegate porphyria and hereditary coproporphyria. Drugs or hormonal changes precipitate attacks. Typically, acute abdominal pain is followed 48–72 hours later by sudden onset of proximal or distal weakness (resembling Guillain–Barré syndrome), with sensory findings less prominent. Tendon reflexes are diminished, but ankle jerks are often retained. Respiratory insufficiency may occur, and autonomic abnormalities are frequent. Pain may present early in the legs or back. Agitation or psychosis is common. Some patients recover rapidly, others have slow improvement of weakness over many months. Acute intermittent porphyria is caused by abnormal porphobilinogen deaminase, and urinary levels of porphobilinogen and aminolevulinic acid are increased.

Treatment

No specific treatment is known for hereditary neuropathy, with the exception of some of the inherited metabolic disorders. Preventive measures can be implemented, such as physiotherapy, orthotics, orthopedic surgery, and technical aids. Stabilizing the ankles by arthrodeses is indicated if foot drop is severe. Regular exercise, but not excessive weight training, is important. Home-based, moderate-intensity resistance training can improve muscle function. In mild and early cases, fitting the legs with light braces and the shoes with springs to overcome foot drop can be helpful. Referral for occupational therapy services is strongly advised to address a variety of activities.

For patients with HSAN, the most important aspect of management is attending to acral ulcers to prevent sepsis and osteomyelitis. For patients with lancinating pain, a similar approach to other painful neuropathies is appropriate. In some patients immobilization of injured limbs and surgical correction of established deformities must be considered. Precautions should be taken to avoid direct exposure to the sun or activities resulting in overheating, because temperature regulation and sweating are impaired. Defective lacrimation requires special attention to dry eyes. Close observation for bone fractures and progressive scoliosis should be integrated into the care of these patients.

In addition to traditional approaches such as rehabilitation medicine, ambulation aids, and pain management, identification of the genes causing CMT has led to improved genetic counseling and assistance in family planning. Delineation of common molecular pathways in multiple forms of CMT may be exploited in future molecular therapies. Scientifically based clinical trials for CMT1A are currently being implemented. Techniques of gene therapy may become feasible options in the future.

Further reading

Braathen GJ, Sand JC, Lobato A, et al. Genetic epidemiology of Charcot–Marie–Tooth in the general population. *Eur J Neurol* 2011;18:39–48.

Chen L, Guo Y, Huang Y, et al. Tomaculous neuropathy of clinic and pathology. *Zhonghua Shen Jing Ke Za Zhi* 1997;30:142–146.

Cui L, Tang X, Li B. Clinical electrophysiological studies of peroneal muscular atrophy: Report of 32 cases. *Zhongguo Yi Xue Ke Xue Yuan Xue Bao* 1989;11:175–179.

El-Abassi R, England JD, Carter GT. Charcot–Marie–Tooth disease: An overview of genotypes, phenotypes, and clinical management strategies. *PM&R* 2014;6:342–355.

Emery AE. Population frequencies of inherited neuromuscular disease: A world survey. *Neuromuscul Disord* 1991;1:19–29.

Murphy SM, Laura M, Fawcett K, et al. Charcot–Marie–Tooth disease: Frequency of genetic subtypes and guidelines for genetic testing. *J Neurol Neurosurg Psychiatry* 2012;83:706–710.

Song S, Zhang Y, Chen B, et al. Mutation frequency for Charcot–Marie–Tooth disease type1 in the Chinese population is similar to that in the global ethnic patients. *Genet Med* 2006;8:532–535.

Vallat JM, Mathis S, Funalot B. The various Charcot–Marie–Tooth diseases. *Curr Opin Neurol* 2013;26:473–480.

Wilmshurst JM, Ouvrier R. Hereditary peripheral neuropathies of childhood: An overview for clinicians. *Neuromuscular Disord* 2011;21:763–775.

102 Acquired neuropathies

Friedhelm Sandbrink

Department of Neurology, Veterans Affairs Medical Center, and Georgetown University, Washington, DC, USA

Immune-mediated neuropathies

Guillain–Barré syndrome

Guillain-Barré syndrome (GBS) is the most common cause of acute flaccid paralysis in Western countries, where acute inflammatory demyelinating polyneuropathy (AIDP) is the most common subtype. The axonal variant of acute motor sensory axonal neuropathy (AMSAN) involves both motor and sensory fibers and is often more severe, with incomplete recovery. The most common form in China is acute motor axonal neuropathy (AMAN). It lacks any sensory disturbance and occurs frequently in children. Variants without predominant weakness include Miller–Fisher syndrome, characterized by areflexia, gait ataxia, and ophthalmoparesis. The related Bickerstaff brainstem encephalitis consists of hyperreflexia, gait ataxia, ophthalmoparesis, and encephalopathy. Other cranial nerve variants are bifacial weakness with distal paresthesias, and sixth nerve palsies with distal paresthesias. Other rare non-motor variants are pure sensory neuropathy and acute (pan-)dysautonomia that affects sympathetic and parasympathetic function. General features of all forms include a rapidly evolving neurological deficit (usually weakness), often preceded by an antecedent infection. Absent reflexes and elevated cerebrospinal fluid (CSF) protein are typical.

Epidemiology

The annual incidence of GBS in Western countries is 1.2–1.9 per 100,000, slightly more common in men than women. GBS may occur at any age, but increases gradually with age. In Europe and North America, the incidence ranges from less than 1 per 100,000 in people younger than 30 years to 4 per 100,000 in those older than 70 years. In contrast, in China GBS affects adults less commonly, with incidence of 0.66 per 100,000 reported for all ages. In Western countries, 80–90% of patients have AIDP and only 5% have axonal subtypes. In Israel, two-thirds of patients have AIDP versus 22% AMAN. In Northern China, 60–80% are AMAN, typically as summer epidemics in children and young adults, and about 20% AIDP. In Japanese patients and in Mexico, the proportions of AIDP and AMAN are similar, with about 30–40% for each. AMSAN and Miller–Fisher syndrome are less common.

Most cases worldwide are sporadic, but as mentioned, summer epidemics of AMAN occur in China. Epidemic AMAN also occurs in Mexico, and small clusters associated with bacterial enteritis caused by contaminated water have been reported in tropical countries.

In two-thirds of patients, the disease follows within weeks of a preceding upper respiratory or gastrointestinal tract infection or, rarely, surgery, vaccination, or drug exposure. *Campylobacter jejuni* is a major cause of bacterial gastroenteritis throughout the world. It is found serologically in one-third of GBS patients in Western countries and more commonly in China. Other patients have serological evidence for anteceding infection with *Mycoplasma pneumonia*, Epstein–Barr virus (EBV), cytomegalovirus (CMV), viral hepatitis, or human immunodeficiency virus (HIV). There is little evidence to support a causal association of GBS with vaccinations, with few exceptions. A slight increase in the risk of GBS was noted after influenza vaccination in 1976–77, with steady decline since then, and more recently after the 2009–10 H1N1 (swine flu) vaccination (estimated as 0.8 cases of GBS per 1 million). A significant risk for GBS was noted after older formulations of rabies vaccination (cultured in mammalian brain tissue; risk 1:1000), but this has been eliminated with the new formulations (cultured in chick embryo material).

Pathophysiology

The anteceding infection presumably triggers an autoimmune response to peripheral nerve antigens by "molecular mimicry." In axonal GBS variants, a primarily antibody-mediated mechanism against motor axolemna is likely. *C. jejuni* lipopolysaccharide and human gangliosides expressed on the motor axolemna of peripheral nerves share homologous epitopes. Serum antibodies against gangliosides GM1, GM1b, GD1a, or GalNAc-GD1a are found in axonal GBS. Autopsy studies in AMAN reveal axonal degeneration of motor fibers without demyelination.

In AIDP, a T-cell-mediated autoimmune response is directed against peripheral nerve myelin and results in myelin stripping, and secondary axon loss in severe cases. Lymphocytic infiltration of the peripheral nerves and macrophage invasion of myelin sheath and Schwann cells are seen. Cellular mechanism is also supported by experimental allergic neuritis (EAN), a rat model for AIDP, which involves T-cell mediated activation of lymphocytes against peripheral nerve myelin components. Antiganglioside antibodies and their target epitopes in AIDP are unknown. Epitopes implicated in Miller–Fisher syndrome are GQ1b and GT1a.

Clinical features

Patients typically present with symmetric weakness that begins in the legs and worsens quickly. Paresthesias may be the initial symptom in AIDP and AMSAN. They typically precede the

---

paralysis by 7–10 days and manifest as paresthesias and radicular pain. The weakness may be more pronounced distally or proximally in the legs, and typically ascends to trunk and arms. Disease severity and progression vary greatly. Some patients have rapidly ascending weakness, resulting in quadriplegia and life-threatening compromise of respiratory function and swallowing within hours. Other patients have only minimal weakness or gradual progression over several weeks. Most patients are maximally weak within 7–10 days, with faster progression in axonal variants (AMAN, AMSAN) than in AIDP. Facial weakness occurs in more than half of patients. Weakness of neck flexor muscles resulting in inability to lift the head against gravity indicates impending respiratory failure. Tendon reflexes may be normal or hypoactive for the first few days, but then are invariably lost (diagnostic criteria). Sensory impairment varies and is often minimal; distally decreased vibration sense may be found. Occasionally, decreased sensation to all modalities in a stocking-and-glove distribution accompanies the weakness, and is regularly present in AMSAN. Autonomic dysfunction occurs frequently (two-thirds of cases of AIDP), including tachycardia, blood pressure fluctuations, sphincter dysfunction, paralytic ileus, and disturbed sweating. Cardiac arrhythmia, hypotension, or pulmonary failure may be life threatening.

Miller–Fisher syndrome begins with diplopia, evolving within days to complete ophthalmoplegia and followed by limb and gait ataxia. Pupillary reflexes are preserved and nystagmus is absent. Mild distal paresthesias and mild muscle weakness may be present.

Investigations

The typical CSF finding is elevation of protein in the setting of a normal cell count (so-called *albuminocytologic dissociation*), frequently above 300 mg/dL. During the first few days after onset of weakness, protein elevation may not be present, and repeat CSF testing 5–7 days later should then be performed. About 10% of patients lack protein elevation even on serial CSF testing. Transient elevation of IgG or positive oligoclonal bands is common. The cell count is usually normal or fewer than 10 cells/μL. Pleocytosis up to 20 cells/μL is well compatible with GBS, whereas more than 50 cells/μL suggest a different diagnosis. In a patient with otherwise typical GBS, infection with HIV and CMV should then be suspected.

Electrophysiological abnormalities may be minor in the beginning of weakness, but then are found in 90%. In AIDP, marked slowing of motor conduction velocities and conduction block document the demyelination. Prolonged or absent F-waves and increased distal motor latencies are typical early findings. Sensory nerve action potentials (SNAPs) show a "normal sural–abnormal median pattern" in one-third of cases of AIDP, (i.e., normal sural SNAP with reduced or absent median or ulnar SNAPs). Evidence of denervation and axonal loss is more pronounced in axonal variants. Due to low sensitivity of nerve conduction studies (NCS) at the time of initial presentation, treatment should not be delayed in patients developing weakness, even if the electrophysiological findings are not supportive, with repeat NCS 3–5 days later.

Spinal magnetic resonance imaging (MRI) may demonstrate gadolinium enhancement of lumbar nerve roots.

Serological testing has limited value. Elevated serum antibodies and positive stool culture for *Campylobacter jejuni* point toward triggering infection. Serological testing (acute and convalescent samples) for EBV, CMV, and *Mycoplasma pneumoniae* are recommended. Antiganglioside antibodies may be present. Antiganglioside IgG antibodies against GQ1b are diagnostic for Miller–Fisher

variant (present in >90%) or Bickerstaff brainstem encephalitis (present in two-thirds of cases). HIV serology may be suggested by clinical context or CSF pleocytosis. Non-specific findings are mild increases in liver transaminases, creatine kinase, or erythrocyte sedimentation rate. In terms of differential diagnosis, GBS needs to be distinguished from other conditions with subacute motor weakness. Diphtheric polyneuropathy has a long latent period between the respiratory infection and subsequent weakness, slower evolution, and frequent paralysis of ocular accommodation. Acute anterior poliomyelitis is distinguished by meningeal irritation, fever, asymmetry of paralysis, and CSF pleocytosis. In acute porphyria, the neuropathy is preceded by abdominal pain, associated cognitive symptoms are common, and CSF is normal. Toxic (*N*-hexane inhalation, acrylamide, organophosphorus compounds, thallium or arsenic intoxication, heavy metals, biological toxins), vasculitic, and critical illness neuropathies may also begin acutely. CSF pleocytosis (more than 50 cells/μL) suggests Lyme disease or HIV-associated polyradiculopathy with superimposed CMV infection. Tick paralysis is an ascending motor paralysis developing 5–6 days after the tick has attached itself to a cutaneous site. Cranial nerve palsies and respiratory paralysis occur. CSF is normal. Symptoms promptly reverse with removal of the tick. Muscle disorders to consider include acute rhabdomyolysis, periodic paralysis, inflammatory myopathy, or severe metabolic disturbances (hypophosphatemia, hypokalemia). Neuromuscular junction disorders may present as subacute weakness. Botulism affects the ocular muscles and pupillary reflexes, and is separated by electrophysiology. Lesions of the central nervous system (CNS), such as acute basilar artery stenosis, spinal cord compression, or transverse myelitis, or hysterical weakness may occasionally present diagnostic difficulties.

Treatment

GBS is best managed in the intensive care setting, as good supportive care is essential. Forced vital capacity (FVC) and negative inspiratory force (NIF) have to be monitored, as they predict impeding respiratory failure well before pulse oximetry. An FVC below 1 liter (15–20 mL/kg), shortness of breath, or retention of carbon dioxide on arterial blood gas measurements are indications for elective endotracheal intubation and assisted ventilation. Treatment of cardiac arrhythmias or severe blood pressure fluctuations is often necessary. Leg stockings and subcutaneous heparin reduce the risk of deep vein thrombosis. Skin breakdown in bedridden patients and exposure keratitis in patients with facial weakness must be prevented. Even with complete quadriplegia, patients remain cognitively intact, and means to communicate should be explored. Treatment of back pain or dysesthesias may require opioid analgesics.

Immunotherapy is recommended for all patients with GBS, especially for patients unable to walk. Randomized studies document equal efficacy of plasma exchange and intravenous immunoglobulin (IVIg). Treatment reduces time to recovery and may decrease residual neurological deficits. There is no proven additional benefit for combining both therapies. Treatment is best instituted early, within 2 weeks of onset, especially in patients with severe or rapidly progressive deficit or respiratory impairment. Delay in treatment should be avoided, but there may be benefit in non-ambulatory patients as late as up to 4 weeks after onset. Plasmapheresis involves removal of 200–250 mL/kg of plasma over 7–10 days. It requires catheter placement for venous access and is not universally available. IVIg (0.4 g/kg/day for 5 days) is usually preferred, especially in adults with cardiovascular instability and in children. Corticosteroids are not beneficial and should be avoided.

Prognosis is generally good, with improvement over weeks to months being the rule. The mean time to onset of recovery is 4 weeks, and the mean time to complete recovery 6–7 months, with 80% of patients being able to walk independently by 6 months. About 20% of patients are left with neurological disability, more common in AMSAN. Older age (>60 years), early progression to maximal deficit (<7 days), severity at nadir, need for ventilatory support, and marked reduction in compound muscle action potential (CMAP) amplitudes indicate poor prognosis. Poor prognosis secondary to severe axonal involvement may be assumed, if NCS document absent motor responses. Preceding *C. jejuni* and CMV infections are unfavorable, whereas EBV is associated with milder forms. The online IGOS GBS prognosis tool may be used to advise patients and their families about the risk of respiratory failure in the first week of admission and risk of being unable to walk 6 months after admission. Even with optimal treatment, mortality is 2–10% from complications including respiratory failure or cardiac arrhythmia, higher in AMSAN than AIDP. Most AMAN patients make a good recovery.

Chronic inflammatory demyelinating polyneuropathy

Chronic inflammatory demyelinating polyneuropathy (CIDP) is clinically similar to GBS, but with a more protracted or relapsing course. CIDP is arbitrarily defined by progression of weakness over at least 8 weeks (or 2 months), whereas progression over 4–8 weeks indicates subacute inflammatory demyelinating polyneuropathy (SIDP). About half of all patients will have an atypical, often multifocal and asymmetric presentation.

Epidemiology

The prevalence is reported as 2–7.7 per 100,000, but it is likely underdiagnosed due to its clinical heterogeneity and rather stringent diagnostic criteria. It occurs at all ages, with peak in the fifth or sixth decade, with a slight male predominance. CIDP is a fairly frequent diagnosis (about 20%) in patients with chronic polyneuropathy referred to neuromuscular centers.

Pathophysiology

A preceding infection is unusual, found in less than 10% of cases. Pregnancy may be a triggering factor (third trimester or postpartum). Immune-mediated mechanisms resulting in peripheral nerve demyelination are postulated, in particular T-cell activation, supported by the finding of lymphocytic infiltration and segmental demyelination in peripheral nerve biopsies and the benefit of immune-modulating therapy. There are, however, no established target epitopes or serological markers in typical CIDP.

Clinical features

CIDP begins insidiously or subacutely, and follows a steady or stepwise progressive (two-thirds of patients) or relapsing–remitting course (one-third, more commonly in younger patients). The classic presentation of CIDP is characterized by motor predominant symptoms with rather symmetric weakness of distal and proximal muscles (strongly suggestive) in upper and lower extremities. Deep tendon reflexes are reduced or absent. Sensory involvement tends to affect the large fiber modalities (numbness, tingling, with on exam impaired vibration and position sense) more than small fiber function (pain or temperature sensation). Initial sensory symptoms

affecting the upper limbs are typical, but sensory symptoms may be minimal or even absent. A distal to proximal sensory gradient is often noted, with fingers as frequently affected as the feet, resulting in numbness or tingling in stocking-and-glove distribution. Cranial nerve involvement is not common, but if present, it suggests CIDP. Constipation and urinary retention occur late.

About half of CIDP patients have an atypical presentation. A multifocal CIDP variant with asymmetric weakness and sensory loss is called *multifocal acquired demyelinating sensory and motor neuropathy* (MADSAM) or Lewis–Sumner syndrome (LSS). This CIDP variant often has gradual onset and slowly progressive course. Motor involvement is usually multifocal (i.e., asymmetric) and affects upper extremities, and thus resembles mononeuropathy multiplex. In MADSAM, in contract to multifocal motor neuropathy (MMN), sensory nerves are affected, and patients typically present with pain and paresthesias. Tinel sign is common at affected nerve sites. Cranial nerves may be affected (optic neuritis, oculomotor, trigeminal, or facial nerve palsy).

It is important to separate MADSAM from MMN due to different treatment options. The diagnosis of MADSAM relies on the objective sensory nerve involvement in addition to motor nerves. Electrophysiology documents an underlying demyelinating disorder with persistent multifocal conduction block in sensory and motor nerves. If the demyelinating neuropathy affects motor nerves only (without sensory loss), the diagnosis is likely MMN.

CIDP may also present with sensory predominant symptoms, including paresthesias, dysesthesias, and proprioceptive ataxia. Patients have usually subclinical motor involvement by electrophysiology. This CIDP variant resembles distal acquired demyelinating sensory neuropathy (DADS), but the latter is considered a separate entity because of IgM paraproteinemia and different treatment response. Other CIDP variants are pure motor presentation, or minimal symptoms with only fatigability and minor paresthesias.

Investigations

All patients with suspected CIDP should be evaluated for monoclonal gammopathy (paraproteinemia), which suggests a lymphoproliferative disorder. CSF protein is usually increased with normal CSF cell count, but less consistently than in GBS. Pleocytosis above 10 cells/μL suggests a different diagnosis such as HIV, Lyme disease, sarcoid, or lymphoma.

Electrodiagnostic evaluation in CIDP documents a demyelinating neuropathy with varying degrees of superimposed axonal degeneration. The electrodiagnostic criteria for demyelination are generally based on NCS of *motor* nerves. In particular, conduction block and temporal dispersion are strongly suggestive of segmental demyelination.

Demyelination is suggested by (1) severe slowing of nerve conduction velocities: conduction velocity reduced by at least 30% below the lower limit of normal (LLN) in nerves with reduced CMAP amplitudes, that is, less than 30 m/s in the arm, 25 m/s in the leg; (2) absence of F-waves, or marked prolongation of F-waves, usually by at least 30% above the upper limit of normal (ULN), and by at least 50% in nerves with significantly reduced CMAP amplitudes; (3) severely prolonged distal motor latencies, at least 50% above the ULN; (4) conduction block: at least 50% CMAP amplitude reduction proximal to distal; and (5) temporal dispersion: at least 30% increase in CMAP duration (specified for motor nerves as median 6.6 ms, ulnar 6.7 ms, peroneal 7.6 ms, and tibial 8.8 ms).

CIDP should also be suspected if the CMAP amplitude is normal in a clinically weak muscle, or if SNAPs are normal despite marked sensory complaints. Strategies to increase sensitivity of NCS include bilateral nerve testing, proximal stimulation of motor nerves, and, if the electrodiagnostic study is not diagnostic initially, a repeat study at a later date.

In some patients with CIDP, routine NCS may not demonstrate demyelination features, such as when conduction block is limited to only proximal nerve segments or nerve roots. Proximal conduction block may be documented by high-voltage percutaneous or needle electrical stimulation of nerve roots; both techniques are technically difficult and associated with risk/discomfort to the patient. Alternatively, the triple stimulation technique (TST) that combines transcranial magnetic stimulation and peripheral electrical stimulation may document conduction block and thus demyelination within the proximal nerve segments (between nerve root and Erb point). Somatosensory evoked potentials can be useful to demonstrate abnormal proximal sensory conduction, particularly in sensory CIDP.

The MRI findings of enhancement or hypertrophy of plexus or nerve roots, including cauda equina, may help confirm the diagnosis (see Figure 102.1).

A nerve biopsy is usually not needed, but may be helpful when other studies are not diagnostic and to rule out other etiologies. Patients who do not meet neurophysiological criteria for a primary demyelinating neuropathy may have evidence of inflammatory demyelination on nerve biopsy. Positive findings on nerve biopsy, however, are not specific, and negative findings do not exclude the diagnosis, as demyelination is seen in only one-half to two-thirds of biopsies.

Several different sets of diagnostic criteria for CIDP are available with varying sensitivity and specificity. According to the European Federation of Neurological Societies/Peripheral Nerve Society (EFNS/PNS) consensus guideline (2010), CIDP should be considered in any patient with a progressive symmetric or asymmetric polyradiculoneuropathy in whom the clinical course is relapsing and remitting or progresses for more than 2 months, especially if there are positive sensory symptoms, proximal weakness, areflexia without wasting, or preferential loss of vibration or joint position sense. The electrodiagnostic criteria by the American Academy of Neurology (AAN) in 1991 have high specificity for patients with classical CIDP and thus are particularly appropriate for research purposes, but are not sufficiently sensitive for clinical use. The EFNS/PNS consensus guideline was designed to increase sensitivity and provides electrodiagnostic criteria for definite, probable, and possible CIDP. Koski and coworkers published criteria to diagnose CIDP based on clinical features alone: symmetric onset or examination; weakness of four limbs; and proximal weakness in at least one limb.

In terms of differential diagnosis, chronic polyneuropathies resembling CIDP occur in chronic active hepatitis (B or C), HIV, lymphoma, diabetes, collagen vascular disorders, thyrotoxicosis, and after organ and bone marrow transplants, nephrotic syndrome, and inflammatory bowel disease. The differentiation may be particularly difficult in diabetes patients, who frequently exhibit more severe slowing of conduction velocities than other axonal polyneuropathies.

Treatment

Comparison studies indicate similar response rates between steroids, intravenous immunoglobulins (IVIg), and plasmapheresis. Two-thirds of patients will respond to initial treatment with one of these therapies, and ultimately 89% of patients will respond to one of these modalities.

Corticosteroids are considered beneficial in classic CIDP and its variants, including MADSAM. Steroids may be more likely to induce a lasting clinical remission. Dosage recommendations range from 60–120 mg oral prednisone daily to pulse methylprednisolone. A typical regimen is prednisone 100 mg/day for 2–4 weeks, gradually tapered by 5 mg/week. Clinical response is expected at around 1.9 months. The dosage is reduced to the lowest effective maintenance dose that prevents relapse. Pulsed high-dose corticosteroids administered intermittently, typically for 6 months,

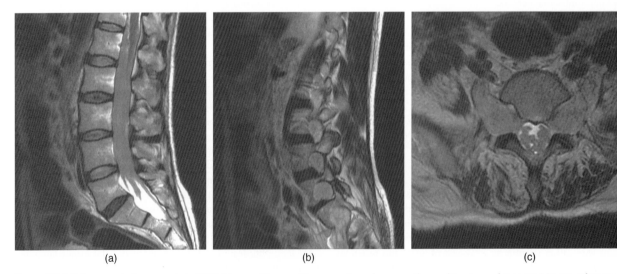

(a)   (b)   (c)

Figure 102.1 Enlargement of nerve roots in CIDP. 64-year-old man with progressive polyneuropathy resulting in quadriparesis. Massive enlargement of lumbar nerve roots and proximal lumbosacral nerves is noted on MRI T2-weighted sagittal and axial images. The patient also had severely enlarged cervical nerve roots, brachial plexuses, and trigeminal nerves. (a) Diffuse thickening of the lumbar nerve roots results in complete obliteration of CSF space from L1 to L5 by the cauda equina. (b) Widening of the neural foramen by the severely enlarged nerve roots at all levels. (c) Severely thickened lumbar nerve roots on both sides with rather symmetric gross enlargement of neural foramina.

achieved comparable improvement to oral steroids with fewer side effects in several studies. The best regimen remains uncertain, with publications reporting use of oral dexamethasone 40 mg daily for 4 days each month, intravenous methylprednisolone 500 mg daily for 5 days each month, or 1000 mg weekly.

IVIg is first-line therapy due to safety and effectiveness, despite cost. It is usually administered as 2 g/kg body weight over 2–5 days (0.4 g/kg/day for 5 days or 1 g/kg/day for 2 days), with clinical benefit as early as 7 days. Most patients tolerate the faster infusion rate over 2 days, but infusion side effects are higher, and the slower infusion regimen is appropriate for patients with diabetes mellitus, impaired renal function, at risk for thrombotic events, or for the elderly. About two-thirds of CIDP patients will improve with IVIg, and time to maximal improvement is 3 months on average. Most patients require repeated administration of IVIg, and a common strategy is to repeat initially with 1 g/kg every 3 weeks for the first 6 months. More than 80% of patients require maintenance infusions of 0.5–1 g/kg every few weeks, with some patients requiring higher dosages, others less frequent infusions. After six months, treatment in patients with stable improvement may be adjusted by decreasing dosage or frequency of infusions. While about half of such patients will remain stable for at least 6 months after stopping IVIg, eventually the majority of patients will relapse. An alternative in patients who experience frequent fluctuations may be administering immunoglobulin therapy subcutaneously at weekly intervals.

In a comparison study of pulsed methylprednisolone versus IVIg, the patients in the IVIg group had a higher response rate by 6 months (88%) and lower side effects than the steroid group (response rate 54%). Over time, most responders eventually relapsed, but at a higher rate and in a shorter time period for the IVIg patients (86% relapsed after median time of 4.5 months) than the steroid group (77% after median time of 14 months).

Plasmapheresis is typically used if IVIg or corticosteroids are ineffective or contraindicated, such as for the patient relapsing on another therapy. If used for maintenance, one regimen is plasma exchange every 2 weeks.

Immunosuppressant therapy may be considered in patients who continue to worsen on standard therapies, and include azathioprine, cyclophosphamide, cyclosporine or tacrolimus, mycophenolate mofetil, rituximab, or interferons.

Treatment in MADSAM is similar to that outlined for CIDP, and both steroids and IVIg are reasonable treatment choices (in contrast to MMN, which should not be treated with steroids).

Multifocal motor neuropathy

MMN is a rare demyelinating peripheral nerve disorder that mimics motor neuron disorder, but needs to be identified, as it responds to treatment.

Epidemiology

The incidence of MMN is about 1 in 100,000. It is more common in men, with first symptoms between age 20 years and 50 years (mean around 40 years).

Pathophyisology

MMN is considered an immune-mediated disorder based on the observation that about half of all patients have autoimmune antibodies, in particular IgM antibodies against the ganglioside GM1. It is not known, however, whether the anti-GM1 antibodies are an epiphenomenon or whether they are involved in the pathogenesis of MMN. The immune hypothesis is further supported by treatment response to IVIg.

Clinical features

MMN presents as slowly progressive, predominantly distal, and asymmetric weakness that typically begins in the upper extremities. It is associated with muscle atrophy and fasciculations, often in the anatomical distribution of individual motor nerves. Muscle cramps are common. Deep tendon reflexes are usually decreased, but tend to be present in unaffected extremities. The disorder is considered purely motor, at least in the beginning. Sensory involvement is controversial, and if present early on suggests the diagnosis of MADSAM, with the exception of possibly decreased vibratory sense in the toes in MMN. In advanced MMN, after several years of progression, patients may develop sensory loss in the territory of affected motor nerves.

Investigations

Many patients (about 40–80%) have IgM antibodies against the ganglioside GM1; a high GM1 titer is specific for the disorder, but GM1 antibody is not required for diagnosis. Occasionally antibodies to other glycolipids (asialo-GM1, GD1a, or GM2) are present.

Electrophysiological testing should be performed on multiple nerves including proximal segments in order to identify focal motor nerve conduction block at sites usually not affected by entrapment. A typical feature of MMN is normal sensory nerve conduction velocity across the same segment, with demonstrated motor conduction block. In some patients, no conduction block may be documented, but other features of demyelination are usually noted with a careful electrodiagnostic evaluation. In patients without demyelination on routine NCS, the triple stimulation technique (TST, described under CIDP) may document conduction block or temporal dispersion in proximal nerve segments. In contrast to MADSAM where motor nerve findings are similar, electrophysiological sensory involvement does not occur in MMN.

Some patients have the typical clinical presentation of MMN, but do not have electrophysiological findings of demyelination, but rather axonal features. These patients are diagnosed with an axonal variant, called multifocal acquired motor axonopathy (MAMA). A few of these patients have GM1 antibodies, and recent cases were found to have antibodies against the ganglioside GD1a.

Treatment

The primary treatment for MMN and MAMA is IVIg. Improvement may begin within days, and most patients show long-term benefit. Subcutaneous immunoglobulins may be an alternative. Some patients lose responsiveness to maintenance IVIg over years. These patients should not be treated with corticosteroids or plasmapheresis, as they are not effective and may even cause worsening. It is controversial whether such patients may benefit from cyclophosphamide or rituximab.

Neuropathies with monoclonal gammopathies

Monoclonal gammopathies are common in the general population and increase with age. Thus, when a patient presents with monoclonal gammopathy and a polyneuropathy, it is often not clear whether it represents an etiological or coincidental association, given the frequency of both conditions. It is therefore important to exclude other treatable causes of polyneuropathy in such patients.

Systemic symptoms accompanying the neuropathy suggest malignancy, amyloidosis, or POEMS syndrome.

Epidemiology

The incidence of monoclonal gammopathy is reported as more than 3% of adults over 50 years of age, and about 5% in the over 70-year-old. The risk of progression to malignancy is estimated as 1–2.7% annually, and may be more common in patients with neuropathy. About 10% of neuropathy patients who have gammopathy are found to have an underlying hematological malignancy, including Waldenström's macroglobulinemia, multiple myeloma, solitary plasmacytoma, and primary amyloidosis.

Paraprotein-associated neuropathies are about 10% of neuropathies with otherwise unknown etiology, with neuropathy often the first symptom of the gammopathy.

Pathophysiology

The most common monoclonal gammopathy is IgG, followed by IgM and IgA. In patients with neuropathy, however, IgM is overrepresented with 48%, versus IgG 37% and IgA 15%, In some patients, the neuropathy is likely caused by the underlying disorder and not directly related to the monoclonal antibody. In this regard, patients with a demyelinating neuropathy and paraprotein of the IgG or IgA type present similarly to CIDP and show a similar response to therapy. In contrast, about half of all patients with IgM and neuropathy have antineural antibodies, in particular against the myelin associated glycoprotein (anti-MAG). In these patients, IgM may bind directly to peripheral nerve myelin and result in separation of the outer layers of compacted myelin.

Clinical features

In patients with monoclonal gammopathy of unknown significance (MGUS) who have neuropathy, the paraprotein is usually IgM (IgM-MGUS). The neuropathy is usually distal, large fiber sensory predominant, and may be associated with sensory ataxia. Electrodiagnostic studies document a demyelinating neuropathy with segmental demyelination and prolonged distal latencies. In contrast, in MGUS without neuropathy the most common type is IgG.

The distal acquired demyelinating sensory (DADS) neuropathy is a slowly progressive symmetric polyneuropathy associated with IgM gammopathy, usually the kappa subtype (DADS-M). Antineural antibodies are commonly found in IgM neuropathy in general, and more than half of DADS patients have antibodies against the Schwann cell-based myelin associated glycoprotein (anti-MAG). The polyneuropathy begins with distal paresthesias and numbness. Weakness is minor, if at all present. After years, patients may develop ataxia, walking difficulty, and tremor. The electrophysiology is demyelinating, with more severe slowing of conduction velocity in distal nerves. Increased CSF protein is common. The prognosis is fair, as the condition is only slowly progressive with predominantly sensory symptoms. Treatment response in patients with DADS-M is generally poor (including for steroids, IVIg, and plasmapheresis). Patients with DADS without a monoclonal gammopathy, however, may show treatment responses similar to CIDP.

Waldenström's macroglobulinemia is a lymphoplasmocytic lymphoma that produces IgM-kappa, and typically presents in the elderly, with a male predominance. The neuropathy is clinically similar to IgM-MGUS, with the most common features distal numbness (feet) and sensory ataxia from large fiber involvement. Occasionally tremor is present. Due to severe anemia and often very high-level IgM, patients often complain of fatigue and may develop complications from hyperviscosity syndrome. Electrodiagnostically, the neuropathy is more common axonal than demyelinative, somewhat in contrast to IgM-MGUS.

In multiple myeloma, the monoclonal gammopathy is more commonly IgG than IgA. Clinical deficits from neuropathy are noted in up to 20% of patients with untreated multiple myeloma. NCS documents a length-dependent and usually sensorimotor polyneuropathy with axonal character. Treatment-emergent polyneuropathy occurs in up to two-thirds of patients after chemotherapy and is related to drug toxicity. Bortezomib and thalidomide commonly cause a length-dependent painful sensory predominant neuropathy.

The polyneuropathy in POEMS syndrome (peripheral neuropathy, organomegaly, endocrinopathy, M-component, and skin changes) is rapidly progressive, with prominent motor involvement and severe disability within 1 year. The gammopathy is frequently IgG or IgA, with low levels of lambda light chain, and an osteosclerotic (myeloma) lesion or Castleman's syndrome is frequently present. Electrophysiological testing shows demyelinating features without conduction block, and severe axonal loss in the legs. POEMS does not respond to typical CIDP treatments. Some patients do well with autologous peripheral blood stem cell transplantation, including clear improvement in neurological deficits.

Amyloidosis is a group of disorders associated with extracellular amyloid deposition. Neurological deficits typically occur in light-chain amyloidosis (AL-amyloid), with deposition in nerves and other tissues, resulting in a progressive length-dependent sensory predominant polyneuropathy. The neuropathy is axonal and usually affects small fiber modalities, thus resulting in pain and symptoms related to autonomic failure (orthostatic hypotension, gastrointestinal dysfunction).

Polyneuropathy in mixed cryoglobulinemia associated with hepatitis C is sensory or sensorimotor, occasionally multifocal, and has axonal character by electrophysiology.

Vasculitic neuropathies

Systemic vasculitides in collagen vascular disease often involve the peripheral nervous system. The typical clinical presentation of peripheral nerve vasculitis is subacute and painful mononeuropathy multiplex, less commonly distal asymmetric or symmetric polyneuropathy. Initially, the condition may present as isolated painful mononeuropathy affecting a single nerve, typically not at one of the usual compression sites. It is important to diagnose peripheral nerve vasculitis in a timely manner, including nerve biopsy if needed, as aggressive immunotherapy may be able to lessen the disability from the otherwise usually severe and progressive neuropathy.

Epidemiology

Neuropathy occurs in about two-thirds of patients with systemic necrotizing vasculitis, including polyarteritis nodosa and Churg–Strauss syndrome (eosinophilic granulomatosis with polyangiitis). In polyarteritis nodosa (PAN), mononeuritis multiplex is the presenting clinical feature in up to 30% of patients. It is also common in microscopic polyangiitis (which resembles PAN) and cryoglobulinemia (associated with hepatitis C). Mononeuropathy multiplex or polyneuropathy occurs in 20–30% of Wegener granulomatosis. Vasculitic neuropathy may develop occasionally in systemic lupus erythematodes, typically presenting as immune axonal sensorimotor polyneuropathy with asymmetric features, and may be associated with CNS involvement. In Sjögren's syndrome, small fiber neuropathy with burning pain and sensory ganglionopathy resulting in sensory ataxia is more common than sensory or sensorimotor polyneuropathy. Vasculitic neuropathy in rheumatoid arthritis occurs occasionally (8%), whereas entrapment neuropathies are often present and axonal sensorimotor polyneuropathy is common after long disease duration. Isolated vasculitic neuropathy occurs occasionally without systemic vasculitis.

A recently recognized immune-mediated axonal neuropathy is postsurgical inflammatory neuropathy, which may affect a single nerve (often the sciatic nerve), multiple nerves (mononeuritis multiplex), or the brachial or lumbosacral plexus. It may be differentiated from a nerve injury due to surgical trauma by delayed onset after surgery (days, sometimes weeks) and a progressive course.

Pathophysiology
Necrotizing vasculitis results in inflammation and necrosis of blood vessel walls, leading to nerve infarction and axonal (Wallerian) degeneration. Typically, the medium to small vessels are affected. The result is an acute or subacute, stepwise progressive neuropathy that may affect large and small nerve fibers, including unmyelinated or thinly myelinated nerves, resulting in autonomic dysfunction and pain.

Clinical features
Clinically, acute onset of pain in one or more cranial or peripheral nerves is followed by motor and sensory deficit in the distribution of the affected nerve. The classic presentation is a focal mononeuropathy that does not seem to localize to one of the typical compression sites, especially if associated with pain and systemic features such as fever, weight loss, or rash. Within days or weeks, additional nerves are affected, resulting in progressive mononeuropathy multiplex. Large fiber involvement may lead to acute weakness or sensory loss from nerve infarction. Small fiber involvement results in pain, often severe, and autonomic dysfunction. With disease progression, the picture of distal asymmetric or symmetric polyneuropathy develops. Less commonly, vasculitic neuropathy presents primarily as symmetric polyneuropathy. Patients often present with signs of systemic involvement (fever, weight loss, anorexia). They should be carefully evaluated for evidence of underlying collagen vascular disorder and infection, including involvement of the skin (rash). End-organ involvement may be present, depending on the underlying vasculitic condition.

Investigations
All patients with suspected vasculitic neuropathy need to be evaluated urgently, due to rapid progression of the disease and response to treatment. Diagnosis is especially difficult in patients with isolated vasculitis of the peripheral nervous system, and depends on histological demonstration of characteristic findings on nerve and muscle biopsies.

Testing for collagen vascular disease may indicate systemic vasculitis, with elevation of erythrocyte sedimentation rate, C-reactive protein, and other features of inflammation. Eosinophilia may be noted. Autoantibody testing includes antineutrophilic cytoplasmic antigen (ANCA) antibodies that occur in microscopic polyangiitis, mainly to myeloperoxidase, and in Wegener granulomatosis (c-ANCA/PR3-ANCA). Routine workup for suspected vasculitic neuropathy includes antinuclear antibody (ANA) and antibodies against double-stranded DNA, C3 and C4, rheumatoid factor, and cryoglobulins. Consider testing for anti-SSA/SSB, angiotensin-

converting enzyme, and porphyria screen. Infectious vasculopathy (usually without definite vasculitis) may be caused by hepatitis B and C virus, HIV, and human T-cell lymphotropic virus (HTLV-I). West Nile virus and cytomegalovirus, and the bacterial infections of syphilis and Lyme disease, cause painful polyradiculopathy. Leprosy is a common cause of infectious neuropathy.

Workup for systemic vasculitis usually includes chest X-ray, and possibly chest computed tomography (CT), sinus X-ray, lumbar puncture, and other tests as directed by the clinical presentation (such as bone scan, paraneoplastic evaluation, or tests for hereditary polyneuropathies).

Electrophysiological testing reveals features of acute axonal nerve lesions; that is, reduced or absent compound motor action potentials and sensory nerve action potentials, with only minor changes in conduction velocity, distal motor latency, or F-waves. Acute onset vasculitis neuropathy may result in focal nerve lesion temporarily mimicking conduction block due to the time required to result in distally reduced nerve excitability from Wallerian degeneration ("pseudo-conduction block").

Nerve biopsy, typically the sural or superficial peroneal nerve, and muscle biopsy should be performed expeditiously in all patients with suspected vasculitis neuropathy. Perivascular and transmural mononuclear cell infiltrates with necrosis of the blood vessel walls and occlusion of epineural blood vessels are pathognomonic.

Treatment
Immunosuppressive treatment should be initiated as soon as the diagnosis is made. Delay in treatment increases the mortality greatly: 15–20% with early treatment versus 80–90% with delayed treatment. Treatment in systemic vasculitis relies on steroids at initially high dosage (induction therapy for 3–6 months) to achieve remission, followed by lower-dosed maintenance therapy. A typical regimen for systemic vasculitis is prednisone 60–100 mg daily (1 mg/kg), with gradual dosage reduction after 1–2 months. In patients with severe vasculitic neuropathy, intravenous methylprednisolone is added initially at 1 g/day for 3–5 days. High-dose steroid therapy is also appropriate for postsurgical inflammatory neuropathy.

For maintenance therapy, oral prednisone is continued at the lowest possible dosage (according to clinical guidance) in combination with azathioprine or methotrexate as steroid sparing agents. Cyclosporine and mycophenolate mofetil are second-line agents for maintenance therapy. In patients with aggressive systemic vasculitis, including polyarteritis nodosa, Churg–Strauss syndrome, microscopic polyangiitis, and Wegener granulomatosis, consider the addition of cyclophosphamide to the induction therapy, especially if there are poor prognostic factors from severe organ involvement. Cyclophosphamide may be given orally (2 g/kg daily) or as intravenous pulse therapy (15 mg/kg or 0.6–0.7 g/m^2 every 2–3 weeks). In patients who do not respond to this therapy or have contraindications, rituximab, IVIg, and plasmapheresis may be considered.

Metabolic neuropathies

Diabetic neuropathy
Neuropathy in diabetes may affect any part of the peripheral nervous system. Most common is diabetic polyneuropathy. Second most common is mononeuropathy, usually nerve entrapment such as carpal tunnel syndrome (Table 102.1).

Table 102.1 Neuropathies associated with diabetes.

Symmetric
(Distal) sensory or sensorimotor polyneuropathy
Small fiber neuropathy
Autonomic neuropathy
Acute painful diabetic polyneuropathy
Focal/asymmetric
Polyradiculoplexopathies
– plexopathy: lumbosacral > brachial
– truncal radiculopathy: thoracic > abdominal
Limb mononeuropathy from nerve infarction
Limb mononeuropathies from nerve entrapment
Mononeuropathy multiplex
Cranial mononeuropathies: III > VI, IV > VII

Epidemiology

A careful history and exam may reveal evidence for diabetic neuropathy at the time of diagnosis of diabetes in 7.5%, and after 25 years in 50%. While it is a common late complication, diabetic polyneuropathy can develop at any time during the course of illness and may occur even in patients with prediabetes. Mean time interval from onset of diabetes to symptoms of neuropathy is 8 years, shorter in diabetes type II than type I.

Pathophysiology

Diabetic polyneuropathy is more common in patients with prolonged hyperglycemia, and tight control of diabetes reduces the risk. According to the metabolic hypothesis, hyperglycemia leads to shunting of glucose into the polyol pathway, resulting in accumulation of sorbitol and fructose in nerve cells. Hyperglycemia causes non-enzymatic glycosylation of structural nerve proteins. The microvascular hypothesis postulates endoneurial hypoxia from capillary damage and increased vascular resistance. An autoimmune neuropathy may emerge from immunogenic alteration of endothelial capillary cells. In addition to hyperglycemia, hyperlipidemia may be a contributing factor.

Clinical features

The most common manifestation (about 70%) is distal sensory or sensorimotor polyneuropathy, often accompanied by autonomic features. It presents as typical length-dependent axonal neuropathy with large and small fiber sensory manifestations beginning in the toes, gradually spreading proximally, in stocking-and-glove distribution. A combination of negative (numbness) and positive sensory symptoms (pain, paresthesias) is common. Diabetic polyneuropathy may present in asymptomatic patients with absent ankle jerks and diminished vibration sense distally. In severe cases, sensory ataxia occurs in combination with distal weakness, diabetic dysautonomia, and Charcot joints and foot ulcers. Most patients have some discomfort related to the neuropathy, and significant neuropathic pain due to small fiber involvement develops in up to one-fourth of patients, often described as burning, sharp/shooting pain in feet, or sensation of continuous coldness distally. In some patients, diabetic neuropathy manifests as rather isolated small fiber neuropathy and/or autonomic neuropathy, typically after long disease duration in diabetes type 2, and earlier in diabetes type 1. Occasionally, an acute painful severe sensory polyneuropathy develops soon after diagnosis and initiation of treatment with tight glucose control. It occurs in both diabetes types 1 and 2 and may be triggered by insulin therapy or oral hypoglycemic

agents. Neuropathic pain is often severe and does not respond well to symptomatic therapy. Autonomic dysfunction is common, especially in patients with diabetes type 1. The condition improves gradually over weeks to months with glucose control and weight gain. An acute painful distal polyneuropathy may also occur spontaneously and is associated with weight loss (diabetic neuropathic cachexia); it may be associated with pain proximally or truncally due to nerve root involvement. It occurs especially in the elderly with poor glycemic control and is partially reversible with diabetes treatment.

Several diabetic neuropathies present with focal or asymmetric symptoms or deficits. Diabetic polyradiculoplexopathy is a proximal diabetic neuropathy and likely of inflammatory vascular etiology. The most common form is diabetic amyotrophy, affecting the lumbosacral plexus (especially femoral and obturator nerves). Typically, asymmetric pain (in thigh, hip, or buttock) is followed days or weeks later by weakness and wasting of pelvic girdle and thigh muscles, with only minor sensory loss. Recovery takes up to 24 months and in many cases mild to moderate weakness persists. Diabetic truncal neuropathy results from ischemic radiculopathy, typically affecting a thoracic dermatome with sensory loss and severely painful dysesthesias. Mononeuropathies of sudden onset (presumably from nerve infarction) may affect a single limb nerve (femoral, sciatic, median, or ulnar), multiple nerves in combination (mononeuritis multiplex), or cranial nerves. The most common cranial neuropathy in diabetes is oculomotor palsy with sparing of the pupillary reflex. It typically has acute onset and is associated with retro- or supraorbital pain. Recovery over weeks to months may be expected. Diabetes may affect also the fourth and sixth cranial nerves, and is the most common cause of isolated fourth nerve palsy. Entrapment neuropathies at typical compression sites are common in diabetes, including carpal tunnel (median nerve) and cubital tunnel (ulnar nerve) syndrome.

Some patients with diabetic polyneuropathy have demyelinating features resembling CIDP. The differentiation may be difficult, as NCS in diabetes polyneuropathy often document somewhat greater slowing in conduction velocity than other axonal neuropathies. In addition, CSF studies in diabetic patients usually show increased protein. It is not clear whether diabetes increases the likelihood of CIDP, but it is important to recognize patients with clinical or electrophysiological features of CIDP in order to treat them according to CIDP guidelines, including IVIg.

Investigations

All patients with unexplained neuropathy need to be checked for diabetes, by measurement of glucose (fasting, if necessary oral glucose tolerance test) and HgbA1c. Nerve conduction studies in diabetic polyneuropathy often reveal diminished amplitudes, with slowing of conduction velocities that tends to be more pronounced than in other axonal polyneuropathies. CSF, if tested, shows mild to moderate increase in CSF protein. Typical polyneuropathy features in the context of longstanding diabetes are usually diagnostic, but 5–10% of diabetic patients may have a different cause. Painless proximal neuropathy is unusual and suggests CIDP.

Treatment

Tight control of diabetes is partially effective in preventing diabetic neuropathy, in both types 1 and 2. Lifestyle intervention including diet and exercise are beneficial in delaying onset of diabetes and progression of small fiber neuropathy in particular. Several studies suggest that treatment with alpha-lipoic acid may reduce severity of diabetic sensory polyneuropathy, such as 600 mg orally given daily over four years. Medications potentially worsening glycemic control should be avoided, and in patients with hypertension, angiotensin-converting enzyme inhibitors or angiotensin-receptor blocking medication are preferred over thiazide diuretics, and may delay onset of cardiovascular and renal complications from diabetes. Symptomatic therapy of painful diabetic neuropathy follows the general recommendations for neuropathic pain in peripheral nerve disorders (outlined in Chapter 100). Patients with entrapment neuropathy benefit from decompressive surgery with guidance as for patients without diabetes. Several reports suggest benefit of IVIg in subcategories of diabetic neuropathy, including diabetic amyotrophy. Patients with polyneuropathy resembling CIDP should be treated with IVIg rather than steroids.

Neuropathy from B$_{12}$ deficiency

Vitamin B$_{12}$ (cobalamin) deficiency may result in neurological, neurocognitive, and neuropsychiatric impairments, in addition to anemia and increased cardiovascular risk. Cobalamin deficiency affects the spinal cord as subacute combined degeneration (referring to combined degeneration of the corticospinal and dorsal column tracts) and the peripheral nervous system as a symmetric axonal sensorimotor polyneuropathy.

Epidemiology

Cobalamin deficiency is more common in the elderly. In a large sample of inpatients (France), functional B$_{12}$ deficiency was found in 9.6% of patients aged 30–60 years and 14.2% in patients over 90 years.

Pathophysiology

A strict vegetarian diet is rarely the cause. In most cases, it results from impaired B$_{12}$ absorption in the gastrointestinal tract, due to inadequate gastric production of intrinsic factor (pernicious anemia, gastrectomy), or from disorders of the terminal ileum (celiac disorders, Crohn's disease, or intestinal resection). Pernicious anemia is an autoimmune disorder involving autoantibody production against gastric parietal cells. Prolonged treatment with antacids (H2-antagonists or proton pump inhibitors) increases risk for B$_{12}$ deficiency. A rare cause is infection with fish tapeworm. Exposure to nitric oxide may precipitate symptom onset by inactivation of cobalamin.

The lack of anemia or macrocytosis does not exclude functional B$_{12}$ deficiency.

Clinical features

The disease begins gradually, with distal paresthesias and weakness. It may present as axonal sensorimotor polyneuropathy with lower motor neuron signs, or due to spinal cord involvement with upper motor neuron findings, often in combination. Subacute combined degeneration refers to involvement of pyramidal tract (spastic paraparesis) and posterior columns (loss of vibration and position sense, sensory ataxia). Deep tendon reflexes may be decreased or increased. Isolated polyneuropathy without any myelopathy is unusual.

Cognitive dysfunction and psychiatric manifestations may be accompanying features.

Investigations

In untreated patients, vitamin B$_{12}$ levels are low. It is important to recognize that patients with B$_{12}$ levels in the low normal range (below 300 pg/ml) may become symptomatic. Methylmalonic acid is a marker for cellular B$_{12}$ levels and, if increased, confirms B$_{12}$ deficiency, even if B$_{12}$ level is low normal. Homocysteine level may also be increased, but is less specific. Macrocytic anemia is often present, but may be masked by treatment with folic acid. Intrinsic factor antibodies and gastrin antibodies establish the diagnosis of pernicious anemia. Schilling test documents B$_{12}$ malabsorption, but is not needed for diagnosis and treatment.

Acquired copper deficiency may present very similar to vitamin B$_{12}$ deficiency with myeloneuropathy and anemia, and copper and zinc levels should be checked in such patients with normal B$_{12}$ level.

Treatment

Treatment with vitamin B$_{12}$ should be given parenterally, at least initially, in a patient with symptoms of B$_{12}$ deficiency or in severe cases. A simple regimen is 1 mg daily for a week, weekly for a month, and then monthly. After restoration of body stores, oral B$_{12}$ administration may be sufficient for maintenance. In patients with borderline to mildly decreased B$_{12}$ levels, oral supplementation with 1 mg B$_{12}$ daily may be sufficient. The normalization of serum B$_{12}$ should be monitored. Symptoms of B$_{12}$ deficiency are often poorly reversible, in part due to spinal cord involvement, and thus treatment should be instituted as early as possible.

Treatment with folic acid only treats the macrocytic anemia, not the neuropathy, and may worsen the neurological deficits.

Other metabolic and endocrine neuropathies

Acquired copper deficiency may present very similar to vitamin B$_{12}$ deficiency with myeloneuropathy and anemia. The condition may be secondary to gastric surgery (as copper is absorbed in the stomach) or zinc exposure (such as from ingestion of denture cream). Zinc competes with copper absorption, and thus both zinc and copper levels should be tested. Treatment is with copper and avoidance of zinc exposure. As with myeloneuropathy from B$_{12}$ deficiency, the neurological deficits are poorly reversible.

In chronic renal failure, a typical sensory predominant axonal polyneuropathy is common. The prevalence is 10–80% depending on duration and severity of uremia. Most bothersome are often dysesthesias in the feet, resulting in "burning feet" and resembling restless leg syndrome. Muscle cramps are common. In advanced uremia, distal weakness and autonomic dysfunction occur. Electrophysiology is axonal, with greater slowing of conduction velocity in patients with creatinine clearance below 10% of normal. Dialysis may prevent or improve the condition. Renal transplantation usually improves even severe uremic neuropathy.

In hepatic insufficiency, symptomatic neuropathy is uncommon and mild, with more common abnormalities on nerve conduction testing.

Hypothyroidism may cause mild axonal polyneuropathy with distal sensory manifestations.

Infectious neuropathies

Detailed descriptions of the most important infectious neuropathies are provided elsewhere, including designated chapters for leprosy (Chapter 65), neurosyphilis (Chapter 66), Lyme disease (Chapter 67), and HIV neuropathy (Chapter 86).

Neuropathy from nutritional causes and alcoholism

Neurological manifestations of malnutrition and alcoholism are discussed in detail in separate chapters. Alcoholic polyneuropathy is outlined here due to its relative frequency (see Chapter 97). Population studies from inner-city hospitals suggest that 10–15% of chronic alcoholics develop a neuropathy. It occurs alone or in combination with other alcohol-related disorders, such as alcohol-related seizures, Wernicke encephalopathy, or the Korsakoff amnestic syndrome. It is subject to controversy whether the neuropathy associated with chronic alcoholism is the result of a direct "toxic" effect of alcohol, or due to associated nutritional deficiencies (thiamine) or chronic liver disease.

The polyneuropathy is typically symmetric and distal in stocking-and-glove distribution. In the legs, decreased sensation to light touch and vibration are usually noted, and ankle jerks are depressed or absent. Painful paresthesias are common. Weakness if present tends to be distal, but proximal weakness and atrophy may occur, and rapidly progressing weakness has been described. Gait disturbance is common, particularly in patients with superimposed alcoholic cerebellar degeneration or Wernicke disease.

Cessation of alcohol consumption is imperative, and nutritional support is essential. Vitamins and minerals should be replaced, especially thiamine 100 mg daily, initially parenterally. Megadose thiamine regimens (such as 500 mg given three times daily) are sometimes advocated for patients with Wernicke encephalopathy or those not responding to usual thiamine supplementation.

Further reading

Ashbury AK, Cornblath DR. Assessment of current diagnostic criteria for Guillain–Barré syndrome. *Ann Neurol* 1990;27(Suppl):S21–S24.

Attarian S, Franques J, Elisabeth J, *et al.* Triple-stimulation technique improves the diagnosis of chronic inflammatory demyelinating polyradiculoneuropathy. *Muscle Nerve* 2015;51(4):541–548. doi:10.1002/mus.24352

Bril V, Katzberg HD. Acquired immune axonal neuropathies. *Continuum* 2014;20: 1261–1273.

Cornblath DR, Feasby TE, Hahn AF, *et al.* Research criteria for diagnosis of chronic inflammatory demyelinating polyneuropathy (CIDP). *Neurology* 1991;41:617–618.

Dimachkie MM, Saperstein DS. Acquired immune demyelinating neuropathies. *Continuum* 2014;20:1241–1260.

Dimachkie MM, Barohn RJ, Katz J. Multifocal motor neuropathy, multifocal acquired demyelinating sensory and motor neuropathy, and other chronic acquired demyelinating polyneuropathy variants. *Neurol Clin* 2013;31:533–555.

Gorson KC, Katz J. Chronic inflammatory demyelinating polyneuropathy. *Neurol Clin* 2013;13:511–532.

Hughes RA, Cornblath DR. Guillain–Barré syndrome. *Lancet* 2005;366:1653–1666.

Mauermann ML. Paraproteinemic neuropathies. *Continuum* 2014;20:1307–1322.

Nobile-Orazio E, Cocito D, Jann S, *et al.* Frequency and time to relapse after discontinuing 6-month therapy with IVIg or pulsed methylprednisolone in CIDP. *J Neurol Neurosurg Psychiatry* 2015;86(7):729–734. doi:10.1136/jnnp-2013-307515

Russell JW, Zilliox LA. Diabetic neuropathies. *Continuum* 2014;20:1226–1240.

Sandbrink F, Klion AD, Floeter MK. "Pseudo-conduction block" in a patient with vasculitic neuropathy. *Electromyogr Clin Neurophysiol* 2001;41:195–202.

Staff NP, Windebank AJ. Peripheral neuropathy due to vitamin deficiency, toxins, and medications. *Continuum* 2014;20:1293–1306.

Van den Bergh PY, Hadden RD, Bouche P, *et al.* European Federation of Neurological Societies/Peripheral Nerve Society guideline on management of chronic inflammatory demyelinating polyradiculoneuropathy: Report of a joint task force of the European Federation of Neurological Societies and the Peripheral Nerve Society – first revision. *Eur J Neurol* 2010;17:356–363.

103 Plexopathies and mononeuropathies

Friedhelm Sandbrink

Department of Neurology, Veterans Affairs Medical Center, and Georgetown University, Washington, DC, USA

This chapter discusses the focal disorders affecting peripheral nerves distal to the nerve roots. For clarity, we will consider the different plexus disorders separately from the most common focal neuropathies affecting individual peripheral nerves.

Plexopathies

The neural plexus are networks of nerve fibers that are formed by the spinal nerve roots, specifically the anterior primary rami of the mixed spinal nerves, and reorganize into peripheral nerves distally. Plexopathies are distinct disorders affecting these neural networks with a wide array of etiologies that are best understood in anatomic correlation. Thus, the cervical, brachial, and lumbosacral plexopathies will be outlined separately.

Epidemiology

Plexopathies occur less frequently than the peripheral nerve disorders affecting the nerve roots or distal nerves, either as focal or generalized peripheral neuropathies. Brachial plexopathies are more common than the other plexopathies, in part due to the greater vulnerability to trauma and the close proximity to other organs with the neck and upper thorax. Thus, injury to the brachial plexus is likely the most common etiology of plexopathy in children and adults. The annual incidence of idiopathic neuralgic amyotrophy, the second most common cause of brachial plexopathy, is estimated as 2–3/100,000 population.

Clinical features: Cervical plexus

Anatomic correlation

The cervical plexus is formed in the lateral neck by the C1–C4 spinal nerves and has communication with the lower cranial nerves X–XII. The phrenic nerve (C4) is the most important nerve derived from the cervical plexus.

Disorders

Cervical plexopathies are rarely diagnosed. Injury occurs during radical neck dissection and from closed violent trauma such as motorcycle accidents, usually in combination with upper brachial plexus lesions. Neoplastic infiltration of the cervical plexus often presents with unrelenting pain in the neck, throat, or shoulder region that worsens with neck movement or swallowing. Clinical examination often does not reveal the mass lesion, but rather neck tenderness and palpable lymph nodes.

Clinical features: Brachial plexus

Anatomic correlation

The brachial plexus receives input from the C5–T1 nerve roots that come together to form three trunks. The upper (C5–C6 root supply), middle (C7), and lower trunk (C8–T1) represent the supraclavicular portion of the brachial plexus. The nerve fibers reorganize into three anterior and three posterior divisions that are situated behind the clavicle. The infraclavicular portion of the brachial plexus includes the cords named in relation to the axillary artery as lateral, posterior, and medial (Figure 103.1). Most terminal nerves derived from the plexus originate from the cords within the axilla.

Brachial plexopathies are the most common plexus lesions, more commonly supraclavicular than infraclavicular. The supraclavicular plexopathies are divided into upper, middle, and lower plexus lesions, indicating involvement of the upper, middle, and lower trunk fibers, respectively. It is often clinically difficult to distinguish supraclavicular plexopathies affecting the trunk from disorders of the corresponding nerve roots or mixed spinal nerves.

Disorders

Trauma is the most common cause of brachial plexopathies. The usual mechanism is traction of the supraclavicular plexus nerve fibers. It tends to damage the upper plexus (trunk) in particular. The burner syndrome occurs in athletes (especially young men in contact sports) who are subjected to forceful depression of the shoulder. It consists of a sudden, intense, burning dysesthesia and anesthesia in the entire arm, often associated with weakness, and usually resolves quickly. Rucksack (pack) palsy is a transient weakness caused by direct compression of the upper trunk or long thoracic nerve by a heavy backpack. More severe injury occurs with excessive separation of the head and shoulder as in motorcycle accidents, which results in traction of the upper trunk, all the trunks, and/or the corresponding nerve roots. A humerus fracture or dislocation may injure the infraclavicular plexus or terminal nerves, especially the axillary nerve. Postmedian sternotomy (open-heart surgery) results in C8 nerve root or lower trunk brachial plexopathy, with weakness, paresthesias, and pain in an ulnar distribution.

The nerve roots, particularly the ventral (motor) roots, are more vulnerable to traction injury than the plexus or

International Neurology, Second edition. Edited by Robert P. Lisak, Daniel D. Truong, William M. Carroll and Roongroj Bhidayasiri
© 2016 John Wiley & Sons, Ltd. Published 2016 by John Wiley & Sons, Ltd.

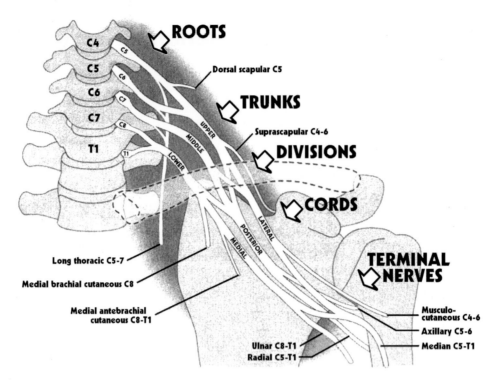

ROOTS

C4
C5
C6
C7
T1

Dorsal scapular C5

TRUNKS

Suprascapular C4-6

DIVISIONS

UPPER
MIDDLE
LOWER

CORDS

LATERAL
POSTERIOR
MEDIAL

Long thoracic C5-7

Medial brachial cutaneous C8

Medial antebrachial
cutaneous C8-T1

TERMINAL NERVES

Musculo-
cutaneous C4-6

Axillary C5-6

Median C5-1

Ulnar C8-T1
Radial C5-T1

Figure 103.1 The brachial plexus. Source: Adapted from Wilbourn 2007. Reproduced with permission of Elsevier.

peripheral nerves because of lesser amounts of collagen and lack of supporting epineurial and perineurial sheaths. Traumatic nerve root avulsion of C5 and C6 roots or upper trunk lesion result in Erb–Duchenne palsy. This may occur during delivery as a result of excessive lateral traction on the fetal head when delivering the shoulder. Motorcycle accidents frequently cause avulsion of upper brachial nerve roots (often combined with middle and lower levels) and result in severe disability from permanent motor and sensory deficits and root avulsion pain. Traumatic avulsion of C8–T1 nerve roots or the lower plexus is less common, resulting in Dejerine–Klumpke palsy. This is caused by traction on the abducted arm or by a fall where the outstretched arm grasps a fixed object to arrest the fall.

Neuralgic amyotrophy is also called idiopathic brachial plexus neuropathy, brachial plexitis, and Parsonage–Turner syndrome. It is considered the second most common cause of brachial plexopathy (after trauma), and is twice as common in men as in women. It may occur at any age including childhood, however the fourth to fifth decades are the most common. The attacks are assumed to be autoimmune in origin, and antecedent events are noted in half of patients, such as viral illness, vaccination, trauma, or surgery. The disorder affects the plexus and/or several individual peripheral nerves and tends to be patchy. Damage in the upper part of the brachial plexus combined with the long thoracic nerve and/or suprascapular nerve is the most common pattern (71% in a recent study), but almost any nerve in the plexus may be affected. The disorder is bilateral in one-third of cases. The attacks typically begin with a severe, continuous pain in the shoulder or neck region that may radiate to the arm. Onset of pain is usually sudden, often overnight, but may be stuttering. Severe weakness in the shoulder girdle muscles typically develops a few days later, with a range from less than 24 hours to

several weeks. Occasionally, the weakness occurs without preceding pain. Fasciculations may be noted. Hypesthesias or paresthesias over the lateral shoulder or upper arm region occur frequently. Vasomotor dysfunction includes skin changes, edema, or increased sweating. Most patients improve at least partially over months to years. The continuous initial pain lasts for days to weeks, and is frequently followed by stabbing or shooting pains elicited by movements or prolonged posturing of the arm. On long-term follow-up (3 years and longer), chronic pain was noted in almost half of patients. After 2–3 years, 10–20% of patients have moderate to severe residual paresis. Recurrent attacks after years are not uncommon.

Hereditary neuralgic amyotrophy (HNA) or familial brachial neuritis is an autosomal dominant disorder linked to mutations in the *SEPT9* gene (a member of the cytoskeleton-related septin family) on chromosome 17q25. Some pedigrees have characteristic facial features, including hypotelorism. Attacks are similar to idiopathic neuralgic amyotrophy. The age at onset is earlier, with the first attack in childhood or young adulthood. Nerves outside the brachial plexus are more commonly affected, such as the lumbosacral plexus, phrenic nerve, intercostal nerves, or recurrent laryngeal nerves (resulting in bilateral vocal cord paresis). Functional outcome is worse, with more severe maximum weakness and greater residual paresis. Repeated attacks are typical, triggered by factors such as stress, infections, or puerperium.

Most malignant *tumors* of the brachial plexus are metastatic lung or breast carcinomas invading the lower plexus, especially lower trunk and medial cord. Severe, persistent pain is the cardinal symptom, usually located in the shoulder and axilla, or radiating along the medial (ulnar) aspect of forearm and hand. Progressive weakness of lower plexus (C8–T1) innervated muscles usually appears later, whereas paresthesias are relatively uncommon. Horner's syndrome indicates invasion of the cervical sympathetic by paravertebral tumor near the first thoracic vertebra, such as caused by "Pancoast" tumor at the apex of the lung.

Radiation-induced brachial plexopathy may follow months to years after radiation treatment, with a median of 1.5 years in breast cancer patients. The overall frequency is cited as 1.8–4.9% of treated patients, likely higher if total dose is >50 Gy, if fewer and higher doses are used (hypofractionation), or if combined with simultaneous chemotherapy. Radiation plexopathy tends to affect the upper plexus or whole plexus. Initial presentation is usually sensory with paresthesias and numbness in lateral cord (median nerve) innervated fingers, followed soon after by weakness and loss of tendon reflexes. Edema of the affected extremity and chronic skin changes in the radiation field are typical. In contrast to neoplastic plexopathy, pain is inconstant and develops late.

Many patients with pain in the shoulder, arm, or hand are labeled as having "*thoracic outlet syndrome*," but do not have a brachial plexus compression. True neurogenic thoracic outlet syndrome is also called cervical rib and band syndrome. It is a rare condition caused by a developmental anomaly. A taut fibrous band extends from the tip of a rudimentary cervical rib or from an elongated C7 transverse process to the first true thoracic rib. Sometimes, the cervical rib articulates directly with the first thoracic rib. Stretching of the distal T1 root or lower trunk fibers results in a predominantly motor syndrome. Typical presentation is unilateral weakness and wasting of hand muscles in a young to middle-aged woman, affecting the thenar eminence in particular. Intermittent, mild aching pain and sensory complaints in the ulnar aspect of forearm and hand may be present, but pain is usually not severe. The entire arm and hand are sometimes developmentally smaller on the affected side. Vascular compression of the subclavian artery is rarely apparent clinically, and the Adson test (decrease in radial pulse with head turning to the affected side and deep inhalation) is often false positive. The congenital bony changes may be noted on X-ray, but the presence of a cervical rib does not prove the condition, and the band is usually radiolucent. Magnetic resonance imaging (MRI) may document the band in some patients or demonstrate distortion of the brachial plexus. Surgical resection or sectioning of the offending band, not the first thoracic rib, is curative.

The *droopy shoulder syndrome* occurs in young women who have low-hanging shoulders and long necks, resulting in chronic stretch of the brachial plexus. Horizontal or down-sloping clavicles on inspection, and visualization of upper thoracic vertebrae on lateral cervical spine films, support the diagnosis. Tapping over the plexus causes pain and paresthesias. Symptoms are worsened by pulling the arms down, relieved by pushing them up. The neurological examination and nerve conduction tests are normal. Treatment consists of exercises to strengthen the shoulder muscles. Surgical resection of the first thoracic rib or the anterior or middle scalene muscles is not indicated in these patients or other patients with arm pain who lack any objective neurological deficit, sometimes labeled "disputed thoracic outlet syndrome."

Clinical features: Lumbosacral plexus

Anatomic correlation

The lumbosacral plexus is anatomically divided into the lumbar plexus (L1–L4) and the sacral plexus, which is formed by the lumbosacral trunk (L4–L5) and S1–S3 roots. Anterior divisions of the lumbar plexus give rise to the obturator nerve and posterior

divisions to the femoral nerve (Figure 103.2). The sciatic nerve is the main nerve of the sacral plexus, with the tibial nerve portion derived from the anterior divisions and the common peroneal nerve from the posterior divisions.

Disorders

Traumatic injuries of the lumbosacral plexus are rare and usually associated with bony fractures of the pelvic ring or dislocations of the sacroiliac joint. A severe stretching force causes intradural nerve root avulsion and tearing of the arachnoid nerve root covering, and is detected on MRI or myelography as a pseudomeningocele or diverticulum-like outpouching.

Malignancy is the most common cause of lumbosacral plexopathy, usually by direct extension from the colorectum or cervix uteri, or from lymphomas and retroperitoneal sarcomas. The sacral plexus is more commonly affected than the lumbar plexus. Metastasis causes 25% of malignant plexopathies and often is bilateral. Pain is usually the first symptom in malignant plexopathies. It is dull, aching, and constant, with worsening in supine position. There is often superimposed sharp radicular pain in the lower back, hip, and thigh with lumbar plexopathy, and posterolateral thigh, calf, and foot in sacral lesions. Paresthesias and weakness follow a few weeks later. During examination, Valsalva maneuver or straight-leg raising may worsen the symptoms. Leg edema may be present, or involvement of sympathetic plexus fibers may cause a "hot–dry foot."

Radiation injury to the lumbosacral plexus is infrequent. It results from treatment of testicular cancer, cervix carcinoma, or lymphomas, with a latency of a few months to decades. As in the upper extremities, it presents initially without much pain, and weakness and paresthesias predominate, sometimes bilateral but asymmetric. Bowel and bladder dysfunction is uncommon.

Diabetic lumbosacral radiculoplexopathy typically occurs in elderly patients with longstanding type 2 diabetes, often superimposed on diabetic polyneuropathy. Typically, rather sudden onset of uni-

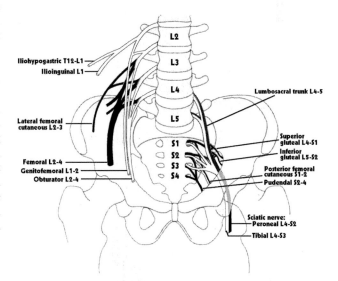

Figure 103.2 The lumbosacral plexus. Schematic representation of the lumbar plexus (on the viewer's left side) and the sacral plexus (right side). The black portions signify the nerves derived from the posterior divisions of the ventral primary rami, and the white portions are derived from either the ventral primary rami or their anterior branches. Source: Adapted from Wilbourn 2007. Reproduced with permission of Elsevier.

lateral, sometimes asymmetric bilateral aching pain in thigh, hip, or buttock regions is followed days or weeks later by weakness and wasting of anterior and lateral thigh muscles. The femoral and obturator nerves seem to be affected predominantly. Minor sensory loss over the anterior thigh is often present. The knee jerk is usually absent on the affected side. The syndrome probably is caused by ischemic nerve injury secondary to microvasculitis. A similar syndrome occurs rarely in non-diabetic patients also. Recovery takes up to 24 months and in many cases mild to moderate weakness persists.

Postoperative lumbosacral plexopathy is a rare but serious complication after total hip arthroplasty, estimated to occur in about 1.5% of surgeries, including revisions. About half of patients recover fully within 2 years, and delayed improvement is possible. Postsurgical neuropathy may be caused by nerve injury related to surgical trauma, patient positioning, hematoma formation, or as anesthesia complication. It was recently recognized that some patients with neurological deficits after surgery have a postsurgical inflammatory neuropathy. The condition is an axonal inflammatory neuropathy that may affect a single nerve (often the sciatic nerve), multiple nerves (mononeuritis multiplex), or the brachial or lumbosacral plexus. It may be differentiated from a nerve injury due to surgical trauma by delayed onset after surgery (days, sometimes weeks) in a progressive course. Electrophysiology documents axonal damage, and nerve biopsy shows ischemic injury and perivascular inflammation. In several patients, treatment with high-dose steroids resulted in neurological improvement.

Lumbosacral plexopathy is occasionally caused by retroperitoneal hemorrhage into the iliacus muscle affecting femoral nerve fibers predominantly, or into the psoas muscle where a large amount of blood may be lost and cause a compartment syndrome. This is a rare but potentially devastating complication of anticoagulant therapy.

Investigations

The most important studies in plexopathies are imaging and electrophysiology. MRI is more sensitive than computed tomography (CT) in documenting brachial or lumbosacral plexus lesions. Tumors are more likely than radiation injury to show root or plexus enhancement on MRI, and positron emission tomography (PET) scanning is frequently positive. In neuralgic amyotrophy, MRI frequently detects signal abnormalities in the affected muscles of the shoulder girdle, and MR neuroimaging documents a thickened and hyperintense plexus.

Electrophysiological studies are more helpful in the evaluation of brachial than lumbosacral plexopathies. In the legs, routine sensory studies only assess the sacral plexus and become unreliable in the elderly. Most plexopathies are axonal in nature and result in decreased sensory and motor nerve potential amplitudes. When present for several weeks, pathological spontaneous activity may be noted on electromyography (EMG). In neuralgic amyotrophy, sensory abnormalities are often limited on nerve testing, due to patchy and predominantly proximal motor nerve involvement. In the arms, stimulation at the supraclavicular Erb point may document conduction slowing or conduction block located distal to the mid-trunk level. In a trauma patient with complete sensory loss of the arm, the presence of sensory nerve action potentials indicates a supraganglionic lesion, thus root avulsion rather than plexopathy. Myokymic EMG discharges are typical of radiation plexopathy.

Treatment

Treatment is directed at the underlying pathology if possible. In neuralgic amyotrophy, high-dose steroids may lessen the time to improvement of pain, but are otherwise of uncertain value. Similarly, in lumbosacral diabetic polyradiculoplexopathy, high-dose intravenous methylprednisolone is sometimes recommended based on improvement in pain and sensory symptoms (but not motor impairment) in one controlled trial. This is rather controversial, however, due to the likelihood of worsening glycemic control. There is little evidence to suggest benefit from intravenous immunoglobin (IVIg) in neuralgic amyotrophy or diabetic lumbosacral plexopathy. In patients with postsurgical inflammatory neuropathy, high-dose steroids are reported as beneficial.

In most instances, treatment of plexopathies is symptomatic, including management of neuropathic pain. Intractable pain in patients suffering from nerve root avulsion is an indication for dorsal root entry zone lesioning.

Mononeuropathies (entrapment neuropathies)

Entrapment neuropathy indicates dysfunction of a peripheral nerve that is compressed, stretched, or angulated by surrounding anatomic structures (Figure 103.3). Only the most common entrapment syndromes are listed. In most instances, initial complaints are intermittent or gradually progressive numbness or paresthesias. The pathophysiology is segmental demyelination that results in slowing of nerve conduction velocity across the affected nerve segment, and if severe in conduction block. Axonal degeneration is usually a secondary event, indicating more severe nerve damage.

Entrapment neuropathies may be triggered by underlying systemic disease or hormonal changes, such as diabetes, hypothyroidism, acromegaly, pregnancy, rheumatological diseases resulting in inflammatory or degenerative arthritis (wrist), previous trauma (elbow), and others.

Epidemiology

Focal peripheral neuropathies due to entrapment occur frequently. The most common mononeuropathy is the median neuropathy at the wrist due to carpal tunnel syndrome, with an estimated clinical prevalence between 1% and 5% of the population, and about twice as common in women than in men. The second most common entrapment neuropathies are ulnar neuropathy at the elbow (sulcus ulnaris) and peroneal neuropathy at the fibular head.

Clinical features

Early symptoms of a focal *median neuropathy* at the wrist (carpal tunnel syndrome) are pain and paresthesias in median nerve distribution (first three digits, lateral half of the fourth digit, and thenar eminence). Painful paresthesias in the hand and arm, sometimes including the upper arm and shoulder region, occur at night and are relieved by shaking the hand or arm. In advanced carpal tunnel syndrome, weakness and atrophy of thenar muscles develop. Examination reveals paralysis of the abductor pollicis brevis and opponens pollicis muscles. Sensory deficit is in the median territory of the hand, but not proximal to the wrist. Tinel sign is positive, when percussion of the median nerve at the wrist causes paresthesias in the nerve's distribution. Phalen maneuver is positive, when flexion of the wrist for 30–60 seconds reproduces or exacerbates the

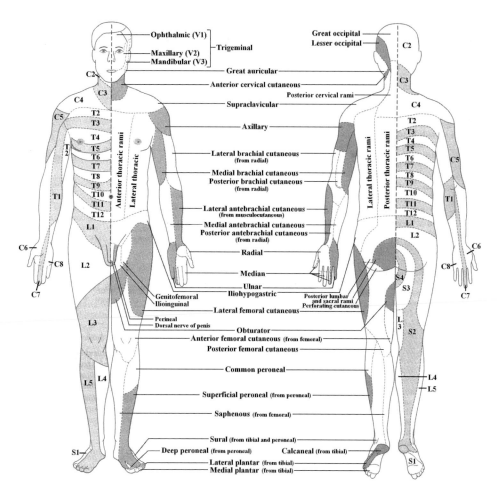

Figure 103.3 Cutaneous innervation. Schematic representation of the dermatomal (radicular) and peripheral nerve innervation from the anterior (left figure) and posterior aspect. Dermatomes are shown on the right side of the body (outer hemibodies), and the peripheral nerve distribution on the left side of the body (inner hemibodies). Source: Adapted from Aminoff 2005 and Haymaker 1945.

symptoms. The differential diagnosis includes proximal median nerve lesions, brachial plexopathy, and C6–C7 radiculopathy.

Ulnar neuropathy at the elbow is the second most common entrapment following carpal tunnel syndrome. Numbness and paresthesias affect digit 5, the medial half of digit 4, and the ulnar aspect of the hand, but not the forearm to any significant extent. The elbow region may be painful and sensitive to touch. Repeated elbow flexion or pressure on the ulnar nerve (such as when leaning on the elbow) exacerbates the symptoms. Weakness, if present, affects intrinsic hand muscles including hypothenar muscles, interossei, and lumbricals. Ulnar innervated forearm muscles (M. flexor carpi ulnaris and M. flexor digitorum profundus) are typically less affected, but may be atrophic in advanced disease. Claw hand (flexion of digits 4 and 5) occurs in severe ulnar neuropathy. Ulnar neuropathy at the elbow occurs at two different entrapment sites that are clinically similar but may be separated by electrophysiology. Compression at the sulcus ulnaris (retroepicondylar groove) is more common than entrapment of the ulnar nerve within the cubital tunnel (humero-ulnar arcade).

In lesions affecting the ulnar nerve at the wrist or palm of the hand, sensory or motor changes in the hand may occur in isolation or in combination, depending on the specific lesion site within the Loge de Guyon. Such lesions may be differentiated from ulnar

neuropathy at the elbow by intact sensation over the dorsal hand on clinical examination and by electrophysiological testing (the dorsal ulnar cutaneous branch is not affected). Sensory deficits in the forearm imply a more proximal lesion, such as lower trunk or medial cord plexopathy and C8–T1 radiculopathy.

The *radial nerve* may be compressed in the axilla by crutches. Injury in the upper arm is caused by prolonged pressure, as seen in alcoholics who have fallen asleep with an arm resting on a hard surface, or by humerus fractures. Weakness of the finger and hand extensors with sparing of the triceps muscle is characteristic, with often only minor associated sensory symptoms affecting the area of the hand between thumb and index finger.

Peroneal neuropathy is the most common entrapment of the lower extremities, usually at the fibular head, secondary to trauma or pressure (sitting with one leg resting over the opposite knee). Weakness affects toe and foot dorsiflexion (anterior tibial muscle) and foot eversion (peroneal muscles), with impaired sensation over the dorsum of the foot and distal leg.

The tarsal tunnel syndrome is a *tibial nerve* entrapment at the ankle inferior and posterior to the medial malleolus. Burning pain over the bottom of the foot, especially at night, is typical and weakness of intrinsic foot muscles may be noted.

In meralgia paresthetica, the *lateral femoral cutaneous nerve* is compressed in the lateral groin (inguinal ligament), resulting in burning pain, paresthesias, and numbness in the anterolateral thigh region. There is no motor involvement. Predisposing factors are pregnancy and sudden weight gain or weight loss.

Investigations

Nerve conduction studies are usually diagnostic by documenting focal slowing at the entrapment site. Denervation on EMG documents axonal degeneration and therefore severe entrapment. Imaging modalities including ultrasound and MRI are increasingly used to diagnose nerve compression syndromes.

Treatment

Avoidance of triggering factors (excessive repetitive wrist flexion and extension or typewriting in carpal tunnel syndrome, leaning on elbows and repetitive elbow flexion in ulnar neuropathy, crossing of legs in peroneal neuropathy) is sometimes sufficient to allow recovery of nerve function. Additional measures include nocturnal wrist splints in carpal tunnel syndrome and elbow pads in ulnar neuropathy.

Pharmacological treatment with a short course of anti-inflammatory agents is often helpful in carpal tunnel syndrome. Steroid injections into the wrist have often only temporary benefit and may be harmful. If deficits are severe or refractory despite conservative treatment, surgical release of the carpal tunnel ligament or ulnar nerve transposition may be indicated.

Further reading

Aminoff MJ, Greenberg DA, Simon RP. *Clinical Neurology*, 6th ed. New York: Lange/McGraw-Hill; 2005.

Ferrante MA. Brachial plexopathies. *Continuum* 2014;20:1323–1342.

Haymaker W, Woodhall B. *Peripheral Nerve Injuries*. Philadelphia, PA: Saunders; 1945.

Jillapalli D, Shefner JM. Electrodiagnosis in common mononeuropathies and plexopathies. *Semin Neurol* 2005;25:196–203.

Moghekar AR, Moghekar AR, Karli N, Chaudry V. Brachial plexopathies: Etiology, frequency, and electrodiagnostic localization. *J Clin Neuromusc Dis* 2007;9:243–247.

Rattananan W, Thaisetthawatkul P, Dyck PJ. Postsurgical inflammatory neuropathy: A report of five cases. *J Neurol Sci* 2014;337:137–140.

Van Alfen N, van Engelen BGM. The clinical spectrum of neuralgic amyotrophy in 246 cases. *Brain* 2006;129:438–450.

Wilbourn AJ. Plexopathies. *Neurol Clin* 2007;25:139–171.

104   Amyotrophic lateral sclerosis

Björn Oskarsson[1], Nanette C. Joyce[2], and Steven P. Ringel[3]

[1] Department of Neurology, University of California, Davis, Sacramento, CA, USA

[2] Department of Physical Medicine and Rehabilitation, University of California, Davis, Sacramento, CA, USA

[3] Department of Neurology, University of Colorado School of Medicine, Aurora, CO, USA

Amyotrophic lateral sclerosis (ALS) is a fatal neurodegenerative disease affecting upper and lower motor neurons. Several other names for ALS are used in different regions of the world, including *maladie de Charcot*, after the great French neurologist Jean Martin Charcot who described the disease in 1874, and in the United States *Lou Gehrig's disease*, after a famous baseball player who succumbed to the disease in 1941. In the United Kingdom and commonwealth countries, the more generic term *motor neuron disease* (MND) is often used and refers to the group of neurodegenerative disorders with selective motor neuron involvement, which includes ALS. Three of these motor neuron disorders have more restricted involvement but may progress to ALS, and are sometimes considered variants of ALS:

- Progressive muscular atrophy (PMA) – a pure lower motor neuron condition (see Chapter 105).
- Primary lateral sclerosis (PLS) – a pure upper motor neuron condition (see Chapter 106).
- Progressive bulbar palsy – which is restricted to the brainstem.

Other less common diseases included in the group of MND are:

- ALS-parkinsonism-dementia complex – a disease seen in the Kii peninsula of Japan and previously in Guam.
- Monomelic amyotrophy – a disease seen mostly in young men.
- Familial Madras motor neuron disease – found in south India.
- Spinal muscular atrophy (SMA) – an autosomal recessive condition affecting lower motor neurons (see Chapter 108).
- Bulbospinal muscular atrophy or Kennedy's disease – an X-linked recessive lower motor neuron disorder (see Chapter 105).
- Hereditary spastic paraparesis – a multigenetic spectrum of upper motor neuron disorders affecting the legs predominantly.

Although ALS primarily involves upper and lower motor neurons, it is a multisystem disorder that to a varying degree involves cognition, behavior, affect, and autonomic function. There is a clinical and pathological overlap between ALS and the most common subgroup of frontotemporal dementia: frontotemporal lobar degeneration with motor neuron disease–type inclusions.

Epidemiology

The incidence of ALS varies between 0.3 and 3.6 per 100,000 person-years. The prevalence is only a few times higher, due to the short life expectancy of those affected by ALS. The disease is gradually progressive, with median time to death of about 3 years, and only 4% of patients surviving longer than 10 years.

Reliable demographic data is lacking for many parts of the world, but in several studies there is a suggestion that Caucasians have a higher incidence than Africans, Asians, and Amerindians. A large part of the variation in crude incidence rates can be explained by variations in age between populations: the highest incidence of the disease is seen in people in their mid-70s, so that prevalence is higher in countries with older populations. Men are 1.5 times more likely than women to develop the disease, and there is a suggestion that male athletes, farmers, and soldiers may have a higher risk of developing ALS.

ALS can be either familial (inherited) or sporadic. Autosomal dominant familial ALS accounts for 10% of all ALS cases. About 40% of familial ALS, and also 7% of apparently sporadic ALS, is explained by a hexa nucleotide repeat in *C9ORF72*. *C9ORF72* mutations are also common in familial frontotemporal dementia (FTD), and these two phenotypes, ALS and FTD, frequently manifest in different individuals of an affected family. Approximately 20% of familial ALS cases are due to mutations in the copper/zinc super oxide dismutase 1 (*SOD1*) gene, albeit with geographic variation. SOD1 familial ALS (ALS1) is clinically identical to sporadic ALS, but the proportion of LMN dominant cases is greater. Many other genes have been shown to cause ALS, but with much lower frequency.

Pathophysiology

The hallmark finding in ALS is degeneration of both upper and lower motor neurons. Extra-ocular motor neurons and the motor neurons of urethral and rectal sphincters in the nucleus of Onufrowicz appear largely spared, but all other motor neurons can be affected.

The cause of sporadic ALS remains unknown, and much of the knowledge we have regarding the pathophysiology of motor neuron degeneration is derived from transgenic animal models with incorporated mutated *SOD1* genes. Motor neuron toxicity in these models appears to be caused by a toxic gain, rather than loss, of *SOD1* function. As in many other neurodegenerative diseases, abnormal accumulations/aggregates of proteins are found and are

International Neurology, Second edition. Edited by Robert P. Lisak, Daniel D. Truong, William M. Carroll and Roongroj Bhidayasiri
© 2016 John Wiley & Sons, Ltd. Published 2016 by John Wiley & Sons, Ltd.

predominantly composed of TAR DNA-binding protein (TDP) 43, but also may include neurofilament, peripherin, and ubiquitin. In SOD1 models, there is also accumulation of SOD1 protein. It is not clear that any of these accumulations are directly toxic, but protein aggregation and misfolding may play an important role in the pathogenesis of ALS.

There are several proposed mechanisms for how aggregates can have a detrimental effect on cells, including inhibition of proteasome activity, loss of protein function through co-aggregation, depletion of chaperone proteins, and dysfunction of mitochondria and other organelles. Structural abnormalities have been observed in mitochondria in both sporadic and familial ALS as well as several SOD1 mouse models. These structural changes are thought to interfere with mitochondria's vital cellular function of energy production, and alter their participation in programmed cell death. Additional mechanisms implicated in the pathophysiology of ALS include evidence of impaired axonal transport, and abnormalities in the inflammatory response with increased inflammatory markers. However, it is not clear whether inflammation is part of the pathogenesis or simply a response to the degenerating neurons. There is also evidence suggesting that the adaptive immune system plays an important role in resolving inflammation and mediating neuroprotection and neuronal repair.

ALS pathology is not limited to motor neurons; microglia, oligodendrocytes, and macrophages also play a role in the development of disease. Astrocytes are vital support cells for motor neurons and play an important role in protecting motor neurons from excitotoxicity. In both sporadic ALS and SOD1 mediated ALS there is reduced ability of astrocytes to remove glutamate, the major inducer of excitotoxicity.

Clinical features

Typically the disease begins with focal or asymmetric weakness in a region along the neuraxis. About one-third of patients are first affected in each of the following: the bulbar, cervical, or lumbosacral regions. A small percentage of patients experience their first symptom in the form of respiratory distress or truncal weakness. Progression of weakness is usually relentless. Although periods of clinical stability may occur, improvement of symptoms is rare. The spread of symptoms is a hallmark of the disease and is normally contiguous, extending initially to the other side of the same spinal segment before progressing to the next region. Upper or lower motor neuron signs and symptoms can be dominant in any region. Upper motor neuron signs and symptoms include spasticity, weakness, spastic dysarthria, dysphagia, laryngospasm, increased tone, hyperreflexia, pathological reflexes, and clonus. Lower motor neuron signs and symptoms are weakness, cramps, fasciculations, atrophy, flaccid dysarthria, and dysphagia.

In addition to corticospinal motor neurons, other cerebral frontal lobe neurons are commonly affected. About half of patients may exhibit inappropriate emotional expression disorder (IEED), also called pseudobulbar affect. This is excessive or completely unprovoked crying, or laughter, lasting only for a few seconds or at most minutes. IEED is often underrecognized and sometimes confused with depression. Cognitive impairment occurs in approximately 30% of ALS patients and a small proportion of patients (5–10%) have frontotemporal dementia, mostly the behavioral variant. In addition, cognitive frontal lobe functions are frequently impaired, especially verbal fluency and executive function. Behav-

ioral changes such as apathy, disinhibition, and irritability are also common.

Respiratory weakness is the most common cause of death, unless mechanical ventilation is implemented. Symptoms of respiratory weakness and hypercapnia are shortness of breath with mild exertion, orthopnea, morning headache, afternoon sleepiness, nightmares, hallucinations, and confusion. Non-invasive ventilation is generally well tolerated, and prolongs the time before invasive ventilation must be instated to sustain life.

Poor nutritional status and weight loss contribute to shorter survival. Dysphagia, especially for thin liquids or mixed consistencies, often limits food intake. Normal individuals produce between 1 and 1.5 liters of saliva per 24 hours. If swallowing is impaired, sialorrhea or drooling results from the inability to swallow saliva efficiently. Excessive yawning can also be seen.

Investigations

Since there is no reliable diagnostic test, ALS remains a clinical diagnosis. The clinical criteria used to establish the diagnosis of ALS were first established at a meeting at the Spanish El Escorial palace/monastery. The current modified El Escorial Awaji clinical criteria separate the body into four segments – bulbar, cervical, truncal, and lumbosacral – and quantify the certainty of diagnosis (see Table 104.1).

Diseases that mimic ALS by causing upper and lower motor neuron symptoms alone or in combination include cervical and lumbar myeloradiculopathies, myasthenia gravis (in particular with muscle specific kinase [MuSK] antibodies), multifocal motor neuropathy (MMN), inclusion body myositis, lead and dapsone neuropathies, and spinal tuberculosis. Diseases with more acute onset that can mimic PMA include poliomyelitis (from West Nile virus, polio virus, or other enterovirus), acute axonal motor neuropathy, and porphyria.

Depending on the particular clinical features in individual patients, diagnostic studies are used to exclude mimickers. Electromyography (EMG) is normally indicated and can show acute and chronic denervation changes from the death of lower motor neurons and decreased activation from upper motor neuron dysfunction. The EMG can also identify other diseases that can mimic ALS, for example conduction block in MMN or a neuromuscular junction defect in myasthenia.

Imaging the brain and spinal regions that are clinically affected is frequently helpful. With modern magnetic resonance imaging (MRI) techniques subtle frontal atrophy or changes in the corticospinal tracts can sometimes be detected, but as a rule imaging mainly serves to exclude other diseases mimicking ALS.

Table 104.1 Awaji diagnostic criteria.

Category of amyotrophic lateral sclerosis (ALS)	Number of body segments involved		
	Upper motor neuron (UMN) findings (by exam)		Lower motor neuron (LMN) findings (by exam or electromyography)
Clinically definite ALS	3	+	3
Clinically probable ALS	2 one rostral to LMN	+	2
Clinically possible ALS	1	+	1
	2	+	0

Analysis of the *C9ORF72* gene should be considered in familial cases and may be considered in sporadic cases to help establish an earlier diagnosis. Additional genetic testing can include *SOD1* gene analysis in familial cases, if *C9ORF72* testing is normal or in cases where lower motor neuron involvement is predominant. Testing of asymptomatic family members should be undertaken with great caution and only if resources are available to address the psychosocial consequences of a positive test.

No other laboratory studies identify ALS, but they can be of use to help exclude other conditions. Creatine phosphokinase is often increased in ALS, but cannot alone be used to differentiate ALS from a myopathy. Antibodies against MuSK and acetylcholine receptors may be useful in patients with bulbar symptoms, to help identify myasthenia gravis. In pure lower motor neuron disease, immunoglobin M (IgM) antibodies directed against GM1 ganglioside can support a diagnosis of an immune mediated neuropathy. Cerebrospinal fluid analysis is usually normal in ALS and abnormalities can suggest infection, malignancy, or nerve root inflammation. Calcium and phosphate can be tested to exclude hyperparathyroidism and thyroid-stimulating hormone (TSH) to exclude hyperthyroidism.

Treatment

After establishing the diagnosis, the results should be shared with the patient in an unhurried and calm environment without interruptions, and with time for questions. It is important to have the patient's family members or friends at this visit, as they can provide psychosocial support between clinic visits and may have many questions of their own. Experienced clinicians try to be as positive as the situation allows, focusing on the many things that can be done to prolong survival and sustain quality of life. Handing out written material, web links, and contact information to local support organizations is often appreciated. Multidisciplinary team care that includes physicians and therapists specialized in ALS has been shown to improve survival and quality of care in the disease. If a local ALS clinic is available, a referral is appropriate.

Treatment remains largely supportive for this progressive, fatal condition. Care is generally palliative, with the goal of maximizing life quality for patients and their families, at some times in favor of extending life. Riluzole, a glutamate antagonist, is the only effective disease-modifying medication. The effect of riluzole is modest, prolonging life in ALS by 2–3 months, without having an effect on quality of life, muscle strength, or respiratory function. Antioxidant vitamins such as vitamins C and E are often recommended, but no good-quality evidence supports their use.

Muscle-related complaints are common in ALS. Cramps can be effectively treated with quinine, which remains in use in many parts of the world. It is worth noting that the US Food and Drug Administration has issued warnings against quinine use due to reports of life-threatening hematological adverse drug-related events. Other possible remedies include hydration, magnesium, potassium, mexiletine, and phenytoin. Gabapentin can also be effective, but it may speed the deterioration of respiratory weakness in ALS. Fasciculations can be bothersome, especially early in the disease, and are typically treatment resistant. Spasticity that is painful or interferes with function can be reduced by muscle relaxants, including baclofen, cyclobenzaprine, and tizanidine. A spastic bladder can be relieved with tolterodine or other anticholinergic agents.

Physical and occupational therapy is beneficial for advice and training on assistive equipment used to improve function and maintain independence and mobility, as well as developing the home range of motion exercises to prevent joint contractures (e.g., frozen shoulders) and reduce spasticity. A multitude of different devices such as ankle foot orthoses, walkers, wheelchairs, lifts, and so on improve the daily function of patients. Physical exercise including mild to moderate-intensity resistance and aerobic exercise is likely beneficial, at least for less disabled patients, and can be addressed during therapy sessions.

Speech therapists can provide recommendations regarding swallow function and safe swallowing techniques, appropriate diet consistency to avoid aspiration, and augmentative communication devices. The weakness from progressive bulbar disease in ALS is not typically amenable to traditional speech therapy exercises, which may worsen speech by causing fatigue. It is very important to assist patients in maintaining communication. If dysarthria becomes a significant problem, writing boards and electronic assistive communication devices can increase quality of life.

Adequate nutrition improves quality of life and prolongs survival in ALS. A body mass index (BMI) of less than 18.5 kg/m^2 has been associated with shorter survival while a higher BMI, around 30 kg/m^2, is associated with improved survival. Many patients experience an increased calorie need and energy-rich foods are often needed to maintain a stable weight. When significant dysphagia is present, eating may lead to aspiration and subsequent pneumonia. Aspiration is normally noticed by the patient as choking; silent, unnoticed aspiration is rare. The severity of dysphagia can be screened by watching the patient drink a glass of water; a barium swallow study offers more details. Inability to feed oneself due to hand and arm weakness also frequently leads to reduced food intake.

Feeding tubes should be considered when a patient has lost 10% of their baseline weight and can be placed by several techniques. The least invasive method is to insert a nasogastric tube manually to provide nourishment temporarily. If one anticipates the need for prolonged tube feeding, then a gastrostomy is a better option. Gastrostomy tubes can be positioned using gastroscopy, fluoroscopic guidance, or open surgery. The risk of anesthesia is high in ALS, especially when the forced vital capacity is less than 50% of that predicted. Minimizing sedation, maximizing local anesthesia, and applying non-invasive ventilation are important interventions for improved safety in more debilitated patients needing gastrostomy tubes; radiographically guided insertion favors these strategies.

Sialorrhea can be treated with anticholinergic medications, including amitriptyline or glycopyrrolate. If swallowing is severely impaired and no feeding tube is in place, then transdermal scopolamine or oral atropine drops can be used. If anticholinergic therapy fails, there are other options. Botulinum toxin A or B injections into the salivary glands reduce salivary production and are effective for several months. Radiation or surgical intervention on the salivary glands or ducts offers a more permanent solution. While these treatments lead to reduced production of secretions, the secretions that are produced often become more viscous. If the secretions are thick, hydration and guaifenesin can make saliva more liquid. Adrenergic beta-blocker drugs also reduce thick secretions. Suction devices and bibs can be helpful for oral secretions. A mechanical insufflator/exsufflator can facilitate coughing to expel secretions lodged deeper in airways and should be prescribed when peak cough flow is reduced to 270 L/min.

In patients with ALS and without severe bulbar involvement, non-invasive positive pressure ventilation (NIPPV) has been shown to improve survival with maintenance of, and improvement in, quality of life. NIPPV should be initiated when signs of nocturnal hypercapnia occur in the form of morning headache and confusion, when the forced vital capacity (FVC) falls to 50% of predicted, or when the maximal inspiratory pressure is less than -60 cmH$_2$O. The respiratory weakness may not be obvious and monitoring of the pulmonary functions should be performed on a scheduled basis, based on the rate of disease progression. The average rate of decline in FVC is 2–3% per month. Supplemental oxygen is in general not indicated, as it can lead to depression of respiratory drive, exacerbate alveolar hypoventilation, and increase carbon dioxide retention along with the risk of respiratory arrest. Supplemental oxygen benzodiazepines and morphinomimetics may be prescribed in the terminal stage of disease as a comfort measure.

Invasive long-term mechanical ventilation can extend life by several years, but does not prevent further physical and cognitive decline. The rate of use varies greatly between countries dependent on physician preference, culture, and healthcare insurance. Japan probably has the highest proportion of ALS patients choosing this intervention, at approximately 36%.

Pain due to physical immobility or other causes is often a feature of ALS, especially late in the disease. Identifying the cause of pain and managing it appropriately are important to sustain quality of life. Caregiver-assisted range of motion exercise, when the patient is no longer able to move independently, can prevent and reduce pain.

Pseudobulbar affect (PBA) or inappropriate emotional expression disorder (IEED) can be treated when it causes social difficulties for the patient. A combination of dextromethorphan and quinidine is effective. Treatment with antidepressants (mostly tricyclic antidepressants, but also selective serotonin reuptake inhibitors) is effective too.

Appropriate recognition and aggressive treatment of depression are important and should not be overlooked. Patients can benefit from counseling as well as from trials of antidepressants.

Fatigue is a common ALS symptom. Reducing sedating medication, maintaining good nutrition, and sleep are the basic tenets of management. Medications such as activating serotonin uptake inhibitors are generally well tolerated, but in select cases stimulants including modafinil and amphetamines are beneficial and appropriate.

Most patients supplement the care they receive from their ALS physician with alternative treatments. It is important to encourage patients to share information about the alternative treatments that they have chosen, and to provide advice against any treatment that is clearly harmful, while not robbing the patient of hope. Many patients find hope and comfort in participating in a clinical trial to increase our understanding of this disease, and should be provided with trial information and given the option to participate when possible.

A minority of patients do wish to choose to die when their symptoms of ALS become overwhelming, but are not yet severe enough to be considered terminal; this is only in part explained by depression. The ability of these patients to act on this choice depends on local legal and cultural norms. It is unusual for ALS patients to commit suicide other than by refusing food and water. In the Netherlands, where euthanasia is legal, a large portion of patients consider its use, and the portion who ultimately use this option has been reported to be as high as 20%. Strictly regulated euthanasia is now also legal in Belgium and Luxemburg. In Switzerland and the US states of Oregon, Montana, Vermont, and Washington, physician-assisted suicide is an option in the terminal phase of the disease.

The timing of end-of-life care discussions requires that the physician be familiar with the patient and family, so there is no standard formula as to when such discussions should be initiated. Different patients have different needs and concerns regarding their approaching death. Fear of pain, choking, and air hunger should be addressed with reassurance of effective treatment. The vast majority of ALS patients have a peaceful and dignified death; this fact should be emphasized.

Further reading

Bensimon G, Lacomblez L, Meininger V. A controlled trial of riluzole in amyotrophic lateral sclerosis. ALS/Riluzole Study Group. *N Engl J Med* 1994;330(9):585–591. doi: 10.1056/NEJM199403033300901

Chio A, Logroscino G, Traynor BJ, et al. Global epidemiology of amyotrophic lateral sclerosis: A systematic review of the published literature. *Neuroepidemiology* 2013;41(2):118–130. doi: 10.1159/000351153

Cronin S, Hardiman O, Traynor BJ Ethnic variation in the incidence of ALS: A systematic review. *Neurology* 2007;68(13):1002–1007. doi: 10.1212/01.wnl.0000258551.96893.6f

de Carvalho M, Dengler R, Eisen A, et al. Electrodiagnostic criteria for diagnosis of ALS. *Clin Neurophysiol* 2008;119(3):497–503. doi: 10.1016/j.clinph.2007.09.143

Forshew DA, Bromberg MB. A survey of clinicians' practice in the symptomatic treatment of ALS. *Amyotroph Lateral Scler Other Motor Neuron Disord* 2003;4(4):258–263.

Miller RG, Jackson CE, Kasarskis EJ, et al.; Quality Standards Subcommittee of the American Academy of Neurology. Practice parameter update: The care of the patient with amyotrophic lateral sclerosis: Multidisciplinary care, symptom management, and cognitive/behavioral impairment (an evidence-based review): Report of the Quality Standards Subcommittee of the American Academy of Neurology. *Neurology* 2009;73(15):1227–1233. doi: 10.1212/WNL.0b013e3181bc01a4

Miller RG, Rosenberg JA, Gelinas DF, et al. Practice parameter: The care of the patient with amyotrophic lateral sclerosis (an evidence-based review): Report of the Quality Standards Subcommittee of the American Academy of Neurology: ALS Practice Parameters Task Force. *Neurology* 1999;52(7):1311–1323.

Morrison RS, Meier DE. Clinical practice: Palliative care. *N Engl J Med* 2004;350(25):2582–2590. doi: 10.1056/NEJMcp035232

Newrick PG, Langton-Hewer R. Pain in motor neuron disease. *J Neurol Neurosurg Psychiatry* 1985;48(8):838–840.

Ravits J, Appel S, Baloh RH, et al. Deciphering amyotrophic lateral sclerosis: What phenotype, neuropathology and genetics are telling us about pathogenesis. *Amyotroph Lateral Scler Frontotemporal Degener* 2013;14(Suppl 1):5–18. doi: 10.3109/21678421.2013.778548

Ravits J, Laurie P, Fan Y, Moore DH. Implications of ALS focality: Rostral-caudal distribution of lower motor neuron loss postmortem. *Neurology* 2007;68(19):1576–1582. doi: 10.1212/01.wnl.0000261045.57095.56

Renton AE, Chio A, Traynor BJ. State of play in amyotrophic lateral sclerosis genetics. *Nat Neurosci* 2014;17(1):17–23. doi: 10.1038/nn.3584

Ringholz GM, Appel SH, Bradshaw M, et al. Prevalence and patterns of cognitive impairment in sporadic ALS. *Neurology* 2005;65(4):586–590. doi: 10.1212/01.wnl.0000172911.39167.b6

Veldink JH, Wokke JH, van der Wal G, Vianney de Jong JM, van den Berg LH. Euthanasia and physician-assisted suicide among patients with amyotrophic lateral sclerosis in the Netherlands. *N Engl J Med* 2002;346(21):1638–1644. doi: 10.1056/NEJMsa012739

105 Progressive muscular atrophy

James Ha[1], Steven P. Ringel[2], Björn Oskarsson[1]

[1] Department of Neurology, University of California, Davis, Sacramento, CA, USA

[2] Department of Neurology, University of Colorado School of Medicine, Aurora, CO, USA

Progressive muscular atrophy (PMA) is a progressive disorder affecting only lower motor neurons (LMNs), in contrast to both amyotrophic lateral sclerosis (ALS), in which both upper and lower motor neurons are affected, and primary lateral sclerosis (PLS), in which only upper motor neurons (UMNs) are affected. Originally described in the mid-1800s by Aran and Duchenne, PMA has been the source of much debate, particularly regarding its classification as a variant of ALS as opposed to a distinct clinical entity. PMA has also been known as progressive spinal muscular atrophy (PSMA), although this term has largely fallen out of favor due to potential confusion with spinal muscular atrophy (SMA), a distinct group of childhood hereditary diseases. The differential diagnosis of pure lower motor neuron syndromes is broader than for ALS and includes several important conditions that should be ruled out due to significant treatment and prognostic implications.

Epidemiology

Similar to PLS, PMA accounts for approximately 5% of patients with motor neuron disease (MND). PMA has a median age of onset of 57 years, but can occur at any age in adults, typically between 25 and 70 years. There is a greater risk for men to develop PMA. PMA has no identified risk factors or known geographic differences. The incidence of PMA is estimated at 0.2 per 100,000 per year. The disease duration of PMA is somewhat more varied than ALS, but on average it is slightly longer.

Pathophysiology

The pathogenesis of PMA remains unknown, as with other forms of MND. Autopsy of patients diagnosed with PMA who never developed clinical UMN signs have shown corticospinal tract degeneration and damage of cortical motor neurons. Inclusions typical of ALS including Bunina bodies and ubiquitinated inclusions containing TDP-43 are also found. *SOD1* mutations have been found in patients with pure LMN disease and the clinical phenotype of PMA, although the majority of patients with *SOD1* mutations have both UMN and LMN involvement clinically.

Clinical features

Patients have typical LMN features such as flaccid weakness, atrophy, fasciculations, and hyporeflexia or areflexia. Generally, weakness and atrophy initially present asymmetrically in one extremity, with spread to the other over months to years. Thoracic involvement leads to respiratory insufficiency. Cramps occur commonly in both weak and unaffected muscles. The progression of disease varies from slow to rapid and survival ranges from less than one year to decades. Individuals with PMA may later develop UMN findings and are then classified as lower motor neuron–onset ALS; such conversions are more common early in the clinical disease course.

Differential diagnosis

A wide range of conditions enter the differential diagnosis, yet all are distinguishable from PMA. Here we list diseases that often warrant consideration.

Multifocal motor neuropathy

Multifocal motor neuropathy (MMN) is an important autoimmune LMN syndrome sometimes associated with GM1 antibodies, affecting motor but not sensory nerves, which must be considered in the differential diagnosis of PMA because in the majority of cases it responds to immunomodulatory therapy such as intravenous immunoglobin (IVIG). Generally, MMN presents with weakness and atrophy of the wrist extensors, but can involve other upper-extremity and even lower-extremity nerves. Fasciculations can be seen and in contrast to PMA, reflexes are often spared. Nerve conduction studies can help differentiate MMN from PMA by showing conduction block.

Multiple radiculopathies

Multiple radiculopathies can cause weakness, atrophy, and fasciculations akin to PMA and may be considered in the differential diagnosis. When radiculopathies cause pain or sensory loss they are readily distinguishable; only rarely is this not the case.

Inclusion body myositis

Inclusion body myositis (IBM) also causes slowly progressive weakness and muscle atrophy later in life. Electromyography (EMG) often shows motor units that appear neurogenic and a muscle biopsy may be required to differentiate the conditions. Genetic variants causing both IBM and MND exist, and an individual patient can have both conditions. Epidemiological data on IBM are incomplete, but the disease may be more common in people of Northern European descent.

International Neurology, Second edition. Edited by Robert P. Lisak, Daniel D. Truong, William M. Carroll and Roongroj Bhidayasiri
© 2016 John Wiley & Sons, Ltd. Published 2016 by John Wiley & Sons, Ltd.

Brachial amyotrophic diplegia (O'Sullivan-McLeod syndrome or flail arm syndrome)

Brachial amyotrophic diplegias are variants of MND with predominant lower motor neuron involvement of both upper extremities (generally with very slow disease progression). The recognition of these subtypes confers useful prognostic information.

Monomelic amyotrophy (Hirayama syndrome)

Hirayama syndrome generally affects younger men between 15 and 25 years of age and is more common in Asians. It presents with unilateral arm weakness and muscle atrophy, due to anterior cervical spine compression in flexion, presumed due to ligamentum flavum hypertrophy.

Lead toxicity

Lead exposure can cause an asymmetric motor neuropathy affecting arms more than legs in adults. A microcytic anemia, constipation, renal failure, hypertension, seizures, and encephalopathy may also ensue. Lead toxicity is more common in developing countries.

X-linked bulbospinal muscular atrophy (Kennedy's disease)

Kennedy's disease is a triplet repeat expansion in the androgen receptor gene that presents in men generally after 40 years of age, with dysarthria and dysphagia followed by fasciculations and proximal limb weakness. Creatinine kinase levels may be elevated and gynecomastia may also be seen. Nerve conduction studies show evidence of neuropathy.

Poliomyelitis and post-polio syndrome

Most infectious anterior horn cell disease is caused by the polio virus, but other enteroviruses and West Nile virus can cause a similar acute paralytic illness with fever and meningitis. Polio remains endemic in three countries – Afghanistan, Nigeria, and Pakistan – with sporadic outbreaks occurring in other regions. The post-polio syndrome evolves decades after recovery has occurred and manifests in slowly progressive weakness and atrophy due to loss of remaining lower motor neurons.

Brachial plexitis

Brachial plexitis tends to be painful, subacute, and self-limiting, but in the early stage can occasionally be hard to differentiate from PMA.

Shingles

Shingles occurs due to reactivation of dormant varicella zoster virus (VZV) and preferentially damages sensory ganglion cells. However, in some cases anterior horn cells are also involved. This disease tends to be painful, subacute, and self-limiting. VZV seroprevalence in adults varies from 50–95%, being lowest in the tropics.

Adult-onset SMA (SMA type 4)

Adult-onset SMA is recessively inherited and by definition occurs after 30 years of age. It presents with limb weakness and can be identified by sequencing of the survival motor neuron gene. SMA carrier frequency is lower in sub-Saharan African, but is otherwise fairly uniform throughout the world.

Adult-type hexosamidase A deficiency (late-onset Tay–Sachs disease)

Late-onset Tay–Sachs disease is a rare, recessively inherited neurodegenerative disease that can cause a pure lower motor neuron syndrome, but generally also causes central nervous system (CNS) dysfunction. The genetic defect is more common in people of Ashkenazi Jewish extraction, but cases without Jewish heritage have been described.

Madras motor neuron disease

Madras motor neuron disease (MMND) has a unique geographic distribution, predominantly occurring in southern India. The disease often presents in the second decade with hearing loss, which is a distinguishing feature. An LMN phenotype can dominate, but the disease can also involve UMN and sometimes the optic nerve.

Hereditary motor neuropathy

Hereditary motor neuropathy is a group of disorders that generally start in childhood, but can develop in the 30s or 40s, usually with foot drop as the initial symptom.

Treatment

Although there is no curative treatment for PMA, riluzole has been used due to its proven beneficial effect on survival in ALS, a condition with some overlapping features with PMA. In addition, assistive devices such as non-invasive ventilators, feeding tubes, walkers, and wheelchairs can be used in patients with PMA, as in those with ALS. Care through multidisciplinary ALS/MND clinics is recommended when available.

Further reading

Riku Y, Atsuta N, Yoshida M, *et al.* Differential motor neuron involvement in progressive muscular atrophy: A comparative study with amyotrophic lateral sclerosis. *BMJ Open* 2014;4(5):e005213. doi: 1o.1136/bmjopen-20140005213

Rowland L. Progressive muscular atrophy and other lower motor neuron syndromes of adults. *Muscle Nerve* 2010;41:161–165.

Visser J, de Jong V, de Visser M. The history of progressive muscular atrophy: Syndrome or disease? *Neurology* 2008;70:723–727.

106 Primary lateral sclerosis

Nanette C. Joyce[1], Björn Oskarsson[2], Yvonne D. Rollins[3], and Steven P. Ringel[4]

[1] Department of Physical Medicine and Rehabilitation, University of California, Davis, Sacramento, CA, USA

[2] Department of Neurology, University of California, Davis, Sacramento, CA, USA

[3] Regional West Physicians Clinic – Neurology, Scottsbluff, NE, USA

[4] Department of Neurology, University of Colorado School of Medicine, Aurora, CO, USA

Primary lateral sclerosis (PLS) is defined as a sporadic primary upper motor neuron (UMN) disorder of several years' duration, characterized by progressive corticospinal dysfunction with sparing of lower motor neurons (LMN). Originally described by both Charcot and Erb, PLS is a rare neurodegenerative disorder accounting for approximately 4% of patients who fall within the motor neuron disease (MND) spectrum. While controversy exists regarding whether PLS is pathophysiologically distinct from amyotrophic lateral sclerosis (ALS), the separation is clinically meaningful, as PLS heralds longer survival. Recent prospective studies support the concept of a "true" PLS phenotype in which progression to an ALS phenotype, with lower motor neuron dysfunction, does not occur. The absence of LMN clinical findings is an important prognostic indicator confirming longer survival.

Epidemiology

PLS has a younger average age of onset than ALS (mean 46.9–53 years vs. 60 years). By definition, familial cases are excluded. However, pure UMN disease cases exist in familial ALS kindreds. Juvenile-onset pure UMN disease cases have been associated with mutations in the *ALS2* gene encoding the protein alsin, and *ERLIN2*, a component of the endoplasmic reticulum.

A large number of MND patients first experience UMN symptoms, but most also rapidly develop LMN deficits. UMN disease must exist in isolation for several years for a PLS diagnosis to be considered, yet LMN involvement and conversion to ALS have been reported up to 27 years after onset. Survival data are incomplete in PLS, but unless conversion to ALS occurs, survival is not necessarily affected.

Pathophysiology

The etiology of motor neuron degeneration and its phenotypic variability remains unknown. Pathological tissue examination in PLS consistently reports loss of Betz cells in layer 5 of the motor cortex, with atrophy in the corticospinal tracts. Spinal anterior horn cells appear to be spared. The typical pathological features of ALS, including Bunina bodies and ubiquitinated inclusions, have been described in autopsy cases of PLS; most reported autopsy cases have shown evidence of mild LMN involvement and thus either do not technically meet criteria for PLS, or provide evidence supporting the hypothesis that PLS is not pathophysiologically a distinct entity from ALS.

Clinical features

Clinical features present at disease onset may help distinguish PLS from upper motor neuron predominant ALS and typical ALS. PLS is more slowly progressive, and more often has limb onset with less weakness, muscle atrophy, and weight loss. PLS patients also have more slowly progressive respiratory dysfunction. Progressive lower extremity spasticity without significant loss of strength is the classic initial symptom. Symptom progression is variable, with both contiguous and non-contiguous patterns of spread. Ocular motor abnormalities, dysarthria, and bladder dysfunction commonly occur as the disease progresses. Although PLS was initially thought to spare cognition, detailed neuropsychological testing shows mild deficits in frontal lobe dysfunction and memory in eight out of nine patients. Involuntary inappropriate emotional expression defect (IEED or pseudobulbar affect) with episodes of unprovoked crying or laughing has been described in approximately half of cases.

Examination reveals increased tone with spastic gait, hyperreflexia, spastic dysarthria, and extensor plantar responses with relative sparing of strength and without significant problems of coordination or sensation.

Clinical diagnostic criteria were proposed by Pringle *et al.* in 1992 and include:

- Insidious onset of spastic paresis, usually beginning in the lower extremities but occasionally bulbar or upper extremities.
- Adult onset in the fifth decade or later.
- Absence of family history.
- Gradually progressive without stepwise loss of function.
- Greater than or equal to 3 years in duration.
- Clinical findings limited to those associated with corticospinal dysfunction.
- Symmetric distribution.

The usefulness of these criteria has been debated. In 2006, Gordon *et al.* argued for a pure PLS syndrome distinct from an UMN dominant ALS, based on a cohort of 29 patients with only UMN signs and a normal electromyography (EMG) on initial evaluation. Of these 29 patients, 13 developed evidence of denervation by EMG or clinical examination within 4 years of follow-up. Disability rating, respiratory function, and life expectancy were best in the pure UMN–PLS syndrome, while the UMN dominant ALS group retained a better life expectancy compared to the combined UMN and LMN ALS group. During the 6.6 years of follow-up of a prospective study based on 50 patients with long disease duration

International Neurology, Second edition. Edited by Robert P. Lisak, Daniel D. Truong, William M. Carroll and Roongroj Bhidayasiri
© 2016 John Wiley & Sons, Ltd. Published 2016 by John Wiley & Sons, Ltd.

diagnosed with PLS according to the Pringle classification, only 3 patients developed evidence of an alternative diagnosis.

Investigations

PLS remains a diagnosis of exclusion. The differential diagnosis includes ALS, hereditary spastic paraplegia (HSP), foramen magnum lesions, spinal cord compression, multiple sclerosis (MS), spinocerebellar atrophy, dentatorubral-pallidoluysian atrophy, adrenomyeloneuropathy, subacute combined degeneration, syphilis, neuroborreliosis, tropical spastic paraparesis, copper deficiency, vitamin E deficiency, hexosaminidase A deficiency, human immunodeficiency virus (HIV), dystonia, and paraneoplastic syndromes. Although superficially resembling PLS, the majority of these conditions demonstrate neurological abnormalities other than the upper motor neuron features that characterize PLS. In addition, two UMN syndromes have been associated with food consumption: on the Indian subcontinent, ingestion of the seed of Lathyrus sativus (chickling or grass pea) is associated with Lathyrism and in Sub-Saharan Africa, consumption of cassava root is associated with konza.

EMG is useful to distinguish PLS from ALS based on the absence of diffuse chronic denervation, although evidence of intermittent and mild focal denervation in PLS has been reported. Diagnostic studies used to exclude disease mimickers include brain and spinal magnetic resonance imaging (MRI), vitamin B_{12}, rapid plasma reagin, Borrelia antibodies, human T-lymphotropic virus (HTLV-1) antibodies, and very long-chain fatty acids. Cerebrospinal fluid (CSF) analysis is usually unremarkable. No biomarker is currently available for definitive diagnosis.

Atrophy of the frontoparietal region of the brain, predominantly in the precentral area, with degeneration of the underlying white matter and selective T2 hyperintensity of the pyramidal tract, is seen with brain MRI. In four PLS patients, cortical positron emission tomography (PET) scan showed decreased metabolism in the motor cortex and right parietal lobe similar to that seen in ALS, with further decrease in the left superior temporal gyrus and the anterior cingulate gyrus. Cortically evoked motor potentials are often absent or prolonged in PLS, while in ALS they are frequently normal or mildly delayed.

It can be problematic to distinguish PLS from HSP. However, in HSP a dominant family history is usually present, with X-linked and recessive forms being less common. Genetic testing is available for a growing number of HSP variants. HSP onset tends to present at a younger age (mean 39 years) and bulbar symptoms including spastic dysarthria and IEED do not occur.

Treatment

No curative treatment is available for PLS. Disease management is symptomatic and includes muscle relaxants such as baclofen, tizanidine, or dantrolene for spasticity; tricyclic antidepressants, glycopyrrolate, or onabotulinum toxin type A (Botox®) for sialorrhea; non-invasive ventilation and in/exsufflation devices (cough assistance) for extra-parenchymal restrictive lung disease; augmentative communication devices for dysarthria; feeding tubes for dysphagia; and mobility devices such as a walker, power wheelchair, and Hoyer lift for gait and transfer impairments. Care is optimally provided by a multidisciplinary clinic team with access to a speech and language pathologist, and physical and occupational therapists who have expertise in treating patients with motor neuron diseases.

Further reading

Al-Saif A, Bohlega S, Al-Mohanna F. Loss of ERLIN2 function leads to juvenile primary lateral sclerosis. Ann Neurol 2012;72(4):510–516.

Brugman F, Veldink JH, Franssen H, et al. Differentiation of hereditary spastic paraparesis from primary lateral sclerosis in sporadic adult-onset upper motor neuron syndromes. Arch Neurol. 2009;66(4):509–514.

Casselli RJ, Smith BE, Osborne D. Primary lateral sclerosis: A neuropsychological study. Neurology 1995;45;2205–2209.

Eymard-Pierre E, Lesca G, Dollet S, et al. Infantile-onset of ascending hereditary spastic paralysis is associated with mutations in the alsin gene. Am J Human Genet 2002;71;518–527.

Floeter MK, Mills R. Progression in primary lateral sclerosis: A prospective analysis. Amyotroph Lateral Scler 2009;10(5–6):339–346.

Gordon PH, Cheng B, Katz I, et al. The natural history of primary lateral sclerosis. Neurology 2006;66:647–653.

Gordon PH, Cheng B, Katz IB, Mitsumoto H, Rowland LP. Clinical features that distinguish PLS, upper motor neuron-dominant ALS, and typical ALS. Neurology 2009;72(22):1948–1952.

Pringle CE, Hudson AJ, Munoz DG, et al. Primary lateral sclerosis: Clinical features, neuropathology and diagnostic criteria. Brain 1992;115:495–520.

Tartaglia MC, Rowe A, Findlater K, et al. Differentiation between primary lateral sclerosis and amyotrophic lateral sclerosis. Arch Neurol 2007;64:232–236.

107 Hereditary spastic paraplegia

Ildefonso Rodríguez-Leyva

Neurology Service, Internal Medicine Department, University of San Luis Potosi, San Luis Potosi, Mexico

Hereditary or familial spastic paraplegia (HSP, FSP, Strümpell–Lorrain syndrome, Strümpell's syndrome) is a group of inherited disorders characterized by progressive spasticity and weakness of the lower extremities, associated with hyperreflexia and extensor plantar responses ("pure"). In addition, various other neurological symptoms and signs may be associated ("complicated"). HSP may be inherited as an autosomal dominant, autosomal recessive, or X-linked recessive trait.

These disorders may be classified based on mode of inheritance. There are more than 50 genetic types. The clinical manifestations can start at any age and usually the disease has a very slow progression over many years. HSP may be caused by mutations of several different genes (genetic heterogeneity), which are designated by the genetic loci 1 through 56 (spastic paraplegia, SPG). Loci for autosomal dominant, autosomal recessive, and X-linked recessive HSP have been identified in various affected families. Multiple proteins encoded by SPG mutations have diverse functions and can explain the phenotype of this disorder (see Table 107.1).

Table 107.1 Hereditary spastic paraplegia disorders. Modified from Salinas 2008 and Fink 2014.

Protein	Gene/ locus	Inheritance	Clinical syndrome Uncomplicated	Complicated	Age of onset
L1 cell adhesion molecule	L1CAM/SPG1 (Xq28)	X-linked		Mental retardation, hypoplasia of corpus callosum, adducted thumbs, hydrocephalus	
Proteo lipoprotein 1	PLP1/ SPG2 (Xq21)	X-linked		Quadriplegia, nystagmus, mental retardation, seizures	
Atlastin-1	ATL1/ SPG3A (14q12-q21)	AD	De novo mutation reported presenting as spastic diplegic cerebral palsy		Typical onset: childhood (may be non-progressive); or adolescence to adulthood (with insidious progression)
Spastin	SPAST/ SPG4 (2p22)	AD	Most common cause of pure AD HSP (~40%)	Occasionally present: late-onset cognitive impairment	Variable onset: from infancy to senescence
Cytochrome P450-7B1	CYP7B1/SPG5A (8p)	AR	Uncomplicated HSP		Variable onset
Non-imprinted in Prader-Willi/ Angelman syndrome region protein 1 (magnesium transporter NIPA1)	NIPA1/ SPG6 (15q11.2-q12)	AD	Rarely, complicated by epilepsy or variable peripheral neuropathy; in 1 case, ALS		Prototypic late adolescent, early adult onset, slowly progressive
KIAA0196 (WASH complex subunit, Strumpellin)	KIAA0196/ SPG8 (8q24)	AD	Uncomplicated HSP, remarkable spasticity		Adult onset
Unknown	SPG9 (10q23.3-q24.2)	AD		Cataracts, gastroesophageal reflux, motor neuronopathy, skeletal abnormalities	
Kinesin family heavy chain, isoform 5A	KIF5A/ SPG10 (12q13)	AD	Uncomplicated HSP	Occasionally complicated by distal muscle atrophy	Early onset
Spatacsin	SPG11	AR		Thin corpus callosum, cognitive impairment, neuropathy	Childhood to early adult onset
Reticulon-2	RTN2/ SPG12	AD	Uncomplicated HSP		Early onset
Chaperonin 60 (heat shock protein 60, HSP60)	HSPD1/ SPG13	AD	Uncomplicated HSP		Onset: adolescent–adult
Unknown	SPG14 (3q27-q38)	AR		Motor neuropathy, mental retardation	Variable onset

continued

International Neurology, Second edition. Edited by Robert P. Lisak, Daniel D. Truong, William M. Carroll and Roongroj Bhidayasiri
© 2016 John Wiley & Sons, Ltd. Published 2016 by John Wiley & Sons, Ltd.

Table 107.1 Hereditary spastic paraplegia disorders. Modified from Salinas 2008 and Fink 2014. (*continued*)

Protein	Gene/ locus	Inheritance	Clinical syndrome		Age of onset
			Uncomplicated	Complicated	
Spastizin	SPG15 (14q)	AR		Kjellin syndrome: pigmented retinopathy, cerebellar signs, mental retardation	Adolescent onset
Unknown	SPG16 (Xq11.2)	X-linked		Aphasia, sphincter disturbance, mental retardation	Onset in infancy
Seipin/ BSCL2 (seipin)	*BSCL2/* SPG17 (11q12-q14)	AD		Amyotrophy of hand muscles (Silver syndrome)	
Unknown	SPG18 (locus reserved)	AD			
Unknown	SPG19 (9q33-q34)	AD	Uncomplicated HSP		Adult onset
Spartin	SPG20 (13q)	AR		Troyer syndrome: amyotrophy, cerebellar signs, developmental delay	Childhood onset
Maspardin	SPG21 (15q)	AR		Mast syndrome: thin corpus callosum, cognitive decline, extrapyramidal features, cerebellar signs	Early adult onset
Unknown	SPG23 (1q24-q32)	AR		Lison syndrome: pigmentary abnormalities, facial and skeletal dysmorhism, cognitive decline	Childhood onset
Unknown	SPG24 (13q14)	AR	Uncomplicated HSP	Occasionally pseudobulbar signs	Childhood onset
Unknown	SPG25 (6q23-q24)	AR			Adult onset
Unknown	SPG26 (12p11.1-q14)	AR			
Unknown	SPG27 (10q22.1-q24.1)	AR			
Unknown	SPG28 (14q21.3-q22.3)	AR			
Unknown	SPG29 (1p31.1-21.1)	AD		Hearing impairment; persistent vomiting due to hiatal hernia (inherited)	
Unknown	SPG30 (2q37)	AR			
Receptor expression-enhancing protein 1	*REEP1/* SPG31 (2p12)	AD	Uncomplicated HSP	Occasionally associated with peripheral neuropathy	
Unknown	SPG32	AR		Mental retardation, thin corpus callosum, pontine dysraphism	Childhood onset
Protrudin	*ZFYVE27/* SPG33	AD	Uncomplicated HSP		
Unknown	SPG34 (locus reserved)	AD			
Unknown	SPG35 (16q21-q23)	AR		Intellectual decline, seizures	Childhood onset
Unknown	SPG36 (12q23-q24)	AD		Motor sensory neuropathy	Onset: age 14–28 years
Unknown	SPG37 (8p21.1-q13.3)	AD	Uncomplicated HSP		
Unknown	SPG38 (4p16-p15)	AD		**In 5 members of a single family Silver syndrome: atrophy of intrinsic hand muscles (severe in 1 subject age 58)	Onset age 16–21 years
Neuropathy target esterase	SPG39	AR		Marked distal wasting in all four limbs	Childhood onset
Unknown	SPG40 (locus unknown)	AD	Uncomplicated HSP		Onset age >35
Unknown	SPG41 (11p14.1-p11.2)	AD		**In a single Chinese family Mild weakness of intrinsic hand muscles	Onset: adolescence
Acetyl-coenzyme A transporter	SLC33A1/ SPG42	Possible instance of incomplete penetrance	Uncomplicated HSP in a single kindred		Onset: age 4–40 years

Epidemiology

The prevalence of HSP varies in different studies, probably due to the use of different diagnostic criteria and geographic factors. A prevalence of autosomal dominant HSP ranged from 0.5–5.5/100,000 and for recessive cases from 0–5.3/100,000, with pooled averages of 1.8/100,000 (95% CI 1.0–2.7/100,000) and 1.8/100,000 (95% CI 1–2.6/100,000), respectively, according to a multisource population-based study from Ruano *et al.*

Pathophysiology

The disorder is known to be associated with several abnormalities of structure or function in axon transport (SPG 4, 10, and 30); endoplasmic reticulum (SPG 3, 4, 12, and 31); mitochondria (SPG 7 and 13); myelin (SPG 2 and 42); folding and stress response (SPG 6, 8, and 17); corticospinal system (SPG 1 and 22); fatty acid and phospholipid metabolism (SPG 28, 35, 39, and 56); and transmembranal traffic (SPG 47, 48, 50, 51, 52, and 53). These alterations cause deterioration in function by axonal degeneration through misfolded protein accumulation with changes of spinal cord tracts, consisting of bundles of myelinated axons. HSP is associated with alterations that are most severe at the ends of the longest tracts and nerve fibers in the central nervous system (CNS). These include descending (corticospinal) and ascending (gracilis and spinocerebellar) systems. There are usually less marked changes of corticospinal tracts that convey motor and sensory (cuneatus) impulses to and from the arms. As a result, most patients do not experience associated symptoms of the upper limbs. Involvement of spinocerebellar tracts is seen in about 50% of cases. The analysis of HSP genes provides insight into the disorder's pathogenesis by permitting pathophysiological molecular and cellular studies of the disorder. These findings should help to understand the molecular functions of the corticospinal tract and to design potential strategies to prevent and treat the disorder and its manifestations.

Clinical features

The onset of stiffness and weakness of hip and leg muscles and associated gait disturbance tends to be insidious, with symptoms typically becoming progressively severe over time. The age at onset is extremely variable even among affected members of the same family. Symptoms have been known to develop as early as infancy to as late as the ninth decade of life. Up to 25% of affected patients are asymptomatic. In some kindred symptoms appear to occur at a younger age with successive generations, with an apparent anticipation.

In those who suffer from HSP without other associated neurological features, often described as uncomplicated or "pure" HSP, initial findings include

spasticity of leg muscles, including the adductors, hamstrings, quadriceps femoris, and calf muscles, causing the characteristic gait of scissoring, circumduction, and toe walking, and weakness of leg muscles with a pyramidal distribution including the ankle extensors, hip flexors, and to a lesser extent the hamstrings. A characteristic feature of HSP is the marked discrepancy between the often severe spasticity and the mild or absent muscle weakness. In childhood-onset HSP, delayed walking (relatively rare) and hyperreflexia of the lower limbs (with extensor plantar responses) and frequently also of the upper limbs may be found.

Uncomplicated HSP may also be associated with additional symptoms and signs such as highly arched feet (pes cavus; see Figure 107.1); muscle spasms and leg cramps; diminished vibration

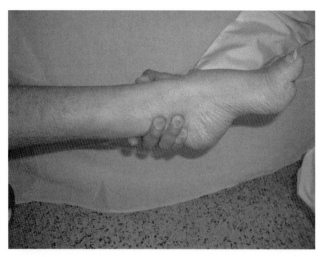

Figure 107.1

sense; paresthesia; and less often diminished joint-position sense in the feet. Sensory impairment is seen in approximately the half of cases of pure HSP (especially in cases with longstanding disease), whereas mild terminal dysmetria, loss of ankle jerks, and relatively mild muscle atrophy are usually spared. Atrophy is usually confined to the small muscles of the feet and the tibialis anterior muscles in wheelchair-dependent patients. Bladder-control problems, like urinary urgency, may progress to incontinence, can occur in up to 50% of patients, and are often a late manifestation. As with the age of onset, the rate of disease progression, symptom severity, and degree of associated disability vary greatly. For example, in some patients with uncomplicated HSP, particularly those with childhood onset, symptoms may become apparent, gradually worsen over a number of years, and eventually stabilize following adolescence. In such cases, patients often maintain an ability to walk with assistive devices. In other cases, once symptoms develop, they slowly become increasingly severe throughout the patient's life. HSP patients rarely experience a complete loss of leg mobility.

Less commonly, families suffering from HSP in association with additional neurological features have been described as "complicated" HSP: features include mental retardation, dementia, epilepsy, peripheral neuropathy, retinopathy, optic neuropathy, deafness, ataxia, dysarthria, nystagmus and movement disorders (characterized by changes in muscle tone, postural abnormalities, impairments in the execution of voluntary actions, and/or the development of abnormal involuntary movements), and sometimes skin disorders (ichthyosis). Interestingly, there is no obvious correlation between clinically "pure" and "complicated" forms and genetic mutations; many HSP genotypes are associated with both pure and complicated phenotypes.

Classification based on genotyping

In the past, classification of HSP was based primarily on whether the symptom onset was before age 35 (type I or early-onset HSP) or after age 35 (type II or late-onset HSP). However, both the early- and late-onset types may occur in the same family, and therefore categorization into pure (uncomplicated) and complicated HSP has been considered a more specific and useful distinction. Such classifications based on clinical findings are gradually being revised as more is learned about the specific underlying genetic mechanisms of HSP. Up to 70% of cases of uncomplicated HSP are transmitted as an autosomal dominant trait.

Multiple genetic loci have been identified in families with autosomal dominant HSP, in chromosomes 2p (known as *SPG4*), 8q (*SPG8*), 12q (*SPG10*), 14q (*SPG3A*), 15q (*SPG6*), and 19q (*SPG12*). Mutations in the spastin gene located on the short arm (p) of chromosome 2 (2p22-p21) are by far the most common cause of uncomplicated autosomal dominant HSP and are responsible for about 40% of cases. Those mutations are considered the prototype of uncomplicated HSP and are associated with mental retardation or dementia, ataxia, and muscle wasting with thin corpus callosum. There may be reduced expression (reduced penetrance) and, as a result, some individuals who inherit a gene mutation for HSP may be asymptomatic. HSP linked to the *SPG3A* locus represents approximately 10% of dominantly inherited cases.

Classification by mode of inheritance and genetic loci is important in order to address questions that have been raised about some clinical features. For example, cognitive impairment – such as learning difficulties, deficits in visuospatial function, memory disturbance, or dementia – have been reported in members of a few families with the most commonly described form of pure uncomplicated HSP (i.e., caused by mutations in the spastin gene). However, the development of cognitive impairment in kindred with this form of HSP is extremely rare, and therefore its expression might depend on additional genetic mechanisms. Complicated autosomal dominantly inherited HSP includes SPG 9 (locus on chromosome 10q, associated with cataracts and amyotrophy), SPG 10 and 12 (loci on chromosomes 12 and 19, respectively, associated with cerebellar signs), and SPG 29 (locus on chromosome 1p, associated with hearing loss). Autosomal recessive HSP is far less common than the dominant form. Genetic loci have been identified on chromosomes 8 (*SPG5A*), 15q (*SPG11*), and 16q (*SPG7*). The latter is caused by mutations in the paraplegin gene and may manifest as pure or complicated HSP. *SPG7* mutations account for fewer than 5% of HSP families compatible with autosomal recessive inheritance.

Two X-linked recessive forms of HSP have also been identified. In one form, the disorder appears to result from mutations in a gene that regulates production of the L1 cell adhesion molecule (*L1CAM*). This gene has been mapped to chromosome Xq28 (*SPG1*). A second X-linked form of HSP is thought to be caused by mutations in a gene that regulates production of a myelin protein (proteolipid protein or PLP). The PLP gene is located on chromosome Xq22 (*SPG2*). A gene duplication is the most common mutation in Pelizaeus–Merzbacher syndrome. In many kindred with HSP, linkage has not been established, suggesting that there are more, currently unknown genetic loci.

Investigations

The diagnosis of HSP is typically based on a careful patient and family history, a thorough clinical evaluation, and assessment of the characteristic symptoms and findings. Diagnostic evaluation may also include various specialized tests. Although DNA analysis may assist in diagnosing certain forms of HSP (e.g., that due to known gene mutations in certain families), such testing is not widely available. As our knowledge of the spectrum of HSP increases, it is expected that such information will lead to further development of laboratory tests that should help confirm the clinical diagnosis. Thus, in most instances, there is currently no definitive test for HSP. Spastic

paraplegia may also result from various other disorders, such as cervical spondylosis, spinal cord injury, or neoplasms, certain infectious diseases – human T-lymphotropic virus (HTLV-1) associated myelopathy, neurosyphilis, human immunodeficiency virus (HIV)/acquired immune deficiency syndrome (AIDS), neuroborreliosis – multiple sclerosis, vitamin B12 deficiency, vitamin E deficiency, copper deficiency, hereditary diseases including adrenomyelopathy and other leukodystrophies, distal hereditary motor neuropathy type V, Charcot–Marie–Tooth syndrome type 2 presenting with predominant hand involvement, Silver syndrome, motor neuron disease, and in particular primary lateral sclerosis, neurolathyrism, arteriovenous malformations, Arnold–Chiari malformation, syringomyelia, mitochondrial disorders, spinocerebellar ataxia, and dopa-responsive dystonia. Therefore, the differential diagnosis of HSP must include certain tests to discard such conditions, particularly if a family history of HSP is not present. Suggested ancillary tests may include the following:

- Extensive laboratory tests.
- Electromyography, nerve conduction tests, and electroencephalography (when clinically there is a suspicious neuromuscular or cortical impairment).
- Neuroimaging studies (computed tomography, magnetic resonance imaging) of the brain and spinal cord.
- Lumbar puncture.
- Other tests to help confirm HSP or to verify or eliminate other disorders, including genetic analysis.

Treatment

Treatment consists of symptomatic and supportive assistance, including physical therapy. Symptomatic therapies used for other forms of chronic paraplegia are sometimes helpful, and physical therapy is important to improve muscle strength and range of motion. Although no available treatment may prevent, slow, or alter the disease progression, therapy with baclofen (oral or intrathecally), dantrolene, or tizanidine (skeletal muscle relaxants) may reduce spasticity in some patients. Benzodiazepines such as diazepam or clonazepam may be tried, although the latter may be associated with more excessive daytime sleepiness. Botulinum toxin can be used for urinary retention secondary to spastic bladder problems. Specific chemical denervation can be useful in HSP patients with botulinum toxin type A injections into the hip adductors or ankle plantar flexors. In selected candidates, injections of phenol into the obturator nerve may be of longer benefit. In some patients with slowly progressive symptoms, neuro-orthopedic surgery to lengthen the ankle plantar flexors or hip adductors may be appropriate.

The prognosis for individuals with HSP varies. Some patients are seriously disabled, whereas others are less incapacitated and can perform activities of daily living without limitations.

The majority of individuals with HSP have a normal life expectancy. However, genetic counseling must be considered, especially when there could be a highly suggestive genetic anticipation (SPG 3 and 4).

The accumulated knowledge and better understanding of these disorders, mainly regarding genetic and epigenetic mechanisms, provide hope for future prevention, diagnosis, and specific treatment for HSP patients.

Further reading

Fink JK. The hereditary spastic paraplegias: Nine genes and counting. *Arch Neurol* 2003;60:1045–1049.

Fink JK. Hereditary spastic paraplegia: Clinico-pathologic features and emerging molecular mechanisms. *Acta Neuropathol* 2013:126:307–328.

Fink, JC. Hereditary spastic paraplegia. GeneReviews 2014;Feb. 6. http://www.ncbi.nlm.nih.gov/books/NBK1509/ (accessed November 2015).

Harding AE. Hereditary "pure" spastic paraplegia: A clinical and genetic study of 22 families. *J Neurol Neurosurg Psychiatry* 1981;44:871–883.

McDermott CJ, White K, Bushby K, Shaw PJ. Hereditary spastic paraparesis: A review of new developments. *J Neurol Neurosurg Psychiatry* 2000;69:150–160.

Neuromuscular Disease Center. 2015. Hereditary motor syndromes (SMA, ALS+ …). http://neuromuscular.wustl.edu/synmot.html (accessed November 2015).

Ruano L, Melo C, Silva MC, Coutinho P. The global epidemiology of hereditary ataxia and spastic paraplegia: Systematic review of prevalence. *Neuroepidemiology* 2014;42;174–183.

Salinas S, Proukakis C, Crosby A, Warner T. Hereditary spastic paraplegia: Clinical features and pathogenetic mechanisms. *Lancet Neurol* 2008;7:1127–1138.

108 Spinal muscular atrophy

Sabine Rudnik-Schöneborn[1] and Klaus Zerres[2]

[1] Sektion Humangenetik, Medical University of Innsbruck, Innsbruck, Austria
[2] Institute for Human Genetics, University Hospital, RWTH Aachen, Germany

The term spinal muscular atrophy (SMA) comprises a clinically and genetically heterogeneous group of diseases characterized by degeneration and loss of the anterior horn cells in the spinal cord, and – depending on type and severity – sometimes also in the brainstem nuclei, resulting in muscle weakness and atrophy.

The criteria used for the subdivision of the SMAs into separate entities (Table 108.1) are age of onset, severity, distribution of weakness, inclusion of additional features, and different modes of inheritance. The classification has been and will be modified with increasing knowledge of the underlying defects.

Epidemiology

This section focuses on the proximal SMAs that can be divided into autosomal recessive and rare autosomal dominant types. According to a rough estimate, less than 2% of cases with disease onset

Table 108.1 Classification of spinal muscular atrophies.

1. Proximal SMA (80–90%)
1.1 Autosomal recessive SMA
– infantile and juvenile SMA (SMA I–III)**
– adult SMA (SMA IV) (mostly sporadic)*
1.2 Autosomal dominant SMA (variable-onset forms)*
1.3 Spinobulbar neuronopathy type Kennedy (XL)**
2. Non-proximal SMA (10–15%)
2.1 Distal SMA
– juvenile distal SMA/hereditary motor neuronopathy (AD, AR, XL)*
– with spasticity (AD, AR)*
– with pyramidal signs (AD, AR)*
– with vocal cord palsy (AD)*
– with respiratory insufficiency (AR)*
– segmental SMA or benign monomelic amyotrophy (mostly sporadic)
2.2 Scapuloperoneal SMA (AD, AR)*
3. Variants of infantile SMA (<2%)
3.1 SMA with respiratory distress (SMARD) (AR)**
3.2 SMA plus pontocerebellar hypoplasia (PCH1) (AR)**
3.3 SMA plus arthrogryposis (AD, AR, XL)*
3.4 SMA with myoclonus epilepsy (AR)*
4. Bulbar palsy (very rare)
4.1 Progressive bulbar palsy of childhood type Fazio–Londe (AR)*
4.2 Bulbar palsy with deafness and distal pareses (Brown–Vialetto–van Laere syndrome) (AR)*
4.3 Adult-onset bulbar palsy (AD)

AD = autosomal dominant; AR = autosomal recessive; XL = X-linked, * = genetic diagnosis possible in some cases; ** = genetic diagnosis available for most cases

before 10 years of age show a parent-to-child transmission, while autosomal dominant transmission is more frequent than autosomal recessive in hereditary adult-onset proximal SMA.

Data for the most severe SMA type I (Werdnig–Hoffmann disease) suggest that the birth incidence among Caucasians varies between 1/25,000 and about 1/10,000. The incidence is much higher in certain inbred communities. Variants of early-onset SMA are very rare, contributing to about 2% of all SMA cases in childhood and infancy.

The more benign forms of the disease (SMA types II and III) have a prevalence among children as high as 1/18,000 and around 1/20,000 in the general population. The overall incidence is 1/10,000 for all types of autosomal recessive SMA; that is, the carrier frequency of 1/50 is valid for genetic counseling in most populations. Adult SMA might account for 8% of all SMA cases, with a prevalence of 0.32/100,000 of the population.

There are only sparse data on prevalences of the non-proximal SMAs. Distal SMA accounts for about 10% of all SMAs, while the definition of scapuloperoneal syndromes is still under debate. Progressive bulbar palsy is extremely rare, while spinobulbar neuronopathy or muscular atrophy (SBMA) type Kennedy has a prevalence of about 1/40,000.

Pathophysiology

Most research results are available for infantile SMA and its pathophysiology. The SMN protein is expressed in all somatic tissues and is highly conserved from yeast to humans. It is involved in RNA processing and is localized in structures called "gems" in the nucleus. The SMN protein acts in concert with several other proteins in the regeneration of the snRNPs, acting as an assemblyosome in the formation of diverse RNP particles. It is still unclear why SMN protein deficiency results in selective motor neuron loss, because the gene is ubiquitously expressed. Studies of cell cultures and animal models have shown that the SMN protein is important for axonal growth and transport of motor neurons. Additional functions are ascribed to the skeletal muscle and to the integrity of the neuromuscular junction.

Clinical features

Proximal SMA

The infantile- and juvenile-onset proximal SMAs (SMA types I-III) are most common (Table 108.1) and are caused by defects of the *SMN1* gene on chromosome 5q13. The clinical picture indicates a

International Neurology, Second edition. Edited by Robert P. Lisak, Daniel D. Truong, William M. Carroll and Roongroj Bhidayasiri
© 2016 John Wiley & Sons, Ltd. Published 2016 by John Wiley & Sons, Ltd.

continuous spectrum, with ages of onset ranging from before birth to adulthood. SMA types I–III follow an autosomal recessive mode of inheritance, and more than 90% of patients show homozygous deletions of the *SMN1* gene, enabling a fast and reliable molecular diagnosis. The situation is different for SMA IV, where the genetic basis is still largely unknown, and most patients have no family history. However, there are some patients with SMA IV with *SMN1* gene deletions. SBMA is X-linked and easily diagnosed by the presence of a CAG repeat expansion in the androgen receptor gene.

SMA type I

The clinical signs of the most severe SMA type I, also referred to as Werdnig–Hoffmann disease or acute SMA, are evident at birth or soon thereafter. Nearly all patients present by 6 months of age. Symptoms are profound hypotonia and generalized weakness. The infants do not kick well and are never able to sit unaided. The tongue fasciculates, and the infant lies in the "frog" position. In the final stages of the disease the child is practically immobile (Figure 108.1a), has a bell-shaped chest with paradoxical breathing, and is tachypneic, indicating imminent respiratory insufficiency. Life span is short, with death occurring at a median age of 7–8 months due to swallowing and respiratory insufficiency. However, 8–10% of patients show an arrested disease course and survive for several years or exceptionally into adulthood.

The differential diagnosis of early-onset SMA type I comprises the whole spectrum of the "floppy infant syndrome." A careful neuropediatric examination is required to exclude other diseases if screening for a deletion in the *SMN1* gene is negative.

SMA type II

The clinical course of SMA type II, also known as chronic childhood SMA or intermediate type SMA, is marked by stable periods and slow progression. The children fail to pass motor milestones because of proximal weakness and hypotonia within the first 18 months of life. There is wide variability of clinical severity, ranging from children who have early difficulties in sitting (Figure 108.1b) or rolling over to patients who are able to crawl or walk with support. For practical purposes, this group is defined by the ability to sit independently, as the children never learn to stand or walk unaided. Hand tremor and fasciculations are characteristic features. Pronounced weakness of trunk muscles gives rise to spine deformities and also causes a reduced lung capacity. Contractures of all major joints occur in the disease course. Most patients survive into adulthood, but life span can vary considerably.

SMA type III

A mild form of childhood and juvenile disease, SMA type III is often referred to as Kugelberg–Welander disease. The age of onset varies widely from the first year of life to the third decade. Patients with SMA type III learn to walk without support, which distinguishes them from those with SMA type II. For prognostic reasons, we separate SMA types IIIa and IIIb, since the prognosis as regards walking probability is markedly different. In SMA type IIIa, the children have early walking difficulties and often fail to pass further motor milestones within the first 3 years (Figure 108.1c). Since many patients are non-ambulatory by school age (50% are wheelchair bound 14 years after onset), there is a considerable handicap in comparison to those whose walking difficulties start in youth or adulthood. Depending on the degree of weakness, spine deformities

and contractures are frequent complications, mainly in the chairbound patients.

In SMA type IIIb, onset is between 3 and 30 years of age. Lower limb involvement causes mainly problems in running, climbing, or sports, with sometimes very slow or even undetectable progression. About 50% of the SMA type IIIb patients are still ambulatory after a 45-year disease duration, and life expectancy is not much reduced.

The clinical picture is often indistinguishable from Becker muscular dystrophy or limb girdle muscular dystrophy, even after neurological investigations. Rarely, patients with SMA type IIIb may have hypertrophic calves and a serum creatine kinase (CK) of more than 10 times the upper limit of normal. If cardiomyopathy is seen in patients with proximal weakness, Emery–Dreifuss muscular dystrophy should be taken into account. Facioscapulohumeral muscular dystrophy (FSHD) can also present like SMA III and can be easily be diagnosed by DNA analysis. Other metabolic myopathies, such as Pompe disease, can be clinically similar with proximal SMA. Rarely, hexosaminidase A deficiency may mimic SMA type III.

SMA type IV

SMA type IV, or adult SMA, comprises a clinically and genetically heterogeneous condition. Usually, onset ranges from 30–60 years, with pronounced proximal weakness, particularly of the limb girdle and thigh muscles. Progression is mostly slow, and the life span is normal. In contrast to SMA types I–III, recurrence of SMA IV within a sibship is rare.

Few genes have been discovered for autosomal dominant adult-onset proximal SMA; nonetheless, in most cases mutations were restricted to single families. It can be expected that new methods in gene sequencing will rapidly increase the number of responsible genes.

The most important differential diagnosis of SMA type IV is Kennedy's disease and amyotrophic lateral sclerosis (ALS), which often starts with pure lower motor neuron signs. Adult acid maltase deficiency shows a similar clinical picture and glycogen accumulation is not always apparent on the muscle biopsy. Proximal myotonic myopathy (PROMM), also known as myotonic dystrophy type 2, has also to be considered, but the presence of myotonia (albeit not always noticeable) and CTTG repeat expansions on chromosome 3 should clarify the diagnosis. Postpoliomyelitis muscular atrophy can cause diagnostic confusion, but has hitherto only rarely been encountered in countries with consequent vaccination programs.

Spinobulbar neuronopathy type Kennedy

Spinobulbar neuronopathy or muscular atrophy (SBMA) type Kennedy is characterized by pronounced muscle cramps and fasciculations accompanying predominantly proximal and symmetric weakness, legs more than arms. Mean age at onset is 30 years (range 15–60). Patients often show signs of partial androgen insensitivity with gynecomastia, impotence, testicular atrophy, and reduced fertility. Frequently, facial and perioral contraction fasciculations and a postural tremor of the hands are observed. Dysarthria, dysphonia, and dysphagia are caused by progressive death of bulbar motor neurons. Serum CK activity can be markedly elevated, especially in early disease stage. Sensory nerve action potentials are mostly reduced. The disease is X-linked and caused by a CAG expansion in the androgen receptor gene, therefore genetic testing enables an easy diagnosis. Female carriers may manifest with cramps and fasciculations.

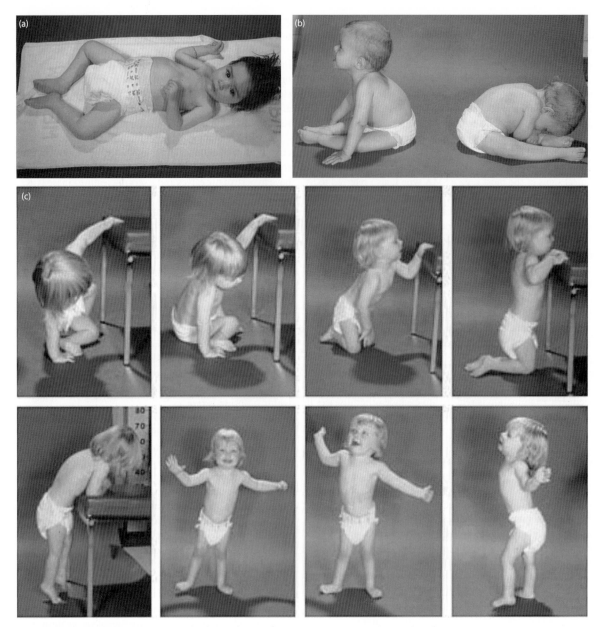

Figure 108.1 (a) Girl with end-stage SMA type I who died at the age of 10 months. (b) Twin brothers with early-onset SMA type II. A sitting position is maintained only for several minutes followed by a "pocket knife" phenomenon. (c) SMA type IIIa in a 2-year-old girl who had delayed motor development. Note difficulties in rising and waddling gait.

Non-proximal SMA

Distal SMA

Distal SMA accounts for about 10% of all SMA cases, and comprises a group of genetically and clinically heterogeneous disorders with a broad spectrum of clinical manifestations. Distal SMAs are also denoted as distal hereditary motor neuronopathies (HMN) and are frequently listed among the Charcot–Marie–Tooth (CMT) neuropathies. Both autosomal dominant and recessive genes cause childhood- and adult-onset forms, and the course is usually chronic and benign. As CMT neuropathy is the main differential diagnosis, it is important to exclude peripheral nerve involvement by electroneurography before diagnosing distal SMA. In non-familial

cases, intraspinal pathology, for instance conus-cauda tumor, has to be excluded. Distal myopathies can normally be distinguished by elevated serum CK activity, muscle biopsy, or DNA studies.

Juvenile segmental spinal muscular atrophy, also known as "monomelic juvenile SMA of the Hirayama type" or "benign monomelic amyotrophy," deserves separate mention. It was first reported in the Japanese literature and later in other populations as well. Almost all patients are male and have no family history; the onset is insidious and is usually between 15 and 25 years. The cardinal features are asymmetric wasting and weakness confined to a single upper limb (hand and forearm) that might spread to the contralateral upper or to a lower limb. The condition is very benign in most cases, with the initial progressive phase coming to a halt within 2–4 years.

Scapuloperoneal SMA

The clinical manifestations of scapuloperoneal SMA are variable, affecting the foot and toe extensors first, and then spreading to the shoulder girdle and proximal muscles of lower limbs. Autosomal dominant and recessive inheritance has been reported. The autosomal dominant form with adult onset was first described by Stark and Kaeser, but the original family turned out to be a desmin myopathy. FSHD is an important differential diagnosis and much more frequent. By identification of the *TRPV4* gene in 2010, a rare and clinically highly variable autosomal dominant SMA was defined, which can present as a congenital form, progressive scapuloperoneal atrophy, laryngeal palsy, or distal SMA. The existence of autosomal recessive scapuloperoneal SMA still has to be confirmed molecular genetically.

Investigations

Neurological investigations disclose progressive muscle weakness and atrophy and reduced tendon reflexes in most of the SMAs. CK activity in the serum is normal or only mildly elevated, except in SBMA where it can be as high as 15 times the upper limit of normal. Electromyography and muscle biopsy studies reveal a neurogenic lesion in the muscle. Peripheral nerve conduction velocities are generally normal, which helps to differentiate SMA from clinically similar motor neuropathies.

Genetic screening is now replacing invasive neurological tests in the diagnosis of SMA types I, II, and III, in some variants of SMA, and in SBMA. Progress in next-generation sequencing methods facilitates the identification of genes, for example by whole exome or whole genome sequencing, and offers better detection rates of rare mutations, such as by targeted gene panel analysis. Current information about identified genes is available in the database of Online Mendelian Inheritance in Man (www.ncbi.nlm.nih.gov/omim). Nonetheless, there is still no routine genetic diagnosis for most non-proximal SMAs and autosomal dominant proximal SMA at the time of writing.

Treatment

Following identification of the SMN gene in 1995, numerous studies focused on the development of gene therapy in infantile SMA. Treatment strategies attempt to increase SMN protein levels either by activating *SMN2* gene expression, increasing inclusion of exon 7 in *SMN2*-derived transcripts, stabilizing SMN protein, or replacing the *SMN1* gene. Some of these trials are in clinical development

(www.clinicaltrials.gov), the most promising to date being based on antisense oligonucleotides that bind specific mRNA sequences and increase exon 7 inclusion of *SMN2*. Research activities are promoted in the United States by Families of SMA (www.fsma.org); in Europe TREAT NMD was founded in 2007 as a network for the development of treatment and clinical care in neuromuscular diseases (www.treat-nmd.eu).

Progress into clinical trials is also seen in SBMA therapeutic strategies. These concentrated on antiandrogen therapies based on the ligand dependency of pathogenic AR accumulation and toxicity, although as yet there is no proven efficacy. Prevention of mutant AR protein aggregation has been another goal of SBMA therapeutics development.

As long as no curative treatment can be offered in SMA, the mainstay of clinical care is symptomatic and multidisciplinary, including physical and orthopedic therapy and ventilatory support if required.

Future prospects

The identification of genes involved in the different forms of SMA will help to define and better differentiate these entities. Moreover, it will provide us with further insights into the pathogenic mechanisms of motor neuron degeneration and might open the way for therapeutic strategies. In those disorders for which the causative gene has been known for many years, such as SMA and SBMA, there has been remarkable progress in clinical therapeutic development. Further work is needed to identify which of these potential therapies offers real promise for clinical efficacy. Since no cure for SMA is yet available, genetic counseling and prognostic assessments are of great importance.

Further reading

Fischbeck KH. Developing treatment for spinal and bulbar muscular atrophy. *Prog Neurobiol* 2012;99:257–261.

Irobi J, Dierick I, Jordanova A, *et al*. Unraveling the genetics of distal hereditary motor neuropathies. *Neuromolecular Med* 2006;8:131–146.

Mercuri E, Bertini E, Iannacone ST. Childhood onset spinal muscular atrophy: Controversies and challenges. *Lancet Neurol* 2012;11:443–452.

Ogino S, Wilson RB. Genetic testing and risk assessment for spinal muscular atrophy (SMA). *Hum Genet* 2002;111:477–500.

Van Meerbeke JP, Sumner CJ. Progress and promise: The current status of spinal muscular atrophy therapeutics. *Discov Med* 2011;65:291–305.

Wang CH, Finkel RS, Bertini ES, *et al*. Consensus statement for standard of care in spinal muscular atrophy. *J Child Neurol* 2007;22:1027–1049.

Zerres K, Rudnik-Schöneborn S, Forrest E, *et al*. A collaborative study on the natural history of childhood and juvenile onset proximal spinal muscular atrophy (type II and III SMA): 569 patients. *J Neurol Sci* 1997;146:67–72.

109 Post polio syndrome

Nils Erik Gilhus

Department of Clinical Medicine, University of Bergen, and Department of Neurology, Haukeland University Hospital, Bergen, Norway

Acute polio is a generalized virus infection. Exposure to poliovirus can lead to four different responses: (1) immunization with no symptoms (>90% of cases); (2) mild illness with fever, sore throat, nausea, abdominal pain, and mild malaise (5%); (3) viral meningitis with fever, headache, and neck stiffness, but with no paresis (1–2%); or (4) paralytic polio with muscle weakness combined with meningitis and signs of generalized disease (1%).

Until approximately 100 years ago, the polio virus was endemic. Improvements in hygiene standards meant that the virus was no longer a constant presence in Western populations. However, when the polio virus reappeared, large and dramatic epidemics occurred. Acute polio was a dominating health issue in Europe and North America in the 1940s and early 1950s. The inactivated polio vaccine was introduced by Salk in 1955 and the attenuated, oral vaccine by Sabin in 1961. Polio epidemics diminished rapidly in the Western world immediately after the introduction of vaccination programs.

A polio survivor is usually left with sequelae manifesting as stable muscle weakness. However, in some patients this is followed many years later by new pareses, termed post-polio syndrome (PPS) or post-polio muscular atrophy. It may be difficult to distinguish new primary muscle weakness from a wide variety of physical and psychosocial problems experienced by former polio patients. Gradual or abrupt onset of new neurogenic weakness should be regarded as the hallmark for PPS.

Epidemiology

In 2013, acute polio was regarded as endemic in three countries – Afghanistan, Nigeria, and Pakistan – and there were 406 case reports from another 6 countries. Since the year 2000 the annual number of cases worldwide has been below 2000. When the World Health Organization (WHO) global polio-eradication initiative was launched in 1988, the polio virus was endemic in more than 125 countries worldwide, and the estimated annual number of acute polio cases was around 400,000, the great majority being children. WHO declared America polio free in 1994, the Western Pacific in 2000, and Europe in 2002. The polio vaccination program is regarded as the largest public health initiative ever. There has been a shift in many countries from live vaccine to inactivated vaccine to avoid the rare cases of vaccine-induced polio, occurring in 4 per million. There is a realistic aim to eradicate acute polio entirely during the next few years.

During the epidemics in Western countries the number of new patients each year was very high. For example, in Norway, the number varied between 1 and 60 cases per 100,000 total population

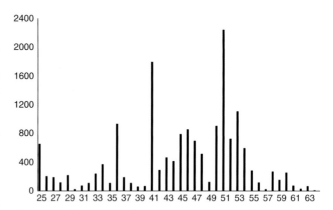

Figure 109.1 Total number of new polio cases per year in Norway, 1925–1964.

per year (Figure 109.1). Two-thirds of patients were younger than 10 years old. In the United States, 640,000 people were estimated to have a history of polio in 1987, in the Netherlands 13,000 in 1999, in France 50,000 at present, and in Norway at least 5,000. The prevalence of previous polio with clinical symptoms in Europe is 0.1%. The total number of patients with polio pareses worldwide has been estimated at 20 million.

The estimated prevalence and incidence of PPS vary based on the PPS definition used and the population evaluated. Most reports consist of selected hospital cases. The frequency of the key complaint, "new weakness," usually ranges from 20–60% of all patients with polio paresis. If adding the more distinct criterion of "new neurogenic weakness," or even "new muscular atrophy," 10–40% of patients fulfill the criteria for PPS. Even patients with non-paralytic acute polio can develop polio-related motor weakness after many years, it being found in 7% of such patients in a small cohort study. These frequencies combined with a large number of polio survivors make PPS by far the most prevalent motor neuron disease, not only in Africa and Asia but also in Europe and America.

Disease mechanisms

The polio virus is a single-stranded RNA enterovirus, 30 nm in diameter, which multiplies in the lymphoid tissue along the gastrointestinal tract. There are three antigenically distinct strains with slightly different capsid proteins, none of which can survive outside the human body. Infection with one type does not give full protection against the other two types. Type 2 poliovirus was eradicated

International Neurology, Second edition. Edited by Robert P. Lisak, Daniel D. Truong, William M. Carroll and Roongroj Bhidayasiri
© 2016 John Wiley & Sons, Ltd. Published 2016 by John Wiley & Sons, Ltd.

in 1999. Persistent viremia is required for entry into the central nervous system, leading to inflammation and cell destruction. The virus infects human cells by binding to an immunoglobulin receptor, CD155, on the cell surface. Its genome can be used as messenger RNA and translated by the host cell, resulting in the production of approximately 10 different viral proteins. The polio virus has a predilection for the spinal cord motor neurons. Mortality during the acute infection is partly due to meningo-encephalitis and partly due to muscle weakness with respiratory failure. Immediate recovery after the acute phase is due to disappearance of inflammation and recovery of motor neurons. Later improvement is due to motor unit enlargement with branching of surviving neurons, combined with adaptation and training.

The new functional deterioration in PPS is focal and slowly progressive. There is an imbalance between degeneration and regeneration of enlarged motor units, and some motor neurons cannot maintain all nerve terminals. Oversized motor units were created in the recovery phase after the acute illness and can no longer be maintained. Muscle overuse and disuse may contribute, and also aging.

Immunological and inflammatory signs have been reported in the cerebrospinal fluid and central nervous tissue of PPS patients. An increased number of cytokine-expressing cells has been reported in the cerebrospinal fluid. The polio virus should be cleared by the immune system in the acute phase of the disease. Although polio virus genomic sequences have been reported in the cerebrospinal fluid decades after the acute infection, the post-polio syndrome is not an infectious process and patients do not shed polio virus.

Clinical features

Clinical features of acute paralytic polio include muscle weakness, muscle pain, meningitis and sometimes meningo-encephalitis, and signs of general infection. Peripheral paresis, often asymmetric and more often in the legs than in the arms, is characteristic. Respiratory muscles can be affected. Improvement in muscle strength may occur for up to 2 years after the acute infection.

Several sets of criteria have been suggested for PPS. Those recently recommended by the European Federation of Neurological Societies are as follows: (1) a confirmed history of polio; (2) partial or fairly complete neurological and functional recovery after the acute episode; (3) a period of at least 15 years with neurological and functional stability; (4) two or more of the following health problems occurring after the stable period: extensive fatigue, muscle and/or joint pain, new muscle atrophy, functional loss, and cold intolerance; (5) gradual or abrupt onset of new neurogenic weakness; and (6) no other medical cause.

The most common symptoms are new weakness, fatigue, and pain. Fatigue is probably the most disabling symptom, both muscular and general. New weakness occurs most frequently in muscles known to have been involved in the acute phase, but can also involve muscles that were subclinically affected. New atrophy is required to fulfill the criteria for post-polio muscle atrophy. In a prospective study, muscle strength was found to be reduced by 1–2% per year in polio survivors, corresponding to the slow deterioration experienced by the patients.

Respiratory function is compromised in a minority of patients, usually in those with impaired ventilation in the acute phase. Respiratory complaints are common, as is subnormal ventilatory capacity. However, hypercapnia and sleep apnea due to previous polio are rare. Degenerative joint disease, skeletal deformities, inactivity osteoporosis, and fractures are common in polio survivors. Radiculopathy, entrapment neuropathies, and myelopathy may occur. Such disorders will contribute to the functional disability and can be difficult to distinguish from a true PPS. Life-long morbidity and mortality are slightly increased in polio patients compared to the non-polio population, especially in those with severe pareses.

Investigations

Exact information about the acute disease is helpful to confirm the polio diagnosis. Clinical neurophysiology is used to establish typical lower motor neuron involvement, to exclude non-polio causes, to find concomitant nerve or muscle disorders such as entrapment, and to assess the degree of motor neuron loss. Neurophysiological parameters cannot be used to define PPS. A thorough examination of respiratory function is often important. Muscle imaging may be helpful to detect abnormalities in subclinically affected muscles. In those with fatigue and loss of function, unrelated neurological and non-neurological disorders represent important differential diagnoses and need to be excluded. There is no specific test for the diagnosis of PPS.

Treatment

Two double blind and placebo-controlled studies showed a positive effect of intravenous immunoglobulin on PPS. The effect was modest, more on pain than on muscular weakness and fatigue. The long-term clinical effectiveness and cost effectiveness are unknown. Studies have shown no significant and confirmed effect of acetylcholinesterase inhibitors, lamotrigine, corticosteroids, amantadine, or modafinil. A Cochrane review published in 2011 found inadequate evidence from randomized and controlled studies for any treatment of post-polio, intravenous immunoglobulin, lamotrigine, muscle-strengthening exercises, and static magnetic fields being slightly promising.

Patients with PPS benefit from a management program, administered by the patient but including health professionals, and having a broad and long-term scope regarding health and function in society. This is probably more important for activities of daily living and social life than for muscle weakness. It has been claimed that muscle overuse and training may worsen the weakness in PPS, but this is unproven in prospective studies. On the contrary, patients with regular physical activity report fewer symptoms and a higher level of function than inactive patients. Significant improvement has been reported from muscle-training programs. Both isokinetic and isometric training are safe and effective in PPS. Periods of rest between exercises are important. Training and rehabilitation in a warm climate have been claimed to be beneficial. Use and adaptation of assistive devices are important. Orthoses, walking sticks, and a wheelchair may facilitate daily life. Weight control is important. Lifestyle modifications regarding work, physical activity, and diet should be discussed. Muscle weakness and chest deformities can lead to hypoventilation, especially during the night. Fatigue, somnolence, and morning headache are more indicative of hypoventilation than shortness of breath. Early introduction of non-invasive ventilatory support delays further decline. Joint and soft-tissue abnormalities should be treated, if necessary, by orthopedic intervention. Non-steroid antiinflammatory drugs may be helpful. Treatment by a multidisciplinary rehabilitation team is often advantageous.

Further reading

Farbu E, Gilhus NE, Barnes MP, *et al*. EFNS guideline on diagnosis and management of post-polio syndrome. *Eur J Neurol* 2006;13:795–801.

Farbu E, Rekand T, Vik-Mo E, *et al*. Postpolio syndrome patients treated with intravenous immunoglobulin: A double-blinded randomized controlled pilot study. *Eur J Neurol* 2007;14:60–65.

Gonzalez H, Sunnerhagen KS, Sjöberg I, *et al*. Intravenous immunoglobulin for post-polio syndrome: A randomized controlled trial. *Lancet Neurol* 2006;5:493–500.

Grimby G, Stålberg E, Sandberg A, Sunnerhagen KS. An 8-year longitudinal study of muscle strength, muscle fiber size, and dynamic electromyogram in individuals with late polio. *Muscle Nerve* 1998;21:1428–1437.

Halstead LS. A brief history of post-polio syndrome in the United States. *Arch Phys Med Rehabil* 2011;92:1344–1349.

Koopman FS, Uegaki K, Gilhus NE, *et al*. Treatment for postpolio syndrome. *Cochrane Database of Systematic Reviews* 2011, Issue 2. Art. No. CD002818 DOI:10.1002/1465 1858.

110   Limb-girdle muscular dystrophies

Anneke J. van der Kooi and Marianne de Visser
Department of Neurology, University of Amsterdam, Amsterdam, The Netherlands

The earliest cases of limb-girdle weakness are ascribed to Leyden and Möbius in 1876 and 1879, respectively. They described adult patients with a pelvic and femoral distribution of weakness and atrophy with a benign course. In 1884, Erb reported a juvenile form characterized by shoulder-girdle weakness and atrophy, with sparing of other muscles of the body and a more benign course than the condition described by Duchenne.

In 1954, the nosological entity of limb-girdle dystrophy was formally established by Walton and Nattrass, who described the disease as a progressive muscle weakness involving predominantly proximal muscles. They described the disease as having expression in both males and females; an age of onset predominantly in the late first or second decade, but sometimes later; variable rates of progression with severe disability within 20–30 years; and usually autosomal recessive, less frequently autosomal dominant inheritance; with muscular pseudohypertrophy and/or contractures uncommon. After the description by Walton and Nattrass, limb-girdle muscular dystrophy (LGMD) became a wastebasket designation. The classification of LGMD has been revolutionized by molecular genetic developments, starting with linkage studies in the 1990s.

Initially, autosomal recessive cases were found to be linked to chromosome 15q, and in autosomal dominant LGMD an association to chromosome 5q was identified. Subsequently other LGMD phenotypes were mapped to other chromosomes. These findings led to a new nomenclature designating autosomal dominant LGMD as LGMD1, and autosomal recessive LGMD as LGMD2. As each distinct gene locus was identified, it received a unique letter – the first dominant LGMD linked to chromosome 5 was termed LGMD1A, the next LGMD1B, and so on. In recessive LGMD the first gene locus was mapped to chromosome15q and designated LGMD2A, the next 2B, and so on. In the ensuing years it became evident that different genotypes can lead to the same phenotype, and that one genotype can cause different phenotypes. Therefore a new classification system is being considered.

Epidemiology

There are always some reservations about accepting figures about prevalence and incidence, because until not long ago diagnostic criteria were too imprecise for a reliable epidemiological study. In 1991, a world survey of population frequencies of inherited neuromuscular disorders was undertaken. The prevalence and incidence rates for mainly adult-onset cases of limb-girdle muscular dystrophies lie between 20 and 40 per million.

Autosomal recessive (Duchenne-like) limb-girdle muscular dystrophy appeared to be a rare disorder, with a prevalence of less than 5 per million. It is, however, more common in certain Arabic communities in North Africa, in Switzerland, in certain inbred communities in North America, and in Brazil. In the Netherlands a prevalence of 8.1 per million was calculated for all cases, and 5.7 per million for autosomal recessive and sporadic cases. Autosomal recessive LGMD (type 2) is more frequent than the dominant forms (LGMD1), the latter representing only about 10–15% of cases (Table 110.1). LGMD2A seems to be the most frequent type of LGMD worldwide, with a relative frequency of 12–33% (United States 12%, Netherlands 21%, Italy 25%, and Brazil 33%). The reported frequency of LGMD2B varies; it is believed to be rare in the Netherlands and other Western countries, but is reported to be as high as 18% in the United States, Italy, and Japan, and 33% in Brazil. The reported frequency of sarcoglycanopathies is 0–35%. LGMD2I was diagnosed in 8% of Dutch patients and 6.4% of Italian patients, whereas in the United Kingdom and Denmark it is considered a frequent cause of LGMD. LGMD2L was identified only recently; it constitutes 10–20% of the autosomal recessive patients. A duplication within exon 5 may be a founder mutation in northern Europe. LGMD2G, 2H, 2J, 2K, and 2M–2S are rare forms described predominantly in inbred families or specific areas of the world.

Pathophysiology

The muscle biopsy demonstrates a dystrophic pattern, which in itself is a rather non-specific pathological reaction of muscle. Various groups of LGMD-associated proteins can be described based on their localization in the muscle cell. These include proteins associated with the sarcolemma, the so-called dystrophin–glycoprotein complex (LGMD 2C-F). Most of the mutations in the genes encoding these proteins destabilize the whole complex at the membrane, resulting in an inability to counteract the mechanical stress generated by contractile activity. Other proteins have a role within the contractile apparatus of muscle, such as titin (LGMD2J) or myotilin (LGMD1A). Myotilin plays an indispensable role in the stabilization and anchorage of thin filaments, hence participating in the organization of the Z disc. Desmin, mutated in LGMD1E and 2R, is also connected to the Z band, and plays a role in the maintenance of structural and mechanical integrity. Mutations lead to abnormal assembly of intermediate filaments and desmin accumulation. Titin, mutated in LGMD2J, is present in the A band, and is associated with telethonin,

International Neurology, Second edition. Edited by Robert P. Lisak, Daniel D. Truong, William M. Carroll and Roongroj Bhidayasiri
© 2016 John Wiley & Sons, Ltd. Published 2016 by John Wiley & Sons, Ltd.

Table 110.1 Classification of limb-girdle muscular dystrophy (LGMD).

Subtype	Gene product	Gene localization	Characteristic feature	
Autosomal dominant				
1A	Myotilin	5q31	Dysarthria	
1B	Lamin A/C	1q21	Cardiac abnormalities	
1C	Caveolin-3	3p25	Childhood onset, rippling	
1D	DNAJB6	7q		
1E	Desmin	6q23	Cardiomyopathy	
1F	Transportin-3	7q32		
1G	HNRPDL	4q21	Limited flexion of fingers and toes	
1H		3p23		
Autosomal recessive				
2A	Calpain-3	15q15	Scapular winging	
2B	Dysferlin	2p12	Little shoulder girdle	involvement, calf involvement
2C	γ-Sarcoglycan	13q12	Scapular winging, calf	hypertrophy
2D	α-Sarcoglycan	17q21	Scapular winging, calf	hypertrophy
2E	β-Sarcoglycan	4q12	Scapular winging, calf	hypertrophy
2F	δ-Sarcoglycan	5q33	Scapular winging, calf	hypertrophy
2G	Telethonin	17q11-12	Including anterior distal weakness,	rimmed vacuoles
2H	TRIM32	9q31-q33	Slowly progressive	
2I	FKRP	19q13.3	Calf hypertrophy, dilated	cardiomyopathy
2J	Titin	2q31	Anterior tibial wasting	
2K	POMT1	9q34	Mental retardation	
2L	Anoctamin-5	11p13	Quadriceps atrophy, asymmetry	
2M	Fukutin	9q31		
2N	POMT2	19q13	Calf hypertrophy, scapular winging	
2O	POMGnT1	1p32		
2P	DAG1	3p21		
2Q	Plectin	8q24		
2R	Desmin	2q35	Scapular winging, cardiomyopathy	
2S	TRAPPC1	4q35	Kyperkinetic movements, ataxia, mental retardation	

2T - (Mannose-1-phosphate 3 guanyltransferase beta GMPPB - 3p21

2U - Isoprenoid synthase domain containing (ISPD) - 7p21

mutated in LGMD2G. Another group of proteins mutated in LGMD include proteins with various enzymatic functions, such as calpain-3 (LGMD2A), a muscle-specific calcium-dependent protease. It is localized in the sarcomere and the nucleus and potentially involved in the regulation of sarcomere plasticity. Other proteins are involved in glycosylation; that is, fukutin-related protein (LGMD2I) and rarely POMT1 (LGMD2K), fukutin (LGMD2M), POMT2 (LGMD2N), POMGnT1 (LGMD2O), and DAG1 (LGMD2P). In LGMD2B dysferlin is located at the plasma membrane and may be involved in membrane fusion or repair. Caveolin-3, the causative gene of LGMD1C, is a transmembrane protein implicated in signal transduction. In LGMD1B there is involvement of a protein of the inner nuclear membrane, lamin A/C, which provides a framework for the nuclear envelope and may interact with chromatin. Lamin A/C deficiency is therefore associated not only with LGMD1B, but with a variety of phenotypes. This also holds true for other LGMD subtypes including LGMD1A, 1C, and 2B. Another nuclear protein, transportin 3 (LGMD1F), transports serine/arginine-rich proteins into the nucleus. The recently discovered LGMD1D is caused by DNAJB6 mutation, a chaperone-related protein disorder. It protects client proteins from irreversible aggregation. In LGMD2G, heterogeneous nuclear ribonucleoprotein D-like protein (HNRNPDL; HN-RPDL) participates in splicing of specific exons in pre-mRNA transcripts. In LGMD2S the transport (trafficking) protein particle complex (TRAPPC11) is involved in endoplasmic reticulum to Golgi vesicle trafficking (ERGIC). The GMPPB protein, affected in LGMD2T, catalyzes formation of GDP-mannose from mannose-1-phosphate & GTP. GDP-mannose is required in 4 glycosylation pathways. ISPD protein Mutations in ISPD involved in LGMD2U impair protein O-mannosylation, which is the first step in synthesis of laminin binding glycan. Novel proteins with various functions are still coming to light, promising to uncover shared pathways that may lead to muscular dystrophy.

Clinical features

LGMDs are a heterogeneous group of disorders characterized by progressive, usually rather symmetric weakness and atrophy of the proximal limb muscles. Asymmetric weakness has been described in LGMD2J and 2L. Involvement of the distal muscles may also occur. Symptoms commonly begin during the first two decades of life, in autosomal recessive LGMD predominantly in childhood, and age of onset may vary both between and within subtypes and even between patients with the same mutation. In LGMD2L men appear to be more severely affected than females. Symptoms gradually worsen, resulting in loss of ambulation 10 or 20 years after onset. Some patients with sarcoglycanopathies, LGMD1B, and with mutations in proteins involving glycosylation may be as severely affected as patients with Duchenne muscular dystrophy. Asymptomatic mutation carriers have been described in LGMD2A, LGMD2B, 2D, 2L, and LGMD1G.

Some of the subtypes of LGMD show specific clinical features. Muscle hypertrophy can be observed quite frequently in caveolinopathy (LGMD1C), sarcoglycanopathies (LGMD2C-F), and LGMD2I (Figure 110.1). Calf hypertrophy is the most common, but other limb muscles and the tongue may also be hypertrophic. Scapular winging is most characteristically seen in LGMD2A and 2C-F. Spinal rigidity, scoliosis, limb contractures, and rippling should be asked about and looked for. Early contractures are not common in LGMD1B, and may occur in a subtype of LGMD2A. Limited flexion of fingers and toes is seen in LGMD2G. Spinal rigidity is often a feature in LGMD1B, LGMD2M, and occasionally in LGMD2A. Scoliosis is most often seen in the early-onset LGMDs, such as LGMD2C-F, particularly when wheelchair dependency occurs. Rippling muscles can be seen in LGMD1C. Intellectual impairment and facial weakness are not frequent, albeit mental retardation is part of the spectrum in LGMD2K and LGMD2P. In LGMD2S hyperkinetic movements, due to central nervous system (CNS) involvement, and hip dysplasia can be present. Dysphagia can occur in some patients with LGMD1D. Myoglobinuria is not uncommon in LGMD2I and LGMD2L.

Cardiac involvement is common in LGMD1A, 1B, LGMD1E, 2C-F, 2G, and 2I. In LGMD1B and 1E rhythm and conduction disturbances are predominantly found, whereas in the other forms dilated cardiomyopathy is part of the clinical spectrum. Respiratory muscle weakness does not necessarily accompany cardiac impairment, and is seen most often in LGMD 2C-F and 2I.

Prognosis for LGMD is not uniform and thus timely intervention through identification of potential complications may improve survival. Nearly 70% of patients are still ambulatory at 40 years of age.

Investigations

Serum creatine kinase (sCK) activity is usually markedly elevated in LGMD2 forms and normal to moderately elevated in LGMD1 types.

Neurophysiological studies are of little value in diagnosing LGMD; electromyography (EMG) usually shows a myopathic pattern.

Muscle magnetic resonance imaging or computed tomography can detect patterns of muscle involvement, which may not be pathognomonic but can be of help in guiding the genetic analysis.

Muscle biopsies usually show a non-specific or dystrophic pattern, consisting of variation in the size of muscle fibers, signs of degeneration and regeneration, increase in the number of fibers with internal nuclei, and increase in endomysial connective tissue. In some LGMDs, such as dysferlinopathy, sarcoglycanopathies, and calpainopathy, lymphocytic mononuclear inflammatory cells can be seen. Rimmed vacuoles are observed in LGMD1A, 1D, and 2J. Immunohistochemical staining for sarcoglycans, caveolin, myotilin, desmin, and α-dystroglycan, and immunobiochemical analysis of calpain-3 and dysferlin in muscle tissue, can be useful to direct genetic analysis specifically to the underlying genetic defect.

A definitive diagnosis is made by molecular identification of the specific abnormal gene or protein product. Specific clinical characteristics (see Table 110.1) can sometimes help to differentiate among the LGMDs, but for a precise diagnosis molecular identification

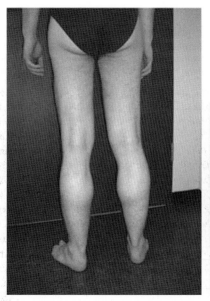
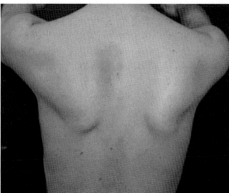

Figure 110.1 Patient with LGMD2I showing firm calves and scapulae alatae.

is required. To date, a classifying diagnosis can be made in approximately 75% of patients and families.

Awareness of symptoms of respiratory insufficiency such as frequent chest infections, morning headache, and daytime somnolence is important. Measurements of sitting and supine forced vital capacity (FVC) can be done at the outpatient clinic. If the FVC is <50%, frequent monitoring is required. In case of symptoms or signs of night-time hypoventilation, overnight pulse oximetry is recommended. Serial monitoring of cardiac function, using electrocardiography (ECG), Holter monitoring, and echocardiography, is advised in patients at risk for developing cardiac involvement.

Differential diagnosis

As already mentioned, a large number of disorders present with weakness in a limb-girdle distribution. "Red flags" include ptosis, extra-ocular muscle weakness, facial involvement, or predominantly distal muscle weakness. Skin rash, sensory symptoms, or progression in weeks or months also suggest a diagnosis other than LGMD.

Metabolic myopathies such as mitochondrial disorders, glycogen storage diseases, and disorders of lipid metabolism can be readily differentiated from LGMD by histological, enzyme-histochemical, and biochemical investigation of a muscle biopsy specimen. If hereditary spinal muscular atrophy (SMA) is in the differential diagnosis, SMN gene screening should be performed. Dystrophinopathies such as Duchenne (DMD), Becker (BMD), and carriers of these disorders are identified by dystrophin analysis and DNA-Xp21 screening. Distinction from inflammatory myopathies and in particular necrotizing autoimmune myopathy may be cumbersome, albeit the latter has subacute onset. Facioscapulohumeral muscular dystrophy is inherited as an autosomal dominant trait and has characteristic early involvement of facial muscles, but there are patients in whom facial weakness is absent. It can be diagnosed by showing a deletion at the telomere of chromosome 4q. Congenital muscular dystrophy (CMD) differs from LGMD by the occurrence of hypotonia or generalized muscle weakness, often associated with joint contractures. Bethlem myopathy, caused by collagen mutations, is characterized by congenital contractures, but hyperlaxity and skin abnormalities are frequently part of the spectrum. X-linked Emery–Dreifuss muscular dystrophy (EDMD) is characterized by scapulohumeral–peroneal distribution of weakness. It can be diagnosed by the absence of emerin on immunohistochemical stain, and mutation analysis of the emerin (STA) gene.

Proximal myotonic myopathy or myotonic dystrophy type 2 (PROMM or DM2) usually starts in the third or fourth decade. Myotonia is present in 75% of patients on clinical or EMG examination. Associated features are cataracts and cardiac abnormalities.

Congenital myasthenia, with mutations in DOK7, ALG2, and ALG12, can also present as a limb-girdle syndrome without fluctuating weakness. Repetitive nerve stimulation shows decrement, and muscle biopsy may show tubular aggregates.

Treatment

There is no proven treatment to cure or significantly delay the disease progression for any of the LGMDs. Several experimental treatments have reached preclinical proof-of-principle tests in rodent models at the level of gene, cell, and pharmacological therapies, especially for the autosomal recessive forms of LGMD. Creatine monohydrate has been shown to have a modest effect on muscle strength. Corticosteroids have been used empirically in some sarcoglycanopathy patients. Treatment of heart failure is undertaken on general principles, with early use of angiotensin-converting enzyme inhibitors and beta blockers. In laminopathies and desminopathies, implantable defibrillators are used to prevent sudden cardiac death. Annual influenza vaccination and prompt treatment of respiratory infections are recommended. Nocturnal home ventilation can be instituted in the case of nocturnal respiratory insufficiency.

Genetic counseling is advised when patients have concern for themselves, relatives, or descendants. Delineation of the LGMD subtype allows knowledge of its autosomal recessive or autosomal dominant pattern to inform genetic counseling appropriately.

A number of the principles of general care for patients with DMD also apply to LGMDs. Supportive treatment remains the standard for now. Prevention of contracture development is important in maximizing functional ability. Ideally, this treatment can be provided by a multidisciplinary team approach, including clinical neuromyologists, physical and occupational therapists, orthopedists for management of contractures and scoliosis, pulmonologists for respiratory complications that may cause nocturnal hypoventilation and eventually require ventilator assistance, cardiologists for assessing cardiac abnormalities and treating of cardiomyopathy, social workers to help with employment opportunities, psychologists to help patients adjust to their environment, and geneticists for genetic counseling. Patients should be advised to join patient support groups.

Further reading

Lo HP, Cooper ST, Evesson FJ, et al. Limb–girdle muscular dystrophy: Diagnostic evaluation, frequency and clues to pathogenesis. *Neuromusc Disord* 2008;18:34–44.

Norwood F, de Visser M, Eymard B, et al.; members of EFNS Guideline Task Force. EFNS guideline on diagnosis and management of limb girdle muscular dystrophies. *Eur J Neurol* 2007;14:1305–1312.

ten Dam L, van der Kooi AJ, van Wattingen M, de Haan RJ, de Visser M. Reliability and accuracy of skeletal muscle imaging in limb-girdle muscular dystrophies. *Neurology* 2012;79:1716–1723.

111 Dystrophinopathies

Chiara S. M. Straathof[1] and Marianne de Visser[2]

[1] Department of Neurology, Leiden University Medical Center, Leiden, The Netherlands
[2] Department of Neurology, University of Amsterdam, Amsterdam, The Netherlands

Dystrophinopathies are inherited in an X-linked recessive pattern and can be distinguished in two classic phenotypes, Duchenne muscular dystrophy (DMD) and Becker muscular dystrophy (BMD). Both disorders manifest with progressive muscle weakness and wasting, which first affects the pelvic girdle and lower limbs and subsequently the shoulder girdle, upper limbs, and respiratory muscles. Pseudohypertrophy of the calf muscles is invariably present in the early stages of the disease and hence formerly the appellation was "pseudohypertrophic muscular dystrophy." Historically, the clinical difference between BMD and DMD was defined by the rate of progression of the muscle weakness. Early natural history studies reported that in general boys with DMD would become wheelchair bound before the age of 13, whereas in boys with BMD ambulation should be preserved at the age of 16 years.

DMD was described in the nineteenth century, first by the English physician Edward Meryon and later by the renowned French neurologist Guillaume Duchenne de Boulogne. The former reported a familial trait of the disease with only males being affected, and he described the pathological substrate for the paralysis in skeletal muscle derived from autopsy: "the striped elementary primitive fibres were found to be completely destroyed, the sarcous element being diffused, and in many places converted into oil globules and granular matter, whilst the sarcolemma or tunic of the elementary fibre was broken down and destroyed." Duchenne was able to obtain muscle specimens in life by means of a needle harpoon and he observed different pathological stages of the disease.

BMD was first described by Kostakow in 1937, and recognized as a novel X-linked muscular dystrophy distinct from Duchenne muscular dystrophy by the German neurologist and geneticist Peter E. Becker and the psychologist Franz Kiener in 1955. They provided detailed clinical descriptions of affected males with an X-linked inheritance pattern among multiple generations within large families; the age of onset was between 12 and 25 years with slowly progressive proximal weakness in the lower limbs associated with calf hypertrophy. The arm muscles were involved approximately 5–10 years later.

Epidemiology

The estimated worldwide prevalence of DMD among males is 4.78 per 100,000 males (95% confidence interval [CI] 1.94–11.81) and the prevalence of BMD is 1.53 per 100,000 males (95% CI 0.26–8.94).

Studies on the incidence of DMD mainly concerned Caucasian populations; the incidence ranges from 10.7–27.8 per 100,000 live-born males. The estimated birth incidence of BMD is about one-third to one-fifth of the incidence of DMD, but the disorder may be underdiagnosed. BMD seems to be more difficult to recognize since only 50% were diagnosed at the age of 15 years and 90% at age 35. Rarely, in BMD, progressive weakness presents in the third until even the sixth decade.

Pathophysiology

Since the identification of the protein dystrophin in 1987, impaired dystrophin synthesis can be assessed by means of immunological investigation of muscle tissue, which enables a dystrophinopathy to be distinguished from limb-girdle dystrophies, and DMD from BMD. In DMD dystrophin is virtually absent and in BMD dystrophin is present but in a decreased amount and/or in altered size. Genetically, DMD and BMD are allelic on the X chromosome and are caused by a mutation in the *DMD* gene, which is the largest human gene, consisting of 79 exons. Approximately 60% of patients have a deletion of one of more exons, and in 5–10% of BMD/DMD patients duplications are found. Besides large rearrangements in the gene, approximately 10% of patients have a small mutation that results in a premature stop of transcription (nonsense mutations), truncating frameshifts, amino acid substitutions (missense and neutral mutations), or affects splicing.

The reading frame hypothesis explains that in DMD the mutations are out of frame, resulting in an early stop of transcription and a protein that is not functional. The mutations in BMD are usually in frame, leading to an altered but still functioning dystrophin. Rarely, exceptions to the reading frame hypothesis are described, including patients with a BMD phenotype but a frame-shift mutation, or patients with DMD with in frame deletions or duplications.

The dystrophin–glycoprotein complex (DGC) is composed of several transmembrane and peripheral components and is highly expressed in the sarcolemma of skeletal muscle. Dystroglycan is a protein central to this complex that spans the sarcolemma and binds to ligands in the surrounding basal lamina through α-dystroglycan and to dystrophin inside the cell through β-dystroglycan. Dystrophin in turn binds to the submembrane actin and intermediate filament cytoskeleton within fibers, thereby completing a link between the cytoskeleton and the extracellular matrix. The function for dystrophin and the dystrophin–glycoprotein complex, at least partially, is in protecting the sarcolemma during muscle contraction. In its absence, the sarcolemma is more susceptible to damage by contractile forces, resulting in increased permeability

International Neurology, Second edition. Edited by Robert P. Lisak, Daniel D. Truong, William M. Carroll and Roongroj Bhidayasiri
© 2016 John Wiley & Sons, Ltd. Published 2016 by John Wiley & Sons, Ltd.

of ions and small molecules, and eventual cell necrosis and muscle degeneration.

Clinical features

Duchenne muscular dystrophy

The mean age at which first symptoms of DMD are noticed is 2.5 years (standard deviation [SD] 1.4, range 0.2–6.1 years). The boys often have an unsteady waddling gait with tiptoe walking. One-third of the boys start to walk after 19 months, but in general all DMD patients will be able to walk before the age of 3 years. Firm calves may be an early sign for the clinician; this is an expression of early involvement of the calf muscles that will become weak and infiltrated by fat. Also the Gowers' sign, in which the child uses his arms climbing up his legs when he rises from sitting on the floor to the standing position, is an important early sign of weakness in proximal leg muscles. Although muscle strength usually improves in toddlers with DMD, they will not be able to run. Following a plateau phase, which is usually reached at age 4–8 years, muscle weakness progresses relentlessly, not only in the upper leg muscles but also in the lower legs, and subsequently the proximal arm and neck muscles. Despite the early symptoms, the reported mean age at diagnosis was around 4.9 years.

All boys will lose ambulation in or before adolescence. In puberty when they grow they are at risk of developing scoliosis due to weakness of the paraspinal muscles. At a later stage of the disease respiratory muscles become weak, resulting in reduced vital capacity. Often the first sign is nocturnal hypoventilation and hypercapnia. Until the introduction of assisted ventilation, most patients died between 15 and 20 years of age in respiratory failure. Life span has increased by 10 years since the introduction of ventilatory support. Cardiac involvement is ultimately present in all patients and is often not symptomatic. Degeneration of cardiac muscle fibers may lead to rhythm disturbances and dilated cardiomyopathy.

The prevalence of cognitive deficit is higher in DMD, with a mean full-scale IQ 1 SD below the normal population. Approximately 30% of boys with DMD have mental retardation, with an IQ <70. In addition, learning problems, especially with reading and spelling, occur more frequently. Behavioral disorders such as attention deficit hyperactivity disorder (ADHD), autism spectrum disorder, and obsessive-compulsive disorder are more prevalent.

Becker muscular dystrophy

In BMD muscle symptoms and signs are more heterogeneous than in DMD, ranging from very mild, such as exercise-induced myalgia or cramps, to severe progressive muscle weakness in the upper legs. Weakness and wasting of the quadriceps femoris muscles can be the only sign for a long time. In some patients the only sign is pseudohypertrophy of the calves, due to fat replacement; however, this is not a specific sign and may be lacking. Usually at a later stage the upper limbs become affected as well. Cardiac involvement that is similar to that in DMD is also frequent and ultimately present in all BMD patients.

As in DMD, a positive family history of X-linked inheritance may be helpful for the diagnosis. However, in patients with a new (de novo) mutation the patient will be interpreted as a sporadic case. Notably, in sporadic cases with a limb-girdle distribution of muscle weakness the differential diagnosis should at least include limb-girdle muscular dystrophies (LGMDs), spinal muscular atrophy (SMA), or Pompe disease (see Table 111.1).

Female carriers of dystrophinopathy

In two-thirds of patients with dystrophinopathy the mutation has been transmitted by the mother, who is the carrier. If the mother carries a mutation in the *DMD* gene her sisters and daughters have a 50% risk of carrying the same mutation and so transmitting the mutation to their offspring.

Table 111.1 Differential diagnosis of limb-girdle muscular dystrophy.

Disorder	Pattern of inheritance	Gene
Limb-girdle muscular dystrophies		
LGMD 1B/Emery–Dreifuss muscular dystrophy	AD	lamin A/C
LGMD 1C	AD	caveolin-3
LGMD 2A	AR	calpain-3
LGMD 2B	AR	dysferlin
LGMD 2C-F (sarcoglycanopathies)	AR	SGCG/SGCA/ SGCD/SGCB
LGMD 2I	AR	fukutin-related protein
LGMD 2K (associated with mental retardation)	AR	POMT1
LGMD 2L	AR	anoctamin-5
LGMD 2M	AR	fukutin
Facioscapulohumeral dystrophy	AD	D4Z4 repeat retraction
Bethlem myopathy	AD	COL6
Myofibrillar myopathies	AD	several genes
Proximal myotonic dystrophy (DM2)	AD	ZNF9
Mitochondrial myopathies	AD/AR	several genes
Congenital muscular dystrophies (CMD)		
Merosin deficient muscular dystrophy	AR	laminin α2
CMD with rigid spine	AR	SEPN1
Glycogen storage disorders	AR	several genes
Acid maltase deficiency (Pompe disease)	AR	acid α-1,4-glucosidase
Limb-girdle myasthenia gravis	AR	Dok-7
Hereditary spinal muscular atrophies		
Proximal SMA with dominant inheritance and late adult onset (Finkel type)	AD	VAPB
Bulbo-spinal muscular atrophy (Kennedy syndrome)	X-linked	androgen receptor
Spinal muscular atrophy with lower limb predominance	AD	DYNC1H1
Early-onset spinal muscular atrophy with contractures	AD	BICD2
Idiopathic inflammatory myopathies	acquired	
Necrotizing autoimmune myopathy		
Dermatomyositis		
Polymyositis		

AD = autosomal dominant; AR = autosomal recessive

In one-third the dystrophinopathy is due to a *de novo* mutation in the affected male. In this case the mother is not a carrier somatically, but she may have germ line mosaicism, with about 9% recurrence risk in a subsequent pregnancy.

Female carriers may be asymptomatic, but about one-quarter have muscle symptoms like myalgia, hyperCKemia, and muscle weakness, and a small proportion have overt cardiomyopathy.

Investigations

Serum creatine kinase (CK) activity is invariably elevated, in DMD usually more than ten-fold the upper limit of normal, especially in the early stages of the disease and diminishing over the years. In BMD CK is usually more than five times elevated. BMD may present with hyperCKemia without clinical symptoms. Electromyography usually does not contribute to the diagnosis, especially not if CK is more than ten times elevated.

Needle or open muscle biopsy is mostly performed in the diagnostic work-up of sporadic patients, especially when there is a differential diagnosis, for example in a male patient with progressive limb-girdle muscle weakness and an elevated CK. Morphological changes include an abnormal variation in muscle fiber size due to atrophic and hypertrophic fibers, focal necrosis and regeneration, and extensive endomysial fat and connective tissue. In BMD the histopathological changes in muscle specimen are similar to those found in DMD. Based on histopathological features alone, BMD cannot be distinguished from DMD. For diagnostic confirmation immunohistochemistry with antibodies raised against different parts of dystrophin is used as a qualitative measure for dystrophin in muscle tissue.

In DMD dystrophin will be absent, although sometimes a minority of the fibers will stain positive. These so-called revertant fibers are explained by recovery of the reading frame through alternative splicing or multiple exon skipping.

In BMD muscle immunohistochemistry may show that dystrophin is distributed normally but globally reduced, or that the staining is discontinuous with either a normal or reduced intensity. However, often this test is not sufficient to confirm the diagnosis of BMD. Western blot analysis, which is a semi-quantitative measurement of dystrophin, can detect abnormal amounts of dystrophin and/or dystrophin with a different molecular weight. A smaller dystrophin may be caused by deletions of one or more exons or by small mutations and a larger size is found in case of duplications of one of more exons.

For genetic classification DNA analysis is needed to elucidate the mutation; the first step is screening for deletion or duplications, for which nowadays multiple ligation-dependant probe amplification (MLPA) is an accurate method. In patients suspected to have a dystrophinopathy in whom no deletion or duplication is found, subsequent sequencing techniques should be performed to search for small mutations. In 2–5% of symptomatic cases with DMD no mutation will be detected, due to mutations in the promoter area or to deep intronic mutations that may affect splicing. Finally, RNA studies can be performed on muscle tissue to give information about the status of the mutation.

Treatment

Targeted treatments aim to restore dystrophin production in DMD. Antisense oligonucleotides (AONs), which induce specific exon skipping during messenger RNA splicing and thus result in correction of the open reading frame, have been shown to restore dystrophin expression in DMD patients when administered locally into the muscle. Systemic delivery of the AON that skips exon 51 was the first AON put on clinical trial. Although the results of the different randomized trials seem conflicting as not all have reached the clinical endpoints, extended non-controlled studies with exon 51 skipping show treatment for >1 year results in stable motor function in ambulant boys with DMD. Clinical trials with other AONs are ongoing.

For about 13% of DMD patients who have a specific (nonsense) mutation that results in a premature stop in the production of normal dystrophin, a treatment has been developed that repairs the effect of premature stop codons, but does not affect normal stop codons; this enables dystrophin expression in DMD boys with nonsense mutations. Preliminary results seem promising and further data should prove that the effect is consistent.

Non-specific treatments do not depend on the genetic mutation and aim to delay the progression of muscle weakness. Meta-analysis has shown that steroid treatment extends the ambulant phase in DMD by 1–2 years. Different regimens are used such as deflazacort 0.9 mg/kg/day or prednisolone 0.75 mg/kg in either daily dosage or intermittently 10 days on, 10 days off, which is thought to have lesser side effects. A randomized controlled trial with head-to-head comparison has started to search for the optimum regimen. In BMD no studies on steroid treatment have been performed.

A multidisciplinary approach is advised and standards of care are proposed for rehabilitation and neuromuscular, respiratory, cardiac, orthopedic, nutritional, and psychosocial aspects of care.

Further reading

Bushby K, Finkel R, Birnkrant DJ, *et al.* Diagnosis and management of Duchenne muscular dystrophy, part 1: Diagnosis, and pharmacological and psychosocial management. *Lancet Neurol* 2010;9:77–93.

Cotton SM, Voudouris NJ, Greenwood KM. Association between intellectual functioning and age in children and young adults with Duchenne muscular dystrophy: Further results from a meta-analysis. *Dev Med Child Neurol* 2005;47:257–265.

Eagle M, Baudouin SV, Chandler C, *et al.* Survival in Duchenne muscular dystrophy: Improvements in life expectancy since 1967 and the impact of home nocturnal ventilation. *Neuromuscul Disord* 2002;12:926–929.

Ginjaar HB, den Dunnen JT, Bakker E. DMD and BMD: Diagnostic principles. In: Chamberlain JRT (ed.). *Duchenne Muscular Dystrophy: Advances in Therapeutics.* New York: Taylor & Francis Group; 2006:77–90.

Manzur AY, Kuntzer T, Pike M, Swan A. Glucocorticoid corticosteroids for Duchenne muscular dystrophy. *Cochrane Database Syst Rev* CD003725, 2008.

Verhaart IE, Aartsma-Rus A. Gene therapy for Duchenne muscular dystrophy. *Curr Opin Neurol* 2012;25:588–596.

112 Facioscapulohumeral muscular dystrophy

George W. Padberg

Department of Neurology, Radboud University Medical Center, Nijmegen, The Netherlands

Facioscapulohumeral muscular dystrophy (FSHD) is an autosomal dominant myopathy with a high mutation rate (~10% of all gene carriers, up to 40% of mitotic origin) that is causally related to the transcription of DUX4 at the D4Z4 locus on chromosome 4q35.

Epidemiology

FSHD is probably the most common neuromuscular disorder, with an estimated prevalence of 12/100,000 in Caucasians. This figure does not include asymptomatic cases, which constitute approximately 30% of all gene carriers in completely examined pedigrees. Taking these mildly affected persons into account as well, the prevalence of clinically recognizable FSHD patients would amount to at least 1/5,600.

Mean onset of the disease is in the second decade, with a large variation from childhood to late adulthood.

Pathophysiology

Over the last couple of years research has resulted in a coherent, although incomplete model of the pathogenesis of FSHD. The disease is caused by a loss of epigenetic repression of the D4Z4 repeat array on chromosome 4q35. This results in a variegated and burst-like transcription of the DUX4 retrogene. DUX4 is a transcription factor with a double homeobox motif and downstream target genes that can be grouped in clusters involved in apoptosis, inflammatory immune responses, and muscle cell regeneration and differentiation. DUX4 can only be transcribed from the last repeat of the array if the telomeric region contains a polyadenylation signal (PAS) necessary to stabilize the transcript. This PAS is present on 4qA alleles and absent on 4qB alleles, which occur in equal frequencies in the normal population. Chromosome 10 contains an almost identical repeat array, but lacks a PAS and therefore a stable transcript. The similarities of the arrays on 4q and 10q were responsible for the many challenges of the FSHD research.

Epigenetic derepression of D4Z4 is characterized by hypomethylation of the repeat and histone modifications. The resulting chromatin relaxation can be brought about by reduction of the number of repeats from 11–150 to 1–10. This leads to FSHD1 and is responsible for 95% of all FSHD cases. The mechanism of repeat reduction appears to be intrachromosomal gene conversion without crossover in the majority of cases.

FSHD2, clinically indistinguishable from FSHD1, is caused by mutations in SMCHD1 (structural maintenance of chromosome hinge domain containing 1 gene) and constitutes about 4% of FSHD patients. Mutations in this gene lead to frequently quite severe hypomethylation of the repeat, suggesting a dominant negative mechanism rather than haploinsufficiency. For the remaining 1–2% of FSHD patients the gene(s) is not known. Details of the derepression machinery, other transcripts of the repeat and their function, and the pathways of downstream genes leading to the weak muscles in their characteristic pattern have yet to be worked out.

Clinical features

FSHD most likely manifests itself first with – often asymmetric (50%) – facial weakness, which frequently goes unrecognized. Initial complaints are usually due to shoulder muscle weakness (80%), while those caused by ankle dorsiflexor (10%), pelvic girdle (5%), and facial (5%) muscle weakness are less commonly mentioned. On clinical examination almost invariably shoulder girdle weakness is present, which is often asymmetric. A proportion of gene carriers do not progress beyond this. At age 60 approximately two-thirds of all gene carriers have developed ankle dorsiflexor weakness and 50% pelvic girdle weakness. At this age 20% of patients are wheelchair dependent outdoors. Females tend to have a milder course.

Dysphagia and dysarthria are rare features; lingual hypoplasia and facial immobility have been reported in severe cases. Respiratory function is related to the severity of the disease, but less than 1% of patients require ventilatory support. Cardiac muscle involvement has been debated for a long time; conduction defects such as right bundle branch block occur slightly more frequently than in the normal population. Muscle pain (50–80%) and fatigue (35–60%) are neglected symptoms in the older literature. Contractures are rare, with the exception of ankle contractures. Pectus excavatum is, because of its frequency (5%), part of the disease spectrum.

Subclinical high-tone hearing loss (75%) and retinal vasculopathy with telangiectasis (60%) only rarely lead to deafness or visual loss, except in the infantile form (onset before age 10 years). The latter represents the more severe end of the clinical spectrum, often with marked facial weakness and early wheelchair dependency. In Japan this form appears to be associated with mental retardation and epilepsy; recently other studies have corroborated the presence of central nervous system involvement in FSHD.

Investigations

Serum creatine kinase (CK) activity usually is mildly elevated in active disease, but as a rule not more than five times the upper limit of normal. Electromyography (EMG) is not specific and occasionally neurogenic features can be found. Muscle biopsies of clinically unaffected muscles might show no abnormalities. Mild changes are

International Neurology, Second edition. Edited by Robert P. Lisak, Daniel D. Truong, William M. Carroll and Roongroj Bhidayasiri
© 2016 John Wiley & Sons, Ltd. Published 2016 by John Wiley & Sons, Ltd.

variation in fiber diameter, some fiber hypertrophy, minimal fibrosis, central nucleation, and moth-eaten fibers. Frequently endomysial and perivascular inflammatory infiltrates can be found, characterized by CD8+ and CD4+ T-cells, respectively. These infiltrates have been correlated with turbo inversion recovery magnitude (TIRM) positive T2-weighted magnetic resonance (MR) images of muscles and the infiltrates have been suggested to be the initiatory mechanism of the morphological changes of the muscle pathology, leading to progressive fatty infiltration and loss of myofibers. As the fat infiltration of the muscles can be quantified and apparently can show significant changes over a 4-month period, MRI might serve as a surrogate marker for disease progression.

Experience with imaging has demonstrated preclinical involvement of the hamstrings, confirmed the often very asymmetric muscle involvement, and led to the recognition of FSHD as a predominant axial/truncal myopathy responsible for the characteristic shoulder girdle weakness, abdominal muscle weakness, hyperlordosis, and occasional dropped head and camptocormia.

The diagnosis of FSHD might not require a muscle biopsy, but otherwise needs genetic confirmation. The D4Z4 reduction at an A-type allele can be safely demonstrated in almost all cases; demonstration of hypomethylation of the repeat and SMCHD1 mutations is at present probably limited to specialized laboratories.

Treatment

No disease-modifying therapies are available. Prednisone, albuterol, and creatine appeared not to be beneficial. Calcium-entry blockers and folic acid have been tested in pilot studies. In a small study aerobic training was found to have a moderate effect on muscle condition, which was confirmed in a recent study where both aerobic training and cognitive therapy had a significant positive effect on muscle fatigue and slowed progression of fatty infiltration, demonstrated by MRI. Other therapeutic strategies being investigated in the model system include PAS knock-out, D4Z4 knock-out, restoring epigenetic repression of D4Z4, interfering with DUX4 mRNA, blocking the DUX4 protein, and targeting downstream genes and proteins.

Further reading

Deenen JCW, Hisse A, van der Maarel S, *et al.* Population-based incidence and prevalence of FSHD. *Neurology* 2014;83:1–4.

Janssen BH, Voet NBM, Nabuurs CI, *et al.* Distinct disease phases in muscles of FSHD patients identified by MR detected fat infiltration. *PlosONE* 2014;9:e85416.

Tasca G, Pescatori M, Monforte M, *et al.* Different molecular signatures in MRI-staged FSHD muscles. *PlosONE* 2012;7:e38779.

Tawil R, van der Maarel S, Tapscott SJ. FSHD: The path to consensus on pathophysiology. *Skeletal Muscle* 2014;4:12–27.

113 Myotonic dystrophies

Giovanni Meola[1,2] and Rosanna Cardani[2]

[1] Department of Biomedical Sciences for Health, University of Milan, Milan, Italy
[2] Laboratory of Muscle Histopathology and Molecular Biology, IRCCS Policlinico San Donato, Milan, Italy

Myotonic dystrophy, also known as dystrophia myotonica, myotonia atrophica, and Steinert disease, is abbreviated as DM according to the International Myotonic Dystrophy Consortium (IDMC). Because of the genetic and phenotypic heterogeneity in this group of disorders, this disease is now called myotonic dystrophies. DM are autosomal dominantly inherited multisystemic diseases with a core pattern of clinical presentation including muscle weakness, myotonia, and distinctive abnormalities of other organ systems. To date two distinct forms caused by repeat expansions have been identified: myotonic dystrophy type 1 (DM1, Steinert's disease) and myotonic dystrophy type 2 (DM2).

Epidemiology

Myotonic dystrophy type 1 is the most common inherited muscular dystrophy in adults, with an estimated prevalence of 1/8,000 in most American and European populations. The highest prevalence was found in the Quebec province of Canada (189/100,000), while it is less common in South East Asia and rare in South and Central (sub-Saharan) Africa.

The prevalence of DM2 is not well established, but is estimated to be similar to DM1 in Eastern European populations.

Pathophysiology

DM1 is caused by an expansion of an unstable CTG trinucleotide repeat in the 3′ untranslated region (UTR) of the myotonic dystrophy protein kinase (*DMPK*) gene on chromosome 19q13.32, while DM2 is caused by an unstable tetranucleotide repeat expansion, CCTG, in intron 1 of the CCHC-type zinc finger nucleic acid-binding protein (*CNBP*) gene (previously known as zinc finger 9 gene, *ZNF9*) on chromosome 3q21.3. The transcription of the expanded allele produces mutant RNA that contains unusually long tracts of CUG or CCUG repeats. The mutant RNAs form imperfect double-stranded structures that accumulate in nuclear foci, leading to deregulation of several RNA-binding proteins, including muscleblind-like 1 (MBNL1) and CUG binding protein 1 (CUGBP1). Deregulation of these splicing regulators alters the alternative splicing of several genes (spliceopathy), explaining at least in part the DM multisystemic disease spectrum. Among the symptoms of DM, myotonia, insulin resistance, and cardiac problems are correlated, respectively, with the disruption of the alternative splicing of the muscle chloride channel ClC-1, of the insulin receptor, and of the cardiac troponin T. However, it is now clear that additional pathogenic mechanism-like changes in gene expression, protein translation, and microRNA metabolism may also contribute to the pathomolecular mechanism.

Clinical features

Myotonic dystrophy type 1

Patients with DM1 can be divided into four main categories, each presenting specific clinical features and requiring specific management: congenital onset; childhood/juvenile onset; adult onset; and late onset/asymptomatic. Congenital myotonic dystrophy (CDM) occurs in 25% of offspring of mothers with DM1. CDM is characterized by profound hypotonia, facial diplegia, eyelid ptosis, a tented upper lip ("carp mouth"), and jaw muscle weakness, in the absence of myotonia. Difficulties in sucking and swallowing and severe respiratory distress are common. Survivors may have delayed motor and speech development, mental retardation, arthrogryposis, and talipes.

The childhood/juvenile-onset form of DM1 is often missed in affected adolescents or children because of uncharacteristic symptoms for a muscular dystrophy and apparently negative family history. These patients have cognitive deficits and learning abnormalities and, as in CDM, degenerative features often develop as these children reach adulthood.

The core features in classic adult-onset DM1 are distal muscle weakness, leading to difficulty with performing tasks requiring fine dexterity of the hands and foot drop, and weakness and wasting of the facial muscles, giving rise to ptosis and the typical myopathic or "hatchet" appearance, and of the sternomastoid muscles. The wasting and weakness of wrist extensors, finger extensors, and intrinsic hand muscles may be the earliest signs of the disease. In the lower extremities distal weakness and wasting involve mainly the anterior tibial and peroneal muscles, leading to foot drop. Disease progression is very slow, with gradual involvement of the proximal limb and truncal muscles. Grip and percussion myotonia are regular features that affect bulbar, tongue, or facial muscles, causing problems with talking, chewing, and swallowing. Cardiac involvement is present in the majority of patients with DM1 and approximately 90% of them show electrocardiographic (ECG) abnormalities. The most common are atrioventricular (AV) as well as intraventricular conduction defects. Sudden death caused by

International Neurology, Second edition. Edited by Robert P. Lisak, Daniel D. Truong, William M. Carroll and Roongroj Bhidayasiri
© 2016 John Wiley & Sons, Ltd. Published 2016 by John Wiley & Sons, Ltd.

complete AV block is the worst cardiac complication in DM1. The finding of QTc interval prolongation and late ventricular potentials correlates with the risk of malignant ventricular arrhythmia and sudden death. Cardiomyopathy and congestive heart failure occur far less frequently than conduction disturbances. The most prevalent echocardiographic changes are mitral valve prolapse and septal and myocardial fibrosis.

Iridescent metachromatic posterior subcapsular cataracts are found by slit-lamp examination in 90% of patients with DM1. Cataract may be present even in completely asymptomatic adult patients. The prevalence of clinical diabetes mellitus is only slightly increased in DM despite the common findings of hyperinsulinemia, hyperglycemia, and insulin insensitivity. Testicular atrophy with hypotestosteronism, oligospermia, reduced libido or impotence, and sterility are frequent manifestations. Early male balding occurs commonly. Women may have a high rate of fetal loss and early menopause. Diaphragmatic and intercostal muscle weakness may be the cause of impaired pulmonary vital capacity and impaired maximum expiratory pressure, resulting in alveolar hypoventilation and chronic bronchitis. Acute respiratory failure and pneumonia are the main causes of death in DM1. Gastrointestinal symptoms occur in as many as 80% of patients. Megacolon and fecal impaction are frequently seen due to reduced colon activity. Skull abnormalities include hyperostosis, enlargement of the paranasal sinuses, decrease in sella turcica size, and prognathism. Hypogammaglobulinemia caused by increased catabolism of immunoglobins IgG and IgM are immune system abnormalities in DM.

Central nervous system involvement includes a mild to moderate degree of mental retardation, dysexecutive syndrome, paranoid personality changes, cerebral ventricular enlargement, and nonspecific focal white-matter lesions as well as diffuse gray-matter atrophy. These symptoms lead slowly but progressively to intellectual and social deterioration. Excessive daytime sleepiness, a common problem, may be mistaken for narcolepsy and is associated with a disturbance of the night-time sleep pattern. Centrally mediated hypoventilation, a sleep-related breathing disorder, is characterized by an absence of the usual hyperpnea as a response to increased carbon dioxide concentration. This is associated with an abnormal sensitivity to barbiturates, morphine, and other drugs that depress the ventilatory drive. Peripheral nerves may also be infrequently involved in DM and present as predominantly motor and axonal polyneuropathy. In late-onset or asymptomatic DM1 patients, myotonia, weakness, and excessive daytime sleepiness are rarely present. In these patients the search for cataracts is helpful for identifying the transmitting person.

A median survival of 59–60 years has been reported for the adult-type myotonic dystrophy and of 35 years for the congenital type.

Myotonic dystrophy type 2

The most important difference between DM1 and DM2 is absence of a congenital form in DM2, and the continuum of clinical presentation from an early adult-onset severe form to a very late-onset mild symptom (paucisymptomatic) form. In contrast to DM1, in DM2 the degree of muscle weakness and atrophy is typically mild until late in the course of the disease, the 4th to 5th decades, affecting predominantly sternocleidomastoid muscles, thumb extensors and deep finger flexors, and hip girdle muscles. The patients have less symptomatic distal, facial, and bulbar weakness, and less pronounced clinical myotonia. Cardiac problems appear to be less severe and frequent than in patients with DM1. Cardiac conduction

alterations are primarily limited to first-degree atrioventricular and bundle branch block. However, sudden death, pacemaker implantation, and severe cardiac arrhythmias have been described in small numbers of patients. Cataracts have an appearance identical to that observed in DM1 and develop before 50 years of age as iridescent, posterior capsular opacities on slit-lamp examination. The type of cognitive impairment is similar to but less severe than that of DM1. Other manifestations, such as hypogonadism, glucose intolerance, excessive sweating, and dysphagia, may also occur and worsen over time in DM2.

Investigations

Routine investigations of blood may reveal a slightly raised serum creatine kinase (CK) activity in some adult DM1 cases and usually mildly elevated CK in DM2. Electromyogram (EMG) reveals electrical myotonia, usually present in adult cases, random spontaneous activity at rest in some muscles, and myopathic features; that is, low-amplitude, short-duration polyphasic motor unit potentials. DM2 has less elicitable waning-type electrical myotonia.

The typical DM1 diagnostic method is mutation verification by genetic tests. In DM1, symptoms and family history are often clear and distinctive enough to make a clinical diagnosis, and the mutation can be confirmed by PCR and Southern blot analysis. In patients affected by DM1 the repeat size ranges from 50–4,000 (150–12,000 base pairs) and is nearly always associated with symptomatic disease, although there are patients who have up to 60 repeats who are asymptomatic into old age, and similarly patients with repeat sizes up to 500 who are asymptomatic into middle age. Healthy individuals have between 5 and 37 CTG repeats. Repeat lengths of 38–50 are considered premutation alleles. Patients with premutations are asymptomatic or present a few mild symptoms, such as cataracts, but are at risk of having children with larger, pathologically expanded repeats. Indeed, the size of the CTG repeat appears to increase over time across generations. Children may inherit repeat lengths considerably longer than those present in the transmitting parent, a phenomenon known as genetic anticipation in which disease severity increases and/or age of onset of disease decreases from one generation to the next. The DM1 mutation length of more than 2,000 repeats causes the congenital form of the disease.

In DM2 the mutation usually contracts in the next generation, being shorter in the children. This may explain some distinct features of DM2 such as the absence of a congenital form, the lack of anticipation, and the later onset. Conventional polymerase chain reaction (PCR) and Southern blot analysis are not adequate for a definitive molecular diagnosis of DM2 due to the extremely large size and somatic instability of the expansion mutation. Several alternative and highly sensitive methods have been developed for DM2 mutation verification, including long-range PCR and a tetraplet-primed PCR. The size of the CCTG repeat is below 30 repeats in normal individuals, while the smallest reported mutation varies between 55 and 75 CCTG and the largest expansions have been measured to be up about 11,000 repeats. A more practical tool to obtain a definitive DM2 diagnosis in a few hours is represented by *in situ* hybridization, which allows the direct visualization of the mutant RNA on muscle biopsy. This approach makes muscle biopsy an essential tool for DM2 diagnosis. The histological features of skeletal muscle biopsy in DM1 and DM2 are very similar, and sufficiently characteristic that a diagnosis of DM can be suggested based on muscle biopsy alone. In both diseases, affected muscles show a high number of central nuclei and a markedly increased variation in fiber diameter. Ring binden fibers and sarcoplasmic masses are generally more frequent in a DM1 muscle biopsy specimen. Severely atrophic fibers with pyknotic nuclear clumps are frequently found in a DM2 biopsy specimen also before the occurrence of muscle weakness, while in DM1 nuclear clumps are present in end-stage muscle biopsy. DM2 is considered a disease of type 2 myofibers, since atrophy and central nucleation selectively affects type 2 fibers and the atrophic nuclear clumps express fast myosin isoform (type 2 fiber).

Treatment

Currently, there are no disease-modifying therapies for patients with DM and treatments are intended only to manage symptoms. Symptomatic therapy by a multidisciplinary rehabilitation team for the progressive muscle weakness includes regular physiotherapy and lightweight orthoses, which stabilize the ankle and knee joints. Cataract surgery is frequently required. Careful cardiac control for conduction disturbances is essential. Pacemaker insertion is strongly recommended for patients with advanced conduction system abnormalities, as are home respirators for patients with respiratory insufficiency. In a cohort of DM1 patients a regular pacemaker is usually not sufficient. Instead, an implantable cardioverter-defibrillator (ICD) should be inserted. Hypersomnia may be treated with methylphenidate or modafinil and depression by imipramine or amitriptyline. Myotonia tends to be less marked and less troublesome in DM2, but in specific circumstances antimyotonia therapy is helpful, especially if muscle stiffness is frequent and persistent

or if pain is prominent. Carbamazepine or mexiletine along with nonsteroidal anti-inflammatory medications or Tylenol ameliorates pain in some patients.

Anesthesia and surgery are hazardous in patients with DM. However, good results can be obtained if there is a preoperative assessment, problems are anticipated and minimized by the choice of the most appropriate anesthetic and surgical techniques, and the vigilance is extended into the postoperative period. Many obstetric risks (miscarriage, ectopic pregnancy, preeclampsia, placenta previa, polyhydramnios, preterm birth ≤36 weeks' gestation) associated with DM1 have been described and are a direct consequence of uterine muscle involvement; they would also be expected less frequently in DM2. Women with DM need constant obstetric monitoring and should be advised to deliver in centers with full perinatal facilities. A better awareness of the clinical picture along with genetic counseling in DM families during pregnancy might help to prevent many of the obstetric complications and the exacerbation of myotonia.

Recently, an antisense drug (ISIS-DMPK$_{Rx}$) has been developed for the potential treatment of DM1 and it is currently being studied in a Phase 1 safety study in healthy volunteers. ISIS-DMPK$_{Rx}$ is designed to target the toxic RNA and reduces its nuclear accumulation, thereby restoring normal cellular functions. In animal studies, it has been demonstrated that the antisense oligonucleotides targeting the mutant RNA entered muscle cells and significantly reduced the toxic RNA, leading to a reversal of the disease symptoms, mainly myotonia (Figure 113.1). Therefore, by removing toxic RNA, ISIS-DMPK$_{Rx}$ could be an effective approach to treating patients with DM1.

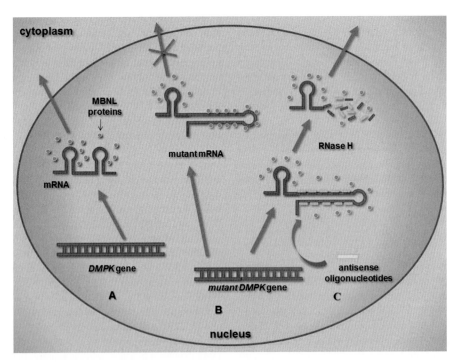

Figure 113.1 (A) The *DMPK* gene is normally transcribed in messenger RNAs (mRNA), which are processed by splicing proteins, such as MBNLs, and then rapidly exported from the nucleus into the cytoplasm, where they are translated into proteins. (B) In myotonic dystrophy type 1, mutant *DMPK* gives rise to mRNA containing CUG repeats, which form long hairpins that accumulate as foci in the nucleus sequestering MBNL proteins. (C) In the HSA^{LR} mouse model, the use of antisense oligonucleotides that selectively target the mutant mRNAs induces their destruction in the nucleus by the enzyme RNase H. Decrease of CUG-containing mRNA leads to a reduction of nuclear accumulation of mutant mRNA, to the release of sequestered MBNL proteins, and thus to the reduction of spliceopathy and to RNA normal translation.

Further reading

Cardani R, Mancinelli E, Sansone V, *et al.* Biomolecular identification of (CCTG)n mutation in myotonic dystrophy type 2 (DM2) by FISH on muscle biopsy. *Eur J Histochem* 2004;48:437–442.

Meola G, Cardani R. Myotonic dystrophies: An update on clinical aspects, genetic, pathology, and molecular pathomechanisms. *Biochim Biophys Acta* 2015;1852: 594–606.

Sansone VA, Brigonzi E, Schoser B, *et al.* The frequency and severity of cardiac involvement in myotonic dystrophy type 2 (DM2): Long-term outcomes. *Int J Cardiol* 2013;168:1147–1153.

Valaperta R, Sansone V, Lombardi F, *et al.* Identification and characterization of DM1 patients by a new diagnostic certified assay: Neuromuscular and cardiac assessments. *Biomed Res Int* 2013; 958510. doi:10.1155/2013/958510

Wheeler TM, Leger AJ, Pandey SK, *et al.* Targeting nuclear RNA for in vivo correction of myotonic dystrophy. *Nature* 2012;488:111–115.

114 Oculopharyngeal muscular dystrophy

Luis A. Chui[1], Tahseen Mozaffar[1,2], and Namita A. Goyal[1]

[1] Department of Neurology, University of California, Irvine, Orange, CA, USA

[2] Department of Orthopaedic Surgery, University of California, Irvine, Orange, CA, USA

Oculopharyngeal muscular dystrophy (OPMD) is a genetically determined adult-onset muscle disease that is associated with progressive eyelid ptosis, external ophthalmoparesis, and bulbar muscle weakness resulting in dysarthria and dysphagia. Inheritance is autosomal dominant, although rare recessive inheritance has been reported. OPMD has unique myopathological features caused by short $(GCG)_{12-17}$ repeat expansions in the poly(A) binding protein nuclear 1 (*PABPN1*) gene. Even though it is a rare condition, the prevalence of OPMD is disproportionately frequent in certain ethnic populations.

OPMD was originally included under the rubric of ocular myopathies; these disorders include ocular myopathies associated with mitochondrial DNA deletions, such as Kearns–Sayre syndrome (KSS). Even though the first reported case of progressive external ophthalmoparesis was described in 1868, it has been difficult to differentiate between different ocular myopathies. The first recognized case report of OPMD was from a French Canadian family, described in 1915. Four members of the family were affected by "progressive vagusglossopharyngealparalysis with ptosis," manifesting with late-onset ptosis and progressive dysphagia, resulting in death from starvation. Subsequently this condition was termed "oculopharyngeal muscular dystrophy" and 10 cases in three generations of a Jewish American family of Eastern European origin were reported. Distinct tubular filaments within the muscle fiber nuclei were identified in French patients with OPMD; these changes have now been confirmed in patients with OPMD of different ethnic origins.

Epidemiology

In North America, French Canadians seem to be the most affected community, with the prevalence of OPMD estimated to be around 1/1,000. It is also particularly common in Bukharan Jews living in Israel (prevalence estimated to be 1/600). Cases of OPMD have been reported in 29 countries of the world to date. Although uncommon even in large Eastern and Midwestern neuromuscular clinics, OPMD is frequently seen in the Southwestern United States, predominantly among Hispanic populations, in New Mexico, Arizona, and southern California. A recent report identified 216 patients seen at two hospitals that serve the entire population of New Mexico. Another cohort was reported in 1998 in California; these subjects were found to have similar mutations in the *PABPN1* gene as in the New Mexico cohort. The origin of the OPMD mutation in New Mexico and California is not known. These cases may be from a new mutation(s) with geographic isolation (founder effect) at a "hot spot" in the genome that has a predilection for limited expansion. This mutation also may have been introduced by Spanish colonists who explored this region in the 1500s, or by French Canadian fur trappers in the 1800s. Many New Mexico patients trace their ancestry to colonial Spanish families that settled in New Mexico in the sixteenth and seventeenth centuries.

Pathophysiology

Autosomal dominant OPMD maps to chromosome14q11.1 and is caused by short $(GCG)_{12-17}$ expansions in the first exon of the poly(A) binding protein nuclear 1 (*PABPN1*) gene. At the protein level this OPMD mutation causes the lengthening of a predicted N-terminus polyalanine domain. *PABPN1* is an abundant, mostly nuclear protein involved in the polyadenylation of all messenger RNAs. The mutation causes a *proteinopathy*, a theme common to other repeat expansion disorders, with a resulting protein that is insoluble and resistant to proteosomal degradation. Gradual accumulation of these insoluble proteins gives rise to the intranuclear inclusions typical of OPMD. The expansion mutation in OPMD interferes with normal cellular trafficking of the *PABPN1* and its role in polyadenylation, thus interfering with crucial cellular processes. Recent findings in muscle biopsies from normal aging control subjects over 40 years of age have shown decreased expression of *PABPN1* by 30–60%, suggesting that patients with the genetic mutation of OPMD are more susceptible to develop severe late-onset myopathy due to accelerated muscle aging.

Clinical features

Most patients become symptomatic in late adulthood, often presenting after the age of 50 years. There are two cardinal symptoms, eyelid ptosis and dysphagia, both of which are slowly progressive. In most cases ptosis is the first symptom, but in some cases dysphagia may manifest first. In families alert to OPMD, these manifestations may be noticed earlier, often by the middle of the third decade, but are often not bothersome until the fifth or sixth decade. Ptosis is always bilateral and can be quite severe. This often results in a compensatory contraction of the frontalis muscle (Figure 114.1) and retrocollis, a pose referred to as Hutchinson's posture or astronomer's sign (Figure 114.2).

International Neurology, Second edition. Edited by Robert P. Lisak, Daniel D. Truong, William M. Carroll and Roongroj Bhidayasiri

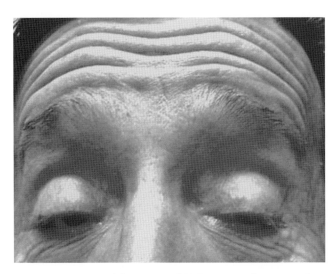

Figure 114.1 Severe eyelid ptosis in an OPMD patient with exaggerated furrowing of the frontalis muscle to compensate for the eyelid ptosis.

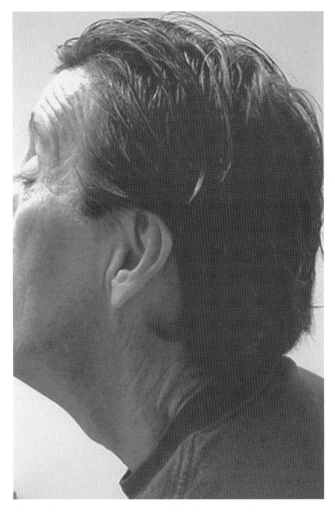

Figure 114.2 Astronomer's sign in an OPMD patient resulting in retrocollis (head tilts back from neck extension) to compensate for the eyelid ptosis.

External ophthalmoparesis is not an early feature of the disease. It usually occurs late, but complete ophthalmoplegia is rare and diplopia is uncommon. Vision is not affected, but visual fields may be restricted because of ptosis. Dysphagia is initially to solids and progresses, with eventual inability to swallow liquids, and can become severe, leading to malnutrition. Palatal hypomotility, pooling of secretions in the tracheobronchial tree, decrease in gag reflex, and palatal and laryngeal weakness with dysphonia are seen usually in the later stages of the disease. Obstructive sleep apnea is encountered frequently in these patients. Facial weakness can be seen as well. Although distal limb muscle weakness is most characteristic in Japanese OPMD patients (in which there are usually no *PABPN1* mutations), most patients outside Japan have predominant proximal muscle weakness. Weakness occurs symmetrically in the presence of atrophy. Cardiac or significant respiratory involvement (external intercostal or diaphragmatic muscle involvement) is not a common feature. The disease has a progressive course, with death occurring due to starvation or aspiration pneumonia. Aggressive medical and nutritional management considerably improves life expectancy in these patients.

Investigations

Serum creatine kinase (CK) activity is generally within normal limits, although CK can be raised up to two or three times the upper limit of normal in some patients, especially early in the disease. Electromyography shows a myopathic pattern. Sensory and motor conduction velocities are usually normal. Cine magnetic resonance imaging (MRI) or manometric studies of the pharyngeal and laryngeal muscles show weak pharyngeal contraction, but are normal in the upper esophageal sphincter; sphincter relaxation, however, is late and incomplete.

Histopathological changes in the muscle fibers are similar to those in other muscular dystrophies, including loss of muscle fibers, increase in the number of internalized nuclei, abnormal variation in muscle fiber size, increased interstitial fibrosis, and infiltration with adipose tissue. Autophagic rimmed vacuoles within muscle fibers are often found, but may be absent in some cases. These vacuoles are more frequent in type 1 than type 2 muscle fibers and are seen more easily in limb than extraocular muscles. Electron microscopy shows characteristic intranuclear tubular filaments with an 8.5 nm outer diameter and 3 nm inner diameter.

The diagnosis of OPMD is confirmed with genetic testing revealing short $(GCG)_{12-17}$ expansions in the first exon of the *PABPN1* gene. When there is a strong clinical suspicion of OPMD, DNA testing can be done first to confirm the diagnosis, which then avoids the need for other less specific and invasive investigations such as electromyography or muscle biopsy.

The differential diagnosis for neuromuscular causes of eyelid ptosis and/or ophthalmoplegia includes myopathies such as mitochondrial myopathies (Kearn–Sayres syndrome or progressive external ophthalmoplegia), myotonic dystrophy, congenital myopathies (myotubular or nemaline), hyperthyroidism/Graves' disease; neuromuscular junction disorders as in myasthenia gravis, botulism, or Lambert–Eaton syndrome; and even peripheral neuropathies as can be seen in Guillain–Barré syndrome or Miller–Fisher syndrome.

Treatment

No treatment has been shown to modify the steady progression of OPMD. Palliative measures improve the ptosis and dysphagia. These include blepharoplasty with resection of the levator palpebrae muscles, primary bilateral silicone frontalis suspension for improvement of levator function, and cricopharyngeal myotomy. In those patients with severe dysphagia, a percutaneous endoscopic gastrostomy feeding tube can be placed for nutrition. The role of chemodenervation of the cricopharyngeal muscles with botulinum toxin to improve dysphagia is currently being explored.

Further reading

Anvar SY, Raz Y, Vermey N., *et al.* A decline in PABPN1 induces progressive weakness in OPMD and in muscle aging. *Aging* 2013;5:412–426.

Becher MW, Morrison L, Davis LE, *et al.* Oculopharyngeal muscular dystrophy in Hispanic New Mexicans. *JAMA* 2001;286:2437–2440.

Brais B. PABPN1 dysfunction in oculopharyngeal muscular dystrophy. In: Karpati G (ed.). *Structural and Molecular Basis of Skeletal Muscle Diseases.* Basel: ISN Neuropath; 2002:115–118.

Brais B, Bouchard JP, Xie YG, *et al.* Short GCG expansions in the PABP2 gene cause oculopharyngeal muscular dystrophy. *Nat Genet* 1998;18:164–167.

Victor M, Hayes R, Adams RD. Oculopharyngeal muscular dystrophy: A familial disease of late life characterized by dysphagia and progressive ptosis of the eyelids. *N Engl J Med* 1962;267:1267–1272.

115 Emery–Dreifuss syndrome and laminopathies

Malcolm Rabie and Yoram Nevo

Neurology Institute, Schneider Children's Medical Center of Israel, Petah Tikva, Israel

Emery–Dreifuss muscular dystrophy (EDMD) is a rare, genetically heterogeneous disease. Together with laminopathies (lamin A/C; *LMNA* gene), it is the first in a broad range of diseases called nuclear envelopathies, which affect mesodermal tissues, mostly skeletal and cardiac muscle. In addition to EDMD, laminopathy phenotypes include various diseases ranging from limb-girdle muscular dystrophy to premature aging. The current classification includes EDMD types 1–3, where commonly Emery–Dreifuss presents with muscular dystrophy, joint contractures, and cardiomyopathy caused by mutations encoding emerin and lamins A and C (Table 115.1). Additional EDMD-like phenotypes may be caused by mutations in nesprin-1, nesprin-2, FHL1, and LUMA (Table 115.2).

Epidemiology

EDMD is very uncommon, with unknown overall prevalence. The estimated prevalence of X-linked recessive EDMD1 is 1/100,000; however, in northern England it was found to be 0.13/100,000.

Table 115.1 Emery–Dreifuss muscular dystrophy types, genes, and inheritance

EDMD type	Gene	Gene product	Inheritance
EDMD 1	*EMD (STA)*, Xq28	Emerin	XR
EDMD 2	*LMNA*, 1q22	Lamin A/C	AD
EDMD 3	*LMNA*, 1q22	Lamin A/C	AR

AD = autosomal dominant; AR = autosomal recessive; EDMD = Emery–Dreifuss muscular dystrophy; XR = X-linked recessive

Table 115.2 Four additional disorders: Emery–Dreifuss muscular dystrophy-like phenotypes, genes, and inheritence

EDMD-like phenotype	Gene	Gene product	Inheritance
EDMD 4	*SYNE1*, 6q25.1-q25.2	Nesprin-1	AD
EDMD 5	*SYNE2*, 14q23.2	Nesprin-2	AD
EDMD 6	*FHL1*, Xq26.3	Four-and-a-half-LIM protein	XR
EDMD 7	*TMEM43*, 3p25.1	Transmembrane protein 43 (LUMA)	AD

AD = autosomal dominant; EDMD = Emery–Dreifuss muscular dystrophy; XR = X-linked recessive

Sporadic emerin mutations are uncommon, but are increasingly recognized for lamin A/C.

Pathophysiology

Most EDMD and laminopathies involve the nuclear lamina, a fibrous meshwork of lamins underlying the inner nuclear membrane, providing a structural framework interacting with inner nuclear membrane proteins, nuclear pore complexes, and chromatin, orchestrating several critical cellular and DNA molecular processes. Exactly how Emery–Dreifuss muscular dystrophy is caused is unknown. The disorder may in part be caused by uncoupling of the nucleoskeleton and cytoskeleton. Most of the proteins causing EDMD occur in the LINC (linker of nucleoskeleton and cytoskeleton) complex of nuclear membrane and associated proteins. These LINC proteins include emerin, lamin A/C, SUN1, SUN2, nesprin-1, and nesprin-2. LINC disruption may cause defects in nuclear mechanics, disorganized chromatin and gene expression, or structural and signaling defects in mechanically stressed tissues (muscle and heart).

Emerin, the inner nuclear membrane protein absent/reduced in EDMD1, tethers chromatin to the nuclear envelope, regulates gene transcription factors (e.g., Lmo7, BAF), controls cell proliferation and cell signaling, and binds nesprins (structural scaffolds), F-actin, and lamins. Transcription factor Lmo7 (Lim-domain-only 7) regulates muscle- and heart-relevant genes, and is inhibited by binding to emerin, suggesting that its dysregulation contributes to Emery–Dreifuss disease.

Lamin A/C filaments involved in EDMD2 and -3 and other laminopathies bind nuclear emerin and nesprins, determining nuclear shape, size, strength, and nuclear pore complex anchoring and spacing, essential for DNA replication and mRNA transcription.

Clinical features

Three EDMD types and four additional disorders that may present with similar clinical findings are shown in Tables 115.1 and 115.2. They all involve the nuclear lamina, except for FHL1.

Typical EDMD is characterized by the following triad:

1 Early elbow and ankle plantar flexor contractures, often associated with inability to fully extend elbows or toe walking before significant weakness. Progressive contractures of the posterior cervical spine cause markedly restricted neck flexion, advancing to rigid spine. Spine and leg contractures may lead to ambulatory loss.

International Neurology, Second edition. Edited by Robert P. Lisak, Daniel D. Truong, William M. Carroll and Roongroj Bhidayasiri
© 2016 John Wiley & Sons, Ltd. Published 2016 by John Wiley & Sons, Ltd.

2 Early humeroperoneal pattern of muscle weakness and wasting of biceps and triceps muscles with relative deltoid muscle sparing is typical. Characteristically initial weakness involves proximal upper limbs and ankle dorsiflexion. The weakness course is moderately benign in the first three decades, with later progression to scapular and pelvic girdle muscles, followed by diffuse weakness, usually without prominent respiratory dysfunction.

3 Life-threatening and potentially treatable cardiac arrhythmias, conduction block, and cardiomyopathy are the most emergent concern in EDMD. They occur in almost all patients by age 30 years. Atrial paralysis is almost pathognomonic of EDMD. EDMD onset, course, and severity show prominent inter- and intra-familial variability.

Age of presentation can vary from neonatal (hypotonia) to the third decade. Characteristically XL-EDMD1 starts in childhood (age 5–15 years), with joint contractures usually as the first sign. Loss of ambulation is rare in XL-EDMD1. XL-EDMD1 and AD-EDMD2 are quite similar clinically. However, AD-EDMD2 may have initial weakness before contractures, more severe cardiac problems, more common scapular winging, and generally a slower course and later onset than XL-EDMD1. Loss of ambulation may occur in AD-EDMD2.

Autosomal recessive EDMD3 is extremely rare, presenting with either early childhood severe muscular dystrophy and contractures, or severe limb-girdle muscular dystrophy later in life. EDMD-like phenotypes 4–7 only have a small number of reported cases, requiring additional data to delineate their exact phenotypes. FHL1 presents with EDMD-like phenotype with joint contractures, spinal rigidity, and cardiac involvement.

Electrocardiogram (ECG) abnormalities are uncommon in the first decade. However, the vast majority of Emery–Dreifuss patients have cardiac arrhythmias by the fourth decade. Conduction system defects and arrhythmias usually evolve with the weakness, and may cause embolic ischemic events and syncope. EDMD may present with sudden death from ventricular bradyarrhythmia or tachyarrhythmia and rarely even in undiagnosed patients with mild or no weakness. ECG findings in this disease may show sinus bradycardia, PR interval prolongation, and bundle branch blocks to complete heart block. In addition, atrial flutter, atrial fibrillation, atrial paralysis, and supraventricular and ventricular arrhythmias may also occur. Most EDMD patients eventually develop a dilated cardiomyopathy with atrioventricular conduction abnormalities.

There is very little differential diagnosis on the classic EDMD phenotype. However, the following diseases may occasionally resemble EDMD: (1) LGMD1B–lamin A/C (pelvic before humeral weakness and mild late contractures distinguishing this disorder from Emery–Dreifuss); (2) collagen VI-related myopathies: Bethlem myopathy (contractures of the last four fingers and rarely of neck–spine, and no cardiomyopathy) and Ullrich congenital muscular dystrophy (proximal contractures and distal joint hypermobility). (3) In addition, LGMD2A, calpainopathy (sparing of hip abductors, cardiomyopathy rare, calf pseudohypertrophy, and contractures), SEPN1-related myopathy (axial weakness, scoliosis, spinal rigidity, and respiratory failure), Fukutin-related protein (FKRP) related myopathies (limb-girdle distribution of muscle weakness, dilated cardiomyopathy is common), and Desmin-related myopathies (scapuloperoneal, limb-girdle, distal muscle weakness, cardiac involvement–i.e., conduction disturbances are common, in some families respiratory involvement) may be considered in atypical cases.

Investigations

EDMD is diagnosed based on the typical clinical triad and supportive family history. Initial evaluation must always include cardiac examination and ECG. Electromyography (EMG) and muscle biopsy are not required in typical cases and in these cases genetic testing is an important non-invasive confirmatory tool. Proportion of Emery–Dreifuss patients with an ascribed causative gene are *EMD* ~61% of XL-EDMD, *FHL1* ~10% of XL-EDMD, and *LMNA* ~45% of autosomal dominant EDMD. Around 45% of EDMD patients do not carry known mutations, and ~64% of patients diagnosed with EDMD and normal emerin immune staining have no identified mutations in *EMD*, *FHL1*, and *LMNA*, implying either mutations in EDMD 4, 5, and 7 or other unidentified new genes.

Negative nuclear emerin stain on muscle biopsy may suggest Emery–Dreifuss in a patient biopsied due to an atypical presentation. Nearly all *EMD* gene mutations cause complete absence of emerin on Western blotting and immunohistochemistry. Emerin detection by immunofluorescence/Western blotting in skin, lymphoblasts, and buccal cells is also possible. Muscle biopsy immunodetection may also be used for EDMD6 (FHL1) diagnosis.

Other investigations include (1) serum creatine kinase (CK) level, usually mild to moderately elevated, sometimes up to 20 times the upper limit in early stages; and (2) muscle magnetic resonance imaging (MRI) may show isolated soleus involvement in initial EDMD1 disease. EDMD2 patients show predominant medial gastrocnemius head involvement and relative lateral head sparing, not seen in EDMD1.

Treatment

There is no specific medication for EDMD. Due to the risk of cardiac conduction defects and sudden death in EDMD with minimal muscle or joint involvement, early cardiac evaluation is vital. Early placement of a permanent ventricular pacemaker with implantable cardioverter-defibrillator may be life saving, as sudden death may occur with just a pacemaker alone. It is important to identify female carriers because of their potentially lethal cardiac risk, requiring yearly monitoring/ECGs. As sudden death may occur with atypical presentation, cardiac evaluation in all undiagnosed muscular dystrophies is recommended. Heart transplantation for end-stage cardiac failure in selected EDMD patients is appropriate.

Management is supportive, with physical therapy and stretch exercises ameliorating early contractures, ambulation assistance (canes, walkers, orthoses, wheelchairs), and at later stages respiratory aids (coughing techniques, respiratory muscle training). Surgery to maintain mobility must be weighed against risk of loss of ambulation. Achilles tenotomy may stabilize ankle contractures, while internal fixation with rods may help neck/spinal contractures. Surgical treatment of elbow contractures is not usually performed.

EDMD surgical–anesthetic issues involve avoidance of myocardial depressants (cardiomyopathy). Some researchers suggest avoidance of malignant hyperthermia triggers, including succinylcholine, halothane, isoflurane, desflurane, and sevoflurane. Cardiac pacing, intubation problems, and epidural anesthesia limitation from spinal contractures must be considered.

Referral is required for cardiac consultation, genetic counseling, prenatal testing, respiratory, and rehabilitation medicine consultation.

Conclusion

EDMD is characterized by slow, progressive muscle weakness and wasting, early contractures, and cardiac conductive and rhythm disturbances. Cardiac involvement is the most critical manifestation of EDMD. Early placement of a cardioverter-defibrillator may be life saving.

Further reading

Attali R, Warwar N, Israel A, *et al*. Mutation of SYNE-1, encoding an essential component of the nuclear lamina, is responsible for autosomal recessive arthrogryposis. *Hum Mol Genet* 2009;18:3462–3469.

Bonne G, Quijano-Roy S. Emery–Dreifuss muscular dystrophy, laminopathies, and other nuclear envelopathies. *Handb Clin Neurol* 2013;113:1367–1376.

Koch AJ, Holaska JM. Emerin in health and disease. *Semin Cell Dev Bio* 2014;29C: 95–106.

Zhang Q, Bethmann C, Worth NF, *et al*. Nesprin-1 and -2 are involved in the pathogenesis of Emery Dreifuss muscular dystrophy and are critical for nuclear envelope integrity. *Hum Mol Gene* 2007;16:2816–2833.

116   Muscle channelopathies

Karen Suetterlin and Michael G. Hanna
MRC Centre for Neuromuscular Diseases, UCL Institute of Neurology, London, UK

The skeletal muscle channelopathies are a rare group of genetic disorders whose muscular manifestations range from pure myotonia to myotonia with episodes of weakness or flaccid paralysis to episodes of weakness or flaccid paralysis alone (see Figure 116.1). They are divided into non-dystrophic myotonias (NDMs) and periodic paralyses (PPs).

Non-dystropic myotonias

The non-dystropic myotonias (NDMs) include myotonia congenita (MC), paramyotonia congenita (PMC), and sodium channel myotonia (SCM). The primary PPs are divided into hypokalemic periodic paralysis (hypo PP), hyperkalemic periodic paralysis (hyper PP), and Andersen Tawil syndrome (ATS), depending on the underlying genetic mutation and response to serum potassium.

The NDMs are differentiated from myotonic dystrophy by the absence of systemic features.

Epidemiology

The skeletal muscle channelopathies have a prevalence that has been estimated to range between 1 and 10 per 100,000 of the population worldwide. However, many of these studies were performed prior to genetic testing. The point prevalence of genetically confirmed NDM in the United Kingdom was recently estimated at 0.75 per 100,000. MC is the most common of the NDMs and has an increased prevalence in consanguineous populations and those with a high frequency of carrier mutations, such as northern Scandinavia. An increased male-to-female ratio has been reported for MC but not for PMC or SCM. NDM patients may report worsening of symptoms in pregnancy. Hypothyroidism has also been reported to exacerbate genetically confirmed myotonia.

Pathophysiology

Mutations causing NDMs result in sarcolemmal hyperexcitability. This impairs muscle relaxation after contraction and manifests as myotonia, which patients tend to describe as stiffness. MC is caused by loss of function mutations in the skeletal muscle voltage-gated chloride channel gene (*CLCN1*). Missense, nonsense, frameshift, base pair deletions, whole exon deletions, whole exon duplications, and splice site mutations have all been reported as causative. Mutations can be inherited in a dominant or recessive manner and for some mutations both modes of inheritance have been observed. This makes genetic counseling complicated.

PMC and SCM are caused by missense mutations in *SCN4A*, the gene encoding the alpha subunit of the skeletal muscle voltage-gated sodium channel. The subsequent gain of channel function may be due to one or a combination of factors, including a shift in the voltage dependence of activation that increases activity in the physiological voltage range, impaired slow inactivation, impaired fast inactivation, and/or faster recovery from inactivation or slowed deactivation. Mutations causing PMC and SCM are inherited in a dominant manner.

Clinical features

The presence of clinical and electrical myotonia combined with an absence of systemic features helps define NDM. Further features that help to distinguish between NDMs include the distribution of myotonia, age of onset, effect of activity, and the presence of associated weakness or exacerbating factors such as diet or cold.

Patients with PMC or SCM tend to have much more prominent facial and eyelid myotonia, while those with MC usually exhibit more prominent limb and truncal myotonia. PMC or SCM usually has the youngest age of onset, from approximately 3 months. For certain *SCN4A* mutations neonatal presentations with laryn-

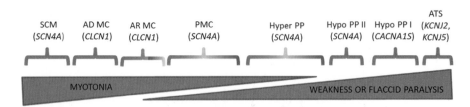

Figure 116.1 The clinical and genetic spectrum of the primary skeletal muscle channelopathies. Non-dystrophic myotonias (to the left) and periodic paralyses (to the right) with the associated genes (second row) are placed on the spectrum of clinical presentations. Source: Suetterlin 2014. Reproduced with permission of Wolters Kluwer.

ADMC = autosomal dominant myotonia congenita; ARMC = autosomal recessive myotonia congenita

International Neurology, Second edition. Edited by Robert P. Lisak, Daniel D. Truong, William M. Carroll and Roongroj Bhidayasiri
© 2016 John Wiley & Sons, Ltd. Published 2016 by John Wiley & Sons, Ltd.

gospasm, stridor, or hypotonia are also documented. MC usually presents later, dominant MC from the age of 2 years and recessive MC from the age of 4 years. However, patients may also present in adulthood – sometimes with worsening of myotonia in pregnancy. MC patients classically exhibit the warm-up phenomenon, whereby their movements become easier and their myotonia reduced with repetitive activity. In contrast, PMC patients classically become stiffer with ongoing activity. Both PMC and recessive MC patients may complain of weakness associated with their myotonia. In recessive MC weakness is transient, tends to occur at the onset of activity, improves with activity, and is short lasting (seconds to minutes). In PMC episodes of weakness are more prolonged, lasting minutes to days and usually following exercise. SCM is not associated with weakness. It is, however, associated with dietary triggers and includes what were formerly described as the "potassium sensitive myotonias." Exposure to cold exacerbates symptoms in PMC; however, patients with MC or SCM may also report worsening of symptoms with cold exposure and therefore this is not a good discriminator. Similarly, those with SCM may report warm-up and may also have muscle hypertrophy, something previously thought classic of recessive MC. Thus, phenotypic overlap exists and can make it difficult to distinguish clinically between SCM and MC in particular.

Investigations

Genetic confirmation is the diagnostic gold standard. However, neurophysiological testing plays a crucial role in the diagnostic workup of NDM. Once myotonia has been demonstrated, short exercise testing is performed to help differentiate between NDMs and to guide genetic testing. This involves measuring compound muscle action potentials (CMAPs) from the abductor digiti minimi before exercise, 2 seconds after maximal isometric contraction, and then every 10 seconds for 50 seconds. This is followed by a 60-second rest and is then repeated. Three trials are performed for each short exercise test. The short exercise test is then performed on the contralateral hand after cooling. The use of cooling and repetitive activity magnifies phenotypic differences between the different NDMs. There are three patterns described. Type 1 is a reduction in CMAP response with repetitive activity and further reduction on cooling. This indicates PMC. Type 2 is an immediate CMAP drop that recovers quickly and improves with exercise (the electrophysiological correlate of transient weakness). This indicates recessive MC. Dominant MC may have a type 2 pattern after cooling. Type 3 is no change in CMAP with repetitive activity or cooling. This indicates SCM or dominant MC.

Magnetic resonance imaging (MRI) is increasingly used to monitor treatment response and disease progression in NDM muscle. However, it may also be of diagnostic use, after the recent finding of a hyperintense stripe in the medial gastrocnemius that was specific to NDM and particularly characteristic of MC.

Treatment

Mexiletine, an old antiarrhythmic sodium channel blocker, is the only evidence-based treatment for NDM. It is very effective in treating myotonia for the vast majority of patients. Electrocardiographic (ECG) monitoring is routinely performed, although the actual incidence of significant cardiac side effects in NDM appears to be low. However, supply has been an issue, as it is no longer routinely used in cardiac practice. If mexiletine is contraindicated, not available, or not tolerated, carbamazepine, phenytoin, and quinine can be used with varying degrees of efficacy. A subset of SCM patients also respond very well to acetazolamide. This group was historically known as the "acetazolamide sensitive myotonias."

Periodic paralyses

Familial or primary PPs result from mutations in the skeletal muscle voltage-gated calcium channel gene (*CACNA1S*), sodium channel gene (*SCN4A*), or inwardly rectifying potassium channel genes (*KCNJ2*, *KCNJ5*); see Figure 116.1. They are subdivided into hypokalemic periodic paralysis (hypo PP), hyperkalemic periodic paralysis (hyper PP), and Andersen Tawil syndrome (ATS). In addition to the muscle symptoms, patients with ATS exhibit important extramuscular features, including potentially fatal cardiac arrhythmias and dysmorphic features. The dysmorphic features may be very subtle and ECG may be normal at presentation. Therefore, ATS should be considered in all patients presenting with PP.

Secondary PPs occur as a result of an underlying disorder that usually causes disturbance in potassium homeostasis. It is the consequent hypokalemia that results in episodes of weakness or paralysis. Endocrine or renal causes are the most commonly described. Thyrotoxic periodic paralysis (TPP), previously considered purely a secondary PP, has more recently been associated with mutations in *KCNJ18* in up to one-third of cases.

Epidemiology

The point prevalence of genetically confirmed primary PPs was recently estimated to be 0.37 per 100,000 in the United Kingdom (0.17 hypo PP, 0.13 hyper PP, 0.08 ATS). This study provided the first estimate of the prevalence of hyper PP and ATS. Hypo PP is the commonest cause of PP in Western countries and TPP is the commonest cause in Asia. Despite the much higher incidence of thyrotoxicosis in females, TPP almost exclusively affects males. Males with PP are also often reported to be more severely affected than females, and asymptomatic female carriers of hypo PP mutations have been identified. The reason for this gender difference is not clear.

Pathophysiology

The common pathomechanism for the attacks of weakness in primary PP is prolonged sarcolemmal depolarization inactivating mutant and wild-type sodium channels with subsequent failure of action potential propagation. Hypo PP mutations affect the S4 voltage-sensing domains of the skeletal muscle voltage-gated calcium channel (hypo PP type 1) or sodium channel (hypo PP type 2). These mutations predispose muscle fibers to paradoxically depolarize when exposed to low levels of potassium. Depolarization is paradoxical as normal muscle fibers, when exposed to the same concentration of potassium, hyperpolarize. Hyper PP mutations usually affect inactivation of the skeletal muscle voltage-gated sodium channel (NaV1.4), causing persistent inward sodium current that, if prolonged, causes sarcolemmal depolarization. Nav1.4 inactivation defects also predispose to sarcolemmal hyperexcitability (as in PMC), and thus a proportion of hyper PP patients also have myotonia. ATS mutations cause loss of function in the inwardly rectifying potassium channel Kir2.1 that plays a crucial role in maintaining muscle resting membrane potential.

Clinical features

There are certain clinical features that help to distinguish between the forms of PP. Dysmorphic features characteristic of ATS include hypertelorism, low-set ears, micrognathia, syndactyly, clinodactyly, and short stature. Shorter attacks triggered by potassium loading, with an age of onset in the first decade, and associated myotonia suggest hyper PP. Longer attacks triggered by carbohydrate loads (e.g., pizza), often occurring in the morning and starting in the second decade, suggest hypo PP. Hypo PP, hyper PP, and ATS can all be triggered by rest after exercise and therefore this is not a helpful discriminator. Diagnostic clues for TPP are patients of Asian origin with systolic hypertension and tachycardia and no family history of PP. However, TPP patients often have no signs or symptoms of thyroid dysfunction on presentation. Episodic attacks of weakness in PP have been reported to reduce in frequency after the age of 30. Around the age of 30–40 (although this may be highly variable), fixed weakness that persists between attacks may develop and a small proportion of patients may even become wheelchair bound in their 60s–70s.

Investigations

An ECG and baseline biochemistry should be performed on all patients presenting with PP. Characteristic features of ATS include QT prolongation, the presence of u-waves, ventricular bigeminy, and bidirectional ventricular tachycardia. Patients with TPP may also have ECG signs including tachycardia, high QRS voltage, or first-degree atrioventricular block. Disturbance in thyroid function, urea, electrolytes, sodium, potassium, magnesium, calcium, or chloride may indicate secondary PP. Creatine kinase (CK) activity in serum may be normal or mildly elevated. If serum CK is significantly elevated, then an alternative pathology should be considered.

The presence of electromyographic (EMG) myotonia in someone with PP suggests hyper PP. However, the key neurophysiological test for PP is the long exercise test. This involves measuring CMAPs from abductor digiti minimi (ADM) before exercise, during 5 minutes of maximal isometric exercise, at 1-minute intervals for the first 6 minutes of rest, and then at 2-minute intervals for the following 45–50 minutes. A positive test is defined as a greater than 40% decrement in CMAP amplitude from baseline or peak for hyper or hypo PP and CMAP area for ATS. A positive test does not discriminate between primary and secondary PP and a negative test does not fully exclude PP. Negative long exercise tests in genetically confirmed patients have been reported. Therefore, genetic confirmation is the diagnostic gold standard.

As with NDM, neuromuscular MRI is proving to be a useful tool in PP. It is particularly helpful in guiding treatment decisions by monitoring disease progression and therapeutic response. Changes observed on MRI include muscle water deposition and/or fatty infiltration of the muscles. The latter is believed to correlate with the development of fixed weakness.

Treatment

Management of an acute attack of primary PP involves correction and monitoring of potassium disturbance and prevention of secondary cardiac dysrhythmia. Although rare, respiratory muscle involvement has been reported in PP and therefore in a severe attack both cardiac and respiratory function should be monitored and the patient transferred to an intensive care setting if necessary. Patients presenting with an acute attack of TPP may be more susceptible to rebound hyperkalemia and subsequent cardiac dysrhythmia. In these patients, non-selective beta blockers should be considered and cardiac monitoring is essential. Currently the carbonic anhydrase inhibitor acetazolamide is the first-line medication for prevention of attacks in PP. This is especially useful prior to genetic confirmation, as it can be used for hyper PP, hypo PP, or ATS patients. Patients must be counseled for the risk of renal stones and renal monitoring should be performed. Dichlorphenamide, another carbonic anhydrase inhibitor, has also been used in PP with good effect, but as with mexiletine, supply has been an ongoing issue.

If carbonic anhydrase therapy fails, the next line of treatment is dependent on the response to serum potassium levels. In hyper PP bendroflumethazide may be used, although reports on its efficacy are limited. A non-diuretic alternative is salbutamol. In hypo PP regular oral potassium may help prevent attacks. Potassium-sparing diuretics such as amiloride or spironolactone have also been used with good effect. In refractory cases combination therapy may be most effective, with acetazolamide, oral potassium supplementation, and potassium-sparing diuretic being used in severe cases and with close monitoring of serum potassium. Bumetanide – a loop diuretic – has been shown to be effective at preventing and even aborting attacks in the animal model of hypo PP and clinical trials are awaited. ATS patients are usually treated as hypo PP as they are more likely to suffer hypokalemic rather than hyperkalemic attacks, and cardiologists advise maintenance of plasma potassium levels between 4 and 5.5 mmoL/L.

Conclusion

Improved phenotypic awareness and refined neurophysiological assessment have improved diagnosis of the skeletal muscle channelopathies. The phenotypic and genetic spectrum of these conditions continues to expand. It is likely to continue to do so as next-generation sequencing facilitates more extensive routine genetic analysis. Improved understanding of the pathogenesis of the skeletal muscle channelopathies has translated into better patient care and new therapeutics are in the developmental pipeline.

Further reading

Chang CC, Cheng CJ, Sung CC, et al. A 10-year analysis of thyrotoxic periodic paralysis in 135 patients: Focus on symptomatology and precipitants. *Eur J Endocrinol* 2013;169:529–536.

Horga A, Raja Rayan DL, Matthews E, et al. Prevalence study of genetically defined skeletal muscle channelopathies in England. *Neurology* 2013;80:1472–1475.

Suetterlin K, Mannikko R, Hanna MG. Muscle channelopathies: Recent advances in genetics, pathophysiology and therapy. *Curr Opin Neurol* 2014;27:583–590.

Tan SV, Matthews E, Barber M, et al. Refined exercise testing can aid DNA-based diagnosis in muscle channelopathies. *Ann Neurol* 2011;69:328–340.

Wu F, Mi W, Cannon SC. Beneficial effects of bumetanide in a CaV1.1-R528H mouse model of hypokalaemic periodic paralysis. *Brain* 2013;136:3766–3774.

117 Congenital dystrophies and myopathies

Young-Chul Choi

Department of Neurology, Yonsei University College of Medicine, Seoul, Korea

Congenital muscular dystrophy (CMD) and congenital myopathy (CM) are a diverse group of diseases that are genetic in origin and frequently present with early-onset weakness.

CMD is a very rare neuromuscular disorder associated with muscle weakness, hypotonia, delayed motor milestones, joint contracture, and dystrophic features on muscle biopsy. CMD is classified into the following five major groups based on the involved gene and function and localization of the protein encoded by the gene: (1) abnormalities of extracellular matrix proteins (*LAMA2, COL6A1, 2, 3*); (2) abnormalities of sarcolemmal proteins (*ITGA7, 9*); (3) abnormalities of dystroglycan and glycosyltransferase enzyme (*POMT1, POMT2, POMGnE1, fukutin, FKRP, and LARGE*); (4) abnormalities at the level of endoplasmic reticulum (*SEPN1*); and (5) abnormalities of nuclear envelope proteins (*LMNA*); see Table 117.1.

CM is also a clinically and pathologically heterogeneous group of skeletal muscle disorders defined by characteristic structural or histological abnormalities on muscle biopsy. They are frequently apparent at birth, usually non-progressive or slowly progressive, and have overlapping clinical features. Central core disease, nemaline myopathy, and centronuclear or myotubular myopathy are the major conditions identified in this group of disorders. The classification of CM was based on muscle histology. Due to advances in immunocytochemical and electron microscopic techniques, a large number of CMs have been identified (Table 117.2). Molecular genetic studies have led to the discovery of new mutations in many genes, and the increased knowledge of their genetic basis has provided new insights and redefined the diagnostic boundaries of both CM and CMD.

Table 117.1 Classification of congenital muscular dystrophies (CMD).

Protein	Gene	Disease phenotype	Inheritance
Extracellular matrix proteins			
Laminin α2	LAMA2	CMD with merosin deficiency (MDC1A)	AR
Collagen VI	COL6A1	Ullrich CMD (Bethlem myopathy)	AR
	COL6A2	Ullrich CMD (Bethlem myopathy)	AR
	COL6A3	Ullrich CMD (Bethlem myopathy)	AR
External sarcolemmal proteins			
Integrin α7	ITGA7	Integrin α7 related CMD	AR
Integrin α9	ITGA9	Integrin α9 related CMD	AR
Dystroglycan and glycosyltransferase enzyme			
Protein-O-mannosyltransferase 1	POMT1	WWS, LGMD2K	AR
Protein-O-mannosyltransferase 2	POMT2	WWS, LGMD2N	AR
Protein-O-linked mannose β1,2-N-acetylglucosaminyltransferase	POMGNT1	MEB, LGMD2O	AR
Fukutin	FKTN	FCMD	AR
Fukutin-related protein	FKRP	MDC1C, LGMD2I	AR
Like-glycosyltransferase	LARGE	MDCD1D	AR
Endoplasmic reticulum protein			
Selenoprotein N	SEPN1	Rigid spine syndrome (RSMD1)	AR
Nuclear envelope protein			
Lamin A/C	LMNA	Emery–Dreifuss muscular dystrophy	AD/AR

AD = autosomal dominant; AR = autosomal regressive

International Neurology, Second edition. Edited by Robert P. Lisak, Daniel D. Truong, William M. Carroll and Roongroj Bhidayasiri
© 2016 John Wiley & Sons, Ltd. Published 2016 by John Wiley & Sons, Ltd.

Table 117.2 Classification of congenital myopathies.

	Gene	Inheritance	Protein
Nemalin (rod) myopathy			
NEM1	TPM3	AD	α-tropomyosin 3
NEM2	NEB	AR	Neblin
NEM3	ACTA1	AR	α-Actin
NEM4	TPM2	AD or AR	β-tropomyosin 2
NEM5	TNNT1	AR	Slow troponin T
NEM6	KBTBD13	AD	Kelch repeat and BTB domain containing 13
NEM7	CFL2	AR	Cofilin 2
NEM8	KHL40	AR	Kelch-like family member 40
Congenital myopathy with central nuclei			
Myotubular myopathy	MTM1	XR	Myotubularin 1
Centronuclear myopathy	DNM2	AD	Dynamin 2
	BIN1	AR	Amphiphysin
	RYR1	AR	Ryanodine receptor 1
Congenital myopathy with cores			
Central core disease	RYR1	AD or AR	Ryanodine receptor 1
Multiminicore disease	RYR1	AR	Ryanodine receptor 1
	SEPN1	AR	Selenoprotein N1
	TTN	AR	Titin
	MYH7	AD	Cardiac β-myosin heavy chain
Hyaline body myopathy	MYH7	AD	Cardiac β-myosin heavy chain
Reducing body myopathy	FHL1	AD	Four-and-a-half LIM domain 1
Cap disease	TPM2	AD	β-tropomyosin 2
	TPM3	AD	α-tropomyosin 3
	ACTA1	AD	α-Actin
Congenital myopathy with fiber size variation			
Congenital fiber type disproportion	ACTA1	AD	α-Actin
	SEPN1	AR	Selenoprotein N1
	TPM3	AD	α-tropomyosin 3
	RYR1	AR	Ryanodine receptor 1
	MYH7	AD	Cardiac β-myosin heavy chain
Congenital neuromuscular disease with uniform type 1 fiber			
	RYR1	AD	Ryanodine receptor 1
	TTN	AR	Titin
Sarcotubular	TRIM32	AR	Tripartite motif-containing 32

AD = autosomal dominant; AR = autosomal regressive

Epidemiology

The exact incidence of CMD and CM is unknown, but they are thought to be rare. The overall estimated prevalence of CMD ranges from 0.68–2.5/100,000. Among the subtypes of CMD, laminin α-2 (*LAMA2*) and collagen VI–related disorders (*COL6A1, 2, 3*), which have abnormality of extracelluar matrix proteins, are the most frequent. The most common form of CM is nemaline myopathy, which occurs in about 1/50,000 live births. Both sexes are affected equally in most CM, with autosomal recessive or dominant inheritance.

Pathophysiology

The etiology and pathogenesis of CMDs and CMs are not fully known, even though most are genetic in origin. The recent interest in CMD and CM has concentrated on defining and classifying distinct disease entities and identifying defective genes. With identification of genetic defects in congenital neuromuscular disorders, there appears to be a clinical and genetic overlap between CMD, CM, and limb-girdle muscular dystrophy.

Clinical features

CMD and CM are clinically and genetically heterogeneous groups of inherited muscle diseases. Most of the patients manifested in early life or infancy and there are clinical and pathological differences between the two disorders.

Congenital muscular dystrophy

CMD usually manifests at birth or within the first year of life. The typical presentation is congenital hypotonia, delayed motor skills, and slowly progressive muscle weakness. CMD may also be associated with contractures or hypermobility of the joints, as well as central nervous system and ocular involvement in some subtypes.

Laminin α-2 (merosin)–deficient CMD

LAMA2-deficient CMD (MDC1A) is caused by mutations in the *LAMA2* gene, which encodes the heavy chain of laminin. The patients present at birth or during the first few months of life with severe muscle weakness with hypotonia, contracture, and respiratory difficulty and feeding problems. The diagnosis of MDC1A can be based on clinical presentation associated with high serum creatine kinase (CK), abnormal white-matter signal on magnetic resonance imaging (MRI), demyelinating neuropathy, and absence of laminin α-2 on muscle tissue or skin biopsy.

Ullrich CMD (collagen VI–deficient CMD)

Descibed by Ullrich in 1930, this is the second most common form of CMD. Mutations in the collagen VI gene (*COL6*) cause different phenotypes, including Ullrich CMD and Bethlem myopathy. Ullrich CMD is usually an autosomal recessive disorder. The classic clinical features of Ullrich CMD are congenital hypotonia, scoliosis or kyphosis of the spine, proximal joint contracture, torticollis, and distal joint hyperlaxity. Congenital hip dislocation may be present. The diagnosis of Ullrich CMD is based on the typical clinical presentation, normal or slightly elevated CK level, muscle biopsy findings, and genetic analysis. Muscle biopsy typically shows myopathic or dystrophic change, with reduction or absence of collagen VI at the sarcolemma. Genetic analysis of the collagen VI gene is important for accurate diagnosis, since there may be an overlap with Bethlem myopathy, which usually has an autosomal dominant trait of inheritance.

Rigid spine congenital muscular dystrophy

Rigid spine CMD (also referred to as rigid spine syndrome) is a rare subtype of CMD caused by a recessive mutation in the *SEPN1* gene that encodes selenoprotein N. Mutations in the *SEPN1* gene have also been identified in other disorders such as multiminicore disease and congenital fiber-type disproportion. Clinical features are characterized by marked axial weakness, rigidity and progressive scoliosis of the spine, and early respiratory insufficiency. CK is normal or mildly elevated.

Congenital muscular dystrophies caused by glycosylation defects of α-dystrophycan (dystroglycanopathy)

The dystroglycanopathies are a group of disorders caused by abnormal glycosylation of α-dystroglycan. Dystroglycan is encoded by *DAG1* and is composed of α-dystroglycan and β-dystroglycan. This complex is an essential component of the dystrophin–glycoprotein complex that links the extracellular matrix to the actin cytoskeleton. α-dystroglycan is a receptor for several proteins in the extracellular matrix, including laminin, neurexin, agrin, biglycan, and perlecan. β-dystroglycan is associated with intracellular proteins including dystrophin. α-dystrophycanopathies include Fukuyama CMD, muscle–eye–brain disease (MEB), Walker–Warburg syndrome (WWS), congenital muscular dystrophy type 1C (FKRP-related or MDC1C), and congenital muscular dystrophy type 1D (LARGE-related or MDC1D). These CMDs are associated with central nervous system pathology and structural eye abnormality. Diagnosis depends on recognition of the clinical phenotype, brain MRI, muscle biopsy, and DNA analysis.

Congenital myopathies

Patients with CM have generalized weakness, hypotonia, hyporeflexia, poor muscle bulk, and dysmorphic features (i.e., chest deformities or high-arched palate), and usually present at birth or in early infancy with a wide variety of symptoms and clinical severity. Muscle weakness is predominantly proximal. In some patients, weakness may involve the axial muscles and face, or even have a distal predominance. The weakness is usually non-progressive or mildly progressive. Lordosis, spinal rigidity, scoliosis, and joint laxity are also frequent. Intelligence is usually normal.

Central core disease

Central core disease (CCD) is a rare congenital myopathy characterized by the presence of a well-defined round area within muscle fibers, called the core, where there is sarcomeric disorganization, lack of mitochondria, and lack of oxidative activity. The core usually extends along the entire length of the fiber. The incidence is unknown, but it is thought to be rare. It is an autosomal dominant disorder, but autosomal recessive and sporadic cases have also been reported.

The clinical features are variable, ranging from asymptomatic to severe. Most patients have non-progressive or slowly progressive proximal muscle weakness and hypotonia during infancy, albeit respiratory failure is not uncommon, in particular in the autosomal recessively inherited forms. Skeletal anomalies such as hip dislocation, kyphoscoliosis, and foot deformity are common findings. Multiminicore diseases (MMD) are defined pathologically by the presence of multiple areas of reduced mitochondrial oxidative activity, so called "minicores." Facial muscle may also be affected, and external opthalmoplegia may be present in ryanodine receptor type 1 (*RYR1*) related CMD with multiminicores. Diagnosis of CCD is confirmed by the presence of the core in the muscle biopsy. On electron microscopy, the core is a circumscribed lesion within which the myofibrils may show structured or unstructured cores with excessive Z-band streaming. CCD is a genetically heterogeneous disease. The main gene associated with this disorder is the ryanodine receptor (*RYR1*) gene, which is also linked to malignant hyperthermia (MH). Both MH and CCD are allelic disorders. Mutations in the *RYR1* and *SEP1* (selenoprotein N1) gene cause MMD.

Nemaline (rod) myopathy

Nemaline myopathy (NM) is a rare, clinically and genetically heterogeneous congenital myopathy characterized by the presence of rod-like structures referred to as nemaline (thread-like) bodies in the muscle fibers (Greek *nema* = thread) and was first described in 1963. To date, more than eight different gene mutations have been identified in α-actin (*ACTA1*), nebulin (*NEB*), tropomyosin 2 (*TPM2*), tropomyosin 3 (*TPM3*), troponin T (*TNNT1*), and Cofilin-2 (*CFL2*) genes (Table 117.2).

NM is the most common form of non-dystrophic congenital myopathy. The clinical spectrum ranges from severe cases with antenatal or neonatal onset and early death to adult-onset cases with slow progression. Muscle weakness mostly affects the neck flexor and proximal limb muscles. Extraocular muscles are usually spared. The most common form of NM is characterized by onset in early infancy or childhood with hypotonia, generalized muscle weakness, and facial involvement leading to an elongated and expressionless face, tent-shaped mouth, and high-arched palate. Feeding difficulties, severe respiratory impairment, and skeletal involvement frequently occur. The mode of inheritance can be autosomal dominant or recessive. Among the eight different genes identified, *ACTA1* mutations are responsible for about 20% of NM cases. Up to 50% of cases with NM are due to *NEB* mutations.

The characteristic pathological feature of NM is a rod-like structure, variable in size, number, and location (Figure 117.1). The rods are often clustered at the periphery of fibers and near nuclei, and even in the nuclei. The rods are found predominantly in type 1 fibers. With electron microscopy, rods are visible as the electron-dense structures originating from the Z discs of sarcomeres.

Centronuclear myopathies

Centronuclear or myotubular myopathy is also a clinically and genetically heterogeneous group of disorders characterized by centrally placed nuclei in the muscle fiber, type 1 fiber predominance, and type 1 fiber hypotrophy. Based on the clinical features, centronuclear myopathy (CNM) is classified into three forms: the severe neonatal form, the childhood-onset form, and the adult-onset form. The severe neonatal phenotype comprises severe hypotonia, muscular weakness, respiratory failure at birth, and early mortality. The muscle fibers are similar to fetal myotubes. There is also a recessive X-linked myotubular myopathy with a mutation of the myotubularin (*MTM1*) gene at Xq28. The childhood-onset phenotype is

characterized by a slowly progressive diffuse muscular weakness. The third or adult-onset form manifests fully in the third decade of life, although incipient clinical signs and symptoms may occur during the first or second decades. Histologically it is identical to the childhood-onset form. In contrast to the severe neonatal form, the inheritance of the latter two forms is not well defined, with most cases being sporadic. The childhood- and adult-onset forms are currently referred to as CNM.

The pathogenesis of CNM is unclear, but mutations in the dynamin 2 (*DNM2*) gene have been shown to cause autosomal dominant CNM. Pathologically CNM has an increased number of centrally nucleated muscle fibers, variation in muscle fiber diameter, type I fiber predominance or atrophy, and a central area of the muscle cell negative for adenosine triphosphatase.

Congenital myopathy with fiber-type disproportion

Congenital myopathy with fiber-type disproportion (CFTD) is a form of CM characterized by a non-progressive neuromuscular disorder that has a relatively good prognosis and type 1 fiber predominance with smallness of the same fiber type. Clinically, patients show hypotonia and delayed motor milestones, often associated with congenital dislocation of the hip, high-arched palate, kyphoscoliosis, and contractures of the elbow and knee associated with hyperinsulinemia and peripheral insulin resistance. The mutations in *ACT1*, *SEPN1*, *TPM3*, and *RyR1* genes can cause CFTD (Table 117.2).

Investigations

Laboratory studies including serum CK activity, electrophysiological studies, brain and muscle imaging, muscle biopsy, and genetic studies are useful for diagnosis; the serum CK test is one of the most useful laboratory tests. Electrophysiological studies including nerve conduction velocity (NCV) and electromyography (EMG) should be part of the routine evaluation of patients with suspected CMD and CM. These studies are useful for differentiating CMD and CM from other neuromuscular disorders. Muscle imaging such as ultrasound and MRI can detect particular patterns of selective muscle involvement, which can contribute to diagnosis and selection of biopsy sites, such as selective sparing of the rectus femoris in *RYR1*-related myopathies, or specific involvement of the central part of the rectus femoris muscle and involvement of the rim between

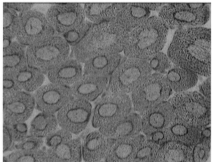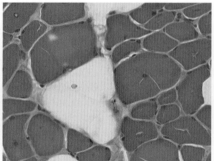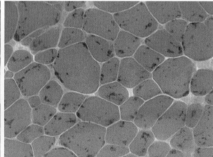

Figure 117.1 The characteristic histological features of congenital myopathies: central core disease (left, NADH-Tr, × 400), centronuclear myopathy (middle, H&E, × 400), and nemaline myopathy (right, Gomori trichrome, × 200). For color details, please refer to the color plates section.

soleus and gastrocnemius in *COLVI*-related muscular dystrophies. Brain imaging studies are also important in differential diagnosis of CMD subtypes, for instance white-matter change abnormalities in merosin-deficient CMD and α-dystroglycanopathies. Muscle biopsy is essential for the diagnosis of CMD and CM, and Western blot and immunocytochemistry can be helpful for the analysis of certain muscle proteins. Because specific molecular genetic defects have been identified for a large number of CMDs and CMs, mutation analysis using peripheral blood or muscle tissue DNA can also aid in the diagnosis of CMD and CM.

Treatment

There is no specific treatment for any of the CMDs and CMs. Therapeutic interventions comprise symptomatic physical therapy, orthopedic treatment of associated skeletal abnormalities, and ventilator support for those with respiratory muscle weakness. Monitoring of developmental state, progression of deficits, and complications is important for early therapeutic management and improvement in quality of life.

Further reading

Bönnemann CG, Wang CH, Quijano-Roy S, *et al.* Diagnostic approach to the congenital muscular dystrophies. *Neuromuscul Disord* 2014;24:289–311.

Gilbreath HR, Castro D, Iannaccone ST. Congenital myopathies and muscular dystrophies. *Neurol Clin* 2014;32:689–703.

North KN, Wang CH, Clarke N, *et al.* Approach to the diagnosis of congenital myopathies. *Neuromuscul Disord* 2014;24:97–116.

Park YE, Choi YC, Bae JS, *et al.* Clinical and pathological features of Korean patients with DNM2-related centronuclear myopathy. *J Clin Neurol* 2014;10:24–31.

Romero NB, Clarke NF. Congenital myopathies. *Handb Clin Neurol* 2013;113:1321–1336.

118 Congenital myasthenic syndromes

Angela Abicht[1] and Ulrike Schara[2]

[1] Neurology Clinic, Friedrich-Baur-Institut, and Medical Genetics Center Munich, Munich, Germany

[2] Department of Neuropediatrics, Developmental Neurology, and Social Pediatrics, Universitätsklinikum Essen, Essen, Germany

Congenital myasthenic syndromes (CMS) are a group of hereditary disorders that display overlapping clinical features and share the etiology of disturbed neuromuscular transmission. The general phenotype is broad and varies with age, as the onset of symptoms can range from birth to mid-adulthood. To date, disease-causing mutations have been identified in at least 18 different genes. It is expected that further genetic defects will be discovered, as an extensive ongoing analysis has identified genetic defects in 50–60% of patients so far. What makes CMS exceptional and their diagnosis essential is the fact that they represent a genetic disorder for which a differential medical treatment is available.

Epidemiology

CMS have been identified in all parts of the world. As most subtypes follow an autosomal recessive pattern of inheritance, they are more frequently seen in populations practicing consanguineous marriage. A few mutations are recurrent and prevalent in restricted populations as a consequence of a founder effect (Table 118.1). Of particular importance in southeastern European countries is the mutation c.1327delG (referred as 1267delG in the literature) in *CHRNE*, the gene encoding the epsilon subunit of the acetylcholine receptor. This mutation has been identified as a Roma founder mutation with a high carrier rate of >4% in this specific ethnic group. The overall prevalence of CMS is estimated to be between 2.8 and 14.8 per million.

Pathophysiology

The fundamental pathomechanism shared by all CMS subtypes is a dysfunction of the neuromuscular junction (NMJ) causing muscle weakness, which increases with exertion. Over the past two decades, underlying germline mutations in an increasing number of genes have been identified. Most of the known genes (*CHRNA1, CHRNB1, CHRND, CHRNE, CHRNG, RAPSN, SCN4A, MUSK, DOK7, PLEC1, LAMB2, COLQ, CHAT, AGRN,* and *LRP4*) encode proteins that primarily function at the neuromuscular junction. According to the localization of the affected protein at the neuromuscular junction, CMS have been classified as presynaptic, synaptic basal lamina associated, and postsynaptic. However, with the recent identification of mutations in genes encoding enzymes critical for glycosylation (*GFPT1, ALG2, ALG14, DPAGT1*), and with mutations in *PREPL*, which encodes a ubiquitously expressed protein

Table 118.1 Summary of known disease-underlying genes in congenital myasthenic syndromes (CMS).

Gene	Overall proportion of CMS attributed to mutations per gene1
AGRN	Rare
CHAT	4–5%
CHRNA1	<1%
CHRNB1	<1%
CHRND	<1%
CHRNE	10–15%
COLQ	10–15%
DOK7	10–15%
GFPT1	2%
MUSK	Rare
RAPSN	15–20%
SCN4A PLEC1 LAMB2	Very rare
ALG2 ALG14 DPAGT1 LRP4 PREPL	Newly identified genes, no frequency data

[1] Estimated percentage based on individuals with CMS investigated at the authors' laboratory and on published data.

involved in trafficking of the vesicular acetylcholine transporter, the molecular basis of CMS has expanded to include molecules that are not confined to the neuromuscular endplate.

Clinical features

According to the common pathomechanism of disturbed neuromuscular transmission, CMS patients share the phenotypic hallmark of exertion-dependent muscle weakness. However, the onset of symptoms, clinical phenotype, and response to treatment vary greatly depending on the precise underlying molecular defect. The age at onset varies from birth to adulthood. The earliest presentation of CMS is *in utero*, with reduced fetal movements resulting in joint contractures in newborns. In newborns, generalized muscle

International Neurology, Second edition. Edited by Robert P. Lisak, Daniel D. Truong, William M. Carroll and Roongroj Bhidayasiri
© 2016 John Wiley & Sons, Ltd. Published 2016 by John Wiley & Sons, Ltd.

weakness manifesting as "floppy infant" with a weak cry, feeding difficulties, as well as neonatal apnea or stridor should include CMS as a differential diagnosis. Motor development may be delayed, but fatigable muscle weakness frequently manifests in early childhood after normal first motor milestones. Except for the recently identified PREPL-associated CMS, cognitive impairment excludes the diagnosis of CMS in infants. Limb-girdle and additional facial weakness are common; bulbar weakness with nasal speech and difficulties in coughing and swallowing may also be present. Not all CMS patients have ptosis or extraocular eye muscle involvement; however, in some patients ptosis and ophthalmoparesis are prominent features.

Infection-related sudden apnea in early infancy and (less frequently) later in childhood are life-threatening events of which parents must be made aware. They are most frequently seen in patients with *RAPSN* and *CHAT* mutations. Muscular weakness can progress, leading to loss of independent ambulation and/or respiratory insufficiency in some patients. In a subtype of CMS – slow-channel CMS (SCCMS) – weakness may affect predominantly neck and finger extensors. In another subtype – limb-girdle CMS (LGCMS) – patients have proximal muscle weakness without ocular involvement. Spinal deformities or mild muscle atrophy may occur, giving rise to a phenotype that overlaps with limb-girdle myopathy. Together with our broader understanding of the molecular basis of CMS, the clinical phenotype is therefore expanding.

Investigations

CMS may be suspected primarily on clinical grounds. The diagnosis is supported by electrophysiological tests showing a decremental response to repetitive nerve stimulation and/or increased jitter in single-fiber EMG recordings. A positive response to acetylcholinesterase (AChE) inhibitors (pyridostigmine and/or edrophonium test) serves as further supporting evidence of CMS. However, a lack of response does not exclude a diagnosis of CMS, because certain subtypes are refractory to or deteriorate with AChE inhibition. Serum creatine kinase (CK) activity may be normal or moderately elevated. No autoantibodies (anti-AChR, anti-muscle specific kinase [MuSK]) are present. A skeletal muscle biopsy does not reveal specific pathology in routine histochemical testing. A type I fiber predominance, type II fiber atrophy, and occasionally minor myopathic changes may be present. Tubular aggregates have been described in specific subtypes (*GFPT1*, *DPAGT1*, or *ALG2* associated limb-girdle CMS). A precise molecular diagnosis defining the specific subtype of CMS is achieved by molecular genetic analysis. The ethnic origin of the patient or specific clinical features may indicate testing of a single gene. Otherwise, a gene panel analysis testing all known CMS genes in parallel is recommended.

Treatment

Therapy is determined by the structural defect of the NMJ and the underlying genetic defect. In practice, it is important to understand that a drug can have a positive effect on one form of CMS (acetylcholinesterase inhibitors in cases of rapsyn deficiency), but show negative effects or even cause symptoms to worsen in another subtype (acetylcholinesterase inhibitors in cases of AChE deficiency).

The assumed mechanisms of therapeutic agents used in treating CMS as well as their side effects are described in this section. For further details concerning the indication for different drugs in different subtypes, see Table 118.2.

AChE inhibitors prolong the activity of acetylcholine (ACh) in the synaptic space by blocking hydrolysis of ACh. The individual dose has to be found in every patient; 4–5 mg/kg body weight/day in 4–6 divided doses is often helpful and well tolerated. Side effects include mainly cholinergic symptoms such as increased bronchial secretion and tear production, hypersalivation, coughing, and diarrhea. AChE inhibitors can exacerbate the clinical course in cases of slow-channel CMS and DOK7 deficiency, and are contraindicated in cases of AChE deficiency due to the severe side effects caused by a hypersensitive muscarinic receptor reaction. 3, 4-diaminopyridine (3,4-DAP) increases quantal release in presynaptic defects. It prolongs the presynaptic action potential by blocking the outward potassium current, leading to increased calcium entry into the nerve terminal. The daily dose is up to 1 mg/kg body weight in 4 divided doses in infancy and childhood; in older patients up to 5–20 mg 4 times a day. Side effects are usually mild and cholinergic; in higher doses the drug may induce seizures and is contraindicated in patients with a history of seizures.

Quinidine sulfate and fluoxetine are long-lived, open-channel blockers of AChR. They shorten the duration of channel opening events and time in a concentration-dependent manner; they therefore show positive effects in cases of slow-channel syndromes. Quinidine sulfate should be administered 15–60 mg/kg body weight/day in children in 4–6 divided doses; adult patients should be treated with 3 × 200 mg/day for 1 week. The dose should then be increased depending on the serum level (normal value 1–2.4 μg/mL or 3–7.5 μm/L). Side effects such as gastrointestinal symptoms, hypersensitivity symptoms, cardiac conduction defects, and inhibition of cytochrome P450IIDA have to be taken into account; the latter impairs several metabolic pathways.

Fluoxetine can be used in patients who cannot tolerate quinidine sulfate, but is less effective. It is eliminated slowly, thus providing a more sustained serum level. The daily dose for adults is 80–100 mg; in children the maximal dose has not been established. Side effects include nausea, nervousness, insomnia, sexual dysfunction, and hyponatremia in adults; in children, fluoxetine can increase the risk of suicide-related behavior. Fluoxetine should therefore not be used in children and adolescents with signs of depression. Both drugs should be monitored by serum-level testing.

In addition to AChE inhibitors, acetazolamide has been reported to be beneficial in a single patient with a CMS caused by mutations in the gene *SCN4A*; it prevented both further attacks and bulbar weakness. The daily dose was 2 × 250 mg/day.

Ephedrine shows positive effects in treating different forms of CMS such as acetylcholinesterase deficiency, DOK7 deficiency, and sometimes in muscle-specific tyrosine kinase deficiency. *In vitro*, it increases quantal release and reduces the opening time of the AChR

Table 118.2 Founder mutations in different congenital myasthenic syndrome (CMS) genes.

Origin	Frequent mutation
Central/Western European origin	*RAPSN* c.264C>A *DOK7* c.1124_1127dupTGCC
Southeastern European or Roma origin	*CHRNE* c.1327delG
Maghreb (Algeria, Morocco, Tunisia)	*CHRNE* c.1353dup

in a dose-dependent manner. In humans, the mode of action is not yet fully understood. Doses in adults vary from 25–50 mg 2–3 times per day. In children, it should be 3 mg/kg body weight/day in 3 divided doses; treatment with ephedrine is often started with 1 mg/kg body weight/day and increased carefully. Side effects include hypertension, nervousness, insomnia, and palpitation.

Albuterol has been described as having positive effects in CMS subtypes such as acetylcholinesterase and DOK7 deficiency. The recommended daily dose for children aged 2–6 years is 0.1 mg/kg body weight/day (maximum 2 mg/day) in 3 divided doses. In children 6–12 years of age, the dose is 2 mg 2–3 times a day; in adults it is 4 mg 1–3 times daily. Side effects are exercise-induced muscle cramps, a burning sensation in the calves and sometimes in other muscles, tightness of the jaw muscles while chewing, mild jitteriness and tremor, insomnia, and an increase in hypertension.

One patient developed atrial flutter, which was reversible after stopping therapy.

So far, CMS therapy is symptomatic and includes medication determined by the underlying genetic defect (Table 118.3). The drugs are usually used as monotherapy; however, a combination of different drugs is sometimes necessary to optimize the positive effect and minimize side effects. If necessary, physiotherapy, speech therapy, orthotics or a wheelchair, a percutaneous gastric tube, or ventilatory support should be used according to the patient's individual situation. It is important to ask about day weakness, headaches, snoring, recurrent respiratory infections, and weight loss as suspicious clinical symptoms, and to perform regular assessments of vital capacity in sitting and supine positions in order to look for increased respiratory distress and hypoxemia and/or hypoventilation. In cases with a vital capacity of less than 40%, polysomnography should be performed.

Table 118.3 Therapy in congenital myasthenic syndromes (CMS) according to the underlying genetic defect. Source: Modified from Schara 2008, Schara 2012.

Defect	Gene	Rational therapy
Choline acetyltransferase	CHAT	1. AChE inhibitors in an individual dosage, often 4–5 mg/kgBW/day in 4–6 divided doses **If necessary additionally** 2. 3,4-DAP 1mg/KgBW/day in 4 divided doses up to 4 × 5–20 mg/day
Acetylcholinesterase deficiency	COLQ	1. Ephedrine 3 mg/kgBW/day in 3 divided doses, begin with 1 mg/kgBW/day and increase carefully, in elder patients: 2–3 × 25–50 mg/day 2. Albuterol in children 2–6 years of age: 0.1 mg/kgBW/day (max 2 mg/day) in 3 divided doses; in children 6–12 years of age: 2 mg 2–3 times daily; in adults 4 mg 1–3 times daily
α-subunit of the AChR β-subunit of the AChR δ-subunit of the AChR ε-subunit of the AChR	CHRNA1 CHRNB1 CHRND CHRNE	**I. Structural defects** 1. AChE inhibitors in an individual dosage, often 4–5 mg/kgBW/day in 4–6 divided doses **If necessary additionally** 2. 3,4-DAP 1mg/kgBW/day in 4 divided doses, up to 4 × 5–20 mg/day 3. Albuterol in children 2–6 years of age: 0.1 mg/kgBW/day (max 2 mg/day) in 3 divided doses; in children 6–12 years of age: 2 mg 2–3 times daily; in adults 4 mg 1–3 times daily **II. Kinetic defects** **a. Slow-channel syndrome** 1. Quinidine sulfate 15–60 mg/kgBW/day in 4–6 divided doses 2. **In case of side effects:** fluoxetine, in adults 80–100 mg/day, in children a maximal dosage has not been established **b. Fast-channel syndrome** 1. AChE inhibitors in an individual dosage, often 4–5 mg/kgBW/day in 4–6 divided doses **If necessary additionally** 2. 3,4-DAP 1 mg/kgBW/day in 4 divided doses, up to 4 × 5–20 mg/day **Quinidine sulfate and fluoxetine should be monitored by serum level measurements**
Rapsyn deficiency	RAPSN	1. AChE inhibitors in an individual dosage, often 4–5 mg/kgBW/day in 4–6 divided doses **If necessary additionally** 2. 3,4-DAP 1 mg/kgBW/day in 4 divided doses, up to 4 × 5–20 mg/day
"Downstream of kinase-7" deficiency	DOK7	1. Ephedrine 3 mg/kgBW/day in 3 divided doses, begin with 1 mg/kgBW/day and increase carefully, in elder patients: 2–3 × 25–50 mg/day 2. 3,4-DAP 1 mg/kgBW/day in 4 divided doses up to 4 × 5–20 mg/day 3. Albuterol in children 2–6 years of age: 0.1 mg/kgBW/day (max 2 mg/day) in 3 divided doses; in children 6–12 years of age: 2 mg 2–3 times daily; in adults 4 mg 1–3 times daily
Muscle specific tyrosine kinase deficiency	MuSK	1. AChE inhibitors in an individual dosage, often 4–5 mg/kgBW/day in 4–6 divided doses **and** 3,4-DAP 1 mg/kgBW/day in 4 divided doses, up to 4 × 5–20 mg/day 2. In some patients ephedrine is helpful, 3. 3 mg/kgBW/day in 3 divided doses, begin with 1 mg/kgBW/day and increase carefully, in elder patients: 2–3 × 25–50 mg/day
Na$_v$1.4	SCN4A	1. AChE inhibitors in an individual dosage, often 4–5 mg/kgBW/day in 4–6 divided doses **and** acetazolamide 2 × 250 mg/day
Agrin deficiency	AGRN	1. **in only single cases reported ephedrine shows positive effects:** 3 mg/kgBW/day in 3 divided doses, begin with 1 mg/kgBW/day and increase carefully, in elder patients: 2–3 × 25–50 mg/day
Glutamine-fructose-6-phosphate transaminase 1	GFPT1	1. AChE inhibitors in an individual dosage, often 4–5 mg/kgBW/day in 4–6 divided doses
Dolichyl-phosphate (UDP-N-acetylglucosamine) N-acetylglucosaminephosphotransferase 1	DPAGT1	1. AChE inhibitors in an individual dosage, often 4–5 mg/kgBW/day in 4–6 divided doses 2. 3,4-DAP 1 mg/kgBW/day in 4 divided doses, up to 4 × 5–20 mg/day
Genes involved in the asparagine-linked glycosylation pathway	ALG2 ALG14	1. AChE inhibitors in an individual dosage, often 4–5 mg/kgBW/day in 4–6 divided doses

3,4-DAP = 3,4-diaminopyridine; AChE = acetylcholinesterase; BW = body weight

In most patients, CMS therapy shows positive results. However, even patients receiving early and appropriate treatment may show continued muscle weakness, swallowing difficulties, or exercise intolerance leading to wheelchair dependency.

For early diagnosis and an optimal result, CMS must be considered for any patient with suggestive clinical symptoms, regardless of age.

Genetic counseling should be offered as a means of informing patients and families about the risk of reoccurrence and the possibility of prenatal diagnosis.

Further reading

Abicht A, Müller JS, Lochmüller H. Congenital myasthenic syndromes. *Gene Reviews* 2003; May 9 (revd 2012; June28). http://www.ncbi.nlm.nih.gov/books/NBK1168/ (accessed November 2015).

Hantaï D, Nicole S, Eymard B. Congenital myasthenic syndromes: An update. *Curr Opin Neurol* 2013;26;561–568.

Schara U, Lochmüller H. Therapeutic strategies in congenital myasthenic syndromes. *Neurotherapeutics* 2008;5;542–547.

Schara U, Della Marina A, Abicht A. Congenital myasthenic syndromes: Current diagnostic and therapeutic approaches. *Neuropediatrics* 2012;43;184–193.

119 Distal myopathies

Phillipa J. Lamont[1] and Nigel G. Laing[2]

[1] Department of Neurology, Royal Perth Hospital, Department of Health, Western Australia, and School of Medicine and Pharmacology, University of Western Australia, Perth, WA, Australia

[2] Centre for Medical Research, University of Western Australia, Harry Perkins Institute of Medical Research and Neurogenetics Unit, PathWest, Department of Health, Western Australia, Nedlands, WA, Australia

The distal myopathies are rare disorders distinguished by their presentation, namely weakness of the distal limb muscles. In some patients the weakness stays confined to these muscles, whereas in others there is spread to proximal muscles. A comprehensive review of the phenotypes, pathological basis, and genetics of distal myopathies has recently been published (see Further reading), so only certain points will be raised for further discussion.

Epidemiology

Distal myopathies are genetic disorders, dominantly or recessively inherited, or arising as a result of *de novo* mutations. The incidence of distal myopathies in large parts of the world remains unknown. For some distal myopathies, particularly those such as Laing distal myopathy with high new mutation rates (30% or more), it is known that the incidence is relatively uniform worldwide. However, some distal myopathies exhibit founder effects and therefore have less uniform prevalence around the world. Founder mutations in genetic isolates have led to higher incidences of Welander distal myopathy in Finland and Sweden, Udd distal myopathy in Finland, and GNE myopathy (also known as Nonaka myopathy, distal myopathy with rimmed vacuoles, or quadriceps-sparing myopathy) in Japan and in certain Middle Eastern populations. Anoctaminopathy is one of the most frequent causes of muscle disease in northern Europe. Six distal myopathies have been described in only one or two families, but are included in Table 119.1 to facilitate identification of other cases. It appears that Laing distal myopathy is the most common distal myopathy in the world.

Pathophysiology

As the causative genes for the distal myopathies have been discovered, the pathophysiology is beginning to be understood for some entities. It remains a mystery why mutations in genes expressed in every muscle fiber in the body can cause weakness confined to certain muscles, but this is the case not only in the distal myopathies, but also in limb-girdle muscular dystrophies, facioscapulohumeral muscular dystrophy, and others. Dysferlin is involved in sarcolemmal repair mechanisms and it has been hypothesized that damage gradually builds in susceptible muscles. The *GNE* gene codes for a double enzyme whose malfunction leads to hyposialation of muscle proteins, and this is currently the target for corrective therapeutic trials. Nebulin and titin are both giant structural protein components of the sarcomere. A single nebulin molecule extends the length of the thin filament, while a single titin molecule bridges from the Z line to the M line. Myofibrillar myopathies, which can present as a distal myopathy, are a genetically diverse group of disorders with the common problem of disintegration of the sarcomeric Z disc and the myofibrils. This leads to abnormal ectopic accumulation of multiple proteins associated with the Z disc, including desmin, dystrophin, and myotilin. However, it is less clear why a mutation in the nuclear matrix gene *MATR3*, or the Kelch-like homologue *KHLH9*, causes a distal myopathy phenotype. In some cases, such as anoctamin 5, the precise function of the protein is still a matter of conjecture.

Clinical, pathological, and genetic features

These are outlined in Table 119.1. The earliest site of muscle weakness is a valuable clue to diagnosis. Welander and Williams distal myopathies preferentially affect the hands first, whereas the rest of the distal myopathies tend to affect the distal legs initially. However, with the exception of Udd distal myopathy, which remains confined to the lower limbs, all eventually affect both the upper and lower limbs. Most affect the anterior compartment of the lower leg, with the exception of Miyoshi, distal anoctaminopathy, and vacuolar neuromyopathy, which usually preferentially affect the posterior compartment. Occasionally the myofibrillar myopathies can affect both the anterior and posterior compartments simultaneously.

Many of the genes involved are also associated with other phenotypes, in addition to distal myopathy. For example, both *ANO5* and *DYS* can cause a limb-girdle muscular dystrophy, either initially or later in the course of the disease. *MYH7* is the commonest cause of familial cardiomyopathy, and can also cause the proximal myosin storage myopathy phenotype. *NEB* is the commonest cause of nemaline myopathy, an early-onset congenital myopathy. Most of the myofibrillar myopathies more commonly give rise to proximal onset of weakness. Cardiac and respiratory involvement is prominent in desminopathies, and often is severe, requiring medical intervention. Although occurring less frequently, this is also true in Laing distal myopathy, alphaB crystallin mutated distal myopathy, and ZASPopathy. In addition, a third of Laing distal myopathy cases have a significant spinal phenotype, either scoliosis or rigidity. The

International Neurology, Second edition. Edited by Robert P. Lisak, Daniel D. Truong, William M. Carroll and Roongroj Bhidayasiri
© 2016 John Wiley & Sons, Ltd. Published 2016 by John Wiley & Sons, Ltd.

Table 119.1 Distal myopathies.

Distal myopathy	OMIM	Protein, gene, and/or location	Age of onset	Initial site of weakness	Muscle pathology
Dominant					
Early onset					
Laing distal myopathy (MPD1)	160500	Slow skeletal/beta cardiac myosin (MYH7) 14q11.2	1–25 years, may delay walking	Ankle dorsiflexion, long toe extension, long finger extension; mild proximal, face, and neck flexion later in disease course	Fiber type disproportion, multiminicores
KLHL9 mutated distal myopathy[+]		Kelch-like homologue 9 (KLHL9) 9p21.3	8–16 years	Ankle dorsiflexion, intrinsic hand muscles	Non-specific myopathic
Adult onset					
Udd myopathy (tibial muscular dystrophy)	600334	Titin (TTN) 2q31.2	>35 years	Ankle dorsiflexion; knee flexion +/- extension later in life	Rimmed vacuoles in atrophic muscles (anterior tibial muscle biopsy)
Welander distal myopathy	604454	TIA1 (TIA1) 2p13	Most >40 years	Index finger extension, other finger extension, wrist flexion, intrinsic hand muscles, ankle and toe dorsiflexion	Rimmed vacuoles with atrophic fibres (affected muscle biopsy)
ZASPopathy (Markesbery–Griggs late-onset distal myopathy)	609452	Z disc alternatively spliced PDZ domain containing protein (ZASP) 10q23.2	>40 years	Ankle dorsiflexion/plantarflexion, finger/wrist extension; proximal limb after 15–20 years of disease	Myofibrillar myopathy with hyaline structures on trichrome which stain for dystrophin, desmin, myotilin, alphaB-crystallin
Desminopathy	601419	Desmin (DES) 2q35	Wide range, from 20–50 years; rarely in childhood	Ankle dorsiflexion/plantarflexion, in combination with dilated cardiomyopathy with or without conduction defects or respiratory failure	Myofibrillar myopathy with excess accumulation of desmin and myotilin, Z-disc alterations with autophagic components
Distal myotilinopathy	182920, 609200	Myotilin (MYOT) 5q31.2	45–60 years	Ankle dorsiflexion/plantarflexion; can progress rapidly over 10 years to give proximal leg weakness and loss of ambulation, arm weakness	Myofibrillar myopathy; myotilin aggregates may be compact, called spheroid bodies
Matrin3 distal myopathy (MPD2, vocal cord and pharyngeal distal myopathy)	606070	Matrin-3 (MATR3) 5q31.2	>50 years	Ankle and toe dorsiflexion, finger extension, dysphonia, and dysphagia	Rimmed vacuoles
VCP-mutated distal myopathy[+]		Valosin-containing protein (VCP) 9p13.3	>40 years	Similar to either Udd or Welander distal myopathy; Paget's disease not present in distal myopathy phenotype, frontotemporal dementia 25 years after onset of muscle weakness	Rimmed vacuoles or multiloculated ring fibers
Distal actin-binding domain filaminopathy (Williams distal myopathy, MPD4)[++]	614065	FilaminC (FLNC) 7q32.1	Teens to 50s	Hand grip, small muscles of hand, ankle plantarflexion	Non-specific, not myofibrillar
Distal myopathy with early respiratory failure[+]	607569	Unknown	32–75 years	Ankle dorsiflexion, respiratory muscles	Eosinophilic inclusions, rimmed vacuoles
Vacuolar neuromyopathy[++]	601846	19p.13.3	Late teens to 50s	Ankle dorsiflexion/plantarflexion	Rimmed vacuoles, filamentous bodies
Distal myopathy 3 (MPD3)[+]	610099	8p22-q11	30–45 years	Ankle dorsiflexion, intrinsic hand muscles	Rimmed vacuoles, eosinophilic inclusions
Autosomal recessive					
Early onset					
Distal nebulin myopathy		Nebulin (NEB) 2q23.3	<10 years	Ankle dorsiflexion, finger and wrist extensors	Grouped atrophic fibers, very small rod structures on EM, rarely nemaline myopathology
Adult onset					
Miyoshi myopathy	254130	Dysferlin (DYS) 2p13.2	Late teens, early 20s	Ankle plantarflexion	Widespread fiber necrosis, with variable other dystrophic changes
GNE myopathy (Nonaka myopathy, distal myopathy with rimmed vacuoles)	605820	UDP-N-acetylglucosamine 2 epimerase/N-acetyl mannosamine kinase (GNE) 9p13.3	>20 years	Ankle dorsiflexion, toe extension	Autophagic rimmed vacuoles
Distal anoctaminopathy	613319	Anoctamin5 (ANO5) 11p14.3	>20 years	Ankle plantarflexion, may be asymmetric	Scattered fiber necrosis

+ = one family described; ++ = two families described

presence of bulbar symptoms suggests a mutation in *MATR3*. There can be marked intrafamilial variability with respect to the severity of the phenotype, particularly in Laing and Udd distal myopathies. Distal muscle weakness can frequently occur in other disorders, and these are outlined in a recent review. In particular, facioscapulohumeral muscular dystrophy (FSHD) can present with isolated footdrop or less frequently with the inability to stand on tiptoe for several years, before the typical winging of the scapulae, or facial weakness, develops. Myotonic dystrophy can also present with isolated hand weakness or footdrop, and that and FSHD are the commonest muscular dystrophies in adulthood.

Investigations

The combination of clinical phenotype, creatine kinase (CK) level, muscle imaging, and histopathological findings on muscle biopsy is the key to diagnosis. CK is markedly elevated in Miyoshi myopathy and anoctaminopathy (20–150-fold normal values). In the remainder of the distal myopathies, CK is only mildly elevated or normal. Electromyography is necessary to exclude motor-predominant neuropathy or distal neuronopathy. However, it has been noted that in distal myopathies affecting the legs, there is often preservation of muscle bulk in the extensor digitorum brevis, whereas there is wasting of this muscle in peripheral neuropathies.

Muscle imaging using magnetic resonance imaging (MRI) or computed tomography (CT) has been recognized as helpful, and sometimes diagnostic. In Udd myopathy there is highly selective fatty degeneration in the anterior compartment muscles of the lower legs, starting in the tibialis anterior. In both ZASPopathy and distal myotilinopathy there are early fatty degenerative changes in the medial gastrocnemius and soleus muscles. In desminopathy, there is greater degeneration in the lateral peroneal muscles than the anterior compartment and medial gastrocnemius and soleus muscles, which is diagnostic. In distal actin-binding domain filaminopathy, MRI shows large-scale fatty-fibrous replacement in all calf muscles, with sparing of the anterior and lateral compartments. The other important benefit of a muscle MRI is that it allows targeting of an affected muscle for biopsy. In many of the distal myopathies, diagnostic features such as rimmed vacuoles will only be found in affected muscles.

Muscle biopsy may show non-specific myopathic features such as variable fiber diameters, increased internal nuclei, or fiber type predominance. However, very specific features can be found, such as rimmed vacuoles in Udd, Welander, and GNE myopathies. The myofibrillar myopathies are united by their pathological appearance, namely myofibrillar disintegration and protein aggregates that stain on immunohistochemistry for dystrophin, desmin, myotilin, and alphaB crystallin, among others.

Molecular genetic analysis has become the gold standard in diagnosis. Previously, the size of several of the genes made routine analysis very difficult, for instance nebulin (183 exons) and titin (363 exons). Increasingly this problem is being overcome by next-generation sequencing technologies, using either whole exome or targeted subexome analysis. It is noteworthy that of the distal myopathies listed in Table 119.1, the only ones where the gene is still not known are three dominant myopathies that have only been identified in one or two families. The FORGE Canada Consortium identified that such families were the most difficult in which to find the mutated genes.

Treatment

To date there are no treatments for the distal myopathies. However, early patient trials are currently assessing the tolerability and efficacy of oral sialic acid in GNE myopathy, targeting the hyposialation. Stop codon readthrough and exon-skipping strategies are being investigated in the treatment of Miyoshi myopathy and others.

Supportive treatment remains the mainstay of caring for people with distal myopathies. Cardiac arrhythmias may require the use of pacemakers or implantable cardioverter-defibrillators. Cardiomyopathy can be treated with medication, or cardiac transplantation if required. In patients with hypercapnia or incipient respiratory failure, continuous or bilevel positive airway pressure ventilation can be used, initially at night and later during the day. Physiotherapy directed toward preventing ankle contractures is important, as are assistive mobility devices such as ankle orthoses.

Conclusions

Progress has been made over the last several years in identifying the molecular basis for the distal myopathies, and this will continue. Other research aimed at understanding the pathophysiology where the genes are known remains important and will lead to the development of effective treatments.

Further reading

Beaulieu CL, Majewski J, Schwartzentruber J, *et al.* FORGE Canada Consortium: Outcomes of a 2-Year national rare-disease gene-discovery project. *Am J Hum Genet* 2014;94:809–817.

Lamont PJ, Wallefeld W, Hilton-Jones D, *et al.* Novel mutations widen the phenotypic spectrum of slow skeletal/beta-cardiac myosin (MYH7) distal myopathy. *Hum Mutat* 2014;35:868–879.

Nishino I, Carrillo-Carrasco N, Argov Z. GNE myopathy: Current update and future therapy. *J Neurol Neurosurg Psychiatry* 2015;86:385–392.

Udd B. Distal myopathies. *Curr Neurol Neurosci Rep* 2014;14:434–442.

120 Polymyositis

Marinos C. Dalakas

Department of Neurology, Thomas Jefferson University, Philadelphia, PA, USA

National University of Athens Medical School, Athens, Greece

Polymyositis (PM) is one of the four main subsets of inflammatory myopathies, the others being dermatomyositis (DM), necrotizing autoimmune myositis (NAM), and inclusion body myositis (IBM). As a stand-alone entity, PM is a rare disease and some writers have even doubted its existence. The exact frequency is unknown, but all four forms occur in approximately 1 in 100,000 adults. PM is often misdiagnosed and requires a careful review of the clinical features, muscle histopathology, and immunopathology to ensure that toxic, metabolic, mitochondrial, or dystrophic muscle diseases are not missed, and that the more common entities such as NAM, overlap myositis, and IBM are not overlooked or misdiagnosed as PM.

Clinical manifestations

PM has no unique clinical features, and it is a diagnosis of exclusion. It is best defined as an inflammatory myopathy of subacute onset (weeks to months) and steady progression that occurs in adults who do not have the rash seen in DM, involvement of eye and facial muscles, family history of a neuromuscular disease, endocrinopathy, exposure to myotoxic drugs, or other myopathies such as dystrophy, metabolic myopathy, IBM (based on unique clinical phenotype), or NAM.

Patients commonly present with subacute onset of proximal and often symmetric muscle weakness; an acute onset should raise the suspicion of NAM. Patients complain of difficulty getting up from a chair, climbing steps, lifting objects, or combing hair. Fine-motor movements that depend on the strength of distal muscles, such as buttoning a shirt, sewing, knitting, or writing, are affected only late in the disease. If these muscles are affected from the outset or early in the course of the disease, IBM should be suspected. In advanced cases, atrophy of the affected muscles takes place. Ocular muscles remain normal even in advanced cases, and if these muscles are affected, the diagnosis of inflammatory myopathy should be doubted. In contrast with IBM, where the facial muscles are affected in the majority of patients, in PM the strength of the facial muscles remains normal except for rare advanced cases. The pharyngeal and neck-extensor muscles can be involved, causing dysphagia and a dropped head state. Tendon reflexes are preserved, but may be absent in severely weakened or atrophied muscles. The respiratory muscles are rarely affected, but respiratory symptoms are common due to interstitial lung disease. Myalgia and muscle tenderness may be present when PM occurs in the setting of a connective tissue disorder or in overlap myositis associated with the antisynthetase syndrome, heralded by the presence of anti-Jo-1 antibodies. In patients with PM who have severe muscle pain, involvement of the fascia should be suspected even without overt signs of skin induration and thickness.

Cardiac abnormalities due to myocarditis related directly to PM are rare. Most often, cardiac abnormalities appear to be secondary to hypertension associated with long-term treatment with steroids, or due to pulmonary hypertension related to interstitial lung disease. Interstitial lung disease, reported in 10–30% of patients, is mostly seen in those with anti-Jo-1 antibodies against various ribonucleoproteins or MDA-4. Associated general systemic disturbances, such as fever, malaise, weight loss, arthralgia, and Raynaud's phenomenon, suggest antisynthetase syndrome, overlap myositis, or the presence of a connective tissue disorder.

PM is extremely rare in childhood, and if a diagnosis is made in patients younger than 16 years, a careful review is needed to exclude another disease, especially inflammatory dystrophy.

Association conditions

PM as an isolated clinical entity is quite uncommon. It is more frequently seen in association with connective tissue disorders, systemic autoimmune diseases, such as Sjögren's syndrome, rheumatoid arthritis, Crohn's disease, vasculitis, sarcoidosis, primary biliary cirrhosis, adult celiac disease, chronic graft-versus-host disease, discoid lupus, ankylosing spondylitis, Behçet's disease, myasthenia gravis, acne fulminans, dermatitis herpetiformis, psoriasis, Hashimoto's disease, granulomatous diseases, agammaglobulinemia, hypereosinophilic syndrome, Lyme disease, Kawasaki disease, autoimmune thrombocytopenia, hypergammaglobulinemic purpura, hereditary complement deficiency, IgA deficiency, and viral infections. Among viruses, human immunodeficiency virus (HIV) and human T-lymphotropic virus (HTLV-1) are the only ones convincingly associated with PM. Claims that other viruses, such as enteroviruses, can be causally connected with PM are unproven. PM is not more frequently associated with cancer compared to other chronic autoimmune disorders treated with immunosuppressants. Cancer is, however, more frequently associated with DM.

Drugs do not cause PM. The main drug that could trigger PM is D-penicillamine. Among the common myotoxic drugs, the antinucleoside analogues like zidovudine cause a mitochondrial myopathy, while the cholesterol-lowering statins have been rarely associated with an antibody-mediated necrotizing myopathy that lacks the features of primary endomysial inflammation, but consists of necrotic fibers with macrophages and MHC-I upregulation rare beyond the necrotic fibers. Most patients with NAM have antibodies against signal recognition particle (SRP) or the 3-hydroxy-3-methylglutaryl-coenzyme A reductase (HMGCR), the pharmacological target of statins. Although anti-HMGCR antibodies were though to be statin-related, they are now seen in NAM due to any cause and more often in statin-naive patients. Because NAM is one of the commonest

International Neurology, Second edition. Edited by Robert P. Lisak, Daniel D. Truong, William M. Carroll and Roongroj Bhidayasiri

© 2016 John Wiley & Sons, Ltd. Published 2016 by John Wiley & Sons, Ltd.

inflammatory myopathies and more than 25% of Americans above 40 years take statins, the association between statins and NAM is likely a chance phenomenon, especially since their role in inducing NAM has not been proven. NAM is seen in all ages but mostly adults, starting either acutely and reaching its peak over days or weeks, or subacutely and progressing steadily, causing severe weakness and very high creatine kinase (CK) levels. NAM occurs alone or after viral infections, in association with cancer, rare in patients taking statins, when the myopathy continues to worsen after statin withdrawal but the connection between the two remains still dubious.

Immunopathogenesis

PM may be one of the best studied or prototypic T-cell-mediated disorders, where cytotoxic T-cells directed against previously unidentified muscle antigens form an immunological synapse with the MHC-I class antigen expressed on the surface of muscle fibers.

The cytotoxicity of the autoinvasive T-cells has been similar to the one studied in IBM and has been supported by the presence of perforin granules, which are directed toward the surface of the muscle fiber and lead to muscle fiber necrosis on their release. The specificity of the T-cells has been further examined by studying the gene rearrangement of the T-cell receptors of the autoinvasive T-cells. In patients with PM, as well as IBM, only certain T-cells of specific T-cell receptor alpha and T-cell receptor beta families are recruited to the muscle from the circulation. Cloning and sequencing of the amplified endomysial T-cell receptor gene families has demonstrated a restricted use of the J-beta gene with conserved amino acid sequence in the CDR3 region, the antigen-binding region of the TCR, indicating that CD8+ cells are specifically selected and clonally expanded in situ by muscle-specific autoantigens. Studies combining laser microdissection, immunocytochemistry, polymerase chain reaction, and sequencing of the most prominent T-cell receptor families have shown that only the autoinvasive, not the perivascular, endomysial CD8+ cells are clonally expanded. Comparison of the T-cell receptor repertoire between PM and DM with spectratyping has confirmed that perturbations of the T-cell receptor families occur only in PM. Further, among the circulating T-cells, clonal expansion occurs only in the cytotoxic CD8+ cells that express genes for perforin and infiltrate the MHC-I-expressing muscle fibers.

The clonally expanded CD8+ T-cells in both PM and IBM, form immunological synapses with the muscle fibers that they invade, as supported by the co-expression of co-stimulatory molecules B7-1, B7-2, BB1, CD40, or ICOS-L on the muscle fibers and the respective counter-receptors CD28, CTLA-4, CD40L, or ICOS on autoinvasive T-cells. Cytokines, chemokines, and metalloproteinases are all upregulated in the muscle tissue. Some of these cytokines, such as γ-interferon, ILI-1β, and TNF-alpha, may exert a direct cytotoxic effect on the muscle tissue. Unique to muscle is the observation that the various cytokines and chemokines can also stimulate the muscle fibers to produce endogenously proinflammatory cytokines, such as γ-interferon, which enhances and perpetuates the immune response. Plasma cells and myeloid dendritic cells, which are potent antigen-presenting cells, have been also seen among the endomysial infiltrates. Although the myeloid dendritic cells may be candidate cells for antigen presentation to surrounding T-cells, their role remains elusive. Based on their immunoglobulin gene isotype, however, the plasma cells appear to mature and expand in situ, implying an antigen-driven response.

In PM as well as in IBM, MHC-I is expressed in all fibers, even in those not invaded by T-cells, often throughout the course of the disease. Such chronic MHC-I upregulation may be deleterious, exerting a stress effect on the endoplasmic reticulum (ER) of the myofiber, independent of T-cell-mediated cytotoxicity. In PM as well as IBM, the muscle fibers are overloaded by MHC molecules and the antigenic peptides cannot undergo proper conformational change to bind to MHC-I complex, leading to ER stress. This contention is supported by upregulation of the chaperone proteins and the activation of NF-kB, a means by which the cells protect themselves from ER stress. Such stressor effects are also seen in MHC-I transgenic mice, suggesting that continuous overexpression of MHC-I alone may be sufficient to induce ER stress and lead to persistence of the chronic inflammatory response.

Factors triggering the T-cell-mediated process in PM remain unclear. Viruses may be responsible for breaking tolerance, but only the retroviruses HIV and HTLV-I have been etiologically connected with the disease in infected individuals. These viruses do not, however, directly infect the muscle fibers; instead, they are only present on some of the infiltrating macrophages. Some of the autoinvasive T-cells are viral specific, carrying viral peptides as demonstrated with tetramers, and may play a role in the disease by cross-reacting with antigens expressed on the surface of muscle fibers.

No specific serum antibodies have been associated with polymyositis, except for antibodies against the histidyl-transfer RNA synthetases in patients with overlap myositis (see Chapter 121). In contrast, in NAM there are two specific antibodies against SRP and HMGCR, as mentioned earlier, that occur irrespective of statin exposure.

Differential diagnosis

Because PM is a diagnosis of exclusion, all diseases that cause an acquired myopathy should be considered before the diagnosis is established. The following myopathies mimic PM and need to be excluded: (1) hereditary neuromuscular diseases, especially inflammatory muscular dystrophies such as dysferlinopathies, fascioscapulohumeral dystrophy, Becker muscular dystrophy, anoctaminopathies, or calpainopathies; (2) metabolic myopathies, endocrinopathies, electrolyte disturbances, or mitochondriopathies; (3) any systemic medical illness, including malabsorption syndromes, alcoholism, cancer, vasculitis, systemic infections, sarcoidosis, granulomatous disease, or treatment with various known myotoxic drugs or a combination of unknown, but potentially myotoxic, drugs or toxins; (4) neurogenic muscular atrophies or neurogenic conditions; (5) biochemical muscle diseases such as McArdle's disease, excluded by muscle enzyme histochemistry; (6) IBM; and (7) necrotizing myopathy, which is characterized by infiltration of macrophages, rather than T-cell infiltrates, abundant necrotic fibers, and, often, prominent expression of MHC-I class antigen.

Diagnosis

In PM the serum muscle enzymes are elevated as much as 30 times higher than normal. Although CK usually parallels disease activity, it can be normal in chronic PM and only slightly elevated in PM associated with connective tissue disease, reflecting the preference of the pathological process for the intramuscular vessels and the perimysium. Along with CK, serum SGOT, SGPT, and LDH (but not gamma-GT) may also be elevated. Needle electromyography (EMG) shows active myopathic discharges that have no unique specificity for PM. The definitive diagnosis of PM is established with muscle biopsy.

In PM, the presence of inflammation is the histological hallmark of the disease (Figure 120.1). The endomysial infiltrates are mostly in foci within the fascicles surrounding healthy muscle fibers, leading eventually to muscle fiber necrosis. Sometimes the inflammatory infiltrates may be so localized and multifocal that they are missed in a small biopsy specimen. Occasionally, inflammation can be better seen in longitudinal sections. As in IBM, the inflammation is primary, a term used to indicate that CD8+ cells invade histologically healthy fibers that express MHC-I antigen. This lesion is termed the "CD8/MHC-I complex" and it is considered to be a specific for PM that secures the histological diagnosis. Eosinophils are rare, but, if abundant, the diagnosis of eosinophilic myositis should be considered. When the disease is chronic, the connective tissue is increased. In PM, there should be no vasculitis, or vacuolated fibers with cytoplasmic inclusions, as seen in IBM. A primary endomysial inflammatory response with upregulation of MHC-I is an invariable feature of PM and its absence early in the illness should raise a critical concern about the diagnosis.

Therapy

Treatment remains empirical, and separate large-scale, prospective, controlled clinical studies have not been performed.

The goal of therapy is to improve functional activities in daily living by improving muscle strength. Although improvement in strength is usually accompanied by a fall in CK, decreases of CK alone need to be interpreted with caution, because most immunosuppressive therapies lower serum muscle enzyme levels without necessarily improving muscle strength. Unfortunately, this has been misinterpreted as "chemical improvement" rather than monitoring muscle strength and has led to unnecessary prolongation of immunosuppressive treatment.

Commonly used drugs are as follows.

Steroids and nonsteroidal immunosuppressive agents

Because the initial response to prednisolone determines whether or not stronger immunosuppressive drugs will be needed, an aggressive approach with high-dose prednisone early in the disease is preferred, with a single daily morning dose of 80–100 mg for an initial period of 3–4 weeks. Prednisolone is then tapered to an every-other-day program. If after 2–3 months there is no objective increase in muscle strength, the patient should be considered unresponsive to prednisolone and the tapering accelerated. In such circumstances, the diagnosis should be reconsidered. The majority of patients with PM respond to steroids to some degree and for some period of time. For those patients responding to steroids, a "steroid-sparing" drug is needed to avoid long-term steroid complications and prevent relapse, which can occur each time the steroid dosage is lowered. The following therapies are used as steroid-sparing agents: (1) azathioprine, up to 3 mg/kg; (2) methotrexate, starting at 7.5 mg weekly for the first 3 weeks and increasing up to a total of 25 mg weekly; (3) mycophenolate mofetil, which has the advantage of working faster than azathioprine and is well tolerated up to 2,500 mg per day; and (4) tacrolimus, which has been promising in difficult cases, especially those with interstitial lung disease. Plasmapheresis, cyclophospamide, and cyclosporine have been disappointing.

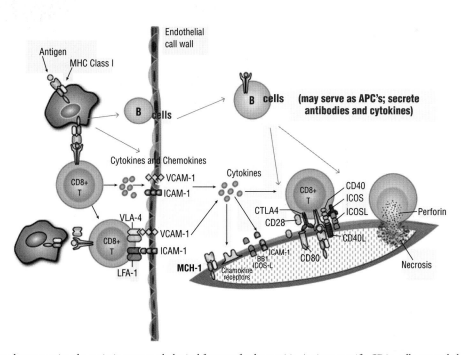

Figure 120.1 A scheme demonstrating the main immunopathological feature of polymyositis. Antigen-specific CD8+ cells, expanded in the periphery and subsequently endomysially, cross the endothelial cell wall and bind directly to aberrantly expressed MHC-I on the surface of muscle fibers via their T-cell receptors. Perforin granules released by the autoaggressive T-cells mediate muscle fiber necrosis. Cytokines released by the activated T-cells enhance MHC-I upregulation and T-cell cytotoxicity. Activated B-cells or plasmacytoid dendritic cells are clonally expanded endomysially and may participate in the process by a still undefined role, either as APC (antigen-presenting cells), or by release of cytokines and antibody production.

Intravenous immunoglobulin

Intravenous immunoglobin (IVIg) is effective in patients with refractory DM and in the majority of PM patients, although a controlled study in PM has not been performed. Because of its safety and efficacy, IVIg is used as second-line therapy after steroid use.

Treatment failures and new agents

New biological agents come in the form of monoclonal antibodies or fusion proteins. Some appear promising, but need controlled trial evidence. Among them, rituximab, a B-cell-depleting monoclonal antibody against CD20, has been tested in a placebo-controlled study in 200 patients with PM and DM, but it did not meet the primary end-point, largely because of study design. Although at week 8 there was no difference between placebo and rituximab, at week 44 when all patients had received rituximab, 83% met the definition of improvement. Patients with anti-Jo-1, Mi-2, or anti-SRP antibodies seem more likely to respond.

When treatment response is suboptimal, the patient should be re-evaluated and the muscle biopsy specimen re-examined. A second biopsy might be considered to confirm the diagnosis. Disorders commonly misdiagnosed as PM include IBM; sporadic limb-girdle muscular dystrophy, which is suspected when the disease has a slow onset and progression and the muscle biopsy specimen does not show primary inflammatory features; metabolic myopathy (e.g., myophosphorylase deficiency); endocrinopathy; and neurogenic muscular atrophies.

Prognosis

The natural history of PM is unknown, because steroids are almost universally applied early after diagnosis. Occasional cases that present as severe acute necrotizing myositis, often after viral infection or in association with cancer or statins, are not typical cases of PM and require aggressive therapy with steroids, IVIg, or rituximab. In general, older age, interstitial lung disease, and frequent pneumonias due to esophageal dysfunction are factors associated with poor prognosis. There are still patients with PM who do not adequately respond to therapies and remain disabled; in these circumstances it is unclear whether the disease is bona fide PM or another disorder misdiagnosed as PM.

Further reading

Dalakas MC. Polymyositis, dermatomyositis, and inclusion-body myositis. *N Engl J Med* 1991;325:1487–1498.

Dalakas MC. Signaling pathways and immunobiology of inflammatory myopathies. *Nature Clinic Practice Rheumatol* 2006;2:219–227.

Dalakas MC. Immunotherapy of myositis: Issues, concerns and future prospects. *Nat Rev Rheumatol* 2010;6:129–137.

Dalakas MC. An update on inflammatory and autoimmune myopathies. *Neuropathol Appl Neurobiol* 2011;37(3):226–242.

Dalakas MC. Inflammatory muscle diseases. *N Engl J Med* 2015;372:1734–1747.

Dalakas MC, Hohlfeld R. Polymyositis and dermatomyositis. *Lancet* 2003;362: 1762–1763.

Luo YB, Mastaglia FL. Dermatomyositis, polymyositis and immune-mediated necrotising myopathies. *Biochim Biophys Acta* 2015;1852(4):622–632.

Wiendl H, Hohlfeld R, Kieseier BC. Immunobiology of muscle: Advances in understanding an immunological microenvironment. *Trends Immunol* 2005;26:373–380.

121 Dermatomyositis

Marinos C. Dalakas

Department of Neurology, Thomas Jefferson University, Philadelphia, PA, USA
National University of Athens Medical School, Athens, Greece

Dermatomyositis (DM) is one of the four main inflammatory myopathies, the other three being polymyositis (PM), necrotizing autoimmune myositis (NAM), and inclusion body myositis (IBM). DM is a disease that affects skin and muscle. As a result, it is cared for not only by neurologists but also by rheumatologists and dermatologists. The role of the neurologist is essential to exclude other myopathies and to initiate or supervise the immunotherapeutic interventions. The exact incidence of dermatomyositis is unknown. The four forms of inflammatory myopathy occur in approximately 4.3–7.9/100,000 person-years, with prevalence ranging from 9.5–32.7/100,000. In other series, the annual incidence is estimated at 5–10 cases per million in adults and 1–5 in children.

Clinical manifestations

DM occurs in both children and adults. It is a distinct clinical entity because of a characteristic rash that accompanies or, more often, precedes muscle weakness. The skin manifestations include a heliotrope rash (blue–purple discoloration) on the upper eyelids with edema, a flat red rash on the face and upper trunk, and erythema of the knuckles with a raised violaceous scaly eruption (Gottron rash). The erythematous rash can also occur on other body surfaces, including the knees, elbows, malleoli, neck, and anterior chest (often in a V shape), or back and shoulders (shawl shape), and may be exacerbated after sun exposure. The initial erythematous lesions may result in scaling desquamation accompanied by pigmentation and depigmentation, giving at times a shiny appearance. Dilated capillary loops at the base of the fingernails are also characteristic of DM. The cuticles may be irregular, thickened, and distorted, and the lateral and palmar areas of the fingers may become rough and cracked, with irregular, "dirty" horizontal lines, resembling "mechanic's hands."

DM in children resembles the adult disease. An early abnormality in children is "misery," defined as an irritable child who feels uncomfortable, has a red flush on the face, is fatigued, does not feel like socializing, and has a varying degree of muscle weakness. A tiptoe gait due to plantar flexion contracture of the ankles is not unusual.

In DM the affected muscles are predominantly proximal, but the degree of weakness varies. It can be mild, moderate, or severe, leading to quadriparesis. Patients complain of difficulty getting up from a chair, climbing steps, lifting objects, or combing hair. Fine-motor movements that depend on the strength of distal muscles, such as buttoning a shirt, sewing, knitting, or writing, are affected only late in the disease. In advanced cases, atrophy of the affected muscles takes place. Ocular and facial muscles remain normal even in advanced cases, and if these muscles are affected, the diagnosis of inflammatory myopathy should be questioned. The pharyngeal and neck-extensor muscles can be involved, causing dysphagia and difficulty holding the head erect. The tendon reflexes are preserved, but may be absent in severely weakened or atrophied muscles. The respiratory muscles are rarely affected, but respiratory symptoms may not be uncommon when there is also interstitial lung disease. Myalgia and muscle tenderness may occur early in the disease, especially when DM occurs in the setting of a connective tissue disorder. In patients with DM who have severe muscle pain, involvement of the fascia should be suspected.

Some patients with the classic skin lesions may have clinically normal strength, even up to 3–5 years after onset. This form of DM, referred to as dermatomyositis sine myositis or amyopathic dermatomyositis, has a better overall prognosis. Although in these cases the disease appears limited to the skin, the muscle biopsy shows perivascular and perimysial inflammation with immunopathological features identical to those seen in the classic DM, suggesting that the "amyopathic" and "myopathic" forms are part of the range of DM affecting skin and muscle to varying degrees.

DM usually occurs alone, but it may overlap with scleroderma and mixed connective tissue disease. Fasciitis and skin changes similar to those found in DM have occurred in patients with eosinophilia-myalgia syndrome caused by the ingestion of contaminated L-tryptophan, and in patients with eosinophilic fasciitis or macrophagic myofasciitis. In up to 10–32% of patients, DM has a paraneoplastic association. Ovarian cancer is most frequent, followed by intestinal, breast, lung, and liver cancer. In Asian populations, nasopharyngeal cancer is more common. The cancer sites usually correspond to those occurring more frequently at the patient's age. Because tumors are often only discovered at autopsy or on the basis of abnormal findings on medical history and physical examination, blind radiological searches are rarely fruitful. A complete annual physical examination, with breast, pelvic, and rectal examinations (including colonoscopy in high-risk patients), urinalysis, complete blood cell count, blood chemistry tests, and chest X-ray, is usually sufficient and is highly recommended, especially in the first 3 years following diagnosis of DM. Some autoantibodies against transcriptional intermediary factor-1 (TIF-1) and nuclear matrix protein NXP-2 have been connected with cancer-associated adult dermatomyositis, but they are influenced by geographic, racial, or genetic factors.

In addition to involvement at the muscles and skin, extramuscular manifestations may be prominent in some patients with DM. These include (1) dysphagia, sometimes as prominent as seen in patients with scleroderma; (2) atrioventricular conduction defects, tachyarrhythmia, low ejection fraction, and dilated cardiomyopathy (either due to the disease itself or, more often, to hypertension or fluid retention associated with long-term steroid use); (3) pulmonary involvement, resulting

International Neurology, Second edition. Edited by Robert P. Lisak, Daniel D. Truong, William M. Carroll and Roongroj Bhidayasiri
© 2016 John Wiley & Sons, Ltd. Published 2016 by John Wiley & Sons, Ltd.

either from the primary weakness of the thoracic muscles, or due to interstitial lung disease, especially in patients who have anti-Jo-1 antibodies, as discussed later; (4) subcutaneous calcifications, sometimes opening onto the skin and causing ulcerations and infections, especially in children; (5) gastrointestinal ulcerations, due to vasculitis or infections; (6) contractures of the joints, especially in the childhood form; and (7) general systemic disturbances, such as fever, malaise, weight loss, arthralgia, and Raynaud's phenomenon, especially when DM is associated with a connective tissue disorder or the antisynthetase syndrome and Jo-1 antibodies.

Imunopathogenesis

In DM there is evidence of a humoral-mediated process based on immunopathological studies performed on muscle biopsy. The primary antigenic targets appear to be components of the endothelium of the blood vessels in the endomysium and probably the skin. Alterations in the endothelial cells consisting of pale and swollen cytoplasm with microvacuoles and tubuloreticular aggregates appear early in the disease. The capillaries undergo active focal destruction, with undulating tubules in the smooth endoplasmic reticulum of the endothelial cells leading to vascular necrosis and thrombi. These changes are caused by immune complexes immunolocalized in the endomysial blood vessels along with the C5b-9 membrane attack complex, the lytic component of the complement pathway. The membrane attack complex and the early complement components C3b and C4b are deposited on the capillaries early in the disease and precede the signs of inflammation or structural changes in the muscle fibers. These complement fragments are also detected in the serum and correlate with disease activity. It is believed that the disease begins when putative antibodies or other factors activate complement C3, C3b, and C4b fragments that lead to formation of membrane attack complex, which is deposited in the endomysial microvasculature and leads to osmotic lysis of the endothelial cells

and capillary necrosis. As a result, there is a reduction in the number of capillaries per muscle fiber, impaired perfusion, and dilatation of the loop of the remaining capillaries in an effort to compensate for the ischemic process. Larger intramuscular blood vessels are also affected similarly, leading to muscle fiber destruction (often resembling microinfarcts) and inflammation. The perifascicular atrophy often seen in more chronic stages is probably a reflection of the endofascicular hypoperfusion that is prominent distally (Figure 121.1).

The activation of complement induces the release of cytokines and chemokines such as IL1, IL6, TNF, TNF-β, CXCL4, and CXCL9, which, in turn, upregulate the expression of VCAM-I and ICAM-I on the endothelial cells and facilitate the transmigration of activated lymphoid cells to the perimysial and endomysial spaces. Immunophenotyping of the lymphocytic infiltrates demonstrates B-cells, CD4+ cells, and plasmacytoid dendritic cells in the perimysial and perivascular regions, supporting the view that a humoral-mediated mechanism plays the major role in the disease. In the perifascicular regions there is also upregulation of cathepsins and STAT-I, probably triggered by interferon-gamma , MxA and Rig-1 triggered by type 1 interferon (see below), as well as TGF-beta and various regenerating molecules. Based on gene arrays, a number of adhesion molecules and cytokine and chemokine genes are upregulated in the muscles of DM patients. Most notable among those genes are the KAL-1 adhesion molecule, and genes induced by α/β interferon. The KAL-I is upregulated by TGF-β and may have a deleterious role in DM by inducing fibrosis. Of interest is that KAL-I along with TGF-β is downregulated in the muscles of DM patients who improve after therapy. Innate immunity also plays a role based on increased expression of type-I interferon-inducible proteins such as myxovirus resistance MxA protein, in the perifascicular regions; whether this effect is triggered by danger signals from the damaged fibers that are sensed by the retinoic acid-inducible gene-1 signaling (Rig-1) and lead to auto-amplification of local inflammation by activating β-interferon and MHC-1, as recently proposed, remains

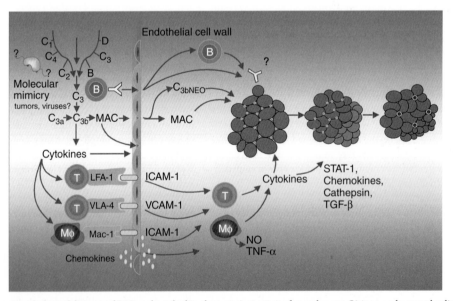

Figure 121.1 The main immunopathological features of DM, as described in the text. Activation of complement C3 is an early event leading to formation of C3b, C3bNEO, and membrane attack complexes (MAC), which are deposited on the endothelial cell wall of the endomysial capillaries, resulting in destruction of capillaries, ischemia, or microinfarcts, most prominent in the periphery of the fascicles, and perifascicular atrophy. Cytokines released by activated complement lead to enhancing the expression of cell adhesion molecules and activation of T-cells, macrophages, B-cells, and 123+plasmacytoid dendritic cells. The perifascicular regions contain fibers in a state of remodeling and regeneration (expressing TGFβ, NCAM, Mi-2), cell stress (expressing HSP 70, 90), immune activation (expressing MHC-1, chemokines, STAT-1), and molecules associated with innate immunity (such as MxA, ISG15, Rig-1).

to be determined. A summary of the immunopathology of DM is shown in Figure 121.1.

The immunopathology of the skin lesions in DM is not fully studied, but perivascular infiltrates consisting mainly of CD4+ cells, and macrophages along with C5b-9 complement deposits, are also noted in the dermis. The basal keratinocytes express CD40 while the neighboring CD4+ T-cells express CD40L, suggesting that the CD40–CD40L system may be involved in the cutaneous manifestations, probably via the upregulation of cytokines and chemokines, in a pattern similar to that described for the muscle.

Autoantibodies against nuclear (antinuclear antibodies) and cytoplasmic antigens (ribonucleoproteins involved in translation and protein synthesis) are also found in up to 60% of DM patients. The antibody directed against the histidyl-transfer RNA synthetase, called anti-Jo-1, accounts for 75% of all the antisynthetases and is clinically useful, because up to 70% of DM or PM patients with anti-Jo-1 antibodies develop interstitial lung disease. Other dermatomyositis-associated antibodies include (1) Mi-2, highlighting the typical skin lesions; (2) melanoma differentiation–associated protein-5 (MDA-5), mostly connected with amyopathic dermatomyositis or interstitial lung disease; and (3) transcriptional intermediary factor-1 (TIF-1) and nuclear matrix protein NXP-2, connected with cancer-associated adult dermatomyositis, but influenced by geographic, racial, or genetic factors.

Diagnosis

The diagnosis of DM is relatively easy because of the characteristic skin changes that appear unique to DM. The diagnosis is, however, aided by determining the level of serum muscle enzymes and the muscle biopsy.

In the presence of active disease, creatine kinase (CK) can be elevated up to 40 times the normal level. Although CK activity usually parallels disease severity, it can be normal in some patients with untreated disease or when DM is associated with a connective tissue disorder, probably reflecting the predominant involvement of the intramuscular vessels and the perimysium. Along with CK, serum glutamic-oxaloacetic transaminase, serum glutamic-pyruvic transaminase, glutamic pyruvic transaminase, lactate dehydrogenase, and aldolase may also be elevated. Needle electromyography (EMG) shows myopathic potentials characterized by short-duration, low-amplitude polyphasic units on voluntary activation and increased spontaneous activity with fibrillations, complex repetitive discharges, and positive sharp waves. Muscle biopsy is the definitive test to exclude other neuromuscular diseases, especially when the skin changes are not clear, and to assess the severity of involvement. The following unique histological features at the light microscopy level are characteristic of DM: (1) endomysial inflammation, predominantly in the perivascular or interfascicular septa and around rather than within the fascicles; (2) fibrin thrombi (especially in children) and obliteration of capillaries; (3) necrosis, degeneration, and phagocytosis, often affecting groups of fibers within a muscle fascicle in a wedgelike shape or at the periphery of the fascicle due to microinfarcts within the muscle; and (4) perifascicular atrophy, which is diagnostic of dermatomyositis, even in the absence of inflammation. The skin biopsy also shows the abnormalities mentioned earlier, but routine skin biopsy samples are not helpful.

Although the diagnosis of DM is very rarely in doubt, sometimes muscle strength is normal (dermatomyositis sine myositis), in spite of clear evidence of subclinical muscle involvement in the muscle biopsy. Other times, the rash may be barely detectable (especially in dark-skinned people) or transient; these cases belong to "overlap myositis." Overlap myositis is often associated with connective tissue diseases or antisynthetase antibodies and its main pathology resembles that of dermatomyositis characterized by inflammation, perifasicular atrophy, and necrotic fibers in the perifasicular, interfasicular, or perimysial areas.

Treatment

The disease is treated with immunosuppressive or immunomodulating agents. Most of the treatment trials have been empirical and non-selective, because the specific target antigens are unknown.

The goal of therapy in DM is to improve function in activities of daily living as the result of improvement in muscle strength, and ameliorate the skin alterations. Although improvement in strength is usually accompanied by a fall in serum CK, a decrease of serum CK alone without a concomitant improvement in strength has to be interpreted with caution in reference to the efficacy of the given drug. For patients with disease limited to the skin, the use of low-dose steroids or hydroxychloroquine sulfate, topical glucocorticoids or calcineurin inhibitors, and sunlight avoidance are recommended first before immunosuppressants are instituted.

Prednisolone is the first-line drug. Because the response to prednisolone, an effective drug for short-term use, determines whether or not stronger immunosuppressive drugs will be needed, an aggressive approach with high-dose prednisolone beginning early in the disease is used by this author, beginning at 80–100 mg/day as a single daily morning dose for 3–4 weeks. Prednisolone is then slowly tapered to an every-other-day dose until the lowest possible dose that controls the disease is reached. Aggressive disease should receive methylprednisolone 1 g intravenously (IV) every day for 3 days first, followed by oral steroid.

Drugs used for "steroid sparing," when a relapse occurs after attempts to lower the high steroid dosage, include (1) azathioprine, up to 3 mg/kg; (2) methotrexate, up to a total of 15-20 mg weekly; (3) mycophenolate mofetil up to 3,000 mg daily; and (4) cyclophosphamide, given intravenously at doses of 0.5–1 g/m^2.

If the response to prednisone is limited, intravenous immunoglobulin (IVIg) at 2 g/kg has been shown to be effective in DM with a controlled trial. In this double blind study, IVIg was shown to be effective in patients with refractory DM, not only by improving the strength and the skin rash, but also by clearing the underlying immunopathology. The improvement begins after the first infusion and is clearly evident by the second monthly infusion. The benefit, however, is short-lived (not more than 8 weeks), requiring repeated infusions every 6–8 weeks to maintain improvement. In DM, IVIg acts by inhibiting the deposition of activated complement fragments in capillaries and by suppressing cytokines and adhesion molecules at the protein, mRNA, and gene level. If IVIg is not effective, rituximab, a monoclonal antibody against CD20 on B-cells at 2 g (divided into 2 bi-weekly infusions) seems effective in a small number of patients. However, a placebo-controlled study in 200 patients with DM and PM did not meet the primary end-point, largely because of study design. Although at week 8 there was no difference between placebo and rituximab, at week 44 when all patients had received rituximab, 83% met the definition of improvement. Patients with anti-Jo-1, Mi-2, or anti-SRP antibodies seem more likely to respond. Plasmapheresis is not effective.

Therefore, a recommended approach to the treatment of DM is as follows:

- *Step 1*: High-dose prednisone (oral or intermittent intravenously in acute cases).
- *Step 2*: Add immunosuppressants, such as azathioprine, methotrexate, or mycophenolate, for steroid-sparing effect.
- *Step 3*: If Step 1 fails, try IVIg at 2g/kg.
- *Step 4*: If these steps fail, consider a trial with rituximab.

Treatment for calcinosis remains difficult; attempts with alendronate, probenecid, or diltiazem are thought to be promising, but offer limited benefit.

Prognosis and complications

The natural history of DM is unknown, as most patients nowadays are treated with steroids. The mortality rates reported 20–30 years ago are outdated. Clinical experience indicates that DM responds to therapy more readily than PM. In children, DM may at times be a monophasic disease with infrequent flares once the disease is under control. Patients with interstitial lung disease may have a high mortality rate, requiring aggressive treatment with cyclophosphamide or tacrolimus. However, there are still a number of patients who do not respond adequately to therapy and remain disabled, especially when subcutaneous calcification has formed, because it cannot be dissolved and appears resistant to all treatment. In these cases, ulceration, infection, and disfiguring scars result when they protrude through the skin.

Further reading

Dalakas MC. Polymyositis, dermatomyositis, and inclusion-body myositis. *N Engl J Med* 1991;325:1487–1498.

Dalakas MC. Immunotherapy of myositis: Issues, concerns and future prospects. *Nat Rev Rheumatol* 2010;6:129–137.

Dalakas MC. Inflammatory muscle diseases. *N Engl J Med* 2015;372:1734–1747.

Dalakas MC, Hohlfeld R. Polymyositis and dermatomyositis. *Lancet* 2003;362: 1762–1763.

Dalakas MC, Illa I, Dambrosia JM, *et al.* 1993. A controlled trial of high-dose intravenous immunoglobulin infusions as treatment for dermatomyositis. *N Engl J Med* 329(27):1993–2000.

Engel AG, Hohlfeld R. The polmyositis and dermatomyositis syndrome. In: Engel AG, Franzini-Armostrong C (eds.). *Myology*. New York: McGraw-Hill; 2005:1335–1383.

Luo YB, Mastaglia FL. Dermatomyositis, polymyositis and immune-mediated necrotising myopathies. *Biochim Biophys Acta* 2015;1852(4):622–632.

122 Inclusion body myositis

Merrilee Needham and Frank L. Mastaglia
Institute for Immunological and Infectious Diseases, Murdoch University, Perth, WA, Australia

Sporadic inclusion body myositis (sIBM) is the most common myopathy in Caucasians over 50 years of age and occasionally also affects younger people. It is traditionally classified as an inflammatory myopathy, but differs from other inflammatory myopathies by having a selective pattern of muscle weakness that is often asymmetric, is resistant to immunosuppressive therapy, and histologically has myodegenerative features with abnormal protein aggregation and inclusion body formation in addition to inflammatory changes. The etiology is unknown, but probably involves a complex interplay between genetic and environmental factors and aging.

Epidemiology

The frequency of sIBM varies in different populations, being highest in northern European, North American Caucasian, and Australian populations, in which prevalence figures of 4.9–14.9 per million have been reported. This contrasts with a prevalence of only ~1 per million in Istanbul, Turkey. In Caucasians, genetic susceptibility is linked to *HLA-DRB1*0301* and the *DRB1*0301/*0101* diplotype, whereas *HLA-DRB4* and *HLA-DRB5* are protective. In Japanese people, *HLA-B*5201* and *DRB1*1502* convey susceptibility. Polymorphism in the mitochondrial *TOMM 40* gene also influences disease risk and age of onset. The importance of genetic factors is also emphasized by the occasional occurrence of IBM in twins and siblings (familial IBM).

Familial IBM differs from the "hereditary inclusion body myopathies" (hIBM), a heterogeneous group of autosomal dominant or recessive disorders with variable clinical phenotypes and pathology resembling sIBM, including rimmed vacuoles and filamentous inclusions, but usually without inflammatory changes. The prototypic recessive forms were first described in Iranian Jews as a "quadriceps-sparing" myopathy and in Japanese as a distal myopathy with rimmed vacuoles (DMRV). Both are caused by mutations in the UDP-N-acetylglucosamine-2-epimerase/N-acetylmannosamine kinase (*GNE*) gene and are allelic with the Japanese form. However, mutations in *GNE* and other hIBM-associated genes have not been found in sIBM.

Pathophysiology

Pathologically, sIBM is characterized by (1) a CD8+ T-cell predominant inflammatory infiltrate, with invasion of MHC-1 expressing non-necrotic muscle fibres by CD8+ cells, macrophages, and myeloid dendritic cells; (2) rimmed vacuoles, congophilic inclusions, and filamentous protein aggregates; and (3) ragged-red

and cytochrome c oxidase (COX) deficient fibers that harbor clonally expanded mtDNA deletions and mutations. In addition to β-amyloid and amyloid precursor protein (APP), a variety of other proteins associated with neurodegenerative diseases, including phosphorylated tau, α-synuclein, prion protein, and apolipoprotein E, are present in the inclusions.

Recent research has led to a better understanding of the possible relationship between inflammatory and degenerative changes. Upregulation of pro-inflammatory cytokines such as interleukin-1 (IL-1), tumor necrosis factor (TNF-α), and interferon (IFN-γ) could be an early upstream event causing upregulation of MHC-1, endoplasmic reticulum (ER) stress, and NFκB upregulation, and further enhancing MHC-1 assembly, leading to a self-sustaining T-cell response. Pro-inflammatory cytokines (particularly IL-1), as well as NFκB, increase APP transcription and β-amyloid production, and could initiate a cascade of ER stress, proteasomal dysfunction, and protein accumulation. Alternatively, it has been suggested that increased APP transcription could itself be an early upstream event.

Clinical features

Sporadic IBM affects males more often than females. The diagnosis is often delayed for many years, and the condition may be misdiagnosed as motor neuron disease, polymyositis, or arthritis. The most common presentation is with insidious onset of quadriceps weakness, resulting in difficulty rising from chairs or climbing stairs and in falls, and less commonly with weakness of the fingers, foot drop, or dysphagia. The weakness is often asymmetric, and more severe on the non-dominant side. Dysphagia and obstructive sleep apnoea are common and respiratory failure also occurs rarely. Clinical examination typically reveals a selective pattern of weakness and atrophy of the quadriceps femoris and forearm muscles, with the flexor digitorum profundus and flexor pollicis longus being preferentially affected in the early stages. Other muscle groups can also be affected as the condition progresses, including the facial and paraspinal muscles, leading to "dropped head" or camptocormia. It is not known whether the clinical phenotype varies in different ethnic groups.

Investigations

The serum creatine kinase (CK) level may be normal or mildly elevated (up to 10 times the upper limit of normal). The condition may be associated with a monoclonal gammopathy, with various autoantibodies or other autoimmune diseases (such as Sjögren's

International Neurology, Second edition. Edited by Robert P. Lisak, Daniel D. Truong, William M. Carroll and Roongroj Bhidayasiri
© 2016 John Wiley & Sons, Ltd. Published 2016 by John Wiley & Sons, Ltd.

syndrome), or with human immunodeficiency virus (HIV-1) or human T-lymphotropic virus (HTLV-1) infections, which should be screened for in at-risk populations. A serum autoantibody to cytosolic 5'-nucleotidase 1A (cN1A) shows early promise as a diagnostic test, with sensitivities of 60–70% and specificities of 83–92% with a low antibody titer. Electromyography demonstrates a combination of short- and long-duration motor unit potentials with spontaneous activity, which may lead to a mistaken diagnosis of a neurogenic disorder such as motor neuron disease. Some cases also have a subclinical peripheral neuropathy. Magnetic resonance imaging (MRI) demonstrates selective involvement of the quadriceps femoris muscles in the thighs (Figure 122.1), medial gastrocnemius in the calves, and flexor muscles in the forearms. Definitive diagnosis traditionally required a muscle biopsy, although due to the highly selective pattern of muscle involvement, there are increasing discussions about the validity of "clinically defined sIBM" (see the 2013 ENMC criteria). The most suitable muscle for biopsy is the vastus lateralis, or, if too severely atrophied, the deltoid, biceps brachii, or tibialis anterior.

In addition to routine stains, stains for β-amyloid (crystal violet or Congo red viewed with Texas red filters) and immunostaining for T-cell subsets and MHC-1 and MHC-2 expression should be performed. There may be diagnostic utility in using immunostains for transactive DNA-binding protein-43 (TDP43) and p62 to help identify protein aggregation. Electron microscopy is required to demonstrate the characteristic 16–20 nm filamentous cytoplasmic or intranuclear inclusions, but is not essential for diagnosis.

Treatment and management

There is currently no therapy that stops the progression of the disease (see the review by Needham and Mastaglia). The protracted natural history has made the results of drug trials difficult to interpret, as few trials have been of adequate duration or sufficiently powered.

Glucocorticoids and cytotoxic agents

Uncontrolled trials of glucocorticoids reported stabilization or short-term improvement in some cases. However, in a prospective trial of high-dose prednisone, muscle strength continued to deteriorate in spite of a fall in CK level, and a reduction in T-cells in repeat biopsies after 6–12 months. This may be because the biopsies also demonstrated an increased number of fibers with vacuoles and amyloid deposits, indicating that the degenerative aspects of the disease failed to respond and continued to progress. In our experience immunosuppressive agents are usually ineffective, however some cases may show temporary stabilization or improvement on methotrexate or mycophenolate mofetil.

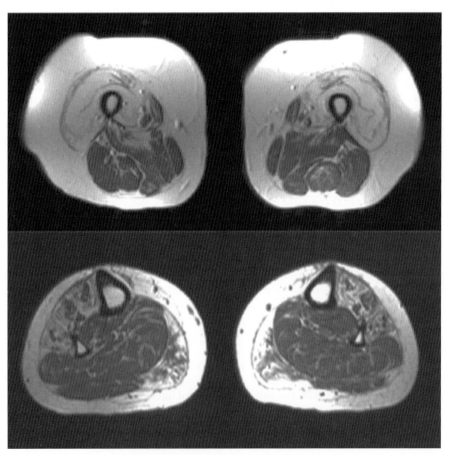

Figure 122.1 T2 axial magnetic resonance imaging scans through the mid-thigh (top two) and mid-calf (bottom two), demonstrating the specific muscle involvement seen in inclusion body myositis. The replacement of the vasti group of muscles with fat and relative sparing of the hamstring muscles can be seen in the thigh, and the selective involvement of the medial head of gastrocnemius and tibialis anterior in the lower leg.

Immunotherapy

Intravenous immunoglobulin therapy (IVIg) may provide short-term benefit in selected cases. A 3-month double blind placebo-controlled trial showed mild improvement in lower limb strength and swallowing. In another 3-month double blind study, the addition of prednisone did not enhance the effect of IVIg. A 12-month double blind trial, although not finding a significant improvement in strength, arrested progression of weakness in 90% of patients. Some patients with severe dysphagia have a good response to IVIg therapy.

A 12-month trial of antithymocyte globulin (ATG) with methotrexate showed a 1.4% increase in muscle strength, compared with 11.1% loss in the control group receiving methotrexate alone. A subsequent proof-of-principle trial of T-cell depletion using alemtuzumab showed evidence of slowing in the rate of deterioration and improvement in strength in some patients, with reduction in inflammation and stressor molecules. These studies indicate that there is a responsive component in IBM and suggest that randomized trials of therapies targeting T-cells may be worthwhile. Two randomized trials of interferon-β1a did not find any significant improvement. A pilot trial of the TNF-α blocker etanercept showed only a slight improvement in grip strength after 12 months of treatment.

Other therapies

Coenzyme Q10, carnitine, clenbuterol, and oxandrolone may provide symptomatic benefit in some patients. In addition to IVIg, swallowing function can be restored by a bougie dilatation, cricopharyngeal myotomy, or botulinum toxin injection into the upper esophageal sphincter in patients with severe dysphagia. Appropriate therapeutic measures should be implemented in patients with obstructive sleep apnoea. Strength training and aerobic conditioning can improve or stabilize muscle strength and functional performance without increasing CK levels or histological changes. However, exercise programs need to be individualized to avoid muscle overloading. Knee-locking braces may be helpful in preventing falls, and ankle-foot orthoses may assist if foot drop is a problem. In patients with severe finger weakness it may be possible to restore opposition of the thumb and index finger by transferring the tendons of the extensor carpi radialis and brachioradialis muscles to the more severely affected flexor tendons.

In addition, there is a current international multicenter phase IIb/III trial of a muscle building drug, bimagrumab (BYM338), which blocks the inhibitory effects of myostatin by binding to the activin II receptor, investigating whether this antibody can maintain muscle strength for longer.

Conclusions

Sporadic IBM is the most important myopathy associated with aging. The etiology is poorly understood, but there is increasing evidence that both HLA and non-HLA genes contribute to susceptibility. There is considerable geographic variation in the prevalence of the disease, and further surveys in different countries and ethnic groups are required to document these differences more fully and determine whether they are due to genetic or environmental influences. Further clarification of the molecular pathogenesis of the disease may lead to the development of more effective therapies targeting the immune response as well as the abnormal protein aggregation in muscle fibers.

Further reading

Dalakas MC. Sporadic inclusion body myositis – diagnosis, pathogenesis and therapeutic strategies. *Nat Clin Pract Neurol* 2006;2:437–445.

Needham M, Mastaglia F. Inclusion body myositis: Current pathogenetic concepts and diagnostic and therapeutic approaches. *Lancet Neurol* 2007;6: 620–631.

Needham M, Mastaglia F. Pathogenesis of sporadic inclusion body myositis: Trying to put the pieces of the puzzle together. *Neuromuscul Disord* 2008;18:6–16.

Needham M, Mastaglia FL, Garlepp MJ. Genetics of inclusion body myositis. *Muscle Nerve* 2007;35:549–561.

Novartis Pharmaceuticals. Efficacy and safety of bimagrumab/503 BYM338 at 52 weeks on physical function, muscle strength, mobility in sIBM patients (RESILIENT) 2014. http://clinicaltrials.gov/show/NCT01925209 (accessed November 2015).

Oldfors A, Lindberg C. Inclusion body myositis. *Curr Opin Neurol* 1999;12:527–533.

Serdaroglu P, Deymeer F, Parman Y. Prevalence of sporadic inclusion body myositis (s-IBM) in Turkey: A muscle biopsy based survey. *Neuromuscul Disord* 2007;17:849.

Rose MR; ENMC IBM Working Group. 188th ENMC International Workshop: Inclusion body myositis, 2-4 December 2011, Naarden, The Netherlands. *Neuromuscul Disord* 2013;23:1044–1055.

123 Immune-mediated necrotizing myopathies

Werner Stenzel[1], Hans-Hilmar Goebel[1,2], Olivier Benveniste[3,4], and Yves Allenbach[3,4]

[1] Department of Neuropathology, Charité – Universitätsmedizin Berlin, Berlin, Germany

[2] Department of Neuropathology, Johannes Gutenberg University, Mainz, Germany

[3] Département de Médecine Interne et Immunologie Clinique, Centre de Référence Maladies Neuro-Musculaires Paris Est, Paris, France

[4] Centre de recherche en myologie, Université Pierre et Marie Curie (UPMC), Paris, France

Immune-mediated necrotizing myopathies (IMNMs) are now considered a sub-entity of the so-called immune inflammatory myopathies (IIM). To date, there are two conditions typically occurring with IMNMs: necrotizing myopathies associated with signal recognition particle (SRP) antibodies, and paradigmatic myopathies that have anti-3-hydroxy-3-methylglutaryl-coenzyme A reductase (HMGCR) antibodies. However, IMNM may also occur in association with neoplastic and other systemic diseases, especially in the antisynthetase syndrome (ASS) or sclerodermia.

Diagnostic procedures to identify IMNM precisely comprise a characteristic clinical syndrome, laboratory markers including a comprehensive panel of autoantibodies, and a muscle biopsy. The latter basically shows necrotic muscle fibers, which give their name to the disease, and minimal to no inflammatory infiltrates. Interestingly, conflicting results have been reported of further biopsy findings, such as major histocompatibility complex (MHC) class I and complement staining.

It should be noted that although IMNM is fairly characteristic clinically and morphologically, it can be difficult to distinguish from genetic muscle disorders, which may also display mild focal inflammation and fiber necrosis on biopsy and may clinically manifest as subacute proximal weakness with high creatine kinase (CK) levels (e.g., dysferlinopathy, anoctaminopathy, or facioscapulohumeral muscular dystrophy). It will be a matter of future debate whether to retain the terms IMNM or autoimmune necrotizing myopathy (ANM) or to define these heterogeneous diseases by different parameters altogether.

Epidemiology

In general, inflammatory myopathies are relatively uncommon, and IMNMs can be considered rare diseases. Depending on the etiological context, some subgroups are even exceptionally rare, such as paraneoplastic IMNM. Anti-SRP and anti-HMGCR-associated IMNM can be found in children and in adults (age ranges from 4–70 years), and women are affected more frequently than men. Both diseases are considered immune mediated since they frequently respond to immunosuppressants, although to date the role of autoantibodies is not well understood. Between 30% and 60% of anti-HMGCR-Ab+-associated IMNM patients have not been exposed to statins, and initial symptoms may be prolonged, mimicking limb-girdle muscular dystrophy. Thus, this immune-mediated condition must not be confounded with statin-induced toxic myopathy.

Pathophysiology

Knowledge of the pathophysiology of these diseases is still very limited, partly due to lack of reliable animal models. However, some solid facts can be presented. Presence and quantity/titer of anti-SRP and anti-HMGCR autoantibodies are closely correlated to clinical disease activity (mainly by muscle weakness) and CK levels. Further, anti-HMGCR autoantibodies were absent in a large cohort of statin-exposed patients, including patients with probably toxic statin effects, arguing that the antibody may be specific for the disease, although this has not formally been proven yet.

The first formal definition of IMNMs was described in a consensus paper in 2003 at the 119th European Neuromuscular Centre (ENMC) workshop. The definition was fulfilling clinical inclusion criteria of adult dermatomyositis (DM) or polymyositis (PM), such as onset over 18 years, subacute or insidious onset of symmetric proximal>distal limb and neck flexor>neck extensor muscle weakness, elevated serum CK levels, and detection of myositis-specific antibodies. Exclusion criteria were clinical features of sporadic inclusion body myositis (sIBM), oculomotor weakness, isolated associated dysarthria and signs of toxic or endocrine myopathy, family history of muscular dystrophy or proximal motor neuronopathies (e.g., spinal muscular atrophy, SMA).

The histology of IMNMs has been described in some detail, but some new data are included here. Necrotic fibers are considered the predominant histological feature, although necrosis of myofibers is particularly difficult to define (Figure 123.1a). Inflammatory cells are sparse or only lightly represented in the perivascular compartment, while a perimysial infiltrate may not be evident. About 20% of cases have significant endo- and perimysial infiltrates of CD3+CD8+ and CD3+CD4+ T-cells in anti-HMGCR- and anti-SRP-Ab+ patients (Figure 123.1b). MHC class I staining of the sarcolemma can be variable (Figure 123.1c). Criteria contained in the consensus paper describe membrane attack complex (MAC, C5b9) deposition on small vessel walls and pipestem capillaries. In our own series, we saw variable but significant deposition of complement, especially on the sarcolemma of myofibers, in all subforms of IMNM (Figure 123.1d). Tubuloreticular inclusions in endothelial cells are not evident in anti-HMGCR- and anti-SRP-Ab+ patients.

A paraneoplastic etiology of necrotizing myopathies different from paraneoplastic dermatomyositis (DM) has been reported earlier, although the link between IMNMs and cancer and thus a paraneoplastic pathogenesis is much less well established than in DM. In contrast to anti-HMGCR- and anti-SRP-Ab+ patients,

International Neurology, Second edition. Edited by Robert P. Lisak, Daniel D. Truong, William M. Carroll and Roongroj Bhidayasiri
© 2016 John Wiley & Sons, Ltd. Published 2016 by John Wiley & Sons, Ltd.

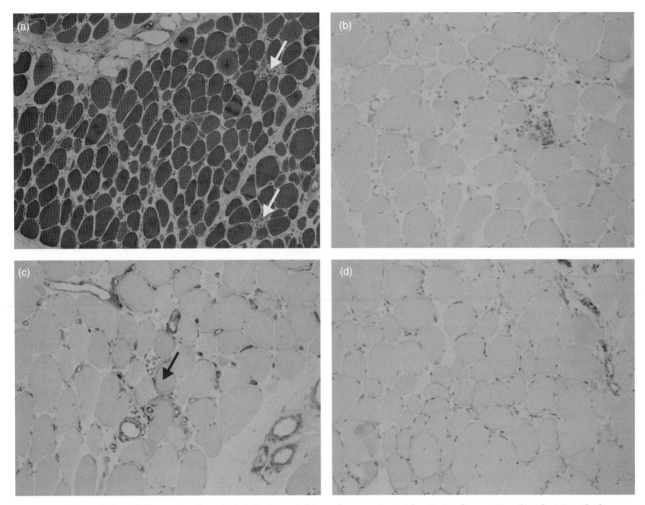

Figure 123.1 Histopathological illustration of a typical skeletal muscle biopsy from a patient with anti-signal recognition particle autoantibodies. (a) Myofiber necrosis at different stages of development and myophagocytosis with diffuse distribution is illustrated by a Gomori trichrome stain. (b) In the proximity of necrotic fibers a conspicuous amount of CD8+ T-cells can be detected. (c) Sarcolemmal staining of major histocompatibility complex class I is positive on a significant amount of myofibers, although with variable intensity. (d) Complement deposition (C5b9) on some myofibers is also a typical feature of most immune-mediated necrotizing myopathy biopsies.

alkaline phosphatase activity is frequently detectable in the endo- and perimysium of paraneoplastic IMNM. IMNM in the context of antisynthetase syndrome (ASS) shows a different local distribution of necrotic fibers comprising a perifascicular predominance. Inflammation can also be very significant, especially in the perimysium, where the interstitial tissue is severely damaged. Complement deposition in patients with ASS-associated autoantibodies is particularly evident on the sarcolemma of myofibers adjacent to the perimysium.

Clinical features

As emphasized earlier, the clinical spectrum of IMNMs is heterogeneous depending on the clinical context and also on the antibody profile. While some symptoms can be considered typical, others are more characteristic of a specific condition like ASS or SRP/HMGCR-associated myositis. Within one group of patients with a defined autoantibody, the clinical presentation is homogenous, emphasizing the importance of antibody testing. There are two main clinical types of presentation: (1) a subacute onset of proxi-

mal weakness that is very symmetric and involves the pelvic as well as the shoulder girdles; and (2) a slowly progressive evolution that may be confounded with limb-girdle muscular dystrophy. As a general rule, if weakness is very severe, dysphagia can also be a features. Early dysphagia is more common in non-immune-mediated muscular disorders with a genetic defect, as are early or predominant involvement of distal muscles, scapular winging, or very slow progression over years, but they can also be described during SRP/HMGCR-associated IMNM. Myalgia may be present in some cases, but painless muscle weakness or only mild myalgia is almost the rule. By contrast, patients may show severe weight loss, reflecting accelerated catabolism. However, if obvious night sweats and mild fever accompany weight loss (the so-called B symptoms), it is important to search for an underlying neoplasm, especially if no autoantibodies can be detected. Signs and symptoms of lung disease (interstitial lung disease, ILD) may provoke a search for an ASS, as will specific skin abnormalities, such as "mechanic's hands" (distal fingers fissuring and cracking of the skin pads) and Raynaud's syndrome combined with arthritis or joint pain. Cardiac involvement may also occur in patients with SRP antibodies, but generally

HMGCR-antibody-associated IMNMs show no involvement of internal organs and only 10% of SRP-antibody-associated IMNMs show ILD. In contrast, ASS-associated IMNM with perifascicular muscle fiber necrosis is associated with a very prominent and characteristic involvement of internal organs, the skin, and joints. Of note is that CK levels are generally markedly elevated.

In addition to ASS, necrotizing myopathy can be found in other systemic diseases such as scleroderma and lupus with presence of "myositis-associated" antibodies and clinical signs of the specific systemic diseases. IMNM with anti-HMGCR antibodies, associated with a gene mutation such as Anoctamin-5, has also been described.

Treatment and management

It emerges that the spectrum of IMNMs is probably much broader than initially recognized. Although IMNMs comprise a number of different diseases, the basic pathological feature is necrotizing myopathy with sometimes prominent, sometimes subtle, but always specific features of activation of the immune system.

There have been no randomized controlled trials or consensus studies on treatment options, since these entities have only been described recently. Therapeutic recommendations are mainly based on case series or even single reports and expert advice. Most experts are currently treating HMGCR- and SRP-antibody-associated IMNMs with corticosteroids using a standard treatment scheme (1 mg/kg body weight). The duration of treatment is monitored by disease/strength evolution and repeated CK measurements. It is very important to remember that frequently IMNM patients show a very severe disease course with significant weakness and a rather acute onset with rapid worsening of the condition. Sometimes, patients may be bedridden a few weeks after onset. Patients with both HMGCR- and SRP-associated IMNMs can show long disease duration with frequent relapses. These considerations should prompt a prolonged treatment plan with a combination of corticosteroids and immunosuppressants, at least as corticoid-sparing agents, from the outset. Immunosuppressants commonly employed include methotrexate and azathioprine in standard doses (AZT 100–150 mg/day (check thiopurin methyltransferase [TPMT] status); MTX 20–25 mg/week). In very severe cases with significant weakness and/or dysphagia, intravenous immunoglobin (IVIg) treatment can be an alternative option to this combination of steroids and immunosuppressants. In this case, we add immunoglobulins to steroid treatment and immunosuppressants. In addition, plasmapheresis can be an option for bedridden patients, since there is emerging evidence for the pathogenic role of autoantibodies in these diseases. In the case of flares of weakness during the disease course, corticosteroids can be augmented again to 1 mg/kg body weight, and corticoid-sparing treatment should be adjusted accordingly. In refractory cases, rituximab may be considered as well. Although no study has proven the benefit of physiotherapy in IMNMs, it is likely helpful, as shown in other IIMs.

In HMGCR$^+$ patients with statin exposure, this medication has to be discontinued, although the situation has to be carefully evaluated for patients who need statin treatment for secondary prevention of ischemic events. There are reports showing that statins can be reintroduced under immunosuppressive treatment without relapse.

When there is a suspicion of neoplasia associated with IMNM, the same therapeutic recommendations are applicable, if anti-cancer treatment allows for immunesuppressive treatment, so this issue has to be considered on a patient-by-patient basis. Since patients suffering from ASS (mainly Jo-1) also present a very high relapse rate of both muscle and pulmonary involvement, treatment combining corticosteroids and immunosuppressants should be introduced early.

Further reading

Allenbach Y, Benveniste O. Acquired necrotizing myopathies. *Curr Opin Neurol* 2013;26:554–560.

Allenbach Y, Drouot L, Rigolet A, *et al.* Anti-HMGCR autoantibodies in European patients with autoimmune necrotizing myopathies: Inconstant exposure to statin. *Medicine* 2014;93:150–157.

Hoogendijk JE, Amato AA, Lecky BR, *et al.* 119th ENMC international workshop: Trial design in adult idiopathic inflammatory myopathies, with the exception of inclusion body myositis, 10–12 October 2003, Naarden, The Netherlands. *Neuromuscul Disord* 2004;14:337–345.

Preusse C, Goebel HH, Held J, *et al.* Immune-mediated necrotizing myopathy is characterized by a specific Th1-m1 polarized immune profile. *Am J Pathol* 2012;181:2161–2171.

Stenzel W, Goebel HH, Aronica E. Review: Immune-mediated necrotizing myopathies – a heterogeneous group of diseases with specific myopathological features. *Neuropathol Appl Neurobiol* 2012;38:632–646.

124 Toxic myopathies

Stefen Brady[1] and David Hilton-Jones[2]

[1] Department of Neurology, Southmead Hospital, Bristol, UK

[2] Nuffield Department of Clinical Neurosciences (Clinical Neurology), University of Oxford, John Radcliffe Hospital, Oxford, UK

A wide range of toxins and prescription and recreational drugs can cause acquired myopathies (Table 124.1). The clinical presentation of such disorders is varied and includes asymptomatic hyper-CKemia (CK = creatine kinase), focal weakness, proximal or generalized weakness (which may be of acute or subacute onset, or insidious) mimicking many other limb-girdle myopathies, cramps and myalgia, rhabdomyolysis, and malignant hyperthermia. Some drugs (e.g., colchicine) can also be toxic to peripheral nerves. The pathological changes observed on muscle biopsy in toxic myopathies can be non-specific or minimal. However, the presence of certain pathological features, for example autophagic vacuoles, may suggest the diagnosis and can help to identify the culprit.

The mechanisms of myotoxicity are diverse and although the pathogenesis of some toxic myopathies is understood, the cause of muscle fiber damage secondary to many commonly used drugs or toxins such as alcohol is uncertain. It is important for clinicians and pathologists to be aware of the commonly used drugs that are myotoxic, as early withdrawal of the offending drug, in most cases, will result in complete recovery. It is not infrequent for an investigation of a suspected drug-induced myopathy to lead to the diagnosis of an underlying primary myopathy, either because the myopathy predisposed to drug sensitivity, or simply coincidentally in that increased medical surveillance led to recognition of a previously subclinical disorder. This chapter focuses on the toxic myopathies most frequently observed in clinical practice: acute and chronic alcohol-associated myopathy, statin myopathy, steroid myopathy, critical illness myopathy, and malignant hyperthermia.

Alcohol-associated myopathy

Alcohol consumption is responsible for 5.1% of the global disease burden and the World Health Organization (WHO) estimated in 2014 that 16% of individuals older than 15 years of age engage in heavy alcohol consumption. Data from the United Kingdom suggest that 24.2% of adults in England drink in a hazardous or harmful way.

Alcohol-associated myopathy is categorized as acute or chronic. Acute alcohol myopathy (AAM) follows an episode of immoderate alcohol consumption, a "binge." The patient typically presents with myalgia, proximal weakness, and muscle swelling and tenderness. Myoglobinuria may precipitate acute renal failure. Serum creatine kinase (CK) is raised and muscle biopsy shows muscle fiber necrosis and phagocytosis. The clinical severity of AAM correlates with the amount of alcohol consumed. Patients typically make a complete recovery, although this may take several months. While considered uncommon, symptoms consistent with AAM were reported by almost one-third of alcoholics in one study.

Chronic alcohol myopathy (CAM) is widely described but poorly understood. Studies indicate that 33–67% of chronic alcohol users have CAM. It is characterized by slowly progressive proximal weakness and muscle atrophy. CK is normal or mildly elevated. Biopsy shows selective atrophy of type IIb muscle fibers. Ultrastructural changes include fiber edema, abnormal mitochondria, dilatation of the sarcoplasmic reticulum, tubular aggregates, and increased lipid and glycogen. Total lifetime ethanol consumption correlates with the severity of CAM. Malnutrition may have an added effect. Women appear to be at equal risk to men of developing CAM, despite average lower lifetime alcohol consumption. Abstinence can lead to an improvement in muscle strength and reversal of pathological changes within months, but recovery is often incomplete. Significant reduction in alcohol consumption may be as effective as abstinence.

The toxic effect of alcohol on skeletal muscle is probably multifactorial. Ethanol disrupts protein synthesis and its metabolite acetaldehyde may impair mitochondrial function. Other pathogenic mechanisms may include disruption of the sarcolemma, inhibition of sarcoplasmic reticulum calcium channels, increased reactive oxygen species, increased autophagy, and apoptosis. Additionally, chronic electrolyte imbalance, such as hypokalemia, may play a role. Alcoholic neuropathy often complicates the clinical picture.

Statin myopathy

Statins substantially lower low-density lipoprotein cholesterol and reduce the risk of cardiovascular disease. They act through inhibition of the hepatic enzyme 3-hydroxy-3-methyl-glutaryl-CoA reductase (HMGCR). Statin-associated myopathies include asymptomatic hyperCKemia, myalgia, rhabdomyolysis, and immune-mediated necrotizing myopathy (IMNM). Clinical experience and observational studies suggest that 10–20% of patients receiving a statin experience musculoskeletal side effects. Although for the individual the risk of severe myotoxicity is very low, the fact that statins are one of the world's most commonly prescribed drugs means that such problems are encountered fairly frequently in clinical practice.

For the non-immune-mediated statin-related myopathies, a number of variables contribute to the risk of toxicity, including

International Neurology, Second edition. Edited by Robert P. Lisak, Daniel D. Truong, William M. Carroll and Roongroj Bhidayasiri

Table 124.1 Myopathies associated with medications and recreational drugs.

	Myalgia and cramps	Vacuolar myopathy	Mitochondrial myopathy	Hypokalemic myopathy	Inflammatory myopathy	Rhabdomyolysis	Myosin-loss myopathy	Malignant hyperthermia
Ethanol (alcohol)	+					+		
Amiodarone		+						
Amphetamines						+		
Amphotericin				+		+		
Beta-adrenergic agonists	+							
Calcium channel blockers	+							
Chloroquine		+						
Ciclosporin	+							
Cimetidine	+				+			
Cocaine								
Colchicine		+						
Depolarizing muscle relaxants	+							+
Diuretics	+			+				
Doxorubicin		+						
Emetine				+				
Epsilon-aminocaproic acid						+		
Fibrates	+					+		
Gold	+							
Heroin						+		
Hydroxychloroquine		+						
Isoniazid						+		
Liquorice				+				
Lithium								
Penicillamine					+			
Perhexiline		+						
Phenytoin					+			
Procainamide					+			
Retinoids						+		
Statins	+				+	+		
Steroids							+	
Tryptophan					+			
Vincristine			+					
Volatile inhaled anesthetics								+
Nucleoside analogues			+					

This table is not an exhaustive list of all medications reported to cause a myopathy. Intramuscularly administered medications causing focal muscle damage are not included.

drug dose, lipophilicity, concomitant use of drugs that affect statin metabolism, renal and liver impairment, hypothyroidism, and genetic polymorphisms. Drugs that are metabolized by, or inhibit, cytochrome P450 3A4 may increase the serum concentration of statins and therefore the toxicity of atorvastatin, fluvastatin, lovastatin, and simvastatin, which are metabolized by this pathway. The PRIMO study found that between simvastatin, fluvastatin, atorvastatin, and lovastatin, fluvastatin was associated with the lowest rate of reported muscle symptoms (5.1%). It has been suggested that the more hydrophilic statins, rosuvastatin and pravastatin, may be better tolerated. A genome-wide association study identified that common variants in *SLCO1B1* on chromosome 12 are strongly associated with an increased risk of statin myotoxicity in patients taking simvastatin. *SLCO1B1* encodes the organic anion-transporting polypeptide, OAT1B1, which regulates hepatic uptake of statins. Currently, there is no evidence to support genotyping to guide statin prescribing.

Statin myopathy typically occurs within the first few months of starting treatment. A baseline CK can be invaluable in determining whether an increased CK identified in a patient established on a statin is treatment related. With isolated hyperCKemia, most specialists recommend continuing the statin if the CK remains less than five times the upper limit of normal. Myalgia is the most common musculoskeletal complaint in patients receiving a statin and it appears to be worse in more physically active patients. In the majority of patients, symptoms will resolve after withdrawal of the statin. If the patient is intolerant of one statin, it is appropriate to consider trying others, using lower doses, and occasionally alternate-day therapy. Rhabdomyolysis is rare, but potentially fatal. It is almost always associated with a recent increase in dose or introduction of other drugs that impair statin metabolism. This risk appears to be lowest with the prescription of fluvastatin.

The mechanism of non-immune-mediated statin myotoxicity is unclear. The most widely accepted theory is that inhibition of cholesterol biosynthesis causes a depletion of downstream intermediaries, leading to disruption of lipid-rich cellular membranes and reduction of mitochondrial respiratory chain function. In addition, the loss of isoprenaline intermediaries impairs multiple cellular functions such as protein synthesis.

The statin-induced problems noted here have a presumed metabolic origin, and resolve on drug withdrawal. In 2007, a necrotizing myopathy was described associated with statin use, which persisted despite statin withdrawal but responded to immunosuppression. Other investigators identified antibodies to an unknown protein in patients with IMNM. These antibodies were discovered to be directed against HMGCR and were predominantly found in patients with a history of statin exposure. Anti-HMGCR antibody levels correlate with clinical features in statin-exposed patients with antibody-positive IMNM, in contrast to statin-unexposed antibody-positive patients. However, despite successful treatment, antibody levels remain elevated, suggesting that they are not directly pathogenic. Anti-HMGCR antibodies appear to be specific for IMNM and therefore they may have a role in identifying those patients with a statin myopathy who will require immunosuppressive treatment.

Clinical experience suggests that statins are safe to use in most patients with primary muscle disease, but it is prudent to discuss potential risks with the patient, monitor serum CK before and during treatment, and initiate therapy at a relatively low dose.

Corticosteroid myopathy

Acute and chronic myopathies are associated with short- and long-term corticosteroid use, respectively. Acute steroid myopathy (ASM), or acute quadriplegic myopathy (AQM), is uncommon, but is one form of critical illness myopathy (see the next section). It is typically associated with high-dose intravenous steroids, often combined with a neuromuscular blocking drug, but has been reported with lower-dose oral steroids or after an increase in the dose of maintenance steroids. Chronic steroid myopathy typically presents with painless proximal weakness affecting the pelvic girdle more than the shoulders. Myalgia may be a feature. Muscle biopsy shows type II fiber atrophy and, rarely, fiber necrosis. CK levels are usually normal or even low.

Critical illness myopathy and malignant hyperthermia

One of the most common causes of weakness affecting patients in intensive care units (ICU) is critical illness myopathy (CIM). It is often noticed for the first time when there is difficulty in weaning

a patient off mechanical ventilation. CIM affects up to one-third of patients in ICU and may be accompanied by a polyneuropathy. Risk factors include the use of corticosteroids and neuromuscular blocking drugs (see earlier), but CIM may occur in the absence of either drug. Patients have a limb-girdle pattern of weakness accompanied by respiratory muscle weakness and sometimes facial weakness. Extraocular muscles are unaffected. CK may be normal or elevated. Muscle biopsy in AQM shows selective loss of myosin filaments. The prognosis of CIM appears to be better than that of critical illness polyneuropathy, with the majority of patients recovering within 6–12 months.

Malignant hyperthermia (MH) is a rare but potentially fatal condition caused by an uncontrolled release of calcium from the sarcoplasmic reticulum, precipitated by the use of specific anesthetic medications, including volatile anesthetics and succinylcholine, in susceptible individuals. Whether succinylcholine alone increases the risk of MH is debated, but it markedly increases the risk when used in combination with volatile anesthetic agents. Symptoms of MH and its severity are highly variable. Characteristic clinical features are hypoxemia, hypercapnia, muscle rigidity, hyperpyrexia, metabolic acidosis, and rhabdomyolysis. The earliest sign of MH is an increase in end-tidal carbon dioxide levels. Management, including the prompt administration of dantrolene, a ryanodine receptor antagonist, and supportive care, has significantly reduced mortality. Prognosis depends on early recognition and treatment. The prophylactic use of dantrolene is not recommended. MH is associated with mutations of the ryanodine receptor (*RyR1*) gene in about 50–70% of patients and of *CACNA1S*.

Functional testing by the *in vitro* contracture test (IVCT), where a fresh muscle sample is exposed to halothane or caffeine, may be performed to help identify individuals at risk of MH and is sensitive and specific. Analysis of the histopathological findings in 399 patients with MH susceptibility confirmed by IVCT found no pathological changes on muscle biopsy in 77% of cases. Although genetic testing is becoming more widely available, it remains problematic because of the genetic heterogeneity of MH, and the interpretation of variants of unknown significance in the very large *RyR1* gene. Safe anesthesia can be administered to patients with MH and involves the avoidance of causative medications. Further information on the investigation and management of MH is available from the European and North American Malignant Hyperthermia Groups.

Further reading

Bruckert E, Hayem G, Dejager S, Yau C, Bégaud B. Mild to moderate muscular symptoms with high-dosage statin therapy in hyperlipidemic patients – the PRIMO study. *Cardiovasc Drugs Ther* 2005;19:403–414.

Mammen AL, Pak K, Williams EK, *et al*. Rarity of anti-3-hydroxy-3-methylglutaryl-coenzyme A reductase antibodies in statin users, including those with self-limited musculoskeletal side effects. *Arthritis Care Res* 2012;64:269–272.

Needham M, Fabian V, Knezevic W, *et al*. Progressive myopathy with up-regulation of MHC-I associated with statin therapy. *Neuromuscul Disord* 2007;17:194–200.

Orlov D, Keith J, Rosen D, *et al*. Analysis of histomorphology in malignant hyperthermia-susceptible patients. *Can J Anaesth* 2013;60:982–989.

Riazi S, Larach MG, Hu C, *et al*. Malignant hyperthermia in Canada: Characteristics of index anesthetics in 129 malignant hyperthermia susceptible probands. *Anesth Analg* 2014;118:381–387.

SEARCH Collaborative Group; Link E, Parish S, Armitage J, *et al*. SLCO1B1 variants and statin-induced myopathy – a genomewide study. *N Engl J Med* 2008;359:789–799.

125 Critical illness neuromuscular disorders

Nicola Latronico and Frank A. Rasulo

Department of Anesthesia, Critical Care Medicine and Emergency, Spedali Civili University Hospital, and Department of Medical and Surgical Specialties, Radiological Sciences and Public Health, University of Brescia, Brescia, Italy

Neuromuscular disorders acquired during an intensive care unit (ICU) stay are common and may have serious clinical consequences. Limb and respiratory muscle involvement may cause limb weakness and paralysis, neuromuscular respiratory failure, prolonged dependency on mechanical ventilation, and long-term physical impairment. Difficulty in swallowing and ineffective cough may combine to cause pneumonia and lung atelectasis, which in turn may precipitate life-threatening acute respiratory deterioration. Immobility, an expected complication of generalized paralysis, contributes to muscle wasting and weakness.

Weakness may result from pathological processes involving the motor neuron with its axon and myelin sheath, the neuromuscular transmission, and the skeletal muscle itself. This chapter focuses on critical illness polyneuropathy (CIP) and myopathy (CIM), because they are the most common neuromuscular complications developing during an ICU stay and the most common cause of ICU-acquired muscle weakness (ICUAW). Muscle disuse atrophy, drugs, and electrolyte abnormalities may have an impact on muscle function and should be considered in the differential diagnosis of muscle weakness in the ICU.

Epidemiology

CIP and CIM reflect the failure of the peripheral neuromuscular system in patients with multiple organ failure (MOF). One-third to one-half of the most severely ill patients in the ICU will develop these complications, more often as combined CIP and CIM; however, incidence varies greatly in relation to the patient case mix, the risk factors, the diagnostic criteria used, and the timing of evaluation. In patients with septic shock or severe sepsis and coma, the incidence approaches 100%.

Pathophysiology

The main defect leading to CIP and CIM during MOF is unknown, as is the case for other failing organs. Electrophysiological changes of peripheral nerves and muscles may have a rapid onset within hours of normal action potential generation. Nerve histology is normal and muscle histology shows minimal changes, with loss of thick filaments in biopsies taken at an early stage of disease. Late biopsies demonstrate muscle fiber necrosis and atrophy, and nerve axonal degeneration. One theory of bioenergetics failure postulates that in a condition of low-energy state such as MOF, the nerves and the muscles can survive by reducing or abolishing the function, as documented by electrophysiological testing. With persisting deficit, the energy supply and/or use is not restored and histological alterations ensue. Disturbed microcirculation and acquired sodium channelopathy with hypoexcitability or inexcitability of nerves and muscles are other potentially relevant mechanisms. The derangement of muscle metabolism with reduced protein synthesis, increased proteolysis, altered glucose utilization, and altered mitochondrial autophagy also play a key role in the pathogenesis of CIM, causing muscle wasting and weakness.

Clinical features

CIP is a distal axonal sensory-motor polyneuropathy affecting limb and respiratory muscles. Facial muscles are usually spared. Limb involvement is diffuse and symmetric, muscle tone is reduced, and sensation is impaired. Deep tendon reflexes can be decreased, but normal reflexes do not exclude CIP. Failed weaning from mechanical ventilation is a common feature, indicating weakness of the respiratory muscles. In alert patients, limb muscle strength can be tested clinically in functional muscle groups using the Medical Research Council (MRC) score or handgrip dynamometry. An MRC score below 48/60 designates ICUAW, which is associated with prolonged mechanical ventilation, increased ICU stay and mortality, and reduced quality of life and increased mortality in survivors of critical illness.

CIM is a primary myopathy characterized by loss of myosin filaments, scattered muscle fiber necrosis, and atrophy. Clinical features are the same as CIP, but sensation is intact.

Investigations

Diagnosis of CIP and CIM necessitates accurate evaluation of medical history, and appropriate clinical and electrophysiological investigations. Muscle weakness of limb and respiratory muscles developing *after* the admission to the ICU and related to critical illness is an essential prerequisite for definitive diagnosis. Facial muscles are spared, which is an important criterion to differentiate CIP from Guillain–Barré syndrome (GBS). Difficult weaning from the ventilator that cannot be explained by lung, cardiac, metabolic, or infectious complications brings attention to CIP and CIM. If a trial of spontaneous breathing is attempted, the patient becomes rapidly distressed and dyspneic, with rapid shallow breathing. Weakness of the diaphragm and other inspiratory muscles results in inadequate lung expansion and microatelectasis, but severe hypoxemia and hypercapnia are late events and are useless as a guide to anticipate impending respiratory failure.

Weakness of the pharyngeal and laryngeal muscles and of the expiratory muscles of the chest wall and abdomen leads to altered swallowing, impaired cough, inadequate clearance of secretions, and increased risk of pulmonary aspiration and pneumonia. Limb weakness can be severe enough to cause flaccid tetraparesis or tetraplegia, which in turn causes immobility and disuse muscle atrophy. This vicious circle exacerbates the ongoing neuropathic and/or myopathic process. Immobility also increases the risk of delirium, a common companion of CIP and CIM.

ICUAW is an important complication causing prolonged mechanical ventilation, lengthy ICU stay, and increased ICU and long-term mortality. It can be caused by several different pathophysiological mechanisms and can be associated with either CIP, CIM, both, or neither. Electrophysiological investigations are essential not only to define the cause, but also to help in outcome prediction. Patients with ICUAW caused by muscle disuse atrophy and deconditioning are clinically indistinguishable from those suffering from CIP or CIM, but mortality can be substantially lower in the former. Similarly, patients with CIM have a better short-term and long-term prognosis than those with CIP.

CIP is an axonal neuropathy, not a demyelinating neuropathy, and hence the nerve conduction velocity is normal or only mildly reduced in nerve conduction studies, whereas the amplitude of compound motor (CMAP) and sensory (SNAP) nerve action potentials is reduced. In CIM, electrophysiological features include reduced CMAP with normal SNAPs, and myopathic motor unit potentials in electromyography (EMG) in patients able to activate their muscles volitionally. In the acute setting, simplified tests with peroneal nerve stimulation can be used to screen at-risk patients. Direct muscle stimulation can diagnose CIM in non-collaborative patients by showing reduced or absent muscle membrane excitability.

GBS, an autoimmune acute polyneuropathy with a distinctive clinical course, is often considered in the differential diagnosis of CIP, but distinction is usually obvious. A flu-like episode or gastroenteritis with diarrhea often precedes the appearance of neurological signs by 2–4 weeks. Infection has subsided by the time neurological signs such as pain, paresthesia, numbness, and weakness in the limbs become evident. Facial muscles, which are unaffected in CIP, are frequently involved. Differential diagnosis can be difficult in the case of rapid progression of neuromuscular respiratory failure in previously undiagnosed GBS. As GBS is amenable to specific treatment with immunoglobulins or plasmapheresis, timely diagnosis is essential. Electrophysiological investigations reveal acute nerve demyelination with greatly reduced nerve conduction velocity; however, axonal GBS forms are also described. Serial electrophysiological investigations are needed to achieve the diagnosis and in gauging response to treatment. Cerebrospinal fluid (CSF) protein content in GBS is typically elevated with a normal white cell count, although CSF can be normal in the first week.

Electrolyte abnormalities affecting muscle function are common in the ICU, and may alter either the neuromuscular transmission as in hypermagnesemia, or muscle excitability as in hypo- and hyperkalemia and hypophosphatemia. Several drugs commonly used in the ICU may aggravate the muscle weakness. These include neuromuscular blocking agents (NMBA), antibiotics (aminoglycosides, polymixin B, clindamycin), drugs with anesthetic-like action (lidocaine, procainamide, quinidine, phenytoin), calcium channel blockers, magnesium, beta blockers, diuretics, and quinolones. In some patients with hepatic or renal dysfunction the block of the neuromuscular junction after the use of NMBA may be prolonged for several hours, but a longer duration of days or weeks is usually caused by CIP or CIM complicating the clinical course. The relation between CIM and corticosteroids is unknown, but use of these drugs is associated with chronic impairment of physical function in survivors of acute lung injury. Propofol at high doses and for prolonged periods may rarely cause a fatal syndrome of cardiac failure, metabolic acidosis, hyperkalemia, hypertriglyceridemia, renal failure, and rhabdomyolysis. With the fully developed syndrome the diagnosis is easy, but incomplete forms can develop with mild early increase in serum creatine kinase; in these cases, prompt recognition is important to stop the propofol infusion and to avoid conversion into the overt syndrome with acute necrotizing myopathy.

Treatment and management

No specific treatment has been shown to reduce the incidence and severity of CIP and CIM. There is moderate evidence that intensive insulin therapy to maintain normal blood glucose concentrations (80–110 mg/dL; 4.4–6.1 mmol/L) may reduce the incidence of electrophysiologically proven CIP and high-quality evidence that it reduces the duration of mechanical ventilation. However, intensive insulin therapy aiming at normoglycemia increases mortality in adult ICU patients. Electrical muscle stimulation and corticosteroids have no beneficial effect, with the latter possibly increasing the risk of long-term functional disability. Supportive treatment with early rehabilitation in the ICU is potentially beneficial for CIP and CIM and is associated with shorter duration of mechanical ventilation. Future studies of appropriate sample size should evaluate the impact of early rehabilitation on long-term measures of physical and mental performance in survivors of critical illness.

Further reading

Fan E, Cheek F, Chlan L, et al.; ATS Committee on ICU-acquired Weakness in Adults; American Thoracic Society. An official American Thoracic Society Clinical Practice guideline: The diagnosis of intensive care unit-acquired weakness in adults. *Am J Respir Crit Care Med* 2014;190:1437–1446.

Hermans G, Van Mechelen H, Clerckx B, et al. Acute outcomes and 1-year mortality of ICU-acquired weakness: A cohort study and propensity matched analysis. *Am J Respir Crit Care Med* 2014;190:410–420.

Kress JP, Hall JB. ICU-acquired weakness and recovery from critical illness. *N Engl J Med* 2014;370:1626–1635.

Latronico N, Bolton CF. Critical illness polyneuropathy and myopathy: A major cause of muscle weakness and paralysis. *Lancet Neurol* 2011;10:931–941.

Latronico N, Nattino G, Guarneri B, et al. Validation of the peroneal nerve test to diagnose critical illness polyneuropathy and myopathy in the intensive care unit: The multicentre Italian CRIMYNE-2 diagnostic accuracy study. *F1000Research* 2014;3:127.

126 Exercise intolerance and myoglobinuria

John Vissing

Copenhagen Neuromuscular Center, University of Copenhagen, Copenhagen, Denmark

Exercise intolerance can be defined as the inability of a person to reach and/or maintain a work intensity that is otherwise expected for the person's age, size, and gender. Exercise intolerance is caused by numerous conditions, many of which are non-neuromuscular, such as arthritis, heart or respiratory failure, recovery from long-standing disease, postinfectious conditions, bone deformities, and many others. Muscle pain, which emerges as exercise is undertaken, can be a reason for exercise intolerance, but chronic syndromes, with pain at rest that limits the initiation of exercise, are typically not categorized as exercise intolerance syndromes.

Since exercise intolerance has many causes, this complaint is very common in the general population. It highlights the importance of being able to distinguish exercise intolerance caused by neuromuscular diseases from the very common symptoms of myalgia and fatigue in people without muscle disease. In many neuromuscular diseases in which there is muscle wasting, exercise intolerance is obvious from the disabling loss of muscle mass, and in such cases the term exercise intolerance is rarely used. The term is generally reserved for conditions in which low work capacity is disproportionate to the muscle mass of the person. Exercise intolerance is considered a hallmark of inborn errors of muscle metabolism, such as metabolic and mitochondrial myopathies, where it is caused by a mismatch between energy demand and supply. However, a number of non-metabolic myopathies, preferentially muscular dystrophies, may also present with a picture characteristic of metabolic myopathies. Thus, exercise-related muscle pain and even myoglobinuria are not rare in certain types of limb-girdle muscular dystrophies (types 2I and 2L) and dystrophinopathies. Exercise-related pain is also commonly found in other muscle diseases such as facioscapulohumeral muscular dystrophy, channelopathies, and myopathy due to thyroid gland dysfunction. In channelopathies, such as myotonia congenita and paramyotonia congenita, the cause of the pain likely relates to the myotonia. In facioscapulohumeral muscular dystrophy and myopathy due to thyroid gland dysfunction, muscle wasting or pain usually explains the exercise intolerance.

Testing of exercise intolerance

In a person with intact muscle mass, complaints of exercise intolerance are often tested with provocative exercise investigations. To differentiate between defects of fat, carbohydrate, and mitochondrial metabolism, it is helpful to interview the patient about when in exercise the symptoms occur and how they do so. At the start of exercise and during strenuous exercise, muscle function depends primarily on energy generated from muscle glycogenolysis and glycolysis. Symptoms evoked by such exercise therefore can suggest an underlying glycogenosis. Painful contractures are typically coupled with the exercise intolerance in these conditions. During prolonged, low-intensity exercise, muscle depends primarily on energy generated from oxidation of fatty acids. Symptoms provoked by such exercise therefore point toward a disorder of muscle lipid metabolism, and these patients do not develop contractures as in glycogenoses, but may experience tightness/stiffness of muscles that have been exercised. In contrast, patients with mitochondrial disease rarely experience contractures, stiffness, or muscle pain, but typically complain about being out of breath, which explains why these patients often have been seen by cardiologists and pulmonologists before referral to neuromuscular centers.

Handgrip exercise tests

Handgrip exercise at maximal work intensity but not necessarily with ischemia, which can produce rhabdomyolysis in affected individuals, is a nice tool to screen for defects of muscle carbohydrate metabolism. Muscle contractures and fatigue in these disorders are well illustrated by the test. The forearm test involves maximal handgrip contractions, every other second for 60 seconds. The test is used diagnostically to demonstrate blocked muscle lactate production and exaggerated production of ammonia in these disorders. The pattern of fatigue is also characteristic. In healthy subjects, maximal voluntary muscle contraction (MVC) typically declines to about 80% of MVC at the end of the test, but in patients with glycogenoses it typically declines to about 20% of MVC.

If a mitochondrial myopathy is suspected, a handgrip test can also be helpful diagnostically. However, the test has to be performed at lower work intensities than for muscle glycogenoses, typically at 20–40% of MVC. This ensures that the work is aerobic, and that the effect parameter does not reflect lactate and ammonia accumulation, but rather oxygen saturation in the venous effluent blood from an exercised forearm. Oxygen extraction is compromised in conditions with respiratory chain insufficiency, and therefore desaturation of venous oxygen is impaired or even absent in these conditions.

Testing of work capacity

A cycle ergometer test is the gold standard to test the oxidative capacity of an individual, and thus the best objective measure of whether a person has exercise intolerance. A maximal oxygen uptake of two standard deviations below the norm for a given age and gender is clearly abnormal. Such a finding does not necessarily tell

International Neurology, Second edition. Edited by Robert P. Lisak, Daniel D. Truong, William M. Carroll and Roongroj Bhidayasiri
© 2016 John Wiley & Sons, Ltd. Published 2016 by John Wiley & Sons, Ltd.

much about the underlying cause, but alone serves as an objective tool to verify exercise intolerance. When performed correctly, subjects have to reach close to their maximal predicted heart rate at exhaustion. Otherwise, a low oxidative capacity could very well just be a question of underperformance. Measures of plasma lactate can also help to verify this. In contrast to the lack of specificity of a maximal cycle test, a lower constant-rate cycle intensity protocol can be diagnostically useful in patients with muscle glycogenoses. As with the handgrip test, blunted or absent lactate responses and exaggerated ammonia responses can be measured during exercise in these conditions, and in patients with myophosphorylase deficiency (McArdle disease) and some patients with phosphoglucomutase deficiency, a second-wind phenomenon develops during exercise. The second-wind phenomenon denotes a sudden, spontaneous marked improvement in exercise capacity after 7–8 minutes of exercise, and is caused by an enhanced uptake and oxidation of glucose and fatty acids. The effect of an intravenous or oral supplement of glucose/sucrose on work capacity during cycle exercise can also be easily observed in McArdle disease, debrancher deficiency, and phosphoglucomutase deficiency.

Myoglobinuria

The term myoglobinuria is used when there is increased urinary excretion of myoglobin. Under normal circumstances, myoglobin is excreted in minimal amounts in urine (less than 5 ng/mL). The excretion gets visible when it exceeds 100–200 μg/mL. This load corresponds to the myoglobin present in 50–100 g of muscle. The urine then takes on an appearance of dark tea or cola. Myoglobin is a small protein (17.8 kDa) made up of 153 amino acids, and the gene encoding myoglobin consists of just 3 exons. Because of the small size of the molecule, a rise in plasma myoglobin precedes elevations of the four times larger creatine kinase (CK) molecule when muscle is injured. Myoglobin is composed of eight helical segments, and with its single heme group has a higher affinity for binding oxygen than hemoglobin. Still, myoglobin is not crucial for cellular oxygen supply. Thus, adult transgenic mice lacking myoglobin expression have normal life expectancy and can exercise, due to adaptive responses such as increased vascularity and overexpression of hypoxia-inducible transcription factors. Rhabdomyolysis is often used interchangeably with myoglobinuria, and describes the dissolution or disruption of striated muscle that leads to loss of muscle proteins, including myoglobin, to the extracellular space.

Irrespective of the mechanism underlying myoglobinuria, it is associated with acute muscle injury, muscle necrosis, swelling of the affected muscles, myalgia, and sometimes weakness. Common to all etiologies of myoglobinuria is direct injury to the sarcolemma, often associated with failure of energy supply to maintain sarcolemmal transport functions, which inevitably will lead to a rise in intracellular calcium. This triggers muscle contraction and the need for more energy, while calcium-dependent proteases and phospholipidases will start to break down essential protein structures of the muscle, and lysosomes will digest the protein debris. Thus, disruption of sarcolemmal integrity starts a vicious circle that may end with disintegration of the muscle fiber.

Causes of myoglobinuria

Myoglobinuria has many intrinsic as well as extrinsic causes. They are commonly divided into genetic and acquired causes. Table 126.1 gives an overview of the many etiologies, indicating the main mechanisms

responsible, and the most common cause(s) for each mechanism. In distinguishing between acquired and hereditary causes, it is helpful to know whether a case of myoglobinuria is recurrent or a first-time incidence. Hereditary causes tend to be recurrent, whereas acquired causes usually occur just once, unless they are coupled with episodic triggering mechanisms, such as generalized epileptic seizures or drug/alcohol abuse. In a neuromuscular clinic, there is a bias toward seeing patients who have recurrent episodes of myoglobinuria due to a genetic disorder, but acquired causes occurring just once constitute the bulk of cases with myoglobinuria. Thus, in a study of 77 patients with myoglobinuria seen in a non-specialty clinic, nearly all had acquired causes; alcohol was the most common, followed in order of frequency by limb immobilization with compression, generalized seizures, direct trauma, and drug abuse.

A number of factors may predispose to myoglobinuria. Low physical fitness decreases the duration and intensity of exercise that can be sustained without muscle injury. Hypokalemia and hypophosphatemia dispose to myoglobinuria, probably because of depolarization of the muscle membrane. Hypo- or hyperthermia and infections, which occasionally may produce myoglobinuria alone, may also act as potentiating factors.

Hereditary causes of myoglobinuria

Recurrent myoglobinuria is the hallmark of metabolic myopathies affecting glucose/glycogen metabolism and fatty acid oxidation (FAO). In 77 muscle biopsies from patients with mostly recurrent myoglobinuria studied in a neuromuscular clinic, 47% had an identifiable enzyme deficiency compatible with a metabolic myopathy, when obvious extrinsic factors had been ruled out beforehand.

Disorders of carbohydrate metabolism

The characteristic symptom preceding myoglobinuria in disorders of muscle carbohydrate metabolism is painful muscle contractures provoked by sudden vigorous exercise. The most common disorder in this group is McArdle disease. The enzyme defect in this condition is typically complete, and therefore exercise capacity is severely reduced. Most other muscle glycogenoses are associated with some residual enzyme activity, and consequently the exercise intensity that provokes myoglobinuria is much higher than in McArdle disease, and the frequency of attacks is lower than in McArdle disease.

Disorders of fatty acid oxidation

These disorders comprise more than 25 enzyme deficiencies of fat metabolism, but many primarily give rise to hepatic manifestations with hypoglycemia, encephalopathy, and seizures. Less than eight of the disorders give rise to myopathic symptoms and myoglobinuria. These disorders can be distinguished from McArdle disease by (1) not having overt contractures, but muscle stiffness/tightness and pain; (2) normal plasma CK levels between episodes; (3) maximal work capacity close to normal; and (4) symptoms provoked by exercise of long duration, and worsened or provoked by emotional stress, cold-shivering, fever, and fasting. Like glycolytic defects, muscle integrity may be disturbed by insufficient ATP production, but in addition non-metabolized fat intermediates behind the metabolic block may also have a direct toxic effect on the sarcolemma. The most common disorder of fatty acid oxidation with myopathic symptoms is carnitine palmitoyltransferase II deficiency. It is also the most common cause of recurrent myoglobinuria. Two other disorders of fatty acid oxidation associated with frequent attacks of

Table 126.1 Causes of myoglobinuria.

Hereditary

Disorders of muscle carbohydrate metabolism

  Myophosphorylase deficiency (McArdle disease)

  Phosphorylase *b* kinase deficiency

  Other muscle glycogenoses (rarely)

Disorders of fatty acid oxidation

  Carnitine palmitoyltransferase II (CPTII) deficiency

  Very long-chain acyl-CoA dehydrogenase (VLCAD) deficiency

  Other disorders of fat oxidation (rarely)

Disorders of mitochondrial respiratory chain function

  Cytochrome *c* oxidase deficiency (COX I-III subunit mDNA mutations)

  Complex III deficiency (cytochrome *b* gene mutations)

  Coenzyme Q10 deficiency

  A number of mutations in mtDNA tRNA genes

  Succinate dehydrogenase deficiency

Malignant hyperthermia susceptibility

Brody's myopathy (sarcoplasmic Ca⁺⁺-ATPase deficiency)

Muscular dystrophies

  Limb-girdle muscular dystrophy type 2I

  Sarcoglycanopathies

  Dystrophinopathies

  Anoctamin 5 deficiency (LGMD2L)

Acquired

Toxic (including drugs)

  Neuroleptic malignant syndrome

  Drugs inducing hypokalemia (thiazides, kaliuretics, laxative abuse, theophylline, amphotericin)

  Cholesterol-lowering drugs (statins, bezafibrate, clofibrate)

  Other drugs (antidepressants, anticholinergics, oxprenolol, opiates, amphetamines, pethidine, ecstasy, lithium, cocaine, barbiturates, antihistamines, vecuronium, succinylcholine, colchicines, cimetidine, zidovudine)

  Alcohol, carbon monoxide, arsenic, ethylene glycol, gasoline, solvents, detergents, herbicides, snake venoms, methanol

Extreme exertion

  Epileptic seizures

  Electric shock

  "March" myoglobinuria

  Status asthmaticus

  Delirium

  Long-distance running

Crush/trauma

  Prolonged immobility (coma, surgery)

  Certain forms of torture

  High-impact deceleration/acceleration trauma

Ischemia

  Compartment syndrome

  Disseminated intravascular coagulation

  Arterial occlusion

Extreme temperatures

  Fever

  Burns

  Hypothermia

Metabolic

  Hypokalemia

  Hypothyroidism

  Diabetic ketoacidosis or hyperosmolar state

  Hyper/hyponatremia

  Hypophosphatemia

Infectious

  Viral (adenovirus, coxsackievirus, influenza virus, measles virus, cytomegalovirus, human immunodeficiency virus)

  Bacterial (campylobacter, clostridia, *E. coli*, listeria, salmonella, staphylococcus, streptococcus)

  Other (toxoplasma, trichinella, aspergillus)

Inflammatory muscle disease (rare cause of myoglobinuria)

  Poly- and dermatomyositis

  Vasculitis

myoglobinuria are very long-chain acyl-CoA dehydrogenase and trifunctional protein deficiencies.

Mitochondrial disorders

Besides the specific mitochondrial disorders mentioned in Table 126.1, myoglobinuria is very rare in patients with mitochondrial myopathy. The underlying mechanism is probably energy failure, as in other metabolic myopathies, but the low incidence of myoglobinuria in these conditions indicates that energy failure alone is probably not the only factor responsible. As with disorders of fatty acid oxidation, build-up of acyl-carnitines may also play a role in disruption of the sarcolemma.

Muscular dystrophies

Recurrent myoglobinuria is being increasingly recognized in a variety of muscular dystrophies, particularly with the advent of better molecular characterization of these muscle diseases. Recurrent myoglobinuria was first recognized in the dystrophinopathies, and may in Becker muscular dystrophy be the presenting symptom. However, myoglobinuria may also be the presenting symptom in 20% of patients with limb-girdle muscular dystrophy types 2I and 2L, and has also been observed in sarcoglycanopathies.

Acquired causes of myoglobinuria

Drugs and toxins

Drugs and toxins probably account for more than 75% of all cases of myoglobinuria in adults. The most common compounds involved are alcohol, illicit drugs (particularly ecstasy, amphetamines, cocaine, opiates), and cholesterol-lowering agents (particularly statins).

Trauma

Myoglobinuria is unfortunately still a major factor in natural and man-made disasters involving compression of musculature. This includes trauma sustained during traffic accidents, falls, war, or other violence. It also includes compression after long immobility, and therefore overlaps with alcohol abuse, compression after prolonged, severe generalized seizures, and as a result of compartment syndromes, which may be either traumatic or exercise induced.

Infections

A number of viral and bacterial agents may cause myoglobinuria (Table 126.1). The most common infectious etiologies are influenza viruses A and B, streptococci, staphylococci, legionella, and salmonella. The pathogenesis of myoglobinuria is still unclear, but may include direct invasion of myocytes by the infectious agent, toxic effects, hyperthermia, and drug therapy in critically ill patients, particularly including muscle relaxants and steroids.

Treatment and prevention

The mainstay of treatment effort in any case of myoglobinuria is to avoid renal failure. It is therefore important to maintain sufficient blood pressure and avoid hypovolemia. Thus, saline infusion is important to maintain urine output and as a means to dilute toxic products released from the necrotizing musculature. Myoglobin crystallizes at low pH, and it may therefore be necessary to alkalinize the urine. If renal failure occurs, hemodialysis must be commenced. Disturbances of plasma calcium and phosphate or potassium levels must be corrected, and if a compartment syndrome is present, fasciotomy may be needed.

After the acute treatment, it is important to identify the correct diagnosis to be able to counsel the patient, and activate preventive measures against repetitive episodes. Besides being careful about engaging in exercise of high intensity in glycolytic defects or of long duration in defects of fatty acid oxidation, a diet high in carbohydrate may protect against muscle injury in both groups of disorders. For acquired causes, it is matter of discontinuing the noxious drug or toxin if possible.

Further reading

Gabow PA, Kaehny WD, Kelleher SP. The spectrum of rhabdomyolysis. *Medicine* 1982;61:141–152.

Haller RG, Vissing J. Spontaneous "second wind" and glucose-induced second "second wind" in McArdle's disease – oxidative mechanisms. *Arch Neurol* 2002;59:1395–1402.

Jensen TD, Kazemi- Esfarjani P, Skomorowska E, Vissing J. A forearm exercise screening test for mitochondrial myopathy. *Neurology* 2002;58:1533–1538.

Sveen ML, Schwartz M, Vissing J. High prevalence and phenotype-genotype correlations of limb girdle muscular dystrophy type 2I in Denmark. *Ann Neurol* 2006;59:808–815.

Tonin P, Lewis P, Servidei S, DiMauro S. Metabolic causes of myoglobinuria. *Ann Neurol* 1990;27:181–185.

Witting N, Duno M, Petri H, *et al.* Anoctamin 5 muscular dystrophy in Denmark: Genotype, phenotype, prevalence, cardiology and muscle protein expression. *J Neurol* 2013;260(8):2084–2093.

127 Muscle cramps

Kimiyoshi Arimura[1] and Raymond L. Rosales[2]

[1] Okatsu Neurology and Rehabilitation Hospital and Department of Neurology and Geriatrics, Kagoshima University, Kagoshima, Japan
[2] Faculty of Medicine and Surgery, Royal and Pontifical University of Santo Tomas and Hospital, Manila, and Saint Luke's International Institute of Neurosciences, Quezon City, Philippines

The term "muscle cramp" is most commonly defined as an involuntary, painful muscle contraction associated with electrical activity (cramp discharge). Muscle cramps usually last for up to a few minutes and gradually cease with residual discomfort and tenderness hours afterward. Muscle cramps are a nearly universal phenomenon and frequently occur during exercise or sleep (e.g., nocturnal leg cramps, especially in elderly people), usually involving the small foot or calf muscles. Among a group of young students recently enrolled in an exercise class, the prevalence of "true" muscle cramps was found at 95% of subjects. Studies of hundreds of elderly outpatients showed a 35–60% prevalence of cramps, 40% having experienced cramps more than three times a week. A largely neglected symptomatology of muscle cramps among diabetics interestingly found an unadjusted prevalence of 75.5% in type 2 diabetes and 57.5% in type 1 diabetes. Based on electrodiagnostic tests, neuropathy was the most important determining factor in cramp development from the same diabetic cohort.

The generic term "muscle spasm" refers to any involuntary abnormal muscle contraction, regardless of whether it is painful or not, that cannot be terminated by voluntary relaxation (e.g., hemifacial spasm). "Muscle stiffness" refers to an involuntary muscle shortening that usually lasts for seconds to minutes, but may be sustained.

Pathophysiology

The pathophysiology of muscle cramps is not fully understood, but two main neural mechanisms have been suggested. One mechanism is hyperexcitability of the distal portion of peripheral nerve. The other mechanism is instability of groups of anterior horn cells due to spinal disinhibition. Muscle cramps usually start with focal muscle twitching (fasciculation), then spread to adjacent muscles, followed by sustained muscle contractions. Electrophysiologically, fasciculations (potentials) are thought to originate from peripheral nerves, especially distal to the motor branch. A recent large case-control study of nocturnal leg cramps found three independent associated factors: muscle twitching, lower limb tingling, and weakness of foot dorsiflexion. Such findings point to hyperexcitability and dysfunction of both the motor and sensory peripheral nerves that correlate with muscle cramps.

A number of involuntary movements mimic muscle cramps (see Table 127.1), and clinical observation alone may fail to distinguish one from the other. Consequently, electromyography (EMG) may have great value in the evaluation of patients with muscle cramps. Cramp discharge refers to the involuntary repetitive firing of motor unit action potentials at a high frequency, along a large area of muscles, and is usually associated with painful contraction. Both the

discharge frequency and the number of motor unit action potentials firing increase gradually during cramp development, and both phenomena also subside gradually through cessation. Table 127.2 indicates involuntary movements and lists the potential lesion sites of origin.

Table 127.1 Involuntary movements that mimic muscle cramp.

Term and definition	Origin	Electromyography findings
Contracture		
Immobility of a joint due to fixed muscle shortening	Muscle	Electrically silent
Fasciculation		
Random, spontaneous twitching of a group of muscle fibers or a motor unit	Nerve	Fasciculation potential
Myoedema		
Focal muscle contraction produced by muscle percussion and not associated with propagated electrical activity	Muscle	Electrically silent
Myokymia		
Continuous quivering or undulating movement of surface and overlying skin and mucous membrane	Nerve	Myokymic discharge
Myotonia		
Clinical observation of delayed relaxation of muscle after voluntary contraction or percussion	Muscle	Myotonic discharge
Neuromyotonia		
Clinical syndrome of continuous muscle fiber activity manifesting as continuous muscle rippling and stiffness	Nerve	Neuromyotonic discharge Myokymic discharge
Tetany		
Clinical syndrome manifesting as muscle twitching, cramps, and carpo-pedal spasm	Nerve	Cramp discharge Myokymic discharge

Clinical features

When obtaining a medical history from a patient reporting muscle cramps, the clinician should obtain a family history of cramps (e.g., familial cramp syndrome, familial dwarfism with muscle cramps, or rippling muscle disease, among others), although familial cases are rare. The clinical approach to cramps is largely based on the following factors: (1) specific nerve/muscle compartments affected (critical

---

International Neurology, Second edition. Edited by Robert P. Lisak, Daniel D. Truong, William M. Carroll and Roongroj Bhidayasiri

Table 127.2 Common etiologies of muscle cramp.

No apparent cause
Nocturnal leg cramps
Exercise related
Lower motor neuron and motor nerve
Motor neuron disorders (amyotrophic lateral sclerosis, post-polio syndrome, Kennedy disease)
Radiculopathy
Neuropathy (diabetic neuropathy, Charcot–Marie–Tooth)
Myopathies
Myotonic syndromes (dystrophic and non-dystrophic)
Lipid storage diseases
Glycogen storage disease
Mitochondrial disease
Inflammatory myopathies (polymyositis, dermatomyositis)
Metabolic derangements
Metabolic disorders
Pregnancy
Uremia
Liver diseases
Hyper- and hypothyroidism
Tetany
Acute extracellular volume depletion
Heat cramps
Hemodialysis
Diarrhea
Medications
Statins and fibrates
Diuretics
Beta-agonists
Cholinergic agents
Steroids
Immune mediated (channelopathies)
Isaac's syndrome
Cramp-fasciculation syndrome
Stiff-person syndrome
Satoyoshi disease
Infections
Tetanus
Botulism

in traumatic and neurovascular etiologies); (2) focal or diffuse muscle weakness; (3) presence of limb posturing; (4) provoking conditions; (5) relationship to movement, stretching, and maneuvers; and (6) presence of spontaneous motor and sensory manifestations.

Investigations

Sustained muscle spasms with or without pain may cause diagnostic confusion, but they should lead one to suspect "central generators." Such would be the case in occupational cramping (e.g., writer's cramp), "off (levodopa) Parkinson dystonia," and pseudo-dystonia (e.g., Satoyoshi's disease). Severe generalized cramps due to tetanus are secondary to involvement of the spinal cord inhibitory interneurons brought about by trans-synaptic spread of the tetanus toxin. Stiff-person syndrome, commonly with truncal involvement, is another case in point, where an antibody to glutamic dehydrogenase may develop.

In addition to a comprehensive medical history and physical and neurological examination, the use of a simple muscle cramp algorithm (see Figure 127.1) can be applied, which points to an initial workup including electrolytes and metabolic and hormonal screening. Tetany has a typical muscle cramp presentation due to low ionic calcium concentra-

tion in the serum. Pregnancy, diabetes mellitus, and abnormal thyroid functions also are frequently associated with muscle cramps. Creatine kinase determination will be needed to screen for myopathies; however, repeated muscle cramps may also lead to this enzyme elevation.

The second step in the diagnosis of muscle cramps is the electrophysiological study. Electrodiagnosis using routine nerve conduction studies (NCS) and EMG will differentiate the origin of muscle cramp from the anterior horn, root, plexus, and the distal peripheral motor nerves and muscles. In lower motor neuron diseases, EMG shows the presence of reinnervation that may have hyperexcitability "spots" along the distal motor branches. Spontaneous discharges including fasciculation potentials, myokymic discharges, and continuous muscle fiber activity are important hallmarks of hyperexcitability of peripheral motor nerves. NCS of both motor and sensory nerves is useful for the diagnosis of focal or diffuse neuropathies, whether demyelinating or axonal in nature.

The third step is to sort out the various causes of muscle cramps in myopathies, especially if there is an elevated creatine kinase. Distribution of muscle weakness minus sensory disturbance and myotonia are important clinical clues leading to the diagnosis of certain myopathies. Pseudomyotonia differs clinically from myotonia because delayed muscular relaxation increases instead of decreases with repetitive activity and percussion myotonia is absent. Myotonic discharges on EMG are an important hallmark of dystrophic and non-dystrophic myotonia. Electrical silence on EMG is a typical finding of muscle contracture that is sometimes seen in myopathies. Cramping myalgia is a prominent feature in the majority of patients with Becker-type dystrophy, as well as in 5% of female carriers of Becker-type and in Duchenne-type muscular dystrophy.

The ischemic forearm exercise test is helpful in approaching metabolic myopathies, wherein a venous canula is placed in the antecubital fossa. Baseline blood is drawn for ammonia and lactate, then the patient opens and closes the hand rapidly and strenuously for a minute while a blood pressure cuff is inflated to above systolic pressure. Immediately after this, the cuff is released and at 1, 2, 4, 6, and 10 minutes post-exercise, further blood is drawn and serum lactate and ammonia levels are documented. A physiological response in a normal individual is a 3–5-fold rise above baseline in lactate and ammonia; if lactate and ammonia do not rise, this suggests that the muscles were not sufficiently exercised, and no conclusion can be drawn; if lactate rises but ammonia is flat, this is diagnostic of myoadenylate deaminase deficiency; and an increase in ammonia with flat lactate is seen in certain glycogen storage diseases (GSDs: myophosphorylase, phosphofructokinase, phosphoglycerate mutase, phosphoglycerate kinase, phosphorylase b kinase, debrancher, and lactate dehydrogenase deficiencies). In mitochondrial myopathy, the ammonia, lactate, and pyruvate will be normal, or slightly increased in the latter two, while fatty acid oxidation defects will have normal levels in all the aforementioned serum parameters. Typified by Pompe's disease (acid maltase deficiency) and McArdle's disease, most of the GSDs are dynamic in that the chief complaints are exercise-induced weakness, cramps, and myoglobinuria. The "second-wind phenomenon" is a specific feature of McArdle's disease. It is characterized by onset of mild exertional cramps, and after a brief rest patients may be able to resume exercise at the previous or a slightly reduced level. The "out-of-wind phenomenon," commonly seen in Tarui's disease (phosphofructokinase deficiency), is decreased exercise tolerance manifested by muscle cramps, and exercise-induced myoglobinuria due to reduction in the availability of free fatty acids and ketones.

Muscle biopsy with immunohistochemistry may be the final option for the investigation of various myopathies. Neuroimaging and antibody testing will add credence to the diagnosis.

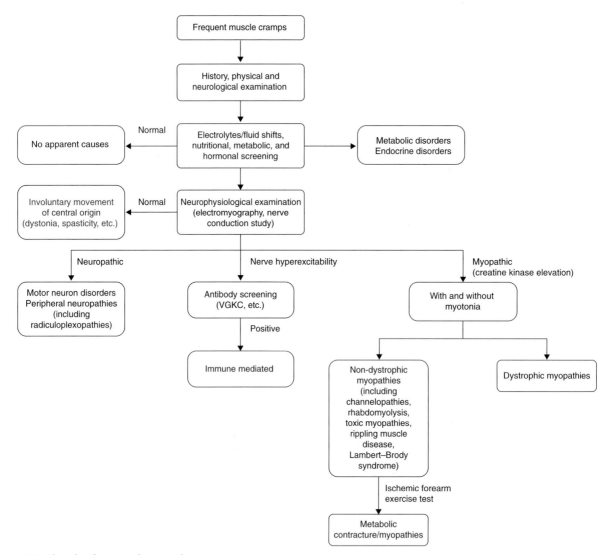

Figure 127.1 Algorithm for approaching muscle cramps.

Treatment

Therapeutic approaches are usually geared toward an established diagnosis of the origin of the muscle cramp, and toward symptom relief of painful muscle cramps and spasms. Withdrawal of offending causative agents, optimal metabolic control, replacement therapy, and immunotherapy are cornerstone treatments. Botulinum toxin therapy is useful in focal dystonia, especially painful task-specific muscle cramping. Physical therapy including nightly stretching before going to bed may be effective in managing or reducing nocturnal leg cramps in elderly people. Quinine sulfate has been reported as an effective drug for muscle cramps, although it is used less commonly than before in clinical practice due to its severe hematological adverse events. Antiepileptic drugs, analgesics, and muscle relaxants are also traditionally used. Mexilletine, which suppresses persistent sodium currents, may also be useful for muscle cramps. Shakuyaku-kanzo-to, a herbal medicine for muscle cramps, has been tried in East Asian countries.

Acknowledgments

Dr. Melanie Leigh Supnet and the CNS staff of the Metropolitan Medical Center assisted in the literature search for this chapter.

Further reading

American Association of Electrodiagnostic Medicine. Glossary of terms in electrodiagnostic medicine. *Muscle Nerve* 2001;Suppl 10:S5–S49.

Donaldson I, Marsden D, Schneider S, Bathia K. *Marsden's Book of Movement Disorders.* Oxford: Oxford University Press; 2012.

Harper CM. Muscle pain, cramps and fatigue. In Engel AG, Franzini-Armstrong C (eds.). *Myology*, 3rd ed. New York: McGraw-Hill; 2004:ch. 63.

Hawke F, Chuter V, Burns J. Factors associated with night-time calf muscle cramps: A case-control study. *Muscle Nerve* 2013;47:339–343.

Hinoshita F, Ogura Y, Suzuki Y, et al. Effect of orally administered shao-yao-gan-cao-tang (Shakuyaku-kanzo-to) on muscle cramps in maintenance hemodialysis patients: A preliminary study. *Am J Chin Med* 2003;31:445–453.

Houston M, Reichman ME, Graham DJ, et al. Use of an active surveillance system by the FDA to observe patterns of quinine sulfate use and adverse hematologic outcomes in CMS Medicare data. *Pharmacoepidemiol Drug Saf* 2014;23(9):911–91. doi:10.1002/pds.3644

Katzberg I, Halpern E, Barnett C, et al. Prevalence of muscle cramps in patients with diabetes. *Diabetes Care* 2014;37:e17–e18. doi:10.2337/dc13-1163

Kimura J. *Electrodiagnosis in Diseases of Nerve and Muscle: Principles and Practice*, 3rd ed. New York: Oxford University Press; 2010.

Kuwabara S, Misawa S, Tamura N, et al. The effects of mexiletine on excitability properties of human median motor axon. *Clin Neurophysiol* 2005;116:284–289.

Miller TM, Layzer RB. Muscle cramps. *Muscle Nerve* 2005;32:431–442.

128 Myasthenia gravis

Richard A. Lewis

Department of Neurology, Cedars-Sinai Medical Center, Los Angeles, CA, USA

Myasthenia gravis (MG) is an autoimmune disorder in which there is a failure of neuromuscular transmission due to binding of antibodies to glycoproteins at the postsynaptic neuromuscular junction (NMJ). MG is the quintessential autoimmune disease, in that it has been demonstrated that antibodies are present at the site of pathology and removal of the antibody is effective therapy. In addition, the disease can be induced in animals by both passive transfer of immunoglobulin from myasthenic patients and immunization of animals with acetylcholine receptor (AChR).

Epidemiology

MG is relatively rare, with an annual incidence of 20–30 per million and a prevalence of about 150–200 per million. Like many other autoimmune disorders, there are two incidence peaks, one between 20 and 40 years of age with predominantly women affected (F:M = 4:1) and the other between 60 and 80 years of age without gender dominance. As many as 15% of cases may present before age 20 years. A transient neonatal MG due to passive placental transfer of maternal AChR antibody occurs in 10% of babies born to myasthenic mothers. This tends to last for 3–4 weeks and does not lead to future development of the disease.

The disease occurs worldwide without specific clustering. There is a strong correlation of young adult MG with HLA genotypes. These have been studied in Japanese, Chinese, Scandinavians, and other Caucasians. There is an increased incidence of MG and other autoimmune disorders in family members of MG patients, but there is no direct Mendelian inheritance. Twin studies have shown disease in both twins in only a minority of twins investigated.

Pathophysiology

Neuromuscular junction transmission and the acetylcholine receptor

Acetylcholine (ACh) is the transmitter at the neuromuscular junction. It is synthesized and stored in vesicles in the distal motor nerve terminal, with each vesicle containing approximately 10,000 ACh molecules, called a quantum. There is spontaneous release of quanta, but depolarization of the nerve terminal produces an inward flux of calcium that causes a large release of ACh quanta. The ACh binds to receptors on the postsynaptic muscle membrane. The AChR is a glycoprotein made up of five subunits that are arranged to form a channel. The two alpha subunits have binding sites for ACh and are the locations for AChR antibody binding (Figure 128.1).

Acetylcholine receptor antibody and the autoimmune disorder

The initial event in MG is unclear, but is related to an autoimmune reaction, predominantly to the main immunogenic region (MIR) on the alpha subunit of the AChR (Figure 128.1). This initial event, particularly in younger patients who are AChR antibody positive and especially those with thymoma, may begin in the thymus. There is evidence that both T and B lymphocytes are important in the development of MG. The immunoglobin G (IgG) AChR antibodies initiate a complement-mediated lysis of the postsynaptic muscle membrane. The resulting reduction in functional AChR causes a reduced effect of ACh on the muscle. Normally, the number of active receptors is more than enough to depolarize the muscle membrane, but with the loss of functional receptors in MG, this safety factor for transmission is lost and some muscle fibers will fail to depolarize during sustained muscular effort.

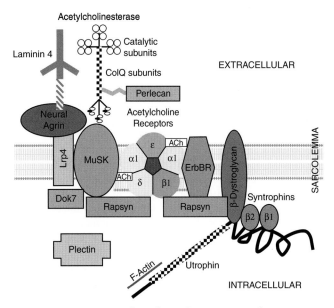

Figure 128.1 Extrajunctional muscle membrane – associated proteins. Source: http://neuromuscular.wustl.edu/musdist/dag2.htm. Reproduced with permission of Dr Alan Pestronk.

International Neurology, Second edition. Edited by Robert P. Lisak, Daniel D. Truong, William M. Carroll and Roongroj Bhidayasiri

The role of the thymus

The association of thymoma and MG has been known for over 70 years. Most patients with thymoma and MG have AChR antibodies. The relationship of thymoma to muscle-specific kinase (MuSK) antibody-related MG is not known (see the Investigations section). Thymoma is present in approximately 15% of MG patients, with a peak incidence at age 50 years in both men and women. The presence of thymoma does not portend a worse prognosis or more severe disease and most patients will have persistent MG after surgical removal of the thymic tumor. Computed tomography (CT) or magnetic resonance imaging (MRI) of the chest will identify a mediastinal mass, but small thymomatous nodules may be identified histologically in radiologically unremarkable mediastinums. Malignant thymomas comprise a small fraction of thymic tumors. In the younger population, the thymus usually shows hyperplasia with increased germinal centers. Older patients who do not have thymoma usually have an atrophic thymus. The thymus contains myoid cells with MIR epitope as well as titin and RyR epitopes, which may have a role in the initiation of the disease, but it is clear that the peripheral immune system becomes involved and in most patients the immunological disorder persists after thymectomy.

Clinical manifestations

Symptoms and signs

The majority of patients present with diplopia and/or ptosis with or without other muscle involvement. Some may only have ocular symptoms, but over 85% develop other symptoms. Those who remain purely ocular for more than 2 years rarely generalize after that. Other manifestations include facial and jaw weakness, speech and swallowing problems, and proximal and/or distal limb muscle weakness. Most concerning is the involvement of respiratory muscles. A clue to the diagnosis is the diurnal fluctuation of the symptoms, with symptoms typically being less on wakening after sleep. Frequently the symptoms become worse with exercise. Respiratory insufficiency and inability to protect the airway are the major life-threatening symptoms. Fortunately, modern intensive care management and immunotherapy have improved the prognosis. Most patients respond to medications and have good function and quality of life, but full remission in which the patient requires no medications occurs in less than 20% of cases.

The examination of the patient with suspected MG should include careful observation for variability of signs. For instance, ptosis may not manifest initially, but be evident intermittently during the examination. Speech may become more nasal as the patient is talking. Repetitive or sustained effort may bring out signs. Sustaining upgaze for 30 seconds may induce ptosis or having the patient raise the arms up for 30 seconds may induce weakness of shoulder abduction. Neck flexion and extension may be particularly weak and jaw closure may be difficult. Some patients with anti-MuSK antibodies have particular problems with bulbar function and neck extension, sometimes with prominent muscle atrophy.

Associated disorders

Patients with MG have an increased incidence of other autoimmune diseases such as rheumatoid arthritis, systemic lupus erythematosus, pernicious anemia, and autoimmune thyroiditis. Some patients present with both MG and hyperthyroidism and it can be difficult to determine which disorder is causing the extraocular muscle problems.

Investigations

Antibody detection

Antibodies (Ab) directed against the AChR are found in 85% of patients with generalized MG and up to 70% in ocular MG. These predominantly IgG polyclonal antibodies are specific for MG, but binding antibody titer does not correlate with clinical severity. Of the 15% of patients who are AChR antibody negative, 40% have antibodies directed against MuSK. It is unclear whether MuSK antibodies are pathogenic, and the incidence of MuSK Ab positivity in the Scandinavian population appears particularly low. Striational antibodies are seen in 30% of MG patients, but in up to 80% of those with thymoma. They are more commonly found in older patients, but they are more predictive of thymoma in the younger patients than those over the age of 50 years. At least two antigens related to striational antibodies have been described, titin and the ryanodine receptor.

Antibodies directed against two other AchR-associated membrane constituents have recently been described. Anti-LRP4 may account for as much as 7% of the MG population. The prevalence of anti-agrin antibodies is unknown.

Electrophysiological studies

The physiological effect of AChR antibodies is to reduce the muscle fiber response to acetylcholine release from the distal nerve terminal. The consequence of this is that there is a reduction in the safety factor of transmission at the postsynaptic muscle membrane. This is manifest in electrodiagnostic studies by a decrement in the compound muscle action potential amplitude with repetitive stimulation at low rates of stimulation (2–5 Hz). This decrement worsens 1–4 minutes after exercise and has been a useful diagnostic test. However, it is not specific for MG, being seen in other neuromuscular junction disorders, and to a lesser extent in motor neuron disease and peripheral nerve disorders. Abnormal decrement usually defined as more than 10% by amplitude is seen in approximately two out of three patients with generalized MG, but less than 50% of patients with ocular MG.

The other consequence of the reduction in the safety factor of transmission is seen in the jitter and blocking that are found on single-fiber electromyography (SFEMG). This technique looks at pairs of muscle fibers from the same motor unit. Normally, they will consistently fire in a closely time-locked fashion. With impaired neuromuscular transmission this firing is less consistent: the interdischarge interval varies or "jitters" and intermittently fibers can fail to fire altogether. These abnormalities occur in over 95% of patients with generalized MG, but are also non-specific.

Diagnosis

A patient who has ptosis and diplopia with or without bulbar, neck, or limb weakness should be suspected of having MG, especially if these are associated with periorbital muscle weakness. Muscle weakness that fluctuates or increases with activity should also raise suspicion. Where tests for AChR antibodies are not available, the diagnosis is dependent on demonstrating the electrophysiological abnormality and/or finding a transient reversal of weakness after intravenous edrophonium (Tensilon®), a short-acting acetylcholinesterase inhibitor. This allows for ACh to remain at the muscle endplate, potentially overcoming the reduced safety factor of transmission. This Tensilon test remains a useful examination tool, but is used less frequently with the availability of laboratory testing for AChR antibodies. In patients with ptosis, placing some ice over the eye for 2 minutes can produce a significant transient improvement in ptosis. This simple bedside test can assist in diagnosis of an NMJ disorder and is based on the recognition that lowering temperature has a beneficial effect on neuromuscular transmission.

AChR antibodies are specific for MG and when detected are pathognomonic for the disease. If these are not detected, MuSK antibodies can be looked for and repetitive stimulation and/or SFEMG can be performed. Testing for antibodies directed against LRP4 and agrin is not yet available commercially.

Other diagnostic studies that are appropriate include laboratory testing for thyroid disease and autoimmune disorders. Creatinine kinase (CK) and antistriational antibody assays are of interest. A chest CT or MRI scan looking for a thymoma is important for patients identified as having MG.

Treatment

Physiological or symptomatic therapy

Acetylcholinesterase inhibitors (AChEI) such as pyridostigmine, directed against AChE at nicotinic receptors, can substantially improve symptoms and in some instances provide complete reversal of symptoms as long as the medication is taken. This, however, does not treat the underlying immunological disorder. Side effects are primarily related to cholinergic muscarinic effects on the gastrointestinal and cardiopulmonary systems. These can be controlled with atropine or similar medications. Excessive amounts of pyridostigmine can cause fasciculations and increased weakness, sometimes leading to cholinergic crisis. The effect of pyridostigmine tends to last for 3–4 hours. There is a slow release form of pyridostigmine that may be useful overnight, but is not recommended for use during waking hours. Pyridostigmine has not been found to be helpful in MuSK antibody MG and may worsen symptoms.

Immunosuppressive and immunomodulatory therapy

If AChEIs are not symptomatically effective, then immunosuppressive agents are utilized. There have been very few large, double blind, placebo-controlled studies, and recommendations are based on the clinical experiences described in the literature.

Corticosteroids have been used for over 40 years and are generally accepted as being effective. The clinical effects are usually apparent within 4–8 weeks and occur in over two out of three patients. There is a potential for clinical deterioration within 5–14 days of initiating high doses and it is usually recommended to gradually increase the dose over a period of 7–14 days, unless the situation is urgent and the patient hospitalized. Some patients may go into remission, but most require continued therapy. The usual side effects of corticosteroids are common, but can be mitigated by alternate-day dosing, the use of biphosphonates, and careful follow-up. Patients with purely ocular MG who do not respond to pyridostigmine may respond to low doses of corticosteroids, avoiding the complications of higher doses.

Azathioprine at doses of 2–3 mg/kg bodyweight has been shown to be an effective steroid-sparing medication. It takes a minimum of 6 months and as much as 18 months before the full immunosuppressive effect is evident. It is usually well tolerated with minimal long-term risk of malignancy, but the patient must be carefully monitored for hepatic and bone marrow toxicity. These are sometimes seen with initiation, but can also be dose related. The effectiveness of azathioprine as a single agent is less clear and has not been adequately studied.

Other immunosuppressives generally accepted as being effective in a significant number of patients include cyclosporine and cyclophosphamide. Both have significant side effects and potential toxicities. Two controlled trials with mycophenolate mofetil failed to find efficacy, but issues with trial length and design have been raised. Other immunosuppressives that have been considered, although with less documented experience, include methotrexate, tacrolimus, and rituximab. Small uncontrolled series of rituximab, a monoclonal antibody directed at the CD20 epitope on B-cells, have shown good effect in both AChR and MuSK antibody-positive patients. The reports are particularly encouraging in anti-MuSK patients, who can be refractory to many of the other immunosuppressant therapies.

Plasma exchange (PLEx), by removing circulating antibodies and other plasma constituents, can have a profound effect within days of initiation, and is therefore a highly effective agent to prevent or reverse myasthenic crisis. Its clinical effect is temporary, usually dissipating in 2–4 weeks, and it has a limited role in long-term management. The major problems with pheresis are venous access and complications of indwelling venous catheters, as well as potential cardiopulmonary effects of fluid and metabolic shifts.

Intravenous immunoglobulin (IVIg) has also been shown to be effective with a slightly lower complication rate, but may not work quite as fast as plasmapheresis. It has the same temporary effectiveness but is more easily given intermittently over months to years. In many countries, patients can be treated at home.

Thymectomy is indicated for patients with CT or MRI evidence of a thymoma. The role of thymectomy in MG without radiological suggestion of thymoma is less clear, although it is commonly utilized. The literature suggests a greater benefit in younger patients with generalized MG who are AChR antibody positive. Thymectomy is not usually recommended for patients who are antibody negative, including those who are anti-MuSK antibody positive or patients over 60 years of age, as thymic pathology including hyperplastic germinal centers has not been found in most instances.

Drugs that can worsen MG

A number of drugs can exacerbate MG. The major ones include aminoglycosides, beta blockers, quinidine, procainamide, and magnesium products, but other medications including antibiotics and antiarrhythmics have been implicated. The most striking drug relationship to MG is with D-penicillamine, which, when given for other disorders such as rheumatoid arthritis, scleroderma, or Wilson's disease, can cause MG with AChR and striational antibodies, but the disease can remit with withdrawal of the drug.

Emergency care of myasthenic patients

Patients with swallowing or breathing problems and those with marked neck weakness and speech problems should be considered to be at risk for respiratory failure or aspiration pneumonia. They should be hospitalized and monitored closely, preferably in an intensive care setting. Respiratory status must be followed closely with parameters that assess respiratory muscle function, usually forced vital capacity, and negative inspiratory force. Oxygen saturation is insensitive to respiratory muscle weakness and is an inadequate guide to respiratory failure. Patients with good swallowing who do not need airway protection may benefit from non-invasive ventilatory support. Plasma exchange or IVIg should be initiated on an urgent basis if one is hoping to prevent intubation or to facilitate early extubation.

Further reading

Jani-Acsadi A, Lisak RP. Myasthenic crisis: Guidelines for prevention and treatment. *J Neurol Sci* 2007;15;261:127–133.

Jayawant S, Parr J, Vincent A. Autoimmune myasthenia gravis. *Handb Clin Neurol* 2013;113:1465–1468.

Kumar V, Kaminski HJ. Treatment of myasthenia gravis. *Curr Neurol Neurosci Rep* 2011;11:89–96.

Querol L, Illa I. Myasthenia gravis and the neuromuscular junction. *Curr Opin Neurol* 2013;26(5):459–465.

Silvestri NJ, Wolfe GI. Myasthenia gravis. *Semin Neurol* 2012;32:215–226.

129 Lambert–Eaton myasthenic syndrome

Emilia Kerty

Neurology Department, Oslo University Hospital/Rikshospitalet, Oslo, Norway

In 1953, Anderson *et al.* described a 47-year-old male presenting with progressive proximal muscle weakness, diminished tendon stretch reflexes, and small cell lung carcinoma (SCLC). Three years later, Lambert, Eaton, and Rooke reported six similar cases with atypical myasthenia, lung carcinoma, and a distinct electrophysiological pattern at repetitive stimulation differing from that seen in myasthenia gravis (MG). To date, such conditions with or without SCLC are named Lambert–Eaton myasthenic syndrome (LEMS). An autoimmune etiology was suggested and proven by passive transfer of LEMS patients' serum to mice by injection. The hypothesis was also confirmed by demonstration of pathogenic antibodies to presynaptic voltage-gated calcium channels (VGCCs) in the serum of LEMS patients. Approximately 50–60% of patients with LEMS have an underlying tumor (T-LEMS) that in 90% of cases is SCLC.

Epidemiology

LEMS fulfills the criteria for a rare disease. Epidemiological analysis in the Netherlands has shown a yearly incidence of 0.75 per million and a prevalence of 3.42 per million, which has increased over the last few decades, probably because of an aging population and improved diagnosis. LEMS is seen in all ages, but only occasionally in children, with a peak age of onset of approximately 35 years and a second, larger peak at age 60 years. Patients without tumor (NT-LEMS) have a lower age of onset than T-LEMS, and women are slightly overrepresented and have a better survival rate. T-LEMS patients are older at onset and 65% are men, usually with a smoking habit. T-LEMS patients have a better survival rate than SCLC patients without neurological dysfunction.

LEMS is not especially prevalent in any part of the world. Although a few epidemiological studies have been reported, none has indicated geographic variation, except that LEMS is less common in countries with a relatively high percentage of children and young people.

Pathophysiology

LEMS is a presynaptic disorder of neuromuscular transmission mediated by antibodies to P/Q-type VGCCs at the motor terminal. In healthy individuals, VGCCs mediate Ca^{2+} influx into the nerve terminal and through several steps lead to quantal release in the synaptic cleft. In LEMS patients, antibodies cause a loss of VGCC function by blocking Ca^{2+} influx during depolarization and/or downregulation of VGCCs, resulting in decreased acetylcholine release from the presynaptic membrane. This causes muscle weakness and areflexia that improve after a few seconds of sustained contraction of the weak muscle. VGCC antibodies presumably are also responsible for the autonomic dysfunction in LEMS patients.

Approximately 10–15% of patients with LEMS have no detectable P/Q VGCC antibodies. In these cases, either antibodies to a different VGCC epitope or antibodies to a different molecule are responsible. The passive transfer of human antibodies from antibody-negative cases to mice also induces disease.

In T-LEMS patients who have SCLC, neuroectodermal antigens expressed by SCLC cells mimic VGCC and induce the production of VGCC antibodies as a paraneoplastic syndrome. In NT-LEMS patients, antibodies are produced as part of a more general autoimmune state.

Clinical features

The clinical triad in LEMS consists of weakness, autonomic dysfunction, and areflexia. Difficulty in walking and standing from a seated position because of proximal leg weakness is nearly always the first symptom, but weakness of the arms is also a common and an early sign. The typical clinical pattern of weakness generally spreads proximally to distally on arms and legs and caudally to cranially, and finally reaching the cranial muscles. Ptosis and bulbar weakness may occur, but are less prominent than in MG. The speed of progression is more pronounced in T-LEMS than in NT-LEMS. The weakness does not show diurnal variation. Although symptoms usually begin insidiously, a rapid onset is not uncommon, especially in T-LEMS. The weakness is painless, but patients may report muscle aching or soreness. Tendon reflexes are usually hypoactive or absent, but may become apparent after voluntary muscle contraction. Post-exercise facilitation of the improvement of muscle strength and transient normalization of tendon reflexes after a brief maximal contraction are present in only half of patients.

Almost all LEMS patients have autonomic dysfunction, which can be mild, including dry mouth, dry eyes, absent sweating, orthostatic hypotension, constipation, and erectile and bladder dysfunction.

The clinical pattern in LEMS is less specific than in MG, therefore diagnostic delay can be long, especially for NT-LEMS. The clinical presentations of LEMS and MG are usually quite distinct. Ptosis and double vision, bulbar weakness, and abnormal fatigue predominate at the initial presentation of MG. The weakness characteristically fluctuates. There have been some reports of patients with features

International Neurology, Second edition. Edited by Robert P. Lisak, Daniel D. Truong, William M. Carroll and Roongroj Bhidayasiri

that overlap between MG and LEMS, but true overlap syndromes with antibodies to both AChR (acetylcholine receptors) and VGCC are very rare. The most frequent misdiagnosis is probably seronegative and atypical MG.

Initial symptoms in LEMS are symmetric and usually mild, and include slowly progressive painless proximal weakness, which suggests myopathy, especially inclusion body myopathy in older patients. However, in LEMS patients muscle enzymes are not elevated and patients have autonomic symptoms. In some tumor-associated cases the symptoms develop subacutely, mimicking Guillain–Barré syndrome (GBS) or amyotrophic lateral sclerosis (ALS). The latter usually starts asymmetrically with hyperreflexia and apparent muscle atrophy. GBS patients have elevated protein in their spinal fluid and usually develop sensory symptoms in addition.

Investigations

A clinical suspicion of LEMS should be confirmed by neurophysiological studies and detection of serum antibodies to VGCC.

Compound muscle action potentials (CMAPs) are small, often 10% of normal, and may fall further with repetitive stimulation at frequencies between 1 and 5 Hz (thus leading to a false diagnosis of MG), but during stimulation at high frequencies of 20–50 Hz or immediately after a brief maximal voluntary contraction, the CMAP increases in size (an amplitude increase of 100% is clearly abnormal). Measurements should be performed for at least one hand and one foot muscle. Single-fiber electromyography shows increased jitter in all patients with LEMS, but it does not distinguish between MG and LEMS.

Antibodies to P/Q VGCC are present in 50–75% of LEMS patients and the positivity rate can approach 100% in T-LEMS patients. The disease is generally associated with high antibody titers. These antibodies are highly specific to LEMS, having only been described in association with paraneoplastic SCLC-related cerebellar ataxia and a small percentage of SCLC patients with pathology lacking neurological findings. An absence of these antibodies does not exclude a diagnosis of LEMS.

Antibodies against SOX protein (Sry-related high-mobility group box) represent an important serological marker for SCLC, but they are not widely available. The presence of this antibody may facilitate earlier tumor diagnosis.

There is a high association between NT-LEMS with histocompatibility complex molecules HLA B8 and HLA DR3 and DQ2, but no relationship has been found for T-LEMS and HLA.

Once a diagnosis of LEMS has been confirmed or is even suspected, an extensive search for associated malignancy is mandatory. More than 90% of T-LEMS patients have SCLC. Screening by computed tomography (CT) thorax, ^{18}F-Fluorodeoxyglucose-positron emission tomography (FDG-PET), and bronchoscopy are required.

SCLC may be too small to detect initially, therefore these investigations need to be repeated every 6 months for at least 2 years. With this approach, 96% of SCLC is found within a year of diagnosing LEMS, while a delay of more than 2 years is extremely rare. Other tumors are associated with LEMS, but it is hard to establish causality. Lymphoma, leukemia, carcinoma of breast, prostate, stomach, colon, bladder, endometrium, and non-small cell and mixed lung carcinoma cases have been reported.

Many NT-LEMS patients have increased occurrence of other autoimmune disease, including thyroiditis, pernicious anemia, celiac disease, juvenile-onset diabetes mellitus, and Sjögren's syndrome.

Treatment

The first therapeutic approach for NT-LEMS patients is 3,4 diaminopyridine (3,4-DAP), a potassium channel antagonist. It is effective and well tolerated, apart from perioral and digital paresthesias, which are common complaints. The most serious (but rare) adverse effects are seizures that appear to have a dose-dependent risk. 3,4-DAP prepared in a phosphate salt formulation for better stability has been recently developed. A new calcium channel agonist (GV-58), alone or in combination with 3,4-DAP, shows promising results. Some patients reported benefits from combined therapy with 3,4-DAP and the cholinesterase inhibitor pyridostigmine. Patients with disabling symptoms not adequately controlled with 3,4-DAP are started on high-dose prednisolone, with subsequent dosage tapering according to clinical responses. The therapeutic effect of azathioprine, a steroid-sparing agent, in combination with prednisolone is best documented. For other immunosuppressive drugs, such as mycophenolate mofetil and cyclosporine, mostly limited series have been reported. Rituximab is also effective for more severe cases. Acute treatment with intravenous immunoglobulin or plasmapheresis is rarely required.

The treatment of associated tumors generally induces significant improvement of neurological symptoms and in some patients no further treatment for LEMS may be necessary. If remission of symptoms is incomplete, prednisolone might induce an improvement.

Further reading

Eaton L, Lambert EH. Electromyography and electric stimulation of nerves in diseases of motor unit: Observations on myasthenic syndrome associated with malignant tumors. *JAMA* 1957;163:1117–1124.

Keogh M, Sedehizadeh S, Maddison P. Treatment for Lambert–Eaton myasthenic syndrome. *Cochrane Database Syst Rev* 2011;2:CD003279.

Lang B, Newsom-Davis J, Wray D, Vincent A, Murray N. Autoimmune aetiology for myasthenic (Eaton–Lambert) syndrome. *Lancet* 1981;2:224–226.

Oh SJ, Kurokawa K, Claussen GC, Ryan HF, Jr. Electrophysiological diagnostic criteria of Lambert–Eaton myasthenic syndrome. *Muscle Nerve* 2005;32:515–520.

Titulaer MJ, Lang B, Verschuuren JJ. Lambert–Eaton myasthenic syndrome: From clinical characteristics to therapeutic strategies. *Lancet Neurol* 2011;10:1098–1107.

130 Neuromuscular transmission disorders caused by toxins and drugs

Zohar Argov

Department of Neurology, Hadassah-Hebrew University Medical Center, Jerusalem, Israel

The neuromuscular synapse is prone to pharmacological blockage by numerous drugs and chemicals and also several naturally occuring toxins. Those most important to the practicing neurologist will be discussed here.

Botulism

Botulism is a synaptic disorder caused by a neurotoxin that inhibits acetylcholine (ACh) release from motor and autonomic nerve endings by cleaving specific proteins essential for ACh vesicle docking. The toxin is excreted by the gram-positive, spore-forming, anaerobic bacillus *Clostridium botulinum*. There are five types of this toxin. Those relevant for human diseases are A, B, and E (very rarely, type F). The spores, prevalent in soils worldwide, are heat resistant, surviving food-preparation methods that do not use temperatures of 120 °C for long enough periods.

There are five forms of human botulism. The "classic" form is food botulism, typically caused by home-canned food like fish, vegetables, and potatoes. In this form the toxin itself is ingested. Infant botulism and occult (adult) botulism occur when spores are ingested and the toxin is slowly released in the gastrointestinal system. Wound botulism has been reported in drug abusers. A rare form is the complication after medical usage of the toxin in low quantities to overcome muscle overactivity. The rarest form is inhalational botulism. The potential use of botulinum toxin as a biological weapon should not be overlooked.

The clinical syndrome of botulism varies by the mode of toxin access into the body. In food-borne cases there is ingestion of the toxin from ill-prepared food and the symptoms appear within hours after the meal. In infant and adult occult botulism the spores residing in the intestinal system slowly release the toxin and symptoms reappear over the course of several days. Similarly, in wound-related cases the spores inhabit the oxygen-free environment of the tissue and the bacilli produce the toxin more slowly; this is also the case for the inhalational form. Botulism after medical use of the toxin is slow to appear due to the low quantities of the toxin injected.

Regardless of access route, once disseminated the toxin produces a rather similar clinical picture of motor paralysis with autonomic failure. Symptoms and signs appear first in the cranial musculature, leading to ptosis, ophthalmoparesis, and speech and swallowing difficulties (the "4Ds": diplopia, dysarthria, dysphagia, and dysphonia). Motor paralysis develops rapidly in a descending pattern, affecting the upper limbs first. Respiratory paralysis may then appear. Autonomic failure manifests commonly as dry mouth, constipation, pupillary abnormalities, and often also urinary retention and hypotension. The fatality rate has markedly decreased in places with modern respiratory support facilities, but is still as high as 10%. Where no critical medical care is present the death rate can reach 50%.

The diagnosis of botulism may be missed if the clinical pattern is not recognized, as the only confirmatory tests include isolation of the bacilli and identification of the toxin in body fluids and tissues. Rarely, the bacilli are grown from tissue cultures and in many instances no biological confirmation can be established, especially if the samples are taken more than 48 hours after disease onset. The main biological sources are serum, stool, and, when relevant, wound. The mode of stool collection (especially in infants) and method of sample storage must be appropriate to prevent diagnosis failure. The toxin is identified and typed in a biological test (a mouse model used in very specialized laboratories only). The main findings in the clinical electrodiagnostic laboratory are small compound muscle action potential and increased jitter on single-fiber electromyogram (SF-EMG). Decremental responses to low-rate repetitive nerve stimulation and spontaneous activity on EMG of paralyzed muscles can sometimes be found.

Infant botulism usually occurs before the age of 6 months and starts mostly with constipation. Feeding difficulties, weak cry, and bulbar weakness with rapidly ensuing limb paralysis should alert the physician to the possible diagnosis. Honey consumption is considered a source of clostridium spores (mainly type B) in 15% of infantile cases and its administration should be avoided before the age of 1 year. Adult intestines are resistant to bacilli growth, but prior abnormalities like surgery, inflammatory bowel disease, and massive antibiotic treatment can reduce resistance.

The main mode of treatment is intensive care with a good respiratory support system until recovery, which may be as long as few months, but usually is 2–8 weeks. Antitoxin administration remains controversial, because this equine-borne treatment is associated with a high rate of serious allergic reactions. When given early, antitoxin reduces the respiratory failure period and fatality rate. The source of contamination should be rapidly recognized in food-borne cases to prevent small epidemics. Human-derived botulinum immunoglobulin has been shown to shorten the disease duration in the infantile form. Other medications like guanidine and aminopyridines have not been sufficiently studied to merit usage. In general, antibiotic use to treat the clostridium infection is considered unnecessary.

International Neurology, Second edition. Edited by Robert P. Lisak, Daniel D. Truong, William M. Carroll and Roongroj Bhidayasiri
© 2016 John Wiley & Sons, Ltd. Published 2016 by John Wiley & Sons, Ltd.

Organophosphate intoxication

Organophosphates (OP) block the activity of acetylcholine esterase (AChE) and thus impair transmission in neuromuscular and other cholinergic synapses. They are mainly used as pesticides. Intoxication can occur in farms, at workplace and manufacturing sites, and at home (by accidental or intentional consumption). OP-modified compounds serve as "nerve gas" for warfare and terror usage; this mandates recognition of the clinical picture and therapy of this intoxication.

The clinical signs and symptoms of acute OP intoxication result from ACh accumulation in nicotinic, muscarinic, and central nervous system (CNS) synapses. The neuromuscular signs include flaccid weakness and fasciculations and are associated with increased gland secretion, autonomic and smooth muscle overactivity, and CNS irritability. Less recognized is the intermediate syndrome that occurs a few days after the acute intoxication (usually not a severe one) and results in proximal muscle weakness, which may lead to respiratory failure and mimic Guillain–Barré syndrome, myasthenic crisis, or unusually severe inflammatory myopathy. Recognition of the clinical picture is the main step in diagnosis; confirmation can be obtained by measuring AChE activity in erythrocytes.

Treatment includes removal of the patient from the contaminated environment (if necessary) and administration of preferably all three types of medication: (1) atropine to block muscarinic synapses, in increasing doses until a therapeutic effect is observed (doses may be extremely high); (2) oximes to reactivate AChE (commonly used but not evidence based); and (3) diazepam to reduce CNS irritability. Supportive therapy, especially mechanical ventilation, is essential, as patients may recover after a prolonged period.

Delayed neuropathy has been described after acute intoxication, but its potential development after low-grade chronic exposure is still debated. Likewise, the prolonged neuropsychological syndrome after exposure (acute or chronic) is controversial.

Medication-induced neuromuscular junction disorders

There is a growing list of drugs implicated in aggravating or inducing myasthenic syndromes. The clinical presentations include the following. (1) Appearance of myasthenia after short exposure to a medication. This condition is attributed to the various drugs' neuromuscular junction (NMJ) blocking properties in susceptible patients (i.e., those with subclinical myasthenia). This complication usually resolves when the offending medication is withdrawn, but in some cases the full picture of myasthenia gravis (MG) continues to evolve. (2) Aggravation of a preexisting NMJ disorder, usually MG, but also Lambert–Eaton myasthenic syndrome (LEMS). The most common situation is the administration of antibiotics to a myasthenic patient. Other drugs have been implicated, usually those with a local anesthetic-like action. (3) Acute weakness or prolonged respiratory depression after uneventful anesthesia. This occurs when a drug with NMJ-blocking properties is given to the patient when the NMJ has not fully recovered from the anesthetic medications. Overuse of magnesium in the treatment of eclampsia can also lead to such an acute event. (4) Development of a chronic immune-mediated myasthenic syndrome after long-term exposure to a medication. This has mainly been described with penicillamine used for rheumatoid arthritis and attributed to its effects on immune control. Recently statin-induced seropositive myasthenia has been postulated, but the role of statins in the evolution of the syndrome remains to be determined. Recognition and withdrawal of a potential offending medication are the main therapeutic approach, but specific therapies that counter the blocking activity may be necessary.

Conclusion

Recognition of toxic neuromuscular disorders is very important for the treatment of patients with these acute, at times life-threatening conditions. It is not always possible to withdraw the offending agent, as can be done with the iatrogenic NMJ disorders, but all the medical emergencies discussed here are potentially treatable if the correct diagnosis is made and suitable therapy is rapidly given.

Further reading

Argov Z. Treatment of myasthenia: Nonimmune issues. *Curr Opin Neurol* 2009;22: 493–497.

Buckley NA, Eddleston M, Li Y, Robertson J. Oximes for acute organophosphate pesticides poisoning. *Cochrane Database Syst Rev* 2011;2:CD005085. doi:10.1002/14651858.CD005085

Costa LG. Current issues in organophosphate toxicology. *Clinica Chim Acta* 2006;366:1–13.

Jokanovic M, Kosanovic M, Brkic D, Vukomanovic P. Organophosphate induced delayed polyneuropathy in man: An overview. *Clin Neurol Neurosurg* 2011;113:7–10.

Mackenzie Ross S, McManus IC, Harris V, Mason O. Neurobehavioral problems following low-grade exposure to organophosphate pesticides: A systematic and meta-analytic review. *Crit Rev Toxicol* 2013;43:21–44.

Rossetto O, Pirazzini M, Montecucco C. Botulinum neurotoxins: Genetic, structural and mechanistic insights. *Nature Rev* 2014;12:535–549.

Zhang J-C, Sun L, Nie Q-H. Botulism, where are we now? *Clin Toxicol* 2010;48:867–879.

PART 14   Neurogenetics

131 | Genetics in neurology

Karen P. Frei and Janice Fuentes
Loma Linda University Medical Center, Loma Linda, CA, USA

Inherited traits have long been of interest. Since the time Gregor Mendel described the heritability of traits in pea plants, we have pursued a modern understanding of our genetic underpinnings. The Human Genome Project, completed in 2003, greatly enhanced this process, providing a comprehensive reference, mapping the entire genome. Many neurological disorders appear to be inherited through a single gene mutation. Others, such as Alzheimer's disease and Parkinson's disease, are thought to be multifactorial in origin, with one or more genes involved as part of their etiology. As the subject of genetic disorders in neurology is so vast, this chapter attempts to describe the basics of genetics using selective neurological diseases as examples. Disorders that are not otherwise covered in the book will be discussed briefly, followed by an update on the treatment of genetic disorders.

Basic definitions
Genes are pieces of DNA that code for the controlled production of proteins. Mutations are abnormalities seen within the DNA of a gene. There are different types of mutations, including substitutions of one base for another, and additions or deletions of DNA. Mutations can produce no change in the protein or they can produce an abnormal or truncated protein. Disease states can be caused by gene mutations, which are then passed on through to the next generation.

Mendelian genetics
Gregor Mendel, known as the father of modern genetics, first described the inheritance of traits in pea plants in 1865. He noted that inheritance of traits follows particular laws. These laws apply to traits such as hair and eye color as well as to disease states resulting from a mutated gene.

Autosomal dominant inheritance
A single mutated gene on one chromosome is all that is required for an autosomal dominant inheritance disease state to be expressed. This means that the disease is present in one of the parents and in 50% of the children. Examples of autosomal dominant inheritance include neurofibromatosis type 1.

Autosomal recessive inheritance
Two copies of the mutated gene are required for this disease state to be expressed. Both parents are carriers of the disease and usually are not affected with the disease. Most of the metabolic single-enzyme deficiency disease states are inherited through autosomal recessive transmission. An example is Gaucher's disease, which is caused by deficiency of the lysosomal enzyme beta glucocerebrosidase. Gaucher type 3 (subacute neuronopathic) patients have neurological features including myoclonic seizures and horizontal supranuclear gaze palsy, in addition to splenomegaly and hepatomegaly.

X-linked dominant inheritance
A single mutation occurring on the X chromosome causes this disease state. Females inherit an X chromosome from each of their parents and males inherit one X chromosome from their mother and one Y chromosome from their father. Because only one X chromosome with the mutation is required to develop the disease state, males and females with a mutation are equally likely to have the disease. However, if the father has the mutation, only his daughters will be affected, since he passes his unaffected Y chromosome to his sons. Rett's syndrome is an example of the X-linked dominant inheritance pattern. Rett's syndrome consists of autism, developmental delay, severe speech and communication impairment, microcephaly, seizures, and stereotypic non-functional hand movements.

X-linked recessive inheritance
Since males have only one X chromosome, a recessive mutation can result in the disease state. Thus, males are more commonly affected than females. Affected fathers will have heterozygous or carrier daughters and normal sons. Carrier mothers will have carrier or normal daughters and affected sons. Duchenne muscular dystrophy and the metabolic disorder Fabry's disease are inherited in this manner. Fabry's disease is a lysosomal storage disorder resulting from a mutation in the alpha galactosidase A gene. There is accumulation of globotriaosylceramide in cells, resulting in cardiac failure, renal failure, and stroke. A painful small fiber neuropathy, dysautonomia, and telangiectasias are also part of this disorder.

International Neurology, Second edition. Edited by Robert P. Lisak, Daniel D. Truong, William M. Carroll and Roongroj Bhidayasiri
© 2016 John Wiley & Sons, Ltd. Published 2016 by John Wiley & Sons, Ltd.

Codominant inheritance

Codominant inheritance involves more than one form of a gene (allele). Each allele is expressed and has an influence on the outward expression (phenotype). Blood types are one example of this type of inheritance with A, B, and O alleles.

Other genetic forms of inheritance

Many disorders are inherited through a complex interaction between several genes and/or the environment. The genetics of these disorders is more difficult to determine. Alzheimer's dementia, dystonia, and Parkinson's disease are examples of these multifactorial disorders. What follows are some of the genetic interactions and other factors influencing the effects of mutations that have been identified.

Reduced penetrance

Penetrance refers to the proportion of people with a mutation who exhibit signs and symptoms of a genetic disorder. Sometimes some of the people who have inherited the mutation do not develop the disease. In this instance, the genetic pattern is said to have reduced penetrance. Reduced penetrance is seen commonly in autosomal dominantly inherited traits. Examples include dystonia due to the *DYT1* gene and Parkinson's disease due to the *LRRK2* gene. Intuitively, reduced penetrance can create difficulties in determining the genetic pattern of a disease state. It is probably due to several influential factors that are unknown.

Variable expressivity

The range of signs and symptoms occurring in people with the same genetic condition is referred to as variable expressivity. Similar to reduced penetrance, variable expressivity also tends to be seen more often in association with an autosomal dominant inheritance pattern; it is likely due to several unknown influential factors and can also interfere with diagnosis of the genetic pattern of the disorder.

An example of reduced penetrance and variable expressivity is the inheritance of dystonia. Oppenheimer's dystonia (DYT1) is inherited in an autosomal dominant pattern with reduced penetrance and variable expressivity. Only approximately 30% of those who inherit this mutation actually show signs of the trait and among family members inheriting the same mutation there is often variability in the types and severity of the dystonia. For example, one family member may have focal dystonia such as writer's cramp and another can have a more severe type such as generalized dystonia, reflecting the variable expressivity of the trait.

Trinucleotide repeats

A trinucleotide repeat is a series of three nucleotides occurring repetitively in a gene. When at an abnormal number of repeats, the gene is unstable and the number of these repeat sequences can change as the gene is passed from parent to child. When the number of repeats enlarges with each generation, it is referred to as trinucleotide repeat expansion. The disease state results when the number of repeats enlarges past a certain number and the gene is no longer functioning normally. With each generation the number of repeats grows, resulting in more severe symptoms and onset of the disease state at an earlier age. This is referred to as *anticipation*. Anticipation is seen in several neurodegenerative diseases, including Huntington's disease, Friederich's ataxia, myotonic dystrophy, spinocerebellar ataxia (SCA), fragile X syndrome (FXS), and Kennedy's disease.

Fragile X syndrome

Fragile X syndrome is a genetic condition associated with developmental problems, including learning disabilities and cognitive impairment, usually by age 2 years. Fragile X syndrome occurs in approximately 1 in 4,000 males and 1 in 8,000 females. In Fragile X syndrome there is expansion of the CGG trinucleotide repeat, affecting the *FMR1* gene on the X chromosome. This expansion results in a failure to express the fragile X mental retardation protein (FMRP), which is required for normal neural development. An allele with normal length of the CGG repeat may be classified as normal (unaffected by the syndrome), with 55–200 repeats classified as a premutation and patients at risk of developing fragile X–associated disorders. A full mutation occurs with 200 or more repeats and patients usually are affected by the syndrome. A definitive diagnosis of fragile X syndrome is made through genetic testing.

Most males with fragile X syndrome have mild to moderate intellectual disability, while about one-third of affected females are intellectually disabled. Patients may also have behavioral problems, including impulsiveness, hyperactivity, attention deficit hyperactivity disorder, and autism. Epilepsy is seen in about 15% of males and about 5% of females. Physical features seen in this syndrome are a long and narrow face, large ears, a prominent jaw and forehead, flexible fingers, flat feet, and, in males, enlarged testicles (macroorchidism) after puberty.

Fragile X–associated tremor/ataxia syndrome

Fragile X–associated tremor/ataxia syndrome (FXTAS) is a neurodegenerative disorder that affects carriers, mostly males, with adult onset and premutation alleles (55–200 CGG repeats) of the *FMR1* gene. Clinical features of FXTAS are highly variable and include progressive intention tremor, gait ataxia, parkinsonism, executive deficits, dementia, neuropathy, psychiatric disturbances, and autonomic symptoms accompanied by characteristic white-matter abnormalities on magnetic resonance imaging (MRI). The neuropathological hallmark of FXTAS is intranuclear inclusions in astrocytes and neurons due to overexpression of the FMR1 mRNA, causing brain atrophy.

There is currently no drug treatment for fragile X syndrome; however, medications are commonly used to treat behavioral problems. Also, supportive management is important and may involve speech therapy, occupational therapy, and individualized educational and behavioral programs.

Kennedy's disease

Kennedy's disease (KD), or spinal and bulbar muscular atrophy (SBMA), is a degenerative disease of the motor neurons that is associated with expansion of polyglutamine-encoding CAG trinucleotide repeats within the androgen receptor (AR). There is currently no treatment or cure for SBMA.

The syndrome has neuromuscular and endocrine manifestations. The neuromuscular signs and symptoms include bulbar signs (i.e., dysarthria, dysphagia), lower motor neuron signs (fasciculations, muscle wasting, muscle cramps, hyporeflexia), primary sensory neuropathy, and intention tremor. The endocrine signs and symptoms include gynecomastia, impotence, erectile dysfunction, reduced fertility, and testicular atrophy.

See Table 131.1 for a list of known neurodegenerative diseases with trinucleotide repeats and anticipation.

Table 131.1 Neurological diseases with trinucleotide repeats and anticipation

Disease name	Mode of inheritance	Trinucleotide repeat	Gene	Protein
Huntington's chorea	Autosomal dominant	CAG	4p16.3 Htt	Huntingtin
Dentatorubralpallidoluysian atrophy	Autosomal dominant	CAG	12p13.31 Atn	Atrophin 1
Spinocerebellar ataxia SCA 1	Autosomal dominant	CAG	6p22.3 ATXN1	Ataxin 1
SCA 2	Autosomal dominant	CAG	12q24.13 ATXN2	Ataxin 2
Machado-Joseph disease SCA 3	Autosomal dominant	CAG	14q32.12 ATXN3	Ataxin 3
SCA 6	Autosomal dominant	CAG	19p13.13 CACNA1A	CACNA1A
SCA 7	Autosomal dominant	CAG	3p14.1 ATXN 7	Ataxin 7
SCA 17	Autosomal dominant	CAG	6q27 TBP	TBP
Kennedy's disease	X-linked recessive	CAG	Xq21.3-22	Androgen receptor
Fragile X syndrome	X-linked	CGG	Xq27.3 FMR1	FMR1
Friedereich's ataxia	Autosomal recessive	GAA	9q13 FRDA	Frataxin
Myotonic dystrophy DM1	Autosomal dominant	CTG	19q13.3 DMPK	Myotonic dystrophy protein kinase
Myotonic dystrophy DM2	Autosomal dominant	CCTG	3q21 Znf9	Zinc finger protein 9

Genomic imprinting

Each person inherits two copies of their genes, one from their mother and the other from their father. Most of the time, both copies of the gene are functional. Sometimes, however, only one copy is functional and the copy that is functional is dependent on the parent of origin. Some genes are functional only when inherited from the mother and others only when inherited from the father. This phenomenon is referred to as genomic imprinting and is related to the presence of methyl groups that "mark" the parent of origin. Methylated genes are non-functional and both addition and removal of methyl groups can be used to control the gene activity. Imprinting is seen in a small percentage of human genes and imprinted genes tend to cluster together in the same regions of chromosomes. Two major clusters of imprinted genes have been identified in humans, one on the short (p) arm of chromosome 11 (at position 11p15) and another on the long (q) arm of chromosome 15 (in the region 15q11 to 15q13). A classic example of genomic imprinting occurs in the inheritance of Prader–Willi and Angelman's syndrome. Both disorders involve the same imprinted region of chromosome 15q11–13.

Angelman's syndrome consists of developmental delay, ataxia, hypotonia, myoclonic epilepsy, absence of speech, and unusual facies. It is also known as "Happy Puppet" syndrome. Angelman's syndrome occurs with deletion of the maternal contribution of the imprinted region of chromosome 15q11–13.

Prader–Willi syndrome consists of obesity, hypotonia, mental retardation, short stature, and hypogonadism, and is inherited through deletion of the paternal contribution of chromosome 15q11–13. Imprinting is also seen in the inheritance of myoclonus–dystonia. The epsilon sarcoglycan gene located at 7q21 is maternally imprinted.

Mutations in this gene result in a marked difference in penetrance depending on the parental origin of the gene mutation, with most clinical disease occurring with paternal transmission.

Mitochondrial disorders

The mitochondria contain their own DNA. Each cell contains many mitochondria existing in the cytoplasm. The mitochondria are not inherited according to Mendelian genetic patterns, but are inherited solely from the mother, being contained in the oocyte. Inheritance patterns may appear to be familial, and may occur in each generation, but are not inherited from the father. Mitochondrial disorders are covered in Chapter 168.

Gene dosage disorders

Genes encode for the production of a protein. With genetic mutations, sometimes a greater amount of protein can be produced with a duplication of the gene and less of the protein can be produced with a deletion of the gene. When this occurs, sometimes a different disorder can result. An example is with the heritable forms of neuropathy. The gene *PMP22* when duplicated results in Charcot–Marie–Tooth type 1A (CMT1A) and when deleted results in hereditary neuropathy with liability to pressure palsies (HNPP). Both disorders are described in Chapter 101 in greater detail.

Susceptibility genes

Susceptibility genes are genes that when mutated can create an environment in which there is a greater tendency toward the development of a disease condition. One example is the glucocerebrosidase gene. Mutations in this gene in the homozygous state produce the lysosomal storage disorder Gaucher's disease. There are a small percentage of patients with Gaucher's disease who also have features of Parkinson's disease. People with the heterozygote mutation in the glucocerebrosidase gene also have an increased rate of development of Parkinson's disease. So it may be that the problem created by the glucocerebrosidase gene may enhance the development of Parkinson's disease. It has been considered that mutations in the glucocerebrosidase gene are the number one genetic risk factor for the development of Parkinson's disease.

Neurocutaneous disorders

The neurocutaneous disorders are also known as phakomatoses, disorders involving the skin and brain. Neurofibromatosis, Von Hippel–Lindau disease, tuberous sclerosis, Sturge–Weber syndrome, xeroderma pigmentosum, and incontinentia pigmenti are considered to be neurocutaneous disorders.

Neurofibromatosis

Type 1

There are two forms of neurofibromatosis: type 1 and type 2. Neurofibromatosis type 1 (NF1), also known as Von Recklinghausen disease, predominantly affects the skin and peripheral nerves. Cutaneous features include café-au-lait spots, freckling, and neurofibromas. Café-au-lait spots are light brown–colored areas of skin discoloration that can be seen anywhere on the body. Six or more café-au-lait spots are supportive of the diagnosis. Skin freckling usually occurs in areas of skin folds or increased friction. Neurofibromas are tumors of the peripheral nerve sheath. Cutaneous and subcutaneous neurofibromas occur mostly in the trunk or upper extremities. Central nervous system (CNS) tumors are usually astrocytomas with a predilection for the optic pathway. Cerebral and spinal cord tumors also occur with a greater frequency in NF1.

The gene involved in NF1 is located on chromosome 17q11.2.7 and is thought to be a tumor suppressor gene. The gene product is known as neurofibromin. An individual with NF1 has a copy of the mutation in all cells. A second somatic mutation in the normal functioning mutated gene is required before the gene becomes nonfunctional. There is a high spontaneous mutation rate at this site and it has complete penetrance.

Type 2

Neurofibromatosis type 2 (NF2) consists of mainly CNS tumors. The hallmark of NF2 is bilateral acoustic neuromas, tumors of the Schwann's cells surrounding cranial nerve VIII. Deafness is the main clinical feature of NF2. Skin involvement is variable, with less frequent café-au-lait spots and infrequent neurofibromas. Other CNS tumors are common and include meningiomas, spinal nerve root schwannomas, trigeminal nerve schwannomas, gliomas, and ependymomas.

NF2 is inherited as an autosomal dominant trait and the gene is located on chromosome 22q11.2. The gene product is known as MERLIN, dysfunction of which has been associated with sporadic meningiomas, sporadic schwannomas, and breast and colon cancer. Treatment of neurofibromatosis is palliative and consists of tumor removal.

Von Hippel–Lindau disease

There is an inherited susceptibility to cerebellar and spinal cord hemangioblastomas in Von Hippel–Lindau disease (VHL). Other features include retinal angiomas, bilateral renal cell carcinoma, pheochromocytoma, and multiple cysts, mainly located in the kidneys, pancreas, and ovaries. Death usually results from renal cell carcinoma.

VHL is inherited in an autosomal dominant manner and the gene is located at the tip of chromosome 3. There are three classifications of VHL: type 1 without pheochromocytoma, type 2a with pheochromocytoma, and type 2b with pheochromocytoma and renal cell carcinoma. Sporadic forms of renal cell carcinoma have been found to have mutations in the VHL gene.

Tuberous sclerosis

Cutaneous symptoms of tuberous sclerosis (TS) include hypomelanotic macules, shagreen patch, ungual fibromas, and facial angiofibromas. Hypomelanotic macules, also known as ash leaf spots, occur in the majority of patients with TS. The shagreen patch is an irregular raised or textured lesion, most commonly found on the back or flank. Ungual fibromas are found underneath or adjacent to the nails. Facial angiofibromas are hamartomas of the vascular and connective tissue elements and are found on the face, predominantly around the nose. Facial angiofibromas, also known as adenomatous sebaceum, are considered to be specific for TS; however, only approximately 75% of patients have these lesions, which may become present later in life.

Neurological manifestations of TS include developmental delay and seizures. Giant cell astrocytomas may occur and are usually located in the anterior horn of the lateral ventricle. Calcified subependymal nodules are characteristic findings on neuroimaging studies. MRI may reveal cortical and subcortical white-matter lesions that correspond to hamartomas, gliotic areas, and neuronal migration defects. Cardiac rhabdomyomata, also considered hamartomas, and renal angiomyolipomas, often a cause of death, may be found in over half of patients with TS.

There are two genes associated with TS: *TSC1* found on chromosome 9q34 and *TSC2* found on chromosome 16. These genes are thought to be tumor suppressor genes and a mutation in both genes is required for tumor formation. TS is inherited in an autosomal dominant manner with variable penetrance. Treatment is palliative with seizure control. A new medication, everolimus, has recently been used to treat TS and has been helpful treating the tumors and seizures.

Sturge–Weber syndrome

Unilateral facial angioma or port-wine stain involving the first branch of the trigeminal nerve is the hallmark of Sturge–Weber syndrome (SW). Seizures and developmental delay are neurological manifestations. Often developmental delay follows intractable seizures. Leptomeningeal vascular malformations occur and produce characteristic neuroimaging findings. Ocular involvement may occur, with vascular malformations occurring in the conjunctiva or choroid and glaucoma in the eye ipsilateral to the port-wine stain. SW is a sporadic disorder with unknown cause. Treatment of the port-wine stain with the argon laser has been successful and seizure control can help to preserve intellectual function.

Xeroderma pigmentosum

Xeroderma pigmentosum (XP) is a rare, recessively inherited disorder involving the ability to repair mutated or damaged DNA. There is striking photosensitivity, with sunburn occurring first, followed by freckling and then telangiectasia and skin atrophy of exposed areas, usually beginning in infancy. Half of affected children have skin cancer by 14 years of age. Corneal scarring, keratitis, and carcinoma can result in vision loss at an early age. Approximately 20% of patients have some form of neurological involvement, which can include progressive neurological deterioration, dementia, abnormal ocular motility, choreoathetosis, ataxia, sensorineural deafness,

spasticity, and microcephaly. Olivopontocerebellar degeneration may be seen on neuroimaging studies. Treatment is aimed at early diagnosis and protection from ultraviolet (UV) exposure through clothing, glasses, and sunblock.

Incontinentia pigmenti

Cutaneous features dominate incontinentia pigmenti (IP) and consist of four phases. The first phase occurs within the first month of life and consists of skin lesions occurring in a whorled, linear, or splash-like pattern over the trunk, scalp, and proximal and flexor surfaces of the limbs. The rash resolves within a few weeks. The second phase can recur during infancy and consists of acanthotic, dyskeratotic lesions in the same distribution as in the first phase. Resolution occurs within a few weeks, with some residual atrophic changes. The third phase consists of melanin deposition outside and within melanophores of the upper dermis, result in striking patterns of variable pigmentation in streaks, whorls, and patterns located on the lateral trunk and proximal extremities, and often in areas not previously involved. These characteristic lesions fade in the second and third decades of life. The fourth phase consists of hypopigmented, hairless, atrophic regions. Seizures, spastic paralysis, and developmental delay are neurological manifestations that occur in approximately 33% of patients. Dental anomalies and strabismus may also occur.

Inheritance is thought to be X-linked dominant transmission with male hemizygote lethality. Two loci, Xp11.21 and Xq28, are thought to be responsible for IP. Treatment is symptomatic and can include dental repair, photocoagulation, cryotherapy of ocular neovascularization, and seizure control.

Other genetic disorders

Ataxia telangiectasia

Ataxia telangiectasia is a rare, autosomal recessive inherited progressive disorder that begins in childhood with ataxia, myoclonus, and choreaform movements and telangiectasias in the eyes and body. Dysarthria and oculomotor apraxia are also seen. Children with this disease are usually wheelchair bound by adolescence. They have immune defects and a tendency toward development of malignancies.

There is a mutation in the ATM gene located at 11q22.3 that is responsible for DNA repair. Patients are abnormally sensitive to ionizing radiation. Treatment with steroids has been helpful in some cases.

Cerebrotendinosis xanthomatosis

Cerebrotendinous xanthomatosis is a rare lysosomal storage disorder characterized by cholesterol and cholestanol deposits in the Achilles tendons and in virtually every tissue. Plasma cholesterol is low normal in affected individuals, but cholestanol is elevated in the serum and is found in the tendons. The disease is characterized by a progressive neurological deterioration, with ataxia beginning after puberty and progression to spinal cord and pseudobulbar involvement. Premature atherosclerosis and cataracts also occur.

This disorder results from mutations in the *CYP27A1* gene located at chromosome 2q35 and is inherited in an autosomal recessive manner. Treatment with cholic acid and chenodeoxycholic acid can improve symptoms dramatically.

Treatment for genetic disorders

Enzyme replacement

Disorders characterized by a single gene mutation resulting in a single enzymatic defect could theoretically be treated by providing the enzyme that is abnormal or deficient. Enzyme replacement therapy (ERT) has been developed for some of the lysosomal storage disorders, including Gaucher's disease, Fabry's disease, and Pompe's disease. Gaucher's disease is characterized by mutations in the glucocerebrosidase gene, resulting in accumulation of glucocerebroside in the liver, spleen, and skeleton. A neurological form of Gaucher's disease (type 3) results in myoclonic seizures and horizontal supranuclear palsy in addition to systemic abnormalities. Fabry's disease results from a mutation in the alpha galactosidase A gene, producing an accumulation of globotriaosylceramide. Fabry's patients suffer from painful small fiber neuropathy, strokes, dysautonomia, and heart and renal disease. In Pompe's disease, excessive amounts of glycogen accumulate and reduce the function of heart and skeletal muscles. The enzyme alpha glucosidase is defective.

Treatment of these three conditions with enzyme replacement infusions have become possible and result in improvement in each condition. In Gaucher's disease anemia, hepatosplenomegaly, and bone fractures improve with ERT. However, neurological abnormalities do not improve. ERT results in improvement in the dysautonomia and neuropathic pain of Fabry's disease, although the renal, cerebrovascular, and cardiac disease do not improve. In Pompe's disease the cardiac hypertrophy, heart failure, skeletal weakness, and respiratory failure improve with ERT, but the lower motor neuron disease does not. In fact, no enzyme given intravenously crosses the blood–brain barrier. In addition, development of antibodies to the enzymes has been found, which reduces the efficacy of the enzyme therapy. So while at present ERT is useful, more research is needed to develop more effective treatment of these disorders.

Mechanism-based therapy

Mechanism-based therapy consists of applying the knowledge of known human disease genes to dissect the genes' function and their mechanism of action in the normal and pathological states in order to design a novel therapy. Our current molecular genetic technology is categorized into two groups: those derived from a gene product or vaccine (expression cloning of normal gene production, production of genetically engineered antibodies, or production of genetically engineered vaccines) and those from genetic material (gene therapy), which will be further discussed in this chapter. Examples of diseases where mechanism-based therapy is applied are mentioned in what follows.

Tuberous sclerosis

TS mutations occur in either of two TS genes, *TSC1* (hamartin) or *TSC2* (tuberin), found in over 85% of patients with TS. TSC genes directly regulate a number of biochemical pathways, such as the "mTOR" pathway, that control cell growth and proliferation. When either TSC1 or TSC2 is deficient, mTOR complex 1 is upregulated, leading to abnormal cellular growth, proliferation, and protein synthesis.

Subependymal giant cell astrocytomas (SEGA) are glioneuronal tumors typically arising near the foramen of Monro in 5–20% of patients with TS. The current standard treatment for SEGA is surgical resection; however, at times resection may be very difficult and associated with multiple complications.

Everolimus is a drug that inhibits mTOR complex 1, correcting the specific molecular defect causing the tuberous sclerosis complex. Several studies have shown a significant reduction in the volume of SEGA and have also been associated with a significant reduction in seizure frequency. Everolimus is a clinically available medication and a promising treatment option for TS patients with SEGA and epilepsy.

Fragile X syndrome

In FXS, as mentioned earlier, the FMR1 gene codes for the fragile X mental retardation protein. This protein, among other functions, regulates the synthesis of the proteins that facilitate synaptic plasticity. Studies with mouse models have been able to show that neuroactive molecules targeting the aberrant pathways seen in this syndrome are able to reverse some of the molecular and behavioral phenotypes of FXS. Preliminary trials with lithium and minocycline in patients with fragile X syndrome have been promising.

Phenylketonuria

Phenylketonuria (PKU) is an autosomal recessive metabolic genetic disorder characterized by a mutation in the gene for the hepatic enzyme phenylalanine hydroxylase (PAH), which is necessary to metabolize the amino acid phenylalanine (Phe) to the amino acid tyrosine. The current treatment for PKU is controlling Phe levels through diet, or a combination of diet and medication. A lifelong diet low in Phe is required for optimal brain development. In addition, tyrosine, which is derived from phenylalanine, must be supplemented.

Tetrahydrobiopterin (or BH4) is a cofactor for the oxidation of phenylalanine. The oral administration of BH4 can reduce blood levels of Phe in certain patients. The compound sapropterin dihydrochloride (Kuvan) is a form of tetrahydrobiopterin. Kuvan is the first drug that can help BH4-responsive PKU patients lower Phe levels to recommended ranges.

Additional treatment options include (1) dietary supplementation with large neutral amino acids (LNAAs) – the LNAAs (e.g., leu, tyr, trp, met, his, iso, val, thr) compete with Phe for specific carrier proteins, decreasing Phe plasma and brain levels; and (2) casein glycomacropeptide (CGMP), a milk peptide naturally free of Phe, which can substitute for the main part of the free amino acids in the PKU diet and contains a high amount of the Phe-lowering LNAAs, which help maintain plasma Phe levels in the target range.

Other therapies are currently under investigation, including gene therapy and enzyme substitution therapy with phenylalanine ammonia lyase (PAL).

X-adrenoleukodystrophy

X-adrenoleukodystrophy (X-ALD) is an inborn X chromosome recessive inherited disorder associated with the abnormal accumulation of saturated very-long-chain fatty acids (VLCFA) in plasma and tissues that leads to central and peripheral nervous system demyelination, adrenal cortex insufficiency, and testis inflammation. There is no cure for X-ALD. However, several treatments seem to slow the disease progression. One of them is Lorenzo's oil in conjunction with a low-fat diet. Lorenzo's oil is a mixture of unsaturated fatty acids (glycerol trioleate and glyceryl trierucate in a 4:1 ratio) that inhibits elongation of saturated fatty acids in the body. Other methods include gene therapy, bone marrow transplant, and anticholesterol drugs.

Maple syrup urine disease

Maple syrup urine disease (MSUD), also called branched-chain ketoaciduria, is an autosomal recessive metabolic disorder affecting branched-chain amino acids. It is one type of organic acidemia. Infants with this disease have a distinctive sweet odor in the urine.

Mutations in the BCKDHA, BCKDHB, DBT, and DLD genes can cause MSUD. These genes provide instructions for making proteins that work together as a complex. The protein complex is essential for breaking down the amino acids leucine, isoleucine, and valine, which are present in many kinds of food (particularly protein-rich foods such as milk, meat, and eggs). Mutations in any of these four genes reduce or eliminate the function of the protein complex. As a result, these amino acids and their byproducts build up in the body, leading to serious neurological problems. A diet with minimal levels of these amino acids must be maintained for life. Synthetic proteins are available that contain substitutes and adjusted levels of the amino acids without causing harm.

Nonsense suppression therapy

In most cases of inherited metabolic diseases there are a substantial number of individuals (10–30%) with nonsense mutations. Nonsense mutations are mutations that produce a truncated protein by introducing a premature termination codon. Truncated proteins are devoid of activity and are considered a severe genetic defect. The discovery that aminoglycoside antibiotics induce nonsense mutation readthrough, producing a full copy of the enzyme in cystic fibrosis, has led to the development of nonsense suppression therapy (NST).

NST utilizes small molecules, known as readthrough drugs, to induce the synthesis of whole copies of the desired protein. Recessive genetic disorders such as inherited metabolic defects are thought to be amenable to NST, as a small amount of enzyme production may be therapeutically relevant. In addition to the currently available aminoglycoside antibiotics, novel compounds based on the aminoglycoside molecular structure with less toxicity have been developed. Non-aminoglycoside compounds such as RTC13 and RTC14 have been discovered to have readthrough properties and are being developed as a potential treatment for ataxia telangiectasia and Duchenne muscular dystrophy. This mutation-specific therapy could be applied to many different genetic disorders irrespective of the pathophysiology resulting from the protein dysfunction.

Gene therapy

Gene therapy is the use of DNA as a drug to treat diseases by providing therapeutic DNA into a patient's cells, to replace a mutated gene, directly correct a mutation, or encode a therapeutic protein to provide treatment. DNA that encodes a therapeutic protein is packaged within a "vector" using either viruses or non-virus methods. Examples of viruses used as vectors include retrovirus, adenovirus, lentivirus, herpes simplex virus, pox virus, and adeno-associated virus. The viruses are inactivated and do not cause disease. Examples of non-virus methods are naked DNA, electroporation, the gene gun, magnetofection, oligonucleotides, sonoporation, lipoplexes, dendrimers, and inorganic nanoparticles. These vectors transport the desired DNA inside cells within the body. Once inside, the DNA becomes expressed by the cell machinery, resulting in the production of therapeutic protein, which in turn treats the patient's disease.

Gene therapy may be classified into two types.

Somatic gene therapy

The therapeutic genes are transferred into the somatic cells of a patient. Any variations and effects will be restricted to the patient only, and will not be inherited by the patient's offspring or later generations. Somatic gene therapy represents the mainstream line of current clinical research. This therapy is promising for treatment, but a complete correction of a genetic disorder or the replacement of multiple genes in somatic cells is not yet possible.

Germline gene therapy

Germ cells (sperm or eggs) are modified by integrating their genomes into functional genes. Germ cells will combine to form a zygote, which will divide to produce all the other cells in an organism, and therefore if a germ cell is genetically modified then all the cells in the organism will contain the modified gene. This would allow the therapy to be heritable and passed on to later generations. Many countries refuse this therapy for technical and ethical reasons.

Gene therapy is a promising treatment option for a number of genetic diseases. Researchers are still studying how and when to use gene therapy. Currently, in the United States gene therapy is available only as part of a clinical trial.

Further reading

Brady RO, Schiffmann R. Enzyme-replacement therapy for metabolic storage disorders. *Lancet Neurol* 2004;3:752–756.

McKusick-Nathans Institute of Genetic Medicine, Johns Hopkins University (Baltimore, MD) and National Center for Biotechnology Information, National Library of Medicine (Bethesda, MD). *Online Mendelian Inheritance in Man*, OMIM™. http://www.ncbi.nlm.nih.gov/omim (accessed April 2008).

National Library of Medicine and National Institutes of Health. *Genetics Home Reference*, www.ncbi.nlm.nih.gov; *Genes and Disease*, http://www.ncbi.nlm.nih.gov/books (accessed April 2008).

Perez B, Rodriguez-Pombo B, Ugarte M, and Desviat LR. Readthrough strategies for therapeutic suppression of nonsense mutations in inherited metabolic disease. *Mol Syndromol* 2012;(3):230–236.

Rosenberg RN, Prusiner SB, Di Mauro S, Barchi RL (eds.). *The Molecular and Genetic Basis of Neurological Disease*. Boston, MA: Butterworth-Heineman; 1997.

PART 15   Neuro-otology

132   Neuro-otology

Kevin A. Kerber
Department of Neurology, University of Michigan, Ann Arbor, MI, USA

Neuro-otology is a multidisciplinary specialty with primary training stemming from either otolaryngology or neurology. The specialty is primarily concerned with evaluating patients who present because of dizziness, balance disturbance, or auditory symptoms. Neurologists focus on the clinical evaluation, diagnosis, and non-surgical management of patients with these symptoms, whereas otolaryngologists emphasize surgical approaches to disorders of the ear.

Epidemiology

A population-based telephone survey in Germany showed that nearly 30% of the population have experienced moderate to severe dizziness. Although most affected persons reported non-specific forms of dizziness, nearly a quarter had vertigo. Dizziness is more common among females and older people. Because of this association with age, the presentation of dizziness is only expected to increase with the aging of the population that is taking place in a number of countries. In the United States, the National Center for Health Statistics reports 7.5 million annual ambulatory visits to physicians' offices, hospital outpatient departments, and emergency departments for dizziness, making it one of the most common principal complaints.

More is known about the prevalence of hearing loss worldwide, because it is a leading cause of burden of disease in high-income countries. Hearing loss affects approximately 16% of adults (age >18 years) in the United States. Men are more commonly affected than women, and prevalence increases dramatically with age, so that by age 75 nearly 50% of the population report hearing loss. The most common type of hearing loss is sensorineural, and both idiopathic presbycusis and noise-induced forms are common etiologies. Tinnitus is less frequent in the US population, with about 3% reporting it, although this increases to about 9% for individuals older than 65 years. Among those with hearing loss, nearly 75% also experience tinnitus. The most common type of tinnitus is a high-pitched ringing in both ears.

International considerations in patients with neuro-otological disorders

When considering international factors regarding neuro-otological symptoms and disorders, one must consider the tremendous variability in how patients of different geographic locations, language backgrounds, and cultures described their symptoms, particularly the symptom of dizziness. In the United States, the symptom of dizziness is generally felt to infer either a spinning sensation (vertigo), some other type of "head" sensation (i.e., lightheadedness, wooziness), or imbalance (unsteadiness when walking). However, some patients reporting dizziness will instead describe a visual phenomenon, general ill-feeling, anxiety, or other symptom. Other important international factors are genetic disorders and communicable diseases, which vary from region to region. As a result, it can be important to identify the patient's geographic and ethnic background.

Pathophysiology

The inner ear is composed of a fluid-filled sac enclosed by a bony capsule with an anterior cochlear part, a central chamber (the vestibule), and a posterior vestibular part (Figure 132.1). Endolymph fills up the fluid-filled sac and is separated by a membrane from the perilymph. These fluids differ primarily in their composition of potassium and sodium, with the endolymph resembling intracellular fluid and the perilymph resembling extracellular fluids. The perilymph communicates with the cerebrospinal fluid through the cochlear aqueduct.

The cochlea senses sound waves after they travel through the external auditory canal and are amplified by the tympanic membrane and ossicles of the middle ear. The stapes, the last of three ossicles in the middle ear, contacts the oval window, which directs the forces associated with sound waves along the basilar membrane of the cochlea. These forces stimulate the hair cells, which in turn generate neural signals in the auditory nerve. The auditory nerve enters the lateral brainstem at the pontomedullary junction and synapses in the cochlear nucleus. The fibers then pass both ipsilaterally and contralaterally up brainstem structures to the auditory cortex of the temporal lobe.

The peripheral vestibular system is composed of three semicircular canals, the utricle and saccule, and the vestibular component of the eighth cranial nerve. Each semicircular canal has a sensory epithelium called the crista; the sensory epithelium of the utricle and saccule is called the macule. The semicircular canals sense

International Neurology, Second edition. Edited by Robert P. Lisak, Daniel D. Truong, William M. Carroll and Roongroj Bhidayasiri
© 2016 John Wiley & Sons, Ltd. Published 2016 by John Wiley & Sons, Ltd.

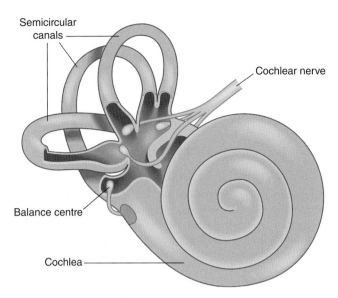

Semicircular
canals

Cochlear nerve

Balance centre

Cochlea

Figure 132.1 Anatomy of the inner ear. Source: Peate 2014. Reproduced with permission of Wiley.

angular movements, whereas the utricle and saccule sense linear movements. Two of the semicircular canals (anterior and posterior canals) are oriented in the vertical plane nearly orthogonal to each other; the third canal is oriented in the horizontal plane (horizontal canal). The crista of each canal is activated primarily by movement occurring in the plane of that canal. When the hair cells of these organs are stimulated, the signal is transferred to the vestibular nuclei via the vestibular portion of the eighth cranial nerve. Signals originating from the horizontal semicircular canal pass via the medial longitudinal fasciculus along the floor of the fourth ventricle to the abducens nuclei in the middle brainstem and the oculomotor complex in the rostral brainstem. The anterior canal (also referred to as the superior canal) and posterior canal impulses pass from the vestibular nuclei to the ocular motor and trochlear nuclei, triggering eye movements roughly in the plane of each canal. A key feature is that once these signals leave the vestibular nuclei, they divide into vertical, horizontal, and torsional components. As a result, a lesion of central vestibular pathways can cause a pure vertical, pure torsional, or pure horizontal pattern of nystagmus.

The primary vestibular afferent nerve fibers maintain a constant baseline firing rate of action potentials. When the baseline rate from each ear is symmetric (or an asymmetry has been centrally compensated), the eyes remain stationary. With an uncompensated asymmetry in the firing rate, resulting from either increased or decreased activity on one side, slow ocular deviation results. By turning the head to the right, the baseline firing rate of the horizontal canal is physiologically altered, causing an increased firing rate on the right side and a decreased firing rate on the left side. The result is a slow deviation of the eyes to the left. In an alert patient, this slow deviation is regularly interrupted by quick movements in the opposite direction (nystagmus), so that the eyes do not become "pinned" to one side. In a comatose patient, the eyes deviate to the side of the slow component, because the corrective fast phases are truncated or absent.

The plane in which the eyes deviate as a result of vestibular stimulation depends on the combination of canals that are stimulated.

If only the posterior semicircular canal on one side is stimulated (as occurs with benign paroxysmal positional vertigo, BPPV), a vertical-torsional deviation of the eyes can be observed, which is followed by a fast corrective response in the opposite direction. However, if the horizontal canal is the source of stimulation (as occurs with the horizontal canal variant of benign paroxysmal positional vertigo), a horizontal deviation with a slight torsional component (because this canal is slightly off the horizontal plane) results. If the vestibular nerve is lesioned (as in vestibular neuritis) or stimulated (as in vestibular paroxysmia), a horizontal greater than torsional nystagmus occurs, because the two vertical canals on one side cancel each other out.

Over time, either an asymmetry in the baseline firing rates resolves (the stimulation has been removed), or the central nervous system compensates for it. This explains why an entire unilateral vestibular system can be surgically destroyed and the patient experience vertigo for only several days to weeks. It also explains why patients with slow-growing tumors affecting the vestibular nerve, such as an acoustic neuroma, generally do not experience vertigo or nystagmus.

Clinical approach to patients with dizziness

The most important processes of care when clinically approaching patients with dizziness are obtaining a focused history and conducting an appropriate examination. The information gathered is key for formulating the case, localizing the lesion, generating a differential diagnosis, and planning the management. Numerous studies have shown that tests do not discriminate non-categorized dizziness from normal controls, and often do not even discriminate one specific vertiginous disorder from another.

History of present illness

Many clinicians focus first on determining the type of dizziness symptom, such as vertigo, lightheadedness, presyncope, or imbalance. However, this effort is often futile, or even misleading, because it has been shown that many patients are not reliable in labeling their type of dizziness, and that types of dizziness actually do not discriminate well among underlying causes of dizziness. The information from the history that is more reliable and useful lies in other characteristics of the present illness, including onset, duration, and triggers. Patients should be specifically queried about whether the symptom is constant or episodic, came on gradually or suddenly, and any other accompanying symptoms (particularly auditory symptoms, neurological symptoms, or palpitations). The patient should also be asked about the duration and frequency of the symptom, aggravating or alleviating factors, and identifiable triggers. Obtaining details about the temporal profile is important as well.

A detailed past medical history, list of medications and allergies, social history, and family history should also be obtained. Medication side effects are one of the most common causes of dizziness. Many times a specific medicine cannot be identified, but the more medications patients take, the more likely side effects become. A complete family history may be a key part of the dizziness evaluation. Many types of dizziness, including benign recurrent vertigo, chronic forms of dizziness, and ataxia syndromes, are now known to be genetic disorders or to have familial patterns.

General medical examination

Details of examination components are listed in Table 132.1. A general medical examination is important in the dizziness patient, because medical disorders such as metabolic, endocrine, or cardiac disorders are common causes of non-vertiginous types of dizziness. Orthostatic blood pressure measurements can provide important information in patients who report the onset of symptoms on standing. Measurement of visual acuity may also provide important information, because poor vision can contribute to or even cause types of dizziness. Arthritis or joint deformity, chronic lung disease, angina, cardiac failure, or peripheral vascular disease can be important factors in balance disorders.

General neurological examination

A mental status examination helps to exclude cognitive impairment as a feature of the patient's presentation. The cranial nerves should be thoroughly inspected. The examiner should determine whether the patient has full ocular movements. A test of the facial nerve strength and symmetry is important because of the close anatomical relationship between the seventh and eighth cranial nerves. Examining palatal elevation, tongue bulk and protrusion, and the trapezius and sternocleidomastoid muscles helps to exclude lower cranial nerve involvement. During the motor examination the tone should be closely assessed, because increased tone or cogwheel rigidity can be the main finding in a patient with an early neurodegenerative disorder. The peripheral sensory examination is important, because a peripheral neuropathy can cause a non-specific dizziness or imbalance. Reflexes should be

tested for their presence and symmetry. However, normal elderly patients often have reduced distal vibratory sensation and absent ankle jerks. Coordination is an important part of the neurological examination in patients with dizziness, because disorders characterized by ataxia can present with the principal symptom of dizziness. Ataxia of the limbs, however, may be very subtle or even absent in ataxia disorders that mainly affect midline cerebellar structures.

Neuro-otological examination

Ocular motor function testing

Assessment of eye movements is a critical part of the evaluation of dizziness patients. Abnormalities found can point to a specific localization and even specific syndromes, whereas normal ocular motor functioning excludes many neurological disorders. The first step is to search for spontaneous involuntary movements of the eyes, mainly nystagmus or saccadic intrusions. Nystagmus is characterized by a slow and fast phase component that can be classified as spontaneous, gaze evoked, or positional. An important type of nystagmus to recognize is the peripheral vestibular pattern. This is readily apparent in acute disorders as a horizontal greater than torsional, unidirectional nystagmus that can be suppressed with fixation. The nystagmus increases when the patient looks in the direction of the fast phase of nystagmus and decreases or stops when the patient looks toward the opposite side. On the other hand, nystagmus that changes direction (e.g., converts from a left-beating nystagmus to a right-beating nystagmus on gaze testing) is a central finding. Some patients may be able to suppress the nystagmus when in a well-lit room, but when fixation is removed the spontaneous component becomes apparent. Techniques to block fixation include evaluating the patient in a darkened environment, using Frenzel glasses, blocking the vision of one eye during a fundoscopic examination of the other, or simply placing a blank sheet of paper up to the patient's nose and observing the eyes from the side.

Saccadic intrusions are spontaneous, non-volitional fast eye movements (i.e., saccades) that do not have the rhythmic fast and slow phases characteristic of nystagmus. The most common type of saccadic intrusion is a square wave jerk, which is a small-amplitude, involuntary saccade that takes the eyes off a target, followed after a characteristic intersaccade delay by a corrective saccade that brings the eyes back on target. Square wave jerks are commonly seen in neurological disorders such as cerebellar ataxia syndromes, Huntington's disease, or progressive supranuclear palsy.

Another type of saccadic intrusion is a saccadic oscillation, which consists of back-to-back saccadic movements that do not have an intersaccade interval. When a burst of saccades occurs in the horizontal plane, the term "ocular flutter" is used. When vertical or torsional components are also present, the term "opsoclonus" is used. Ocular flutter and opsoclonus are pathological findings typically encountered in several types of central nervous system diseases that involve brainstem and cerebellar pathways. Paraneoplastic disorders should be considered in patients who present with these saccadic oscillations.

Gaze testing

After searching for spontaneous movements of the eyes, the examiner then searches for gaze-evoked nystagmus by instructing the patient to look in each direction. Many normal patients have

Table 132.1   Key components to the examination of the dizzy patient

Examination component	Description
General medical examination	
Vital signs	Blood pressure, orthostatic blood pressure, pulse rate
Head and neck examination	External ear vesicles, external auditory canal
Cardiac examination	Heart rhythm
General neurological examination	
Mental status testing	Level of alertness, orientation, concentration, memory
Cranial nerves	Cranial nerves 2–12 in detail
Motor	Tone, strength
Sensory examination	Distal sensory loss, reflexes
Neuro-otological examination	
Ocular motor exam	Spontaneous movements (nystagmus, saccadic intrusions), gaze testing, smooth pursuit, saccades, optokinetic nystagmus, fixation suppression of the vestibular-ocular reflex
Vestibular nerve exam	Head-thrust test, doll's-eye test
Positional testing	Head-hanging positions (Dix–Hallpike), supine positional testing
Fistula testing	Pneumatoscopy, Valsalva maneuver, tragal compression
Gait assessment	Gait initiation, heel strike, stride length, base width, tandem gait, Romberg position
Auditory evaluation	Whisper test, tuning forks, finger rub

a few beats of non-sustained nystagmus with gaze greater than 30° off-center, and this is called end-gaze nystagmus. The most common cause of gaze-evoked nystagmus is a medication side effect, typically an antiepileptic drug. However, brainstem and cerebellar abnormalities are also common causes of gaze-evoked nystagmus.

Smooth pursuit

When patients track objects that move back and forth in their visual field, the eye movements should be smooth as long as the target is not moving too quickly. This movement of the eyes is called smooth pursuit and it is a central nervous system function. This type of eye movement serves to keep moving objects on the fovea to maximize vision, but it inevitably breaks down when the target moves at a high enough velocity. Patients with impaired smooth pursuit will be observed to have frequent small saccades when trying to keep up with the target. Because of this characteristic, the term saccadic pursuit is used to describe this type of impairment. Abnormalities of smooth pursuit occur as a result of disorders throughout the central nervous system, and also with the use of tranquilizing medicines or alcohol. Patients with early or mild cerebellar degenerative disorders often present complaining of dizziness (typically imbalance), and usually will have impaired smooth pursuit even when truncal and/or limb ataxia is only minimally apparent.

Saccades

Saccadic eye movements are fast eye movements that are used to bring the image of an object quickly onto the fovea. These movements are generated by the burst neurons of the pons (horizontal movements) and the midbrain (vertical movements). A lesion or neuronal degeneration of these regions will lead to slowing of saccades. Slowing of saccades can also occur with lesions of the ocular motor neurons or extraocular muscles. Severe slowing can be readily appreciated at the bedside by instructing the patient to look back and forth from one target to another. When testing saccades, the examiner observes both the velocity of the saccade and also the accuracy. Overshooting saccades (missing the target by passing it) typically indicates a lesion of the cerebellum. Undershooting of saccades is less specific and to a small degree will occur even in normal persons.

Optokinetic nystagmus and fixation suppression of the vestibular ocular reflex

Optokinetic nystagmus (OKN) and fixation suppression of the vestibular ocular reflex (VOR) can also be informative when examining dizzy patients at the bedside. OKN combines both saccadic and smooth pursuit movements. Although it is best tested using a full-field stimulus, moving a striped cloth in front of the patient can approximate OKN at the bedside. Fixation suppression of the vestibulo-ocular reflex (VOR suppression) can be tested at the bedside by having the patient sit in a swivel chair with an arm extended in the "thumbs up" position out in front. The patient is instructed to focus on the thumb and to allow the extended arm to move with the body, so that the visual target (i.e., the patient's thumb) remains directly in front of the patient. The chair is then rotated from side to side and the patient's eyes are observed. Normally, patients should be able to suppress the nystagmus that is stimulated by the rotation of the chair. If nystagmus is observed during the rotation movements, then there is an impairment of VOR suppression, which is analogous to an impairment of smooth pursuit.

Vestibular nerve examination

The head-thrust test is a bedside test that directly assesses the vestibular ocular reflex. The physiology involved in this test is analogous to that of the test for an afferent pupillary defect. To perform the head-thrust test, the physician stands directly in front of the patient seated on the examination table. With the patient's head held in the examiner's hands, the patient is instructed to focus on the examiner's nose. The head is then quickly moved about 5–10° to one side. In patients with an intact vestibulo-ocular reflex, the eyes will move in the direction opposite to the head movement. Therefore, the patient's eyes will remain fixated on the examiner's nose after the sudden movement. The test is then repeated in the opposite direction. If the examiner observes a corrective saccade required to bring the patient's eyes back to the examiner's nose after the head thrust, impairment of the VOR in the direction of the head movement is identified. Although the doll's-eye test also can assess the vestibulo-ocular reflex, this test is not specific to the VOR, because fully conscious patients can also generate the compensatory slow movements of the eyes in response to the slow rotation of the head by using the smooth pursuit system. However, the smooth pursuit system does not operate at high velocities, which is why the head-thrust test is used specifically to test the VOR. The doll's-eye test, the head-thrust test, and the VOR-suppression test can be helpful in identifying impairment of the smooth pursuit system, vestibulo-ocular reflex, or both.

Positional testing

Although typically only thought of in terms of triggering benign paroxysmal positional vertigo, positional testing can also be extremely helpful in identifying central causes of dizziness. BPPV is caused by free-floating calcium carbonate debris, usually in the posterior semicircular canal, but occasionally in the horizontal canal or, rarely, the anterior canal. To test for posterior canal BPPV, the patient is taken from the sitting position to the head hanging left or head hanging right position (Dix-Hallpike test; Figure 132.2). If BPPV is present, a burst of upbeat-torsional nystagmus will be triggered on the side that is involved. This nystagmus will last less than 30 seconds. If the patient is then brought back up to the sitting position, the debris will move in the opposite direction in the canal, so that a burst of downbeat-torsional nystagmus will be seen. Placing these patients through the modified Epley maneuver is more than 80% effective at 24 hours in treating patients with posterior canal BPPV, compared with the 10% effectiveness of a sham procedure. If the debris is in the horizontal canal, a horizontal nystagmus is triggered by either the head-hanging position or by turning the patient's head to either side while the patient lies supine. The nystagmus of this variant can be either paroxysmal geotropic (beating toward the ground) or persistent apogeotropic (beating away from the ground). Importantly, a characteristic of the horizontal canal variant is that the nystagmus will change direction after the patient's head is turned to the opposite side. The side with the stronger nystagmus is typically the side with the debris in the horizontal canal. Various techniques have been reported for removing the debris in the horizontal canal, including rolling the patient toward the normal side and the forced prolonged position.

Central types of nystagmus can also be triggered by positional testing. Chiari malformations, mass lesions of the posterior fossa, or cerebellar ataxia syndromes are the most common central nervous system disorders that can present with positional nystagmus. The most common pattern of central positional nystagmus is a

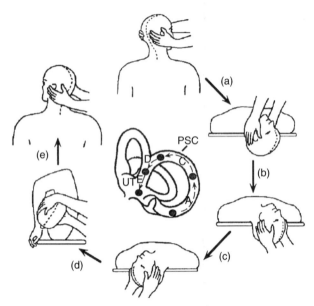

Figure 132.2 Treatment maneuver for benign paroxysmal positional vertigo affecting the right ear. The procedure can be reversed for treating the left ear. The drawing of the labyrinth in the center shows the position of the debris as it moves around the posterior semicircular canal (PSC) and into the utricle (UT). The patient is seated upright, with head facing the examiner, who is standing on the right. (a) The patient is then rapidly moved to head-hanging right position (Dix–Hallpike test). This position is maintained until the nystagmus ceases. (b) The examiner moves to the head of the table, repositioning hands as shown. (c) The head is rotated quickly to the left with the right ear upward. This position is maintained for 30 seconds. (d) The patient rolls onto the left side, while the examiner rapidly rotates the head leftward until the nose is directed toward the floor. This position is then held for 30 seconds. (e) The patient is rapidly lifted into the sitting position, now facing left. The entire sequence should be repeated until no nystagmus can be elicited. Following the maneuver, the patient is instructed to avoid head-hanging positions to prevent the debris from reentering the posterior canal. Source: Rakel 1995. Reproduced with permission of Elsevier.

persistent downbeat nystagmus that is readily distinguished from BPPV patterns of nystagmus, although the very rare anterior canal variant of BPPV can closely mimic this central pattern of nystagmus. Positional nystagmus also may be prominent in patients with migraine-associated dizziness or multiple sclerosis.

Fistula testing
In patients reporting sound- or pressure-induced dizziness, testing for a defect of the bony capsule of the labyrinth can be performed by pressing and releasing the tragus and observing the eyes for brief associated deviations. Pneumatoscopy or Valsalva maneuver performed against pinched nostrils or closed glottis can also trigger associated eye movements. The direction of the triggered nystagmus helps identify the location of the fistula.

Gait assessment
Since imbalance is a common type of dizziness and is also present in many other types of dizziness, a formal gait assessment is important. The patient's casual gait is closely observed for ability to initiate gait, heel strike, stride length, base width, and general steadiness. The Romberg test and tandem walking are also important tests. A

wide-based gait with inability to tandem walk is characteristic of truncal ataxia caused by midline cerebellar dysfunction. Patients with acute vestibular loss are unsteady and often veer or fall toward the side of the affected ear for several days after the event. A parkinsonian gait is characterized by small shuffling steps, narrow base, flexed posture, reduced arm swing, *en bloc* turns, festination, and postural instability. Patients with peripheral neuropathy or bilateral vestibulopathy may be unable to stand in the Romberg position with eyes closed.

Auditory examination
The external auditory canal and tympanic membrane can be visualized during otoscopy. Some of the middle ear components can also be observed through a translucent tympanic membrane, but the inner ear cannot be visualized. Since the advent of antimicrobial medications, pathology of the external and middle ear is only rarely associated with dizziness disorders. The Ramsay–Hunt syndrome is a viral disorder caused by the varicella zoster virus. In addition to vestibular nerve and facial nerve involvement, patients with this disorder usually have vesicles around the outer ear or in the external auditory canal. A fresh vesicle can be unroofed and the base of the vesicle can be swabbed. The cellular material is then rolled onto a sterile glass slide and tested for viral antigens using direct immunofluorescence.

The finger-rub and whisper tests can be a useful way to screen for hearing loss at the bedside. Tuning fork tests, such as the Weber and Rinne tests, are commonly used at the bedside to test for sensorineural or conductive hearing loss. However, a standard audiogram is much more sensitive in picking up all types of hearing loss, because it more accurately assesses the wide spectrum of the auditory system.

Common presentations of dizziness
An effective strategy for diagnosing causes of dizziness is first to place patients into specific categories of dizziness based on information obtained from the history and physical examination. The management of the patient, including testing and treatment, can be directed by the category of dizziness.

Acute severe dizziness
The patient presenting with new-onset severe dizziness probably has vestibular neuritis, a presumed viral/postviral disorder analogous to Bell's palsy, but stroke should also be a concern. An abrupt onset with accompanying focal neurological symptoms or signs suggests an ischemic stroke. A number of studies now demonstrate how closely a small stroke can mimic vestibular neuritis. Making the proper diagnosis is important, because the management is drastically different, and because stroke is a potentially life-threatening disorder. The patient's age and accompanying risk factors for stroke, particularly diabetes, should be considered. If no abnormalities are noted on the general neurological examination, attention should be directed to the neuro-otological evaluation.

The clinician should search for spontaneous nystagmus and if none is observed, a technique to block visual fixation should be applied. The characteristics of the nystagmus should be noted and the effect of gaze on the nystagmus should be assessed. If a peripheral vestibular pattern of nystagmus is identified, a positive result on the head-thrust test localizes the lesion to the vestibular nerve. In patients who are not at risk for stroke, the diagnosis can be presumed to be vestibular neuritis. Additional reassurance can be obtained if the patient also does not have a skew deviation. When a patient has central ocular motor abnormalities or the head-thrust test is negative, then the possibility of a brainstem or cerebellar stroke should be seriously considered. If hearing loss accompanies the episode, labyrinthitis is the most likely peripheral disorder, but auditory involvement does not exclude a vascular cause, because the anterior inferior cerebellar artery supplies both the inner ear and the brain. When hearing loss and facial weakness accompany acute-onset vertigo, the examiner should closely inspect the outer ear for vesicles characteristic of varicella zoster (Ramsay–Hunt syndrome). An acoustic neuroma is a slow-growing tumor and thus would not be expected to cause acute-onset dizziness. Migraine can mimic vestibular neuritis, although the diagnosis of migraine-associated vertigo hinges on recurrent episodes and lack of progressive auditory symptoms.

Recurrent attacks of dizziness

In patients with recurrent attacks of dizziness, the key diagnostic information lies in the details of the attacks. Ménière's disease is characterized by recurrent attacks of dizziness that generally last for hours and are associated with unilateral auditory symptoms. If Ménière's-like attacks manifest in a fulminant fashion, the diagnosis of autoimmune inner ear disease should be considered. Transient ischemic attacks (TIA) should be suspected in patients who report brief episodes (minutes) of dizziness, particularly when the patient is at risk for stroke and when other neurological symptoms, such as dysarthria, are reported. Case series of patients with rotational vertebral artery syndrome demonstrate that the inner ear and possibly central vestibular pathways have high energy requirements and are therefore susceptible to levels of ischemia tolerated by other parts of the brain. Spontaneous recurrent attacks of dizziness lasting seconds may be caused by scarring, compression, or irritation of the vestibular nerve on one side, a condition referred to as vestibular paroxysmia. Benign recurrent vertigo, characterized by a history of recurrent episodes of vertigo without prominent hearing loss or auditory features, is most likely a migraine equivalent, because patients with this presentation typically have a history of other migraine features, normal findings on examination, a positive family history of migraine headaches, or other features characteristic of migraine.

Recurrent positional dizziness

Positional vertigo syndromes are characterized by the symptom being triggered, not simply worsened, by certain positional changes. The typical history of a patient with BPPV is recurrent brief (<1 minute) episodes of dizziness that are triggered by rolling over in bed to one side, getting in and out of bed, or tilting the head back to look up ("top shelf" dizziness). The general medical and neurological examinations are normal in these patients, and the neuro-otological examination is normal until positional testing uncovers the positionally triggered nystagmus. The posterior canal is the most commonly involved canal in BPPV and is readily treated by the Epley maneuver. Other potential causes should be considered when the findings are not typical of BPPV or when the patient does not respond to the treatment. However, central causes of positional vertigo generally do not have a burst of nystagmus and the nystagmus is typically down beating in the head-hanging position. If the head-hanging tests (Dix–Hallpike testing) are negative, the examiner should search for the horizontal canal variant of BPPV.

Central positional nystagmus occurs as the result of disorders (e.g., tumors, cerebellar degeneration, Chiari malformation, or multiple sclerosis) that involve posterior fossa structures. The positional nystagmus of these disorders typically is down beating and persistent, although pure torsional nystagmus may also occur. Following the loss of one vertebral artery, vertigo or significant dizziness after head turns to the direction opposite the intact artery may develop, because the bony structures of the spinal column can pinch off the remaining vertebral artery. Finally, migraine can also mimic BPPV. Patients with migraine as the cause typically report a longer duration of symptoms once the positional vertigo is triggered, and the nystagmus may be of a central or peripheral type.

Non-specific dizziness

Non-specific dizziness refers to types of dizziness other than vertigo, imbalance, or presyncope. Because patients may have a difficult time describing their dizziness, characterizing the symptom and performing a thorough examination are important processes, as central vestibular or peripheral vestibular disorders can be identified even when the patient denies true vertigo.

When the symptom is episodic, one should consider a similar differential diagnosis to patients who have recurrent episodes of vertigo. However, anxiety or panic attacks should also be strongly considered. Patients with panic attacks can present with non-specific dizziness accompanied by other symptoms such as a sense of fear or doom, palpitations, sweating, shortness of breath, or paresthesias. The patient's medication list should be thoroughly reviewed when the complaint is non-specific dizziness, because medication side effects can cause episodes of dizziness or constant dizziness. Other medical conditions such as cardiac arrhythmias or metabolic disturbances, for instance hypoglycemia, can also cause non-specific episodes of dizziness. Chronic types of dizziness commonly occur in patients who also have migraine headaches or other migraine features. Although the underlying mechanisms leading to migraine-associated dizziness are not yet clear, evidence suggests that it can stem from either peripheral or central disturbances. In the elderly, confluent white-matter hyperintensities have a strong association with dizziness and balance problems. Presumably the result of small vessel arteriosclerosis, decreased cerebral perfusion has been identified in these patients even when blood pressure taken at the arm is normal. Patients with dizziness associated with white-matter hyperintensities typically also have impaired balance and they usually feel better sitting or lying down.

Imbalance

Common causes of imbalance include sensory loss syndromes, musculoskeletal conditions, cerebellar disorders, parkinsonian syndromes, frontal cortex and subcortical white-matter lesions, and fear of falling. Loss of somatosensory, vestibular, and/or visual systems comprises sensory loss syndromes because impairment of any of these afferent systems leads to reduced information about the position of the head and body in space. Because so many genetic causes of hearing loss are now known, bilateral vestibular loss due to genetic causes is probably underrecognized. Musculoskeletal disorders remain a major cause of imbalance simply based on the prevalence of arthritis and injuries. Abnormalities of the joints can usually be identified and patients typically have an antalgic gait. However, spinal stenosis caused by degenerative changes in the cervical spine can lead to cervical spondylotic myelopathy (CSM), which can present principally with imbalance. Patients with CSM usually have increased reflexes and may have other signs of spasticity, including increased tone and a spastic gait; however, sensory findings are variable and incontinence is surprisingly rare.

Cerebellar causes of imbalance usually have an obvious ataxic gait pattern and also associated ocular motor signs that could include spontaneous vertical nystagmus, gaze-evoked nystagmus, central positional nystagmus, saccadic dysmetria, and impaired smooth pursuit. When ataxia is acute in onset, a stroke of the cerebellum should be considered. When an ataxic presentation is subacute in onset but rapidly progressive, an autoimmune ataxia, postinfectious cerebellitis, paraneoplastic disorder, cerebellar tumor, or even the Brownell–Oppenheimer variant of Creutzfeldt–Jakob disease should be considered. The spectrum of genetic ataxias continues to expand. There are now more than 30 autosomal dominant spinocerebellar ataxia (SCA) syndromes that have either been reported or have a designation reserved. Significant overlap among these disorders is common and variability also occurs even in patients with the same mutation. Most of the SCA subtypes have only been described in single families. SCA1, SCA2, SCA3, SCA6, and SCA7 are the most common autosomal dominant subtypes worldwide, but there is variation, so that some SCA types aggregate in certain geographic locations. Other important genetic causes of ataxia include Friedreich's ataxia and the fragile X tremor-ataxias syndrome.

Parkinsonian syndromes that can present with non-specific dizziness or imbalance include Parkinson's disease, progressive supranuclear palsy, and multiple systems atrophy. However, over time other features will develop, including a characteristic gait disorder, ocular motor abnormalities, or autonomic failure, so that a more specific classification can be made. Frontal gait disorders are similar to parkinsonian disorders, but the gait is characterized by impaired initiation and a magnetic-type gait. In addition, these patients typically do not develop a rest tremor or cogwheel rigidity. The most common cause of this disorder is probably the multi-infarct syndrome. Patients with this syndrome will have prominent and confluent white-matter hyperintensities on brain magnetic resonance imaging (MRI) and presumably these hyperintensities interrupt long-loop reflexes that are important for gait and balance. Patients with this syndrome typically have cardiovascular risk factors, but genetic factors likely play a major role in subgroups without prominent cardiovascular risk factors. Patients with normal pressure hydrocephalus (NPH) can also present with a frontal type of gait disturbance. These patients also typically have cognitive impairment and urinary incontinence. A required finding for the diagnosis of NPH is enlargement of the lateral ventricles out of proportion to the degree of generalized atrophy.

Finally, fear of falling is common among older people and studies have demonstrated an association between the fear of falling and poor balance performance. Although many of these patients likely have an underlying reason for the fear of falling (e.g., a previous injury from a fall), some individuals who have never fallen and who do not demonstrate impaired balance have a high level of fear of falling.

Management of the patient with dizziness

Symptomatic dizziness can be reduced with the use of medications such as meclizine, benzodiazepines, or antiemetics. These medicines are generally only effective in reducing the symptom and are not preventive.

The management of the patient with dizziness must be driven by the information gathered from the history and physical examination. When a specific disorder is identified, treatments should be directed toward that disorder. Although a randomized controlled trial found that oral corticosteroids can improve vestibular system recovery in patients with vestibular neuritis, subsequent studies have not demonstrated functional or symptomatic improvement. Patients with stroke or TIA should undergo an appropriate assessment to identify the cause and also to prevent a recurrence. Patients with Ménière's disease may improve with a low-salt diet. Although diuretics are usually tried, the benefit of diuretics has yet to be shown in Ménière's disease. Benign recurrent vertigo or chronic dizziness that is presumed to be a migraine phenomenon should first be addressed by instructing the patient in lifestyle factors such as adequate quality of sleep, stress-reduction techniques, regular exercise, and identifying and avoiding any food triggers. If these measures are not effective, migraine-preventive medications can be tried, but formal clinical trials of these medicines for treating dizziness are lacking. The repositional maneuvers are highly effective and guideline-supported treatments for treating benign paroxysmal positional vertigo.

Patients with non-specific chronic dizziness who are taking several medications should probably undergo trials of reducing medications as an initial step. Anxiety or panic attacks can be treated with general lifestyle measures and also with serotonin-acting medications. No specific treatment is known to help improve the symptoms of dizziness in patients with severe white-matter hyperintensities, but since a flow-related phenomenon could be a factor, patients taking blood pressure–lowering medications may note reduced dizziness when those medications are reduced.

Patients with imbalance demonstrated on examination will usually benefit from a formal physical therapy program. Patients with a parkinsonian syndrome may benefit from a trial of levodopa, but this medication has not been shown to improve balance performance, and any benefit in patients other than those with Parkinson's disease is generally short-lived. Treating painful joints can help improve the balance of patients who have arthritis as the cause of the gait disorder. Some patients with cervical spondylotic myelopathy will improve or stabilize after surgery to correct it. Patients with a presumed autoimmune ataxia have the potential to benefit from treatments aimed at reducing the immune response, although formal trials are lacking. There is no high-level evidence to support treatment for patients who have genetic or degenerative spinocerebellar ataxia syndromes. These patients should be instructed in fall-prevention strategies and encouraged to exercise regularly and stay as healthy as possible.

Investigations

Tests in clinical medicine should be selected based on the patient's clinical presentation and the likelihood of identifying a clinically relevant finding. If neither a positive nor a negative result of a test will change management, the test is probably not warranted. For both new and old tests, properly designed studies are critical for determining the range of normal results, diagnostic accuracy, variability, and the potential role of the testing clinical medicine.

Imaging studies

Imaging studies are the gold standard for identifying and often diagnosing structural lesions of the brain. Although computed tomography (CT) can rule out a large mass, small lesions and acute ischemia cannot be excluded by CT because of artifacts and poor resolution in the posterior fossa. Due to these limitations, MRI is the imaging modality of choice, but it is expensive and may not be readily available in many areas. Determining which patients should have an MRI can be difficult. Patients diagnosed with BPPV, vestibular neuritis, or Ménière's disease do not require an imaging study. Patients with normal neurological and neuro-otological examinations reporting dizziness dating back more than several months are unlikely to have a pertinent abnormality on MRI. For any patients experiencing focal neurological symptoms, having unexplained neurological deficits, or with an otherwise rapid unexplained progression of symptoms, an MRI may be the critical factor in identifying a tumor or other structural disorder. MRI of the cervical spine is the test of choice when cervical spondylosis is suspected, although plain radiographs, CT of the cervical spine, or CT myelogram could also provide the key information.

Vestibular laboratory tests

Vestibular laboratory testing can help to identify and quantify a unilateral or bilateral vestibulopathy and ocular motor abnormalities. The usefulness of the test is highly dependent on test administration, patient cooperation, and test interpretation. Artifacts are common and there is generally a wide range of normal values. Abnormal findings on these tests must be put in the context of the patient's presentation and clinical findings. Vestibular testing does not typically add additional value to the management of patients with BPPV, patients diagnosed with vestibular neuritis having a positive head-thrust test, or patients with bedside central nervous system findings, unless quantifying the abnormality is important. The caloric test has traditionally been considered the most sensitive and readily available laboratory test for identifying and quantifying a unilateral vestibulopathy. The rotational chair test has traditionally been the test of choice for identifying and quantifying a bilateral vestibulopathy. However, a relatively new method to measure the vestibular-ocular reflex is a portable goggle system that uses the head-impulse test to quantify both unilateral and bilateral vestibular function.

Auditory testing

Because of well-established standards and formal certified training programs, audiograms are a reliable and reproducible test. Auditory testing is not subject to as many artifacts and subjective interpretations as vestibular testing. Because the hearing and balance organs are in close proximity, are connected as part of the labyrinth, share overlapping vascular supply, and have key nervous system components with a common trunk entering the brainstem, a lesion of one system generally affects the other. For patients complaining of vertigo, with or without hearing loss, obtaining an audiogram may be helpful in making a diagnosis or at least in establishing the patient's baseline hearing for later comparison. Although Ménière's disease is characterized by hearing loss in addition to vertigo and tinnitus, the auditory symptoms may not develop in the early stages, or patients may not perceive the hearing loss.

Common presentations of hearing loss

Patients with the primary complaint of hearing loss do not generally present to neurologists for an evaluation, but hearing loss can be an important finding in patients who complain of dizziness or imbalance. Therefore, it is important for the neurologist to be familiar with common types of hearing loss.

Asymmetric sensorineural hearing loss

Evaluation of patients identified as having an asymmetric hearing loss is primarily the search for a tumor in the area of the internal auditory canal or cerebellopontine angle, or more rarely other lesions of the temporal bone or brain. With an asymmetry of hearing defined as 15 dB or greater in two or more frequencies, or 15% or more asymmetry in speech discrimination scores, approximately 10% of patients will have lesions identified on MRI. When the hearing loss is in the low frequencies and the patient also has recurrent episodes of vertigo, a diagnosis of Ménière's disease can be made.

Sudden sensorineural hearing loss

The etiology of sudden sensorineural hearing loss is similar to that of both Bell's palsy and vestibular neuritis. A viral cause is presumed in the majority of cases, but proof of a viral pathophysiology in a given case is difficult to obtain. The hearing loss in this situation is generally unilateral and it usually evolves over several hours. Sudden sensorineural hearing loss can result in permanent severe hearing loss, although most patients' hearing will improve with time. Focal ischemia affecting the cochlea, cochlear nerve, or root entry zone can also cause abrupt loss of hearing over several minutes. In a patient at risk for stroke, this should be considered early on, because it can be the harbinger of basilar artery occlusion.

Hearing loss with age

Presbycusis is the bilateral hearing loss commonly associated with advancing age. It is not a distinct entity, but rather represents multiple effects of aging on the auditory system. It may include conductive and central dysfunction, but the most consistent effect of aging is on the sensory cells in the neurons of the cochlea. The typical audiogram appearance in patients with presbycusis is that of symmetric hearing loss, with the tracing gradually sloping downward with increasing frequency. The most consistent pathological condition associated with presbycusis is a degeneration of sensory cells and nerve fibers at the base of the cochlea.

Genetic hearing loss

Genetic research into hearing loss is probably among the most advanced research in any genetic condition. Likely because of a sensitive marker (i.e., audiogram) and also a phenotype that can be associated with disability, affected families are readily identifiable and phenotypable. Most hereditary hearing loss disorders are autosomal recessive, but autosomal dominant causes are common, and X-linked and mitochondrial forms are also described. Much heterogeneity exists among the many genetic causes and some variability also occurs among patients with the same genetic cause. The non-syndromic hereditary hearing loss disorders typically present with sensorineural hearing loss that can persist in a mild form or progress to profound deafness. Autosomal recessive types typically are severe to profound deafness, prelingual and non-progressive, whereas autosomal dominant types are usually postlingual and progressive from mild to severe. Surprisingly, vestibular involvement has been reported only in two subtypes.

Common presentations of tinnitus

Tinnitus is a noise in the ear that usually is audible only to the patient, although occasionally the sound can be heard by the examining physician. It is a symptom that can be associated with a variety of disorders that may affect the ear or the brain. The most important piece of information is whether the patient localizes it to one or both years, or whether it is not localizable. Tinnitus that localizes to one ear has a much higher likelihood of having an identifiable cause than tinnitus that localizes to both ears or that is non-localizable.

The characteristics of the tinnitus can provide helpful information. For example, the typical tinnitus associated with Ménière's disease is described as a roaring sound, like listening to a seashell. The tinnitus associated with an acoustic neuroma typically is a high-pitched ringing or resembles the sound of steam blowing from a tea kettle. If the tinnitus is rhythmic, the patient should be asked whether it is synchronous with the pulse or with respiration. Recurrent rhythmic or even non-rhythmic clicking sounds in one ear can indicate stapedial myoclonus. The most common form of tinnitus is a bilateral high-pitched sound that usually is worse at night when it is quiet, with less background noise to mask it. It may worsen when the patient is under stress, or with the use of caffeine.

Conclusion

Neuro-otological symptoms are a very common reason for patients to seek medical care and accordingly have been shown to be highly prevalent in population-based studies. A detailed description of the patient's symptom must be obtained, because patients often use terms for dizziness interchangeably and will use "dizziness" to report any feeling of illness. When considering international aspects of dizziness, delineating the terms that are used in various geographic locations and cultures is of paramount importance. Similar terms may radically differ in their connotations from one region to another. The examination is also critical because it localizes the lesion. From this information, the management can be determined.

Further reading

Baloh RW, Honrubia V, Kerber KA. *Baloh and Honrubia's Clinical Neurophysiology of the Vestibular System*, 4th ed. Philadelphia, PA: Oxford University Press; 2011.

Bhattacharyya N, Baugh RF, Orvidas L, *et al*. Clinical practice guideline: Benign paroxysmal positional vertigo. *Otolaryngol Head Neck Surg* 2008;139:S47–S81.

Fife TD, Iverson DJ, Lempert T, *et al*. Practice parameter: Therapies for benign paroxysmal positional vertigo (an evidence-based review): Report of the Quality Standards Subcommittee of the American Academy of Neurology. *Neurology* 2008;70:2067–2074.

Hilton MP, Pinder DK. The Epley (canalith repositioning) manoeuvre for benign paroxysmal positional vertigo. *Cochrane Database Syst Rev* 2014;12:CD003162.

Kerber KA, Brown DL, Lisabeth LD, Smith MA, Morgenstern LB. Stroke among patients with dizziness, vertigo, and imbalance in the emergency department: A population-based study. *Stroke* 2006;37:2484–2487.

Kerber KA, Burke JF, Skolarus LE, *et al*. Use of BPPV processes in emergency department dizziness presentations: A population-based study. *Otolaryngol Head Neck Surg* 2013;148:425–430.

Kerber KA, Zahuranec DB, Brown DL, *et al*. Stroke risk after nonstroke emergency department dizziness presentations: A population-based cohort study. *Ann Neurol* 2014;75:899–907.

Neuhauser HK, von Brevern M, Radtke A, *et al*. Epidemiology of vestibular vertigo: A neurotologic survey of the general population. *Neurology* 2005;65:898–904.

Newman-Toker DE, Kerber KA, Hsieh YH, *et al*. HINTS outperforms ABCD2 to screen for stroke in acute continuous vertigo and dizziness. *Acad Emerg Med* 2013;20:986–996.

Peate I, Nair M, Wild K. *Nursing Practice: Knowledge and Care*. Chichester: John Wiley & Sons; 2014.

Rakel RE (ed.). *Conn's Current Therapy*. Philadelphia: WB Saunders; 1995.

Tarnutzer AA, Berkowitz AL, Robinson KA, Hsieh YH, Newman-Toker DE. Does my dizzy patient have a stroke? A systematic review of bedside diagnosis in acute vestibular syndrome. *CMAJ* 2011;183:E571–E592.

PART 16   Neuro-ophthalmology

133   Neuro-ophthalmology

Anuchit Poonyathalang
Ramathibodi Hospital, Mahidol University, Bangkok, Thailand

Neuro-ophthalmology, a subspecialty of both ophthalmology and neurology, deals with disorders of the visual, oculomotor, and pupillary systems. The treatment of the purely ophthalmological disorders should be carried out by ophthalmologists, ophthalmological specialists, or neuro-ophthalmologists.

Clinical approach to visual loss

Transient visual loss
Patients with transient visual loss should be approached by characterizing the visual loss, including duration and pattern of visual obscuration, the patient's age, and associated symptoms and signs (Table 133.1). Common causes of transient visual loss are cardiovascular disorders, migraine, vasospasm, and optic nerve head disorders.

Duration
Binocular visual loss for less than 10 seconds may occur in papilledema with or without postural change. Visual field tests

reveal enlarged blind spots with normal visual acuity and normal color vision in the early phase. In the late stage, there is peripheral constriction of the visual field. True edema of the optic nerve head can be confirmed with magnetic resonance imaging (MRI) or ocular ultrasonography. Disc anomalies such as optic disc drusen, high myopia, and coloboma are sometimes confused with edema. In optic disc drusen, discs are scalloped but have a clear edge, are elevated but small in diameter, with whitish-yellow refractile bodies without vascular congestion. Visual field tests often show an enlarged blind spot or arcuate scotoma. Ultrasound examination of the optic nerve head and fundus fluorescein angiography (FFA) are usually used to confirm the buried drusen. Optic disc drusen is rare in some countries, such as Thailand. Orbital tumors, especially optic nerve sheath meningiomas, can compress the nerve when the eye moves in a certain direction and cause visual loss in specific directions of gaze. Mild proptosis, subtle relative afferent pupillary defect (RAPD), visual field loss, optociliary shunt vessels, and choroidal fold are common findings. Imaging studies help differentiate the lesion.

Table 133.1 Clinical aspects of transient visual loss

	Optic nerve head disorders		Cardiovascular disorders	Migraine	Vasospasm
	Papilledema	Drusen			
Period of visual loss	<10 seconds	10-30 seconds	Few minutes to half an hour	20-30 minutes	Seconds to 1 hour
Laterality	Bilateral	Asymmetrical (bilateral-80%)	Ocular:unilateral Brain: bilateral	Ocular: unilateral Brain: bilateral	Bilateral
Pattern of visual field loss	Enlarged blind spot	Enlarged blind spot or arcuate scotoma	Shading down and up, iris diaphragm	Scintillating scotoma	Blackout of all fields
Age of patient	Any age	Average 22 years (7-70 years)	>50 years	<50 years	
Fundus findings	Large, blurred, congested disc	Scalloped edge, normal vessels	Emboli, cotton wool spot, hemorrhage	Retinal artery spasm or normal	Normal or cherry-red spot
Testing	Ultrasound 30° test	Ultrasound, high spike	FFA delayed filling	N/A	Nail capillaries
Treatment	Reduce ICP	None	Antiplatelets, carotid surgery	Tryptans for acute attack, etc.	Vasodilator

FFA = fundus fluorescein angiography; ICP = intracranial pressure

International Neurology, Second edition. Edited by Robert P. Lisak, Daniel D. Truong, William M. Carroll and Roongroj Bhidayasiri
© 2016 John Wiley & Sons, Ltd. Published 2016 by John Wiley & Sons, Ltd.

Young patients with migraine or vasospasm may have visual disturbances lasting seconds to hours. Scintillating scotoma in migraine usually lasts about 15–30 minutes. Headache and nausea are common associated symptoms. Retinal migraine has been reported on rare occasions; transient monocular visual loss with demonstrated visual field defect and correlated retinal artery spasm were temporary findings. Amaurosis fugax, with visual loss lasting for several minutes to half an hour, is caused by retinovascular and cerebrovascular disorders. Platelet or cholesterol emboli can be found in retinal arteries, commonly at bifurcations. Carotid bruit may be audible, but plaque and degree of stenosis should be confirmed by carotid ultrasound and Doppler, magnetic resonance arteriography (MRA), computed tomographic arteriography (CTA), or angiography.

Pattern of visual loss

Pattern of visual loss and recovery of vision can be useful in defining the cause of the lesion. An altitudinal pattern with black shade closing down the vision and gradually lifting up while returning vision over several minutes is seen with carotid artery disease (emboli from the proximal carotid artery). Gradual constriction of the visual field resembling a camera diaphragm closing in and then opening out from the center during recovery is associated with cardiac arrhythmia or severe stenosis of the great vessels. In patients with vascular risk factors, usually in individuals over 50 years of age, the amaurosis fugax may also precede non-arteritic ischemic optic neuropathy or central retinal artery occlusion. Investigation and preventive treatment should be carried out in those patients. Younger patients may develop brief episodes of binocular visual loss from involvement of the occipital cortex commonly associated with migraine. In patients with migraine, visual loss usually involves a partial field defect during the attack, while in other disorders there is generally loss of the entire visual field. Rarely, in patients with frequent recurrent episodes of migraine the visual field defect can become permanent. MRI should be performed to rule out cerebral arteriovenous (AV) malformations. Vasoconstriction of retinal vessels and transient loss of vascular supply of the optic nerve and visual pathways have been reported. Other systemic vascular-related disorders that may decrease blood supply to the eye include systemic lupus erythematosus (SLE), antiphospholipid syndrome, hyperviscosity syndrome, hypercoagulable disorders, and, in patients over 60 years old, extracranial giant cell arteritis. Cortical transient ischemic attacks characterized by symmetric bilateral fleeting blindness associated with ataxia, vertigo, or double vision occur with vertebrobasilar insufficiency.

Ocular disorders

Ocular disorders causing transient visual loss can be painless or painful. Painful transient visual loss can be found in acute episodes of closed angle, acute uveitis, and glaucomatocyclic crisis. Visual losses in those patients are described as foggy or blurry; visual deficits are not entirely dark, as in vascular obstruction. Non-painful ocular disorders that can cause transient visual loss include vitreous floaters, in which the area of decreased visual field moves with the eye movement; corneal punctate epithelial erosion; or dry spots on the cornea, which improve by blinking or topical tears supplement. Other causes include recurrent hyphema in uveitis–glaucoma–hemorrhage syndrome; here the patient usually describes blurred red vision. In macular-retinal diseases, blurring after exposure to bright light is reported. Patients who have central retinal vein occlusion (CRVO), venous stasis retinopathy, or ocular ischemic syndrome can also experience amaurosis fugax. The fundus of patients with CRVO may have an appearance mimicking papilledema.

Venous stasis retinopathy and ocular ischemic syndromes may have fundus resembling diabetic retinopathy. Fundus fluorescein angiogram (FFA) is a helpful diagnostic aid. Investigation to detect any underlying compromise of circulation such as hypertension, dural arteriovenous malformations (DAVM), or carotid artery stenosis should be performed. Patients with DAVM usually have low-flow vascular reversal and a small number of patients may also have venous stasis retinopathy.

Sudden visual loss

Monocular sudden visual loss

Patients with sudden visual loss may experience their symptoms when they awaken or while awake. A common disorder is anterior ischemic optic neuropathy (AION). AION typically presents with profound painless monocular visual loss. In patients over 60 years of age, AION from giant cell arteritis, although less common (5–10% of all AION), must be considered until it can be ruled out. Since 20% of patients with AION have no systemic symptoms, investigations should be carried out in every AION patient over 55 years of age. Another form of AION is non-arteritic anterior ischemic optic neuropathy (NAION). NAION is less severe than arteritic AION; the usual patient is younger, 50–60 years of age. Altitudinal blindness on waking up is a common presentation. Associated risk factors are hypertension, diabetes mellitus (DM), dyslipidemia, and smoking. Nocturnal hypotension, sleep apnea syndrome, and treatment with sildenafil or related medications are reportedly associated factors.

Altitudinal pale segment with a partly hyperemic swollen disc, cotton-wool spot, flame-shaped hemorrhage, and attenuated retinal vessels are typical fundus findings. The non-affected fellow eye usually has a disc at risk that is characterized by a small ratio of disc–vein width, diameter less than 1500 μm, and no physiological cup. Visual field tests demonstrate an altitudinal field defect in the affected eye and a small blind spot in the non-affected fellow eye. FFA demonstrates delay and slow filling of the optic nerve head without choroidal ischemia.

There is no proven effective treatment for the affected eye. A combination of high-dose corticosteroids, aspirin, and pentoxifylline has been associated with significant improvement of the visual field, but not visual acuity. In the acute phase, administration of oral prednisone 80 mg/day (or equivalent) for 2 weeks and then tapering the dose down to zero over 15 days resulted in a significant improvement in visual acuity and visual fields when compared to an untreated group of patients.

Cause and effect have not been demonstrated. Prevention of an attack in the second eye by aspirin during the subsequent 2 years has been reported. NAION in younger patients, approximately 40–50 years old, has a similar presentation and similar risk factors, but antiphospholipid antibodies have been proposed as an additional risk factor.

Central retinal artery occlusion (CRAO) typically presents as painless monocular blindness. Profound visual loss is common, with visual acuity reduced to hand motion or even no light perception. Markedly impaired pupillary light reaction, RAPD, pale optic disc, pale and edematous retina with foveal sparing (so-called cherry-red spot), and retinal vessel attenuation with possible emboli are typical findings. Associated severe headache and neck pain should raise the possibility of carotid dissection.

Common sources of emboli are the carotid artery and heart. Rare entities such as vasospasm, hypercoagulability, and antiphospholipid syndrome may be the etiology. Emboli are visible in about 10% of cases, compared to 70% in branch retinal artery occlusion (BRAO). Systemic vasculitis and giant cell arteritis should be considered (see Chapter 17). Immediate treatment is required. Anterior chamber paracentesis, ocular massage, sublingual vasodilator, antiglaucoma medications, and anticoagulants are employed, but proof of efficacy is limited. There is no established period for retinal tolerance time in humans.

Cortical occipital or subcortical lesions are common causes of sudden binocular loss of vision. Symptoms are homonymous visual field loss, typically congruous homonymous hemianopia; other patterns are tubular visual field, checkerboard, and keyhole appearances. The homonymous hemianopia from the occipital cortical lesion has a sharp vertical midline and a symmetric pattern rather than asymmetric tilted hemianopia of the optic tract lesion. Pituitary apoplexy can cause sudden bitemporal hemianopic visual field loss by acute compression of the optic chiasm.

Acute to subacute visual loss

Visual loss, progressing for days or weeks, is acute to subacute. Etiologies are inflammation with or without degeneration, acute compression, and toxins.

Optic neuritis

Optic neuritis is characterized by inflammation, demyelination, and axonal loss, and results in acute to subacute visual loss. Demographic data in the Optic Neuritis Treatment Trial (ONTT) showed that 77% of patients were female, between the ages of 20 and 50 years, with a mean age of 32 years. Visual acuity is variable, from 20/20 to no light perception. A large central scotoma is common and patients may describe preservation of peripheral vision. In the ONTT study the most common reported visual field defect was a diffuse scotoma. Dyschromatopsia is also noted by patients; objects appear as if there is a gray filter in front of the object, or red becomes orange or pink, or rarely black or white. Optic neuritis causes demyelination and axonal loss and results in type 2 red–green defect, which is more accurately detected by special tests. The degree of poor pupillary reaction to light and dyschromatopsia is often out of proportion to the degree of visual loss. Orbital pain or supraorbital pain, particularly with eye movement, is characteristic. Prolonged latency time of visual evoked potential (VEP) confirms the decreased ability of nerve conduction by demyelination and can be useful to determine prior optic neuritis (ON) in the uninvolved eye.

Based on location, there are two types of ON: anterior or papillitis and retrobulbar. About two-thirds of patients with ON have retrobulbar ON. Since retrobulbar ON is a common presentation of demyelinating diseases, MRI scan of the brain to detect white-matter lesions should be performed. The risk of multiple sclerosis (MS) is higher in patients with white-matter lesions than without. In some non-Western countries, the risk of MS is still considered low using available criteria. Atypical ON is considered if there is lack of improvement in 3 months or if there is severe pain, ocular inflammatory signs, or disc swelling with exudates.

In atypical ON laboratory tests for collagen vascular disease and vasculitis – anti-DNA, antinuclear antibody, erythrocyte sedimentation rate (ESR), syphilis (Venereal Disease Research Laboratory [VDRL]), and sarcoidosis (chest X-ray or computed tomography [CT] scan, gallium scan, serum angiotensin-converting

enzyme [ACE]) – should be performed in some clinical settings. Other rare causes of optic neuritis are neuromyelitis optica spectrum disorder (Devic's disease), human immunodeficiency virus (HIV), cytomegalovirus, herpesvirus, *Cryptococcus*, toxoplasmosis, tuberculosis, aspergillosis, and Dengue virus. Bilateral ON is common in children; infection and postviral reaction are more likely etiologies than an attack of MS. In children with bilateral or unilateral retrobulbar ON, imaging study of the sphenoid and ethmoid sinuses should be performed. Treatment of idiopathic demyelinating ON is based on visual acuity of the affected and the non-affected eye, systemic disorder, and pain. With initial visual acuity better than 20/40 visual outcome is generally excellent, and thus no treatment may be required.

When the patient has more severe visual loss, involvement of the only functional eye, or severe discomfort, intravenous methylprednisolone 1g/day for 3–5 days and possibly oral corticosteroid taper should be strongly considered. Benefits of methylprednisolone treatment are shortening the time of visual recovery and perhaps reduction of clinical definite MS development in the first 2 years. Systemic disorders such as poorly controlled diabetes, systemic infections, active peptic ulcer disease, marked gastroesophageal reflux disease (GERD), and early pregnancy may be relative contraindications.

Neuromyelitis optica spectrum disorder

Diagnosis of this less common form of optic neuropathy has been increasing in recent years, particularly in Asian and African American populations. This may be the result of better imaging and laboratory testing. Visual loss in neuromyelitis optica (NMO) are usually more severe than in typical optic neuritis. Bilateral involvement or sequential involvement are common. There appear to be two types of presentation. The first is relapsing and is seen in the majority of cases. Females are affected four times more often than males. The other presentation is monophasic, with one severe attack and with no predilection for either sex. Autoantibodies to aquaporin 4 (AQP4) is a reliable test with a specificity of 90–100% and sensitivity of 70–91%, depending in part on laboratory techniques used to detect the antibodies. This antibody was found positive in about 50% of atypical optic neuritis patients in Thailand and China. NMO tends to involve the hypothalamus, brainstem, and periventricular regions, areas rich in AQP4.

Conventional MRI studies revealing long-segment involvement of optic nerves/chiasm associated with acute swelling and gadolinium enhancement strongly suggest NMO. In many patients clinical involvement of the spinal cord occurs. In addition, it is now appreciated that there can be other types of clinical manifestations in AQP4 seropositive patients; (see Chapter 91).

Treatment of optic neuritis in NMOSD consists of intravenous methylprednisolone with 1 g/day for 3–5 days, followed by oral corticosteroids for at least 6 months. Plasma exchange is recommended concurrently with methyl prednisolone in bilateral attacks or in those monocular cases who fail to respond to steroids. For seropositive optic neuritis or seronegative relapsing optic neuritis with appropriate MRI appearances Azathioprine or mycophenylate mofetil may be used.

Leber's hereditary optic neuropathy

Another cause of acute to subacute central visual field loss is Leber's hereditary optic neuropathy (LHON). Males (80–90%) are affected more than females. It occurs mainly in the second or third decade of life. Apart from some reports of associated disorders such as cardiac conduction abnormalities or muscle anomalies, most of the patients are otherwise healthy. This painless visual loss usually reduces vision to 20/200–5/200, with a subtle decrease of pupillary light reaction. The interval between first and second eye involvement is weeks to months. In this period between attacks, RAPD may be present. A deep small central scotoma (about 10–15 degrees) on visual field testing helps to differentiate LHON from malingering with tubular visual field defects. Two-thirds of male patients have typical disc appearance of disc swelling without fluorescein leakage (pseudoedema) on FFA, peripapillary telangiectasia, dilated surface capillaries, tortuosity of medium-sized retinal arterioles, and haziness of nerve fiber layers.

Genetic mitochondrial transmission passes from mother to offspring. High percentages of mutated mitochondrial DNA cause overt clinical disease (heteroplasmy). Why males should have more clinical occurrence than females is unknown (see Chapter 131). Patients with mutation at 14484 are less prone than those with mutation at 11778 to develop LHON, but have a better chance of some recovery of vision. Overall, partial visual recovery is about 10–20%. No treatment has been proven effective.

Decrease in disability in the second eye with immediate treatment with coenzyme Q10 has been reported in some studies.

Neuroretinitis

Neuroretinitis is inflammation of the disc and the retina with a macular star on examination. Fluid leakage from optic disc capillaries accumulates and forms a white streak, radiating a sunburst pattern of exudates around the fovea within 1–2 weeks. Visual defects include acuity of 20/40–20/200, decreased color vision, and visual field defect. RAPD and vitreous cells are frequently present. Infections such as syphilis, toxoplasmosis, Lyme disease, and cat scratch disease should be ruled out.

Syphilitic optic neuropathy treatment includes antibiotics such as penicillin. Administration of oral minocycline results in higher concentrations in ocular vitreous humor than tetracycline or doxycycline.

In varicella zoster infection, acute severe visual loss may be caused by ischemic vasculitis of the retina or optic nerve or optic neuritis. Prompt treatment with high-dose steroid and high-dose systemic antiviral agents has been reported to be beneficial.

Idiopathic orbital inflammatory syndrome

Idiopathic orbital inflammatory syndrome (IOIS) or orbital pseudotumor causes visual loss by three mechanisms. First, diffuse inflammation compresses the proximal optic nerve. In this setting, patients may experience combinations of acute pain, vascular congestion, chemosis, lid swelling, ptosis, violaceous injection, limitation of eye movements, proptosis, and optic disc swelling. Second, a posterior scleritis can cause visual loss by associated papillitis, choroiditis, uveitis, or exudative retinal detachment. Inflammation of the optic nerve sheath (perioptic neuritis) is the third mechanism. In this setting, optic nerve sheath inflammation results in disc swelling and retinal vascular congestion. Other disorders that can cause perioptic neuritis are syphilis, *Cryptococcus*, tuberculosis, carcinomatous meningitis, and Wegener's granulomatosis. MRI and ultrasound can be useful for diagnosis.

Treatments include high-dose systemic steroids in early phases along with medications for associated infections. Systemic steroid and immunosuppressive agents are used for tapering; long-term low doses are used in recurrent disease. In children, orbital

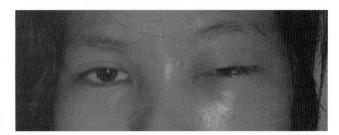

Figure 133.1 External appearance of orbital apex syndrome from gnathostomiasis with optic nerve compression.

cellulitis is more common than IOIS. Infection usually spreads from adjacent sinuses, and from root canal abscess. Rarely, parasitic infection can cause orbital cellulitis with optic neuropathy (Figure 133.1).

Thyroid-associated orbitopathy

In the inflammatory form of thyroid-associated orbitopathy (TAO), acute optic nerve compression can occur and present with the orbital apex syndrome or solely optic nerve dysfunction. Acute central scotoma or diffuse visual field defect along with optic disc edema and RAPD can be observed. Other signs of TAO such as lid retraction, limitation of upward gaze, mild proptosis, lid edema, and conjunctival chemosis help confirm the diagnosis. MRI may show the so-called four-leaf-clover-like enlargement of the four rectus muscles compressing the optic nerve.

Intravenous high-dose steroids should be administered on an urgent basis. Orbital radiation or orbital decompression is considered if the steroid treatment is ineffective. After recovery and tapering of steroids, if the optic neuropathy recurs, antithyroglobulin antibody and other thyroid antibodies should be tested to rule out thyroid-associated autoimmune optic neuropathy. Long-term steroid treatment is indicated.

Acute glaucoma

Patients usually present with very painful, acute to subacute as opposed to sudden visual loss. Some complain of severe headache with pain-induced hypertension, and may be mistakenly thought to have headache associated with hypertension or stroke. Foggy vision, corneal haziness, semi-dilated fixed pupil, ciliary injection, very high ocular pressure, and contralateral shallow anterior chamber are clues to the diagnosis. Urgent treatment by an ophthalmologist is critical. In a patient with monocular visual loss described as a shade slowly coming down, the pupil should be dilated to search for retinal detachment. Flashing lights and floaters are common preceding symptoms. The extent of loss of visual acuity depends on the area of detachment, with macular involvement causing the greatest deficit. RAPD may not be present if the detached area is small. Examination by direct ophthalmoscope reveals a pale wavy retina, but with shallow detachment the retina may appear normal. With opaque media, ultrasound is always used to detect the obscured retinal detachment.

Radiation optic neuropathy

Radiation optic neuropathy (RON) also presents with subacute severe painless visual loss. Symptoms may develop from 18 months to 10 years, with an average of 1 year, after radiation treatment of sellar and parasellar tumors, nasopharyngeal, or intraocular tumors. Anterior RON shows disc edema and radiation retinopathy, with cotton-wool spots and hemorrhages. Retrobulbar RON is difficult to differentiate from recurrent tumor or empty sella syndrome. Treatment with high-dose systemic steroids is commonly employed, but efficacy is still unproven.

Methanol toxicity

Methanol ingestion can cause profound visual loss even with ingestion of small amounts. Vomiting, abdominal pain, bilateral visual loss, reduced level of consciousness, or coma may develop over 18–48 hours. Patients usually have a history of consuming homemade alcoholic beverages. Since the marked bilateral disc swelling resembles papilledema, increased intracranial pressure should be ruled out. Treatment includes dialysis, bicarbonate for metabolic acidosis, and intravenous ethanol to interfere with methanol metabolism.

Chronic visual loss

Ocular disorders

Cataract causes opacity of the lens and subtle decline of vision over years. The majority of cases can be detected by penlight, except for posterior subcapsular cataract (PSC). PSC has a thin layer of opacity deep in the lens and can be missed even with a slit lamp. Visual acuity of PSC in bright light is far worse than in room light. After pupillary dilation this type of cataract can be detected more easily. Decreased red reflex through the direct ophthalmoscope is an important clue. However, vitreous hemorrhage with dense brown or black cataract (cataract nigra) can also give a very dark red reflex. Ultrasonography is generally used to differentiate the nature of the opacity, whether it is in the anterior or posterior segment.

Chronic open angle *glaucoma* is an optic neuropathy caused by slowly increasing intraocular pressure (IOP), ganglion cell death, and nerve fiber layer loss. Enlarged optic disc cup in glaucoma is more likely to be vertical than horizontal. Visual field defects begin with arcuate scotomas; double arcuate scotomas may result in a tubular field of vision in late stages. The optic disc rim is not pale in glaucomatous optic neuropathy. Normal-tension glaucoma occurs in patients who do not have increased intraocular pressure. Several mechanisms are proposed, such as chronic ischemia and compression by a dolichoectatic carotid artery.

Early symptoms of *toxic or nutritional optic neuropathy* are very subtle, with blurring or clouding of the fixation point, which can be confirmed by Amsler grid. Rapid progressive painless bilateral symmetric central visual loss and/or dyschromatopsia is a common presentation. Common reported substances that induce toxic optic neuropathy are ethambutol, isoniazid, chloramphenicol, hydroxyquinolones, disulfiram, cisplatin, and vincristine. In ethambutol ON, the earliest symptom is dyschromatopsia, commonly in the blue–yellow axis. Visual acuity is usually around 20/200. Cecocentral and central scotoma are the most common visual field defects; bitemporal field defect is also observed. The disc and retina are usually normal at first, or temporal optic atrophy develops in later stages. Toxicity is dose related and bodyweight related. Renal function should be monitored, along with the D 15-hue color vision test, AOHRR (American Optical Hardy–Rand–Rittler) color plate, and visual field test. Treatment is immediate cessation; no other treatment has proved effective. However, zinc supplementation may assist in recovery in ethambutol optic neuropathy cases. Prognosis

is unpredictable. In reversible cases, the period of recovery usually starts in 3–8 months, with slow improvement.

Nutritional optic neuropathy also occurs, with pernicious anemia, some gastrointestinal disorders, and rarely poor nutrition leading to vitamin B_{12} deficiency. Symptoms and signs are visual acuity loss, central or cecocentral scotoma, and pale discs. Optic neuropathy secondary to thiamine (vitamin B_1) deficiency occurs in patients who are generally malnourished, such as alcoholics, and those on starvation diet, dialysis, and chronic parenteral diet without sufficient vitamin supplements and gastric plication. With severe B_1 depletion patients develop Wernicke's syndrome, which includes encephalopathy, eye movement disorders, and gait ataxia. Optic nerves usually are normal, but swelling occurs in some cases. With parenteral administration of hydroxycobalamin (in the case of B_{12} deficiency) and thiamine (in the case of B_1 deficiency) early in the course of the disease, vision may improve in a few days.

Orbital tumors

Orbital tumors slowly compress the optic nerve, resulting in disc pallor, usually without disc swelling, retinochoroidal (optociliary) shunt vessels, mild proptosis, and RAPD. Visual field defect can be central, arcuate, or diffuse.

Optic nerve sheath meningioma is the second most common primary optic nerve tumor. Women are affected three times more than men, with the most frequent age of onset between 40 and 50 years of age. Because of the very slow growth of the tumor, patients usually notice their visual loss when a large portion of their visual field has already been lost. Because optic nerve sheath meningiomas begin around the optic nerve, the compression leads to a progressively constricted visual field defect. Imaging generally leads to the diagnosis. Bilateral optic nerve sheath meningioma suggests neurofibromatosis. Stereotactic conformal radiation is the treatment of choice when a patient still has vision. Surgical excision is indicated when a patient has no useful vision, with cosmetic concern, and to prevent involvement of the contralateral optic nerve or pressure on the frontal lobes.

Optic nerve gliomas are uncommon orbital tumors, but they are the most common primary optic nerve tumor. Most of the cases present in childhood and adolescence. In children with proptosis, leukocoria, monocular nystagmus, and RAPD, optic nerve glioma should be differentiated from retinoblastoma. Because optic gliomas originate from the nerve, visual loss is early and becomes severe by the time proptosis is prominent. Optic nerve gliomas are very slow growing or self-limited. The diagnosis can be made with MRI; fusiform enlargement, elongation of optic nerve kinking, smooth sheath margin, and no calcification are typical. Biopsy is not suggested, because optic glioma has similar pathology to nerve sheath and biopsy can cause further damage to the nerve. Patients with neurofibromatosis are 25% of cases.

Many regimens for chemotherapy have been studied. Chemotherapy helps delay radiation treatment, which may affect intellectual, neurological, and endocrine function. Surgical excision is indicated when there is no useful vision, with unpleasant proptosis, or with extension toward the chiasm or brain.

Cavernous hemangiomas are the most common benign orbital tumors in adults. Progressive proptosis, hyperopia, retinochoroidal striae, increased intraocular pressure, strabismus, and optic nerve compression may be present. They are more common in women than men, commonly starting in middle age. Imaging studies such as CT and MRI can help confirm the diagnosis. Unlike capillary hemangioma in children, this tumor has limited feeders from the systemic circulation; thus angiogram or venogram is not necessary or helpful. Treatment by surgical excision is indicated when ocular functions are disturbed.

In terms of *metastases and tumor invasion*, local invasion from sinuses is not uncommon, with squamous cell carcinoma from maxillary sinuses the most common epithelial tumor invading the orbit. Patients present with proptosis, globe displacement, and limitation of eye movement, pain, and compressive optic neuropathy. Differential diagnoses are orbital pseudotumor, orbital apex syndrome, or orbital cellulitis. Imaging studies and tissue biopsy are diagnostic. Treatment includes surgical excision combined with irradiation or chemotherapy in some cases. Orbital mucormycosis presents with violaceous hue of skin and rapid progression of orbital inflammation, more often with pain in diabetics. Tissue biopsy demonstrates fungus invasion of blood vessel walls, which confirms the diagnosis. Treatment by wide local excision and amphotericin B is required, but with a poor survival rate.

Retinal vascular disorders

Presenting symptoms and signs of central retinal vein occlusion (CRVO) are divided into two types, ischemic and non-ischemic. In the non-ischemic presentation, patients may have a vague complaint of mild to moderate visual dullness or blurring, with uncertain onset. Examination of the fundus shows venous engorgement and tortuosity and retinal hemorrhage with or without macular edema. In ischemic presentation, visual acuity is more acute, with severe visual loss. Retinal vein engorgements are more severe, there are flame-shaped and dot hemorrhages, and cotton-wool spots are numerous and obscure most of the macula area. FFA demonstrates areas of retinal capillary non-perfusion causing retinal infarction. Branch retinal vein occlusion usually presents with a strip of black shadow. Visual field tests confirm partial arcuate visual field loss. With macular edema, visual acuity may decrease.

Carotid artery and cavernous sinus fistulas (C–C fistulas)

C–C fistulas usually present with corkscrew arterialized conjunctival blood vessels, proptosis, and hearing sounds within the head. Eyelid vessels are engorged; in some cases the pulsating superior orbital vein can be palpated. Bruit is common in the high-flow type, which is usually associated with severe head trauma. Vision can deteriorate due to optic nerve compression, venous stasis retinopathy, choroidal effusions, or glaucoma.

Dural arterial venous malformations (DAVM) connect the carotid artery to the cavernous sinuses through small collateral vessels of the cavernous sinus wall. Clinical presentations of DAVM are less severe and some may spontaneously close.

Treatment for low-flow DAVM depends on the severity and findings of angiographs. Manual carotid artery compression (Higashida technique) is recommended in some cases. Most cases of direct C–C fistula and DAVM can be successfully treated with endovascular embolization.

Central visual field loss from macular disorder

Central serous chorioretinopathy (CSCR) is most common in young adults, especially men, and is often associated with stress, lack of sleep, and excessive use of vision. Visual loss is subtle to mild, usually 20/30–20/50, rarely less than 20/70. Examination of the fundus demonstrates a round swelling of the retina in the macular area with fluid retention, causing a change of refractive power to mild hyperopia. This macular edema is difficult to detect by monocular viewing ophthalmoscope. The Amsler grid is a very useful test. Color vision is normal. Pupil reaction to light is normal and RAPD is generally absent. Optical coherence tomography (OCT) is a convenient instrument to detect the fluid in different retina layers. In CSCR, fluid is confined in the space between the retinal pigment epithelium (RPE) and the retina. FFA is also helpful in demonstrating fluid leakage to the subretinal space, identifying the point of leakage, which can be treated with laser therapy and may shorten the course of the disorder. CSCR is self-limiting in the majority of patients.

Macular edema is a swelling of the central retina caused by accumulation of fluid and blood components leaking from retinal vessels. Diabetic macular edema is one common form of maculopathy, found in the preproliferative stage of diabetic retinopathy. Other disorders that can cause macular edema are uveitis, CRVO, postoperative ocular surgery, neuroretinitis, and optic neuritis. Macular edema is a rare side effect of treatment with fingolimod. Visual loss is slowly progressive with variable severity. If this edema does not resolve after treating the underlying disease, laser photocoagulation should be performed. Intravitreal injection of bevacizumab is considered an effective treatment option for cystoid macula edema in CRVO and in some other causes of macular edema.

Age-related macular degeneration (AMD) is a common retinal lesion in older patients. Soft drusen and geographic atrophy of RPE are typical findings in the dry type, and RPE detachment, choroidal neovascularization, and disciform scar indicate the wet type. AMD is now one of the leading causes of blindness in the elderly. Ultraviolet (UV) exposure and smoking are risk factors. Presenting symptoms are blurred vision, metamorphopsia, and central acuity loss. Investigations include FFA, indocyanine green angiography (ICGA), and OCT. The aim of various newer treatments is to inhibit new vascular formation and reduce subretinal neovascular membrane.

Cone dystrophy is a progressive central visual loss with only cone functions affected. Autosomal dominant transmission, autosomal recessive transmission, and sporadic cases have been reported. Mild visual loss with decreased color vision is a common early presentation, with photophobia and day blindness, making it difficult to diagnose. The most common age of presentation is in the first and second decades of life. Visual acuity in the late phase is usually reduced to about 20/400. The macula and disc are normal at first, with late macular depigmentation, areolar atrophy of RPE, and bull's-eye appearance. Multifocal electroretinography (ERG) is very useful for diagnosis. Differential diagnoses include sick RPE syndrome, central choroid dystrophy, and Stargardt's disease.

Macular hole is a full-thickness round loss of the retina layer in the fovea region. Early thin and elevated retina is difficult to observe at the onset. OCT of the macula can aid in the demonstration of the early phase of a macular hole. After slow thinning of the retina, a full-thickness macular hole develops. The visible underlying choroid is relatively red compared to the yellow–white-colored surrounding retina.

Paraneoplastic syndromes

Cancer-associated retinopathy (CAR) is an autoimmune disorder of the photoreceptors associated with autoantibodies. The antigen identified in most CAR patients is recoverin. Patients usually complain of bilateral dark peripheral vision and difficult night adaptation over weeks to months. Ring scotoma (paracentral scotoma) is confirmed in a 120-degree visual field test. Appearance of the fundus appears normal in the early phase, ERG demonstrates markedly decreased amplitudes, while multifocal ERG may give more details. In the late phase, there is a mottling pattern of the retina in the paracentral area developed with attenuated vessels and optic atrophy. CAR precedes identification of the occult cancer. Small cell carcinomas of the lung, breast, colon, uterus, and cervical cancer have been reported. Treatment includes systemic corticosteroids, intravenous immunoglobulins, and plasmapheresis, with poor prognosis for recovery.

Clinical approach to double vision

There are some steps to help evaluate the patient with double vision (diplopia). First, cover each eye; if diplopia persists the open eye may have one of the following optical problems: corneal disorder, cataract, lens dislocation, large iris hole, or retinal irregularities. Second, ask the patient if the diplopia is vertical or horizontal. With horizontal diplopia, either lateral rectus (CN VI) or medial rectus function is impaired. If the patient has vertical diplopia, a helpful clue is the presence or absence of ptosis. Without ptosis, the superior oblique may be suspected. Third, if there is variable or intermittent diplopia, *myasthenia gravis* should be considered.

Horizontal diplopia

Isolated lateral rectus palsy is most commonly caused by ischemia. Patients who have systemic risks for ischemia such as diabetes, hypertension, hypercholesterolemia, or vasculitis are most at risk. Improvement is generally seen in 6 weeks to 3 months and no further studies are needed, although non-invasive imaging is frequently performed where available. Increased intracranial pressure may cause unilateral or bilateral sixth nerve palsies with optic disc edema. Sixth nerve palsy with intermittent diplopia suggests Duane's retraction syndrome. Co-contraction of the lateral rectus with adduction causes retraction of the globe and narrowing of the palpebral fissure, which resembles ptosis. Isolated medial rectus weakness with ptosis often points to myasthenia gravis, which can be confirmed by ice-pack compression over the ptotic eyelid for 2 minutes (ICE) test (improvement of ptosis or reversal of diplopia). Additional testing is described in Chapter 128. Isolated medial rectus weakness (slow saccades) that improves with convergence with or without abducting nystagmus represents internuclear ophthalmoplegia (INO). MRI scans often demonstrate a lesion in the brainstem. MS is a common cause during the second through the fifth decades of life, particularly with bilateral INO.

Horizontal diplopia with other neurological symptoms

Sixth nerve palsy that is associated with facial palsy, facial hypoesthesia, and anterior tongue dysgeusia is caused by intra-axial lesions, so-called Foville syndrome. Millard–Gubler syndrome consists of contralateral hemiplegia, ipsilateral facial palsy, and sixth nerve palsy. Sixth nerve palsy with Horner's syndrome suggests a lesion in the cavernous sinus.

Vertical diplopia without ptosis

In vertical diplopia without ptosis, if the patient cannot look up, restrictive myopathy of the inferior rectus should be confirmed by the force duction test. With lid retraction and painless exophthalmos, TAO should be suspected. With a history of trauma, a fracture of the orbital floor or intramuscular hemorrhages are possible diagnoses. A CT scan is recommended to evaluate such patients. Another cause of vertical diplopia without ptosis is fourth nerve palsy. Patients usually complain of diplopia when walking down stairs or reading. The superior oblique muscle has a rather a small range of contraction; its normal function is best observed when the patient has a complete third nerve palsy. In fourth nerve palsy, slight asymmetry of eye movement is found when the paretic eye looks down and in. Since the etiologies of isolated fourth nerve palsy are usually benign, some writers suggest that imaging studies should be done when the condition persists for longer than 3 months. On rare occasions bilateral fourth nerve palsies can be caused by compression from pineal tumors.

Vertical diplopia with ptosis

Presentation of vertical diplopia with ptosis from isolated third nerve palsy is a common syndrome. Third nerve palsy can present with complete or incomplete paralysis of the medial, inferior, or superior rectus, levator palpebrae, and inferior oblique muscle with or without paralysis of the iris sphincter and ciliary muscles. Complete ptosis and large-angle exotropia are the typical appearance of a complete palsy. Third nerve palsy with pupil involvement is not common. Aneurysms from a posterior communicating artery and internal carotid artery can compress the third nerve either before or after it ruptures. Pupil involvement may develop as much as 7–10 days later. Therefore, a third nerve palsy with initial spared pupil must be closely observed and investigated early. Pupil involvement includes dilated fixed pupil, slow reaction to light, or slow consensual light reflex without dilatation. CT angiogram or MR angiogram are effective in detecting small aneurysms ([3]2–3 mm). Third nerve palsy with pupil sparing is commonly caused by ischemia, including that associated with diabetes mellitus (DM). After close observation for 7–10 days (every day for younger patients 20–40 years old without DM or hypertension), if the complete or incomplete third nerve palsy is still pupil sparing, some experts feel that no imaging is needed. Pain around the eye to the head can happen in both diabetic ophthalmoplegia and aneurysms.

If a patient does not improve in 2 months, a compressive lesion should be ruled out by an imaging study. Another indication for imaging is aberrant regeneration; the paretic muscle is reinnervated with the wrong branch. Ischemic third nerve palsy does not cause aberrant degeneration. Other disorders that can lead to vertical diplopia and ptosis are myasthenia gravis, orbital pseudotumor, Tolosa–Hunt syndrome, orbital tumor, infiltrative lesions of cavernous sinuses and the orbital apex, Fisher syndrome, and carotid-cavernous fistula.

Vertical diplopia with bilateral ptosis

On rare occasions, the third nerve nuclei are involved in causing bilateral ptosis, bilateral superior rectus paresis, and ipsilateral paresis of the medial and inferior rectus and inferior oblique.

Vertical diplopia with other neurological disorders

Brainstem lesions that involve the third nerve fascicles can cause ipsilateral third nerve palsy with other neurological findings. Associated disorders are contralateral hemiparesis in Weber's syndrome, contralateral hemiparesis with tremor in Benedikt's syndrome, contralateral tremor in Claude's syndrome, and skew deviation and ocular torsion with head tilt in ocular tilt reaction.

Treatment of diplopia

In ischemic ocular motor nerve paresis, strict control of blood glucose levels and blood pressure are recommended. Antiplatelet agents are generally prescribed. Ischemic oculomotor nerve paresis may begin to recover in 3–6 weeks. If it does not recover by 6 months, MRI scan of the brain and orbit are strongly recommended if not already performed, something that is often done earlier in settings where imaging is readily available. Eye patching is recommended by many writers, but there is no study demonstrating an effect on the time to recovery or degree of recovery toward single vision. Eye exercise helped reduce diplopia recovery time in primary position compared to a non-exercise control group. However, eye exercises should not be advised for thyroid-associated diplopia, because intraocular pressure can increase when the patient performs the upward gaze. The recovery from the palsy depends on the survival of the nerve and the extraocular muscles. Prism correction with both "press on" and prism eyeglasses is expensive and has limited access in many countries, as well as limited usefulness in cases with rapid recovery.

Botulinum toxin can be used in particular cases that need to have early single vision. However, unwanted ptosis is commonly found after retrobulbar botulinum toxin injection. Surgical correction of extraocular muscles should be done after the angle of diplopia is stable, more than 6 months subsequently. Compressive lesions such as posterior communicating artery aneurysm are successfully embolized by modern neuroradiological intervention techniques, although direct surgical clipping is sometimes an alternative approach.

Recommended treatments of myasthenia gravis depend on several factors such as extent, severity, concomitant disease, and age of patient, and should be individualized.

Clinical approach to pupillary abnormalities

Examination of the pupil should include size, function, and shape. The resting size of the pupil becomes smaller with age. Average pupil size is between 4 mm and 6 mm. Pupils smaller than 4 mm and larger than 6 mm may require attention.

Small pupil

An "occluded" pupil is a condition when synechia from the iris occlude the pupil. The pupil is very small and filled in with synechiae that attach from the iris to the lens. Because of severe synechia, pupils do not react either to light or to near objects. In early uveitis, a patient may have intense photophobia, ciliary injection, decreased vision, and ocular pain. The small pupil is helpful in distinguishing uveitis from acute glaucoma, which has similar symptoms except for the presence of a semi-dilated fixed pupil.

Unilateral small pupil

Visible physiological anisocoria is common, from 0.4–1 mm. The differences are unchanged in dim light and bright light. In dim light, if the smaller pupil does not dilate or slowly dilates, pathological anisocoria should be suspected. These pupils can be more easily observed in the dark using a blue or green filter covering a penlight. Horner's syndrome, or oculosympathetic disruption, has more anisocoria in dim light because the fellow normal pupil will fully dilate.

Clinical presentations include miosis, ptosis, and an elevated lower lid, and in some cases anhydrosis. A lighter iris color indicates the congenital type, which is usually benign. The cocaine test (topical 10% cocaine eye drops into both eyes) confirms Horner's syndrome when the difference in pupil diameter is 1 mm or more after 60–90 minutes. After 24–48 hours, one can help localize the site of oculosympathetic disruption by 1% hydroxyamphetamine eye drops. If the pupil fails to dilate and anisocoria increases by 1 mm or more, a postganglionic lesion is present. Since false positive and false negative results of the hydroxyamphetamine test have been reported, other clinical findings should be used to localize the lesion in Horner's syndrome. First-order neuron lesions can be lesions in the brainstem or cervical spinal cord based on other findings. Second-order neuron lesions may be caused by apical lung tumor. Postganglionic (third-order neuron) lesions are often benign, especially an isolated case. Horner's syndrome with involvement of cranial nerves III, IV, and/or VI or second or third divisions of the fifth nerve indicate lesions in the cavernous sinus. MRA, MRI, and CT may be needed to define the nature of the lesion. Acquired childhood Horner's syndrome can be associated with neuroblastoma. In conclusion, patients who have Horner's syndrome accompanied by severe or chronic pain, pulmonary symptoms, cranial nerve abnormalities, or cancer-related symptoms require imaging studies of the suspected locations.

Bilateral small pupils

Bilateral small pupils are commonly found in older individuals, those with DM, and patients treated with eye drops for glaucoma. Pupils get smaller with age, from 6–7 mm in teenagers to 5–6 mm in middle age, and 4–5 mm around age 60 years. About two-thirds of diabetic patients have smaller pupils than the average for their age; however, a pupil size of 3 mm or less is uncommon. One-third of diabetic patients have sluggish pupils, which is otherwise rare in patients under 40 years old. Pilocarpine or phospholine iodide, now rarely prescribed antiglaucoma drugs, usually cause very small pupils (about 2 mm or less) with very poor light or near reaction. Argyll Robertson's (AR) pupils are very small, often irregular, with light and near dissociation (loss of light reflex but normal near reflex). AR pupils are suggestive of tertiary neurosyphilis. Another common bilateral small pupil syndrome, accommodative spasm, is now commonly found in computer vision syndrome (CVS). With prolonged use of a computer, accommodative reflexes are sustained, and patients may have temporary myopia, small pupils, and dull eye pain. Similar to muscle cramp, ciliary muscles and dilator muscles are unable to relax. When patients then change their sight from computer to distance, their vision becomes blurred. This improves with a minus lens. Mydriatic drops at bedtime and periodic rest after 45–60 minutes' use of a computer are recommended. Other causes of bilateral small pupils are hypothalamic lesions, pontine lesions, metabolic encephalopathies, and opiate use.

Large pupil

Unilateral large pupil

Differential diagnoses of large pupils with normal or mildly reduced vision include compressive third nerve palsy, internal ophthalmoplegia, Adie's pupil, iris trauma, and instillation of mydriatic eye drops. Patients with large pupils may have visual symptoms such as photophobia (or glare reaction) and difficulty focusing, especially near focusing. Acute closed-angle glaucoma can also cause a large pupil and mid-dilated fixed positions are common. Patients present with marked visual loss, severe eye pain, nausea, and vomiting, and see a halo around light with very high intraocular pressure.

Adie's pupil is a tonic pupillary disorder and occasionally occurs in healthy individuals. Young women are more affected. Patients may complain about a unilateral large pupil in their photographs, photophobia (without pain), or blurred near vision. This large tonic pupil has poor reaction to light, slow redilatation, and light-near dissociation. The lack of constriction in paralytic segments causes pupils to appear oval or scalloped. Tonic relaxation can also cause difficulty in distance refocusing and far objects become blurred after reading. This tonic pupil is called Adie's syndrome when it is accompanied by an absence of deep tendon reflexes. Injuries to parasympathetic ganglia and dorsal root ganglia may be the cause. Topical low concentration (0.1%) pilocarpine is used to confirm diagnosis. Denervation hypersensitivity facilitates pupil constriction with the diluted solution compared to the normal pupil.

Treatment of Adie's pupil is with 0.1% pilocarpine to reduce photophobia. In accommodative paresis, plus lenses are needed to aid in near visual tasks specifically in bilateral cases (10% of cases). Laboratory and imaging studies are directed to find systemic causes, especially in bilateral tonic pupils. Orbital trauma, viral infections, vasculitides, tumor, and orbital surgery are possible etiologies for Adie's pupil. Autonomic dysfunction may occur. The Fisher variant of the Guillain–Barré syndrome, cancer, amyloidosis, and other autoimmune disorders have been reported as rare associated factors.

Trauma-related large pupil

Blunt trauma and ocular surgery can injure the iris sphincter. Pupils are irregularly dilated, with poor or no response to miotic drops. Iris pigments can be lost, causing transillumination or iris holes. In certain ocular surgeries such as corneal graft implantation or refractive surgery such as LASIX, patients may experience pupil dilatation with or without accommodative paralysis. Ciliary nerve injuries by laser photocoagulation treatment for diabetic retinopathy, orbital trauma, and strabismus surgery have also been reported to cause dilated pupils. The pupil may be fixed and non-reactive to light or near stimulations.

RAPD are reductions of pupil reaction to light in the affected eye compared to the non-affected eye. RAPD can be classified into four grades. In a 1+ RAPD the pupil is initially constricted with subsequent dilatation; 2+ means that there is no initial constriction followed by subsequent dilatation; 3+ is immediate dilatation; and 4+ means that the pupil is totally deafferented and the eye is completely blind. The correct method to test RAPD involves the subject looking into the distance, with dim room illumination and an oblique light source. Then carry out a swinging flashlight test, allowing 3–5 seconds of light shining on the first side, letting the pupil complete its cycle. Repeated tests in one direction, starting from the patient's right eye and moving to the left eye, are less confusing. Then reverse the direction of the tests to confirm the site and characteristics of the pupillary defect. RAPD may be mildly positive with amblyopia or retina lesions and usually obvious in optic nerve lesions, especially in optic neuritis. In monocular cataract patients, RAPD may be positive in the fellow eye, possibly caused by light diffusion or reduced retinal sensitivity in the cataract eye. In rare occasions, optic tract lesions can cause contralateral RAPD. Homonymous incongruous visual field defects and bow-tie disc atrophy are associated findings in such lesions.

In the emergency room, unconscious patients with a unilateral dilated pupil are problematic. With traumatic mydriasis, a small level of hyphema or uveitis may be present. The pupil may have notches and does not respond to miotic drops. Normal contralateral RAPD helps rule out afferent loop trauma. Prominent relative afferent defect (3+ and 4+ RAPD) with a history of trauma around the forehead may suggest traumatic optic neuropathy (TON). If CT scan of the optic canal demonstrates fracture of the adjacent bony structures, optic nerve compression should be performed. Unilateral pupil enlargement and an altered level of consciousness with associated brainstem signs such as negative oculocephalic or progressive third nerve involvement require emergency imaging studies to detect uncal herniation.

Many types of mydriatic eye drops are commonly used in ophthalmological therapy. Tropicamide is a short-acting (4–5 hours of dilatation) mydriatic agent, which produces mydriasis and accommodative paresis. It is used in outpatient clinics for fundus examinations. Pupil dilatation and paralysis of accommodation are more pronounced and prolonged (7–10 days of dilatation) with atropine, which is often prescribed in uveitis patients to prevent synechia. Cyclopentolate is preferred in childhood refraction because it has more blocking effect on accommodation than dilatation. Phenylephrine and adrenaline have potent effects on ocular sympathetic systems, resulting in large pupils, increased palpebral fissures, and conjunctival vasoconstriction, without affecting accommodation. Phenylephrine and neosynephrine are commonly used for preoperative ocular surgery. Any contamination with these eye drops can cause pharmacological mydriasis that does not respond to light or near stimulation and is unable to be reversed by miotic eye drops.

Bilateral large pupils

Bilateral large pupils can be caused by bilateral blindness from ocular disorders, anoxic brain injury from midbrain ischemia, generalized tonic–clonic seizures, and other syndromes, including the aforementioned Adie's pupil.

Abnormal shape of pupils

Congenital anomalies that cause irregular-shaped pupils are iris coloboma, corectopia, aniridia, anterior chamber cleavage syndrome, ectropion uvea, polycoria, congenital miosis, and persistent pupillary membrane. Acquired disorders resulting in abnormal pupillary shapes include uveitis and iritis, idiopathic or secondary infections or infestations, traumatic iridodialysis, traumatic pupillary tear, surgical iridectomy, tonic pupils, tadpole pupils, iris tumor, laser photocoagulation, laser iridoplasty, and ruptured cornea with anterior synechia.

Further reading

Alvarez E, Wakakura M, Khan Z, Dutton GN. The disc–macula distance to disc-diameter ratio: A new test for confirming optic nerve hypoplasia in young children. *J Pediatr Ophthalmol Strabismus* 1998;25:151–154.

Hayreh SS1, Zimmerman MB. Non-arteritic anterior ischemic optic neuropathy: Role of systemic corticosteroid therapy. *Graefes Arch Clin Exp Ophthalmol* 2008;246(7):1029–1046.

Lisak RP. Myasthenia gravis. *Curr Treat Options Neurol* 1999;1(3):239–250.

Poonyathalang A, Boon-Gasem B. Treatment of AION by megadose steroid plus ASA and pentoxifylline. *Neuro-ophthalmol Jpn Asian Section* 2002;19:369–374.

Poonyathalang A, Sukavatcharin S, Sujirakul T. Ischemic retinal vasculitis in an 18-year-old man with chickenpox infection. *Clin Ophthalm* 2014;8:441–443.

Preechawat P, Poonyathalang A. Bilateral optic neuritis after dengue viral infection. *J Neuroophthalmol* 2005;25:51–52.

Poonyathalang A, Suksuratchai M. Optic neuritis in Ramathibodi Hospital. *Thai J Ophthalmol* 1996;10:139–146.

Poonyathalang A, Preechawat P, Janvimaluang V. Effect of eye exercise on clinical outcome of noncompressive ocular motor nerve palsy. In: Leigh RJ (ed.). *Advances in Understanding Mechanisms and Treatment of Infantile forms of Nystagmus*. Oxford: Oxford University Press; 2008:ch. 16.

Poonyathalang A, Preechawat P, Laothammatat J, Charuratana O. Four recti enlargement at orbital apex and thyroid associated optic neuropathy. *J Med Assoc Thai* 2006;89:468–472.

Preechawat P, Sukawatcharin P, Poonyathalang A, Leksakul A. Aneurysmal third nerve palsy. *J Med Assoc Thai* 2004;87:1332–1335.

Preechawat P, Wongwatthana P, Poonyathalang A, Chusattayanond A. Orbital apex syndrome from gnathostomiasis. *J Neuroophthalmol* 2006;26:184–186.

Toyama S, Wakakura M, Chuenkongkaew WL. Optic neuropathy associated with thyroid-related auto-antibodies. *Neuro-ophthalmol* 2001;25:127–134.

Wingerchuk D, Hogancamp W, O'Brien P, Weinshenker B. The clinical course of neuromyelitis optica (Devic's syndrome). *Neurology* 1999;53:1107–1114.

Yang Y, Huan DH, Wu WP, *et al*. The role of aquaporin-4 antibodies in Chinese patients with neuromyelitis optica. *J Clin Neurosci* 2013;20(1):94–98.

PART 17 Neuro-oncology

134 Neuro-oncology overview

Marc C. Chamberlain

Department of Neurology and Neurological Surgery, University of Washington, Seattle, WA, USA

Neuro-oncology is a subspecialty that is concerned with the treatment of both primary and metastatic brain tumors, spinal cord disorders related to cancer and treatment, paraneoplastic disorders affecting the nervous system, as well as cancer treatment–related complications that pertain to the central and peripheral nervous system. The following 13 chapters are divided into four sections: glial neoplasms, non-glial tumors, metastatic tumors, and paraneoplastic complications relevant to the nervous system.

In Chapter 135, Chinot and Chamberlain discuss high-grade gliomas that are operationally defined as World Health Organization (WHO) Grade 3 and 4 gliomas. WHO Grade 3 gliomas (so-called anaplastic gliomas, AG) are subdivided into three histological categories: anaplastic astrocytoma, anaplastic oligodendroglioma, and anaplastic oligoastrocytoma. Molecular genotyping defines these tumors as either codeleted for 1p19q (an unbalanced translocation of chromosomes 1 and 19 that is characteristic of oligodendroglial lineage) or not, as well as manifesting the ATRX (alpha thalassemia/mental retardation X-linked gene) mutation (which defines astrocytic lineage) or not. Codeleted AG have the best survival and respond best to radiotherapy (RT) and PCV (procarbazine, CCNU, vincristine) chemotherapy, whereas currently non-deleted AG are treated with either RT only or an alkylator-based chemotherapy (PCV or temozolomide, TMZ). By contrast, WHO Grade 4 tumors (termed glioblastoma, GB) in non-elderly patients are customarily treated with RT and concomitant and adjuvant TMZ. The role of alternating currents generated by the Novocure external device applied to the scalp may, as recently presented, have a new role in the up-front management of GB. Elderly patients with GB are best managed with either hypofractionated RT or TMZ-only chemotherapy, depending on the presence or absence of methylation of the DNA repair enzyme MGMT (methylguanine methyltransferase) promoter. Recurrent GB is managed with re-resection, re-irradiation, CCNU, or bevacizumab. In Chapter 136, van den Bent discusses low-grade gliomas (LGG; WHO grade 2 tumors) and outlines a strategy of early surgery followed by observation and deferred RT in low-risk LGG (defined as age <40 years or complete resection). In high-risk LGG (age >40 years or incomplete resection), RT + PCV appears superior to RT only. In Chapter 137, Cabrera, Maurice, and Mason discuss oligodendroglial tumors, including both WHO Grades 2 and 3 oligodendrogliomas. There appears to be a similar outcome in patients with either histology if both are codeleted

for 1p19q and when treated with RT + PCV, which appears to be superior to RT only. In Chapter 138, Dunkel and Souweidane discuss brainstem gliomas, with particular attention to diffuse intrinsic pontine gliomas that are invariably high grade and fatal, with RT only still the most effective therapy. Last in this section, in Chapter 139, Chamberlain discusses ependymomas, wherein the extent of resection is the most important prognostic variable, such that second completion surgeries are often contemplated following an incomplete initial resection.

In Chapter 140, Ranalli et al. review nerve sheath tumors comprising neurofibromas and schwannomas, which are mostly found as either vestibular or spinal cord intradural extramedullary tumors. Surgery is the primary therapy, although bevacizumab appears to have a clinically meaningful role in surgery and RT-refractory recurrent vestibular schwannomas. In Chapter 141, Raizer and Singh discuss meningiomas, where the mainstay of treatment remains surgery and RT, with targeted therapies (i.e., somatostatin analogues and angiogenic inhibitors) reserved for surgery and radiotherapy-refractory recurrent tumors. In Chapter 142, Brandes, Jakacki, and Franceschi present a new molecular categorization of medulloblastoma such that these tumors are now subdivided into four groups (Wnt/b-catenin signaling, sonic hedgehog signaling, and groups 3 and 4) that have both biological and prognostic relevance. In Chapter 143, Blumenthal and Ben-Horin summarize new therapies for primary central nervous system (CNS) lymphoma, emphasizing the increasing trend to use a high-dose methotrexate regimen and deferring RT in the initial treatment of these tumors.

In Chapter 144, Jyoti et al. summarize data on the treatment of brain metastases (BM), the most common CNS metastatic complication of cancer. Increasingly, stereotactic radiotherapies are utilized to treat both solitary and oligometastatic BM. Whole-brain RT is generally administered to patients with polymetastatic BM, patients failing stereotactic RT, or in patients with compromised performance in whom palliative treatment is warranted. Surgery is used in BM that are solitary and in non-eloquent brain, or in instances of multiple BM with a dominant lesion resulting in neurological dysfunction. In Chapter 145, LeRhun, Taillibert, and Chamberlain discuss leptomeningeal metastases (LM), the third most common CNS metastases that are underrecognized and consequently undertreated. Recognizing the pleomorphic neurological manifestations of LM is critical so as to treat early, before neurological deficits become

International Neurology, Second edition. Edited by Robert P. Lisak, Daniel D. Truong, William M. Carroll and Roongroj Bhidayasiri
© 2016 John Wiley & Sons, Ltd. Published 2016 by John Wiley & Sons, Ltd.

fixed and permanent. Treatment is primarily with intra-cerebrospinal fluid (CSF) chemotherapy using one of several available agents by either lumbar puncture or preferably a ventricular access device. In Chapter 146, Rudà and Soffietti review spinal cord metastasis, of which the most common manifestation is epidural spinal cord compression. Spinal cord compression in cancer presents with evolving pain well before neurological deficits manifest. Early recognition and treatment are critical, as post-treatment ambulation is determined by pre-treatment ambulatory status. Treatment for the majority of patients entails involved-field RT, although selective patients may be considered for resective (vetebrectomy and spinal instrumentation) surgery.

Finally, in Chapter 147, Rosenfeld and Dalmau consider paraneoplastic disorders of the nervous system. These disorders, although rare and occurring in <1% of all patients with cancer, are clinically relevant, as when recognized they often predict cancer before manifestations of systemic cancer are apparent. The syndromes most commonly affect the CNS and are mechanistically categorized as either cytotoxic T-cell-mediated (defined in part by cytoplasmic or nuclear antigens and characteristic oncofetal proteins found in blood and CSF) or antibody-mediated (defined by cell surface antigens and characteristic serum/CSF antibodies that are pathogenic) disorders. Treatment differs between these two categories, wherein cytotoxic T-cell-mediated disorders are best treated by treating the underlying cancer with minimal response to immune-based therapies, whereas pathogenic antibody-mediated disorders respond best to immune-based therapies such as intravenous immunoglobin G, plasmapheresis, and cyclophosphamide.

While relatively brief, these various chapters provide a contemporary overview of neuro-oncology by experts in the field that hopefully is both instructive and stimulates interest in this hybrid discipline of neurology and oncology.

135 High-grade astrocytomas

Olivier L. Chinot[1] and Marc C. Chamberlain[2]

[1] Neuro-oncology Department, Aix-Marseille University, Marseille, France

[2] Department of Neurology and Neurological Surgery, University of Washington, Seattle, WA, USA

High-grade astrocytomas (HGA), occurring primarily in the cerebral hemispheres, include anaplastic astrocytoma (AA; World Health Organization [WHO] grade 3 gliomas) and glioblastoma (GB; WHO grade 4 gliomas) and are the most frequent gliomas. Prognosis is dependent on age, performance status, and tumor location, as well as several molecular markers that increasingly influence glioma classification and treatment decisions. While a standard of care is defined for GB consisting of maximal safe resection followed by radiotherapy (RT) and adjuvant and concomitant temozolomide (TMZ), the optimal treatment of AA remains relatively undefined and currently consists of RT or TMZ only. A large international trial, CATNON, is exploring the role of RT + TMZ in the treatment of AA. Other novel treatment modalities including the NovoCure (Optune) device and immunotherapy (predominantly vaccine-based therapy) are under investigation for the treatment of GB.

Epidemiology

High-grade astrocytomas encompass 35% of all adult primary brain tumors, with an incidence rate of 5/100,000 adults affected per year. While the peak of incidence of GB is 63 years of age, this peak is observed one decade earlier for AA. An increasing incidence of HGA globally has been described, primarily in the elderly population.

Genetics

Hereditary genetic syndromes account for less than 3% of all gliomas and include Li–Fraumeni syndrome (*TP53* gene), Turcot's syndrome (*HMLH1*, *HPSM2* genes), neurofibromatosis type 1 (*NF1* gene), and neurofibromatois type 2 (*NF2* gene). The rarity of these syndromes obviates the need for a genetic investigation in the overwhelming majority of patients. Similarly, the risk for other family members following diagnosis of an HGA in an index case is negligible.

Clinical features

Symptoms of HGA may include increase in intracranial pressure (ICP) manifesting as headache, nausea and vomiting, seizures, and focal neurological deficits. Headache occurs in approximately 75% of patients and constitutes the initial symptom in 40% of patients. Headache can result from increase in ICP or be the result of traction on pain-sensitive structures such as meninges or blood vessels.

Increase in ICP may result from cerebral edema (related to tumor mass), vasogenic edema (produced by leakage of the brain vasculature), obstruction of cerebrospinal fluid, or obstruction of venous outflow. Symptoms of ICP include headache, nausea, vomiting, drowsiness, and visual abnormalities (e.g., papilledema or diplopia).

The incidence of seizures at presentation is approximately 30% in HGA; both secondarily generalized and focal seizures are observed.

Focal neurological signs are dependent on tumor location and may include motor or sensory deficits, language disturbances, cognitive deficits, or personality change.

Investigations

Radiological assessment

Magnetic resonance imaging (MRI) with gadolinium (contrast) administration is the standard method to determine tumor location, extent of disease, and edema. MRI is superior to computed tomography (CT), except when acute hemorrhage is suspected. The typical appearance of GB by MRI is a supratentorial, heterogeneously contrast-enhancing mass associated with extensive vasogenic edema. Diffuse non-contrast-enhancing infiltration of tumor is frequently observed and is best identified with T2 or fluid-attenuated inversion recovery (FLAIR) MRI sequences. Intratumoral hemorrhage is frequently observed (10–20% of cases). While the majority of GBs are solitary lesions, multifocal or multicentric tumors are seen in 5% of newly diagnosed GB patients. Anaplastic astrocytomas present as infiltrative tumors with indistinct margins and variable enhancement (one-third are non-enhancing). Other imaging techniques such as MRI perfusion, MRI spectroscopy, and positron emission tomography (PET), with radioisotopes such as 18FDG, F-DOPA, or methionine, although not established in the management of brain tumors, may help to differentiate HGA from brain abscess or other non-neoplastic processes, and may also contribute to evaluating iatrogenic effects such as radionecrosis.

Pathology and molecular biology assessment

Histological examination of tumor tissue is recommended in every case so as to verify a pathological diagnosis and exclude other entities such as a brain abscess, a solitary brain metastasis, or a primary central nervous system (CNS) lymphoma. When only a stereotactic biopsy is performed, limited sampling of tumor may result in underrepresentation of pathological features such as endothelial proliferation and necrosis (key features of GB), and thereby underscore

International Neurology, Second edition. Edited by Robert P. Lisak, Daniel D. Truong, William M. Carroll and Roongroj Bhidayasiri
© 2016 John Wiley & Sons, Ltd. Published 2016 by John Wiley & Sons, Ltd.

the tumor grade. More challenging is the pathological determination of AA, where there are several overlapping entities that need to be excluded, including low-grade glioma or anaplastic oligodendroglial tumors. Such difficulties may be resolved in part by integrating molecular markers such as *IDH1* (isocitrate dehydrogenase 1) and *ATRX* (alpha thalassemia mental retardation X-linked) mutations and codeletion of chromosomes 1p and 19q into the classification of gliomas.

The genetic instability of HGA is reflected by the high number and frequency of genetic alterations. Mutations of *IDH1* and in rare cases *IDH2* occur early in the gliomagenesis. As a consequence, *IDH1* mutations, frequently observed in WHO grades II and III (70–80%), characterize secondary GB, although it has been also reported in 3–7% of GB *de novo*. *IDH1* mutation, which can be reliably detected by immunohistochemistry, is associated with a better prognosis regardless of histological type and grade. In addition to *IDH1/2* mutations, AA may harbor *TP53* mutations, which are mutually exclusive with the 1p/19q codeletion observed in oligodendroglial tumors. Additionally, AA are characterized by mutations in the *ATRX* gene (seen in 60–70%), a chromatin-modifying protein, which when present confers a better prognosis. Other frequent alterations include loss of chromosome 10q (80% of GB), homozygous deletion of *P16/CDKN2A* gene (50%), and mutations of *PTEN/MMAC* tumor-suppressor gene (20%).

The Cancer Genome Atlas project classified GB into four subtypes according to gene expression profiling, although the clinical relevance of this classification has not yet been established. Epigenetic silencing of the *MGMT* (O6-methylguanine-DNA methyltransferase) DNA repair gene by promoter methylation has been observed in 30–40% of GB. Overexpression of *MGMT* results in enhanced chemotherapy-induced lesion repair activity and so confers a resistant phenotype to alkylating agents. *MGMT* gene promoter methylation, assessed by methylation-specific polymerase chain reaction (PCR) or pyrosequencing, is associated with a better outcome in both AA and GB, irrespective of treatment modalities. Moreover, *MGMT* promoter methylation is predictive of TMZ benefit in patients with GB. Alteration of the epidermal growth factor receptor (*EGFR*), which includes gene amplification (40%) or over-expression (60%), is observed in primary GB. Gene rearrangement of the *EGFR* gene results in a truncated constitutionally activated receptor (EGFRvIII) that is observed in 50% of *EGFR*-amplified GB and is the target of a vaccine (rindopepimut) currently in clinical trials for GB. The prognostic value of these *EGFR* alterations is uncertain.

Prognostic factors

Overall survival in GB is poor, with a median survival of 10 months and a 2-year survival rate of 10% in cohort studies. Survival associated with AA is slightly better, with a mean survival of 2–3 years. Apart from histological grade, age and functional performance status are the strongest prognostic factors in high-grade astrocytomas. Age may be considered as a continuous variable, although patients over the age of 65–70 years have an even more impoverished survival (median 6–8 months). Performance status is generally evaluated according to the Karnofsky Performance Score (KPS) scale, with distinct risk groups defined by a score of <70 or ≥70. Additionally, cognitive status as evaluated by neurocognitive testing also appears to influence survival. While tumor location does not have a clear impact on survival, tumors that cross the midline or are in

eloquent brain and are unresectable appear to have a shorter survival. The benefit of extent of resection has not been prospectively determined, but is consensually accepted as influencing survival. As mentioned earlier, *MGMT* promoter methylation, *IDH1*, or *ATRX* mutations are associated with a favorable outcome.

Prognostic groups of HGA were defined by the Radiation Therapy Oncology Group (RTOG) using a recursive partitioning analysis (RPA). The RPA created a regression tree according to prognostic variables including age, KPS, histology, mini-mental status (a surrogate for cognition), and extent of surgery, which classified HGA patients into six homogenous subsets by survival. By example, groups 3–6 constitute GB wherein group 3 are young patients (age <50 years) with no neurological deficits having undergone complete tumor resections and with a median survival of 18 months. By contrast, group 6 represents elderly patients with a compromised performance status and often with biopsy as the initial surgery, who have a median survival of 4–6 months.

At the time of recurrence, expected median survival of either AA or GB is poor, averaging 6–12 months. Histology (GB vs. AA), age, KPS, steroid dose, tumor size, and number of salvage therapies have been identified as important prognostic factors. The expected proportion of patients free of progression at 6 months is 15% in GB and 30% in AA. These analyses have been performed in populations included in clinical trials, and so likely do not reflect survival rates of the general HGA population.

Treatment

Because HGA are incurable and associated with a limited survival, the treatment challenge has been to increase survival and to maintain or improve neurological function and cognition without adversely affecting quality of life. Treatment of both AA and GB shares common principles, as both entail surgery and radiotherapy; however, chemotherapy strategies are better defined for GB than for AA.

Symptomatic management

Corticosteroids, primarily dexamethasone, control vasogenic edema and thereby improve clinical symptoms within 1–2 days. Doses should be monitored and decreased to the minimum effective dose so as to minimize steroid-related side effects. Although widely used, antiepileptic drugs (AEDs) should be restricted to patients with a history of seizure, as there are no data demonstrating a benefit of AEDs in HGA patients who have not had a seizure. When AEDs are used, non-enzyme-inducing AEDs are preferred so as to mitigate interactions with chemotherapy. Because of the high incidence (20–40%) of venous thromboembolism in patients with HGA, anticoagulants are frequently required and do not appear to increase the risk of intratumoral hemorrhage. Low molecular weight heparinoids are the preferred treatment due to their better efficacy in cancer patients.

Rehabilitation (physical, occupational, and speech therapies) is often useful and psychosocial support is crucial for both patients and their families.

Surgery

Surgery provides diagnostic tissue for pathology and molecular analysis, improves neurological symptoms by excising mass, and thereby rapidly improves quality of life. Maximal safe surgery is recommended, although evidence for the value of complete surgical resection is still primarily based on retrospective studies. Methods have been developed to improve tumor resection, including surgical navigation systems, intraoperative MRI, and intraoperative visualization of glioma by means of the fluorescent dye 5-aminolevulinic acid (5-ALA). Early (1–3 days) postoperative MRI should be performed to evaluate residual disease objectively. Development of local therapies using techniques such as implantation of biodegradable carmustine polymers or administration by convection-enhanced delivery of various biotoxins has been the subject of numerous clinical trials. To date, only carmustine implants have shown limited efficacy in the management of HGA. However, the benefit of adding carmustine implants to the standard of care (RT and TMZ) in patients with newly diagnosed GB has not been demonstrated.

Radiotherapy

Radiotherapy provides a significant improvement in survival for both AA and GB. A total dose of 59–60 Gray (Gy) delivered in 30–35 fractions of 1.8–2 Gy/fraction and to limited brain volume is considered the optimal schedule. The RT target volume includes both the T1 contrast-enhanced tumor and the non-enhancing tumor visualized on T2 or FLAIR MRI. Additionally, an added margin of 0.5–2 cm beyond the T2 or FLAIR abnormality is included in the final RT treatment volume. The risk of toxicity, particularly for delayed late reaction, is increased by protracted RT schedules, large volume of brain irradiated, and higher doses of RT (both fraction and total dose), as well as advanced age and vascular risk factors. Radiotherapy with or without TMZ may result in the so-called pseudoprogression phenomenon, seen mostly 1–3 months following radiotherapy. This transient increase of tumor contrast enhancement by MRI may or may not be associated with neurological symptoms and is observed in 10–15% of cases. Currently there is no imaging modality that reliably distinguishes pseudoprogression from a true early tumor progression. As a consequence, the diagnosis of pseudoprogression is made after continuation of planned therapy and a repeat MRI that shows radiographic improvement or stability in 1–2 months.

First-line treatment

For patients with GB age ≤70 years and with a good functional status (KPS ≥70), standard of care following surgery consists of concomitant and adjuvant TMZ plus radiotherapy (Table 135.1). This regimen improves median survival from 12 to 14.5 months over RT alone and increases late survival by 10%. Temozolomide is administered orally and daily (dose 75 mg/m²/day) during RT. Post-RT TMZ is administered for 5 consecutive days (150–200 mg/m²/day) every 28 days for up to 6 cycles. The extension of TMZ beyond 6 cycles has no proven benefit. The benefit of adding TMZ to RT is mainly observed in patients with MGMT methylated tumors. However, considering a limited benefit of TMZ in unmethylated MGMT tumors and the lack of alternative treatments, TMZ is still added to RT irrespective of MGMT status. Two randomized Phase 3 studies have shown that adding the antiangiogenic agent bevacizumab (Avastin) to this regimen extends progression-free survival by 3–4 months, although no improvement in overall survival was observed. Interpretation of these results remains controversial and there is no consensus to integrate this agent into first-line treatment.

In patients with poor general and functional condition (KPS <70), the benefit of administering both RT and TMZ has not been

Table 135.1 Contemporary randomized up-front glioblastoma trials.

Trial	Regimen	Median overall survival (months)
EORTC/NCIC	RT	12.1
	RT + TMZ (SOC)	14.6
RTOG 0525	SOC	16.6
	RT + TMZ with dose-dense post-RT TMZ	14.9
RTOG 0825	SOC	15.7
	SOC + bevacizumab	16.1
AVAglia	SOC	16.8
	SOC + bevacizumab	16.7
Centric (MGMT methylated only)	SOC	26.3
	SOC + cilengitide	26.3

RT = radiotherapy; SOC = standard of care; TMZ = temozolomide

shown. Alternative options include hypofractionated RT (40 Gy in 15 fractions), TMZ only, or supportive care only. For the growing population of elderly patients defined as age >70 years with either AA or GB, the benefit of RT only as compared to best supportive care has been proven to increase survival without affecting functional status or quality of life. Based on two randomized trials comparing RT to TMZ in this population, the value of MGMT testing is germane, as patients with tumor lacking MGMT promoter methylation benefit most from RT, while patients with methylated MGMT benefit most from TMZ only. A study that examines the role of adding TMZ to hypofractionated RT is ongoing.

For patients with AA, RT alone is the standard of care, although the addition of concomitant and adjuvant TMZ is often utilized notwithstanding the lack of a prospective trial. An ongoing EORTC/RTOG trial, CATNON, will determine the benefit of adding concomitant and/or adjuvant TMZ to RT in patients with AA.

Treatment at recurrence

No standard of care has been established at recurrence, although several strategies are used, including enrollment in a clinical trial, re-resection in patients felt likely to benefit from re-operation, re-radiation in patients with limited tumor volume, and use of chemotherapy. However, re-operation and re-radiation have not been shown in randomized trials to benefit patients with recurrent HGA, notwithstanding their frequent utilization. Up to 40% of patients with recurrent AA or GB decline further therapy or are not candidates for further therapy and are referred to supportive care only.

Systemic chemotherapy is offered to the majority of patients with recurrent HGA. Lomustine (CCNU) is most often utilized in Europe and is associated with a 5% response rate, a progression-free survival at 6 months (PFS6) of 20%, and median overall survival of 7 months. Rechallenge with temozolomide (given in the standard 5-day schedule) is often considered in patients with a late recurrence (>6 months after completing adjuvant TMZ). There appears to be no role for a dose-intensive TMZ schedule. Bevacizumab is the most common agent used in recurrent HGA in the United States and demonstrates a radiographic response rate of 30–40% and a PFS6 of 35–50%, which appear to be superior to historical controls, but with limited comparative trials. Additionally, bevacizumab has also been associated with an improvement in functional status and a steroid-sparing effect. Whether bevacizumab should be used as monotherapy or combined with a cytotoxic agent such as lomustine is under investigation in a large randomized trial conducted by the European Organization for Research and Treatment of Cancer.

Conclusion

Increased understanding of gliomagenesis has the potential to improve the current classification and treatment of HGA. Tumors with favourable molecular markers – that is, *MGMT* promoter methylation and *IDH1* and *ATRX* mutated tumors – are primarily the subgroups showing an improvement with current therapies. What remains a significant challenge in patients with HGA is the impact of both the tumor and treatment on quality of life, an issue of profound concern given the frequently compromised condition of patients during their survival with this disease.

Further reading

Chinot OL, Wick W, Mason W, *et al*. Bevacizumab plus radiotherapy-temozolomide for newly diagnosed glioblastoma. *N Engl J Med* 2014;370(8):709–722.

Curran W, Scott CB, Horton J, *et al*. Recursive partitioning analysis of prognostic factors in three radiation therapy Oncology Group malignant glioma trials. *J Natl Cancer Inst* 1993;85:704–710.

Hegi ME, Diserens AC, Gorlia T, *et al*. MGMT gene silencing and benefit from temozolomide in glioblastoma. *N Engl J Med* 2005;352(10):997–1003.

Keime-Guibert F, Chinot O, Taillandier L, *et al*. Radiotherapy for glioblastoma in the elderly. *N Engl J Med* 2007; 356(15):1527–1535.

Ricard D, Idbaih A, Ducray F, *et al*. Primary brain tumours in adults. *Lancet* 2012;379(9830):1984–1996.

Stupp R, Mason WP, van den Bent MJ, *et al*. Radiotherapy plus concomitant and adjuvant temozolomide for glioblastoma. *N Engl J Med* 2005;352(10):987–996.

Weller M, van den Bent M, Hopkins K, *et al*. EANO guideline for the diagnosis and treatment of anaplastic gliomas and glioblastoma. *Lancet Oncol* 2014;15(9):e395–e403.

Wen PY, Macdonald DR, Reardon DA, *et al*. Updated response assessment criteria for high-grade gliomas: Response assessment in neuro-oncology working group. *J Clin Oncol* 2010;28:1963–1972.

Wick W, Platten M, Meisner C, *et al*. Chemotherapy versus radiotherapy for malignant astrocytoma in the elderly. *Lancet Oncol* 2012;13:707–715.

Yan H, Parsons DW, Jin G, *et al*. IDH1 and IDH2 mutations in gliomas. *N Engl J Med* 2009;360(8):765–773.

136   Low-grade astrocytomas

Martin J. van den Bent
Brain Tumor Center at Erasmus MC Cancer Institute, Rotterdam, The Netherlands

Diffuse astrocytomas represent a continuum, with grading dependent on the presence or absence of anaplastic features. According to the World Health Organization (WHO) classification, a low-grade astrocytoma (grade II) is defined as an astrocytic neoplasm with a high degree of cellular differentiation, slow growth, and diffuse infiltration of neighboring brain. Most textbooks on primary brain tumors lump the grade II astrocytomas together with the oligoastrocytomas and oligodendrogliomas in one chapter on low-grade gliomas. The rationale for this is that these tumors pose similar clinical problems (young adults presenting with seizures only, and an unenhancing lesion on computed tomography or magnetic resonance imaging), share a better prognosis compared to their anaplastic counterparts, and, perhaps most importantly, guidelines on the treatment of these tumors are obtained from studies that include all three histologies. It is increasingly clear, however, that these low-grade gliomas carry distinct genetic profiles, with most low-grade gliomas having mutations in the gene encoding for isocitrate dehydrogenase 1 and 2 (*IDH1* and *IDH2*), and astrocytomas often showing mutations in the gene encoding for alpha-thalassemia/mental retardation syndrome X-linked (*ATRX*) and *TP53*. A separate subgroup of astrocytomas exists without *IDH* mutations, which as a rule have a worse prognosis. On the molecular level, mixed low-grade oligoastrocytomas do not exist, and this entity points to the difficulties of the histological classification of gliomas.

Despite their former name, "benign gliomas," low-grade astrocytomas are by no means benign tumors. With 2- and 5-year survival rates of 80–85% and 50–55%, respectively, in large prospective trials most patients die of recurrent disease, at which time 65% of tumors are transformed into a high-grade tumor. Little is known about the cause of astrocytomas. Most cases of astrocytoma are sporadic, although familial predispositions do exist.

Epidemiology and clinical features

Astrocytomas constitute about 5–15% of all diffuse gliomas. Within the diffuse astrocytomas, there is a strong association between tumor grade and age at presentation. Astrocytomas have a peak incidence at the age of 30–40 years. The clinical presentation of brain tumors depends on the localization of the tumor and the rate of growth. Many low-grade glioma patients present with seizures only, which may be related to the lower growth rate of low-grade gliomas, including astrocytomas. Focal deficits may arise depending on the site of the lesions. With larger lesions or lesions interfering with cerebrospinal fluid (CSF) flow, signs of raised intracranial pressure may arise. Low-grade astrocytomsa tend to dedifferentiate over time into high-grade lesions.

Pathophysiology and molecular biology

Three histological subtypes of grade II astrocytoma are recognized: fibrillary astrocytomas, gemistocytic astrocytomas, and the rare protoplasmic astrocytomas. This distinction has little clinical relevance, although it is generally assumed that gemistocytic astrocytomas have a more aggressive course than the more common fibrillary astrocytomas. A caveat in the histological diagnosis of grades II and III gliomas is the high interobserver variability (up to 25–33%) in the histopathological diagnosis of these tumors. Especially in biopsied patients, sample error may easily lead to the erroneous diagnosis of an astrocytoma, while a tumor of oligodendroglial lineage or an anaplastic tumor is actually present.

Recent studies have shown that 60–80% of all grades 2 and 3 gliomas carry *IDH* mutations, which are associated with a more favorable outcome. *IDH* mutated tumors with astrocytic morphology and without 1p/19q codeletion usually also have *ATRX* mutations and *TP53* mutations. *IDH* mutated tumors also have a CpG island methylated phenotype (CIMP), in which as a rule the *MGMT* promoter gene is methylated. This may confer sensitivity to alkylating chemotherapy. A subgroup of low-grade histology tumors do not have *IDH* mutations; it has been assumed that these may be low-grade precursors of lesions that may readily transform into glioblastomas. Trisomy or polysomy of chromosome 7 (or 7q) occurs in 50–65% of grade II astrocytomas and has been correlated with poor survival. The simultaneous overexpression of the platelet derived growth factor receptor (PDGFR) and its ligand PDGF is also frequent, indicative of the presence of autocrine loops. Most mixed oligoastrocytomas carry either typical oligodendroglial genetic lesions (1p/19q loss) or *TP53* and *ATRX* mutations, suggestive of an astrocytic lineage. Thus, there is compelling evidence that mixed oligoastrocytomas are not true mixed tumors, but are either of astrocytic or of oligodendroglial lineage. If the histological findings are suggestive of a low-grade tumor but molecular findings suggest a higher-grade tumor (e.g., *EGFR* amplification), this should be considered in further treatment decisions.

Investigations

On computed tomography (CT) scan, low-grade astrocytomas present themselves as low-density lesions with or without mass effect. These lesions can easily be mistaken for ischemic vascular lesions. On T1 magnetic resonance imaging (MRI) the lesions are often

International Neurology, Second edition. Edited by Robert P. Lisak, Daniel D. Truong, William M. Carroll and Roongroj Bhidayasiri
© 2016 John Wiley & Sons, Ltd. Published 2016 by John Wiley & Sons, Ltd.

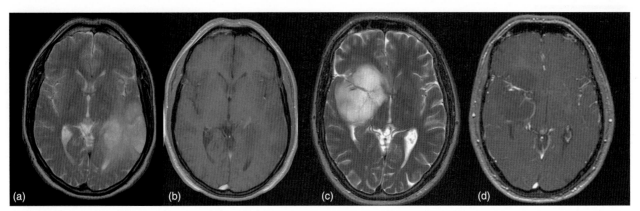

Figure 136.1 T2-weighted images (a, c) and T1-weighted images after contrast administration (b, d) of patient A (a, b) and patient B (c, d). Both young patients presented with seizures and were followed for years before initiation of treatment, were diagnosed with a grade II astrocytoma at the time of progression, and responded well to radiotherapy. The magnetic resonance scans are typical for low-grade astrocytoma: lesions with limited mass effect, high signal intensity on T2 images either diffuse (a) or more circumscribed (c), and low signal intensity on T1-weighted imaging without enhancement (b, d). T2-weighted images provide superior tumor delineation compared to T1-weighted images.

hypointense, and hyperintense on T2-weighted images (Figure 136.1). The margins on T2 may be either sharp or somewhat diffuse. Although the area with abnormal signal intensity often appears rather homogenous, this is not always the case. Most astrocytomas arise supratentorially and do not show enhancement, but exceptions occur. Still, if histological examination of an enhancing tumor suggests a grade II astrocytoma, this should raise suspicion. In the presence of clear enhancement, such a tumor should be treated as a high-grade tumor, especially if the diagnosis was obtained by biopsy and sample error is likely. The differential diagnosis of the neuroimaging findings is in particular ischemic lesions and white-matter diseases. Radioactively labeled amino acid (methionine, tyrosine) positron emission tomography (PET) imaging may help to guide biopsies and allow sampling of more anaplastic areas of the tumor. It may also identify patients with a poor prognosis and rapid malignant transformation. The final diagnosis of a low-grade glioma always rests on the histological and molecular diagnosis, either obtained through a biopsy or through a resection of the lesion. However, imaging findings consistent with a high-grade lesion (clear enhancement nodular) should prompt treatment according to a high-grade tumor.

Prognosis

Large phase III studies on low-grade glioma have identified astrocytic histology (versus oligodendroglial or mixed), >6 cm tumor diameter, midline involvement, presence of neurological deficits, and age >40 years as poor prognostic factors. In the presence of three or more of these factors survival decreased to 3–4 years, while survival was more than 7 years in patients with fewer than 3 factors present. These studies included oligodendroglial tumors, however, and the size and extent of the tumor were assessed with CT scanning. Other studies have identified cognitive function (assessed by the Mini Mental Status Examination), enhancement of the tumor, and extent of resection as prognostic factors. A more recent prospective study on low-grade gliomas with an observation-only arm for patients under 40 years of age who had undergone a gross total resection identified both tumor diameter over 4 cm and astrocytic histology to be poor prognostic factors for progression. After 2 years and 5 years of follow-up, 67% and 34%, respectively, of patients with an astrocytoma larger than 4 cm in diameter were still

free from progression. Several series have shown that radioactively labeled amino acid (methionine, tyrosine) PET imaging can identify patients with a poor prognosis and rapid dedifferentiation. On the molecular level, the presence of *IDH* mutations is an important favorable prognostic parameter.

Treatment and management of astrocytomas

Although recent studies have shown that adjuvant chemotherapy following radiotherapy improves outcome in low-grade gliomas regardless of histology, many aspects of the management of low-grade astrocytomas remain unresolved. First of all, there is a debate on the optimal treatment in the good-prognosis subset of patients, namely young patients presenting with seizures only. Because these patients may do well for a prolonged period of time without any treatment, many physicians defer diagnostic procedures and treatment as long as possible, whereas others advocate early treatment consisting of an extensive resection (or even a so-called radical resection beyond the macroscopic boundaries of the tumor if possible) with or without adjuvant therapy. Arguments against early treatment including surgery are derived from the observation that many patients remain asymptomatic (apart from the seizures) for a prolonged period of time, and may deteriorate following treatment. Arguments for early treatment are uncertainty about the diagnosis and a potentially longer survival after early treatment. Moreover, even so-called stable untreated low-grade gliomas show a constant tendency for growth over time (on average 4 mm per year).

Overall approach

With respect to clinical decision making, two situations must be distinguished: (1) patients presenting with a presumed low-grade glioma; and (2) patients with a histologically proven astrocytoma. For the management of these patients several issues must be considered.

What is the reliability of the neuroradiological diagnosis "presumptive low-grade glioma"?

In larger series about one-third of patients with unenhancing intra-axial lesions are diagnosed after surgery with a high-grade glioma (usually an anaplastic astrocytoma), and patients over 40 years of age may have a greater likelihood of having a high-grade lesion. Conversely, 30% of anaplastic astrocytomas and even some glioblastomas multiforme were non-enhancing on contrast-enhanced CT scan. Some writers see this as an argument for early histological verification in cases with a presumed low-grade glioma, but the assumption that an early diagnosis (and treatment) will improve outcome has never been proven in clinical trials. Moreover, regular neuroradiological follow-up will identify those patients with progressive lesions requiring treatment.

What evidence is available to decide at what moment diagnosis should be obtained and treatment should be initiated?

Small retrospective studies have suggested that early treatment, including radiotherapy of young patients presenting with seizures only, does not improve outcome and may actually decrease quality of life and cognitive function. A larger study with long-term follow-up of cognitive deficits in low-grade glioma patients using several non-glioma control groups found an association between prior radiotherapy and cognitive deficits. A randomized trial comparing early radiotherapy versus radiotherapy at the time of progression showed that early radiotherapy improves progression-free survival (PFS) without affecting overall survival. This shows that with respect to overall survival, delaying radiotherapy does not adversely affect outcome.

Which patients should undergo early diagnosis and treatment?

In young patients with an unenhancing intracerebral lesion suspected for a low-grade glioma without mass effect and without signs other than well-controlled seizures, a wait-and-see policy can be followed provided that the patient is carefully monitored. A first follow-up scan should be obtained within 2–3 months of the first scan to detect early progression of an unenhancing but high-grade tumor. In those cases that are being followed, histological confirmation can be postponed until the start of treatment is clinically indicated. Clear radiological progression or new – even subtle – enhancement during follow-up also provides an indication for treatment, as this will herald focal deficits or a rise in intracranial pressure. Also, tumors that grow relatively rapidly during follow-up are more likely to dedifferentiate early. Intractable seizures may also constitute an indication for treatment, as treatment may improve seizure control. Although some advocates of early surgery in low-grade glioma consider a wait-and-see policy in patients with a presumed low-grade glioma a strategy that may adversely affect survival, there are no data from well-controlled trials that support this view.

In view of the worse prognosis, the higher risk of malignant transformation, and the higher risk of a high-grade tumor in unenhancing lesions in elderly patients, most physicians will recommend initiation of treatment in patients over 45–50 years of age with presumed or proven low-grade gliomas. However, no strict cutoff level with regard to age can be used; the effect of age on prognosis increases each year.

Patients with focal deficits, raised intracranial pressure, or with lesions showing a mass effect also require treatment without undue delay.

Surgery

There are three objectives for surgery in astrocytoma: (1) histological confirmation of the nature of the lesion; (2) improvement of the neurological condition of the patient; and (3) improvement of sur-

vival by preventing progression and malignant transformation. The first of these objectives is obvious. With regard to the second, small retrospective case series suggest that surgery may improve neurological condition and control of seizures. There are no randomized trials, however, on the significance of the extent of resection in low-grade glioma with regard to the third objective, survival of the patient, and patient selection may be at stake here. Several large retrospective case series have identified the extent of resection in multivariate analysis as an important prognostic factor, but others were unable to confirm this. Resected low-grade gliomas with a residual lesion of more than 2 cm had a higher risk of radiological progression than those with a smaller residual lesion, but this did not affect overall survival. However, survival in low-grade glioma is generally better in patients with smaller tumors that do not cross the midline – a subset of patients that is much more likely to undergo extensive surgery. Thus, one might argue that the improved outcome of more extensively operated tumors is due to patient selection.

Nevertheless, in view of the observed improved outcome in many retrospective series, there is a general trend toward early extensive resection in low-grade glioma patients, even those with a favorable profile (young patients, presenting with seizures only). Once surgery is considered, the resection should be as extensive as safely possible. To obtain this goal, specialized procedures like awake craniotomy, functional neuroimaging, and intraoperative ultrasound or MRI evaluation of extent of resection are to be considered in patients with tumors in eloquent areas.

Radiation therapy

A large randomized trial showed that early radiotherapy increased time to progression from 3.4 years in control patients who were observed (and not irradiated until the time of progression) to 5.3 years for patients treated with early radiation therapy. However, early radiation therapy did not improve overall survival, because of the efficacy of salvage radiotherapy given at the time of progression in the control arm. The overall picture that emerges from this trial is that the timing of radiotherapy is less relevant as long as it is given. In addition, at 1 year seizures were better controlled in the radiotherapy arm.

Another prospective trial observed a clear radiological response to radiation therapy in almost one-third of patients with low-grade gliomas, and small retrospective surveys have suggested improvement of neurological function or improved seizure control after radiation. Higher dosages of radiotherapy (59–64 Gy) do not lead to better tumor control than lower doses and may cause more toxicity. It is generally advised to treat these tumors to a dose of 50–54 Gy in fractions of 1.8 Gy.

Chemotherapy

The long-term follow-up of a US randomized phase III study on adjuvant chemotherapy with procarbazine, CCNU (lomustine), and vincristine (PCV) after RT in low-grade glioma shows increased overall survival from 7.8 to 13.3 years. With an increase in overall survival from 4.4 to 7.7 years even low-grade astrocytoma patients appeared to benefit, although the benefit was statistically non-significant in this small subgroup. In terms of overall survival, with the present data the optimal treatment for patients requiring post-surgical treatment is radiotherapy followed by chemotherapy. A first analysis of a European phase III study comparing temozolomide to radiotherapy shows radiotherapy-treated low-grade glioma patients without 1p loss had a slightly longer PFS than those treated with temozolomide chemotherapy (41 months versus 30 months); overall survival data from this study are not yet mature.

Many physicians currently postpone radiotherapy in low-grade tumors in order to delay radiotherapy-induced cognitive deficits, and treat with chemotherapy first. It is questionable, however, whether this will delay further (radiotherapy) treatment in 1p/19q intact patients for a significant amount of time. For progressive astrocytomas, after radiotherapy chemotherapy is often the only remaining treatment option. Trials have shown a 30–60% response rate to temozolomide of 6–12 months' duration. Temozolomide is the drug of choice, as other drugs have either not been systematically evaluated or were proved to be ineffective.

Further reading

Douw L, Klein M, Fagel SS, *et al.* Cognitive and radiological effects of radiotherapy in patients with low-grade glioma: Long-term follow-up. *Lancet Neurol* 2009;8(9):810–818.

Pignatti F, van den Bent MJ, Curran D, *et al.* Prognostic factors for survival in adult patients with cerebral low-grade glioma. *J Clin Oncol* 2002;20:2076–2084.

Shaw E, Arusell RM, Scheithauer B, *et al.* A prospective randomized trial of low versus high dose radiation in adults with a supratentorial low grade glioma: Initial report of a NCCTG-RTOG-ECOG study. *J Clin Oncol* 2002;20:2267–2276.

van den Bent MJ, Afra D, De Witte O, *et al.* Long term results of EORTC study 22845: A randomized trial on the efficacy of early versus delayed radiation therapy of low-grade astrocytoma and oligodendroglioma in the adult. *Lancet* 2005;366:985–990.

137 Low-grade and anaplastic oligodendrogliomas

Sergio Cabrera, Catherine Maurice, and Warren P. Mason

Department of Neurology, Division of Neuro-Oncology, University of Toronto, Pencer Brain Tumor Centre, Toronto, Canada

Oligodendrogliomas (OD) are well-differentiated, diffusely infiltrating, primary brain tumors of presumed glial origin that involve most frequently hemispheric cerebral white matter and the overlying cortex. They differ from other glial tumors by their unique molecular profile, their generally indolent behavior, and marked chemosensitivity, both of which contribute to the prolonged survival typically associated with this disease. Oligodendroglial neoplasms represent 5–19% of all intracranial tumors and 25% of all gliomas. The World Health Organization (WHO) classifies OD as low grade (grade II) or anaplastic (grade III). The presence of histopathological features of both oligodendroglial and astrocytic morphology is classified as oligoastrocytomas (OA) or anaplastic oligoastrocytomas (AOA). Despite recent advances in our understanding of the molecular genetic features of OD and therapeutic advances that have demonstrated clear benefit from radiochemotherapy as initial treatment, OD remains an incurable and fatal disease.

Epidemiology

Oligodendroglial tumors typically afflict young to middle-aged adults. Low-grade OD occurs at an earlier age (median age 41 years) than anaplastic OD (median age 49 years). In contrast, glioblastoma (GB), the most common primary brain tumor in adults, arises in older individuals (median age 62–64 years). Oligodendroglial tumors can develop at any age, but are distinctly uncommon in childhood, where they represent only 6% of gliomas. OD are more common in males (male-to-female ratio 2:1) and Caucasians (white-to-black incidence rate ratio 2.69). The average 5-year survival rate is 72% for OD, 58% for OA, and 45% for anaplastic OD. The 10-year survival rate of oligodendroglial tumors is 51%.

Historically, anaplastic OD has a worse prognosis than OD, where reported median survival in the range of 4–5 years compares poorly to the 10–15 years reported for OD. Prognosis for patients with oligodendroglial tumors is influenced by many variables, including clinical presentation, histological and molecular features of the tumor, and treatment administered (Table 137.1). Although extensive surgical resection likely increases overall survival (OS) and progression-free survival (PFS) in patients with low-grade OD, surgery does not appear to alter time to malignant progression, and this observation has been reported for both for 1p/19q codeleted and intact tumors.

Table 137.1 Characteristics of the tumor, clinical manifestations, and treatment influencing a better prognosis

Tumor characteristics	1p/19q codeletion *IDH1* mutation Absence of an astrocytic component Absence of endothelial proliferation and necrosis Tumor location in the frontal or parietal lobe Tumor size less than 4–5 cm
Clinical manifestations	Young age High Karnofsky performance status Absence of neurological deficits at presentation Seizures as symptom of presentation Long-standing history of seizures
Treatment	Extensive surgical resection Radiological absence of residual tumor after surgery

Pathophysiology

Macroscopic features

Macroscopically, OD are well-circumscribed, soft grayish or pinkish lesions associated with mild peritumoral edema. A gelatinous consistency can reflect mucinous changes within the tumor. Because of their infiltrative nature, they can expand a gyrus, erode the skull, or disseminate in the subarachnoid or subpial space as a creamy white mass. One-fifth of oligodendroglial tumors are cystic; less frequently foci of hemorrhage are identified. The microscopic appearance of an OD is characterized by sheets of regular cells with uniform round nuclei, distinct small nucleoli, and a perinuclear halo, an artifact of fixation, giving a "fried-egg" appearance. Microscopically, OD are highly vascular and typically contain a complex network of arborizing thin capillaries, giving the "chicken-wire" appearance; 70–90% harbor microcalcifications (Figure 137.1). Tumoral cells can cluster around blood vessels or neurons, creating the phenomenon of satellitosis. Some oligodendroglial tumors demonstrate mini gemistocytes or gliofibrillary oligodendrocytes. In contrast, anaplastic oligodendrogliomas are dense, hypercellular lesions with a high mitotic index, nuclear pleomorphism, endothelial proliferation, and focal tumor necrosis. As the natural evolution of low-grade tumors is a slow progression to a higher-grade neoplasm, the distinction between grade II and grade III tumors can be challenging.

International Neurology, Second edition. Edited by Robert P. Lisak, Daniel D. Truong, William M. Carroll and Roongroj Bhidayasiri
© 2016 John Wiley & Sons, Ltd. Published 2016 by John Wiley & Sons, Ltd.

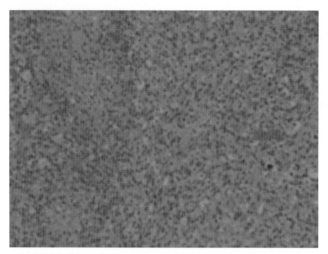

Figure 137.1 1p/19q codeleted anaplastic oligodendroglioma with necrosis (left), frequent perinuclear haloes and occasional microcalcifications (20x magnification, H&E stain). Source: Reproduced with permission of Dr. Rasmus Kiehl.

While OA by definition demonstrate histological features of astrocytic and oligodendroglial differentiation, these uncommon tumors are always astrocytic or oligodendroglial in lineage when characterized by molecular features. Although there are no standard criteria for the diagnosis of a mixed glial or oligoastrocytic neoplasm, EORTC (European Organization for Research and Treatment of Cancer) and RTOG (Radiation Therapy Oncology Group) require that an oligodendroglial neoplasm displays at least 25% astrocytic morphology for this diagnosis.

Molecular features

Oligodendroglial neoplasms harbor distinct and exclusive molecular genetic derangements and these biomarkers have prognostic and therapeutic significance. Low-grade gliomas almost universally express isocitrate dehydrogenase 1 (*IDH1*) mutation, and this appears to be a primordial event in gliomagenesis. *IDH1* mutations (and rarely *IDH2* mutations) are encountered in 60–80% of grades II and III oligodendroglial tumors with or without 1p/19q codeletion, suggesting that *IDH* mutation precedes 1p/19q codeletion. Mutation of *IDH* has been identified as a favorable prognostic factor for gliomas and a predictor of response to alkylating-agent chemotherapy and radiotherapy, even in patients with OD who do not harbor 1p/19q codeletion. Additionally, *IDH1* mutation appears to lead to the CpG-island methylated phenotype (CIMP+), accounting for the widespread occurrence of *MGMT* (O^6-methyl-guanine-DNA-methyltransferase) promotor hypermethylation in low-grade gliomas. It is believed that epigenetic modulation by 2-hydroxyglutarate (2-HG), a putative oncometabolite of aberrant a-ketoglutarate metabolism by mutant *IDH1*, accounts for the CIMP+ phenotype. *MGMT* promotor hypermethylation is associated with favorable outcome and response to alkylator chemotherapy in gliomas; however, the role of this molecular genetic biomarker in the behaviour of gliomas is not clear, as it is intimately linked to *IDH1* mutation and the genesis of the CIMP+ phenotype.

Although most low-grade gliomas have *IDH1* mutation and CIMP+ phenotype, 1p/19q codeletion is the sine qua non of oligodendroglial neoplasms. This unique genetic signature, a consequence of an unbalanced translocation between chromosomes 1q and 19p, has become the cornerstone for the diagnosis of an oligodendroglial neoplasm. Approximately 60–80% of tumors classified as oligodendroglial by histological criteria have 1p/19q codeletion. Recently mutation of the *CIC* gene, located on chromosome 19q, and *TERT* promotor mutation have been identified in the vast majority of 1p/19q codeleted OD; the significance of these observations remains unclear. Codeletion of 1p/19q, in addition to defining a tumor as oligodendroglial in lineage, denotes tumors with favorable prognosis and predictable response to radiotherapy and alkylator chemotherapy. Furthermore, the presence of 1p or 19q deletion alone is favorable, albeit it diminishes prognostic significance. Codeletion of 1p/19q is a primordial and persistent event in gliomagenesis, with two-thirds of primary brain tumors with 1p/19q codeletion maintaining this profile after progression. Rarely, oligodendroglial tumors harbor loss of heterozygosity for chromosome 10q, and shorter survival has been observed in patients with OD expressing this molecular characteristic more commonly encountered in astrocytic neoplasms.

Clinical features

The clinical presentation of a patient with an oligodendroglial neoplasm is influenced by tumor location and rapidity of growth. Low-grade OD characteristically has an indolent course and infiltrative nature; associated brain plasticity minimizes symptoms and most patients present with seizures and no signs of focal neurological deficits. Many patients with OD can remain asymptomatic for years. The presentation of an OD may occur more rapidly if the tumor involves eloquent areas (e.g., motor cortex, speech area). However, partial seizures are the most frequent mode of presentation (80% of patients present with seizures) and the morphology of the seizures reflects the function of the cerebral lobe involved. OD arise more frequently in the supratentorial area (85%) and are distributed among the frontal, parietal, temporal, and occipital lobes with a ratio of 3:2:2:1. Rarely, OD arise in the cerebellum, brainstem, or spinal cord. OD infrequently arise intraventricularly and these tumors must be distinguished from a central neurocytoma. Anaplastic OD are more likely to present with symptoms of intracranial hypertension as decubitus headaches, cognitive dysfunction, and focal neurological deficits. Despite a natural history in the range of one to two decades, OD rarely metastasize outside the central nervous system; they cannot be surgically cured and residual disease, despite responding to radiotherapy (RT) and chemotherapy, cannot be eradicated, making these neoplasms ultimately fatal.

Radiographic features

Typically an OD appears on computed tomography (CT) imaging as a non-enhancing hypodense mass (Figure 137.2). High-attenuation areas within the tumor may represent calcifications or, rarely, hemorrhagic foci. Intratumoral calcifications are more common in tumors with 1p/19q codeletion, can arise centrally or at tumor margins, and sometimes display a "ribbon-like" pattern. The overlying skull may show signs of pressure erosion, a feature that reflects the slow-growing nature of the tumor. Cystic degeneration is common, and occasionally multiple cysts coalesce to form a larger cyst associated with a solid nodule, creating the appearance of a "honeycomb." While anaplastic OD are more likely to show increased enhancement, the absence of contrast enhancement does not exclude

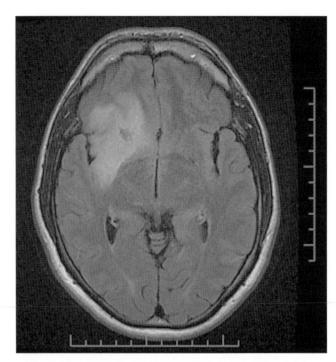

Figure 137.2 Axial T2/FLAIR brain magnetic resonance image demonstrating a right fronto-temporal infiltrative oligodendroglioma. There is local mass effect with effacement of the overlying sulci, without midline shift or hydrocephalus.

anaplasia; in oligodendroglial tumors, enhancement is of limited significance as patchy enhancement occurs in 50% of OD. A retrospective French study of 927 histologically proven WHO grade II gliomas confirmed contrast enhancement (patchy or nodular-like pattern) in 16%. In a univariate analysis, this radiographic feature did not influence prognosis.

On MR imaging, the typical oligodendroglial tumor is hypointense on T1 and hyperintense on T2, excluding areas of calcification that appear as "blooming" artifact on the T2* sequence. FLAIR images are particularly helpful for delineating oligodendroglial tumors, as on this sequence they appear more intense than CSF and brain parenchyma. It is reported that 1p/19q codeleted tumors are more heterogeneous, with a mixed signal intensity on T1 and T2 images, and their borders are less distinct on MR imaging than 1p/19q intact tumors.

Diffusion sequences can assist in distinguishing an OD from a higher-grade neoplasm. The latter demonstrates increased restriction, reflecting a more cellular tumor. In OD, increasing grade is characterized by increased vascularity and a relative elevation of cerebral blood volume. Consequently, MR perfusion imaging can distinguish low-grade from anaplastic OD with a reported sensitivity of 95% and a positive predictive value of 87%. Grade II and grade III oligodendroglial tumors can also be distinguished by positron emission tomography (PET) imaging utilizing [C]-methionine as the radioisotope. PET imaging utilizing fluorodeoxyglucose is less useful, as uptake resembles normal white matter for low-grade tumors and normal gray matter for high-grade tumors. However, advanced imaging is not considered standard of care and remains controversial as a modality for distinguishing low-grade gliomas from high-grade gliomas.

Treatment

The management of OD depends on grade and location. Options for low-grade OD include surgery, radiotherapy, and chemotherapy.

Low-grade oligodendroglioma

Surgery

In the absence of completed trials exclusively dedicated to low-grade OD, the recommendations in this section are extrapolated from data regarding all low-grade glioma trials.

While it has been established that initial tumor size and extent of the surgical resection have an impact on long-term prognosis in low-grade gliomas, the value of immediate surgery versus deferring surgery in low-grade tumors until there is evidence of clinical or radiological progression in patients with minimal symptoms remains controversial. Early surgical intervention is indicated for patients with large tumors associated with intracranial hypertension, for tumors that have progressed radiographically, and for tumors associated with intractable seizures. The goals of surgery are to confirm pathology prior to further therapy and to alleviate seizures and symptoms related to mass effect. As with all gliomas, oligodendroglial tumors are infiltrative neoplasms and complete surgical resection is rarely feasible.

However, three more recent retrospective cohort studies, involving 577 patients with low-grade gliomas, have furnished evidence that a more aggressive resection predicts significant improvement in overall survival (OS) and progression-free survival (PFS), and decreases the risk of malignant degeneration compared with a simple debulking procedure. Patients with at least 90% tumoral resection had 5- and 8-year OS rates of 97% and 91%, while patients with a resection of less than 90% had 76% and 60% OS rates, respectively. New postoperative deficits were seen in 1.8% of patients. The extent of surgery was independently associated with increased OS (P = 0.017) and PFS (P = 0.043). Despite the results of these retrospective studies, there has never been a controlled clinical trial evaluating prospectively the role of surgery in low-grade gliomas. Additionally, a recent study assessing the impact of extent of resection on malignant transformation of pure OG (WHO grade II) concluded that while extent of surgery is associated with an improved survival, it does not influence the interval to tumor transformation, and this observation is not influenced by 1p/19q codeletion status. These results raise questions about the nature of the biological mechanisms influencing malignant transformation following surgical resection. Nonetheless, when a decision is made to operate, a maximum safe resection is recommended; a postoperative MRI within 24–72 hours is recommended to document residual disease.

Radiotherapy

Radiotherapy is an effective treatment for low-grade gliomas, but its timing remains controversial. The EORTC 22845/BR04 trials assessing this question revealed that early RT immediately after surgery prolongs PFS, but does not affect OS (OS in the RT group was 7.4 years vs. 7.2 years in the control group, p=0·872). Based on an analysis of the two EORTC trials (EORTC 22844 and EORTC 22845), Pignatti et al. divided patients in two groups with different prognosis: low-risk and high-risk. High-risk patients require at least three of the following criteria: (1) age ≥40 years; (2) largest preoperative tumor diameter ≥6 cm; (3) tumor crossing midline; (4) tumor of astrocytoma histology; and (5) preoperative neurological deficit. However, RTOG defines low risk as a patient younger than 40 years who underwent a gross total resection, and high risk as a patient older than 40 years who underwent a subtotal resection or a biopsy. The RTOG 0424 study compared the 3-year survival of a regimen of concurrent and adjuvant temozolomide (TMZ) and RT in the high-risk, low-grade glioma group following Pignatti *et al.*'s criteria to historical controls. The preliminary results indicate a 3-year OS rate of 73.1%, which is significantly higher than the results reported by studies involving historical controls (54%).

In addition, further trials failed to demonstrate an advantage of high-dose versus low-dose radiation within the range of 45–64.8 Gy in patients with low-grade gliomas. Indeed, patients who received higher doses reported lower performance status and more side effects following the completion of RT.

There may be a role for higher doses of RT (>50 Gy) in the group of patients who underwent partial tumor resection (<50%). However, predictive factors of patients who could benefit from early RT postsurgery are not yet well defined.

Chemotherapy

The efficacy of alkylating agents as an initial treatment in newly diagnosed and recurrent low-grade OD is well established. While the use of TMZ is widespread due to a very favorable toxicity profile, PCV (combination of procarbazine + CCNU + vincristine) is historically the chemotherapy of choice for oligodendroglial tumors. Phase II trials have documented the efficacy of TMZ in the treatment of OD, achieving control in 90% of patients. The phase III RTOG trial 9802 studied the impact of RT alone versus RT followed by PCV for the treatment of low-grade gliomas. The analysis showed that the addition of PCV conferred an OS (from 7.8 to 13.3 years) and PFS advantage, despite the fact that 77% of patients who progressed after RT alone were treated with salvage chemotherapy. Patients with favorable characteristics (younger than 40 years and gross total resection) demonstrated an increased OS at 2 and 5 years (99% and 93%, respectively) compared to the higher-risk group (85% and 72%, respectively). However, PFS was similar for both groups. RTOG trial 0424 evaluated the role of TMZ and RT in high-risk low-grade gliomas. A randomized phase III intergroup study by the EORTC (22033-26033) investigated the role of primary chemotherapy versus RT on PFS and OS in progressive, symptomatic, or "high-risk" patients diagnosed with a low-grade glioma. The first-line treatment with TMZ compared to RT did not improve PFS, and there was a trend for inferior PFS in the subgroup with intact 1p. However, preliminary results suggest that OS is superior in the 1p-deleted subgroup treated with TMZ upfront.

Most neuro-oncologists choose to observe patients with low-risk OD; treatment with an alkylating agent is often administered at progression. In high-risk patients, surgery should be followed by chemotherapy alone or with RT. To avoid late neurotoxicity from RT, chemotherapy is an attractive option in patients with larger tumors, particularly if they have favorable molecular features such as 1p19q codeletion. While recent trials have provided evidence to support the addition of PCV chemotherapy to RT for high-risk low-grade gliomas, and to support a policy of using TMZ before RT in 1p19q codeleted tumors, the choice and timing of chemotherapy for low-grade gliomas remain an area of intense controversy.

High-grade oligodendroglioma

Initial management

Recent updates of large phase III trials evaluating the addition of PCV chemotherapy to RT for newly diagnosed anaplastic oligoden-

droglial neoplasms have established a role for chemotherapy in the initial management of this disease. Initial analyses of EORTC 26951 (six standard PCV cycles administered immediately after radiotherapy; each cycle consisted of lomustine 110 mg/m^2 orally on day 1, procarbazine 60 mg/m^2 orally on days 8–21, and vincristine 1.4 mg/m^2 intravenously on days 8 and 29) and RTOG 9402 (radiotherapy prescribed following intensive PCV chemotherapy; four PCV cycles were given every 6 weeks before RT, as follows: lomustine 130 mg/m^2 orally on day 1; procarbazine 75 mg/m^2 orally daily, days 8–21; and vincristine 1.4 mg/m^2 intravenously on days 8 and 29) determined that adjuvant PCV chemotherapy improved median PFS with no OS benefit at 5 years. A 10-year analysis of RTOG 9402, however, revealed that while the addition of PCV to RT did not extend OS (4.6 years PCV + RT vs. 4.7 years RT), a favorable subgroup of patients with 1p19q codeletion had a significantly longer survival with PCV chemotherapy (codeleted 14.7 years PCV + RT, 7.3 years RT; non-codeleted 2.6 years PCV + RT, 2.7 years RT). Regardless of therapy administered at progression, 1p/19q codeleted patients had inferior survival if the initial treatment consisted of RT alone.

A retrospective multi-institutional study reviewing therapies administered to 1,013 patients with newly diagnosed anaplastic OD not enrolled in the EORTC and RTOG trials has suggested that 1p19q non-codeleted tumors also benefit from chemotherapy plus RT. These results will be prospectively confirmed by the CATNON (Concurrent and Adjuvant Temozolomide Chemotherapy in Non-1p/19q Deleted Anaplastic Glioma) trial, which examines the role of TMZ chemotherapy when added to standard RT for newly diagnosed 1p/19q non-codeleted anaplastic gliomas.

The NOA-04 (Neuro-Oncology Working Group) trial comparing monotherapy with RT, PCV, or TMZ in newly diagnosed anaplastic gliomas revealed that the three regimens are equally effective as initial therapy for patients with this disease. TMZ is favored because of its better tolerability profile, but the effectiveness of TMZ versus PCV in high-grade gliomas following RT appears to be similar. Although controversial in the management of AOA, the decision to initiate a monotherapy with an alkylating agent to delay RT and potentially minimize its late neurotoxicity is an option for some patients based on several factors, including the tumor size, location, and its molecular profile. Delayed toxicity may occur several months to years following radiation therapy and implicates cerebral necrosis, atrophy, hemorrhage, infarction, or neoplastic transformation. The initial management of patients with anaplastic gliomas will likely be determined by the results of two ongoing international trials that are driven by molecular profiling. The CODEL Trial 26081-22086 (Phase III Intergroup Study of Radiotherapy versus Temozolomide Alone versus Radiotherapy with Concomitant and Adjuvant Temozolomide for Patients with 1p/19q Codeleted Anaplastic Glioma) compares initial treatment with RT versus TMZ versus RT with concomitant followed by adjuvant TMZ for newly diagnosed anaplastic OD or anaplastic mixed glioma patients with 1p/19q codeletion. The EORTC CATNON phase III trial evaluates the role of concurrent and adjuvant TMZ in non-codeleted anaplastic gliomas. These large studies will take years to complete and analyze, but should provide definitive guidelines for the initial management of anaplastic gliomas.

Management at progression

There is no standard of care for the management of recurrent AOD. Given the prolonged survival of many patients with oligodendroglial tumors, surgery and even re-irradiation have a role. However, the cornerstone of management for patients with recurrent oligodendroglial tumors remains chemotherapy, and common choices are still PCV chemotherapy, TMZ, etoposide, irinotecan, Taxotere (docetaxel), and platinum analogues. Bevacizumab may have a role as well, with PFS at 6 and 12 months of 68% and 23%, respectively.

Conclusion

In neuro-oncology, oligodendroglial neoplasms are a unique entity. They differ from other gliomas in their unique and exclusive molecular genetic features. They are remarkably responsive to therapy and are the most chemosensitive gliomas. Recently updated trial results have demonstrated an unprecedented impact of chemotherapy on survival, particularly for patients who have 1p19q codeleted tumors. Despite remarkable developments in our understanding of the molecular biology and our ability to treat these tumors, they remain ultimately fatal diseases. Ongoing therapeutic controversies will ensure that these diseases will continue to fascinate and preoccupy basic and clinical neuro-oncologists for years to come.

Further reading

Baumert BG, Mason WP, Ryan G, *et al*. Temozolomide chemotherapy versus radiotherapy in molecularly characterized (1p loss) low-grade glioma: A randomized phase III intergroup study by the EORTC/NCIC-CTG/RTOG/MRC-CTU (EORTC 22033-26033). *J Clin Oncol* 2013;31(suppl):abstr 2007.

Cairncross G, Wang M, Shaw E, *et al*. Phase III trial of chemoradiotherapy for anaplastic oligodendroglioma: Long-term results of RTOG 9402. *J Clin Oncol* 2013;31(3):337–343.

Fisher BJ, Lui J, Macdonald DR. A phase II study of a temozolomide-based chemoradiotherapy regimen for high-risk low-grade gliomas: Preliminary results of RTOG 0424. *J Clin Oncol* 2013;31(suppl):abstr 2008.

Pignatti F, van den Bent M, Curran D, *et al*.; European Organization for Research and Treatment of Cancer Brain Tumor Cooperative Group; European Organization for Research and Treatment of Cancer Radiotherapy Cooperative Group. Prognostic factors for survival in adult patients with cerebral low-grade glioma. *J Clin Oncol* 2002;20(8):2076–2084.

Snyder LA, Wolf AB, Oppenlander ME *et al*. The impact of extent of resection on malignant transformation of pure oligodendrogliomas. *J Neurosurg* 2014;120(2):309–314.

Van den Bent MJ, Afra D, de Witte O, *et al*; EORTC Radiotherapy and Brain Tumor Groups and the UK Medical Research Council. Long-term efficacy of early versus delayed radiotherapy for low-grade astrocytoma and oligodendroglioma in adults: The EORTC 22845 randomised trial. *Lancet* 2005;366(9490):985–990.

138 Brainstem glioma

Ira J. Dunkel[1] and Mark M. Souweidane[2]

[1] Department of Pediatrics, Memorial Sloan Kettering Cancer Center, and Department of Pediatrics, New York Presbyterian Hospital Weill Cornell Medical College, New York, USA

[2] Department of Neurosurgery, Memorial Sloan Kettering Cancer Center, and Department of Neurological Surgery, New York Presbyterian Hospital Weill Cornell Medical College, New York, USA

Brainstem tumors are heterogeneous. They range from diffuse intrinsic pontine gliomas (DIPGs), which are almost invariably fatal despite all known therapies, to lower-grade focal or exophytic tumors, which often have a very good prognosis with surgery or observation only.

DIPGs, while rare, are a significant contributor to mortality among pediatric oncology patients. Diagnosis in typical cases is made via magnetic resonance imaging (MRI) scan, without biopsy. No highly effective standard treatment exists and so inclusion of eligible patients in well-designed clinical research studies is extremely important. If an appropriate trial is not available, conventionally fractionated external beam radiation therapy can provide good short-term palliation to a significant proportion of patients. Finally, autopsy should be considered for patients who die of DIPGs, with the goal of obtaining tumor tissue for biological studies that may in the future lead to novel therapies.

Epidemiology

About 30,000–40,000 children worldwide develop brain tumors each year. Data from the population-based German Childhood Cancer Registry reveal that 1 in 2,500 children will be diagnosed with a central nervous system tumor within the first 15 years of life, and from their data we can estimate that about 1 in 23,000 children will develop a DIPG by 15 years of age.

While rare, DIPGs represent a significant portion of deaths due to childhood cancer. The German registry included 16,826 pediatric oncology patients enrolled over a 10-year period. If we assume that 75% of the children were cured, then about 4,200 children died of all forms of cancer. There were 351 patients with tumors of the brainstem (not otherwise specified) and pons, and if we assume that 90% of those died, then they represent about 8% of total deaths due to childhood cancer.

Pathophysiology

Recent studies involving whole-genome DNA sequencing of DIPG tumors have revealed that mutations of the histone gene *H3.3* are common, occurring in about 80% of tumors. Other molecular aberrations that may be important include N-myc and PDGFR amplification and p53 and ACVR1 mutation.

Clinical features

Patients with DIPGs usually present with a short history (weeks) of signs or symptoms. The most common symptoms include double vision and gait instability. Physical examination typically reveals long tract signs, ataxia, and cranial neuropathies, particularly afflicting the sixth cranial nerve.

While this chapter focuses on DIPGs, it is important to realize that there are other types of brainstem tumors that should not be categorized with the highly lethal DIPGs. Cervicomedullary, dorsally exophytic, and focal brainstem tumors are usually grade I tumors and are associated with a better prognosis. Similarly, tumors in patients with a longer antecedent history of signs or symptoms and brainstem lesions in patients with neurofibromatosis type 1 often behave less aggressively.

Investigations

Brain MRI scan with and without gadolinium typically reveals infiltrative expansion of the pons, with high signal on T2 and fluid-attenuated inversion recovery (FLAIR) weighted images, little or no enhancement, and no significant exophytic component. Cystic changes are infrequently seen, while envelopment of the basilar artery is commonly present. Hydrocephalus is rarely present at the time of diagnosis.

Treatment

While treatment aims, of course, to provide a cure, the reality to date has been that therapy for DIPGs has almost always been palliative only. The current extremely poor prognosis of patients with DIPGs suggests that autopsies should be strongly considered to obtain tumor tissue that may allow us to improve our understanding of biological features of the tumor that may translate into new biologically based therapies.

Surgery

DIPGs are not surgically resectable and even diagnostic biopsy is not indicated for patients presenting with typical signs and symptoms and unequivocal MRI evidence of such a tumor. Prior to the advent of MRI, biopsy was performed, with the majority of tumors being World Health Organization (WHO) grade II–IV fibrillary astrocytomas. Autopsy series have demonstrated that at the time of death DIPGs are usually high-grade astrocytomas.

In contrast, biopsy should be considered if there is any suspicion that the lesion has atypical characteristics for a DIPG. Exophytic primary neuroectodermal tumors of the brainstem and focal low-grade brainstem tumors are two examples that would demand a different therapeutic approach.

Additionally, the recent recognition that DIPGs frequently harbor histone mutations and other molecular alterations may make biopsy reasonable when appropriate targeted therapies become available.

International Neurology, Second edition. Edited by Robert P. Lisak, Daniel D. Truong, William M. Carroll and Roongroj Bhidayasiri
© 2016 John Wiley & Sons, Ltd. Published 2016 by John Wiley & Sons, Ltd.

Radiation therapy

External beam radiation therapy is the standard therapy for DIPGs, but several cooperative group (Pediatric Oncology Group [POG] and Children's Cancer Group [CCG]) trials published in the early 1990s indicated that only approximately 10% of patients achieve 3-year survival despite dose escalation as high as 7800 cGy via hyperfractionation.

POG 9239 was a phase III trial of conventional radiation therapy versus hyperfractionated radiation therapy in children with newly diagnosed DIPGs. Conventionally treated patients received 5400 cGy in 180 cGy daily fractions, while patients on the experimental arm received 7020 cGy in 117 cGy fractions administered twice daily. Two-year survival rates were 7.1% and 6.7%, respectively.

Accelerated fractionation (conventional fraction doses administered twice daily, resulting in shorter total treatment duration) was studied in the United Kingdom. While the treatment was tolerable, it was also associated with very poor survival.

Multiple agents have been used in conjunction with radiation therapy, often as putative radiation sensitizers. Examples of this include high-dose tamoxifen, topotecan, and etanidazole. None has yet been demonstrated to be superior to radiation therapy alone, but clinical research in this area continues. There is some evidence that the combined use of external beam radiation therapy and radiosensitizers may actually be worse than radiation therapy alone. POG investigators non-randomly compared patients with DIPGs treated with hyperfractionated radiation therapy alone (7020 cGy) on POG 8495 with those treated with the same radiation therapy plus concurrent cisplatin on POG 9239. A strong trend was noted toward inferior 1-year survival among patients treated with combined therapy.

Outside of a clinical research protocol, standard radiation therapy should be considered as a single daily fractionated treatment (about 180 cGy/day) to a dose of approximately 5400–5940 cGy.

Chemotherapy

Conventional-dose chemotherapy (usually administered in conjunction with external beam radiation therapy) has not been effective for DIPGs.

Children's Oncology Group (COG) ACNS 0126 was a phase II trial of external beam radiation therapy (5940 cGy) and temozolomide chemotherapy for children with newly diagnosed DIPGs. In the trial, 63 patients received temozolomide (90 mg/m2/day × 42 days) during radiation therapy and 4 weeks post-radiation therapy began temozolomide (200 mg/m2/day × 5 days every 28 days) × 10 cycles. The 1-year event-free survival and overall survival were 14% (+/− 4.5%) and 40% (+/− 6.5%), respectively. The treatment was not considered to be more effective than previously studied regimens.

Additionally, high-dose thiotepa-based chemotherapy with stem cell rescue has been investigated and has not proven to be effective for DIPGs.

Adults

Adults may rarely present with brainstem tumors. The literature relevant to such patients is sparse, but there has been some suggestion that adults may survive significantly longer than children.

Emerging therapies

The blood–brain barrier presents a significant obstacle to achieving high tissue concentrations of therapeutic agents delivered systemically. Convection-enhanced delivery (CED) is a method of local delivery that bypasses the blood–brain barrier. CED is typically accomplished by inserting a small-bore cannula directly into a tumor, followed by infusion through the cannula. Experimental studies have revealed that local drug concentration exceeds that achieved with systemic administration several thousand-fold, while systemic exposure by way of efflux into the vasculature is negligible. CED can also be used for the delivery of large macromolecules such as monoclonal antibodies or targeted toxins, a feat not possible by systemic administration. The authors are currently conducting a phase I clinical study of 124-I-8H9 (a radiolabeled monoclonal antibody) in children with non-progressive DIPGs 4–14 weeks post-completion of external beam radiation therapy (NCT01502917).

Other lines of investigation are currently being studied in active clinical trials. Investigators at the Children's Hospital of Pittsburgh are studying a peptide vaccine in HLA-A2(+) children with DIPGs post-radiation therapy (NCT01130077). Investigators at the Dana-Farber Cancer Institute are leading a phase II trial based on biopsy results. Following biopsy of the DIPG, all of the participants are treated with external beam radiation therapy (5940 cGy) and bevacizumab; additionally, those whose tumors are O6-methylguanine-DNA methyltransferase (*MGMT*) hypermethylated receive temozolomide and those whose tumors express epidermal growth factor receptor (*EGFR*) receive erlotinib (NCT01182350). The Pediatric Brain Tumor Consortium is performing a phase I/II study (PBTC 033) of external beam radiation therapy (5400 cGy) with ABT-888 (a PARP inhibitor) followed by post-radiation temozolomide and ABT-888 (NCT01514201). It is too early to know whether any of these investigational approaches will prove to be beneficial, but we strongly support the participation of all children with DIPGs in well-designed clinical research trials that may allow progress to be made to improve the very inadequate therapies currently available.

Further reading

Albright AL, Packer RJ, Zimmerman R, *et al.* Magnetic resonance scans should replace biopsies for the diagnosis of diffuse brain stem gliomas: A report from the Children's Cancer Group. *Neurosurgery* 1993;33:1026–1030.

Buczkowicz P, Hoeman C, Rakopoulos P, *et al.* Genomic analysis of diffuse intrinsic pontine gliomas identifies three molecular subgroups and recurrent activating ACVR1 mutations. *Nat Genet* 2014;46:451–456.

Cohen KJ, Heideman RL, Zhou T, *et al.* Temozolomide in the treatment of children with newly diagnosed diffuse intrinsic pontine gliomas: A report from the Children's Oncology Group. *Neuro-Oncology* 2011;13:410–416.

Fisher PG, Breiter SN, Carson BS, *et al.* A clinicopathologic reappraisal of brain stem tumor classification: Identification of pilocytic astrocytoma and fibrillary astrocytoma as distinct entities. *Cancer* 2000;89:1569–1576.

Landolfi JC, Thaler HT, DeAngelis LM. Adult brainstem gliomas. *Neurol* 1998;51:1136–1139.

139 Intracranial ependymoma

Marc C. Chamberlain

Department of Neurology and Neurological Surgery, University of Washington, Seattle, WA, USA

Ependymomas arise from the ependymal cells of the cerebral ventricles, the central canal of the spinal cord, and cortical rests. Ependymomas constitute 8–10% of brain tumors in children and 1–3% of brain tumors in adults; 60% of ependymomas occur in children under 16 years of age and 25% occur in children under 4 years of age. Tumors arising in the supratentorial compartment (50–60% of adult ependymomas; 30% of pediatric ependymomas) most often are hemispheric or occur in relation to the third ventricle. Posterior fossa tumors either are seen in a midline fourth ventricular location (40–50%) or are located in the cerebellopontine angle (50–60%).

The World Health Organization (WHO) classification of tumors separates ependymomas into subependymomas (grade 1), myxopapillary ependymomas (grade 1), ependymomas (grade 2), and anaplastic ependymomas (grade 3). Ependymoblastomas are considered a different type of tumor, classified under embryonal primitive neuroectodermal tumors (PNET).

Approximately 30% of all intracranial ependymomas are anaplastic, although the prognostic significance of anaplasia is controversial. Part of this uncertainty relates to the lack of uniform histological criteria for diagnosing anaplastic ependymomas. Defining tumors as anaplastic based on proliferation indices such as Ki67 staining more than 1% may permit stratification of patients at high risk for recurrence and decreased survival.

Cerebrospinal fluid (CSF) dissemination occurs in 3–12% of all intracranial ependymomas and is most frequent with infratentorial anaplastic ependymomas. Because a small but measurable risk for CSF dissemination exists for all patients with newly diagnosed ependymoma, an extent of disease evaluation including CSF cytology and craniospinal magnetic resonance imaging (MRI) is required following surgery. Staging permits stratification of patients into those with (M+) or without (M0) metastasis and with or without residual disease following surgery, the two most important clinical parameters affecting outcome.

Chromosomal number alterations have been described (6p, 9p, and 22q loss; 9q, 15q, and 18 gain) in ependymomas and appear to have prognostic significance. In addition to copy number alterations, gene expression analysis suggests that subdivision of ependymoma into genomic subgroups (three categories in supratentorial and two in infratentorial ependymoma) is prognostic and may in the future define novel molecular targets for drug therapy.

Treatment

Intracranial ependymomas often present with signs and symptoms of raised intracranial pressure (headache, alteration in level of consciousness, nausea/vomiting, diplopia, gait instability, papilledema, meningismus) due to either tumor mass or obstructive hydrocephalus.

Surgery

Treatment is primarily surgical, as essentially all analyses have determined that completeness of surgical resection is the most important covariate affecting progression-free and overall survival. As a consequence, if initial surgery is found to be incomplete or at time of tumor recurrence, reoperation is advocated if complete resection is achievable.

Postoperative complications are not uncommon and should be anticipated. It has been estimated that about 33% of adult patients develop new cranial nerve abnormalities after resection of infratentorial ependymomas, often with dysphagia requiring gastrostomy tube placement. Most deficits resolve with time and support. The posterior fossa syndrome (cerebellar mutism) following an infratentorial craniotomy in children is a well-defined yet infrequent complication.

Following surgery, the issue of how often to image patients is unclear. It is generally accepted that surveillance neuroimaging can reveal asymptomatic recurrences and that its use has a favorable impact on survival and subsequent treatment, in particular the ability to perform a reoperation with complete resection.

Radiotherapy

After resection, radiotherapy represents the most frequently utilized adjuvant treatment for ependymomas, despite the lack of a randomized clinical trial showing benefit and the belief that ependymomas are radioresistant. Furthermore, there are no data regarding a dose–response relationship in ependymomas and, as such, total tumor dose has varied. By consensus, many radiation oncologists believe that a tumor dose exceeding 45 Gray (Gy) is necessary and most advocate a dose of 54–55 Gy for ependymomas and 60 Gy for anaplastic ependymomas. Because of the possibility of CSF spread, one controversy regarding the radiotherapeutic management of ependymomas is the volume of brain that needs to be treated. Notwithstanding early enthusiasm for craniospinal irradiation (CSI), several recent studies support limited-field radiotherapy for M0 tumors and reserve CSI for M+ tumors. There are advocates for observation only following complete resection for supratentorial ependymomas (withholding radiotherapy); however, this is based on case series and has not been rigorously evaluated. Conformal radiotherapy including stereotactic radiotherapy is increasingly utilized despite few studies showing survival or quality-of-life benefits. A radiotherapy boost following conventional radiotherapy (most often administered by linear accelerator [LINAC] radiosurgery, gamma knife, or cyberknife) is increasingly utilized outside of clinical trials. This is based on the assumption that the radioresistance of ependymomas is relative and that by increasing dose to the tumor, radioresistance may be overcome. Also, given that the majority of ependymoma treatment failures are local, augmenting tumor radio-

International Neurology, Second edition. Edited by Robert P. Lisak, Daniel D. Truong, William M. Carroll and Roongroj Bhidayasiri
© 2016 John Wiley & Sons, Ltd. Published 2016 by John Wiley & Sons, Ltd.

Table 139.1 Chemotherapy trials in newly diagnosed and recurrent ependymoma. Source: Chowdhary 2006. Reproduced with permission of Springer

No. of patients	Chemo regimen	Progression-free survival	Overall survival
66	CYC+VCR/CDDP+VP16	41% at 1 year	NR
19	CBDCA+VCR/IFOS+VP16	74% at 5 years	NR
32	Randomized to CCNU+VCR+PRED or 8 in 1 regimen	50% at 5 years	64% at 5 years
73	PCZ+CBDCA/VP16+CDDP/VCR+CYC	22% at 4 years	59% at 4 years
83	PCZ+CBDCA/VP16+CDDP/VCR+CYC	48% at 5 years	46% at 10 years
		68% at 5 years	47% at 10 years
8	CYC+VCR+VP16	13% at 3 years	32% at 3 years

No. of patients	Chemo regimen	Response rate	Stable disease
12	PCV	15%	NR
16	HDC+ABMT	0%	63%
5	Etoposide	40%	NR
15	HDC+ABMT	0%	0%
16	Platinum or nitrosurea	67% and 25%	30% and 50%
12	Etoposide	17%	30%
13	Paclitaxel	6%	37%
10 (SCE)	Etoposide	20%	50%
13	Cisplatin	30%	46%
8	Bevacizumab	75%	0%

8 in 1 regimen: VP16+CBDCA+PCV+MOPP (mechlorethamine+vincristine+prednisone+procarbazine) alternating with CYC+VCR+CDDP+VP16+ABMT; ABMT = autologous bone marrow transplantation; CBDCA = carboplatin; CCNU = lomustine; CDDP = cisplatin; CYC = cyclophosphamide; HDC = high-dose chemotherapy; IFOS = ifosfamide; NR = not reported; PCV = procarbazine, CCNU, and vincristine; PCZ = procarbazine; PRED = prednisone; SCE = spinal cord ependymoma; VCR = vincristine; VP16 = etoposide

therapy dose may improve long-term control. Despite an appealing construct, the lack of an established dose–response relationship for ependymomas following radiotherapy and the empirical observation that measurable neuroradiographic responses are rare suggest that more is not necessarily better.

Chemotherapy

The role of chemotherapy in the management of ependymomas is controversial (Table 139.1). In newly diagnosed adults or children, most studies suggest either no additional benefit after surgery and CSI or only modest efficacy. Patients who received postsurgical chemotherapy in lieu of radiation have poorer survival than those who received adjuvant radiation, also supporting the absence of a primary role for chemotherapy in this disease.

Recurrent ependymoma

The management of recurrent ependymoma has not received much attention, despite the fact that nearly 50% of patients will have a recurrence. In general, median time to recurrence is about 3 years and in the majority of cases the relapse is local, with a small percentage having local recurrence with concomitant distant metastasis. Reoperation should be considered, followed by radiation, if possible. Most patients will also receive chemotherapy at relapse. Numerous regimens have been explored, with cisplatin often felt to be the most active agent among the four commonly used chemotherapeutics (cisplatin, procarbazine, 1-(2-chloroethyl)-3-cyclohexyl-1-nitrosourea (CCNU), and vincristine).

Conclusion

Optimal management of ependymomas includes surgical resection and evaluation of the extent of central nervous system (CNS) involvement using both CSF cytology and craniospinal contrast-enhanced MRI. In patients not considered for further surgery and with residual disease, limited-field radiotherapy is usually administered. Craniospinal irradiation is reserved for patients with CSF-disseminated disease. The majority of tumor recurrences are local and at the site of the primary tumor. No clear role for adjuvant chemotherapy has been demonstrated. Recurrent ependymomas are managed by reoperation of tumors that are surgically accessible, by radiotherapy (either conformal re-radiation or stereotactic radiotherapy), and by salvage chemotherapy.

Further reading

Chowdhary, et al. Ependymomas. In. *Curr Treat Options Neurol* 2006; 8 (4): 309–318.

Mack SC, Witt H, Wang X, *et al.* Emerging insights into the ependymoma epigenome. *Brain Pathol* 2013;23(2):206–209.

Nagasawa DT, Trang A, Choy W, *et al.* Genetic expression profiles of adult and pediatric ependymomas: Molecular pathways, prognostic indicators, and therapeutic targets. *Clin Neurol Neurosurg* 2013;115(4):388–399.

Paulino AC, Wen BC, Buatti JM, *et al.* Intracranial ependymomas: An analysis of prognostic factors and patterns of failure. *Am J Clin Oncol* 2002;25:117–122.

Raghunathan A, Wani K, Armstrong TS, *et al.* Histological predictors of outcome in ependymoma are dependent on anatomic site within the central nervous system. *Brain Pathol* 2013;23(5):584–594.

Reni M, Gatta G, Mazza E, Vecht C. Ependymoma. *Crit Rev Oncol Hematol* 2007;63(1):81–89.

140 | Nerve sheath tumors

Nathan J. Ranalli[1], Zarina S. Ali[2], Gregory G. Heuer[2], and Eric L. Zager[2]

[1] University of Florida Health Science Center – Jacksonville and Division of Pediatric Neurological Surgery at Lucy Gooding Pediatric Neurosurgery Center, Jacksonville, FL, USA

[2] Department of Neurosurgery, University of Pennsylvania, Philadelphia, PA, USA

Nerve sheath tumors represent an intriguing group of tumors that may affect any peripheral, cranial, or autonomic nerve. There is great variation in terms of tumor location, clinical presentation, and treatment strategy. It is important to separate nerve sheath tumors into two categories: (1) benign nerve sheath tumors, which include most commonly schwannomas and neurofibromas; and (2) malignant peripheral nerve sheath tumors (MPNSTs). Although most nerve sheath tumors are solitary lesions arising from single nerves, they may also be associated with global genetic disorders, such as neurofibromatosis type one (NF-1) or type two (NF-2), in which case there may be multiple tumors involving different nerves. During the past half-century, the introduction of the operative microscope and intraoperative neurophysiological monitoring along with the wide availability of magnetic resonance imaging (MRI) have contributed significantly to improvement in surgical outcomes. Here, we present a review of the characteristics, diagnosis, and treatment options for common nerve sheath tumors.

Epidemiology and pathophysiology

The incidence, etiology, and effects of nerve sheath tumors differ greatly between benign and malignant, as well as sporadic versus inherited, subtypes. As such, we will discuss schwannomas and neurofibromas, MPNSTs, and neurofibromatosis individually.

Benign nerve sheath tumors

Schwannomas

The schwannoma is one of the two most common histological types of benign nerve sheath tumors affecting the nervous system. These lesions can occur at any age, but are most common in the third to sixth decades, are seen equally in men and women, and represent 5% of all benign soft-tissue neoplasms. Over 50% of all schwannomas are located in the head and neck and they may originate from any of the cranial, peripheral, or autonomic nerves. Most of these tumors are indolent and generally painless, although patients may present with a radiculopathy or paresthesias secondary to compression of an adjacent nerve. Schwannomas arise from Schwann cells, occurring within the endoneurium, and are surrounded by a capsule of perineurium and fibrous epineurium; they do not contain axons. Most schwannomas are solitary, although multiple or plexiform schwannomas may be found in association with neu-

rofibromatosis and schwannomatosis. In schwannomatosis, these tumors occur without concomitant involvement of the vestibular nerves and may occur by distinct molecular mechanisms.

Microscopically, schwannomas are composed of a distinctive pattern of Schwann cells arranged into sections of Antoni A (spindle-shaped cells oriented in sheets and palisades within pathognomonic Verocay bodies) and Antoni B (loose myxoid matrix with collagen fibrils and rare spindle cells and lymphocytes) areas.

Neurofibromas

The neurofibroma is the other most common nerve sheath tumor, having a peak incidence in the third to fifth decades with equivalent predilection for men and women. Recently, a high prevalence of autism spectrum disorder has been associated with NF-1. Neurofibromas arise from the perineurial cells of the nerve sheath and are not encapsulated. They may occur in isolation, but are frequently multiple, especially in cases associated with NF-1 (Figure 140.1). Solitary neurofibromas can occur on peripheral nerves throughout the body and are often visible as small subcutaneous nodules.

Generally, neurofibromas can be divided into three subtypes: localized, diffuse, and plexiform. The first of these represents nearly 90% of all neurofibromas in patients without NF-1. Diffuse neurofibromas are rarely seen, but occur almost exclusively in children and young adults. Plexiform neurofibromas, which have the appearance of a thick, convoluted bulbous mass, are pathognomonic for NF-1. Histologically, neurofibromas are composed of intercalated bundles of fusiform, elongated cells with darkly staining nuclei surrounded by a matrix containing collagen fibrils, mucoid deposits, lymphocytes, and xanthoma cells.

Malignant peripheral nerve sheath tumors

MPNSTs are highly malignant, rare tumors with an incidence of 0.001% in the general US population. More than 50% of patients with MPNSTs have NF-1 and the ratio of men to women affected is equal. MPNSTs are really a form of soft-tissue sarcoma and account for 5–10% of these tumors overall. The World Health Organization (WHO) has defined MPNSTs as any malignant tumor arising from a peripheral nerve or exhibiting nerve sheath differentiation, excluding those originating from the epineurium or from peripheral nerve vasculature. Older terms for these lesions have included neurofibrosarcoma, malignant neurilemmoma, malignant schwannoma,

International Neurology, Second edition. Edited by Robert P. Lisak, Daniel D. Truong, William M. Carroll and Roongroj Bhidayasiri
© 2016 John Wiley & Sons, Ltd. Published 2016 by John Wiley & Sons, Ltd.

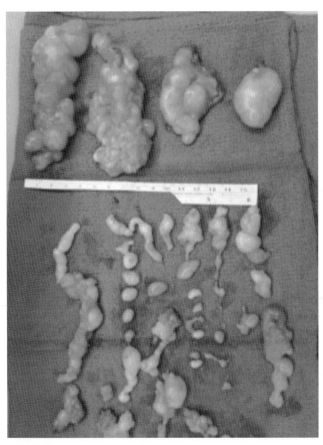

Figure 140.1 Multiple plexiform neurofibromas resected from a patient with NF-1.

and neurogenic sarcoma. These neoplasms usually present as a painful, enlarging mass, most typically located deep in the trunk, extremities, or head and neck region.

Two major risk factors for developing MPNSTs are NF-1 and a prior history of radiation. Patients with NF-1 typically develop tumors in the third and fourth decades, while those with sporadic MPNSTs are more frequently affected in the fifth and sixth decades. The average latency period for development of a radiation-induced MPNST is 15 years.

Microscopically, most of the MPNSTs are comprised of spindle cells with markedly increased cellularity, nuclear pleomorphism, mitotic figures, hemorrhage, and necrosis.

Neurofibromatosis

Neurofibromatosis is one of the most common genetic disorders, occurring in nearly 1 in 3,000 live births. The disease can be classified based on gene locus and associated characteristics into two major subtypes: NF-1 (Von Recklinghausen's disease) and NF-2.

NF-1

NF-1 has an incidence of 1 in 2,500 at birth regardless of gender and accounts for 90% of all neurofibromatosis patients. The *NF1* gene has been localized to chromosome 17 and the syndrome can be caused by an inherited or new mutation in this gene. NF-1 is characterized clinically by neurocutaneous findings (café-au-lait spots, axillary freckling), superficial neurofibromas, and iris hamartomas (Lisch nodules). This disease also has a variety of effects on the ocular,

musculoskeletal, endocrine, and vascular systems. Nearly all individuals with NF-1 will develop peripheral neurofibromas (any of the three subtypes) at some time and are at increased risk for MPNSTs, optic gliomas, and childhood leukemia.

NF-2

NF-2 is much less common than NF-1, occurring in 1 in 33,000 live births. The *NF2* gene has been localized to chromosome 22 and the inactivation of a tumor suppressor leads to the generation of multiple neural tumors seen in this disorder. Another type of nerve sheath tumor, a perineurioma, has been described as a benign tumor of neuroplastic perineural cells, according to the current WHO classification of nervous system tumors; initial molecular findings also implicate chromosome 22 abnormalities, although perineurioma is not considered part of the NF-2 disease spectrum. The diagnostic hallmark of NF-2 is the presence of bilateral eighth cranial nerve schwannomas, which occur in over 95% of NF-2 cases. These patients often have multiple cranial and spinal schwannomas as well as meningiomas; spontaneous malignant transformation of a schwannoma to an MPNST rarely occurs.

Clinical features and investigations

Signs and symptoms in a patient with a nerve sheath tumor are variable and depend on the location of the tumor as well as the extent of nerve compression or mass effect that it causes. Presenting complaints include local or radiating discomfort, paresthesias, weakness, autonomic dysfunction, and cosmetic deformity. Key features of the history include the rate of growth of the lesion, the presence of neurological complaints or severe pain, a personal or family history of neurofibromatosis or any of its stigmata, and the presence of other masses or systemic diseases. Physical examination should focus on the size and location of the tumor, the extent of tenderness and ease of mobility, Tinel's sign (which can be present in both benign and malignant processes), and neurological deficit. Pigmentary abnormalities such as café-au-lait spots and skinfold freckling are the most obvious clinical features of NF-1. A rapidly enlarging, deep, or very painful lesion is more suggestive of a malignant tumor, particularly in the presence of significant neurological deficits.

With regard to radiographic evaluation, MRI is currently the most important imaging modality in the evaluation of the anatomic and pathological characteristics of peripheral nerve sheath tumors. MRI is particularly helpful in delineating the relationships among the lesion, the nerve of origin, and the surrounding vessels, bone, and soft tissues. Neurofibromas frequently show inhomogenous enhancement with gadolinium, while small schwannomas tend to enhance uniformly. Degenerative cyst formation may be seen in schwannomas; this finding does not necessarily indicate malignancy. In some cases the ragged, invasive margin of an MPNST can be demonstrated on MRI, but this finding is not reliably present. A recent modification of MRI, known as MR neurography, can be useful in select cases in discriminating between intraneural and perineural masses. Preoperative electromyography (EMG) may provide evidence of nerve involvement and help define the baseline function of the target nerve. Ultrasonography can support clinical and electrophysiological testing for the detection of a nerve sheath tumor as a hypoechoic lesion with well-defined contours, but it is usually not as helpful as MRI in providing anatomic detail around the tumor itself. In cases of deep nerve sheath tumors, ultrasound can be used intraoperatively to localize the lesion for incision placement.

Treatment

Options for the treatment of nerve sheath tumors include conservative management, surgical resection, radiation, and chemotherapy. Small, non-painful, indolent tumors that cause neither neurological dysfunction nor cosmetic concern can be monitored. For patients with neurofibromatosis or schwannomatosis, these asymptomatic tumors should be monitored with serial MRI studies, typically on an annual basis. Surgery is indicated for lesions that cause deficits or pain, or for any rapidly growing tumors that raise suspicion of malignancy. Surgical resection is the treatment of choice for most benign nerve sheath tumors and complete resection usually results in a cure. Surgical goals include the resolution of pain, preservation of neurological function, correction of a cosmetic deformity, and attainment of a diagnosis. Recently, there has been an emphasis on optimizing patient-reported outcomes in patients with nerve sheath tumors. Specifically, a recent international trial identified that the most important endpoint domains for neurofibromatosis clinical trials are pain, functional ability, disease-specific quality of life (QOL), and general QOL.

The surgical approach is optimized to preserve the nerve of origin and to avoid any additional nerve injury. If a functional nerve fascicle has to be sacrificed during tumor removal, grafting should be considered to achieve good functional recovery (alternatively, a small portion of tumor should be left in place and followed in order to preserve nerve function). Sacrifice of an entire nerve segment should virtually never occur in the setting of a benign tumor. Benign solitary symptomatic neurofibromas and schwannomas can usually be completely resected and that results in a cure, especially with the refinement of microsurgical techniques.

MPNSTs carry a high risk of local invasion, recurrence, and metastasis to lung, liver, bone, and soft tissue. Therefore, if a lesion is suspicious for malignancy, the recommended procedure is an open biopsy to obtain tissue diagnosis and to guide further therapy. Percutaneous needle biopsy is also a viable option, but there are notorious problems with sampling error, non-diagnostic tissue, nerve injury, and exquisite pain during and/or after the procedure. If the diagnosis of MPNST is confirmed, treatment involves wide resection (occasionally including appendicular amputation) followed or preceded by adjuvant chemotherapy and radiation to help provide local control and delay the onset of recurrence. The prognosis of MPNST is poor; tumor size is a significant predictor of survival. In the future, biological therapies directed at relevant genetic alterations and new pharmaceutical agents will ultimately lead to novel therapeutic strategies to treat these difficult tumors.

Further reading

Gutmann DH, Aylsworth A, Carey JC, *et al.* The diagnostic evaluation and multidisciplinary management of neurofibromatosis 1 and neurofibromatosis 2. *JAMA* 1997;278(1):51–57.

Huang JH, Zaghloul K, Zager EL. Surgical management of brachial plexus region tumors. *Surg Neurol* 2004;61(4):372–378.

Perrin RG, Guha A. Malignant peripheral nerve sheath tumors. *Neurosurg Clin N Am* 2004;15(2):203–216.

Pilavaki M, Chourmouzi D, Kiziridou A, *et al.* Imaging of peripheral nerve sheath tumors with pathologic correlation: Pictorial review. *Eur J Radiol* 2004;5(3):229–239.

Tiel R, Kline D. Peripheral nerve tumors: Surgical principles, approaches and techniques. *Neurosurg Clin N Am* 2004:15(2):167–175.

141 Meningiomas

Jeffrey Raizer and Simran Singh
Department of Neurology, Northwestern University, Chicago, IL, USA

Meningiomas are typically slow-growing dural-based tumors arising from arachnoid cap cells. They are frequently an incidental finding when a magnetic resonance imaging (MRI) or computed tomography (CT) scan of the brain has been ordered for other neurological evaluations, or are found on autopsy. Meningiomas are the most common type of all primary intracranial tumors. Although the vast majority (70–80%) of these tumors are benign, they can recur and cause significant morbidity depending on the location.

Epidemiology

The overall incidence of intracranial meningiomas is 2–6/100,000, representing 13–30% of all primary intracranial tumors in adults. Spinal meningiomas make up about 10% of all meningiomas. Meningiomas occur predominantly in patients in their fifth to eighth decades of life and are twice as common in women as in men. Multiple meningiomas are seen in approximately 8% of patients.

The etiology of meningiomas is not clearly understood, but patients who have had prior cranial radiation seem to be at risk; usually they present after a couple of decades with multiple meningiomas, mainly of grade II or III. Patients with some familial and genetic disorders, in particular neurofibromatosis (NF) type 2, are also at risk. Sporadic meningiomas are typically associated with one or more focal chromosomal deletions. Atypical and malignant grades tend to have multiple chromosomal alterations.

Pathophysiology

Meningiomas are thought to arise from arachnoid cap cells, which form the outer layer of the arachnoid mater and the arachnoid villi. The most frequent genetic abnormality in meningiomas is the loss of the chromosomal region (22q, 12.2) of the *NF2*, gene as seen in patients with NF, but also in patients with sporadic meningiomas. This gene codes for a protein called Merlin or Schwannomin, which regulates cell growth and motility. Other genetic aberrations in the signaling pathways are well described and more prevalent with higher-grade meningiomas. These genetic changes are part of the transformation that occurs from a grade I to a grade III meningioma. In addition, 6q and 14q loss is associated with recurrent or atypical meningiomas.

Gonadal hormones

Cell growth and multiplication are controlled by growth factors, hormones, and their receptors. The role of gonadal hormones in meningioma development and growth is suggested by the higher incidence in females. Meningiomas may increase in size during pregnancy and increased incidence has been seen in women who use hormone replacement therapy. Low concentrations of estrogen receptors are seen in approximately 30% of meningiomas and 70% have progesterone receptors. Progesterone receptors tend to decrease in meningiomas that undergo malignant transformation. Somatostatin receptors are also found in 70–100% of meningiomas; their role is unknown. Although there appears to be an association between the use of hormone replacement therapy and increased meningioma risk, there is no definitive evidence of risk with the use of oral contraception.

Histology

Meningiomas can exhibit both epithelial and mesenchymal features that can be diagnostically useful. For example, the epithelial phenotype is most prominent in the secretory variant of meningioma. Epithelial cells express epithelial membrane antigen (EMA). In contrast, the mesenchymal phenotype is most prominent in fibroblastic subtypes of benign meningiomas. Mesenchymal cells have spindle-cell morphology and produce collagen.

The World Health Organization (WHO) has distinguished 16 histological variants of meningiomas falling into three grade designations. WHO grade I (benign meningiomas) account for approximately 60–75% of cases. Meningothelial, fibrous, and transitional meningiomas are the most common grade I meningiomas. WHO grade II (atypical meningiomas) make up 15–20% of meningiomas and are based on greater than four mitoses per high-powered field (HPF). If the mitotic rate is not elevated, then at least three of the following other characteristics are required for a grade II diagnosis: sheet architecture, high nuclear-to-cytoplasmic ratio, hypercellularity, or necrosis. Of note is that brain-invasive meningiomas, even if otherwise benign in appearance, should be regarded as WHO grade II. WHO grade III (anaplastic meningiomas) account for 3–5% of cases. These tumors have either more than 20 mitoses per HPF or the presence of frank anaplasia. The average survival is less than 2 years.

Clinical presentation

Meningiomas are often asymptomatic and have slow growth. The most common presenting symptoms are seizures (seen in 30–70% of patients) and headaches. The location of the meningioma determines the neurological symptoms. Tumors compressing the cerebrum can cause focal symptoms such as weakness or visual field deficits. Meningiomas compressing the cerebellum may cause ataxia or symptoms related to increased intracranial pressure. Meningiomas of the skull base can cause cranial neuropathies.

International Neurology, Second edition. Edited by Robert P. Lisak, Daniel D. Truong, William M. Carroll and Roongroj Bhidayasiri
© 2016 John Wiley & Sons, Ltd. Published 2016 by John Wiley & Sons, Ltd.

Investigations

On head CT, the typical appearance of meningioma is a well-defined extra-axial mass that displaces normal brain tissue. The lesions may exhibit calcification, a smooth contour, and uniform enhancement with contrast. The presence of indistinct margins, marked edema, or deep parenchymal infiltration suggests aggressive behavior. MRI is the preferred method of imaging. Meningiomas on MRI are usually isointense to gray matter on T1- and hyperintense on T2-weighted images. There is homogenous enhancement with gadolinium. The characteristic sign of most meningiomas is the tapered thickening called a "dural tail" (Figure 141.1). MR venogram may show occlusion when a meningioma abuts a dural sinus. On catheter angiography, meningiomas classically exhibit tumor blush.

Treatment

The treatment may include active observation, surgical resection, radiotherapy, chemotherapy, or a combination of these. The choice of therapy depends on performance status, medical comorbidities, the presence of symptoms, and tumor characteristics (location, size, and grade). Observation may be indicated in cases of asymptomatic, small tumors.

Surgery

For tumors deemed non-resectable, biopsy only may be done for histological grading. Surgical resection, either partial or complete, is preferred for meningiomas with disease progression, mass effect, and those causing symptoms. Longer survival has been observed among patients who undergo complete resection compared to those who undergo partial resection. For large vascular meningiomas, an

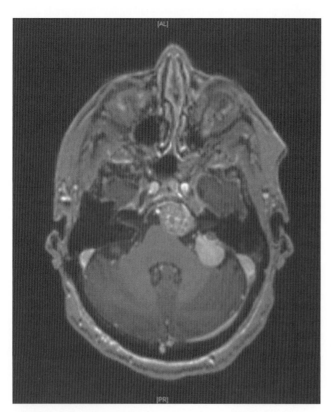

Figure 141.1 Postcontrast T1 magnetic resonance image showing 2 meningiomas abutting the left-side brainstem and cerebellum.

angiogram with embolization of the arterial feeders is often done to minimize bleeding. The complete removal of the tumor cures most patients with WHO grade I (benign) meningiomas. The probability of recurrence is less than 5% 5 years after the operation. Patients with grade III meningiomas should have as much tumor removed as feasible, given the very high rate of recurrence. Current data also support surgery for recurrent tumors.

Radiation

The method of radiation therapy (RT) employed for the treatment of meningiomas includes external beam (EBRT), stereotactic radiosurgery (SRS), and intensity modulated radiation therapy (IMRT). The purpose of RT is to slow the growth of the tumor. Adjuvant RT is indicated in cases of incomplete surgical resection and/or grade II or III meningiomas due to the greater risk of local recurrence. SRS is a technique that delivers a single-fraction dose with rapid decline of radiation around the target volume, thereby protecting adjacent tissues. To be a candidate for SRS, the tumor should be smaller than 3 cm and well circumscribed.

Chemotherapy

Grade II and III meningiomas have a high rate of recurrence despite surgical removal and radiotherapy. Less often, even grade I tumors can progress to high-grade lesions when they recur. These more aggressive, recurrent tumors may require medical therapy beyond surgery and radiation. Classes of agents used against meningiomas include cytotoxic agents, hormonal agents, targeted molecular agents, and angiogenesis inhibitors.

Hydroxyurea has been a standard therapy for meningiomas refractory to resection and radiation based on several small studies that have shown modest benefit, but recent data suggest limited activity. Hydroxyurea arrests meningioma cell growth in the S phase of the cell cycle and induces apoptosis. Results from trials investigating other chemotherapy agents including temozolomide and irinotecan have been disappointing.

Based on the variable expression of hormone receptors in meningiomas, chemotherapy-based regimens against such receptors have been studied. Estrogen receptor inhibitors, specifically tamoxifen, have had disappointing results. Similarly, mifepristone, a progesterone receptor inhibitor, failed to demonstrate benefit. Somatostatin receptors are expressed in almost 90% of meningiomas. Somatostatin or its analogues may have promise in the subset of patients demonstrating somatostatin receptor positivity on octreotide scintigraphy.

More recently, targeted molecular therapies against platelet-derived growth factor (PDGF), epidermal growth factor (EGF), and vascular endothelial growth factor (VEGF) receptors have been investigated. Therapies directed against the PDGF receptor (such as imatinib) and EGF receptor have not demonstrated proven efficacy. VEGF inhibitors may have an impact on meningioma growth because of the known hypervascularity of these tumors. Bevacizumab (a VEGF inhibitor) and sunitinib (a VEGF and PDGF inhibitor) are currently undergoing clinical study to determine whether there is benefit in the recurrent setting. For recurrent meningiomas requiring medical therapy, the United States CNS National Comprehensive Cancer Network guidelines recommend three agents: hydroxyurea, IFN-a, and monthly long-acting somatostatin (Sandostatin), although the data supporting the guidelines are weak. Molecular profiling of meningiomas is a relatively new area of research that will likely identify new targets for therapy.

Outcomes

Ten-year overall survival and progression free survival for WHO grade I meningiomas are 90% and 87%, respectively. Rates of recurrence increase with increasing grade. The recurrence rate for benign (grade I) meningiomas is 7–20%, for grade II meningiomas 20–40%, and for anaplastic meningiomas (grade III) it is 50–78%. Survival decreases with increased grade; grade I meningiomas are cured in most cases, while patients with grade III meningiomas survive less than 2 years after diagnosis.

Further reading

Mawrin C, Perry A. Pathologic classification and molecular genetics of meningiomas. *J Neurooncol* 2010;99:379–391.

Moazzam AA, Wagle N, Zada G. Recent developments in chemotherapy for meningiomas: A review. *Neurosurg Focus* 2013;35(6):E18,1–10.

Nader G, Sebastiao M, Miranda F, *et al.* Meningioma: Review of the literature with emphasis on the approach to radiotherapy. *Expert Rev Anticancer Ther* 2011;11(11):1749–1758.

Sherman WJ, Raizer JJ. Chemotherapy: What's its role in meningioma? *Expert Rev Neurother* 2012;12(10):1189–1196.

Wiemels J, Wrensch M, Claus EB. Epidemiology and etiology of meningioma. *J Neurooncol* 2010;99:307–314.

142 Adult medulloblastoma

Alba A. Brandes[1], Regina I. Jakacki[2], and Enrico Franceschi[1]

[1] Department of Medical Oncology, Bellaria Hospital, Azienda USL – IRCCS Institute of Neurological Science, Bologna, Italy
[2] Neuro-Oncology Program, Children's Hospital of Pittsburgh, Pittsburgh, PA, USA

Medulloblastoma is the most common central nervous system (CNS) tumor in children, while it is extremely rare in adults.

Few evidence-based guidelines are available for the treatment of adult medulloblastoma. Therapeutic regimens, typically modeled following pediatric protocols, consist of surgical resection followed by radiotherapy with or without adjuvant chemotherapy. Because of the rarity of this disease in adults, any treatment undertaken is based mainly on small and retrospective studies. An important challenge for the future will be the biological characterization of medulloblastoma in adults, with the identification of specific genetic patterns of patients with different prognosis and different response to targeted treatments.

Epidemiology

The incidence of medulloblastoma in adults (>18 years of age) has been estimated around 0.6–1 patient per million. Thus, this tumor type is extremely rare in adults, representing 1% of CNS tumors, whereas it is the most common malignant brain neoplasm in childhood, accounting for between 15% and 25% of all childhood CNS neoplasms. The difference in incidence between adult and pediatric patients is the reason for the different amount of data available from pediatric and adult studies, as well as the lack of evidence-based approaches; thus only a few centers have achieved sufficient expertise to treat this type of rare tumor in adults.

Since 1981, adult 5-year overall survival (OS) has increased up to 67%. These data seem to be consistent with those obtained from a large retrospective series that evaluated adults showing a 5-year OS in the range of 70%. Similarly, data from the only prospective trial in adults showed a 5-year OS of about 75%.

Clinical features

At magnetic resonance imaging (MRI), medulloblastoma typically appears iso- to hypointense depending on white matter on T1-weighted images. The T2 signal is variable, ranging from hyperintense to hypointense in relation to gray matter. Contrast enhancement of medulloblastoma is usually present to a heterogeneous degree and extent.

Medulloblastoma is found in the midline cerebellum in more than 75% of pediatric patients, while it is more likely to be found within the cerebellar hemispheres in older children and adults.

Investigations

Staging

Standard staging procedures include diagnostic imaging with brain MRI, which should be performed before surgery to evaluate location, dimension, and/or intracranial metastases. Cerebrospinal fluid (CSF) cytology and MRI of the spinal canal are necessary to detect possible metastatic spread, and to avoid misinterpretation of the postsurgical neuroradiological picture (i.e., bleeding). Surgical information and imaging data allow staging to be carried out according to the Chang system (Table 142.1). If CSF cytology was found to be positive within the first 7–10 days after surgery, a repeat spinal tap should be performed 3 weeks after surgery to avoid false positive results.

Tumor biology

Adult and pediatric patients display significant differences in terms of tumor biology, chemotherapy tolerance, and potential long-term side effects, which led to the development of distinct treatment approaches.

Table 142. Chang's staging system. Source: Chang 1969. Reproduced with permission of RSNA.

T stage	
T1	Tumor < 3 cm in diameter
T2	Tumor > 3 cm in diameter
T3a	Tumor > 3 cm with extension into aqueduct of Sylvius or foramen of Luschka
T3b	Tumor > 3 cm with unequivocal extension into the brainstem
T4	Tumor > 3 cm with extension past aqueduct of Sylvius or down past foramen magnum
M stage	
M0	No evidence of gross subarachnoid or hematogenous metastasis
M1	Microscopic tumor cells found in CSF
M2	Gross nodular seeding intracranial^ beyond the primary site (in cerebellar/cerebral subarachnoid space or in third or lateral ventricle)
M3	Gross nodular seeding in spinal subarachnoid space
M4	Metastasis outside cerebrospinal axis

Abbreviation: CSF, cerebrospinal fluid.

International Neurology, Second edition. Edited by Robert P. Lisak, Daniel D. Truong, William M. Carroll and Roongroj Bhidayasiri
© 2016 John Wiley & Sons, Ltd. Published 2016 by John Wiley & Sons, Ltd.

During the past few years, transcriptional profiling has uncovered the existence of distinct molecular subgroups and substantial alterations have been identified between pediatric and adult medulloblastoma patients, overall identifying four molecular subtypes: sonic hedgehog (SHH); WNT; group 3 (also known as subtype C); and group 4 (also known as subtype D).

Remarkably, subtype C tumors are not found in adults and should be considered almost exclusively confined to pediatric or adolescent patient cohorts.

When evaluating clinicopathological variables, data from an international meta-analysis suggest that large cell anaplastic (LCA) histology predicts a very poor outcome in all age categories.

SHH group

In adults the majority of medulloblastomas (60%) are classified as SHH tumors. The 5-year overall survival rate is about 75%, and SHH-driven adult tumors show progression-free survival (PFS) similar to that obtained in pediatric patients. Genetic features are also correlated with morphology; all medulloblastomas with nodular/desmoplastic histology belong to the SHH subtype, although not all SHH-subtype tumors have desmoplastic histology.

Other groups in adults

The WNT subtype represents 15% of adult tumors, with a 5-year OS of 100%. Subtype D affiliation was identified in 25% of tumors and in these patients the 5-year OS was 47%.

Confirming these data, a meta-analysis of seven studies showed that SHH tumors were most prominent in adults and infants, but not in children, while group 3 tumors were almost absent in adults. Group 4 was mainly represented in childhood, and patients in this group have an intermediate prognosis similar to the SHH subgroup. Adults with Group 4 medulloblastoma may do significantly worse.

Treatment

In the past it was assumed that medulloblastomas in adults had the same properties as those in children. Adult patients therefore were frequently treated with pediatric protocols, with simple variations in drug dosages and schedules. More recently it has been recognized that medulloblastomas in adults harbor genetic and clinical differences, so that specific protocols need to be used or developed in this population.

Surgery

Findings made in several recent studies confirm the prognostic importance of achieving a total or near total surgical excision. Today, developments in neurosurgical skills have increased the proportion of tumors falling into this category, and peri- or postoperative complications and neurological deficits following surgery are now rare occurrences.

Radiation therapy

As for pediatric patients, in adults surgery alone is associated with a high recurrence rate, thus adjuvant radiotherapy is required. Postoperative radiotherapy consists of craniospinal irradiation (CSI) followed by a boost to the posterior fossa. The dose–response relationships for treatment of tumors within the posterior fossa have been clearly documented in pediatrics as well as in adults. In adults, a dose of >54 Gy provide a 5-year disease control rate in the range of 70–90%, compared to 40% with doses of less than 50 Gy. Dose reductions in the adjacent areas of the neuraxis appear to be critical. In particular, in girls and young women, irradiation of the ovaries may lead to premature ovarian failure and subsequently to sterility. Thus, novel radiotherapy techniques provide potential to decrease toxicity by limiting the radiation dose to normal structures.

Since CSI in children with medulloblastoma increases the risk of neurological, cognitive, and endocrinological sequelae, there have been attempts to reduce the dose of CSI for children without apparent disseminated disease. However, treatment with reduced-dose CSI (23.4 Gy) without chemotherapy has resulted in a higher likelihood of early isolated neuroaxis relapse. A 5-year OS of 79% after treatment with reduced-dose CSI and chemotherapy during and after radiotherapy has been reported in average-risk patients. In the same setting, similar results were obtained in a phase III trial that compared two different chemotherapy regimens after reduced-dose radiotherapy, thus reinforcing the evidence that CSI dose reductions were feasible together with chemotherapy in average-risk pediatric patients. In adults, the only retrospective data available report an increase in the recurrence rate after dose reductions.

Chemotherapy
Average-risk medulloblastoma

Five-year OS for average-risk adult patients is in the range of 80%. Although medulloblastoma remains a chemosensitive disease in adults, cytotoxic tolerance, especially after CSI, limits its use. A large retrospective study suggested that in average-risk patients there was no OS difference between patients treated with axial doses of >34 Gy and those treated with craniospinal doses of <34 Gy plus chemotherapy. In the only published data from a prospective trial in adults with medulloblastoma, 10 low-risk patients (T1–T3a, no residual, and M0) received radiotherapy alone and 26 high-risk patients were treated with chemotherapy before and after CSI. The 5-year OS and PFS were not significantly different between the risk groups. Of note is that data with long-term follow-up from this trial demonstrated that the risk of recurrence increased markedly after 7.6 years of follow-up in average-risk patients, raising the issue of a role for chemotherapy in average-risk patients.

Additional data comes from an observational study of adults with non-metastatic medulloblastoma who were treated within the prospective multicenter trial HIT 2000 by postoperative CSI and maintenance chemotherapy. This study showed that maintenance chemotherapy did not significantly improve 4-year PFS or OS. However, the follow-up of 3.7 years has to be considered too short to draw significant conclusions. Interestingly, the authors reported data regarding toxicity among patients treated with chemotherapy with a cisplatin, lomustine, and vincristine regimen. Neurotoxicity was the most common toxicity and included peripheral neuropathy (grade 2–3 in 69%), while grade 3–4 hematological toxicity was found in 58%. Moreover, cisplatin was replaced by carboplatin in 15 (32%) patients, mainly due to ototoxicity.

The recommendation for average-risk patients is surgery followed by postoperative radiotherapy (CSI followed by a boost to the entire posterior fossa) without dose reductions. To date, adjuvant chemotherapy cannot be recommended, since its effect and possible toxicity when administered for this disease are unknown.

High-risk medulloblastoma

Five-year OS for patients with high-risk medulloblastoma is about 60–70%, indicating that the efficacy of chemotherapy in adults is similar to that in children. However, because of the heterogeneity of patients and protocols, one regimen cannot be considered preferable to another, although some agents such cisplatin/carboplatin and etoposide have frequently constituted the backbone for chemotherapy in this setting, both in adults and in children.

Another issue relates to the timing of chemotherapy, since pre-CSI chemotherapy may provide several advantages (i.e., better tolerability because bone marrow reserves are not compromised by craniospinal radiotherapy), but also concerns regarding the potential harm from the delay of radiotherapy. In pediatric patients prospective randomized trials using effective chemotherapy regimens pre-radiotherapy did not show detrimental effects.

In adults, data from the prospective trial conducted by Brandes *et al.* suggest that in high-risk patients upfront chemotherapy (cisplatin, etoposide, and cyclophosphamide) followed by CSI is feasible and safe, since no patient experienced disease progression during this treatment. This approach provided a 5-year OS rate of 80% in average-risk patients and 73% in high-risk patients.

Future strategies

New strategies are under investigation in this setting and novel subgroup-specific therapies are being explored in clinical trials, particularly for the SHH subgroup.

The SHH pathway can be activated by mutations in *PTCH1*, *SUFU*, or *SMO* that lead to ligand-independent, constitutive signaling. Thus, oral SHH-pathway inhibitors (vismodegib, sonidegib – LDE225) are currently under active investigation.

Data from phase I studies showed pronounced tumor shrinkage with these agents, even after multiple chemotherapy lines. Thus, despite the fact that resistance to these agents has been found, further studies have been conducted or are ongoing.

Interestingly, patients who responded to LDE225 treatment were found to have activated SHH, as determined by a 5-gene SHH signature assay. Thus, specific trials for medulloblastoma patients are ongoing.

Further reading

Brandes AA, Ermani M, Amista P, *et al.* The treatment of adults with medulloblastoma: A prospective study. *Int J Radiat Oncol Biol Phys* 2003;57:755–761.

Brandes AA, Franceschi E, Tosoni A, *et al.* Long-term results of a prospective study on the treatment of medulloblastoma in adults. *Cancer* 2007;110:2035–2041.

Chang CH, Housepian EM, Herbert C, Jr. An operative staging system and a megavoltage radiotherapeutic technic for cerebellar medulloblastomas. *Radiology* 1969;93:1351–1359.

Northcott PA, Korshunov A, Witt H, *et al.* Medulloblastoma comprises four distinct molecular variants. *J Clin Oncol* 2011;29:1408–1414.

Padovani L, Sunyach MP, Perol D, *et al.* Common strategy for adult and pediatric medulloblastoma: A multicenter series of 253 adults. *Int J Radiat Oncol Biol Phys* 2007;68:433–440.

Rudin CM, Hann CL, Laterra J, *et al.* Treatment of medulloblastoma with hedgehog pathway inhibitor GDC-0449. *N Engl J Med* 2009;361:1173–1178.

143 Primary central nervous system lymphoma

Deborah T. Blumenthal and Idan Ben-Horin

Neuro-oncology Service, Tel-Aviv Sourasky Medical Center, Tel-Aviv, Israel

Primary central nervous system lymphoma (CNSL) is a relatively rare brain neoplasm that is of growing importance due to its increased incidence and favorable response to conventional treatments. Although CNSL is similar histologically to systemic diffuse large B-cell lymphomas (DLBCL), it has a different biology and natural history, and its location in the central nervous system dictates a different approach in both diagnostic workup and therapy. These differences may be correlated to specific gene expression profiles that can be distinguished from systemic B-cell lymphoma. Therefore, CNSL is considered a separate disease entity according to the 2008 World Health Organization (WHO) classification of lymphoid neoplasms.

Epidemiology

The incidence of CNSL has increased from a rate of 1% before the 1980s to 3–8% in the 1990s and 2000s. Part of the increased incidence is related to the AIDS (acquired immune deficiency syndrome) epidemic, but there is also a less understood increase seen in the "immune-competent" population. There are several hypotheses to explain this increase in incidence, including observation bias and population shift toward the elderly. The median age at diagnosis in the non-HIV (human immunodeficiency virus) patient group is in the fifth decade, with men and women equally affected.

Overall, incidence rates are similar between racial groups, although African Americans have a higher incidence rate in patients diagnosed before age 50 years and a lower rate in those diagnosed over age 50 years. When evaluating by age group, incidence rises with advanced age, with the highest rate of incidence in the 75+ group. Advanced age, male sex, and HIV-positive status are independent negative prognostic markers.

Pathophysiology

Unlike the varied histological classification in systemic lymphoma, the classification of CNSL is typically that of diffuse large B-cell origin, with a much smaller percentage (2% to as high as 8% reported in Japan) being T-cell. Histological examination usually reveals a vasocentric neoplasm with invasion of the perivascular spaces, thus contributing to the disruption of the blood–brain barrier.

Considerable effort has been directed at understanding the genetic and mutational basis of CNSL. This has led to the identification of several genes and pathways that might serve as possible therapeutic targets, such as B-cell receptors, NFkB, the JAK/STAT pathway, and BCL-6. Elements of the tumor microenvironment, such as chemokine pathways and T-cell responses, might also be exploited in future treatment regimens.

Clinical features

As the apparent biology of CNSL differs from most systemic lymphomas, so do its appearance and its treatment. Mass lesions involving the deep parenchyma of the brain are more likely to be primary versus systemic lymphoma. While primary CNSL can also involve the cerebrospinal fluid (CSF), nervous system metastasis of systemic lymphoma typically follows a subdural-meningeal pattern and/or dissemination via the leptomeninges.

Investigations

Since CNSL is a treatment-sensitive tumor, surgical intervention, with its inherent risks, should be restricted to biopsy for the purpose of definite diagnosis. Outcomes are also not improved by an aggressive resection. Additionally, as CNSL typically responds to treatment, but also grows quickly, it is imperative to begin therapy as soon as the diagnosis is definite. The longer the neurological symptoms worsen, the more the patient is at risk for suffering irreversible neurological deficits. Post-treatment imaging may show excellent response to therapy, but the patient may remain disabled by neurological damage if therapy is delayed.

A caveat in securing the definite diagnosis is performing the biopsy without exposure to steroids. Steroids are tumor cell lytic in the case of lymphoma, and steroid exposure can cause the enhancing mass to disappear completely, rendering a biopsy non-diagnostic.

The workup of CNSL also includes consideration of the systemic immune status of the patient. A thorough history should be taken for any autoimmune disorder or exposure to immune-suppressive treatment or environmental agents. It is recommended to stop the immune-suppressive agent in question, which may assist in managing the CNSL. It is standard practice to check for HIV status even if the patient has no obvious risk factors.

Magnetic resonance imaging (MRI), the imaging study of choice, assists greatly in making the diagnosis of CNSL. Lymphoma typically appears densely contrast-enhancing on computed tomography (CT) or MRI. The exception is central, "ring-enhancing" necrosis, which can be seen in HIV-associated CNSL. As the tumor is densely cellular,

International Neurology, Second edition. Edited by Robert P. Lisak, Daniel D. Truong, William M. Carroll and Roongroj Bhidayasiri
© 2016 John Wiley & Sons, Ltd. Published 2016 by John Wiley & Sons, Ltd.

T2 MR images are typically iso- to hyperintense in the area of the lesion, while diffusion-weighted sequences show restrictive signal. More than 30% of CNSL lesions are multicentric, often appearing in a periventricular pattern, involving the deep white-matter parenchyma. The frequency of multiple lesions is increased among immunosuppressed patients. The more commonly involved brain regions are frontal, temporal, deep nuclei, occipital, and cerebellar. Slightly more than 60% of cases are solitary enhancing lesions, either with measurable borders (Figure 143.1) or more diffuse in nature. Only 10% of patients present with seizures, as most lesions involve the deeper white matter. Microscopically, although a lesion may appear well defined on imaging, lymphoma cells are known to infiltrate widely throughout apparently radiographically uninvolved brain areas. More extensive disease than would be suspected by MRI has been confirmed histologically and correlated with autopsy. Hence, CNSL should be treated as a diffuse, not focal, disease. MRI of the spine is indicated in patients who have spinal or radicular symptoms. Primary spinal lymphoma has been reported, but is an exceedingly rare entity.

Unless there is a pressure-related threat of tonsillar or uncal herniation, a spinal tap should be performed for examination of the CSF and for cell count, cytology and flow cytometry, protein, glucose, and immunoglobulin heavy-chain gene-rearrangement studies. The finding of monoclonal lymphocytes in the CSF is diagnostic for CNSL. Tests for protein, cell count and differential, and glucose can be supportive, but are not specific for CSF involvement. Lowered glucose, increased protein, and pleocytosis are usually seen if the CSF is involved. Elevated lactic dehydrogenase (LDH) isoenzymes and ß-2 microglobulin are suggestive of CNSL involvement of the CSF, but can also be seen in infections and other illnesses.

Newly published data suggest that the CSF detection of soluble CD19, a protein found on the surface of B-cells, can serve as both a diagnostic and a prognostic marker, as increased levels are correlated with poorer overall survival. Similarly, CSF levels of specific microRNAs (miRNA), regulatory RNA molecules that are deregulated in many disease types, rise compared to controls with inflammatory CNS disorders. Combined miRNA analyses improved diagnostic accuracy. Furthermore, there is an apparent difference in miRNA expression between primary CNSL and nodal DLBCL. CSF levels of interleukin-10 (IL-10) and IL-6 have been reported to be higher in primary CNSL patients compared to other brain tumors and to decrease after therapy, thus possibly serving as a diagnostic marker.

Slit-lamp examination by an ophthalmologist should be performed in the initial evaluation, as intraocular involvement of CNSL occurs in 10–25% of patients at presentation. However, primary intraocular lymphoma spreads to the CNS in over 80% of cases and therefore requires neuroaxis imaging. Chest/abdomen/pelvis CT scanning is accepted as part of the evaluation for newly diagnosed CNSL, while bone marrow biopsy, testicular ultrasound for men over 60 years, and fluorodeoxyglucose-positron emission tomography (FDG-PET) scan are less likely to add to the diagnostic results. A comprehensive systemic evaluation is recommended if histology of the nervous system lesion is other than large B-cell.

Treatment

The prognosis of CNSL without treatment is dismal, with survival being less than 4 months; some individual patients, however, can respond for extended periods with steroid treatment alone. Increased age (over 60 years), decreased Karnofsky performance status (KPS less than 70), elevated serum lactate dehydrogenase or CSF protein concentration, and the spread of disease outside of the hemispheres (CSF, orbits) have a negative impact on prognosis. Unlike gliomas, the initial KPS at diagnosis should not dictate the decision to treat, as if started in a timely fashion, CNSL therapy may lead to a rapid clinical recovery. It is the authors' observation that even in cases of good radiographic response to therapy, patients may still suffer from neurological deficits. It is debated whether these deficits are disease-related or therapy-induced.

Until the 1980s, whole-brain radiation treatment (WBRT) was the accepted standard therapy for CNSL despite the lack of prospective randomized trials to determine optimal fields and/or doses. Tumors responded quickly in almost all cases, but invariably recurred in a resistant fashion within 12 months. Furthermore, most patients whose tumors were controlled often suffered from disabling neurotoxicity, in some cases beginning less than a year after their treatment. Patients with a KPS less than 40 despite corticosteroid treatment can still be considered candidates for primary WBRT with a standard treatment volume including the brain, eyes, and optic nerves, while protecting the lens.

The standard chemotherapy regimens used for high-grade systemic lymphoma are not efficacious in CNSL, likely due to poor CNS penetration. The chemotherapy of choice for CNSL since the 1970s is methotrexate (MTX); when used in a "high-dose" regimen (at least 3.5 g/m^2) it has a high rate of CNS penetration. Most accepted chemotherapy regimens for CNSL today are MTX-based, often combined with alkylators, antimetabolite agents, monoclonal

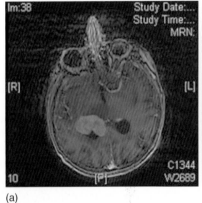
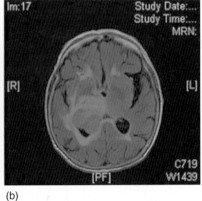

(a)　　　　　　　　　　　　　(b)

Figure 143.1 Primary central nervous system lymphoma. (a) Axial T1 gadolinium-enhanced magnetic resonance imaging (MRI) shows a densely enhancing solitary mass in the area of the right temporal trigone. (b) Axial fluid-attenuated inversion recovery (FLAIR) MRI shows a hypointense mass (due to increased cellular density), with surrounding (hyperintense) edema.

antibodies (e.g., rituximab, a monoclonal anti-B-cell antibody), and at times radiation. The optimal dose of MTX during induction has not been defined, although most regimens use 3.5 g/m^2 in combination with other agents or 8 g/m^2 if used as monotherapy.

Intrathecal chemotherapy for patients with newly diagnosed disease is less frequently recommended, especially if the CSF is initially negative, as similar outcomes with decreased toxicity may be obtained using a high dose of systemic MTX. For patients who cannot tolerate MTX, other chemotherapy regimens can be considered. Recent small series have showed responses to lower doses of MTX in combination with oral temozolomide.

Anecdotal responses have been seen by the authors in elderly, frail candidates with reduced-dose WBRT (24 Gy) combined with a low dose (50 mg/m^2) of temozolomide. The regimen of temozolomide and rituximab also seems to have activity for CNSL. In cases of leptomeningeal involvement, intrathecal chemotherapy is typically recommended. Intrathecal rituximab may be useful in this setting and is currently under study in several trials.

There is controversy regarding the optimal treatment of ocular disease due to its rarity. The 2011 International CNSL Collaborative Group recommended systemic treatment if disease involves the CNS and local treatment if only one eye is involved. High-dose systemic MTX, possibly with rituximab, can evoke responses in intraocular lymphoma, but with relapse seen in half of the cases. Local approaches include ocular radiation and intravitreal therapy. In cases of bilateral ocular disease, both systemic and intravitreal therapies are suggested. Radiation therapy using opposed lateral beams is well tolerated and the local recurrence rate is low. Treatment-related side effects include cataracts, dry eyes, and radiation retinopathy. Intravitreal injection of MTX or rituximab may also be viable treatment options for intraocular disease. Initial studies show possibly improved responses with less morbidity than is seen with radiation to the orbit. Such treatments should be performed at a center with an ophthalmologist experienced with the injection technique to minimize possible complications, including vitreous hemorrhage, endophthalmitis, and retinal detachment. In cases of refractory disease to initial systemic intravenous therapy, most centers rely on direct radiation to the orbits. Two ongoing trials are investigating the role of thalidomide derivatives, lenalidomide and pomalidomide, in recurrent/refractory intraocular lymphoma with rituximab or as single agents. Prospective randomized studies are also investigating the role of intense chemotherapy with thiotepa, busulfan, and cyclophosphamide combined with stem cell rescue.

Salvage therapy

Salvage regimens for recurrent CNSL disease include repeated treatment with high-dose MTX if initial response was favorable and sufficient time since cessation of treatment has elapsed (early recurrence suggests MTX-resistance). The use of temozolomide and rituximab for salvage appears to have a useful role and patients can tolerate further therapy after recurrence. WBRT alone or at a reduced dose with temozolomide is an option, although data are only anecdotal. Topotecan and cytarabine have been studied as salvage agents, but these drugs can cause significant adverse events. Pemetrexed has also shown benefit in relapsed CNSL with primarily hematological and infectious toxicities.

High-dose chemotherapy with hematopoietic cell transplantation has been studied as salvage therapy in patients with complete response to salvage chemotherapy, with limited success. Transplant can be considered an option for selected relapsed patients, although systemic chemotherapy and re-irradiation are typically preferred.

Treatment-related toxicity

It was recognized in the late 1980s–1990s that a significant proportion of CNSL patients who survived for 6 months or longer developed a neurological degenerative syndrome characterized by progressive dementia, gait apraxia, and incontinence ("NPH-like"). This neurological syndrome is related to toxic treatment effects thought to be primarily related to radiation injury, with a possible additive component of MTX-toxicity in some cases. Imaging shows brain atrophy and white matter changes. Although it is felt that all patients suffer some degree of radiation-induced neurotoxicity, increased patient age is associated with a more significant risk. Concurrent treatment with MTX or treatment shortly following WBRT increases the syndrome's severity and the likelihood of cognitive impairment. Intrathecal chemotherapy can cause leukotoxicity independently, and increases the neurological damage from radiation. Some patients with this "NPH-like" syndrome have responded at least temporarily to ventriculoperitoneal shunt placement.

High-dose methotrexate can lead to acute renal failure despite aggressive hydration, urine alkalinization, and avoidance of agents that interact with MTX, such as penicillin derivatives. Third-space effusions must be drained before MTX administration and leucovorin rescue started 24 hours after the MTX chemotherapy infusion. Intravenous glucarpidase can be employed on an emergency basis to circumvent renal failure and dialysis, through effectively decreasing MTX levels by cleaving the drug and forming the amino acid glutamate and 2,4-diamino-N^{10}-methylpteroic acid, compounds that are primarily excreted by the liver.

HIV/AIDS-related central nervous system lymphoma

CNSL is recognized as an AIDS-defining illness in an HIV-positive patient. CNSL affects advanced HIV patients whose CD4 count is 50 mm^3 or less. AIDS-related CNSL is an example of a true "oncovirus," in that Epstein–Barr virus (EBV) incorporates itself cellularly and triggers a clonal expansion of the neoplasm. The definitive diagnosis of CNSL in the case of a suspicious mass in an HIV-positive patient can be made by CSF DNA analysis. The sensitivity and specificity of EBV polymerase chain reaction (PCR) in such a patient are 80% and 100%, respectively. EBV DNA is usually negative in immunocompetent patients.

There have been anecdotal reports of regression of CNSL after combination highly active antiretroviral therapy (HAART) is initiated and the lymphocytic immune status restored. The AIDS patient is usually more susceptible to the toxic effects of chemotherapy, and although the tumor may respond radiographically, the patient may succumb to a myriad of infectious complications from overly aggressive chemotherapy. Hence, the approach to CNSL in this setting is often palliative and median survival for AIDS-CNSL is under 6 months. Standard treatment involves WBRT combined with HAART. There are small series supporting the feasibility and efficacy of high-dose MTX for selected AIDS patients and case reports on rituximab- and MTX-based chemotherapy with autologous stem cell transplantation.

Treatment guidelines, clinical trials, and future direction

CNSL is a disease sensitive to chemotherapy and radiation. It should be approached with a multimodality, preferably MTX-based chemotherapy regimen, with radiation used judiciously on a case-by-case basis (e.g., initial consolidation versus salvage, reduced-dose radiation); see Table 143.1. Initial data using reduced-dose WBRT with immunochemotherapy

Table 143.1 Clinical trials for primary central nervous system lymphoma (CNSL).

Trial	No. of patients	Protocol	CR (%)[a]	PFS (years)	OS (years)
Morris PG	52	R-MPV if CR: rdWBRT+cytarabine no CR: WBRT+cytarabine	60	3.3	6.6
Rubinstein JL	44	MT-R if CR: EA	66	2.4	not reached
Kasenda B	43	HD-MTX+HD carmustine/thiotepa+ASCT ±WBRT	79	N/A	8.7
Wieduwilt MJ	31	MT-R if CR: EA	52	2.0	6.9
Fritsch K	28	R-MCP	64	1.3	1.5
Thiel E*	551	*HD-MTX±WBRT or HD-MTX+ifosfamide ±WBRT	35	with WBRT 1.5 without WBRT 1.0	with WBRT 2.7 without WBRT 3.1
Chamberlain MC	40	HD-MTX+rituximab + HD-MTX (as maintenance)	60	1.8	2.4
Ferreri AJM	79	MTX±cytarabine all received WBRT	MTX only 18% MTX+cytarabine 46%	3y-PFS MTX only 21% MTX+cytarabine 38%	3y-OS MTX only 32% MTX+cytarabine 46%
Yamanaka R	112	WBRT or MVP+WBRT or ProMACE-MOPP+WBRT or R-MTX+WBRT	N/A	1.5	2

[a] after induction, when appropriate; * the only phase III trial for CNSL to date.
ASCT = autologous stem cell transplantation; CR = complete response; EA = etoposide, cytarabine; HD-MTX = high-dose methotrexate; MT-R = methotrexate, temozolomide, rituximab; MVP = methotrexate, vincristine, prednisolone; N/A = not available; OS = overall survival; PFS = progression-free survival; ProMACE-MOPP = cyclophosphamide, pirarubicin, etoposide, vincristine, procarbazine, prednisone, methotrexate; rdWBRT = reduced-dose whole-brain radiotherapy; R-MCP = rituximab, methotrexate, procarbazine, lomustine; R-MPV = rituximab, methotrexate, procarbazine, vincristine; R-MTX = rituximab, methotrexate, pirarubicin, procarbazine, prednisone; WBRT: whole-brain radiotherapy.

appear promising, showing improved survival responses and decreased neurotoxicity. Series of patients treated with immunochemotherapy (rituximab, carboplatin, and methotrexate) and blood–brain barrier disruption or intraventricular administration of rituximab show promising early results. Likewise, the use of a chemotherapy-based consolidation therapy for patients who achieve complete response to induction chemotherapy is now being explored, with findings indicating comparable results to regimens involving WBRT.

Current large, multinational randomized phase II clinical trials are evaluating several key controversial issues, including the role of temozolomide in the multiagent regimen; the use of high-dose chemotherapy with stem cell transplant; and a reduced-dose and changed fractionation scheme (36 Gy given in hyperfractionated twice-daily doses), or reduced-dose WBRT (2340cGy) versus withholding radiation altogether in cases of complete response to initial chemotherapy.

Impressive activity of ibrutinib in central nervous system spread of mantle cell (systemic) lymphoma has been recently reported. Pharmacokinetic analysis of cerebrospinal fluid and plasma levels show that this tyrosine kinase inhibitor penetrates the blood-brain barrier. Accordingly, several early phase trials using ibrutinib for CNS lymphoma are ongoing.

The role of surgery in the treatment of CNSL has been limited to biopsy. An unplanned subgroup analysis of the G-PCNSL-SG-1 trial demonstrated a statistically improved complete response rate at 6 months in patients undergoing gross or subtotal resection compared to biopsied patients. However, there was no difference in progression-free or overall survival.

Further reading

Bernard S, Goldwirt L, Amorim S, *et al.* Activity of ibrutinib in mantle cell lymphoma patients with central nervous system relapse. *Blood* 2015;126(14):1695-8.

Chamberlain MC, Johnston SK. High-dose methotrexate and rituximab with deferred radiotherapy for newly diagnosed primary B-cell CNS lymphoma. *Neuro Oncol* 2010;12(7):736–744.

Ferreri AJM, Reni M, Foppoli M, *et al.* High-dose cytarabine plus high-dose methotrexate versus high-dose methotrexate alone in patients with primary CNS lymphoma: A randomised phase 2 trial. *Lancet* 2009;374(9700):1512–1520.

Fischer L, Hummel M, Korfel A, *et al.* Differential micro-RNA expression in primary CNS and nodal diffuse large B-cell lymphomas. *Neuro Oncol* 2011;13(10):1090–1098.

Fritsch K, Kasenda B, Hader C, *et al.* immunochemotherapy with rituximab, methotrexate, procarbazine and lomustine for primary CNS lymphoma (PCNSL) in the elderly. *Ann Oncol* 2011;22(9):2080–2085.

Kasenda B, Schorb E, Fritsch K, *et al.* Prognosis after high-dose chemotherapy followed by autologous stem-cell transplantation as first-line treatment in primary CNS lymphoma – a long term follow-up study. *Ann Oncol* 2012;23(10):2670–2675.

Morris PG, Correa DD, Yahalom J, *et al.* Rituximab, methotrexate, procarbazine, and vincristine followed by consolidation reduced-dose whole-brain radiotherapy and cytarabine in newly diagnosed primary CNS lymphoma: Final results and long-term outcome. *J Clin Oncol* 2013;31(31):3971–3979.

Ponzoi M, Issa S, Batchelor TT, *et al.* Beyond high-dose methotrexate and brain radiotherapy: Novel targets and agents for primary CNS lymphoma. *Ann Oncol* 2014;25(2):316–322.

Rubinstein JL, His ED, Johnson JL, *et al.* Intensive chemotherapy and immunotherapy in patients with newly diagnosed primary CNS lymphoma: CALGB 50202 (alliance 50202). *J Clin Oncol* 2013;31(25):3061–3068.

Shah GD, Yahalom J, Correa DD, *et al.* Combined immunochemotherapy with reduced whole brain radiotherapy for newly diagnosed primary central nervous system lymphoma. *J Clin Oncol* 2007;25(30):4730–4735.

Theil E, Korfel A, Martus P, *et al.* High-dose methotrexate with or without whole brain radiotherapy for primary CNS lymphoma (G-PCNSL-SG-1): A phase 3, randomised, non-inferiority trial. *Lancet Oncol* 2010;11(11):1036–1047.

Wang CC, Carnevale J, Rubenstein JL. Progress in central nervous system lymphomas. *Br J Haematol* 2014;166:311–325.

Wieduwilt MJ, Valles F, Issa S, *et al.* Immunochemotherapy with intensive consolidation for primary CNS lymphoma: A pilot study and prognostic assessment by diffusional weighted MRI. *Clin Cancer Res* 2012;18:1146–1155.

Yamanaka R, Morii K, Shinbo Y, *et al.* Results of treatment of 112 cases of primary CNS lymphoma. *Jpn J Clin Oncol* 2008;38(5):373–380.

144 Brain metastases

Babita Jyoti[1], Farida Balkhi Alam[2], Silvia Hofer[3], and Michael Brada[2,4]

[1] Health Proton Therapy Institute, University of Florida, Jacksonville, FL, USA
[2] Department of Radiation Oncology, Clatterbridge Cancer Centre NHS Foundation Trust, Wirral, UK
[3] Division of Oncology, Luzerner Kantonsspital, Luzern, Switzerland
[4] Department of Molecular and Clinical Cancer Medicine, University of Liverpool, UK

Brain metastases are a common manifestation of malignancy, affecting 20–40% of patients with solid tumors. The majority develop in the context of known primary or metastatic disease and a small proportion of patients present with intracranial lesions as the first feature of malignancy. The approach to management of brain metastases has consisted of corticosteroids, brain irradiation, and surgery for solitary lesions. With developments in radiotherapy and systemic treatment the range of treatment options has increased, even though the evidence base for management alternatives is limited.

Epidemiology

The frequency of brain metastases reflects the incidence of primary malignancy as well as the propensity for central nervous system (CNS) dissemination. The overall risk of developing brain metastases in patients with solid tumors is about 10%. The reported incidence for patients with lung cancer is 20%, melanoma 7%, renal carcinoma 7%, breast cancer 5%, and colorectal cancer 2%. Patients with breast cancer aged 20–39 years have the highest proportional risk of brain metastases.

Pathophysiology

The development of brain metastases is through a metastatic cascade. The dissemination of tumor cells is either via an early event when tumor cells are released from the primary tumor site to become circulating tumor cells (CTC) and dormant cells within a metastatic site in the brain, or as a late event when tumor cells are released either from an advanced primary tumor or from another metastatic site. The release of tumor cells from the primary tumor includes steps of tissue invasion, vascular intravasation, and release into the circulation as CTCs. These steps are common to systemic dissemination to all metastatic sites. For tumor cells to become viable intracerebral metastases requires three principal steps: arrest of tumor cells (CTCs) in the capillary bed, extravasation into brain parenchyma, followed by proliferation. The metastatic cascade can be interrupted by a number of agents (metastases suppressors, e.g., caspases and cadherins) tested in preclinical models. However, their efficacy in the clinical setting requires the steps of development of CTCs to occur after the diagnosis and treatment of the primary tumor, which is in some doubt. The potential alternative strategy is eradication of CTCs and dormant cells by "prophylactic" therapy approaches.

Clinical features

Patients present with features characteristic of single or multiple space-occupying brain lesions (brain tumors). These consist of features of increased intracranial pressure (ICP), and of neurological dysfunction specific to the location of the metastases and seizures. The classical triad of presenting features of a brain tumor consisting of raised ICP (with headache, nausea and vomiting, and papilledema), focal neurological deficit, and seizures is relatively infrequent at the time of the diagnosis of brain metastases. As brain metastases are not infrequently multiple, the focal features may be multiple and subtle and may include more global deficit such as cognitive impairment. Raised ICP is more common in the presence of secondary hydrocephalus and would be unusual with early diagnosis of brain metastases. Therefore, patients with known malignant disease, presenting with features indicating an intracranial problem that could be subtle or unusual, should have a low threshold for brain imaging.

Prognosis

Median survival in patients with multiple brain metastases is 3–4 months, with 10–15% survival at 1 year. Independent prognostic factors for survival are performance status (PS), age, the presence and activity of systemic disease (both primary and metastatic), and the number of brain metastases. Prognosis is also primary tumor specific.

Performance status, age, and the presence and activity of primary and metastatic disease and the number of lesions are embodied in the graded prognostic assessment (GPA), which is also dependent on primary tumor type. Patients with a GPA score of 3.5–4.0 – Karnofsky performance status (KPS) >70, age <65, and absence of extracranial metastases with controlled primary tumor and one or few brain metastases – have a median survival of approximately 11 months; patients with a GPA score of 0–1.0 have a median survival of 2.6 months. The median survival in patients with brain metastases from breast cancer ranges (highest to lowest GPA score) from 25–3.4 months and from non-small cell lung cancer (NSCLC) from 15–3 months.

The prognostic factors for survival in patients with solitary brain metastases are the same as in patients with multiple brain metastases. The dominant adverse prognostic factor for survival is poor performance status; patients with poor PS and marked disability have survival rates similar to patients with multiple brain metastases.

International Neurology, Second edition. Edited by Robert P. Lisak, Daniel D. Truong, William M. Carroll and Roongroj Bhidayasiri
© 2016 John Wiley & Sons, Ltd. Published 2016 by John Wiley & Sons, Ltd.

Investigations

Brain metastases are typically iso- or hyperdense on computed tomography (CT) and iso- or hyperintense on magnetic resonance imaging (MRI), usually with surrounding low-density area assumed to represent edema, and they generally enhance with intravenous contrast. The difficulty in differential diagnosis arises in the presence of hemorrhage into the lesion, which does not allow for visualization of the underlying tumor. While the majority of brain metastases lie within the brain parenchyma, they may be meningeally based and may occasionally mimic tumors such as meningioma or acoustic neuroma.

In the presence of known systemic malignancy and metastatic disease, there is no indication for biopsy of intracranial lesions unless there is a high index of suspicion for an alternative diagnosis such as an atypical infection. In patients presenting with lesions in the brain, without previous history of primary malignancy, histological confirmation is generally required, preferably from an extracranial site.

Treatment

Medical management

The aim of treatment is to improve neurological deficit and thereby quality of life (QoL) and to control the growth of brain metastases to prolong progression-free survival and survival. Mass effect from the combination of tumor mass(es) and surrounding edema is treated with corticosteroids. This improves the features of increased ICP and frequently focal neurological deficit. Oral dexamethasone is generally the drug of choice and can be administered in a single daily dose of 4–16 mg.

One randomized trial compared daily dexamethasone doses of 4–12 mg. Improvement in function at 1 week was the same regardless of the dose, with higher doses causing more severe Cushingoid side effects.

In patients with features of increased ICP, higher loading doses (16 mg) are frequently used, although there is no clear evidence for benefit of this strategy other than in life-threatening situations. After clinical benefit has been achieved, the dose should be titrated to the lowest necessary to maintain improvement in symptoms. Corticosteroids should be reduced and discontinued after definitive treatment to avoid long-term corticosteroid side effects. In patients with no or minimal symptoms, corticosteroids should not be automatically administered. They are also not recommended as a prophylactic treatment prior to cranial irradiation or chemotherapy.

The management of seizures in patients with brain metastases is the same as that of patients with primary brain tumor; the indication for the use of anticonvulsants is the presence of seizures. There is no evidence that prophylactic anticonvulsants confer any benefit. If chemotherapy is part of the management and anticonvulsants are indicated, it is preferable to avoid enzyme-inducing anticonvulsants (e.g., phenytoin), which increase the metabolism of many chemotherapeutic agents, leading to lower effective doses.

Surgery

Surgery is the appropriate treatment for accessible solitary brain metastases in non-eloquent locations. In patients with multiple brain metastases, surgical excision is generally not indicated, unless one easily accessible lesion is responsible for the majority of symptoms. Although resection of multiple brain metastases has been recommended by some researchers, the apparent favorable survival seen was most likely due to patient selection rather than the efficacy of surgery.

The survival benefit of surgical resection of solitary brain metastases has been tested in three small randomized trials comparing surgery and whole-brain radiotherapy (WBRT) with WBRT alone. Two studies showed prolongation in survival, and this was not confirmed in the third study. The consensus opinion is that surgery is appropriate for patients with accessible solitary brain metastases. Radical excision should be reserved for patients with favorable prognostic factors, particularly without progressive systemic disease.

Radiotherapy

Whole-brain irradiation has been the mainstay of treatment of patients with brain metastases. One recent randomized trial (QUARTZ trial) compared supportive care (corticosteroids alone) with WBRT in poor-prognosis patients with non-small cell lung cancer (NSCLC) and showed no clear survival or QoL benefit. There are no randomized studies of WBRT in favorable-prognosis patients and the general consensus is to offer treatment particularly to symptomatic patients. The preferred WBRT for patients with multiple brain metastases is 20 Gy in 5 fractions or 30 Gy in 10 fractions. No randomized studies have shown benefit from more intensive radiation dosing.

In summary, it is generally accepted that patients with good PS (KPS > 70), younger age, and controlled extracranial disease may benefit from WBRT in terms of both survival and neurological function/QoL, although this is lacking high-level evidence. The value of radiotherapy in patients with marked disability and poor performance status remains questionable.

Patients with brain metastases sensitive to systemic therapy are appropriately treated with primary chemotherapy or targeted therapy. On the basis of presumed residual microscopic disease following completion of chemotherapy or targeted therapy, patients can be offered consolidation WBRT, although randomized studies assessing the additional value of irradiation are not available.

In diseases with a high incidence of intracranial dissemination, brain irradiation is used as prophylaxis. Prophylactic cranial irradiation (PCI) improves intracranial tumor control and survival in patients with limited and advanced-stage small cell lung cancer (SCLC), who achieve complete or good partial remission, although the magnitude of gain in life expectancy is not large. There is no proven benefit of PCI in patients with other solid tumors, including locally advanced NSCLC.

Radiation therapy and radiosensitizers

A number of radiation sensitizers have been tested in addition to radiotherapy, but to date none has demonstrated benefit in randomized studies.

Radiosurgery

Stereotactic radiotherapy/radiosurgery (SRS) delivers localized radiation for lesions less than 4 cm in diameter. Following single-fraction radiosurgery to a dose of 15–25 Gy, the probability of reduction in the size of a solitary metastasis is 80–90%; complete disappearance is uncommon. In patients with MRI-confirmed solitary brain metastases, the addition of radiosurgery to WBRT improves overall survival and tumor control. Radiosurgery does not prolong survival in patients with two or more brain metastases. The present recommendation is to offer radiosurgery to patients with a solitary brain metastasis and good performance status. Nevertheless, radiosurgery is increasingly used in patients with oligometastatic disease (up to 3 metastases) with controlled primary disease, no other sites of dissemination, and good PS. The increasing popularity of SRS as an alternative to WBRT is based on the assumption that localized treatment is associated with less cognitive decline, although the evidence to support this is limited.

Routine addition of WBRT to local treatment continues to be practiced on the assumption that it improves intracranial disease control. However, when tested in a large randomized study, routine addition of WBRT to local treatment failed to show either a survival benefit or a prolongation of "quality survival," measured as maintenance of good performance status. Our current policy is not to offer WBRT following successful local treatment and to continue close monitoring.

Systemic treatment
The blood–brain barrier (BBB) has been considered a block to the delivery of systemic agents that are not lipid soluble. Nevertheless, the enhancing characteristics of brain metastases indicate leaking BBB and the administration of both lipid-soluble and lipid-insoluble drugs, which cannot cross an intact BBB, results in regression of brain metastases. Therefore, the BBB should not be considered the reason for withholding potentially effective chemotherapy.

The response rate of brain metastases to chemotherapy tends to reflect the chemoresponsiveness of the malignant disease. In patients with brain metastases from untreated chemosensitive tumors such as non-Hodgkin's lymphoma, SCLC, and germ cell tumors, the appropriate first-line treatment is chemotherapy. Patients with common solid tumors such as breast cancer who have systemic and brain metastases not considered chemo/targeted/hormone therapy resistant, can also be treated with appropriate systemic therapy first.

Targeted agents are increasingly explored as primary therapy in patients with specific sensitizing mutations (e.g., BRAF in melanoma and sensitizing EGFR mutations in NSCLC) and targeted agents have been shown to be effective in achieving high response rates and control of brain metastases.

Chemotherapy has been considered as an additional treatment to WBRT, although several randomized phase II studies showed no additional survival benefit and at best a small difference in response rate and progression-free survival, both of which are of questionable clinical significance. Concomitant and adjuvant chemotherapy with agents such as temozolomide, used successfully in primary brain tumors, is therefore of no known additional value.

Management in common solid tumors

Non-small cell lung cancer
The actuarial 2-year cumulative risk of developing brain metastases in patients with locally advanced (stage III) adenocarcinoma and squamous cell carcinoma following combined modality treatment is 22% and 10%, respectively, and nearly half present within 4 months of completion of treatment. Chemotherapy reduces the risk of extracranial failure, but has no effect on the incidence of CNS relapse. In patients with locally advanced NSCLC, PCI may reduce the risk of developing disease in the brain without survival benefit, and the routine use of PCI is not recommended.

Patients with brain metastases from NSCLC tend to be heavily pretreated and therefore have less chance of responding to second- or third-line agents; they should receive short palliative WBRT as the treatment of choice. The response rate of brain metastases to

platinum-based chemotherapy is as would be expected in systemic NSCLC. In asymptomatic chemo-naïve patients, chemotherapy or targeted agents (in patients with appropriate mutations) can be considered as first-line treatment, particularly in the presence of disseminated or locally advanced and progressive disease, with radiotherapy reserved for progressive intracranial disease. There is increasing evidence that patients with poor performance status and brain metastases from NSCLC do not benefit from radiotherapy and should be considered for supportive care alone.

Small cell lung cancer
The incidence of brain metastases is particularly high in SCLC. In patients with limited disease who achieve complete/good remission, PCI has become part of the initial treatment. PCI decreases the incidence of brain metastases and has a modest survival benefit. Even in responding patients with extensive disease, PCI reduces the incidence of brain metastases and improves survival, albeit at a cost of some acute toxicity. Although there is concern regarding the impact of PCI on QoL and cognitive function, there is no consistent difference between patients with or without PCI on these measures.

Intracranial metastases from SCLC respond to chemotherapy as disease at other sites. In newly diagnosed chemo-naïve patients the response of brain metastases to chemotherapy (without irradiation) is 70–80%, while at relapse it is 40–50%. The use of additional WBRT does not translate into improved survival, suggesting that extracranial disease is the principal determinant of outcome in these patients.

Breast cancer
Due to the high incidence of breast cancer, nearly a quarter of patients presenting with brain metastases have underlying primary breast cancer. The risk of developing brain metastases is higher in younger patients with negative estrogen receptor status, grade 3 disease, and large tumors; it is also more common in the presence of visceral metastases, especially in the lung. Time from primary diagnosis to the development of brain metastases correlates with tumor subtype, with the basal triple negative subtype showing the shortest time followed by HER-2, Luminal B, and Luminal A. In patients with HER-2 overexpressing tumors, the incidence of brain metastasis is not reduced by the HER-2 monoclonal antibody trastuzumab.

Breast cancer is both chemo- and radioresponsive. WBRT is considered the standard of care in the majority of symptomatic patients. However, patients with metastatic disease at other sites can be considered for primary systemic therapy, including chemotherapy, hormone therapy, or targeted therapy; such an approach can also be used in patients with isolated brain metastases considered sensitive to systemic treatment, with a response rate similar to that obtained in systemic disease.

The current recommendation in HER-2 positive patients who develop brain metastases while on (or after the use of) trastuzumab is the combination of capecitabine and lapatinib or trastuzumab emtansine.

Malignant melanoma
Although radiotherapy is perceived to be poorly effective, patients with primary melanoma brain metastases have not shown significantly worse survival with radiotherapy than other tumors and WBRT remains the treatment of choice. Chemotherapy with dacarbazine (DTIC), temozolomide, or fotemustine results in brain tumor response rates of 7%. Although a more aggressive approach

using platinum and DTIC combined with IL-2 and interferon may result in marginally better response rates, it does not prevent the development of brain metastases. Replacing DTIC with temozolomide does not result in improved survival. A small retrospective study suggested a higher response rate for ipilimumab given prior to radiotherapy.

The use of BRAF inhibitors (e.g., vemurafenib) is associated with a high response rate of brain metastases in patients with BRAF V600 mutation and is considered the first-line treatment, particularly in the presence of systemic disease.

Germ cell tumors

Approximately 10% of all patients with advanced gonadal germ cell tumors present with brain metastases and CNS disease may also appear as part of systemic relapse. The primary treatment in patients with brain metastases is chemotherapy, as used in advanced disease.

Conclusion

Nearly a quarter of patients with malignant disease develop brain metastases and this is generally a hallmark of incurable disseminated disease. In this context, the primary aim of management is palliative and can be achieved with symptomatic management and a range of oncological treatments, of which WBRT remains the most commonly used. More aggressive treatments with surgery, radiosurgery, and combined therapies are best reserved for patients with solitary brain metastases with minimal neurological deficit and absent or static systemic disease. Intensive local treatments are inappropriate for patients with multiple brain metastases, particularly in the context of other metastatic disease. The development of targeted systemic therapies has led to increasing use of targeted agents in patients with appropriate mutations and brain metastases.

Palliative care services have an important and often primary role in the care of patients affected by brain metastases and their families. The aim in all patients with brain metastases should be to allow symptom-free independent life at home or in a palliative care setting, with the focus on support and not oncological treatment alone.

Further reading

Andrews DW, Scott CB, Sperduto PW, *et al*. Whole brain radiation therapy with or without stereotactic radiosurgery boost for patients with one to three brain metastases: Phase III results of the RTOG 9508 randomised trial. *Lancet* 2004;363(9422):1665–1672.

Barnholtz-Sloan JS, Sloan AE, Davis FG, *et al*. Incidence proportions of brain metastases in patients diagnosed (1973 to 2001) in the Metropolitan Detroit Cancer Surveillance System. *J Clin Oncol* 2004;22:2865–2872.

Eichler AF, Chung E, Kodack DP, *et al*. The biology of brain metastases – translation to new therapies. *Nat Rev Clin Oncol* 2011;8(6):344–356.

Kocher M, Soffietti R, Abacioglu U, *et al*. Adjuvant whole-brain radiotherapy versus observation after radiosurgery or surgical resection of one to three cerebral metastases: Results of the EORTC 22952-26001 study. *J Clin Oncol* 2011;29:134–141.

Pinkham MB, Whitfield GA, Brada M. New developments in intracranial stereotactic radiotherapy for metastases. *Clin Oncol* 2015;27(5):316–323.

Ramakrishna N, Temin S, Chandarlapaty S, *et al*. Recommendations on disease management for patients with advanced human epidermal growth factor receptor 2-positive breast cancer and brain metastases: ASCO clinical practice guideline. *J Clin Oncol* 2014;32:2100–2108.

Sperduto PW, Berkey B, Gaspar LE, Mehta M, Curran W. A new prognostic index and comparison to three other indices for patients with brain metastases: An analysis of 1,960 patients in the RTOG database. *Int J Radiat Oncol Biol Phys* 2008;70:510–514.

Sperduto PW, Kased N, Roberge D, *et al*. The effect of tumour subtype on the time from primary diagnosis to the development of brain metastases and survival in patients with breast cancer. *J Neurooncol* 2013;112:467–472.

Thiolloy S, Rinker-Schaeffer CW. Thinking outside the box: Using metastasis suppressors as molecular tools. *Semin Cancer Biol* 2011;21(2):89–98.

145 Leptomeningeal metastases

Emilie Le Rhun[1], Sophie Taillibert[2], and Marc C. Chamberlain[3]

[1] Department of Medical Oncology, Centre Oscar Lambret, Lille, Department of Neurooncology, Hopital Roger Salengro, Lille, and PRISM laboratory, INSERM U1192, Villeneuve d'Ascq, France

[2] Department of Neurology Mazarin and Department of Radiation Oncology, Pitié-Salpêtrière Hospital University Pierre et Marie Curie, Paris, France

[3] Department of Neurology and Neurological Surgery, University of Washington, Seattle, WA, USA

Leptomeningeal metastases (LM) results from metastastic infiltration of the leptomeninges (the pia, ararchnoid, and contained cerebrospinal fluid [CSF] space) by tumor cells. Its incidence is increasing with more effective anticancer treatments that have resulted in prolongation of survival. However, many of these new therapies do not readily cross the blood–brain barrier, and the failure to cross the blood–brain barrier has manifested as an increase in late metastatic spread to the central nervous system (CNS). LM is diagnosed in approximately 5% of all patients with cancer. Most LM occurs in patients with widely disseminated and progressive systemic disease (>70%). Breast cancer, lung cancer, and melanoma are the most common solid tumors that cause LM, although any type of cancer can result in LM.

Pathophysiology

The leptomeninges and CSF may be invaded though different pathways: hematogenous; endoneural/perineural and perivascular lymphatic spread; direct extension from the brain parenchyma; choroid plexus; or iatrogenic spread during neurosurgical procedures. Once malignant cells enter the CSF, tumor disseminates throughout the neuraxis by convective CSF flow to distant sites in the CNS.

Clinical features

Neurological symtoms and signs of LM may be pleomorphic and multifocal, although most patients present with isolated and subtle neurological findings. Signs and symptoms are classically divided into three domains: cerebral, cranial nerve, or spinal. Cerebral dysfunction is mainly manifested by headache, change in mental status, difficulty in walking, nausea, and vomiting. Diplopia and facial paresis are the most frequent manifestations of cranial nerve involvement. Lower motor weakness, limb paresthesia, back or neck pain, and radiculopathy are the leading spinal manifestations. Raised intracranial pressure due to CSF resorption disorders (i.e., communicating hydrocephalus) is also a common presentation of LM. Neck stiffness (meningismus) is uncommon (<15% of all cases), as are seizures (<10%). Clinical features of LM need be distinguished from those due to parenchymal brain metastases, complications of antineoplastic treatment, metabolic and toxic encephalopathies, chronic meningitis, or other concurrent diseases.

Investigations

Imaging

Gadolinium-enhanced magnetic resonance imaging (MRI) of the entire CNS, with 90% sensitivity to detect LM, represents the imaging technique of choice. Brain contrast-enhanced computed tomography (CT), with a 23–38% sensitivity, should be reserved for patients unable to undergo MRI. Brain and spine MRI abnormalities are observed in 40–75% and 15–25%, respectively, at the time of diagnosis. The most frequent MRI findings include subarachnoid and parenchymal-enhancing nodules (10–35%) and diffuse or focal pial enhancement (10–20%). Nerve root enhancement or hydrocephalus can also be observed. Any irritation of the leptomeninges, such as infection, inflammation, subarachnoid blood, or lumbar puncture (LP), can result in enhancement of MRI.

CSF examination

The standard CSF analysis is abnormal in >90% of cases of LM, with increased opening pressure in 46%, increased leukocyte count in 57%, elevated protein in 76%, and decreased glucose in 54%. The standard diagnostic feature of LM is the identification of malignant cells in CSF. The LP may need to be repeated, as the sensitivity of a first tumor cell analysis by CSF cytology is estimated at only 45–55%, but is increased to 80% with a second CSF examination. A third CSF examination has little benefit and is not recommended. A simple methodology can improve the sensitivity of the cytological analysis, including submission of a non-hemorrhagic and large-volume (>10 ml) CSF sample and processing the CSF specimen in a timely manner (only 10% of cells remain viable after 90 minutes). Obtaining CSF from an asymptomatic or radiographically negative site may result in a false negative CSF cytology. The role of CSF fixation in dedicated tubes for CSF cytology needs to be validated. A variety of CSF biomarkers have been evaluated. One of the most promising methods may be the application of the Cellsearch® (Janssen Diagnostics, USA) technology that allows identification and quantification of malignant cells by the use of flourescent probes directed at tumor cell surface markers.

Prognosis

The median survival of untreated patients with LM is 4–6 weeks. Despite aggressive treatment, the median survival of breast cancer, non-small cell lung cancer (NSCLC), and melanoma is 3.3–5 months,

International Neurology, Second edition. Edited by Robert P. Lisak, Daniel D. Truong, William M. Carroll and Roongroj Bhidayasiri.
© 2016 John Wiley & Sons, Ltd. Published 2016 by John Wiley & Sons, Ltd.

3–4.3 months, and 2.5 months, respectively. The US National Comprehensive Cancer Network (NCCN) CNS guidelines describe risk factors in LM and have identified as good risk patients with LM (and a group considered for treatment) by the following: excellent performance status (Karnoskfy performance status ≥ 60), absence of major neurological deficits, minimal systemic disease, reasonable systemic cancer treatment options, and absence of CSF block or compartmentalization. Nonetheless, deciding which patients to treat remains challenging. The objective of LM management is to improve or stabilize neurological status, maintain quality of life, and ideally prolong survival.

Treatment and management

Symptomatic treatment

Supportive care is required in every patient with LM. The contribution of steroids in the treatment of LM is at best modest. Non-enzyme-inducing antiepileptic drugs (AEDs; e.g., levetiracetam, lacosamide, lamotrigin) are usually selected for the management of seizures. Prophylactic administration of AEDs is not recommended. Appropriate physiotherapy, antidepressant medication, and pain medications are often required.

Surgery

Ventriculoperitoneal shunting may be required for symptomatic hydrocephalus. The placement of a ventricular access device (e.g., an Ommaya reservoir) is often useful to facilitate the administration of intra-CSF chemotherapy.

Radiotherapy

Craniospinal irradiation, which treats the entire neuraxis and therefore potentially LM, is rarely used, as it further compromises bone marrow reserve and is generally eschewed as too toxic. The benefit of WBRT (whole-brain radiotherapy; 30 Gy in 10 fractions) on overall survival in LM is not clearly established. Involved-field radiotherapy is, however, indicated for sites of symptomatic disease regardless of MRI findings (e.g., lumbosacral irradiation for cauda equina syndrome or skull-base radiation for cranial neuropathies), sites of bulky disease seen by MRI, or sites of CSF flow blocks defined by radioisotope ventriculography. Radiotherapy can provide relief of pain and stabilize neurological symptoms, but rarely improves neurological signs due to LM.

Chemotherapy and targeted therapy

Intra-CSF treatment

Intra-CSF therapy is the mainstay of treatment for LM, although its benefit has never been established in prospective randomized trials. The rationale for using intra-CSF treatment includes limited CNS penetration (<5%) of most systematically administered anticancer agents. A limitation of intra-CSF chemotherapy is the limited diffusion into tumors, consequently intra-CSF chemotherapy is most effective for relatively low tumor burden disease. The presence of CSF flow obstruction in LM can result in uneven distribution of intra-CSF agents due to compartmentalization and can increase the risk of treatment-related neurotoxicity.

Intra-CSF treatment can be administered by LP or by a ventricular access device. The ventricular route of administration ensures uniform distribution of the drug in the CNS and the certainty that the drug has not been administered outside of the CSF compartment, as seen in 10% of all lumbar injections. Additionally, the ventricular access device can be used safely in patients with thrombocytopenia. Intraventicular administration is furthermore simple for the patient and time efficient for both patient and physician. In one randomized study, intraventricular administration of methotrexate was associated with a better progression-free survival when compared to intra-lumbar administration (19 vs. 43 days, p = 0.048).

Methotrexate, liposomal ara-C, and thiotepa are the three primary intra-CSF chemotherapy agents currently used for LM. These drugs are, however, ineffective in the majority of solid cancers. Regimens of intra-CSF chemotherapy are illustrated in Table 145.1. Methotrexate (MTX) is a folate antagonist, with a 4.5–8-hour CSF half-life that is eliminated from the CSF by CSF/venous resorption. Renal insufficiency, the presence of pleural or peritoneal effusions, or the coadministration of drugs that displace MTX from albumin may increase MTX toxicity. The neurological complications of MTX (or any other xenobiotic administered into the CSF space) include a transient aseptic meningitis (most common), acute or delayed encephalopathy, and transverse myelopathy.

Table 145.1 Intra-cerebrospinal fluid regimens.

	Induction		Consolidation		Maintenance	
	Bolus	CxT	Bolus	CxT	Bolus	CxT
Methotrexate	10–15 mg twice weekly (total 4 weeks)	2 mg/day for 5 days every other week (total 8 weeks)	10–15 mg once weekly (total 4 weeks)	2 mg/day for 5 days every other week (total 4 weeks)	10–15 mg once a month	2 mg/day for 5 days once a month
Cytarabine	25–100 mg twice weekly (total 4 weeks)	25 mg/day for 3 days weekly (total 4 weeks)	25–100 mg once weekly (total 4 weeks)	25 mg/day for 3 days every other week (total 4 weeks)	25–100 mg once a month	25 mg/day for 3 days once a month
DepoCyt®	50 mg every 2 weeks (total 8 weeks)				50 mg every 4 weeks (total 24 weeks)	
Thiotepa	10 mg twice weekly (total 4 weeks)	10 mg/day for 3 days weekly (total 4 weeks)	10 mg once weekly (total 4 weeks)	10 mg for 3 days every other week (total 4 weeks)	10 mg once a month	10 mg/day for 3 days once a month
α-interferon	1 × 10⁶ U twice weekly (total 4 weeks)		1 × 10⁶ U three times every other week (total 4 weeks)		1 × 10⁶ U three times weekly 1 week per month	

	Induction		Consolidation		Maintenance
Etoposide		0.5 mg/day for 5 days every other week (total 8 weeks)		0.5 mg/day for 5 days every other week (total 4 weeks)	0.5 mg/day for 5 days once a month
Topotecan	0.4 mg twice weekly (total 4 weeks)		0.4 mg twice weekly every other week (total 4 weeks)		0.4 mg twice weekly once a month
Rituximab	25 mg twice weekly (total 4 weeks)		25 mg twice weekly every other week (total 4 weeks)		25 mg twice weekly once a month
Trastuzumab	20–50 mg once weekly (total 4 weeks)		10–100 mg once every other week (total 4 weeks)		20–100 mg once a month

CxT = concentration × time

Liposomal cytarabine (Depocyte®), a pyrimidine nucleoside analogue with a long CSF half-life of 141 hours, is another commonly used intra-CSF chemotherapy. Concomitant administration of oral dexamethasone is recommended to prevent a treatment-related chemical meningitis.

Thiotepa, an alkylating agent with a 20-minute CSF half-life, is most often used as a second-line intra-CSF therapy. The most frequent adverse event is a leukoencephalopathy and myelosuppression due to rapid transcapillary uptake of thiotepa. The superiority of using a combination of intra-CSF drugs has never been demonstrated. The exact duration of intra-CSF treatment has also never been established and often a prolonged treatment is proposed. Novel intra-CSF agents have been evaluated most unfortunately, with only modest activities. Intra-CSF trastuzumab may be a promising new intra-CSF agent for HER-2/neu positive cancers and is currently being evaluated.

Systemic treatment

The choice of a systemic agent is based on the presumed tumor chemosensitivity of the primary tumor and the ability of the drug to achieve effective CSF concentrations. High-dose MTX or cytarabine regimens achieve effective concentrations in the CSF, but have limited benefit in LM from solid tumors, with the exception of breast cancer–related LM. Notably, high-dose regimens require hospitalization and also induce significant myelotoxicity. Agents used to treat brain metastases are often used to treat LM, although they have only been reported in small case series. Examples include capecitabine in breast cancer; epidermal growth factor receptor inhibitors (erlotinib and gefitinib) in non-small cell lung cancer; immune checkpoint inhibitors (anti-CTLA4 monoclonal antibody ipilimumab; anti-PD1 monoclonal antibody nivolumab) and BRAF inhibitors (vemurafenib and dabrafenib) in melanoma.

Conclusion

LM represents an increasing challenge in oncology. The prognosis of LM remains poor with median survival of 3 months and <15% of all patients survive 1 year after initial diagnosis and treatment. New clinical trials based on tumor-specific histology are an unmet need in this challenging disease.

Further reading

Chamberlain MC. Comprehensive neuraxis imaging in leptomeningeal metastasis: A retrospective case series. *CNS Oncology* 2013;2(2):121–128.

Chamberlain MC, Glantz M, Groves MD, Wilson WH. Diagnostic tools for neoplastic meningitis: Detecting disease, identifying patient risk, and determining benefit of treatment. *Semin Oncol* 2009;36(4 Suppl 2):S35–S45.

Chamberlain M, Soffietti R, Raizer J, *et al.* Leptomeningeal metastasis: A Response Assessment in Neuro-Oncology critical review of endpoints and response criteria of published randomized clinical trials. *Neuro Oncol* 2014;16(9):1176–1185.

Groves MD. New strategies in the management of leptomeningeal metastases. *Arch Neurol* 2010;67(3):305–312.

Le Rhun E, Taillibert S, Chamberlain MC. Carcinomatous meningitis: Leptomeningeal metastases in solid tumors. *Surg Neurol Int* 2013; 4(Suppl 4): S265–S288.

146   Spinal epidural metastases

Roberta Rudà and Riccardo Soffietti

Department of Neuro-oncology, University of Turin, Turin, Italy

This chapter outlines the epidemiology, pathophysiology, presentation, diagnostic workup, treatment, and prognosis of epidural metastases (metastatic epidural spinal cord compression, MESCC) and discusses the broad differential diagnosis from an international perspective.

Epidemiology

The incidence of MESCC is 5–10% of patients with cancer. While metastatic tumor from any primary site can produce ESCC, cancers of breast, lung, and prostate are the most common culprits, accounting for 20%, 13%, and 9% of cases with MESCC, respectively. Although epidural disease arises most often in patients known to have systemic cancer, ESCC is the initial manifestation of malignancy in up to 30% of patients. This is most often seen in cancers of unknown primary, myeloma, lung cancer, and non-Hodgkin's lymphoma.

Cancers of the prostate, breast, lung, and colon dominate in much of North America, Europe, and Australia. Stomach and cervical cancer predominate in Central and South America, whereas cancer of the liver, bladder, and Kaposi's sarcoma are commonly found in Africa. Countries of southern and southeastern Asia have significantly higher incidences of esophageal, stomach, and liver carcinoma. Nasopharyngeal cancer, common in southwest Asia and the Mediterranean basin, commonly metastasizes to the bony skeleton.

Pathophysiology

Since the 1940s, cancer cells were thought to enter the vertebral column through Batson's vertebral venous plexus. However, recent studies suggest that arterial seeding of the vertebrae may be a more common mechanism. This occurs largely in the hematopoietic bone marrow, and thus the posterior vertebral body is invaded first, followed by the pedicle and laminae. Less commonly, tumors such as lymphomas spread from the paraspinal region through the intervertebral foramina.

The neurological deficit of ESCC may be produced by direct mechanical compression of the spinal cord, cauda equina, or nerve root by tumor itself; by interruption of the vascular supply to the spinal cord by tumor; or by direct vertebral compression or collapse due to pathological fracture (so called spinal instability).

Clinical features

Approximately 70% of spinal epidural metastases occur in the thoracic vertebrae, 20% the lumbosacral spine, and 10% the cervical spine. Multiple metastatic lesions are reported in about one-third of patients.

Early recognition of ESCC is crucial, as treatment success is directly related to the severity of neurological deficits at presentation. Studies have shown that overall survival is directly related to ambulatory status at diagnosis, but unfortunately about two-thirds of patients are not ambulatory at diagnosis of ESCC.

In over 90% of patients, pain is the initial symptom. Back pain from epidural metastases is often aggravated with recumbency, Valsalva maneuver, or spinal percussion. Radicular pain is less common than local pain; however, thoracic epidural lesions can produce a band-like sensation around the anterior trunk. Usually a pain syndrome precedes neurological disturbances, but occasionally patients present with sudden neurological deficits.

ESCC produces upper motor neuron weakness if localized at or above the conus medullaris, manifested by symmetric weakness of the lower extremities, hyperreflexia, hypertonicity, and extensor plantar responses. Proximal leg weakness is most severe with thoracic ESCC. More commonly, motor dysfunctions precede sensory disturbances.

Sensory symptoms are almost as common as motor findings at diagnosis. Early symptoms include ascending numbness and paresthesias. If a spinal sensory level is found, it is usually one to five levels below the site of cord compression. Cauda equina lesions may produce saddle anesthesia. Autonomic dysfunction is a late finding and most often manifests as painless urinary retention.

Investigations

Contrast-enhanced magnetic resonance imaging (MRI) is the most sensitive and specific diagnostic tool for MESCC. Plain radiographs are easily available and can demonstrate classic signs of ESCC such as vertebral body collapse or pedicle erosion. However, they have an unacceptably high false negative rate (up to 17%), because 50% of cortical bone must be destroyed before the radiograph becomes abnormal. Similarly, radiation ports planned on the basis of radiographs alone are commonly insufficient.

Radionuclide bone scanning is more sensitive than plain radiographs, but less specific in detecting bone metastasis, correctly predicting the presence and location of epidural spinal lesions in about two-thirds of subjects. However, there is evidence that patients with cancer who present with back pain but have negative bone scans and spinal radiographs have a very low incidence of ESCC.

Myelography, often combined with postmyelogram CT, can define the level and extent of epidural compression. However, myelography is invasive, may not visualize paravertebral soft tissue involvement, and can rarely precipitate neurological deterioration in patients with complete spinal subarachnoid block above the level of lumbar puncture ("spinal coning"). For these reasons,

International Neurology, Second edition. Edited by Robert P. Lisak, Daniel D. Truong, William M. Carroll and Roongroj Bhidayasiri
© 2016 John Wiley & Sons, Ltd. Published 2016 by John Wiley & Sons, Ltd.

MRI has replaced myelography as the gold standard. MRI can also detect intramedullary and leptomeningeal metastases, and multiple epidural lesions that if present may alter the treatment plan. Therefore, most experts agree that patients with suspected MESCC should undergo MRI of the entire spine, or at least the thoracic and lumbosacral spine, as asymptomatic epidural deposits are rarely found in the cervical spine.

Computed tomography (CT) is used when concerns of spinal instability are suggested by MRI or the etiology of vertebral body collapse is uncertain (metastasis vs. osteopenic vertebral body collapse).

In patients with no known site of metastases or no history of cancer, pathological confirmation is required and is most often obtained by percutaneous biopsy.

Differential diagnosis

The differential diagnosis of back pain with or without neurological dysfunction in patients with cancer includes malignant and non-malignant etiologies. In patients with systemic cancer, vertebral metastases with or without epidural extension can be differentiated from intramedullary spinal cord metastases (ISCM) via neuroimaging. Other complications to consider include leptomeningeal metastases and neoplastic plexopathy. Radiation myelopathy usually follows treatment by one or more years, and presents with ascending sensory deficits, weakness, and hemicord symptoms. This can be distinguished from ESCC by MRI.

A detailed discussion of specific infections is beyond the scope of this section, but a few key regional infections are important to consider in the differential diagnosis of ESCC. In general, when there is a history of systemic cancer, the probability of an ESCC is definitely higher than that of an infectious complication; however, the differential diagnosis is particularly important when the systemic cancer is controlled and the prognosis is extended.

Risk factors for spinal epidural abscesses (SEA) include intravenous drug use, diabetes, and spinal trauma, while fever, back pain, spinal tenderness, and peripheral leukocytosis should raise clinical suspicion. Localization is most often thoracic, followed by cervical. The diagnostic method of choice is contrast-enhanced MRI, while cultures often yield a microbiological diagnosis. *Staphylococcus aureus* is most common worldwide.

Spinal involvement with *M. tuberculosis* (Pott's disease) can include discitis, epidural abscess, or osteomyelitis. TB spondylitis is the most common cause of non-traumatic paraplegia in developing countries. TB myelopathy is characterized by its predominantly thoracic location, painless leg weakness, and frequent co-occurrence with HIV. Plain radiographs are often but not always abnormal.

With 40 million people worldwide infected with human immunodeficiency virus (HIV) and the largest number of affected people in sub-Saharan Africa, HIV-associated myelopathy (HAM) is an important entity to consider. Patients present with slowly progressive painless spastic paraparesis, urinary incontinence, and gait ataxia. MRI is typically normal, and HAM is a diagnosis of exclusion. HIV infection predisposes to bacterial SEA, bone metastases from Kaposi sarcoma, intramedullary lymphoma and radiculomyelitis from cytomegalovirus (CMV), herpes simplex virus (HSV), varicella zoster virus (VZV), and human T-cell lymphotropic virus (HTLV), among others.

Acute viral myelitis presents with motor weakness, sensory loss, and autonomic dysfunction evolving over days, but rarely involves pain. Etiologies include HSV-1 and HSV-2, VZV, CMV, EBV, enteroviruses, West Nile virus, and Japanese B encephalitis. Poliovirus presents with proximal greater than distal flaccid areflexic paralysis. Despite nearly worldwide eradication, close to 1500 cases were reported in India in 2002.

HTLV-associated myelopathy/tropical spastic paraparesis (HAM/TSP) develops in less than 5% of the estimated 20 million people worldwide infected with the retrovirus. HAM/TSP presents similarly as HIV-associated myelopathy. Contrasted MRI may or may not show abnormal enhancement and spinal cord edema at affected sites.

Schistosomiasis is endemic to Africa, the Middle East, and southeast Asia. In sub-Saharan Africa, neuroschistosomiasis causes 1–5% of non-traumatic spinal cord lesions. Schistosomal myelopathy most commonly involves *S. mansoni* localized to the conus medullaris and presents with flaccid paraplegia, lumbar radiculopathy, and autonomic dysfunction weeks to months after initial infection. Eosinophilia and the schistosomal ova in biopsy specimens lead to the diagnosis.

Brucella species cause 2–5% of all spondylodiscitis in Mediterranean countries, most often localized to the lumbar region. Complaints of systemic brucellosis dominate early and include fever, malaise, and polymyalgia. Unlike spinal tuberculosis, brucella infection preserves the vertebral architecture despite diffuse spondylodiscitis.

Lyme neuroborreliosis causing acute painful radiculoneuritis is more common in Europe than in North America. The tapeworm *Echinococcus granulosus*, endemic to the Mediterranean basin, Middle East, central Asia, and eastern Africa, spares the intervertebral discs and usually remains confined to one vertebral body. *Coccidioides immitis* preferentially affects the thoracic spines of Filipinos, African Americans, and the elderly of the southwest United States, Central America, and parts of South America, while *Blastomyces dermatitidis* is found in the Mississippi and Ohio river basins of the United States. Neurocysticercosis very rarely involves the spine by causing inflammation in the subarachnoid space, leading to cerebrospinal fluid obstruction. Neurosyphilis can cause either thrombosis of spinal vessels, resulting in a syndrome similar to transverse myelitis, or tabes dorsalis, which manifests years to decades after initial infection. Rarely, osteomyelitis has been attributed to *Aspergillus* species, *Salmonella typhi*, and *Bartonella henselae*.

Treatment

The treatment of ESCC is palliative, with the goals of providing pain relief, maintenance or recovery of neurological function, local durable tumor control, and spinal stability. Pain control often requires opiate analgesics. Anticoagulation should be considered in non-ambulatory patients to prevent venous thromboembolism. Corticosteroids reduce vasogenic edema and improve pain scores and clinical outcome. Doses between 16 and 96 mg of dexamethasone as an initial bolus are acceptable, usually followed by 16 mg daily in divided doses, tapered over days to weeks.

Definitive therapy includes radiation therapy (RT) with or without surgery. RT is preferred for patients with a radiation port extending two levels above and below the symptomatic lesion. While pretreatment neurological function is the strongest predictor of outcome, tumor histology is an important prognostic factor. Radiosensitive tumors, such as lymphomas, myelomas, breast, prostate, ovarian, and neuroendocrine carcinomas (compared to the more radioresistant melanomas, renal cell, colon, and non-small cell lung carcinomas) have a better response and prognosis. Recurrence rates after RT range from 7.5–20%, and almost half of recurrences will be at a site distant from the initial lesion. In a modern approach to

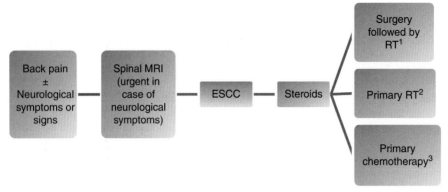

Figure 146.1 Treatment algorithm of newly diagnosed epidural spinal cord compression (ESCC).

[1]Radioresistant tumors, spinal instability, single site of compression
[2]Radiosensitive tumors, absence of spinal instability, multiple sites of compression, medical and/or oncological contraindications for surgery
[3]Chemosensitive tumors (lymphomas, germ cell tumors, myelomas in the absence of myelopathy)
MRI = magnetic resonance imaging; RT = radiotherapy

ESCC, patients with radiosensitive tumors are treated with a conventionally fractionated RT (more commonly intensity-modulated radiotherapy) regardless of ESCC grade, while patients with radioresistant tumors are better treated with stereotactic radiosurgery (which can allow higher doses) with or without previous surgery.

Surgery is reserved when the diagnosis is in doubt, for spinal instability, when vertebral body collapse has caused bony impingement on the cord or nerve roots, for radioresistant tumors, or for failure after spinal radiotherapy. Historically, posterior approaches including decompressive laminectomy were utilized; however, this method often further destabilizes the spinal column. Given that the anterior vertebral elements are most often involved in MESCC, vertebral corpectomy with instrumentation via an anterior approach is becoming more commonplace. However, aggressive tumor resections are associated with prolonged anesthesia and greater potential morbidity; therefore, the goal of modern surgery for ESCC is increasingly to provide a separation of the tumor from the spinal cord to optimize the radiosurgical dose to the tumor volume (so-called separation surgery). Mechanical instability represents an independent indication for surgical stabilization or percutaneous cement augmentation (vertebroplasty or kyphoplasty) regardless of the ESCC grade and radiosensitivity of the tumor.

Systemic chemotherapy can be effective for ESCC caused by chemosensitive tumors such as Hodgkin's and non-Hodgkin's lymphomas, germ cell tumors, neuroblastomas, and breast cancers. Hormonal therapy has been employed successfully in ESCC secondary to prostate and breast cancer (Figure 146.1).

Prognosis

The overall median survival following diagnosis of ESCC is 3–6 months. However, survival is closer to 4 weeks in those patients who remain non-ambulatory after treatment. Prognosis appears to be best in breast and prostate cancers, and significantly worse in lung cancer or in cases of multiple epidural spinal cord metastases. If radiotherapy is initiated while the patient is still ambulatory, a large majority will maintain the ability to walk. However, fewer than 1 in 10 paraplegics will regain ambulation despite adequate treatment. Therefore, prompt diagnosis and initiation of treatment before permanent neurological sequelae develop from MESCC are key.

Pediatric epidural metastases

The most common pediatric tumors associated with MESCC include sarcoma (especially Ewing's sarcoma), neuroblastoma, germ cell neoplasms, and Hodgkin's disease. Neurological complications of neuroblastoma and non-Hodgkin's lymphoma are not uncommonly the initial manifestation of systemic malignancy. Plain radiographs of pediatric epidural metastases are often normal, because the mechanism is usually invasion of the epidural space through vertebral foramina, forming paravertebral masses without producing bony lesions. Overall prognosis is thought to be better than in adults due to the radio- and chemosensitivity of neuroblastoma, germ cell tumors, and Hodgkin's lymphoma.

Further reading

Chamberlain MC. Neoplastic meningitis and metastatic epidural spinal cord compression. *Hematol Oncol Clin North Am* 2012;26(4):917–931.

Laufer I, Rubin DG, Lis E, *et al.* The NOMS framework: Approach to the treatment of spinal metastatic tumors. *The Oncologist* 2013;18(6):744–751.

Loblaw DA, Perry J, Chambers A, Laperriere NJ. Systematic review of the diagnosis and management of malignant extradural spinal cord compression: The Cancer Care Ontario Practice Guidelines Initiative's Neuro-Oncology Disease Site. *J Clin Oncol* 2005;23(9):2028–2037.

Scheld WM, Marra CM, Whitley RJ (eds.). *Infections of the Central Nervous System.* Philadelphia, PA: Lippincott Williams & Wilkins; 2004.

147 General approach to the diagnosis and treatment of paraneoplastic neurological disorders

Myrna R. Rosenfeld and Josep Dalmau

Department of Neurology, Hospital Clínic/IDIBAPS, Barcelona, Spain

Paraneoplastic neurological disorders (PND) are immune-mediated disorders that may affect any part of the nervous system. Although the exact pathogenesis of PND is unclear, the current concept is that the expression of neuronal proteins by a tumor breaks immune tolerance and provokes an immune response against both the tumor and the nervous system. This hypothesis is supported by the frequent detection in the serum and cerebrospinal fluid (CSF) of antibodies reacting with antigens expressed by the tumor and nervous system. Some antibodies have a direct pathogenic role in causing the neurological dysfunction, while other antibodies occur in association with cytotoxic T-cell responses that are the main effectors of the neuronal degeneration.

Paraneoplastic neurological disorders are rare and it is estimated that they occur in less than 1% of all patients with cancer. Regional variations in incidence and prevalence will mirror regional differences in rates of cancers and also cancer types, as some cancers are more commonly associated with PND than others.

Diagnosis

The diagnosis of PND is based on recognizing the neurological syndrome, demonstrating the presence of an associated cancer, and detecting serum and CSF paraneoplastic antibodies. Recognizing the syndrome can be difficult, since PND precede the cancer diagnosis in about 60% of patients and similar syndromes may occur in the absence of cancer. Some syndromes (e.g., acute or subacute cerebellar dysfunction in an adult or opsoclonus-myoclonus in a child) are highly characteristic and so often associated with cancer that their presence should immediately lead to the suspicion of a paraneoplastic etiology. Other syndromes (e.g., brainstem dysfunction, myelopathy) result from paraneoplastic mechanisms, but occur more frequently in the absence of cancer and therefore require a more extensive differential diagnosis. An initial clue is the mode of onset, as most PND present in an acute or subacute manner compared with the chronic progression of non-inflammatory neurodegenerative disorders (Table 147.1).

PND usually develop at early stages of cancer and therefore the tumor (or its recurrence) may be difficult to demonstrate. In most instances, the tumor is revealed by computed tomography (CT) of chest, abdomen, and pelvis. Combined CT and fluorodeoxyglucose-positron emission tomography (FDG-PET) are useful in demonstrating occult neoplasms; cancer serum markers are helpful. Patients with a neuropathy of unclear etiology should be examined for a monoclonal gammopathy in the serum and urine, and if positive undergo a skeletal survey and bone marrow biopsy.

The specificity of paraneoplastic antibodies for certain PND or some types of cancer makes them useful diagnostic tools. In the appropriate clinical context, the detection of a paraneoplastic antibody helps diagnose the PND and focus the search for the neoplasm. For antibody-positive patients, if a cancer is not discovered, the presence of an occult neoplasm is assumed. Although almost any cancer can associate with PND, the tumors most commonly involved are small cell lung cancer (SCLC), cancers of the breast or ovary, thymoma, neuroblastoma, and plasma cell tumors. The presence of paraneoplastic antibodies in the CSF is diagnostic of PND; however, it is important to keep in mind that some antibodies are detectable at low titers in the serum of some patients with cancer without PND.

The diagnosis of PND is more difficult in patients who develop less characteristic symptoms (e.g., brainstem dysfunction, myelopathy), especially if no antibodies are found. In a patient known to have cancer, metastases and non-metastatic neurological complications of cancer should be considered and can often be ruled out with neuroimaging. The CSF of patients with PND of the central nervous system often suggests an inflammatory process: pleocytosis, increased protein concentration, intrathecal synthesis of immunoglobulin G, and oligoclonal bands. Biopsy of an abnormal brain region identified by magnetic resonance imaging (MRI) or FDG-PET may be considered if a neoplastic process is suspected or if the clinical, CSF, and MRI findings are unusual. Abnormalities supporting, but not specific to, PND include infiltrates of mononuclear cells, neuronophagic nodules, neuronal degeneration, microglial proliferation, and gliosis.

For patients in whom no cancer is found but the suspicion for a PND is high, periodic cancer screening for at least 5 years is recommended, keeping in mind that in 90% of patients the underlying tumor will be uncovered within the first year of PND symptom onset. Patients whose cancer is in remission who develop PND should be examined for tumor recurrence.

Treatment

The first approach for treating any PND is to promptly identify and treat the tumor. Based on the syndrome and associated immune responses, for treatment purposes PND can be divided into those

---

International Neurology, Second edition. Edited by Robert P. Lisak, Daniel D. Truong, William M. Carroll and Roongroj Bhidayasiri

Table 147.1 Paraneoplastic syndromes and antibody associations.

Syndromes of the central nervous system (possible antibody associations)
Paraneoplastic cerebellar degeneration (isolated or predominant cerebellar symptoms: anti-Yo, anti-Tr, anti-VGCC with or without association with LEMS; in the context of encephalomyelitis or brainstem encephalitis: anti-Hu, anti-CV2/CRMP5, anti-amphiphysin, anti-Ri, anti-Ma2)
Paraneoplastic encephalomyelitis (anti-Hu, anti-CV2/CRMP5, anti-amphiphysin)
Limbic encephalitis (usually in the context of encephalomyelitis or brainstem encephalitis: anti-Hu, anti-CV2/CRMP5, anti-amphiphysin, anti-Ma proteins. Isolated or predominant limbic dysfunction: antibodies to neuronal cell-surface proteins*)
Paraneoplastic opsoclonus-myoclonus (anti-Ri)
Stiff-man syndrome (anti-amphiphysin)
Syndromes of the peripheral nervous system
Paraneoplastic sensory neuronopathy (anti-Hu)
Vasculitis of the nerve and muscle
Subacute and chronic sensorimotor neuropathies (anti-CRMP5)
Sensorimotor neuropathy associated with plasma cell dyscrasias and B-cell lymphoma
Peripheral nerve hyperexcitability (anti-Caspr2, rarely anti-LGI1)
Autonomic neuropathy (anti-nAChR)
Brachial neuritis
Acute polyradiculoneuropathy (Guillain–Barré syndrome)
Syndromes of the neuromuscular junction and muscle
Lambert–Eaton myasthenic syndrome (anti-VGCC)
Myasthenia gravis (anti-AChR)
Dermatomyositis
Acute necrotizing myopathy
Paraneoplastic visual syndromes
Retinopathy (anti-recoverin; anti-bipolar cell)
Optic neuritis
Uveitis (usually in association with encephalomyelitis; anti-CV2/CRMP5)

* Includes antibodies to AMPAR (alpha-amino-3-hydroxy-5-methyl-4-isoxazolepropionic acid receptor); GABA(B)R (gamma-aminobutyric acid-B receptor); LGI1 (leucine-rich glioma inactivated protein-1); mGluR5 (metabotropic glutamate receptor 5)

AChR = acetylcholine receptor; LEMS = Lambert–Eaton myasthenic syndrome; VGCC = voltage-gated calcium channel

in which the paraneoplastic antibodies are pathogenic and those in which cytotoxic T-cells are the likely mediators of the neurological dysfunction. In the former category are disorders such as Lambert–Eaton myasthenic syndrome associated with anti-voltage-gated calcium channel (VGCC) antibodies, myasthenia gravis with anti-acetylcholine receptor (AChR) antibodies, a subset of autonomic neuropathies with antibodies to the ganglionic AChR, and the autoimmune encephalitis associated with antibodies to neuronal cell-surface or synaptic receptors (the latter discussed in further detail in Chapter 80). In these disorders, removal of the antibodies with plasma exchange or modulation of the immune response with intravenous immunoglobulins (IVIg) often results in neurological improvement.

For those PND that are likely T-cell mediated, immunosuppression or immunomodulation is recommended, although these disorders are often refractory to therapy unless instituted when there is still active central nervous system (CNS) inflammation. For these cases stabilization or mild improvement can occur. For patients who may be receiving chemotherapy, simultaneous corticosteroids, IVIg, or plasma exchange may be considered. Patients with progressive symptoms who are not receiving chemotherapy should be considered for more aggressive immunosuppression that may include cyclophosphamide, tacrolimus, cyclosporine, or rituximab.

The remainder of this chapter briefly describes several syndromes that are highly characteristic and so frequently associated with cancer that their identification should lead to an immediate suspicion of a paraneoplastic etiology.

Specific syndromes

Paraneoplastic cerebellar degeneration

Paraneoplastic cerebellar degeneration (PCD) usually presents with dizziness, gait unsteadiness, and oscillopsia, and evolves in a few days or weeks to severe cerebellar dysfunction. Most patients become wheelchair bound, with dysarthria, dysphagia, blurry vision or diplopia, and absent or very mild impairment of sensation and reflexes. Cognitive functions are usually preserved, but about 25% of patients show mild impairment. Almost all well-characterized paraneoplastic antibodies have been reported in association with PCD. Serological markers that associate with "pure" PCD include Yo, Tr, VGCC, and infrequently Zic4 and Ma2 antibodies. Between 30% and 40% of patients with PCD do not have detectable paraneoplastic antibodies; in these patients the diagnosis relies on the exclusion of other etiologies and demonstration of the cancer. PCD rarely responds to treatment. An exception is the group of patients with anti-Tr antibodies and Hodgkin's lymphoma; approximately 20% show improvement after tumor treatment and corticosteroids, IVIg, or plasma exchange.

Paraneoplastic encephalomyelitis

Patients with paraneoplastic encephalomyelitis (PEM) may develop dysfunction of any part of the CNS, dorsal root ganglia (causing paraneoplastic sensory neuronopathy), and autonomic nerves. Symptoms develop rapidly and progress over weeks or months until stabilization or death. The CSF usually shows a mild to moderate lymphocytic pleocytosis, increased protein and normal glucose concentrations, and oligoclonal bands or increased IgG index. Brain MRI often shows fluid-attenuated inversion recovery (FLAIR) or T2 sequence hyperintensities in involved and at times clinically silent regions. Patients with PEM and SCLC often have anti-Hu, and less frequently anti-CV2/CRMP5 antibodies, or both. Management of PEM is based on prompt treatment of the tumor along with immunosuppression. Although the standard of care remains to be established, the use of corticosteroids and IVIg combined with chemotherapy may help to stabilize or improve the neurological symptoms during the period of time for which the tumor is treated. Afterwards, if the neurological symptoms have stabilized or improved, patients should be considered for prolonged treatment with immunosuppressive therapies that target not only the antibodies but also the T-cell immunity (e.g., cyclophosphamide combined with corticosteroids, among other strategies).

Limbic encephalitis and brainstem encephalitis

Patients with paraneoplastic limbic encephalitis (LE) present with anxiety, depression, confusion, delirium, hallucinations, seizures, or short-term memory loss. In approximately 80% of patients the MRI T2 and FLAIR sequences show hyperintense abnormalities in one or both medial temporal lobes. Almost all patients have an abnormal electroencephalogram (EEG) that includes uni- or bilateral temporal lobe epileptic discharges, or slow background activity.

Patients with brainstem encephalitis (BSE) develop diplopia, dysarthria, dysphagia, and gaze abnormalities, usually accompanied by symptoms of cerebellar dysfunction. Patients with Hu antibodies usually present with predominant lower brainstem dysfunction, while patients with Ma2 antibodies have predominant initial involvement of the upper brainstem. The brainstem encephalitis related to Ri antibodies often is accompanied by opsoclonus and other movement disorders, and may result in life-threatening laryngospasm. Symptoms of LE and BSE may overlap in some patients.

LE associated with antibodies to intracellular antigens (e.g., Hu, Ma2, CV2/CRMP5) is likely mediated by cytotoxic T-cell responses and in general these disorders are poorly responsive to treatment. An exception is LE/BSE associated with Ma2 antibodies, in which 30% of patients respond to treatment of the tumor and immunotherapy (usually corticosteroids and IVIg). LE also occurs in the autoimmune encephalitis syndromes associated with antibodies to the neuronal cell surface (e.g., AMPA receptor, GABA(B) receptor, LGI1, and mGluR5). Due to the pathogenicity of the associated antibodies, these disorders are often responsive to immunotherapies.

Paraneoplastic sensory neuronopathy

Paraneoplastic sensory neuronopathy (PSN) results from an immune attack against the neurons of the dorsal root ganglia.

Patients develop pain, numbness, and sensory deficits that can affect limbs, trunk, and cranial nerves. The presentation is frequently asymmetric, associated with decreased or abolished reflexes, and relative preservation of strength. All types of sensation can be affected, but loss of proprioception is often predominant, resulting in sensory ataxia and pseudoathetoid movements of the extremities (predominantly hands). PSN may occur in isolation, but often precedes or coincides with the development of PEM. While most types of cancers may occur in association with PSN, almost 80% of patients have SCLC. Therefore, PSN should be suspected in a patient with a history of smoking who develops the subacute onset of asymmetric sensory symptoms. Prompt treatment of patients with corticosteroids and IVIg along with treatment of the tumor may result in stabilization or mild improvement of the dorsal root ganglia dysfunction.

Paraneoplastic opsoclonus-myoclonus

Paraneoplastic opsoclonus-myoclonus, often with ataxia, usually occurs in association with neuroblastoma in children, while in adults several underlying tumors have been reported, most commonly SCLC and cancers of the breast and ovary. Almost all well-characterized paraneoplastic antibodies have been reported in isolated case reports; however, the majority of patients are antibody negative. An exception is a small subset of adults, predominantly with breast and ovarian cancer, who develop anti-Ri antibodies. A small proportion of patients with SCLC and 5% of children with neuroblastoma have anti-Hu antibodies.

Children with neuroblastoma-associated opsoclonus-myoclonus respond to tumor treatment along with immunomodulatory therapies such as prednisone, adrenocorticotropic hormone, IVIg, rituximab, or cyclophosphamide, although in many patients the response is partial. Adults whose tumors are treated promptly have better neurological outcomes than those whose tumors are not treated. In the latter cases the disorder often progresses to death.

Further reading

Giometto B, Grisold W, Vitaliani R, *et al.* Paraneoplastic neurologic syndrome in the PNS Euronetwork database: A European study from 20 centers. *Arch Neurol* 2010;67:330–335.

Giometto B, Vitaliani R, Lindeck-Pozza E, Grisold W, Vedeler C. Treatment for paraneoplastic neuropathies. *Cochrane Database Syst Rev* 2012;12:CD007625.

Graus F, Dalmau J. Paraneoplastic neuropathies. *Curr Opin Neurol* 2013;26:489–495.

Graus F, Delattre JY, Antoine JC, *et al.* Recommended diagnostic criteria for paraneoplastic neurological syndromes. *J Neurol Neurosurg Psychiatry* 2004;75:1135–1140.

Skeie GO, Apostolski S, Evoli A, *et al.* Guidelines for treatment of autoimmune neuromuscular transmission disorders. *Eur J Neurol* 2010;17:893–902.

Titulaer MJ, Soffietti R, Dalmau J, *et al.* Screening for tumours in paraneoplastic syndromes: Report of an EFNS task force. *Eur J Neurol* 2011;18:19–e3.

Vedeler CA, Antoine JC, Giometto B, *et al.* Management of paraneoplastic neurological syndromes: Report of an EFNS Task Force. *Eur J Neurol* 2006;13:682–690.

148   Insomnia

Delwyn J. Bartlett[1] and Colin A. Espie[2]

[1] University of Sydney Central Clinical School, Medical Psychology/Sleep & Circadian Group, Woolcock Institute of Medical Research, Sydney, Australia

[2] Sleep and Circadian Neuroscience Institute, Nuffield Department of Clinical Neurosciences, University of Oxford, Oxford, UK

Insomnia is the most common sleep disorder and is central to a number of medical, neurological, and psychiatric disorders representing an increasing public health concern. Insomnia is a repeated, distressing difficulty in initiating sleep, maintaining sleep, or waking early (greater than 30 minutes), which is chronically non-restorative despite adequate sleep opportunity. It is associated with impairment of daytime functioning, with symptoms being present for at least 3 months and occurring at least 3 times per week. The most recent version of the *Diagnostic and Statistical Manual of Mental Disorders* (DSM-5) defines insomnia as a disorder, which is a paradigm shift in removing a causal pathway and possibly blocking comorbid treatment options. However, within the neurological field insomnia may present as a hypersomnia such as narcolepsy and/or as a sleep-related movement disorder, including restless legs syndrome (RLS) and period limb movement (PLM; see Table 148.1). This chapter summarizes insomnia and lists evidence-based management.

Epidemiology

Insomnia affects one-third of adults episodically, and 9–12% on a chronic basis, with some reports as high as 18.5%. It is more commonly reported in women, in shift workers, and in patients with medical and psychiatric disorders. Among older adults prevalence has been estimated at 25% or higher, with comorbid conditions and hypnotic drug co-presenting.

Pathophysiology

Sleep disruption is often unreported until insomnia is well established. It is unclear whether the physiological changes associated with insomnia precede onset or are a consequence. High-frequency electroencephalogram (EEG) activity is exaggerated in individuals with insomnia. These findings suggest a central nervous system arousal, supporting previous research of increased cortisol or reduced morning cortisol and adrenocorticotrophic hormone, possibly reflecting an adaptation to poor quality sleep. Objective performance is not necessarily impaired.

Clinical features

Subjectively, sleep is non-restorative. Individuals are overwhelmingly concerned about sleep onset, return to sleep, and the unpredictability of sleep. The clinical presentation is commonly one of a frustrated patient, trapped in a vicious circle of anxiety and poor sleep, reporting having "tried everything" and generally unable to "downregulate" arousal levels at bedtime.

While some cognitive and performance effects are present, fatigue is more common, along with inattention and mood problems, including anxiety and irritability. The presence of sleepiness is unusual in insomnia and investigations for other sleep disorders (obstructive sleep apnea syndrome, narcolepsy, periodic limb movement disorder, and restless legs syndrome), head injury, or depression are prudent.

Insomnias due to drug or substance abuse can also include hypnotic dependent sleep disorder, commonly associated with benzodiazepine (BZ) drugs where fast withdrawal exacerbates the primary insomnia problem, reinforcing hypnotic dependency. Psychiatric conditions, particularly depression, have an established bi-directional relationship with insomnia. Sleep disturbance often precedes depression, being an independent risk factor for a first episode or recurrence of depression. The role of anxiety is less clear, but other studies emphasize the relationship between ruminations and an overarousal response. In the updated International Classification of Sleep Disorders there is also an emphasis on persistent sleep difficulties, adequate sleep opportunity, and daytime impairment. Comorbid medical and psychiatric disorders are frequently seen to accompany insomnia along with other sleep disorders. Recent research found that 20% of individuals presenting with obstructive sleep apnea (OSA) also had insomnia. In a prospective 3-year study of the natural course of insomnia, 46% of individuals with severe insomnia at baseline experienced persistent insomnia at all time points. Age alone does not cause insomnia if the individual is healthy, but comorbid medical conditions are often precipitating factors. Circadian rhythm disorders, shift work, parasomnias, and inadequate sleep hygiene can all be triggers for insomnia.

Investigations

A thorough history, incorporating screening questions for mood, lifestyle, restlessness, limb movements, and breathing, is important. Sleep diary monitoring is the most useful form of assessment, with additional questionnaires on beliefs and mood. Wrist actigraphy estimates sleep/wakefulness based on body movement and is worn for 10–14 days consecutively; it can identify paradoxical insomnia and circadian anomalies. Polysomnography is undertaken only

International Neurology, Second edition. Edited by Robert P. Lisak, Daniel D. Truong, William M. Carroll and Roongroj Bhidayasiri
© 2016 John Wiley & Sons, Ltd. Published 2016 by John Wiley & Sons, Ltd.

Table 148.1. Diagnosis and differentiation of the insomnias: International Classification of Sleep Disorders (ICSD-3).

Classification	Essential features of insomnia	Other features
Chronic insomnia disorder	1. Difficulty with sleep initiation and/or maintenance problems 2. Despite adequate opportunity to sleep 3. Daytime consequences as per other features 4. Present for at least 3 months 5. Occurring >3 times per week	Fatigue/malaise; attention, concentration, or memory impairment; impaired social, family, occupational, or academic performance; mood disturbance/irritability; daytime sleepiness; behavioral problems (e.g., hyperactivity, impulsivity, aggression); reduced motivation/energy/initiative; proneness for errors/accidents; concerns about or dissatisfaction with sleep

	Behavioral insomnia of childhood now included under this heading
	Other previous primary insomnia disorders are now listed under chronic insomnia cisorder:
	  Psychophysiological insomnia
	  Idiopathic
	  Paradoxical insomnia
	  Insomnia due to a mental disorder
	  Inadequate sleep hygiene
	  Insomnia due to a medical disorder
	  Insomnia due to drug or substance
		Inappropriate sleep associations or inadequate limit setting

Short-term insomnia	Insomnia symptoms of less than 3 months	Adjustment disorder or acute with a specific stressor
Other insomnia disorder	Neither of the above	
Sleep-related breathing disorders	Obstructive sleep apnea syndrome Complex sleep apnea Sleep-related hypoventilation disorders	Excessive sleepiness, obstructed breathing in sleep; symptoms snoring and a dry mouth Persistent or residual symptoms following effective treatment Sustained hypoxemia during polysomnography
Sleep-related movement disorders	Periodic limb movement disorder	Episodes of repetitive, highly stereotyped limb movements occurring in sleep
	Restless legs syndrome	Strong, nearly irresistible urge to move legs, relieved by walking; circadian effect
	Also includes sleep-related leg cramps; sleep-related bruxism; sleep-related rhythmic movement disorder; and other movement disorders related to medical/medicine/substance and unspecified	
Central disorders of hypersomnolence	Narcolepsy with or without cataplexy (sudden loss of muscle tone during highly emotive situations) Idiopathic hypersomnia	Excessive daytime sleepiness (EDS) not attributable to another sleep disorder. Episodes of "irrepressible need to sleep or daytime lapses into sleep." Paradoxically can have poor night-time sleep quality EDS not explained by another condition
Circadian rhythm sleep–wake disorders (CRSD)	CRSD: Delayed sleep phase type	Phase delay of major sleep episode, initial insomnia, excessive sleepiness in morning
	CRSD: Advanced sleep phase type	Phase advance of major sleep episode, inability to stay awake in evening, early wakening
	Also includes irregular sleep–wake rhythm disorder; non-24-h sleep–wake rhythm disorder; shift work disorder; jet lag disorder; circadian sleep–wake disorder not otherwise specified	
Parasomnias Undesirable physical events	NREM	Confusional arousals; sleep walking; sleep terrors; sleep-related eating disorder; sleep-related movement disorders
	REM	REM behavior disorder; recurrent isolated sleep paralysis; nightmare disorder
	Other	Exploding head syndrome; sleep-related hallucinations; sleep enuresis; parasomnia due to a medical condition; parasomnia due to a medication or substance; parasomnia unspecified

when another sleep disorder is suspected, but can be undertaken to reassure an individual that they can sleep even if it is an exception.

Treatment
Drug therapy

BZ compounds superseded barbiturates, and although effective in the short term, potential problems are tolerance and withdrawal. Contemporary hypnotic therapy includes benzodiazepine receptor agonists (BzRAs; "z"-drugs) zopiclone and zolpidem, which were introduced in the 1980s with fewer side effects and maintained slow-wave sleep, compared with the benzodiazepines associated with prolongation of N2 sleep. A recent meta-analysis explored 20 studies and found negative effects on verbal and working memory

for zopiclone, and attention and speed of processing for zolpidem. Even a single dose of these z-drugs in healthy adults tested the following morning is associated with negative effects on cognitive function. More recently, melatonin receptor agonists have been used (MeRAs). BzRAs offer fewer adverse effects, although long-term effectiveness is less clear. Increasingly (off-label) sedative antidepressants and more recently antipsychotics such as quetiapine are also being used for their sedating side effects. However, a 2014 review stated that there are no current studies to support the efficacy or safety of these in the treatment of insomnia.

Melatonin, the pineal hormone, triggers sleep onset by lowering core body temperature and is a useful chronobiotic for reducing sleep latency in delayed sleep phase syndrome (DSPS). Circadin is a slow-release melatonin derivative used to treat over 55-year-olds with sleep maintenance insomnia, although there is currently only questionnaire data to support its efficacy.

Psychological and behavioral therapy

Psychological treatment in the form of cognitive behavioral therapy (CBT) has demonstrated large effect-size changes in primary outcomes that are maintained at long-term follow-up. CBT is also effective in general practice and can be adapted for other settings. The combination of hypnotic therapy in conjunction with CBT is effective in the first week, with consequential tapering as CBT interventions predominate.

Overall management strategies in the treatment of insomnia

Factual information sets boundaries and challenges inaccurate sleep attributions. Understanding what sleep is, how sleep changes with age, good sleep hygiene practices (reducing caffeine and alcohol etc.), and some facts about sleep loss form the starting point for self-management.

Bright light is a potent stimulus for human circadian rhythm, resetting sleep times in advanced sleep-phase syndrome (ASPS) and DSPS. Sleep-initiation insomnia is improved with morning light and avoidance of evening light.

Exercise can positively influence sleep quality, particularly in the late afternoon or early evening. Morning exercise with light exposure suppresses melatonin-enhancing circadian rhythm and sets a constant waking time.

Relearning sleep is about enabling the individual to perceive that the environment is now safe to let sleep happen and includes examination of external factors (heating, noise, violent others) and internal factors relating to previous experiences.

Specific behavioral treatments

Stimulus control

Stimulus control is a reconditioning treatment forcing discrimination between daytime and sleeping environments. For the poor sleeper, the bedroom triggers associations with being awake and aroused. Treatment involves removing all stimuli that are potentially sleep incompatible (reading and watching television) and excluding sleep from living areas. The individual is instructed to get up if not asleep within 15–20 minutes or if wakeful during the night for approximately the same time frame.

Sleep restriction therapy

Sleep restriction relates to the ratio of time asleep with time in bed, and involves recording average nightly sleep duration. The aim is slowly to reduce time in bed to match recorded sleep duration, which increases sleep efficiency and confidence.

Cognitive control

Intrusive thoughts are addressed before bedtime. Setting aside 15–20 minutes in the early evening to rehearse the day and to plan for tomorrow allows the day to be put to rest. Thought stopping attempts to interrupt the flow of thoughts via "blocking" techniques, such as repeating the word "the" every 3 seconds. This procedure occupies the short-term memory store used in the processing of information and, by not demanding attention, potentially allows sleep to happen. Cognitive restructuring challenges faulty beliefs that maintain both wakefulness and helplessness. By challenging

such thoughts as "I shall be useless at work tomorrow," high levels of preoccupation and anxiety are reduced along with inaccurate thinking, thereby aiding sleep onset.

Relaxation methods include progressive relaxation, imagery training, biofeedback, meditation, hypnosis, and autogenic training, with little evidence to indicate the superiority of any one approach. At the cognitive level, these techniques may act through distraction.

Paradoxical intention

Attempting to remain wakeful rather than "trying" to fall asleep decatastrophizes the wakefulness (confronting the worst-case scenario – e.g., "What if I do not go to sleep? I have managed this in the past!") and strengthens the sleep drive, reducing performance effort. Relaxation techniques for reducing insomnia symptoms have an effective track record in lowering the overarousal and wired response. There is less evidence in relation to third-wave therapies such as mindfulness, which appear to be clinically effective along with CBT.

Finally, prevention needs to be extended to known extrinsic causes of certain sleep disorders and to alcohol, stimulants, or proprietary drugs that interfere with sleep. Encouraging individuals to seek advice *early* rather than self-administering treatment is critical in reducing long-term complications. Avoiding the use of hypnotic agents, both in general practice and during acute admissions to hospital, as the first line of treatment without CBT would substantially reduce the number of iatrogenic cases of chronic insomnia.

Conclusion

Chronic insomnia disorder in most clinical situations is both multidimensional and complex. It is characterized predominantly by fatigue and poor-quality sleep, where the individual often presents believing that their sleep has "gone away." Early treatment of the insomnia, whether it is associated with other psychiatric or medical disorders, is crucial in prevention of long-term chronicity and exacerbation of the other disorders. CBT alone is the treatment of choice, both short term and long term. However, in the initial treatment phase hypnotic medication can be useful in helping individuals commence the behavioral interventions, gain confidence, and then with assistance taper this while maintaining the CBT parameters.

Further reading

American Academy of Sleep Medicine. *International Classification of Sleep Disorders (ICSD-3): Diagnostic and Coding Manual*, 3rd ed. Westchester, IL: AASM; 2014.

Espie C. The daytime impact of DSM-5 insomnia disorder: Comparative analysis of insomnia subtypes from the Great British Sleep Survey. *J Clin Psychiatr* 2012;73:e1478–31484.

Morin C. Combined therapeutics for insomnia: Should our first approach be behavioural or pharmacological? *Sleep Med* 2006;7(Suppl 1):S15–S9.

Morin CM. *Insomnia: A Clinical Guide to Assessment and Treatment*. New York: Kluwer Academic/Plenum Publishers; 2003.

Morin CM, Ivers H, Vallières A, Guay B, Savard J. Speed and trajectory of changes of insomnia symptoms during acute treatment with cognitive–behavioral therapy, singly and combined with medication. *Sleep Med* 2014;15:701–707.

Morin CM, LeBlanc M, Ivers H, *et al.* The natural history of insomnia: A population-based 3-year longitudinal study. *Arch Intern Med* 2009;169:447–453.

Morin C, Rodrigue S, Ivers H. Role of stress, arousal, and coping skills in primary insomnia. *Psychosomat Med* 2003;65:259–267.

Ohayon M, Hong S. Prevalence of insomnia and associated factors in South Korea. *J Psychosomat Res* 2002;53:593–600.

Perlis M, Aloia M, Millikan A, *et al.* Behavioral treatment of insomnia: A clinical case series study. *J Behav Med* 2000;23:149–161.

149   Narcolepsy

Marcel Hungs

Department of Neurology, University of Minnesota, Minneapolis, MN, USA

Narcolepsy is a common sleep disorder characterized by excessive daytime sleepiness, cataplexy (episodes of muscle weakness triggered by emotions), hypnagogic hallucination, sleep paralysis, fragmented night sleep, and automatic behaviors. It is generally separated into two pathophysiological subtypes: narcolepsy with or without cataplexy (defined as sleepiness with rapid sleep onset into rapid eye movement [REM] sleep). Narcolepsy was first reported by Westphal in 1877 and the term was coined by Gélineau in 1880. Along with obstructive sleep apnea (OSA) and idiopathic hypersomnia, narcolepsy is one of the leading causes of excessive daytime sleepiness (EDS). The discovery in 1999 that narcolepsy with cataplexy was caused by a hypocretin/orexin deficiency in the hypothalamus led to a major advance not only in the insights related to this condition, but also in the general understanding of the sleep–wake system. In contrast, much less is known regarding narcolepsy without cataplexy.

Epidemiology

The prevalence of narcolepsy with cataplexy in North America and Europe averages 0.02–0.05%. Similar prevalence estimates have been reported in Hong Kong. Prevalence data from other countries suggest a higher prevalence in Japan (0.16%) and a lower prevalence in Israel (0.002%), although these figures may be confounded by differences in epidemiological methods and other factors, such as reduced access to healthcare and limited awareness of healthcare providers regarding sleep disorders. Incidence data are limited; one US study reports an incidence rate of 0.74 per 100,000 person-years for narcolepsy with cataplexy.

Few studies have reported the prevalence of narcolepsy without cataplexy due to the requirement of a sleep study for diagnosis. In one study, the prevalence of diagnosed cases was observed to be 0.02%, with an incidence of 1.37 per 100,000 person-years. However, many cases meeting the diagnostic criteria may go undiagnosed. In two studies, where sleep studies were performed in a population-based sample, approximately 2–4% of the population met international criteria for narcolepsy without cataplexy.

Pathophysiology

When cataplexy is present, narcolepsy in humans is almost always caused by a deficiency of hypocretin (also called orexin), a neurotransmitter produced by 50,000–100,000 neurons located in the posterior hypothalamus. Hypocretin receptors are located in various areas of the brain, including the cerebral cortex, hypothalamus, brainstem, and spinal cord. Input from the limbic system and interaction with metabolic signals such as leptin and glucose allow hypocretin neurons to play a role in emotion, energy homeostasis, reward, addiction, and arousal. The hypocretin system has effects on midbrain dopaminergic systems other than the nigral–striatal pathway. Interestingly, patients with hypocretin deficiency are less susceptible to stimulant abuse, suggesting a role for hypocretin in the regulation of drug addiction. Hypocretin neurons interact with the cholinergic and monoaminergic systems, which modulate the sleep–wake cycle. In narcolepsy, it is suggested that the loss of excitatory hypocretin input to monoaminergic cell groups mediates sleepiness and short REM sleep latency. This parallels the observation that indirectly stimulating monoaminergic transmission, using amphetamine-like compounds and antidepressants, improves narcolepsy symptoms.

The occurrence of narcolepsy involves genetic predisposition and environmental triggers. Multiplex families are rare, but a 10- to 40-fold increase in relative risk is reported in first-degree relatives. The strong association of narcolepsy with the human leukocyte antigen (HLA) system suggests an autoimmune mechanism responsible for hypocretin cell loss. Most patients with typical cataplexy carry *HLA-DQB1*0602*, an HLA subtype found in 12% of Japanese, 25% of Caucasians, and 38% of African Americans. The HLA association and associated hypocretin deficiency are robust (>90%) in patients with definite cataplexy. In patients without cataplexy, a weaker HLA association is observed, with approximately 40% of patients positive for *DQB1*0602*. A 2009 pandemic H1N1 influenza virus in China was followed by a higher rate of narcolepsy, suggesting that in genetically susceptible individuals, narcolepsy might be triggered by a similarity between a region of hypocretin and a portion of a protein from the pandemic H1N1 virus or the H1N1 vaccine. This concept, known as "molecular mimicry," could explain that T-cells of the immune system primed to attack H1N1 could also cross-react with hypocretin and potentially cause the destruction of hypocretin-producing neurons.

Clinical features

Narcolepsy can be best described as a disorder of wakefulness, sleep consolidation, and abnormal REM sleep. Narcolepsy typically begins in adolescence and early adulthood, although late adult onset or onset in prepubertal children is described in approximately 10% of cases. The following symptoms are the primary clinical features of narcolepsy.

International Neurology, Second edition. Edited by Robert P. Lisak, Daniel D. Truong, William M. Carroll and Roongroj Bhidayasiri
© 2016 John Wiley & Sons, Ltd. Published 2016 by John Wiley & Sons, Ltd.

Excessive daytime sleepiness

Excessive daytime sleepiness is often the first symptom of narcolepsy and is frequently the presenting complaint requiring medical attention. Sleepiness in narcolepsy is often severe. It frequently culminates with sudden sleep attacks (an overwhelming urge to sleep within minutes). The resulting sleep episode is usually brief, often associated with dreaming, and, in contrast to naps in other sleep disorders, frequently refreshing. Sleepiness in narcolepsy is not always distinguishable from sleepiness due to other sleep disorders, in that it typically occurs after lunch or in the absence of external stimulation.

Cataplexy

When cataplexy is present in combination with sleepiness, the diagnosis of narcolepsy is almost certain, and confirmatory tests are optional, although still advisable. Cataplexy is characterized by sudden and transient episodes of bilateral loss of muscle tone, without loss of consciousness, often triggered by an emotional stimulus such as laughter, surprise, anger, fear, or humorous situations. Early in the course of narcolepsy, cataplexy may only affect facial muscles or cause knee buckling. Severe cataplectic attacks can lead to falls and temporary loss of striated muscle tone in the extremities. The events can last from seconds to minutes. Other clinical events that can cause falls (such as syncope, sleep attacks, or generalized seizures) can be differentiated from cataplexy, as they are associated with a loss of consciousness. In true cataplexy, the episodes of muscle weakness are reasonably frequent (more than once a month), and are often triggered by strong emotions such as laughter or joking.

Sleep paralysis

Patients with narcolepsy often experience sleep paralysis and an inability to move for seconds (or even longer) at the onset of sleep or on waking. Sleep paralysis is considered normal REM sleep atonia that occurs without other features of REM sleep. Sleep paralysis can occur in normal individuals when sleep deprived or on waking from a dream. It can also be associated with depression in patients without narcolepsy.

Hallucinations

Hypnagogic (while falling asleep) or hypnopompic (on awakening) hallucinations occur in narcolepsy. They are usually visual, sometimes tactile or auditory, and reflect an immediate transition from wake to dreaming, without loss of consciousness. In severe cases, hallucinations can occur while drowsy, and can be difficult to distinguish from reality. Hypnagogic hallucinations can also occur in individuals without narcolepsy. In these cases, however, they are often less vivid in nature.

Sleep fragmentation

Individuals with narcolepsy usually lack the difficulty of falling asleep at bedtime, but experience frequent nocturnal awakenings. Spontaneous micro-arousals lead to sleep fragmentation and reduced deeper sleep stages. Sleep fragmentation contributes to non-restorative overnight sleep, the severity of cataplexy, and EDS. Periodic leg movements (PLM), REM behavior disorder, and nightmares are also frequent in narcoleptic patients.

Automatic behaviors

Automatic behaviors are a semiautomatic continuation of activities, with multiple mistakes and no memory of the event. Automatic behaviors may include driving, carrying on basic conversation, and performing most activities of daily living with virtually no impairment.

Investigations

Narcolepsy with cataplexy can often be diagnosed based on a detailed history and physical examination of the patient. The interview must focus on the detection and confirmation of typical cataplexy, if present. Narcolepsy without cataplexy requires a sleep study; International Classification of Sleep Disorders (ICSD-3) diagnostic criteria for narcolepsy were recently published (see Table 149.1). In some cases, a biochemical determination of low cerebrospinal fluid (CSF) hypocretin-1 can also provide a definitive diagnosis.

The most common differential diagnoses are sleep apnea, insufficient sleep, psychiatric hypersomnia, and circadian rhythm sleep disorders. Moreover, a combination of these diagnoses is not infrequent, further confusing the picture. Assessments for these diagnoses are included in Chapter 150. Anemia, hypothyroidism, infection, and various cardiovascular problems should be ruled out. A careful interview of the patient may reveal history of a brain trauma, central nervous system (CNS) infection, medication effects from drugs such as sedatives, anxiolytics, and antihistamines (such as those used in decongestants), and encephalopathy due to various causes, including renal or liver dysfunction.

Once clinical suspicion of narcolepsy is raised, confirmatory testing including overnight polysomnogram (PSG) and a Multiple Sleep Latency Test (MSLT) should be completed to identify comorbid sleep disorders causing fragmented sleep. The MSLT, used to quantify daytime sleepiness objectively, consists of five 20-minute

Table 149.1. Criteria for narcolepsy from the *International Classification of Sleep Disorders*, 3rd edition. Source: *International Classification of Sleep Disorders*, 3rd edition. Reproduced with permission of AASM.

Narcolepsy Type 1 (formerly known as narcolepsy with cataplexy)
Criteria A and B must be met.
A. The patient has daily periods of irrepressible need to sleep or daytime lapses into sleep occurring for at least three months.
B. The presence of one or both of the following:
   • Cataplexy (as defined under Essential Features) and a mean sleep latency of ≤8 minutes and two or more sleep onset REM periods (SOREMPs) on an MSLT performed according to standard techniques. A SOREMP (within 15 minutes of sleep onset) on the preceding nocturnal polysomnogram may replace one of the SOREMPs on the MSLT.
   • CSF hypocretin-1 concentration, measured by immunoreactivity, is either ≤110 pg/mL or <1/3 of mean values obtained in normal subjects with the same standardized assay.

Narcolepsy Type 2 (formerly known as narcolepsy without cataplexy)
Criteria A–E must be met.
A. The patient has daily periods of irrepressible need to sleep or daytime lapses into sleep occurring for at least three months.
B. A mean sleep latency of ≤8 minutes and two or more sleep onset REM periods (SOREMPs) are found on a MSLT performed according to standard techniques. A SOREMP (within 15 minutes of sleep onset) on the preceding nocturnal polysomnogram may replace one of the SOREMPs on the MSLT.
C. Cataplexy is absent.
D. Either CSF hypocretin-1 concentration has not been measured or CSF hypocretin-1 concentration measured by immunoreactivity is either >110 pg/mL or >1/3 of mean values obtained in normal subjects with the same standardized assay.
E. The hypersomnolence and/or MSLT findings are not better explained by other causes such as insufficient sleep, obstructive sleep apnea, delayed sleep phase disorder, or the effect of medication or substances or their withdrawal.

CSF = cerebrospinal fluid; MSLT = Multiple Sleep Latency Test

Table 149.2. Pharmacological management of narcolepsy.

	Compounds	Daily dosage	Notes
Stimulants	Modafinil	100–400 mg	Few sympathomimetic effects
	Armodafinil	150–250 mg	Few sympathomimetic effects
	Methylphenidate	10–60 mg	Short duration of action
	Dextroamphetamine	5–60 mg	Variable duration of action
	Methamphetamine	5–60 mg	More potent
Anticataplectic compounds	Venlafaxine	75–225mg	Slow-release formulation, acting on both the serotoninergic and adrenergic systems
	Atomoxetine	10–80 mg	Norepinephrine reuptake inhibitor
	Protriptyline	5–80 mg	Anticholinergic effects, mild stimulant
	Imipramine	10–100 mg	Anticholinergic effects
	Desipramine	25–100 mg	Same as imipramine but more adrenergic
	Clomipramine	1–150 mg	Very effective
	Fluoxetine	20–60 mg	Well tolerated, less weight gain
Hypnotic compounds	Sodium oxybate	4.5–9 g	Short duration of action, resulting anticataplectic effects during daytime, also alleviates daytime sleepiness

daytime naps at 2-hour intervals. Sleep latency along with the occurrence of REM sleep should be recorded.

A mean sleep latency (MSL) of less than 8 minutes and two or more sleep onset REM periods (SOREMPs) is diagnostic for narcolepsy. A SOREMP (within 15 minutes of sleep onset) on the preceding nocturnal polysomnogram may replace one of the SOREMPs on the MSLT. If there is no cataplexy, an MSLT (preceded by PSG) is indispensable. Special considerations in arranging the MSLT are as follows:

- The MSLT should be preceded by a PSG to rule out other causes of short MSL or SOREMPs such as sleep apnea, insufficient sleep, or delayed sleep phase syndrome.
- Psychotropic medications that affect REM sleep, especially antidepressants, should be avoided for 2 weeks prior to the study.
- In the 15% of patients with cataplexy in whom the MSLT is not diagnostic, measurement of cerebrospinal fluid (CSF) hypocretin-1 levels may assist in diagnosing narcolepsy. Low CSF hypocretin-1 levels (less than or equal to 110 pg/mL or one-third of mean normal values) are found in over 90% of patients with narcolepsy with cataplexy and almost never in controls or in patients with other pathologies.
- A urine toxicology screen may be used to screen for sedatives, stimulants, and antidepressants that may influence PSG and MSLT.

Treatment

The management and treatment of narcolepsy include life-modifying interventions and medications targeting the most disabling symptoms, typically EDS and cataplexy (Table 149.2). Life-modifying interventions include scheduled napping for 20 minutes, once at noon and once in the later afternoon, to decrease EDS, minimizing the use of stimulants, and reducing the frequency and severity of cataplexy.

Pharmacological treatment choices for EDS include stimulants and other wake-promoting agents. Commonly prescribed stimulant agents include but are not limited to modafinil, armodafinil, dextroamphetamine, and methylphenidate. Side effects include insomnia, hypertension, palpitations, and worsening of psychiatric conditions (such as mania), and, very rarely with amphetamines,

psychosis. Modafinil and the newer armodafinil are the drugs of choice because they are safer than other traditional stimulants and have less potential for abuse.

Hypnagogic hallucinations, sleep paralysis, and cataplexy respond to tricyclic antidepressants and monoamine reuptake inhibitors. A drug of choice is venlafaxine, a dual noradrenergic/serotoninergic uptake inhibitor. Venlafaxine and related drugs are rapidly effective for cataplexy. It is important to emphasize to patients the need for compliance, as sudden cessation of these drugs leads to a rebound of cataplexy. Atomoxetine, an adrenergic reuptake inhibitor used for attention deficit hyperactivity disorder (ADHD), can be helpful to treat cataplexy and mild daytime sleepiness.

Sodium oxybate, a hypnotic used twice during the night, is now increasingly used to consolidate sleep and reduce sleep fragmentation. It is a drug of choice in narcolepsy/cataplexy, as it can reduce the symptoms of narcolepsy. It is suggested that the increased amount of deep sleep induced by sodium oxybate leads to decreased EDS, reduced frequency and severity of cataplexy, and a reduced need for stimulants. In many cases, sodium oxybate alone or in combination with a small dose of venlafaxine and/or modafinil confers adequate coverage for patients with narcolepsy/cataplexy. In patients without cataplexy, typical treatments may involve modafinil or atomoxetine, with careful use of amphetamine-like stimulants.

Further reading

American Academy of Sleep Medicine. *International Classification of Sleep Disorders (ICSD-3): Diagnostic and Coding Manual*, 3rd ed. Westchester, IL: AASM; 2014.

Bassetti C, Billiard M, Mignot E (eds.). *Narcolepsy and Hypersomnia*. New York: Informa Health Care; 2007.

Dauvilliers Y, Arnulf I, Mignot E. Narcolepsy with cataplexy. *Lancet* 2007;369(9560):499–511.

Hungs M, Mignot E. Hypocretin/orexin, sleep and narcolepsy. *Bioessays* 2001;23:397–408.

Lin L, Hungs M, Mignot E. Narcolepsy and the HLA region. *J Neuroimmunol* 2001;117:9–20.

Mignot E, Lin L, Finn L, *et al.* Correlates of sleep-onset REM periods during the Multiple Sleep Latency Test in community adults. *Brain* 2006;129(Pt 6):1609–1623.

Morgenthaler TI, Kapur VK, Brown T, *et al.*; Standards of Practice Committee of the AASM. Practice parameters for the treatment of narcolepsy and other hypersomnias of central origin. *Sleep* 2007;30(12):1705–1711.

Partinen M, Kornum BR, Plazzi G, *et al.* Narcolepsy as an autoimmune disease: The role of H1N1 infection and vaccination. *Lancet Neurol* 2014;13(6):600–613.

150   Idiopathic hypersomnia

Marcel Hungs

Department of Neurology, University of Minnesota, Minneapolis, MN, USA

Idiopathic hypersomnia (IH), along with obstructive sleep apnea (OSA) and narcolepsy, is a frequent condition presenting with excessive daytime sleepiness (EDS). Patients experience difficulty waking up in the morning and sleep drunkenness (a difficulty with waking), daytime sleepiness, an overwhelming urge to nap, and occasionally autonomic dysfunction. The total sleep time at night may be normal or longer than 10 hours. Despite significant impairment in quality of life due to daytime sleepiness, little is known about the epidemiological and pathophysiological background or ethnic and regional variations of IH. Treatment includes education and the use of wake-promoting agents.

Epidemiology

The evolving clinical concept of IH, with the search for a proper clinical and pathophysiological definition, lacks widespread epidemiological data. International studies are lacking, but some researchers suggest that narcolepsy is three times more common than IH.

Pathophysiology

In contrast to narcolepsy, there are no animal models available for IH, and basic scientific data are limited. Destruction of noradrenergic neurons in cats leads to a hypersomnia resembling IH. There is no *HLA-DQB1*0602* association, as seen in narcolepsy, but the possibility of an *HLA-Cw2* and *DR11* association is reported without other evidence of an autoimmune-mediated mechanism. Interleukin-6 and tumor necrosis factor-α are elevated in IH, but are also elevated in other disorders with excessive daytime sleepiness, such as sleep apnea and narcolepsy.

γ-aminobutyric acid (GABA) receptors have been associated with endogenous ligands contributing to sleepiness, while antagonism of GABA receptors improves vigilance in some patients. One ligand in the cerebrospinal fluid (CSF) of patients with IH is thought to act as a positive allosteric modulator of synaptic GABA receptors, leading to the observation that flumazenil normalizes vigilance in some patients with IH.

CSF studies reveal decreased monoaminergic metabolites and histamine levels, as well as normal hypocretin-1 levels. Brain imaging studies are normal. Although a few studies suggest a genetic relationship in IH, a definitive determination of a mode of inheritance is not substantiated.

Clinical features

The symptoms of IH are characterized by excessive daytime sleepiness, with non-refreshing prolonged naps and sleep drunkenness. Historically, IH lacked objective diagnostic approaches (such as an overnight sleep study or Multiple Sleep Latency Test) and absent pathophysiological concepts. IH is often misdiagnosed as narcolepsy, sleep apnea, depression, or circadian rhythm disorder (Table 150.1). Our understanding of IH has primarily emerged in the last decade and is characterized by the following features.

Excessive daytime sleepiness

The hallmark of IH presenting to healthcare providers is excessive daytime sleepiness with prolonged unrefreshing daytime naps. Individuals with IH, despite sufficient and sometimes prolonged night sleep, experience reduced daytime alertness and, on awakening, feelings of sleep drunkenness (difficulty in awakening completely accompanied by confusion, disorientation, poor motor coordination, and slowness). Overnight sleep is rarely refreshing, and individuals with IH tend to doze off in monotonous situations such as dark rooms, offices, or even at traffic lights. Daytime naps are common but non-refreshing and do not increase alertness (in contrast to the often refreshing effect of napping in narcolepsy). The detailed history of an individual with IH will reveal that he/she does not experience cataplexy, an element frequently seen in narcolepsy. However, it is difficult to distinguish IH from narcolepsy on the basis of daytime sleepiness patterns alone.

A monosymptomatic form of IH is characterized by isolated sleepiness, while the polysymptomatic (also called classic) form

Table 150.1. Causes of hypersomnia.

- Narcolepsy (without or with cataplexy)
- Obstructive sleep apnea
- Delayed sleep phase syndrome
- Depression
- Periodic limb movement disorder
- Behaviorally induced insufficient sleep syndrome
- Hypersomnia due to medical condition, drug, or substance
- Hypothyroidism
- Brain trauma
- Central nervous system infections
- Encephalopathy
- Periodic hypersomnia, e.g., Kleine–Levine syndrome
- Sleeping sickness
- Hypersomnia not due to substance or known physiological condition

International Neurology, Second edition. Edited by Robert P. Lisak, Daniel D. Truong, William M. Carroll and Roongroj Bhidayasiri

includes other symptoms, such as autonomic dysfunction. The polysymptomatic form of the disorder is rare and is classified as "IH with long sleep time." Nocturnal sleep may or may not be of long duration (10 or more hours). An important feature of IH is normal overnight sleep without sleep fragmentation, while in sleep apnea or periodic limb movement (PLM) sleep fragmentation is common.

Autonomic dysfunction

Some patients experience autonomic dysfunction with fainting episodes, orthostatic hypotension, and peripheral vascular complaints of the Raynaud type. Migraine or tension-type headaches are also observed.

Other features

IH is a life-long disorder without remission or significant fluctuations in the clinical presentation. The onset of EDS is less apparent than in narcolepsy and usually presents between adolescence and age 30 years. Sleep paralysis and hypnagogic hallucinations are described in individuals with IH; dreams are less bizarre than in narcolepsy. The socioeconomic impact of the disease can be significant, affecting social, academic, and personal achievement.

Differential diagnosis

IH is characterized by EDS, unexplained by other conditions, and is essentially a diagnosis of exclusion (Table 150.1). A main consideration is narcolepsy, a condition with EDS, sleep paralysis, hypnagogic hallucinations, and cataplexy (loss of muscle tone while awake triggered by emotional stimulus). Patients with narcolepsy have a normal overnight sleep test with short sleep latency, two or more rapid eye movement (REM) episodes, and a mean sleep latency ≤8 minutes on the Multiple Sleep Latency Test (MSLT). Insufficient sleep, as seen in chronic sleep deprivation, can be excluded using sleep logs. PLM during sleep, conditions with significant sleep fragmentation, or sleep-disordered breathing (such as obstructive sleep apnea [OSA] or upper airway resistance syndrome) can be identified in an overnight sleep study. EDS associated with conditions such as depression, Parkinson's disease, or post-traumatic stress should be considered.

Diagnostic assessment

While well-defined clinical, polysomnographic, or immunogenetic features mark narcolepsy and sleep apnea, IH is mainly diagnosed by exclusion (Table 150.1). The hallmark of IH, excessive daytime sleepiness, should be experienced daily with periods of irrepressible need to sleep or daytime lapses into sleep, occurring for at least 3 months. A careful review of the patient's history, comorbidities, and physical examination leads to the diagnosis of IH with or without long sleep time. It is imperative that the hypersomnolence in IH is not explained by any other sleep disorder, medical or psychiatric disorder, or the use of drugs or medications. Normal or prolonged overnight sleep with short sleep latency is an important feature of IH. The total sleep time usually exceeds 660 minutes (typically 12–14 hours) during 24-hour observation. In an overnight polysomnogram (PSG), normal sleep stage distribution and lack of clear sleep fragmentation are observed. In contrast to narcolepsy, with IH a mean sleep latency of ≤8 minutes is seen on the MSLT *without* occurrence of two or more REM sleep episodes.

Treatment

In contrast to narcolepsy, naps may not be refreshing for patients with IH; therefore, patients avoid napping. Treatment parallels that of EDS in narcolepsy patients, but the response to medication is variable. The drug of choice is modafinil (100–200 mg in the morning and in the early afternoon) or its successor armodafinil (150–250 mg in the morning). Stimulant drugs, such as dextroamphetamine (5–60 mg), methylphenidate (10–60 mg), and pemoline (20–115mg), are used, but are often less effective in IH than in narcolepsy.

Further reading

Black JE, Brooks SN, Nishino S. Narcolepsy and syndromes of primary excessive daytime somnolence. *Semin Neurol* 2004;24(3):271–282.

Dauvilliers Y. Differential diagnosis in hypersomnia. *Curr Neurol Neurosci Rep* 2006;6(2):156–162.

Morgenthaler TI, Kapur VK, Brown T, *et al.*; Standards of Practice Committee of the AASM. Practice parameters for the treatment of narcolepsy and other hypersomnias of central origin. *Sleep* 2007;30(12):1705–1711.

Rye DB, Bliwise DL, Parker K, *et al.* Modulation of vigilance in the primary hypersomnias by endogenous enhancement of GABAA receptors. *Sci Transl Med* 2012:4:161–151.

Young TJ, Silber MH. Hypersomnias of central origin. *Chest* 2006;130(3):913–920.

151   Obstructive sleep apnea

Janesh Patel and Christian Guilleminault
Stanford University Sleep Medicine Division, Stanford Outpatient Medical Center, Redwood City, CA, USA

Obstructive sleep apnea (OSA) is characterized by repeated episodes of upper airway collapse and obstruction during sleep. It is associated with a constellation of symptoms and objective findings.

Epidemiology

Recent population-based studies report a wide range of prevalence estimates for OSA in the adult Western population, from 2–28%. Mild OSA likely affects 1 in 5 adults, while 1 in 15 adults has at least moderate OSA. In the adult population, the most significant risk factors are obesity and male gender. Other risk factors for OSA include age between 40 and 65 years, cigarette smoking, use of alcohol, and poor physical fitness.

The prevalence of OSA peaks between the fifth and seventh decades and plateaus thereafter. In the Cleveland Family Study, the prevalence of moderate OSA (apnea-hypopnea index [AHI] >15 events per hour) for subjects more than age 60 years was 32% in women and 42% in men. The prevalence in adults less than 60 years of age is 4% for women and 22% for men.

Both epidemiological and sleep clinic-based studies indicate that the prevalence of OSA is approximately 8 to 1, while in the population-based studies the ratio is closer to 2 to 1. The Wisconsin Sleep Cohort Study evaluated the association between OSA and premenopause, perimenopause, and postmenopause states, and found that the odds ratio for having OSA in perimenopausal women compared to premenopausal women was 1.2, and 2.6 for postmenopausal women, after adjusting for age, body habits, smoking, and other potentially confounding factors. In fact, menopausal women have similar prevalence and incidence of OSA to men.

Reported prevalence rates in different ethnic groups vary. OSA was found to be more prevalent in African Americans than in the white population after controlling for body mass index (BMI), alcohol use, and tobacco exposure. In the Sleep Hearty Health Study, however, the prevalence of OSA was not higher in African Americans compared to Caucasians, after adjusting for age, sex, and BMI. Unfortunately, there are no data on OSA prevalence in the black population of African countries.

Pacific Islanders and Mexican Americans have been reported by some researchers to have a higher incidence of OSA than Caucasians. However, a study in New Zealand comparing sleep apnea severity among Maori, Pacific Islanders, and Europeans reported that race was not an important predictor of OSA severity when adjusted for factors such as neck size, BMI, and age.

In a study of middle-aged men in Hong Kong, the estimated prevalence of OSA was approximately 5%, and the prevalence of OSA syndrome (AHI >5 with excessive daytime sleepiness) was estimated to be approximately 4%. Chinese women in Hong Kong have a reported prevalence of 2% for OSA syndrome. In the population of Singapore, sleep apnea affects about 15% of adults. The relatively higher prevalence of OSA in the Asian population, despite their lower prevalence of obesity, suggests the presence of other predisposing factors such as craniofacial anatomy.

Pathophysiology

Sleep-disordered breathing is caused by increased upper airway resistance secondary to narrowing at one or more sites of the upper airway. Locations of narrowing include the nose, retropalatal region, retroglossal region, or, less commonly, the hypoglossal region.

With sleep onset, there is an increase in the resistance due to a natural decrease in the upper airway muscle tone. In those with narrow airways, the upper airway dilators are unable to oppose the negative pharyngeal intraluminal pressure to maintain minute ventilation and normal gas exchange. In these cases, inspiratory effort is increased. With this increase, there is a further decrease in the diameter of the upper airway, as upper airway dilators are unable to overcome the inspiratory negative pressure. At some point, an abnormally negative pressure is reached, tidal volume is reduced for one to three breaths, and an arousal response is triggered.

Risk factors

Studies have shown that OSA prevalence increases with age, usually with a plateau around the sixth and seventh decades of life. Males tend to be at a higher risk of OSA, but women have a similar risk once menopause is reached. Obesity has a strong concordance with OSA irrespective of gender. In population studies, an increase in 10% of body weight increases the risk of OSA six-fold. Severe obesity also has a concomitant risk of obesity hypoventilation syndrome. Craniofacial anatomy features such as high-arched, narrow hard palate, macroglossia, and increased mallampati scores have a higher preponderance for OSA; as mentioned earlier, this has been seen in the Asian population studies. Soft tissue structures such as the tonsils and adenoids may also contribute to OSA, especially in the pediatric population. Other risk factors include nasal congestion, which increases OSA risk two-fold when compared to control, although treatment may not completely ameliorate it. Smokers are at a higher risk for OSA compared to non-smokers.

International Neurology, Second edition. Edited by Robert P. Lisak, Daniel D. Truong, William M. Carroll and Roongroj Bhidayasiri
© 2016 John Wiley & Sons, Ltd. Published 2016 by John Wiley & Sons, Ltd.

Clinical features

Snoring, witnessed apneas, snorting, and gasping during sleep, recurrent awakenings from sleep, and unrefreshing sleep are the most common nocturnal symptoms of OSA. Loud guttural snoring, at its worst in the supine position, punctuated by choking sounds and followed by cessation of breathing, is virtually pathognomonic. Nocturnal diaphoresis may be seen in association with the increased effort required to inspire against resistance during the night.

Dry mouth or drooling during the night is a sign of mouth-breathing, and is commonly associated with OSA. Many sleep apneics have sleep bruxism, which is often eliminated by continuous positive airway pressure use. Increased intra-abdominal pressure from exaggerated inspiratory attempts against a closed upper airway is thought to contribute to enuresis and nocturnal esophageal acid reflux. Non-rapid eye movement (NREM) parasomnias such as sleep walking, sleep eating, and nocturnal confusional spells can be the presenting symptoms in adults as well as in children with OSA.

The cardinal daytime symptom of OSA is excessive daytime sleepiness (EDS), which manifests as a tendency inadvertently to fall sleep during quiet or passive activities, to take intentional naps, or to experience short but repetitive attention lapses while doing monotonous tasks. Such sleepiness is the consequence of sleep fragmentation.

Cognitive complaints from nocturnal hypoxemia and sleep fragmentation are common, and may be the only clue to OSA in those who misperceive their sleepiness. Studies have shown that OSA patients have abnormal neuropsychological test results in attention, executive function, visuospatial learning, motor performance, and constructional ability.

Investigations

A full-night polysomnography (PSG) study in the sleep laboratory is the main method of evaluation. An entire night of study is generally recommended, as opposed to a partial night, because substantial changes in respiratory disturbances typically occur from one sleep cycle to another across the night. Because rapid eye movement (REM) sleep predominates toward the end of the night, REM sleep–related respiratory disturbances might easily be missed without a full night of study.

Although a portable study is a convenient, cost-effective, and accessible alternative to standard PSG, there are important limitations. The absence of trained personnel to intervene In the event of technical difficulty or medical emergency is one of the primary shortcomings. Concern has also been raised about the precision and accuracy of some portable units for the evaluation of more subtle cases of sleep-disordered breathing, such as those with a predominance of hypopneas or upper airway resistance syndrome. The practice parameters regarding portable PSG studies, published in 2003 by the American Academy of Sleep Medicine, the American Thoracic Society, and the American College of Chest Physicians, conclude that there is insufficient evidence to recommend the use of portable PSG. Since more data have been available, the most negative finding is often the absence of electroencephalogram (EEG) recordings that eliminate any possibility of recognizing hypopnea leading to EEG arousals without important oxygen saturation drops. Such a finding is common in younger subjects and normal-weight individuals. A negative study with a portable monitor does not eliminate the presence of OSA.

Treatment

Positive airway pressure

The pinnacle of therapy starts with continuous positive airway pressure (CPAP) to eliminate upper airway obstruction during sleep and is considered the treatment of choice for OSA. It abolishes obstructive events by increasing the pressure in the pharyngeal airway, thereby eliminating the negative intraluminal pressures that make airway collapse possible.

A subgroup of sleep apnea patients, even when obstructive respiratory events are eliminated by CPAP, will continue to have increased AHI (mainly because of central apneas or hypopneas) and will also continue to experience significant oxygen desaturation (mainly due to hypoventilation). These patients are considered to have a reduced ventilator drive, often with daytime hypercapnia, and may benefit from bilevel positive airway pressure ventilation instead of CPAP. Bilevel positive airway pressure is also used to help with patient compliance. Effective bilevel positive airway pressure titration depends on not only appropriate inspiratory pressure (IPAP), but also expiratory pressure (EPAP). Studies show that upper airway resistance increases during end-expiration, particularly during the three to four breaths preceding an apneic or hypopneic event. This narrowing of the airway may be an active, rather than passive, effect of the expiratory pharyngeal constrictor and dilator muscles. Thus, even though IPAP may be equivalent to therapeutic CPAP, inadequate EPAP may result in residual apneas and hypopneas.

Automatic positive airway pressure (AutoPAP) units measure upper airway obstruction by detecting a reduction or flattening of flow, or an increase in airway impedance. Median AutoPAP levels are lower than fixed CPAP levels, while being equally effective at ameliorating sleep apnea and preserving sleep architecture. AutoPAP has been shown to decrease common side effects associated with pressure intolerance and to increase compliance, particularly in patients requiring CPAP greater than 10 cm of water.

Surgery

In general, surgical success for OSA is unpredictable and not as effective as CPAP. Procedures addressing nasal obstruction include septoplasty, turbectomy, and radiofrequency ablation of the turbinates. These procedures, while providing better nasal breathing, often do not suffice for treating OSA, and are frequently used in adjunct to CPAP.

Surgical procedures to reduce soft palate redundancy include uvulopalatopharyngoplasty (UPPP), laser-assisted uvulopalatoplasty, lateral pharyngoplasty, and radiofrequency soft palate ablation. Surgery directly on the pharyngeal tissues is associated with severe pain, hemorrhage, and airway edema in the postoperative period. Such surgeries may also result in permanent velopharyngeal insufficiency, nasopharyngeal stenosis, voice change, and dysphagia. There is also a high recurrence rate of OSA, even after initial improvement. If UPPP is no longer recommended, pharyngoplasty with tonsillectomy may be performed in appropriate cases, as it brings improvement of the syndrome.

Surgical options for retrolingual obstruction in patients with OSA include tongue suspension, genioglossal advancement with mandibular osteotomy, hypoepiglottoplasty, and radiofrequency tongue ablation. Tongue suspension and genioglossal advancement stabilize the tongue without modifying tongue position or volume, and produce appreciable results when performed on non-overweight patients suffering from severe OSA. Such surgeries have had limited long-term benefits.

Maxillomandibular advancement, which "pulls forward" the anterior pharyngeal tissues attached to the maxilla, mandible, and hyoid to enlarge the entire velo-orohypopharynx, is the most effective surgical treatment for OSA (excluding tracheostomy, which bypasses any upper airway obstruction), with reported success rates in selected patients of over 90%. This procedure requires a multidisciplinary approach with surgeons, sleep specialists, and dentists, who need to determine the appropriate degree of advancement while making sure that teeth alignment, bite, and aesthetics remain intact.

Tissue reduction using radiofrequency energy has been the most valuable development in the field of surgery on nasal turbinates; results are much less significant when directed to the uvula and tongue. This procedure has been shown to be effective and minimally invasive. In the last 5 years, other new surgical techniques have not been attempted. Instead, development in this area appears to concentrate on combining previously known methods (so-called multilevel surgery) and optimizing methods of patient selection. Combined surgical procedures can achieve success rates of about 70–95%.

Oral appliances

Oral appliances are a relatively recent development and act by positioning the mandible in a protruded position during sleep. This creates a structural change in the upper pharyngeal anatomy, and enhances the caliber of the airway by triggering stretch receptors that activate the airway support muscles. Up to one-quarter of patients are unable to tolerate this particular device due to temporomandibular joint pain, teeth pain, excessive salivation, dry mouth, gum irritation, and/or next-morning occlusion changes. Although this device has been recommended for use in patients with mild to moderate OSA or in those who have failed a trial of CPAP, there is a paucity of data about its effectiveness, utility, and long-term outcomes.

Hypoglossal nerve stimulators

One of the latest treatment options that is continuing to be studied is hypoglossal nerve stimulation. The nerve implantation is a purposed mechanism to help maintain a physiological upper airway patency. Phase III trials have shown promising results, but will need to be studied further for mainstream use.

Further reading

Li KK, Kushida C, Powell NB, *et al.* Obstructive sleep apnea syndrome: A comparison between Far-East Asian and white men. *Laryngoscope* 2000;110:1689–1693.

Young T, Palta M, Dempsey J, *et al.* Burden of sleep apnea: Rationale, design, and major findings of the Wisconsin Sleep Cohort study. *WMJ* 2009;108:246–249.

Young T, Skatrud J, Peppard PE. Risk factors for obstructive sleep apnea in adults. *JAMA* 2004;291:2013–2016.

Wetter DW, Young TB, Bidwell TR, *et al.* Smoking as a risk factor for sleep-disordered breathing. *Arch Intern Med* 1994;154:2219–2224.

152

Restless legs syndrome and periodic limb movement disorders

Birgit Högl[1], Birgit Frauscher[1], Claudio Podesta[2]
[1] Department of Neurology, Medical University of Innsbruck, Innsbruck, Austria
[2] Sleep Medicine Unit, FLENI Foundation, Buenos Aires, Argentina

Restless legs syndrome (RLS), now also known as Willis-Ekbom Disease (WED), is a frequent neurological disorder that is often underdiagnosed by neurologists. Patients with RLS frequently present with unspecific leg problems or insomnia, and often have difficulties describing the symptoms. Only approximately 1 out of 8 RLS sufferers who sought consultation for RLS symptoms was correctly diagnosed. Epidemiological studies show that none of the RLS patients identified was on first-line RLS treatment and that approximately 2 out of 3 were initially misdiagnosed with a vascular disorder.

Epidemiology

RLS occurs 1.5–2 times more commonly in women than in men. The prevalence of idiopathic RLS is estimated to be approximately 10% in Europe and Northern America. Studies in other countries have shown varying prevalence rates, from 0–1% in India, Singapore, and Japan up to 4% in Korea and 5% in Japan. Similarly, in South America, prevalence estimates range between 2% in native South Americans in Ecuador to 13% in Chile, a population of predominantly European origin. In African Americans, a prevalence of about 5% was found. Differences in prevalence may be due to the genetic variability in different ethnic groups or to a lack of consistent diagnostic criteria across studies. As a general estimate, approximately one-third of those affected with RLS will require treatment ("bothersome RLS"); the other two-thirds have sporadic or mild RLS.

Idiopathic RLS has two phenotypes based on age of onset. In comparison to late-onset RLS, early-onset RLS has a younger age of onset, a slower progression, and frequently a family history of RLS. Secondary RLS is associated with an underlying disorder or condition such as iron deficiency, end-stage renal disease, polyneuropathy, pregnancy, multiple blood donations, and Parkinson's disease. Whether these secondary associations are causally related or coincident with RLS remains controversial. There are also medications reported to induce or aggravate RLS. The most important ones are dopamine receptor antagonists, mirtazapine, tricyclic antidepressants, and selective serotonin reuptake inhibitors. The selective serotonin reuptake inhibitors and venlafaxine have been reported to induce periodic leg movements (PLM).

Pathophysiology

Dopaminergic mechanisms are hypothesized to play a key role in the pathophysiology of RLS. However, although dopaminergic drugs are very effective in RLS, a structural dopaminergic deficit has not been found, and it is hypothesized that there may be a functional impairment of the dopaminergic system in RLS.

Impaired brain iron metabolism is another principal factor in the pathogenesis of idiopathic RLS. Magnetic resonance imaging (MRI) and brainstem sonography reported correlates of reduced iron in the substantia nigra. In the cerebrospinal fluid (CSF), reduced ferritin levels and increased transferrin levels were found. In postmortem studies of the substantia nigra in RLS patients, multiple signs of iron deficiency were reported. Paradoxically, transferrin receptors were decreased instead of being upregulated. This suggests impaired cellular regulation of iron in RLS. Because iron deficiency can affect dopaminergic neurotransmission, it may be that the dopaminergic hypoactivity in RLS is downstream to iron deficiency.

Spinal structures are the final pathway for periodic leg movements and the primary input stage for sensory symptoms. RLS and PLM have been reported in patients with spinal cord lesions, spinal cord ischemia, or transiently after undergoing spinal anesthesia. Moreover, investigation of the flexor reflex resembling PLM suggests an increased spinal cord excitability in the pathogenesis of RLS.

In RLS, several studies have reported significant linkage on different chromosomes. Recently, common variants in several genomic regions (*MEIS1, BTBD8, MAP2K5, LBXCOR1, PTPRD*) have been reported to be associated with RLS. They are also associated with iron metabolism and PLM, and *MEIS1* has been reported to play a role in the development of the murine telencephalon, specifically the embryonic ganglionic eminences, the prospective basal ganglia.

Clinical features

RLS

RLS is diagnosed by history. The neurological examination is normal. The new diagnostic criteria for RLS are given in Table 152.1. All essential criteria must be fulfilled for the diagnosis of RLS. Supportive clinical features include a positive family history of RLS,

International Neurology, Second edition. Edited by Robert P. Lisak, Daniel D. Truong, William M. Carroll and Roongroj Bhidayasiri
© 2016 John Wiley & Sons, Ltd. Published 2016 by John Wiley & Sons, Ltd.

Table 152.1 Diagnostic criteria of restless legs syndrome.

- An urge to move the legs, usually accompanied with or caused by uncomfortable and unpleasant sensations in the legs (sometimes the arms or other body parts are involved in addition to the legs)
- The urge to move or unpleasant sensations begin or worsen during periods of rest or inactivity such as lying or sitting
- The urge to move or unpleasant sensations are partially or totally relieved by movement, such as walking or stretching, at least as long as the activity continues
- The urge to move or unpleasant sensations are worse in the evening or night than during the day or only occur in the evening or night (when symptoms are very severe, the worsening at night may not be noticeable but must have been previously present)

response to dopaminergic treatment, and PLM during wakefulness (PLMW) or sleep (PLMS). The natural history of RLS varies, and remissions can occur. Sleep-onset or sleep-maintenance disturbances are often associated.

The diagnosis of RLS in children or the cognitively impaired elderly can be problematic because a typical RLS history is often difficult to obtain. In children, a family history of RLS in a first-degree relative, the presence of a sleep disturbance, and a PLMS >5/ hour during polysomnography can support the diagnosis, although a definite diagnosis requires the child to describe RLS symptoms in her/his own words. In the cognitively impaired elderly, a diagnosis of probable RLS demands the presence of visible or behavioral signs of leg discomfort and excessive motor activity in the lower extremities during periods of inactivity or in the evening.

Diagnostic criteria (ICSD-3, 2014)
The diagnostic criteria for RLS are:

A An urge to move the legs, usually accompanied by or thought to be caused by uncomfortable and unpleasant sensations in the legs. These symptoms must:
  1 Begin or worsen during periods of rest or inactivity such as lying down or sitting;
  2 Be partially or totally relieved by movement, such as walking or stretching, at least as long as the activity continues; and
  3 Occur exclusively or predominantly in the evening or night rather than during the day.
B The above features are not solely accounted for as symptoms of another medical or a behavioral condition (e.g., leg cramps, positional discomfort, myalgia, venous stasis, leg edema, arthritis, habitual foot tapping).
C The symptoms of RLS cause concern, distress, sleep disturbance, or impairment in mental, physical, social, occupational, educational, behavioral, or other important areas of functioning.

Criterion B is an important addition to the previous diagnostic criteria. In the past, it was shown that several other conditions with leg symptoms could confound the diagnosis, and in fact imitate RLS ("RLS mimics"). Mimics now need to be actively excluded prior to making a diagnosis of RLS, and this is achieved with criterion B. Criterion C has caused some discussion, as patients with only sporadic and mild symptoms of classic RLS will no longer be diagnosed as RLS. The advantage is that only patients who fulfill criterion C, with bothersome symptoms or other impairment, will be treated. Therefore, in the clinical context this criterion is useful, and it can be omitted for genetic or other studies, when mild phenotypes are also included.

Periodic leg movements (PLM) and periodic limb movement disorder (PLMD)
PLM are defined as stereotyped limb movements of a duration between 0.5 and 10 seconds, an intermovement interval between 5 and 90 seconds, and at least 4 movements in a row. Although PLMS are frequently associated with RLS, they are not specific and are frequently found in normal elderly persons. PLMD can only be diagnosed when there is PLM plus an additional sleep disturbance or a complaint of daytime fatigue not explained by any other sleep disorder. PLMD can only be diagnosed in the absence of RLS, and another sleep disorder (e.g., narcolepsy or REM behavior disorder) needs to be excluded prior to making a diagnosis of PLMD.

Investigations
Diagnosis of RLS is based on history. Patients with idiopathic RLS do not have neurological findings, such as peripheral neuropathy, but may have comorbid disorders. To exclude factors that may aggravate RLS, laboratory testing to assess iron status (iron, ferritin, transferring, and transferring saturation) is necessary. Additional testing should be done as indicated. Polysomnography is only indicated if there is uncertainty in the diagnosis or an additional sleep pathology is suspected.

Treatment
Not all patients with RLS will need or seek pharmacological treatment. If RLS is associated with a reduced serum ferritin less than 50 μg/L, iron replacement should be done and the possible causes of iron deficiency evaluated. Oral iron replacement is sometimes not well tolerated. Iron preparations given together with vitamin C in the morning fasting state for 2–3 consecutive months are recommended. In severe iron deficiency, intravenous iron substitution is recommended. In oral and intravenous iron substitutions, regular laboratory workup of iron parameters needs to be done to avoid iron overload.

If RLS symptoms are frequent and bothersome, drug treatment is indicated. Dopaminergic agents are considered first-line therapy in RLS. Large double-blind, placebo-controlled clinical trials demonstrate the efficacy of levodopa and dopamine agonists.

However, after several years of experience with dopaminergic treatment of RLS, it became apparent that augmentation is frequent with those substances and, after an initial positive response, often severely complicates the long-term treatment. Because of levodopa's short plasma half-life and high risk of augmentation, levodopa is only rarely used now for daily treatment of RLS, and should not be used in doses higher than 200 mg/day. Although the dopamine agonists pramipexole and ropinirole have been shown to be efficacious, a significant proportion of patients will experience loss of efficacy with a need for dose increase, or augmentation over time.

The transdermal application of rotigotine as a patch has been shown to have a good sustained efficacy for up to 5 years in those who tolerate the patch without local skin problems. The ergot dopamine agonists, pergolide and cabergoline, are no longer used for the treatment of RLS because of their association with cardiac valvulopathy. Patients on all dopamine agonists need to be warned, and at each visit carefully questioned for the development of any impulse control disorder. For each dopamine agonist, the initial dose is low and slowly titrated upward until benefit, but kept as low

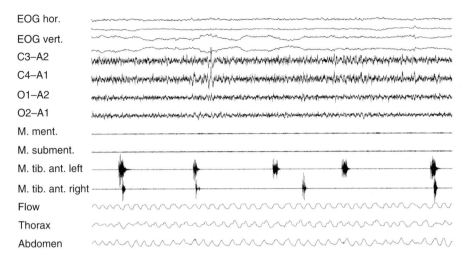

EOG hor.
EOG vert.
C3–A2
C4–A1
O1–A2
O2–A1
M. ment.
M. subment.
M. tib. ant. left
M. tib. ant. right
Flow
Thorax
Abdomen

Figure 152.1 This is a 2-minute polysomnography example of stage 2 sleep in a patient with restless legs syndrome. In the tibialis anterior muscles, bilateral periodic leg movements during sleep occur with different periodicity.

as possible. Generally, the doses are much lower than the doses used in Parkinson's disease, for example for rotigotine patch 1–3 mg, for pramipexole 0.18–0.54 mg/day, and so on. Opioids (e.g., low-dose oxycodone or methadone) and alpha-2-delta ligands (gabapentin, gabapentin enarcabil, and pregabalin) have long been used as alternative therapy, and recent double-blind placebo-controlled studies have shown that augmentation is not a problem with pregabalin or prolonged-release oxycodone-naloxone or methadone. Pregabalin might be considered as an alternative therapy if dopaminergic augmentation has occurred, or as primary therapy if RLS goes along with severe sleep disturbance. The high-potency opioid oxycodone prolonged release has been shown to be highly useful for patients with severe and treatment refractory RLS, and efficacy is sustained up to 1 year.

Augmentation

Augmentation is the major long-term complication of dopaminergic therapy in RLS. Basically, one should always think of augmentation when RLS gets worse despite increasing treatment (paradoxical response). A typical sign of augmentation is also the occurrence of RLS symptoms >4 hours earlier than at the beginning of treatment (e.g., in the afternoon instead of the evening), or an increase or a spread of symptoms to previously unaffected body parts, shorter latency to symptoms at rest, and so on. Augmentation has been reported both with levodopa and with dopamine agonists. To pre-

vent augmentation, the dopamine agonist dosages should be kept low and ferritin levels should be checked regularly. Treatment of augmentation implicates a switch to another substance, often a longer-acting dopaminergic drug or an opioid. The recently revised criteria for augmentation are given in Further reading.

Further reading

Allen RP, Picchietti DL, Garcia-Borreguero D, *et al.* Restless legs syndrome/Willis-Ekbom disease diagnostic criteria: Updated International Restless Legs Syndrome Study Group (IRLSSG) consensus criteria – history, rationale, description, and significance. *Sleep Med* 2014;15(8):860–873. doi:10.1016/j.sleep.2014.03.025

Garcia-Borreguero D, Allen RP, Kohnen R, *et al.* Diagnostic standards for dopaminergic augmentation of restless legs syndrome: Report from a World Association of Sleep Medicine-International Restless Legs Syndrome Study Group consensus conference at the Max Planck Institute. *Sleep Med* 2007;8:520–530.

Garcia-Borreguero D, Kohnen R, Silber MH, *et al.* The long-term treatment of restless legs syndrome/Willis-Ekbom disease: Evidence-based guidelines and clinical consensus best practice guidance: A report from the International Restless Legs Syndrome Study Group. *Sleep Med* 2013;14(7):675–684. doi:10.1016/j.sleep.2013.05.016

Trenkwalder C, Beneš H, Grote L, *et al.* Prolonged release oxycodone-naloxone for treatment of severe restless legs syndrome after failure of previous treatment: A double-blind, randomised, placebo-controlled trial with an open-label extension. *Lancet Neurol* 2013;12(12):1141–1150. doi:10.1016/S1474-4422(13)70239-4. Erratum in *Lancet Neurol* 2013;12(12):1133.

Spieler D, Kaffe M, Knauf F et al: Restless Legs Syndrome-associated intronic common variant in *Meis1* alters enhancer function in the developing telencephalon Genome Res. 2014 April; 24(4): 592–603. doi: 10.1101/gr.166751.113

153 Circadian rhythm sleep–wake disorders

Sergio Tufik, Lia R. A. Bittencourt, and Monica L. Andersen

Department of Psychobiology, Universidade Federal de São Paulo (UNIFESP-EPM), São Paulo, Brazil

Sleep timing and duration are rhythmic behaviors regulated by complex physiological and psychological factors. Times selected to go to bed and awaken are clearly influenced by genetic factors, sleep homeostasis, age, circadian rhythm, subjective needs, and ambient influences, but the tendency to sleep at night and to be active during the day is under physiological control and specific to the human species. The pattern of sleeping at night and being awake during the day is referred to as a diurnal pattern.

Because the secretion of melatonin occurs at night, at the same time as humans need to sleep, the pineal gland, which is responsible for the secretion of melatonin, has long been suspected of being involved with the regulation of sleep. Although melatonin secretion is influenced by the light–dark cycle, the diurnal rhythm of the pineal gland is directly controlled by an endogenous synchronizer, probably the suprachiasmatic nucleus (SCN) of the anterior hypothalamus. The SCN is the central biological synchronizer of the brain, which controls its overt biochemical, physiological, and behavioral rhythms. Determination of melatonin rhythm may therefore reflect the internal perception of external conditions and provide a means of assessing the temporal organization of the organism.

While circadian rhythms are endogenous and part of normal physiology, some individuals have an irregular sleep–wake pattern or are fully arrhythmic to it. The arrhythmicity is very disruptive to familial and social life, and to successful employment. Circadian rhythm sleep–wake disorders (CRSWD) are characterized by disruption of the internal circadian timing system or a misalignment between this system and the 24-hour social and physical environments, resulting in chronic symptoms of excessive sleepiness and insomnia.

Epidemiology

Studies on the prevalence of circadian rhythm sleep disorders are scarce. They have been found in 0.13–10% of the population and the number of cases seems to have increased in the past few decades. The prevalence of the different types of CRSWD is linked to the age, gender, ethnicity, and socioeconomic status of the studied population. Disruptions in the timing of sleep and wakefulness are often associated with symptoms of insomnia or excessive sleepiness that cause patients to seek medical attention. Thus, in clinical practice, CRSWDs are often under-recognized, yet they should be considered in the differential diagnosis of any patient presenting with symptoms of insomnia or hypersomnia.

Pathophysiology

According to the recent International Classification of Sleep Disorders (ICSD-3, 2014), measurement of endogenous circadian timing is important for the accurate diagnosis of CRSWD. In the new classification, there are 7 types of CRSWD.

CRSWDs are one of 8 categories of sleep disorders. The main characteristic of this category is that the desired optimal sleep time fails to match the timing of the circadian rhythm of sleep and wake propensity, which can lead to chronic conditions of sleep disturbance. These may be due to alterations of the circadian timing system, or a misalignment between the timing of the individual's circadian rhythm of sleep propensity and the 24-hour social and physical environments. These disorders may arise when the physical environment is altered relative to internal circadian timing (for example, shift work disorder and jet lag disorder), or the circadian timing system is altered relative to the external environment (for example, delayed and advanced sleep–wake phase disorder, irregular sleep–wake rhythm disorder, and non-24-hour sleep–wake rhythm disorder).

Physiological and environmental factors, as well as maladaptive behaviors, might also influence the presentation and severity of CRSWDs.

Clinical features

The clinical presentation of these diseases depends on the CRSWD type and can affect older people, as in advanced sleep–wake phase disorder, or younger people, as in delayed sleep–wake phase disorder. These complaints are often just diagnosed as insomnia or excessive sleepiness.

Investigations

For diagnosis, the chronotypic questionnaire is the most important tool, but multiple other tools are also available to assess sleep–wake patterns. Sleep log and actigraphy are essential instruments in the evaluation of CRSWDs and should be conducted for at least 7 days, preferably for 14 days, to capture work and non-work days. Measures of endogenous circadian timing (salivary or plasma dim light melatonin onset and urinary 6-sulfatoxymelatonin) can also provide important diagnostic information (ICSD-3, 2014).

All disorders described in the following sections imply a sleep difficulty that meets each of the criteria below. The specific features

International Neurology, Second edition. Edited by Robert P. Lisak, Daniel D. Truong, William M. Carroll and Roongroj Bhidayasiri
© 2016 John Wiley & Sons, Ltd. Published 2016 by John Wiley & Sons, Ltd.

that characterize each type of CRSWD are included within the individual diagnostic criteria.

Diagnostic criteria that must be met for all CRSWD

A A chronic or recurrent pattern of sleep–wake rhythm disruption primarily due to alteration of the endogenous circadian timing system or misalignment between the endogenous circadian rhythm and the sleep–wake schedule desired or required by an individual's physical environment or social/work schedules.

B The circadian rhythm disruption leads to insomnia symptoms, excessive sleepiness, or both.

C The sleep and wake disturbances cause clinically significant distress or impairment in mental, physical, social, occupational, educational, or other important areas of functioning.

Classification of rhythm sleep–wake disorders

Delayed sleep–wake phase disorder

Delayed sleep–wake phase disorder is characterized by a stable, chronic (at least 3 months), or recurrent pattern of habitual sleep–wake times that are delayed relative to conventional or socially acceptable times. There is some disagreement, but the prevalence of this disorder in the general population is between 7% and 16%. Genetic factors could be present.

Advanced sleep–wake phase disorder

Advanced sleep–wake phase disorder is a stable, chronic (at least 3 months), or recurrent pattern of advance of the major sleep period, characterized by habitual sleep onset and wakeup times that are several hours earlier, relative to conventional/desired times. The prevalence of this disorder in the general population is unknown. Genetic factors may also influence the development of the condition.

Irregular sleep–wake rhythm disorder

Irregular sleep–wake rhythm disorder is characterized by a chronic (at least 3 months) or recurrent temporally disorganized sleep–wake pattern so that sleep and wake periods are variable throughout a 24-hour period. This disorder is more commonly observed in neurodegenerative disorders, such as dementia, and in children with developmental disorders.

Non-24-hour sleep–wake rhythm disorder

Non-24-hour sleep–wake rhythm disorder is characterized by chronic sleep symptoms (at least 3 months) that occur because the intrinsic circadian pacemaker is not entrained to a 24-hour period, or is free running with a non-24-hour period. Most individuals presenting non-entrained circadian rhythms are totally blind, and the failure to entrain circadian rhythms is related to the lack of photic input to the circadian pacemaker.

Shift work disorder

Shift work disorder is characterized by complaints of insomnia or excessive sleepiness temporarily associated with a recurring work schedule of at least 3 months that overlaps the time for sleep and leads to a reduction in total sleep time. In addition to an impairment of performance at work, reduced alertness may be associated with consequences for safety. An estimated prevalence of 2–5% of the general population is reasonable.

Jet lag disorder

Jet lag disorder is characterized by complaints of insomnia or excessive daytime sleepiness, accompanied by a reduction of total sleep time, associated with transmeridian jet travel across at least two time zones.

Circadian sleep–wake disorder not otherwise specified

Circadian sleep–wake disorder not otherwise specified (NOS) consists of disorders that depend on an underlying neurological or medical disorder. Patients may present with a variety of symptoms, including insomnia and excessive sleepiness. These disorders that (1) satisfy the criteria of a circadian rhythm sleep disorder; (2) are not due to drug or substance misuse; and (3) do not meet the criteria for other CRSWD are classified by ICSD-3.

Treatment

Treatment should be tailored to the severity of symptoms, comorbid psychopathology, school schedules, work obligations, social pressures, and the ability and willingness of the patient/family to comply with treatment. Current treatment options for CRSWDs include sleep hygiene education, timed exposure to bright light and avoidance of bright light (at the wrong time of the day), planned sleep schedule and naps, and chronobiotic pharmacological approaches, such as ralmeteon and melatonin (which is not currently Food and Drug Administration–approved for treatment of CRSWDs).

Conclusions

TheICSD-3 publication provides a more detailed framework concerning diagnostic criteria, associated and essential features, clinical and pathophysiological subtypes, demographics, predisposing and precipitating factors, as well as familial patterns.

The detrimental effects caused by the impossibility of reconciling sleep needs with social demands have far-reaching consequences. As a result, scientific productivity in the field has been intense and sleep loss will most likely continue to be a major affliction, although its treatment remains a challenge for the patients. Hopefully, new evidence will bring new approaches to these disorders.

Acknowledgments

Our studies have been supported by AFIP. All the authors are recipients from CNPq (Conselho Nacional de Desenvolvimento Científico e Tecnológico).

Further reading

American Academy of Sleep Medicine. *International Classification of Sleep Disorders (ICSD-3): Diagnostic and Coding Manual*, 3rd ed. Westchester, IL: AASM; 2014.

Barion A, Zee PC. A clinical approach to circadian rhythm sleep disorders. *Sleep Med* 2007;8(6):566–577.

Dunlap JC, Loros JJ, DeCoursey PJ. The relevance of circadian rhythms for human welfare. In: Dunlap JC, LorosJJ, DeCoursey PJ (eds.). *Chronobiology: Biological Timekeeping*. Sunderland, MA: Sinauer; 2004:325–358.

Pandi-Perumal SR, Smits M, Spence W, *et al.* Dim light melatonin onset (DLMO): A tool for the analysis of circadian phase in human sleep and chronobiological disorders. *Prog Neuropsychopharmacol Biol Psychiatry* 2007;31:1–11.

Reid KJ, Zee P. Circadian disorders of the sleep-wake cycle. In: Kryger MH, Roth T, Dement WC (eds.). *Principles and Practice of Sleep Medicine*, 4th ed. Philadelphia, PA: WB Saunders; 2005:691–701.

154 Arousal disorders

Li Ling Lim

Singapore Neurology & Sleep Centre, Gleneagles Medical Centre, Singapore

Disorders of arousal (arousal disorders, AD) belong within the spectrum of parasomnias that refer to undesirable sleep-related movements, behaviors, or experiences that cause sleep disruption and other adverse health effects. Common ADs include confusional arousals, sleepwalking, and sleep terrors. These usually occur in non-rapid eye movement (NREM) slow-wave sleep, but can also occur in stage 2 NREM sleep.

Epidemiology and risk factors

ADs are more common in children than in adults. Childhood prevalence estimates: are confusional arousals 17.3%; sleepwalking 17%; and sleep terrors 1–6.5%. Adult prevalence estimates are: confusional arousals 2.9–4.2%; sleepwalking 2–4%; and sleep terrors 2.2%. In adults, sleepwalking associated with violence is more commonly reported in men. Sleepwalking peaks by age 8–12 years. Sleep terrors peak at about 5–7 years and usually resolve by adolescence.

AD can be triggered by sleep deprivation, forced awakenings, physical or emotional stress, anxiety, fever, psychotropic drugs, antihistamines, alcohol, environmental stimuli, and primary sleep disorders such as obstructive sleep apnea (OSA). In adults, associated psychiatric problems (depression, anxiety, or bipolar disorder) have been reported, although significant psychopathology is usually not present.

Pathophysiology

ADs tend to run in families and are believed to be a result of faulty transitions between slow-wave and lighter stages of sleep, with a sleep–wake state dissociation. This faulty transition is reflected by episodes of electroencephalogram (EEG) activity comprising an admixture of slower sleep and faster wake-like frequencies. Other factors contributing to the complex behaviors include dissociation of locomotor centers (from the state of NREM sleep) and inherent instability of slow-wave sleep. Structural lesions in the brain's normal wake centers (posterior hypothalamus and reticular activating system) have been reported to cause AD; however, most cases present with normal brains.

A positive family history in a first-degree relative is found in 60% of children. One study reported the prevalence of sleepwalking and sleep terrors being 10 times higher in first-degree relatives of sleep terror patients than in the general population. The rate of sleepwalking in children with a family history increases to 45% with one parent and 60% with both parents affected.

Clinical features and differential diagnoses

AD patients act out complex behaviors while in deep sleep, typically remaining amnestic of their actions. Episodes tend to occur in the first third of the night when slow-wave sleep predominates. Forced arousals from sleep can also induce episodes.

Confusional arousals occur most frequently in infants and toddlers, but are also seen in young adults (age 15–24 years), decreasing with age. Episodes are characterized by disorientation, slowed mentation, agitation, crying, thrashing, and combative behavior, lasting 5–15 minutes or as long as 30–40 minutes.

Sleepwalking consists of walking around in a state of altered consciousness, either calmly or agitated, after partial arousal from slow-wave sleep. It can vary in duration and complexity. Safety is a major concern, as falls, environmental exposure, and injury may occur.

In contrast to sleepwalking, in which the child usually remains calm, sleep terrors generally begin with a piercing cry or scream, associated autonomic arousal (tachypnea, mydriasis, tachycardia, and diaphoresis), behavioral manifestations of intense fear, and prominent motor activity (running or hitting). The child is typically inconsolable and difficult to arouse, and may later recall feeling threatened or scared.

Sleep disorders that cause recurrent arousals – such as OSA and periodic limb movement disorder (PLMD) – can trigger AD. Physical examination is usually normal, but should include a comprehensive evaluation of clinical features of associated conditions.

The diagnosis of childhood arousal parasomnias can usually be made by the witnessed description of events (given by a parent). Movements and behaviors, when they occur shortly after sleep onset, can be recorded in sleep diaries and on home videos. Conditions that mimic AD include nocturnal seizures (frontal lobe epilepsy and complex partial seizures), sleep-related movement disorders, panic attacks, and nightmares.

A scale to assess the severity of arousal disorders was recently published, based on a controlled study, to be used to screen and stratify patients who are at risk of injury to self and to others (including violent behavior and "automatic" driving while unaware). The Paris Arousal Disorders Severity Scale (PADSS) comprises three parts, including an inventory of behaviors (PADSS-A), the frequency of episodes (PADSS-B), and the general consequences of the disorder (PADSS-C). The PADSS has been reported to be a potentially useful clinical and research tool as a valid and reliable self-administered scale for arousal disorders.

International Neurology, Second edition. Edited by Robert P. Lisak, Daniel D. Truong, William M. Carroll and Roongroj Bhidayasiri
© 2016 John Wiley & Sons, Ltd. Published 2016 by John Wiley & Sons, Ltd.

Investigations

Polysomnography (PSG) is not routinely required for AD, but is useful in providing corroborative documentation as well as excluding associated primary sleep disorders. If epilepsy is suspected, an expanded EEG montage is required (ideally with time-synchronized video-EEG recording). Multiple arousals from slow-wave sleep are classic PSG findings in AD. EEG may show a mixture of alpha, theta, and delta waves, reflecting the sleep–wake state dissociation characteristic of AD.

Treatment

Parents should be reassured that ADs are common and generally benign. Often, therapy is not required; however, sensible safety precautions should be discussed, such as padding the bedroom environment, securing doors and windows, and installing alarm/monitoring systems. Using good sleep hygiene, avoiding sleep deprivation, and discontinuing stimulants (caffeine and triggering medications) should also be recommended. Parents should be advised not to wake the child during an episode, or to discuss the events of the night with the child. This is because it is typically difficult to awake the child, and trying to do so may actually prolong the episode or frighten the child. It may be best, for example in confusional arousals, which may last for several minutes, to let the child calm down and return to restful sleep spontaneously. If episodes become predictably recurrent, scheduled awakenings just before the typical time of a sleepwalking episode have been reported to eliminate sleepwalking successfully. Relaxation therapy may also be useful.

Parasomnias that pose a risk of injury to the patient (or bed partner) and those that are triggered by treatable conditions (OSA and PLMD) require specific therapy. For frequent or potentially injurious arousal parasomnias, benzodiazepines and tricyclic antidepressants are helpful. Clonazepam has been used successfully, starting at low doses (0.25 mg at bedtime) and titrating according to effect and tolerability.

Clinical course

Pediatric parasomnias are generally benign and self-limited, and usually do not persist into late adolescence or adulthood. Confusional arousals decrease after the age of 5 years, but may progress to sleep walking in adolescence. The adult variant may persist and is associated with sleep-related injury and impaired performance.

Conclusion

Classic arousal parasomnias form a spectrum of common features, including abnormal transition from slow-wave sleep, complex automatic behaviors, and amnesia following episodes. Injury to self and to others, and sleep disruption with daytime dysfunction, are important clinical consequences of AD. The severity of arousal disorders may be assessed using recently developed self-administered scales such as the PADSS. Management should focus on accurate diagnosis, exclusion of treatable associated conditions, and simple behavioral interventions to reduce the risk of physical injury and psychosocial problems.

Further reading

Arnulf I, Zhang B, Uguccioni G, *et al.* A scale for assessing the severity of arousal disorders. *Sleep* 2014;37(1):127–136.

Frank NC, Spirito A, Stark L, Owens-Stively J. The use of scheduled awakenings to eliminate childhood sleepwalking. *J Pediatr Psychol* 1997;22(3):345–353.

Kales A, Soldatos CR, Bixler EO, *et al.* Hereditary factors in sleepwalking and night terrors. *Br J Psychiatry* 1980;137:111–118.

Mahowald M, Schenck C, Basetti C, *et al.* Parasomnias. In: Sateia M (ed.). *The International Classification of Sleep Disorders*, 2nd ed. Westchester, IL: American Academy of Sleep Medicine; 2005:137–147.

Mason TBA, Pack AI. Pediatric parasomnias. *Sleep* 2007;30(2):141–151.

Ohayon MM, Guilleminault C, Priest RG. Night terrors, sleepwalking, and confusional arousals in the general population: Their frequency and relationship to other sleep and mental disorders. *J Clin Psychiatry* 1999;60(4):268–276.

Pressman MR. Disorders of arousal from sleep and violent behavior: The role of physical contact and proximity. *Sleep* 2007;30:1039–1047.

Schenck CH, Mahowald MW. A polysomnographically documented case of adult somnambulism with long-distance automobile driving and frequent nocturnal violence: Parasomnia with continuing danger as a noninsane automatism. *Sleep* 1995;18:765–772.

Schenck CH, Milner DM, Hurwitz TD, Bundlie SR, Mahowald MW. A polysomnographic and clinical report on sleep-related injury in 100 adult patients. *Am J Psychiatry* 1989;146:1166–1173.

155   REM sleep behavior disorder

Li Ling Lim
Singapore Neurology & Sleep Centre, Gleneagles Medical Centre, Singapore

Rapid eye movement (REM) sleep behavior disorder (RBD) is the most common REM sleep parasomnia. RBD is characterized by the absence of muscle atonia, which permits acting out of dreams, often resulting in physical injury. RBD was first described as a distinct clinical entity in a series of adults manifesting violent behaviors while acting out dreams during sleep and injuring themselves or their spouses in the process. RBD is characterized by a loss of normal REM atonia, loss of chin muscle atonia, and excessive muscle twitching on polysomnography (PSG). RBD is often associated with neurodegenerative disease and is responsive to clonazepam.

Epidemiology and risk factors

The estimated overall prevalence of RBD is about 0.5%, with a reported range from 0.38% to as high as 0.8%. The majority (approximately 90%) of RBD patients are older men, although any age group or gender can be affected.

RBD has been associated with a range of neurological conditions, most notably parkinsonism and degenerative dementia, often reflecting an underlying synucleinopathy. RBD may precede the onset of parkinsonism or dementia in patients with Parkinson's disease (PD), multiple system atrophy (MSA), or dementia with Lewy bodies (DLB) by years or decades. Thus, "idiopathic" RBD may represent the initial manifestation of an evolving neurodegenerative disorder. A higher incidence of RBD is also seen in narcolepsy. This probably reflects the REM sleep-related dyscontrol common to both conditions in which the elements normally regulating REM sleep are not present.

Many commonly used drugs (e.g., selective serotonin reuptake inhibitors [SSRIs], monoamine oxidase inhibitors, and tricyclic antidepressants) can induce or aggravate RBD symptoms in patients at risk.

Pathophysiology

The pathophysiology of RBD is believed to be analogous to that described in animal models in which damage to pontine tegmental pathways mediating REM atonia (and those structures that normally suppress the phasic locomotor drive in REM sleep) result in complex behaviors as seen in RBD. Positron emission tomography (PET) and single photon emission computed tomography (SPECT) studies have shown dysfunction in the nigrostriatal dopaminergic pathways in patients with idiopathic RBD. In humans, RBD may precede the onset of the motor symptoms of parkinsonism. This suggests that the first clinical symptoms to appear may correspond to the brainstem regions first affected by neuronal degeneration (RBD when beginning in the mesopontine junction or parkinsonism when beginning in the midbrain).

Clinical features and differential diagnoses

RBD typically manifests as complex dream-enacting behaviors that are often vivid, unpleasant, or violent, such as being attacked or chased. Typically, the abnormal movements include vocalizations, flailing, punching, kicking, swearing, gesturing, leaping, and running. These movements lead to sleep disruption and sometimes injuries to the patient or bed partner. The episodes typically occur approximately 90 minutes after sleep onset, coinciding with the timing of the first REM cycle, and may recur with subsequent REM sleep cycles.

RBD is usually a chronic and progressive disorder that is either idiopathic or associated with a range of neurological disorders – including the synucleinopathies such as PD, MSA, and DLB. Various studies have suggested that in as many as two-thirds of patients, RBD may precede (by a few years or decades) later development of neurodegenerative disorders characterized by alpha-synuclein deposition. In PD, RBD is associated with akinetic–rigid phenotype and falls as well as with non-motor symptoms, such as increased depressive symptoms, other sleep disturbances, and fatigue. RBD can also occur with cerebrovascular disease, neoplasm (such as brainstem and cerebellopontine angle tumors), and inflammatory conditions (such as Guillain–Barré syndrome and multiple sclerosis). RBD has also been noted in patients with narcolepsy, mitochondrial disorders, Tourette syndrome, autism, normal pressure hydrocephalus, and spinocerebellar ataxia. An acute form of RBD can occur during REM sleep rebound states, such as withdrawal from alcohol or sedative-hypnotic agents, and may be triggered by medications, including serotonergic antidepressants.

The diagnosis of RBD is based on a clinical history of injurious or potentially injurious dream-enacting behavior that disrupts REM sleep. Diagnosis requires a PSG. PSG shows REM sleep without atonia, excessive tonic and phasic electromyogram (EMG) activity recorded from the chin, excessive phasic EMG activity in the limbs, and abnormal REM sleep behaviors. This occurs in the absence of electroencephalogram (EEG) epileptiform activity during REM sleep.

International Neurology, Second edition. Edited by Robert P. Lisak, Daniel D. Truong, William M. Carroll and Roongroj Bhidayasiri
© 2016 John Wiley & Sons, Ltd. Published 2016 by John Wiley & Sons, Ltd.

Differential diagnoses encompass other causes of abnormal behavior in sleep, such as NREM parasomnias (sleepwalking, sleep terrors), nocturnal epilepsy, and obstructive sleep apnea (OSA), which may mimic RBD.

Investigations
PSG with time-synchronized video-EEG recording is needed to document the typical PSG features of RBD and to exclude disorders that may mimic RBD. Periodic limb movements in sleep (PLMS) can be seen in about 75% of RBD patients during NREM sleep.

Treatment
Clonazepam (beginning dose of 0.5 mg at night, increasing to 1 or 2 mg) is very effective in treating RBD and is considered first-line treatment. It is generally well tolerated and produces rapid (within the first week) and sustained (up to several years) improvement in the majority of patients, with little evidence of tolerance or abuse. Beneficial effects may be related to suppression of motor manifestations and partly to clonazepam's serotonergic properties.

Alternatively, melatonin (dosing between 3 mg and 12 mg at night) works as monotherapy for patients who may not tolerate long-acting benzodiazepines, or who have OSA. The mechanism of melatonin is not well understood, but has been reported to be effective for RBD, especially in patients with low melatonin levels. Studies have reported that melatonin reduces motor activity during sleep and partially restores REM sleep muscle atonia. Postulated mechanisms of melatonin include restoration of RBD-related desynchronization of the circadian rhythm and mechanisms producing REM sleep muscle atonia.

The effectiveness of other drugs including dopaminergic agents (pramipexole or levodopa), acetylcholinesterase inhibitors (donepezil or rivastigmine), and antiepileptic agents (carbamazepine or gabapentin) remains unclear. Dopamine receptor agonist therapy using pramipexole, while improving symptoms of parkinsonism in PD, has not been shown in a small, prospective, uncontrolled study to reduce RBD symptoms, suggesting that dopamine mechanisms may not play a central role in the pathogenesis of RBD. A recently published placebo-controlled, cross-over pilot study using rivastigmine in 25 consecutive patients suggested that in patients with mild cognitive impairment and RBD resistant to conventional therapies (including benzodiazepines or melatonin), treatment with rivastigmine may induce a reduction in the frequency of RBD episodes compared to placebo.

Improving sleeping environment safety, removing potentially dangerous objects, and allotting separate sleeping arrangements for bed partners are also useful measures.

Clinical course
RBD is slowly progressive and is rarely associated with spontaneous remissions, although symptoms may subside in the advanced stages of an underlying neurodegenerative condition. Drug-induced RBD should improve on withdrawal of the offending medication.

Conclusion
RBD, the most common REM parasomnia, is a striking clinical entity associated with neurodegeneration, affecting primarily older men. Evaluation should include a comprehensive clinical history detailing sleep behaviors and medication use, neurological examination, and PSG. Prompt recognition is important to reduce potential complications, including physical injury and marital discord arising from trauma and sleep disruption. Treatment with clonazepam is safe and effective in the majority of cases.

Further reading
Boeve BF, Silber MH, Ferman TJ. Melatonin for treatment of REM sleep behavior disorder in neurologic disorders: Results in 14 patients. *Sleep Med* 2003;4(4):281–284.

Boeve BF, Silber MH, Parisi JE, *et al*. Synucleinopathy pathology and REM sleep behavior disorder plus dementia or parkinsonism. *Neurology* 2003;61(1):40–45.

Brunetti V, Losurdo A, Testani E, *et al*. Rivastigmine for refractory REM behavior disorder in mild cognitive impairment. *Curr Alzheimer Res* 2014;11(3):267–273.

Gagnon JF, Postuma RB, Montplaisir J. Update on the pharmacology of REM sleep behavior disorder. *Neurology* 2006;67(5):742–747.

Kumru H, Iranzo A, Carrasco E, *et al*. Lack of effects of pramipexole on REM sleep behavior disorder in Parkinson disease. *Sleep* 2008;31(10):1418–1421.

Neikrug AB, Avanzino JA, Liu L, *et al*. Parkinson's disease and REM sleep behavior disorder result in increased non-motor symptoms. *Sleep Med* 2014;15(8):959–966. doi:10.1016/j.sleep.2014.04.009

Schenck CH, Mahowald MW. Polysomnographic, neurologic, psychiatric, and clinical outcome report on 70 consecutive cases with REM sleep behavior disorder (RBD): Sustained clonazepam efficacy in 89.5% of 57 treated patients. *Cleve Clin J Med* 1990;57(Suppl):S9–S23.

Schenck CH, Bundlie SR, Ettinger MG, Mahowald MW. Chronic behavioral disorders of human REM sleep: A new category of parasomnia. *Sleep* 1986;9(2):293–308.

156 Paroxysmal nocturnal dystonia

Cynthia L. Comella

Department of Neurological Sciences, Rush University Medical Center, Chicago, IL, USA

Paroxysmal nocturnal dystonia (PND) is one of a group of clinically heterogeneous disorders included under the category of nocturnal frontal lobe epilepsy (NFLE). The clinical presentation of NFLE includes paroxysmal arousals, partial arousals with sleep walking, sleep terrors or confusional arousals, repetitive stereotypic behaviors, and paroxysmal nocturnal dystonia or dyskinesias. PND was initially described in the early 1980s in 5 patients in whom brief, stereotypic movements occurred during non-rapid eye movement (NREM) sleep. Although scalp electroencephalography (EEG) did not show epileptiform discharges, all responded to carbamazepine. Subsequently, sphenoidal and zygomatic electrodes showed epileptic discharges in mesiotemporal and orbital or mesial frontal regions. However, there remains controversy over the terminology of NFLE as there are no standard diagnostic criteria, with the events often being similar to the parasomnias, and findings that suggest that epileptiform activity may originate outside of the frontal lobe.

Clinical features

NFLE is a rare disorder. Epidemiological studies are lacking because there is no systematic method for case ascertainment. NFLE has diverse presentations that have been categorized into four general types. Paroxysmal arousal is a very brief, abrupt, recurrent arousal from NREM sleep. Patients may look around, appear frightened, and have vocalizations. PND is a sudden arousal with movements that may be dystonic with twisting of the head, neck, torso, and limbs, or ballistic and last up to 100 seconds. PND may be preceded by a paroxysmal arousal. During an episode, there is often autonomic activation. Asymmetric bilateral tonic seizures can also occur. Episodic nocturnal wanderings often appear as more violent motor behaviors, with getting out of bed, screaming, and fear. These episodes may last up to 3 minutes. The episodes appear very similar in the same patient from night to night, but may vary from patient to patient.

Episodes of NFLE are frequent, and may occur several times a week, and recur several times a night. The age of onset is usually in childhood or adolescence, although onset as late as 64 years of age is reported. Up to 35% of NFLE patients have occasional seizures during daytime wakefulness. Family history is positive for a parasomnia or daytime epilepsy in 25–40% of patients. Neurological examination and brain imaging are usually normal.

Genetics

Most NFLE is primary, without an underlying cause. In some families, NFLE is autosomal dominant, but with considerable heterogeneity. There have been linkage studies that have identified mutations in the *CHRNA2* gene coding for the α4 and β2 subunits of the neuronal nicotinic acetylcholine receptor. Additional loci have been identified, but no causative mutations have yet been found. However, these genes have been excluded in many families, indicating the heterogeneity of the disorder despite a similar phenotype.

Differential diagnosis

The differential diagnosis of NFLE includes a variety of parasomnias that occur in NREM sleep and REM sleep. These include confusional arousals, sleep terrors, and sleep walking. REM parasomnias include REM sleep behavior disorder and nightmares. Other disorders that can cause episodic movements during the night include bruxism, sleep starts, and propriospinal myoclonus at sleep onset.

Investigations

The evaluation of a patient with sleep-associated movement disorders includes a careful history from the patient and a bed partner. Additional clinical assessments include a home video of several occurrences of the nocturnal movements. Video polysomnography is the most important diagnostic test. However, EEG with scalp electrodes often does not show abnormal activity, even during the ictal period. Deep electrodes (sphenoidal or zyagomatic) are more sensitive, but not always revealing.

Treatment

NFLE is a chronic disorder with few spontaneous remissions. The treatment of NFLE with carbamazepine may significantly reduce the number and severity of the episodes, although 30–50% of patients do not benefit. Levetiracetam and topiramate have also been used. Although a minority of patients become seizure free, more than half will have a reduction in episode frequency. There are no large controlled trials for this disorder and the efficacy of many anticonvulsants has not been assessed.

International Neurology, Second edition. Edited by Robert P. Lisak, Daniel D. Truong, William M. Carroll and Roongroj Bhidayasiri
© 2016 John Wiley & Sons, Ltd. Published 2016 by John Wiley & Sons, Ltd.

Further reading

American Academy of Sleep Medicine (AASM). Sleep related epilepsy. *International Classification of Sleep Disorders, 2nd ed: Diagnostic and Coding Manual.* Westchester, IL: AASM; 2005:232–235.

Bisulli F, Vignatelli L, Provini F, *et al.* Parasomnias and nocturnal frontal lobe epilepsy (NFLE): Lights and shadows – controversial points in the differential diagnosis. *Sleep Med* 2011;12(Suppl 2):S27–S32.

De Marco EV, Gambardella A, Annesi F, *et al.* Further evidence of genetic heterogeneity in families with autosomal dominant nocturnal frontal lobe epilepsy. *Epilepsy Res* 2007;74:70–73.

De Paolis F, Colizzi E, Milioli G, *et al.* Effects of antiepileptic treatment on sleep and seizures in nocturnal frontal lobe epilepsy. *Sleep Med* 2013;14:597–604.

Lugaresi E, Cirignotta F. Hypnogenic paroxysmal dystonia: Epileptic seizure or a new syndrome? *Sleep* 1981;4:129–138.

Provini F, Plazzi G, Montagna P, Lugaresi E. The wide clinical spectrum of nocturnal frontal lobe epilepsy. *Sleep Med Rev* 2000;4:375–386.

Provini F, Plazzi G, Tinuper P, *et al.* Nocturnal frontal lobe epilepsy: A clinical and polygraphic overview of 100 consecutive cases. *Brain* 1999;122(Pt 6):1017–1031.

Tinuper P, Bisulli F, Provini F, Montagna P, Lugaresi E. Nocturnal frontal lobe epilepsy: New pathophysiological interpretations. *Sleep Med* 2011;12(Suppl 2):S39–S42.

Tinuper P, Provini F, Bisulli F, *et al.* Movement disorders in sleep: Guidelines for differentiating epileptic from non-epileptic motor phenomena arising from sleep. *Sleep Med Rev* 2007;11:255–267.

Vignatelli L, Bisulli F, Giovannini G, *et al.* Prevalence of nocturnal frontal lobe epilepsy in the adult population of Bologna and Modena, Emilia-Romagna Region, Italy. *Sleep* 2015;38(3):479–485.

157 Sleep abnormalities in neurological disorders

Margaret Park[1] and Cynthia L. Comella[2]

[1] Chicago Sleep Health, Chicago, IL, USA

[2] Department of Neurological Sciences, Rush University Medical Center, Chicago, IL, USA

Sleep and alertness are complicated processes mediated by the neurological system. Thus, patients with neurological disorders often have comorbid sleep disorders. For example, pathology in the brainstem regions may alter respiratory control centers, adversely affecting ventilation and gas-exchange mechanisms. Additionally, pathology within the brainstem and spinal cord can lead to unusual movements during sleep, ranging from simple motor phenomena as seen with periodic limb movements to complex behaviors as with REM behavior disorder. Along with alterations in sleep, central nervous system diseases can affect arousal and alertness systems, leading to excessive sleepiness in disease states such as narcolepsy.

The following is intended as a brief overview of sleep disorders and some common comorbid neurological disease states.

Sleep-disordered breathing

Sleep-disordered breathing (SDB) includes obstructive sleep apnea-hypopnea syndrome (OSA), complex sleep apnea, and central sleep apnea (CSA). Obstructions cause absence of airflow despite respiratory effort. Hypopneas are characterized by reduced airflow despite respiratory effort. In contrast, central sleep apnea represents complete airflow absence. Polysomnography (PSG) is a sleep study evaluating various physiological parameters, including breathing events, during sleep. Respiratory events that occur during sleep are scored and averaged across the sleep period on a per-hour basis, called the apnea-hypopnea index (AHI). More than 5 events per hour (AHI >5) is considered diagnostic for SDB. Continuous positive airway pressure (CPAP) is considered the primary treatment of choice for OSA, while other PAP ventilation modes (e.g., bilevel PAP) and/or oxygen may be useful for other SDB. SDB is frequently comorbid with the following neurological conditions.

Stroke

SDB is prevalent in stroke, with shared risk factors including hypertension. SDB is both a risk factor for and a consequence of stroke, but an unclear cause-and-effect relationship exists. SDB in stroke is associated with worsening functional impairment, increased hospital stay, and increased future stroke risk. Studies are needed to determine whether treating SDB reduces stroke risk and improves outcome.

Neuromuscular disease

Neuromuscular disease (NMD) compromises diaphragmatic function, whether due to motor neuron disease (e.g., poliomyelitis, amyotrophic lateral sclerosis [ALS]), phrenic nerve involvement (e.g., Guillain–Barré), or neuromuscular junction alterations (e.g., myasthenia gravis). NMD generally interferes with rapid eye movement (REM) sleep, as REM is heavily dependent on the diaphragm. However, central respiratory involvement, pharyngeal-bulbar weakness, craniofacial dysmorphisms, and musculoskeletal deformities also compromise ventilation, causing SDB-related nocturnal hypoxemia. Treating SDB improves quality of life in NMD and may delay the need for intubation or tracheotomy. This, in addition to the high prevalence of SDB in NMD, warrants a low threshold for obtaining evaluation.

Headache syndromes

Headache syndromes (HA) are common in OSA, but there is an uncertain pathophysiological link. Possible mechanisms include intermittent hypoxia and/or hypercarbia, causing fluctuations in cerebral blood flow and intracranial pressure. In addition to morning HA, OSA also triggers migraines and cluster headaches, usually during or around REM sleep, and particularly after oxyhemoglobin desaturation. HA improvement can occur when OSA is successfully treated.

Restless legs syndrome and periodic limb movement disorder

Clinical diagnostic criteria for restless legs syndrome (RLS) include non-specific sensory disturbances in the legs (e.g., "creepy crawly" sensation), association with an urge to move, relief with movement, and a nocturnal component (i.e., worse in the evening, particularly at bedtime). Unlike RLS, periodic limb movement disorder (PLMD) is a polysomnographic disorder, evaluated by counting periodic limb movements (PLMs) during sleep. PLMs are repetitive, stereotypic limb movements and are scored per hour of sleep, called the PLMS index (PLM-I). PLMs can occur with (PLM-AI) or without arousals. PLMD is diagnosed by a total index greater than 15 (PLM-I >15) or an index with arousals greater than 5 (PLM-AI >5).

RLS and PLMD are often grouped together because they are frequently comorbid. Approximately 80–90% of RLS patients also have PLMD, but only about 30% of patients who have PLMD fulfill clinical criteria for RLS. Pathophysiologically, there is a presumption of a shared dopaminergic dysfunction, with exacerbation from low ferritin levels (less than 75 ng/mL). Treatment goals consist of iron supplementation (goal ferritin >75 ng/mL), dopaminergic medications, sedative-hypnotics, and gabapentin or gabapentin-like

International Neurology, Second edition. Edited by Robert P. Lisak, Daniel D. Truong, William M. Carroll and Roongroj Bhidayasiri
© 2016 John Wiley & Sons, Ltd. Published 2016 by John Wiley & Sons, Ltd.

derivatives. In addition to idiopathic/primary forms, which are generally considered genetic in origin, secondary RLS/PLMD occurs in the following neurological disorders.

Neuropathy

Neuropathic disturbance is associated with RLS/PLMD, possibly due to shared sensorimotor disturbance. Theoretically, abnormal sensory stimuli from small or large fiber neuropathy, axonal neuropathy, or radiculopathy may inappropriately activate movement generators in the brainstem or spinal motor dopaminergic cells. This may explain why medications that stimulate dopamine receptors or improve neuropathic pain can successfully treat RLS/PLMD, although secondary forms of RLS/PLMD may differ in pathophysiology from primary forms.

Parkinson's disease

Patients with Parkinson's disease (PD) frequently have RLS/PLMD. Because these disease states respond to dopaminergic medication, there is an assumed pathophysiological relationship. However, the increased prevalence of RLS in PD may be due to lower ferritin levels in these patients rather than a true pathophysiological link. Additionally, it has been hypothesized that idiopathic PLMs and PD-related PLMs may differ with regard to brainstem versus spinal pathophysiology. Studies are too few to conclude whether physiological differences exist between idiopathic versus PD-related RLS/PLMD.

Parasomnias

Parasomnias are undesirable behavioral phenomena that occur during sleep, classified according to whether they occur during non-REM (NREM) or REM sleep periods. However, overlap syndromes frequently occur.

NREM parasomnias

NREM parasomnias are "arousal disorders" due to their tendency to occur after an arousal from N3 (slow-wave) sleep. Common examples include confusional arousals, sleep terrors, and sleep walking. NREM parasomnias generally occur during and resolve after childhood, but persistence into adulthood is common. Resolved NREM parasomnias may recur with different triggers, including substances such as alcohol, sleep deprivation, and other sleep disorders including OSA and PLMD. Treatment consists of both behavioral modification and potentially pharmacotherapy. Behavioral measures include avoidance of alcohol and sleep deprivation. Comorbid sleep disorders should be treated accordingly. Medication may not be necessary and is left to clinical discretion; however, if episodes are frequent, potentially injurious, cause social dysfunction, or cause excessive daytime sleepiness (EDS), benzodiazepines are generally prescribed.

REM behavior disorder

REM behavior disorder (RBD) is characterized by loss of the normal physiological muscle atonia that occurs during REM sleep, allowing patients to "act out" dreams. Dream enactment can often result in serious injuries to both patient and bed partner. PSG is diagnostically helpful even in the absence of clinical events, as loss of muscle atonia is evident during REM. RBD typically occurs in older adults and is associated with other disorders, including OSA, narcolepsy, and neurodegenerative disorders, particularly synucleinopathies (PD, Lewy body dementia, multiple systems atrophy). Idiopathic RBD may precede neurodegenerative disorders; thus frequent neurological follow-up is advised. While clonazepam is considered the treatment of choice, melatonin has also been reported to be beneficial. Behavioral modification is necessary, including avoidance of alcohol and of sleep deprivation, along with general safety precautions during sleep.

Pathological hypersomnias

Pathological hypersomnias are disorders of sleep and wake states. Complaints of excessive daytime sleepiness (EDS) are the cardinal symptom of these disorders. In order to diagnose pathological hypersomnias accurately, it is imperative to correct the underlying causes of the sleep deficiency, including ensuring treatment of behaviorally induced insufficient sleep and other sleep disorders such as OSA.

Narcolepsy

Narcolepsy is the instability of sleep–wake states, likely due to mutations in the hypothalamic hypocretin/orexin system. The "tetrad" of narcolepsy includes EDS, cataplexy, hypnogogic/hypnopompic hallucinations, and sleep paralysis. However, these symptoms often occur independently or in different combinations. The hallmark symptom of narcolepsy is EDS, while the remaining symptoms are attributed to REM intrusion into wakefulness. Patients with narcolepsy often have fragmented nocturnal sleep, exacerbating EDS and REM intrusion into wake periods. Diagnostically, PSG and a next-day Multiple Sleep Latency Test (MSLT) show shortened sleep latencies and 2+ sleep-onset REM periods. Treatment is a mixture of behavioral modification and pharmacotherapy. EDS is typically treated with wake-promoting or stimulant medications, and/or frequent napping schedules. REM intrusion can be treated with sodium oxybate or antidepressants. Comorbid sleep disorders often accompany narcolepsy, including OSA, PLMD, and RBD.

Idiopathic hypersomnia

Idiopathic hypersomnia (IH) is characterized by EDS, with non-refreshing sleep despite prolonged sleep episodes. PSG/MSLT shows high sleep efficiency and shortened sleep latencies. Despite attempts to characterize IH further, pathophysiology is still unclear. IH thus remains a diagnosis of exclusion. Treatment with stimulants has variable response. Prolonged sleep schedules are generally not beneficial.

Further reading

American Academy of Sleep Medicine. *International Classification of Sleep Disorders*, 3rd ed. Westchester, IL: AASM; 2014.

Avidan A (ed.). *Sleep in Neurological Practice*. New York: Thieme; 2005.

Diagnostic Classification Steering Committee of the American Sleep Disorders Association. *The International Classification of Sleep Disorders: Diagnostic and Coding Manual*. Rochester, MN: American Sleep Disorders Association; 1997.

Iber C, Ancoli-Israel S, Chesson A, Quan SF; for the American Academy of Sleep Medicine. *The AASM Manual of the Scoring of Sleep and Associated Events: Rules, Terminology and Technical Specifications*. Westchester, IL: AASM; 2007.

Meir H, Kryger T, Dement W (eds.). *Principles and Practice of Sleep Medicine*. Philadelphia, PA: Elsevier; 2006.

158   Spinal cord disorders

David B. Vodušek[1], Miran Jeromel[2], and Simon Podnar[3]

[1] Medical Faculty, University of Ljubljana, and Division of Neurology, University Medical Centre Ljubljana, Ljubljana, Slovenia
[2] Department for Neuroradiology, University Medical Centre Ljubljana, Ljubljana, Slovenia
[3] Division of Neurology, University Medical Centre Ljubljana, Ljubljana, Slovenia

"Spinal pain" is estimated to be one of the most prevalent morbid conditions, leading to absenteeism from work and early retirement. The lifetime prevalence of spinal pain both in the neck and in the lower back has been reported to be as high as 80%.

Two adjacent spinal vertebrae are joined by paired facet joints and the intervertebral disc, and form the "motion segment." The disc is formed by the collagenous outer annulus fibrosus and the gel-like nucleus pulposus. Only the outer layer of the annulus has nerve and blood supply and the other parts are dependent on diffusion exchange of nutrients. By middle age, the annulus develops fissures, and through these, disc protrusion, prolapse, or even sequestration may occur, with the possibility of mechanical compression of nerve roots, spinal cord, or blood vessels within the spinal canal and the nerve root exit foramina (Figure 158.1). From the second decade onward, the degeneration process becomes more and more

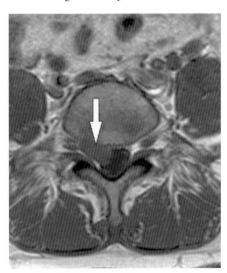

Figure 158.1 This 43-year-old patient presented with acute right sciatica accompanied by paresthesias of the dorsal aspect of the right foot and weakness of foot and particularly big toe dorsiflexion, indicating L5 nerve root involvement. T1-weighted MRI showed a L5–S1 disc herniation with extrusion of nucleus pulposus toward the right lateral recess (S1 root) and right neural foramen (L5 root). The patient was treated surgically with discectomy and nerve root decompression.

frequent; degeneration of the superior and inferior margins of the vertebral bodies accompanied by the formation of osteophytes, osteoarthritic changes of the facet joints (i.e., spondylosis), and hypertrophy of the longitudinal ligament invariably lead to the extremely prevalent changes seen on plain X-ray, computed tomography (CT), and magnetic resonance imaging (MRI), which in the majority of persons and most of the time are asymptomatic. The changes may cause pain without actually involving and injuring neural structures. In a minority of patients structural changes damage nerve roots or the spinal cord, through either compression of the nervous tissue or its vascular supply; inflammatory mechanisms possibly contribute.

In adults, the spinal cord occupies the spinal canal to the level of the L1/L2 interface (with some individual variability). The anterior and posterior roots are attached to the spinal cord, the spinal ganglion on the posterior root being situated just before the two roots unite into the spinal nerve. The anterior root and the posterior root with the ganglion are intradural, exiting individually and uniting into the spinal nerve root extradurally, but before leaving the spinal canal through the intervertebral foramen. Nerve roots are accompanied by arteries and veins. In the neck, the spinal ganglion lies within the intervertebral foramen. From L2, it moves more medially. The L5 spinal ganglion lies at the inner aperture of the foramen, and the spinal ganglia below that level move into the spinal canal. The cervical roots exit from foramina lying above the respective vertebrae (the C8 root thus being situated above T1). From root C4 down the roots have a more and more steep downward course. They also increase in length, with the lowermost roots reaching 25 cm. Conus medullaris represents the lowest part of the spinal cord (sacral segments S3–S5), which is usually positioned behind the L1 vertebral body. Below the conus medullaris the assembly of L2–S4 spinal roots, known as the cauda equina, pass to their respective foramina and contain peripheral nerve fibers passing between the respective spinal cord segments and the target segments. The steep downward course of lumbar and sacral roots means that a disc prolapse typically compresses the root of the segment below (the L5–S1 disc prolapse compresses the S1 root; see Figure 158.1), but also two adjacent roots may be compressed. Prolapse of the cervical (and rarely the thoracic) disc may injure only the respective root if the direction of prolapse is lateral (mostly posterolateral), but compresses the spinal cord if it is posteromedial. In the most commonly

International Neurology, Second edition. Edited by Robert P. Lisak, Daniel D. Truong, William M. Carroll and Roongroj Bhidayasiri
© 2016 John Wiley & Sons, Ltd. Published 2016 by John Wiley & Sons, Ltd.

affected segments in the back (L4–L5, L5–S1, and L3–L4), postero-lateral protrusion will affect only one or two roots, while postero-medial protrusion will compress the cauda equina.

Root compression by disc or spondylosis causes demyelination of the nerve fibers within the root, or axonal injury; in the latter case, axonal degeneration takes place. In the case of the motor axons this will lead to denervation of the respective motor units (a motor unit comprises all muscle cells innervated by a single lower motor neuron). Dorsal root compression may cause preganglionic axonal injury of the primary sensory neuron; this leads to degeneration of the proximal but not the distal neurite.

Pathological processes affecting the "mobile spinal segment" (even though not compromising the roots) cause pain, and the pain may radiate in the affected segment (known as referred pain). Referred pain does not as a rule irradiate to the most distal segments of the upper or lower limb, and is – of course – not accompanied by segmental neurological deficit. The distribution of "neurogenic" pain (a typical consequence of root compression) is related to the segmental innervation of skin, muscles, and bones (dermatome, myotome, and the sclerotome, respectively).

Cervical disc disease

The most commonly affected segment in the neck is the C6–C7 level (a lateral disc herniation will affect the C7 root). The next most common cervical radiculopathy is C6 (herniation at level C5–C6), and then C5 (herniation at C4–C5). Patients usually complain of neck pain radiating to the shoulder and upper arm (C5) and into the lower arm and hand into the thumb (C6), or the second, third, and fourth fingers (C7). Root involvement is accompanied by paresthesias and dysesthesias affecting the dermatome (in its distal part). Motor symptoms are usually not prominent, although needle electromyography (EMG) of the muscles belonging to the particular myotome may show abnormalities (see later). Notably, the deltoid will be paretic in the C5 syndrome, the biceps and brachioradialis in the C6 syndrome, the pectoralis major, the triceps brachii muscle, and the finger extensors in the C7 syndrome, and the intrinsic hand muscles and index finger extensor in the C8 syndrome. C5 radiculopathy weakens the biceps reflex, which may be absent in C6 radiculopathy. The triceps brachii reflex is affected particularly in the C7 syndrome. Cervical radiculopathy is not accompanied by vegetative symptoms, as autonomic fibers do not leave the spinal cord via cervical roots.

An acute posteromedial disc herniation in the cervical region may lead to spinal cord compression, causing myelopathy. This is clinically manifested by more or less pronounced long-tract signs with paresthesias in lower limbs, accompanied by a spastic tetra- or paraparesis (according to the level of the lesion) with lower urinary tract, anorectal, and sexual dysfunction. Cervical myelopathy due to cervical spondylosis occurs as a slowly progressive disorder, unless it is precipitated unmasked by (minor) neck injury.

Lumbar disc disease

The most commonly affected individuals are middle-aged men, but a functionally significant episode of low back pain may be encountered by up to 80% of the adult population over a lifetime. The typical presentation is with low back pain, which may be accompanied by referred pain. The term "sciatica" is used for pain referred to the lower limb, but this is not necessarily indicative of nerve root involvement.

In a minority of patients, there is spinal nerve/radicular involvement with "root pain" and neurological symptoms. As the most often involved nerve roots are L5 or S1, pain in these instances typically radiates down the whole lower extremity to its distal parts (i.e., dorsum of the foot and big toe, or heel, lateral side of foot, and the lateral toes, respectively). "Proof" of nerve root involvement is in paresthesias in the appropriate segmental distribution. In the case of radiculopathy, pain may begin in the back and "move" downward. It may also be restricted to the lower limb. Onset may be spontaneous or associated with mechanical stress to the spine. The pain may be excruciating and make the patient more or less immobile, with accompanying paraspinal muscle spasm. Radicular neurological deficit (sensory, motor, and reflex) may be discrete or prominent, and may occur (or be revealed) after the acute pain episode. Local tenderness to palpation or percussion over the spinous processes may be present, and the patient often adopts a fixed posture, somewhat tilted away from the affected side. Passive hip flexion with the lower limb extended at the knee exacerbates the pain in L5 and S1 root involvement (Lasègue sign), particularly if the foot is passively dorsiflexed when the extended leg is raised. Pain may be exacerbated by increases in intra-abdominal pressure (coughing, sneezing, defecating, etc.).

Most commonly the L4–L5 and L5–S1 interspaces are affected, with the L5 or S1 and less commonly L4 roots being compressed. Other interspaces and other roots are rarely affected. A posteromedial protrusion may affect several roots and lead to a cauda equina syndrome.

The radiculopathies produce typical sensory-motor syndromes, but individual variability in segmental innervation exists. L4 radiculopathy leads to pain radiating down the distal lateral thigh and the anteromedial leg. The pain in L4 root compression is exacerbated by the patient lying on his or her stomach with the knee flexed and the hip extended. L5 radiculopathy leads to pain radiating to the anterolateral leg and the dorsum of the foot and hallux. Pain in the S1 syndrome radiates down the posterior leg to the heel, and the lateral aspect of the foot to the third to fifth toes. The L4 syndrome may partially weaken the quadriceps muscle, with hyporeflexia of the knee jerk and sensory loss along the anteromedial leg. The L5 syndrome leads to weakness of the ankle and particularly big toe dorsiflexion; walking "on heels" may be affected and weakness of ankle inversion also helps localize an L5 syndrome. The absence of the tibialis posterior reflex is helpful only in individuals with brisk jerks, which will allow the unequivocal demonstration of the contralateral reflex. The L5 dermatome is typically affected – the dorsal foot and the anterolateral leg. In S1 radiculopathy walking "on toes" may be affected (due to paretic plantar flexors) and the ankle jerk is absent or very reduced. The sensory loss involves the heel, lateral surface of the foot, and the fifth toe.

A cauda equina lesion is recognized by bilateral symptoms (which, however, are as a rule asymmetric). Pain radiates from the lower back to both legs and paresthesias may be bilateral and typically involve the perineal region. Distal lower limb paresis may or may not be present, but ankle jerks are asymmetrically reduced or absent. Urinary retention usually precedes urinary incontinence, which is of the overflow type. Urinary symptoms are the leading autonomic dysfunction in the acute stage, with anorectal and sexual dysfunction revealed in due course. The sensory deficit involves the affected segments and typically the lower sacral segments. The upper posterior parts of the thighs and buttocks (S2), the perineal and perianal regions, as well as the region overlying the coccygeal bone (S3–S5) are affected, resulting in so-called saddle anesthesia. The anal reflex is absent unilaterally or bilaterally; in most healthy subjects, pricking the perianal skin with a pin causes visible anal sphincter contraction.

In a patient presenting with bilateral neurological symptoms and signs attributable to sacral segments, the question of a cauda equina versus conus medullaris lesion arises. In theory, conus medullaris lesions should demonstrate a combination of upper and lower motor neuron signs, but usually the signs of a lower motor neuron lesion predominate. Cauda equina lesions tend to be more asymmetric, with radicular pain and more pronounced lower limb deficits. Dissociated sensation, when found, distinctly diagnoses a (vascular) conus medullaris lesion. Sacral function (bladder, bowel, and sexual) deficits, and saddle sensory loss, are usually found in both. Cauda equina lesions are more common than those of the conus medullaris, with estimated annual incidence rates of 3.4 and 1.5 per million, and prevalence rates of 8.9 and 4.5 per 100000 population, respectively. The most common etiologies are lumbar intervertebral disc herniations for cauda equina lesions, and T11–L1 spinal fractures for conus medullaris lesions.

Natural course of disc herniation

Prognosis of acute disc disease is good and it has been demonstrated by MRI that disc protrusion and prolapse tend to recede with time. The prognosis of nerve root demyelination is excellent. Root lesions of the axonal type probably get little true regeneration of the destroyed axons, but collateral reinnervation of the partially denervated muscle from the remaining axons can result in good functional recovery. On the sensory side, central axons probably do not regenerate.

Diagnosis

The clinical picture of acute neck pain radiating to one limb with neurological deficit should be readily recognizable. The clinical examination defines the neurological deficit and thus the particular root syndrome. Plain radiography only helps to exclude serious disease (malignant, infectious), the readily and expectedly demonstrable degenerative changes being rarely of diagnostic relevance. Thus MRI is the diagnostic procedure of choice. Care should be taken not to miss radicular compression in the lateral recess or foramen by a strictly lateral disc herniation (Figure 158.1). In patients with isolated pain (even if radiating) but without a neurological syndrome, inflammatory causes and bone-destructive lesions should be ruled out. MRI in patients with segmental spinal pain is used routinely as part of the diagnostic workup, but findings of disc and other "degenerative" changes have to be interpreted cautiously in the context of the clinical picture; over half of demonstrated disc herniations are said to be asymptomatic.

In the acute stage electrodiagnostic testing is not indicated – the diagnostically relevant abnormal spontaneous ("denervation") muscle activity detected by needle electromyography (EMG) takes 3 weeks to develop. After the period of acute muscle denervation, reinnervation processes manifest themselves by "remodeling" of motor units. This process is mirrored in the change of motor unit potentials (which become large, polyphasic, and of prolonged duration), as detected by needle EMG. The residual abnormality in radiculopathy is recognized by a myotomal distribution of abnormal EMG findings. In practice, electrodiagnostics is particularly useful to exclude involvement of plexus and limb nerves, often a relevant differential diagnostic consideration, particularly since therapy for a median neuropathy at the wrist (carpal tunnel syndrome), for instance, if promptly instituted, will abolish the symptoms.

Treatment

The generally good prognosis of disc disease dictates conservative treatment as the primary approach. Emergency surgery is indicated in acute spinal cord compression and the cauda equina syndrome. Similarly, early surgery may be contemplated in acute radiculopathy with a severe and functionally relevant motor deficit matched by appropriate MRI radicular injury and in some instances by myotomal fibrillation potentials on needle EMG.

Treatment approaches to radiculopathy vary considerably in different centers and countries, and there are no generally agreed guidelines. In many hospitals (delayed) surgery is commonly performed for a variety of indications. A common indication is the situation when the symptoms (with significant pain) do not recede in weeks or months. However, there are no large-scale controlled clinical trials demonstrating surgery to be superior to other treatments in the long term.

Conservative treatment comprises an explanation of the usual benign and self-limiting course of the disease, and appropriate analgesia (primarily with non-steroidal anti-inflammatory drugs), which may be combined with (temporary) striated muscle relaxants. Relative immobilization in the acute stage may be necessary, but the patient should be encouraged to remain mobile as much as possible. Physical therapy to abate pain and physiotherapy to improve mobility may be helpful. Appropriate positioning in bed (at night-time) is important. Nightly soft neck immobilization is often appropriate and necessary in the acute stage. Ventral or ventrolateral positioning in bed (with appropriate positioning of cushions) is often helpful in the patient with severe lumbar radicular pain. Local infiltration with analgesics and steroids (including CT-guided nerve root sleeve injection) may provide short-term symptomatic benefit. Manual manipulation in the presence of neural system involvement should not be attempted.

Chronic radicular symptoms may occasionally gain a neuropathic pain quality and should be treated as such.

Chronic spinal pain (as a rule without neurological symptoms) is the more common and much more therapy-resistant problem, which may require a multidisciplinary approach with behavioral treatment, and is often only complicated by surgery.

Cervical spondylosis

Symptoms due to cervical spondylosis develop mostly after middle age and more commonly in men. Although the overall clinical picture may be similar to that of disc disease, both the onset and intensity of the symptomatology are less dramatic and sensory-motor deficits are usually less marked. Pain is increased on head movement. Although the morphological changes are not expected to recede, symptomatology often fluctuates. Repeated exacerbations of symptoms occur, but with a decreased range of spine movement due to progressive spondylotic changes, pain episodes may decrease.

Spondylotic changes may deform the spinal canal and the intervertebral foramina, leading to root irritation and radiculopathy. The sixth and seventh cervical roots are most commonly affected; C8 is only occasionally involved.

Spondylotic changes may also encroach on the spinal canal. Protrusion of discs, hypertrophy of facet joints, and thickening of the ligamentum flavum lead to both stenotic changes of the intervertebral foramina as well as the spinal canal itself. Below a canal width of 12 mm myelopathy may develop, with slowly progressive long tract signs (spastic paraparesis with sensory ataxia), leading to a broad-based uncertain gait. Urinary symptoms may appear. The segmental involvement of cervical spinal cord and concomitant radiculopathy can cause a segmental cervical sensory-motor deficit with muscle atrophy.

MRI is the diagnostic procedure of choice, as it demonstrates not only the osseous and non-osseous components of the spinal stenosis, but also intramedullary signal intensity changes in the spinal cord (myelopathic change); see Figure 158.2.

The progression of the disease is unpredictable and may comprise prolonged static intervals punctuated by episodic deterioration. An expectant conservative approach is appropriate in mild and non-progressive cases, while progressive neurological deficits should be treated early rather than late, because, once developed, functional impairment tends not to recede after surgery.

Lumbar spinal stenosis

Spondylotic changes of the lumbar spine along with other degenerative changes lead – particularly in the presence of a congenitally narrow spinal canal – to encroachment on lumbosacral roots, causing radiculopathy or at worst a specific clinical picture: neurogenic claudication (claudication of the cauda equina). This comprises discomfort and pain in the back radiating downward, usually bilaterally, and exacerbated by stance and walking. Pain slowly increases on walking and becomes too uncomfortable to bear after a certain distance. Other sensory symptoms in the lumbar and sacral segments may appear (numbness, paraesthesia). Motor weakness and

occasionally autonomic symptoms occur (urinary incontinence, but also urgency of micturition and persistent penile erection/priapism, due possibly to lower sacral root irritation). If the patients are followed up, the distance they can walk without symptoms gets progressively shorter. Typically walking downhill is more difficult for the patient than uphill, because it is the extension of the lumbar lordosis that causes buckling of the ligamentum flavum and leads to an up to 20% additional narrowing of the spinal canal. Somewhat paradoxically, these patients may cycle for long distances even though they are unable to walk even short distances without becoming symptomatic. Symptoms can also appear during prolonged standing in the upright position and particular in a "back leaning" position of the body (such as reaching to shelves above the head).

Typically in most patients the neurological examination during rest will not reveal significant abnormalities, and EMG may be non-informative.

In mild cases, conservative/expectative treatment (ensuring that the patient understands the nature of the problem) is appropriate. Patients may remain reasonably mobile with a rational alteration of their lifestyle. With progressive problems and if the limitation of their mobility is unacceptable, surgery will relieve the symptoms, particularly if there is discrete and focal narrowing of the spinal canal.

Paget's disease

In Paget's disease there is excessive bone resorption coupled with abnormal new bone formation resulting in altered bone structure, increased vascularity, and mechanical weakness. The disease has a predilection for the axial skeleton. Back pain has been described in up to 43% of patients with spinal Paget's disease. The involved vertebrae are increased in width and reduced in height. Particularly (mid) lumbar (58%), low thoracic (42%), and cervical (14%) segments are involved. The disease manifests itself in the elderly, affecting

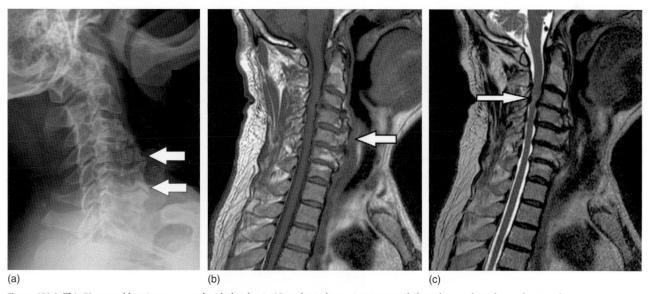

(a)   (b)   (c)

Figure 158.2 This 72-year-old patient presented with dysphagia. Neurological examination revealed no abnormality of cranial nerves, but upper extremity weakness and a positive Babinski sign. (a) A plain radiograph of cervical spine in lateral view revealed massive ventral spondylophytes (arrow) protruding from C3–C6 level. (b) MRI of cervical spine in sagittal plane demonstrated displacement and mechanical compression of pharynx and esophagus caused by ventral spondylophytes (arrow) seen on T1-weighted image. (c) The examination also revealed severe cervical spinal canal stenosis caused by dorsolateral spondylophytes with spinal cord edema (arrow) – a sign of compressive myelopathy. The patient was treated with surgical resection and stabilization.

up to 3% of the population above 55 years of age in Europe and North America. In up to 14% of patients there is a family history, but the etiology is poorly understood. Although changes may be prominent, most patients are asymptomatic. Most commonly local pain occurs. The overlying skin may be warmer due to increased bone vascularization. The pain is typically worse at rest. Fractures may occur. Creeping neurological symptoms may develop due to encroachment of the changed bone on the spinal canal, compressing either single roots, spinal cord, or cauda equina. Acute neurological syndromes may occur with pathological fractures. Neural compromise may occur also through vascular causes; epidural hematoma causing acute compressive myelopathy has been described.

Spinal stenosis occurs in 10–20% of patients with Paget's disease. Extradural ossification of the ligamentum flavum and epidural fat may result in spinal cord or root compression, but myelopathy and the cauda equina syndrome may occur without evidence of direct compression on neuroimaging. Because neurological symptoms respond to medical treatment with calcitonin (which reduces the abnormal skeletal blood flow to normal), an arterial "steal phenomenon" has been suggested as a cause in such instances.

The diagnosis is usually made by imaging, with findings of increased serum alkaline phosphatase and increased urinary hydroxyproline. However, alkaline phosphatase levels have been described as normal in almost one-third of patients with Paget's disease and spinal stenosis. Radionuclide scans localize disease activity (Figure 158.3).

The treatment of choice for symptomatic spinal stenosis is medical (a bisphosphonate) and results in improvement of myelopathy or cauda equina syndrome. Unfortunately, relapses occur, but may be treated by repeating the therapy. Oral bisphosphonates are recommended for patients with slowly progressive symptoms, and intravenous bisphosphonates are indicated in rapidly progressive neurological deterioration before surgery to minimize bone hemorrhage. Surgical treatment of spinal disease is difficult also because involvement is often at multiple levels. Clinical monitoring of neurological function with repeated imaging, serum alkaline phosphatase, and urinary hydroxyproline determinations every 6–12 months has been recommended if surgery can be delayed.

Fibrous dysplasia

Fibrous dysplasia of bone is a mesenchymal disease affecting single or multiple bones, and in most cases is already diagnosed in childhood. It is caused by activating missense mutations of the *GNAS1* gene, encoding the α subunit of the stimulatory G-protein, Gsα. These mutations are postzygotic, are not inherited, and result in a mosaic state. Diagnosis is based on clinical, radiographic, and histopathological features. Markers of bone turnover are usually elevated. Total body bone scintigraphy determines the extent of bone involvement.

In the polyostotic form, fibrous dysplasia may be accompanied by pigmented skin areas (patches) and endocrinological abnormalities (much more frequently in girls).

The disease may appear and progress in adults and uncommonly affects the lumbar and thoracic vertebrae. Scoliosis occurs in approximately 50% of patients with the polyostotic form of the disease. In addition to deformity, pain may be prominent and pathological fractures occur, as do neurological complications, often due to compression. Expansion of the vertebral body, the arches, or the articular processes has been described, with the potential to involve nerve roots and spinal cord.

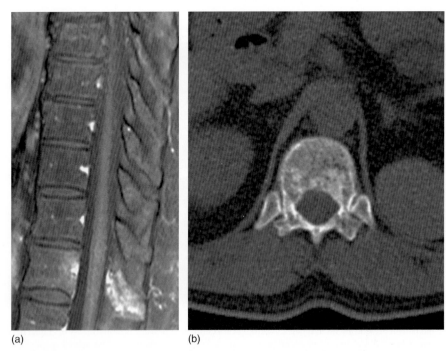

(a)   (b)

Figure 158.3 This 42-year-old patient presented with persistent low back pain. (a) The T12 vertebral body (posterior part, including posterior vertebral elements and spinous process) showed contrast enhancement on T1-weighted image with fat suppression. No extension into the spinal canal was noticed. (b) The lesion appeared sclerotic on CT examination. Scintigraphy showed signs of osteoblastic activity in the lesion. Percutaneous bone biopsy was performed and a diagnosis of Paget's disease was histologically proven.

Therapy is surgical if warranted by symptoms. Treatment with bisphosphonates has been advocated, but there have been no controlled studies.

Other compressive disorders

In the spinal canal there is little free space outside the cord and the nerve roots. Neural compression most often arises anteriorly, particularly from the intervertebral joint and disc, which, through mechanical stress of the mobile segments of the lower cervical spine and the weight-bearing lumbar spine, develop degenerative changes. The clinical picture of spinal pain with root or spinal cord symptoms may of course occur with any type of developmental disorder affecting the spine (achondroplastic dwarves are prone to all forms of vertebrogenic spinal disease), and by any type of compressive, traumatic, or inflammatory lesion. Trauma usually has a clear-cut history, and will not be further discussed, but minor injuries can lead to a severe neurological deficit in patients with cervical stenosis, and from pathological vertebral fractures of any cause including osteoporosis (osteoporotic fractures are by no means always "benign"). Intraspinal new bone formation with myelopathy may occur in hypophosphatemic osteomalacia (particularly in the mid to low thoracic, but also in the cervical region), in osteopetrosis, and in diffuse idiopathic skeletal hyperostosis.

Infection will usually but not always give additional symptoms and cause "atypical" local pain. Root compression with pain may be caused by an extradural tumor, such as secondary carcinoma, neurofibroma, and reticulosis. Posteriorly located tumors may at first cause only a sensory deficit. Intradural extramedullary tumors (meningioma, neurolemmoma) commonly arise within the vicinity of dorsal roots and cause radicular pain. They progress and compress both roots and spinal cord. In other locations tumor(s) will cause a different sequence of neurological deficit. Intradural intramedullary tumors (glioma, ependymoma) rarely cause radicular pain, but may cause a neuropathic burning or dull, more diffuse pain in the segments below the lesion. Tumors, especially typically neurofibroma, may grow in the intervertebral foramen, achieving an "hourglass" shape and compressing first the root and then the spinal cord. Rarely, an extradural hematoma (particularly in patients with defects in coagulation) gives rise to a local pain syndrome with neurological deficit.

In addition to these diverse compressive pathologies that may cause both a pain syndrome (local and irradiating referred pain) and radiculopathy (without or with myelopathy), the most common differential diagnostic considerations to discopathic or spondylotic radiculopathy are pain syndromes originating in one of the structures of the mobile spinal segment itself. These are (if not malignant or inflammatory) rather trivial as far as the medical issues involved, but may cause prolonged and recurrent symptoms.

A final important diagnostic consideration is that of painful clinical conditions accompanied by localized neurological symptoms, arising from involvement of structures peripheral to the root. The diagnostic possibilities range from plexus involvement – of different etiologies – to distal neuropathy, which is most commonly caused by entrapment.

Investigation

In considering the differential diagnosis of discopathic and spondylotic radiculopathy, two basic clinical syndromes can be conceptualized. On the one hand, there is the "typically" localized pain syndrome without (clinically obvious) neurological involvement and, on the other hand, there is a "localized" neurological syndrome accompanied (or not) by pain. In the first, it is necessary to rule out malignant and infectious spinal disease (pyogenic epidural abscess, tuberculous abscess, acute discitis), and readily curable disease such as carpal tunnel syndrome (which may not be accompanied by any neurological deficit, even in patients with bothersome symptoms). The other group comprises patients with clinically relevant (and particularly progressive) neurological symptomatology with (or without) pain. These patients usually need more diagnostic attention to clarify the problem. A typical situation would be a patient with irradiating pain from the shoulder to the fifth finger and paraesthesia, in whom in due course a Pancoast tumor compressing the lower brachial plexus is demonstrated. Generally speaking the investigations recommended for suspected spinal compressive disorders are blood tests (full blood count, sedimentation rate, C-reactive protein, fasting glucose, serum proteins, calcium phosphatase) and a spinal tap for cerebrospinal fluid testing (for infection/inflammation). MRI is excellent for cord and root lesions, combined with gadolinium enhancement for neoplastic and inflammatory processes. CT is very good for osseous lesions, and if MRI is not possible or available. Isotope scans are helpful for bone metastases and infective lesions. Electrodiagnostic testing is helpful to extend and refine the clinical examination and to follow up peripheral nervous system involvement. EMG helps to diagnose recent denervation and reinnervation in muscles. It helps to distinguish between the radicular, plexus, and nerve syndromes, and generalized disease, particularly if appropriately combined with testing parameters of conduction in both proximal and distal parts of the motor nerve fibers, and recording sensory neurograms. Nerve conduction studies help to diagnose compression neuropathy and other neuropathies. Evoked potential studies have limited value in the diagnosis of compressive and inflammatory lesions, because the nervous system involvement is mostly characterized by axon loss, and is thus less easy to demonstrate with conduction studies.

Further reading

Binder DK, Schmidt MH, Weinstein PR. Lumbar spinal stenosis. *Semin Neurol* 2002;22:157–166.

Carette S, Fehlings MG. Clinical practice: Cervical radiculopathy. *N Engl J Med* 2005;353:392–399.

Healy JF, Healy BB, Wong WH, Olson EM. Cervical and lumbar MRI in asymptomatic older male lifelong athletes: Frequency of degenerative findings. *J Comput Assist Tomogr* 1996;20:107–112.

Jacobs WCH, Rubinstein SM, Willems PC, et al. The evidence on surgical interventions for low back pain disorders: An overview of systemic reviews. *Eur Spine J* 2013;22:1936–1949.

Leet AI, Magur E, Lee JS, et al. Fibrous dysplasia in the spine: Prevalence of lesions and association with scoliosis. *J Bone Joint Surg* 2004;86:531–537.

Mulleman D, Mammou S, Griffoul I, Watier H, Goupille P. Pathophysiology of disk-related sciatica. I. Evidence supporting a chemical component. *Joint Bone Spine* 2006;73:151–158.

Podnar S. Epidemiology of cauda equina and conus medullaris lesions. *Muscle Nerve* 2007;35:529–531.

Ralston SH, Langston AL, Reid IR. Pathogenesis and management of Paget's disease of bone. *Lancet* 2008;372:155–163.

159 Ischemic and congestive myelopathies

Simon Podnar[1], Miran Jeromel[2], and David B. Vodušek[3]

[1] Division of Neurology, University Medical Centre Ljubljana, Ljubljana, Slovenia
[2] Department for Neuroradiology, University Medical Centre Ljubljana, Ljubljana, Slovenia
[3] Medical Faculty, University of Ljubljana, and Division of Neurology, University Medical Centre Ljubljana, Ljubljana, Slovenia

Ischemic and congestive myelopathies form two broad groups of rare neurological conditions, each caused by several individual etiologies.

Basic knowledge of the spinal cord vascular supply is essential for understanding spinal vascular disorders. The spinal cord is supplied by a single anterior and a pair of posterior spinal arteries, whose rostral origin is from the vertebral arteries and which anastomose caudally at the level of the conus medullaris. The spinal arteries anastomose with the pial plexus, and the posterior spinal arteries may be linked together. At each level the anterior spinal artery provides central arteries entering the spinal cord and supplying the anterior horn and the anterior part of the lateral columns. The spinal arteries also receive supply from the radicular arteries, thus forming several functional regions of the spinal cord: C1–T3 (vertebral artery branch at C3 level, and a branch from ascending cervical arteries at C6–C7 level), T3–T7 (sometimes a branch from the intercostal artery), and T8–conus medullaris (a branch from the intercostals artery at T9–T12 level – artery of Adamkiewicz – and sometimes a conus-feeding artery originating from the internal iliac artery, most often at L5 level – artery of Desproges–Gotteron). Inadequate perfusion and resulting ischemia of the spinal cord may be produced by interruption of blood flow through critical arteries, by hypotension in the relevant vascular bed, or – indirectly – by venous hypertension. The latter typically occurs in spinal arteriovenous fistulas, but may be a consequence of other vascular malformations.

The more obvious manifestation of arteriovenous malformations (AVM) in the spinal canal is an acute neurological syndrome due to hemodynamic or hemorrhagic problems (in the case of perimedullary fistulas and intramedullary angiomas). However, vascular malformations of the spinal cord can appear as isolated intramedullary lesions with apparently normal surface vessels that may be difficult to distinguish from spinal cord neoplasms (Figure 159.1). Hereditary hemorrhagic telangiectasia (Osler–Weber–Rendu disease) is an autosomal dominant vascular dysplasia that is associated with a diverse array of neurological disorders; myelopathy secondary to AVM may occur. Indeed, all AVM within the spinal canal may lead to progressive myelopathy (i.e., venous congestive myelopathy). Congestive myelopathy is the main clinical manifestation of spinal dural arteriovenous fistula, the most common AVM of the spinal canal.

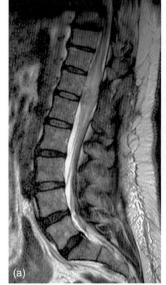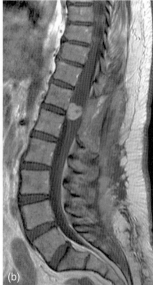

Figure 159.1 This 46-year-old patient presented with progressive lower urinary tract and anorectal dysfunction and sacral paresthesias. (a) T2-weighted MRI showed a pathological formation in the conus medullaris with hyperintense signal in the distal medulla (myelopathy). (b) T1-weighted contrast-enhanced MRI showed a well-delineated tumor-like lesion with homogenous contrast accumulation. Open biopsy was performed and the lesion was diagnosed as a capillary hemangioma.

Acute ischemic myelopathy

Ischemic cord infarction is a rare condition when compared to all acute myelopathies (5–8%), as well as all vascular neurological pathologies (1–2%). Therefore, the pathogenesis and natural history of this disorder are difficult to study. In patients with acute ischemic myelopathy, symptoms usually develop in less than 2 minutes, but can in some extend to several hours. Most patients have acute, monophasic symptoms, reaching a nadir in <24 hours, and feel acute pain at the lesion level before other signs and symptoms appear. Clinical symptoms and findings include motor, spinothalamic, and lemniscal sensory deficits depending on the spinal level and the pattern of ischemic myelopathy. In general, in clinically and radiologically proven anterior spinal artery (uni- or bilateral) and posterior spinal artery (uni- or bilateral) occlusions, central

International Neurology, Second edition. Edited by Robert P. Lisak, Daniel D. Truong, William M. Carroll and Roongroj Bhidayasiri
© 2016 John Wiley & Sons, Ltd. Published 2016 by John Wiley & Sons, Ltd.

and transverse patterns are observed. Unilateral patterns are explained by the duplication of the anterior system and by the incomplete linking of the posterior systems. Profound and prolonged arterial hypotension usually results in central and transverse spinal cord lesions, caused by global hypoperfusion of the spinal cord.

The etiology of the spontaneous spinal cord ischemia is often unclear, as only a small proportion usually have vascular risk factors (e.g., diabetes, hypertension). Mechanical stress may be a triggering factor. The spinal arteries run along a mobile spinal column, which makes them prone to mechanical damage. Ischemic symptoms often occur immediately after some movement. Central intervertebral disc herniations may compress the anterior spinal artery, and lateral herniations may occlude radicular arteries. A special case of the latter is occlusion of the conus (Desproges–Gotteron) artery by intervertebral disc at L4–L5 or L5–S1 level. The condition may result in a conus medullaris syndrome, which may be reversible.

The neurological deficit arising with the anterior spinal artery syndrome as a rule involves the anterior parts of the cord bilaterally and exhibits the following: segmental lower motor neuron lesion with flaccid paresis in involved myotomes, pyramidal tract signs below the segmental lesion with spastic paraparesis (and also bladder and bowel dysfunction), and damage to decussating anterior spinothalamic tracts with analgesia and thermalgesia in the involved dermatomes (the so-called dissociated sensory loss, as commonly there is no loss of fine touch and other dorsal column sensation). Anterior spinothalamic tract lesions in the affected segments cause dissociated sensory loss in body parts below the lesion. Unilateral anterior spinal artery territory infarcts occur, and also spare lemniscal sensory fibers within the dorsal columns of the spinal cord.

Due to separate perfusion by anterior and posterior spinal arteries, vascular cord lesions generally do not result in a hemicord or Brown–Sequard syndrome (which includes ipsilateral segmental lower motor neuron signs, ipsilateral pyramidal involvement, and ipsilateral posterior column sensory deficits below the level of the lesion, combined with a contralateral spinothalamic sensory deficit). This syndrome is most often due to trauma, but may be also caused by demyelination plaque, tumor, disc herniation, and so on.

Only a minority of patients, such as those with ischemia of the cervical cord, report identical previous transitory symptoms – transient ischemic attacks (TIAs). At the onset of symptoms patients often report back or neck pain localized to the level of the spinal cord lesion (59% in one study), with a radicular component in the majority of these patients (81%). Paresthesias are rare and, as with pain, usually resolve spontaneously within a few days.

Laboratory studies are usually normal, with the exception of increased cerebrospinal fluid (CSF) protein concentration in a proportion of patients (up to 44%).

Acute spinal cord ischemia has a typical course on magnetic resonance imaging (MRI): findings are usually normal in the acute phase, but spinal cord swelling and T2 abnormality are expected after 1–2 days, while gadolinium enhancement appears even later after symptom onset (2–11 days). The sensitivity and specificity of MRI can be increased by repeated imaging. Diffusion-weighted MRI (DWI) of the spinal cord, although technically difficult to perform in the spinal region, can help in early diagnosis of acute infarction within hours after symptom onset.

To improve the patient's outcome after spinal cord ischemia, a variety of medications (antiplatelet agents, anticoagulants, corticosteroids) and interventions (hyperbaric therapy) have been tried. No prospective therapy trials have so far been published. In iatrogenic spinal myelopathy due to endovascular aortic repair, early detection and treatment with blood pressure augmentation alone or in combination with CSF drainage is the treatment proposed.

Initial severe weakness and a young age at onset are correlated with poor recovery of motor functions. Preoperative renal insufficiency was identified as a risk factor for the development of myelopathy after thoracic endovascular aortic repair.

In spite of the general belief in the ominous prognosis of spinal cord ischemia, the outcomes are not always unfavorable. Complete or incomplete recovery occurs in a high proportion of patients (70% in one study), with about half of patients having significant gait impairment on leaving the hospital. Motor deficits show better recovery than sensory and sacral deficits. Thus, long-term prognosis depends largely on the degree of conus medullaris involvement. Neuropathic pain may appear following hypesthesia after several months.

Congestive myelopathy

Congestive myelopathy was described by Foix and Alajouanine in 1926; it is rare (annual incidence of 5–10/million). It has been shown to be due to venous hypertension, most often resulting from a dural arteriovenous fistula – a tiny connection between a radicular artery and vein that impedes venous drainage of the spinal cord. Ensuing spinal pathology consists of congestive edema followed by necrosis, predominantly of the gray matter. Damage most often starts at the conus medullaris, and spreads slowly up the spinal cord to the level of the fistula. The resulting clinical picture is a chronic progressive myelopathy (sensory loss, paraparesis, uroanogenital symptoms). The mechanism by which the arteriovenous fistula itself forms remains unclear, but it is assumed to be an acquired condition. Most often arteriovenous fistulas are intradural, occurring in the intervertebral foramen on the dorsal surface of the dural root sleeve, where the radicular vein and dural branch(es) of the radicular artery pierce the dura. Most fistulas are located in the thoracolumbar region, but they can occur at any craniospinal level, including intracranially. The condition is underdiagnosed, as it is rare and presents with non-specific symptoms and the diagnosis may not be made for months or years, because dural fistulas never bleed and clinical deterioration is slow. Disk disease and intraspinal space-occupying lesions are among the common differential diagnoses.

Congestive myelopathy occurs more commonly in men than women (ratio 5:1), with a peak age of 55–60 years, and very rarely before 30 years of age. It usually presents with gait difficulties (50–81%), paresthesias in one or both feet, diffuse or patchy sensory loss (sensory disturbances, 17–72%), radicular pain (13–64%), and micturition (4–75%) and defecation (0–38%) problems. The condition progresses slowly, often has a "claudicatory" component, and it usually takes 1–3 years before it is diagnosed. On examination, both central and anterior sensory and upper motor neuron signs are found in the lower limbs.

Apart from history and clinical neurological examination, MRI and catheter angiography are most useful in making the diagnosis (Figure 159.2). As a rule, MR angiography is able to demonstrate abnormal vessels within the spinal canal in the majority of patients with spinal vascular malformations. MR angiography allows identification of the arterial feeder in patients with intramedullary arteriovenous malformations and perimedullary arteriovenous fistulas, but is less useful in identification of the source of intradural draining vein in patients with dural arteriovenous fistula. Homogenous

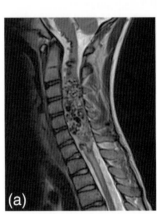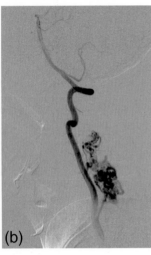

(a) (b)

Figure 159.2 This 14-year-old patient presented with a three-month history of a progressive right-sided hemiparesis. (a) Multiple flow void phenomena presented in the cervical spinal canal on T2-weighted MRI extending from C2 to the C7 segment. The spinal cord is distended in the affected segments, and the hyperintense signal extends to the T3 level. A diagnosis of arteriovenous vascular malformation and spinal cord edema (congestive myelopathy) was made. (b) Digital subtraction angiography (DSA) confirmed the vascular malformation fed by arteries originating predominantly from the right vertebral artery. Malformation drained in the caudal direction via the internal jugular vein and also in the cranial direction (intracranially) to the anterior medullary venous plexus (not shown). The patient was successfully treated with endovascular embolization, without appearance of new deficits.

changes in the signal intensity (hypo on T1- and hyper on T2-weighted images) extending over an average of 5–7 vertebrae, often occurring in the spinal cord center with peripheral sparing, which may extend to involve the conus medullaris, are most characteristic. Lesions may show some enhancement, most often 45 minutes

after gadolinium injection. Enlarged "flow void phenomena" over the surface of the spinal cord are also characteristic, which MR angiography typically shows to be serpentine perimedullary dilated venous structures in up to 100% of patients, which may also give an indication about the level of fistula. This is important for planning catheter angiography, which remains the gold standard for the diagnosis. It must, furthermore, determine whether the arterial feeder is only a dural branch or is also a tributary to the anterior spinal artery. The latter situation prohibits endovascular therapy, which is otherwise an alternative to microsurgery. The outcome of both methods depends on the success of occlusion of the vein draining the fistula. The main determinant of the patient's outcome is pretreatment disability, but neurological deficit may improve after early successful treatment. Gait difficulties and muscle strength respond better than micturition, pain, and muscle spasms. Gait improved in 64% and muscle strength in 56% of patients in one recent study.

Most neurologists will see only a few patients with congestive myelopathy during their career, but the condition should be recognized and duly incorporated into differential diagnosis of progressive myelopathy, particularly in older men. Regardless of its etiology, congestive myelopathy is potentially reversible if properly diagnosed and treated early enough.

Further reading

Alblas CL, Bouvy WH, Lycklama À, Nijeholt GJ, Boiten J. Acute spinal-cord ischemia: Evolution of MRI findings. *J Clin Neurol* 2012;8:218–223.

Jellema K, Tijssen CC, van Gijn J. Spinal dural arteriovenous fistulas: A congestive myelopathy that initially mimics a peripheral nerve disorder. *Brain* 2006;129:3150–3164.

Nedeltchev K, Loher TJ, Stepper F, *et al.* Long-term outcome of acute spinal cord ischemia syndrome. *Stroke* 2004;35:560–565.

Novy J, Carruzzo A, Maeder P, Bogousslavsky J. Spinal cord ischemia: Clinical and imaging patterns, pathogenesis, and outcomes in 27 patients. *Arch Neurol* 2006;63:1113–1120.

Robertson CE, Brown RD, Jr, Wijdicks EF, Rabinstein AA. Recovery after spinal cord infarcts: Long-term outcome in 115 patients. *Neurology* 2012;78:114–121.

Ullery BW, Cheung AT, Fairman RM, *et al.* Risk factors, outcomes, and clinical manifestations of spinal cord ischemia following thoracic endovascular aortic repair. *J Vasc Surg* 2011;54:677–684.

160 Syringomyelia

Alla Guekht

Moscow Research and Clinical Center for Neuropsychiatry and Russian National Research Medical University, Moscow, Russia

The term syringomyelia was suggested in 1827 by the French physician Ollivier d'Angers after the Greek *syrinx* (a cavity of tubular shape) and *myelos* (marrow). A syrinx is a fluid-filled cavity within the spinal cord that can be an incidental finding or it can be accompanied by symptoms of pain and temperature insensitivity (Figure 160.1).

Later, the term hydromyelia was used to indicate a dilatation of the central canal, and syringomyelia referred to cystic cavities separated from the central spinal canal.

Syringomyelia is a chronic disorder characterized pathologically by the presence of long cavities, surrounded by gliosis, situated in the central part of the spinal cord and sometimes extending up into the medulla (syringobulbia). These cavities are filled with fluid that is identical or similar to cerebrospinal (CSF) and extracellular fluid (ECF).

Epidemiology

Syringomyelia occurs in approximately 8 out of every 100000 individuals in Western countries and approximately 2 out of every 100000 individuals in Japan. Information about the occurrence of syringomyelia in different races/ethnic groups is scarce. Some studies suggest a higher prevalence of syringomyelia in African Americans, Maori, and Pacific people than in Caucasians.

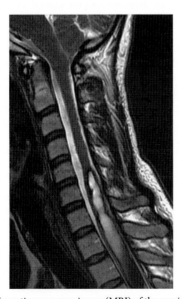

Figure 160.1 Magnetic resonance image (MRI) of the cervical spine showing a syrinx on T2-weighted MR image. Source: Reproduced with permission of Dr. R. Sakovich.

The pathological condition is probably more common, since the widespread availability of magnetic resonance imaging (MRI) has identified that some individuals can have small asymptomatic syringes. The onset of syringomyelia is most commonly observed between the ages of 25 and 40 years, but symptoms can appear at any age between 10 and 60 years. Males are considered to be affected more often than females, but this was not found in the Japanese patients. The condition has been rarely described in more than one member of a family and other congenital malformations, including spina bifida, have been found in families containing affected members.

Pathophysiology

The typical pathological changes associated with syringomyelia are most frequently found in the lower cervical and upper thoracic regions of the spinal cord. Extension to the medulla is common and, rarely, the process may reach the pons. The affected region of the cord may be enlarged, mainly in the transverse plane. A transverse section of the cord reveals a cavity surrounded by a zone of translucent gelatinous material that, microscopically, contains glial cells and fibers. The expanding cavity and surrounding gliosis affect the less resistant gray matter more severely than the more dense white matter and invades the anterior horns of the gray matter, thus causing atrophy of anterior horn cells and degeneration of their axons in the ventral roots and peripheral nerves. The pathophysiology of syringomyelia development is not fully understood.

There are four main types of syringomyelia that may be described in descending order of frequency and are associated with (1) Chiari I malformations; (2) vertebral trauma or (late complication) of subrachnoid hemorrhage; (3) basilar invagination; and (4) hydrocephalus. Recently, the advancement of imaging techniques has revealed more incidental idiopathic syringes that are not associated with Chiari, trauma, or other causes.

Syringomyelia is regarded as a state in which ECF is trapped in the spinal cord due to obstruction of CSF flow, spinal cord tethering, or an intramedullary tumor. Extracellular space and subarachnoid space are two parts of a single fluid compartment, and the only anatomical barriers between the two are the pia mater on the surface of the central nervous system and the ependymal cells of ventricles and the central canal of the spinal cord. Depending on local flow resistances and presumed pressure differentials, ECF may accumulate predominantly in the central canal or in the spinal cord extracellular space itself.

International Neurology, Second edition. Edited by Robert P. Lisak, Daniel D. Truong, William M. Carroll and Roongroj Bhidayasiri
© 2016 John Wiley & Sons, Ltd. Published 2016 by John Wiley & Sons, Ltd.

Clinical features

Segmental amyotrophy, dissociated segmental sensory disturbances, spasticity, scoliosis, weakness, bladder dysfunction, and pain all have been reported in patients with syringomyelia. The onset is usually insidious. Occasionally, the first symptoms may follow an episode of coughing, sneezing, or straining. Wasting and weakness of the small muscles of the hands are common early symptoms, but, alternatively, the patient may notice loss of feeling in the hands or the resulting injuries. Less often, pain or trophic lesions appear first. The index of clinical suspicion for syringomyelia should be raised in children with scoliosis, as its incidence is 50% in those children.

Patients can have fairly extensive and otherwise asymptomatic lesions if the process is very slow, and these are only found by incidental MRI.

Sensory signs

Sensory signs are usually the most prominent clinical feature and manifest as a consequence of the progressive lesion in the central region of the spinal cord. At the earliest stage there is a predominantly unilateral syrinx in the central gray matter, extending longitudinally through several segments, usually in the lower cervical and upper thoracic cord. It interrupts decussating sensory fibers derived from several consecutive dorsal roots. As these fibers conduct pain, heat, and cold sensitivity, these forms of sensation are impaired while others are preserved. Accordingly, pain and temperature sensory loss with preservation of position, vibration, and touch (dissociated sensory loss) is characteristic. It usually appears along the ulnar border of the hand, forearm, and arm, and on the upper part of the chest and back on one side, in a "half-cape" (unilateral) distribution, with a lower border across the chest wall.

When the lesion is situated centrally, or has extended from one side of the cord to the other, the area of dissociated sensory loss is bilateral. As the lesion extends upward and downward in the cord, the area of sensory impairment reaches the radial side of the hand, forearm, and arm and downward over the thorax.

On reaching the upper cervical segments, the lesion begins to involve the spinal tract and nucleus of the trigeminal nerve, with the formation of the area of dissociated sensory loss extending in a concentric manner from behind forwards on the face.

The progressive extension of the spinal lesion later causes compression of the lateral spinothalamic tracts on one or both sides, leading to loss of sensation of pain, heat, and cold over the lower parts of the body. Such thermoanaesthesia and analgesia expose the patient to injuries, especially burns to the fingers, which, being painless, are not noticed at the time.

Pain is a prominent feature in 50–90% of adult patients with established syringomyelia. Patients typically present with complaints of radicular pain (often in a band-like distribution), headache, neck, or interscapular pain. In addition to the more common clinical pain syndromes, approximately 40% of patients with syringomyelia experience significant dysesthetic pain, which is variously described as a burning sensation, pins and needles, or stretching of the skin. Other common characteristics include dermatomal patterns of hypersensitivity, as well as trophic changes such as shiny or glossy skin, coldness, paleness, and abnormal sweating.

Motor signs

The earliest motor manifestations are usually muscular weakness and wasting in the small hand muscles due to compression or destruction of the anterior horn cells. As the lesion extends, the wasting spreads to involve forearms and later the arms, shoulder girdles, and upper intercostals. In contrast to motor neuron disease, fasciculation and severe wasting are uncommon. Contractures may develop, especially in hand and forearm muscles. Extension of the lesion to the posterolateral medulla often involves the nucleus ambiguus, causing paresis of the soft palate, pharynx, and vocal cord, occasionally leading to laryngeal stridor. Compression of the corticospinal tracts in the spinal cord causes weakness, with slight spasticity and extensor plantar responses in most cases in the later stages. The tendon reflexes are exaggerated in the lower limbs, but are diminished and lost early in the upper limbs, particularly on the side of the dissociated anesthesia.

Cranial nerve involvement becomes apparent with development of syringobulbia.

Autonomic signs

Impairment of autonomic pathways can cause Horner's syndrome, trophic changes of the skin, and neurogenic bladder. Trophic changes in the skin include cyanosis and hyperkeratosis. Loss of sweating or excessive sweating may occur, usually over the face and upper limbs.

Neuropathic osteoarthropathy, also known as Charcot neuroarthropathy (usually with involvement of the shoulder and elbow), is exhibited in 20% of patients. Ulceration, whitlows, and necrosis of bone are not uncommon. The scars of former injuries are usually evident on the palmar surface of the fingers.

Investigations

MRI is the leading diagnostic tool used in determining syringomyelia. T1-weighted sagittal and axial spin-echo images reveal the low signal central cavity in the spinal cord; the lesion is hyperintense on T2. When the syrinx is associated with a Chiari malformation, the latter is also readily demonstrated on sagittal T1-weighted images that include the level of the foramen magnum. Where the differential diagnosis includes intrinsic spinal cord tumor, gadolinium enhancement may identify enhancing tumor tissue (enhancement is not seen in syringes). It is important to look at disturbances in CSF flow, as well as structural abnormalities including arachnoid webs, cysts, and scars.

Myelography, followed by immediate and delayed computed tomography (CT) scanning, is used now only if MRI is contraindicated or unavailable.

The CSF usually shows no abnormality unless the cavity is large enough to cause a block, when the protein content of the fluid is raised.

Involvement of anterior horn cells in the cervical segments can be demonstrated by concentric needle electromyography (EMG).

Treatment

An etiology-driven approach is recommended in the diagnosis and management of syringomyelia. In the absence of symptoms, syringomyelia should probably not be treated, but carefully monitored.

As its natural history is not understood, conservative management suffices for most cases. Patients are advised to avoid straining. Protection of analgesic areas and early treatment of cutaneous lesions in order to promote healing are essential. Symptomatic treatment for pain and spasticity may be required. Physical therapy may be needed to maximize muscular function.

Surgical intervention remains controversial and is individualized to those patients with progressive spinal cord damage to maximize residual function. Surgical procedures are performed if there is an identifiable mass compressing the spinal cord. Surgical options to minimize the syrinx include correction of spinal deformities and various CSF-shunting procedures. In cases involving a Chiari malformation, the main goal of surgery is to provide more space for the cerebellum at the base of the skull and upper cervical spine. Successful surgery should stabilize the condition and may result in a modest improvement in symptoms.

Further reading

Greitz D. Unraveling the riddle of syringomyelia. *Neurosurg Rev* 2006;29(4):251–263.

Klekamp J, Samii M. *Syringomyelia: Diagnosis and Treatment*. New York: Springer Verlag; 2001.

Miller D. Spinal cord disorders. In Donaghy M (ed.). *Brain's Diseases of the Nervous System*. Oxford: Oxford University Press; 2001:620–631.

Ravaglia S, Bogdanov EI, Pichiecchio A, *et al*. Pathogenetic role of myelitis for syringomyelia. *Clin Neurol Neurosurg* 2007;109(6):541–546.

Roy AK, Slimack NP, Ganju A. Idiopathic syringomyelia: Retrospective case series, comprehensive review, and update on management. *Neurosurg Focus* 2011;31(6):E15.

161 Neonatal neurology

Mary Payne[1] and Ann Tilton[2]

[1] Department of Neuroscience, Marshall University, Huntington, WV, USA

[2] Department of Neurology, Louisiana State University Health Sciences Center, New Orleans, LA, USA

Improvements in neonatal intensive care worldwide have increased the survival rate of premature infants and ill term infants. Thus, many children who have suffered intracranial hemorrhage, asphyxia, infection, and seizures survive to be cared for by the neurologist. This chapter will highlight common causes of neurological deficits occurring in infancy and continuing through adulthood.

Hypoxic ischemic encephalopathy

Perinatal asphyxia occurs in premature and term newborns. Diagnosing asphyxia is based on cord blood acidosis, low Apgar scores, such as 6 or below, or other metabolic abnormalities that may suggest damage to other organs besides the brain (e.g., heart, liver, kidneys). Asphyxia exposes the brain to low oxygen, decreased blood flow, and hypercarbia. In a state of prolonged hypoxic-ischemic injury, cardiac output fails, systemic hypotension occurs, and cerebral blood flow decreases. Healthy brain vasculature is able to compensate by autoregulation to maintain adequate blood flow to the brain. However, premature brains and infants with cardiorespiratory illness have poor autoregulation. The cerebral circulation is pressure passive, meaning that a fluctuating arterial blood pressure causes an associated fluctuating pattern of cerebral blood flow velocity due to the poor ability of the cerebral vessels to compensate for these alterations. As a result, levels of many neurotransmitters are unbalanced, including glutamate, excitatory amino acids, and aspartate, and there may be an influx of sodium, calcium, and chloride into cells. Cell death then occurs.

Sequelae of hypoxic-ischemic injury are determined by the extent and area of the ischemia. A global hypoxic-ischemic injury produces infarction in the watershed areas of the brain, whereas a more focal injury from localized vascular compromise leads to focal infarction. Affected white matter causes spasticity in corresponding limbs. Often, the basal ganglia, a region in which active metabolism increases susceptibility to periods of relative ischemia, is injured and may produce a concomitant movement disorder such as dystonia or athetosis with spasticity. Gray-matter damage causes seizures and cognitive dysfunction. Hypothermia for 72 hours followed by slow rewarming in neonates with moderate to severe encephalopathy has been shown to reduce morbidity.

Intraventricular hemorrhage

Periventricular and intraventricular hemorrhage (IVH) are most likely to occur in the infant born before 32 weeks gestational age. The incidence has been reported to be as high as 50% in the United States for births less than 35 weeks gestational age. Internationally, the incidence of hemorrhage is directly related to the incidence of prematurity. The germinal matrix is very cellular and highly vascularized and supports the differentiation of glial cells until about 32 weeks of gestation. The capillary bed in the subependymal germinal matrix is composed of thin endothelial-lined vessels lacking a developed adventitia. The combination of poor autoregulation and fragile vessels predisposes premature infants to intraventricular and periventricular hemorrhage in this area. Bleeds range in severity, as listed in Table 161.1.

IVH is frequently accompanied by global hypoxic-ischemic injury and periventricular leukomalacia, as these diseases also occur in the setting of variable pressure changes (most notably low pressure states leading to ischemia) and occur more frequently in infants with cardiorespiratory illness. The periventricular white matter adjacent to the germinal matrix becomes ischemic from hypoperfusion and hemorrhagic from ventricular blood impairing venous drainage.

IVH causes hydrocephalus from decreased absorption of cerebral spinal fluid (CSF) due to blockage of blood and debris in the arachnoid villi. Chronic obstruction from arachnoiditis impairs outflow of the fourth ventricle, causing hydrocephalus.

Table 161.1 Grades of intracranial hemorrhage.

Grade I	Blood in subependymal region
Grade II	Blood extends into lateral ventricles
Grade III	Blood extends into lateral ventricles with ventricular dilatation
Grade IV	Intraparenchymal hemorrhage

International Neurology, Second edition. Edited by Robert P. Lisak, Daniel D. Truong, William M. Carroll and Roongroj Bhidayasiri
© 2016 John Wiley & Sons, Ltd. Published 2016 by John Wiley & Sons, Ltd.

Infection

Infection may occur in the prenatal, perinatal, or postnatal period. Prenatal infections acquired by the mother and transmitted to the fetus that can cause brain damage include cytomegalovirus, toxoplasmosis, rubella, human immunodeficiency virus (HIV), varicella zoster virus, parvovirus B19, and syphilis. Brain calcifications are commonly seen in cytomegalovirus and toxoplasmosis. Microcephaly, seizures, and thrombocytopenia are common in all of these infections. Mental retardation is a common outcome, as is sensorineural hearing loss (most common in congenital rubella).

Herpes, Listeria, E. coli, Group B streptococcus (GBS) and other gram-negative or gram-positive organisms present in the birth canal may be transmitted to the newborn during birth. Infection with these organisms may lead to meningoencephalitis with seizures, coma, cerebral edema, ventriculitis, and infarction. Chronic changes resulting from these insults include encephalomalacia, hydrocephalus, and gray- and white-matter atrophy.

Inborn errors of metabolism

Inborn errors of metabolism include disorders of amino acids, organic acids, and carbohydrates, and present in the neonatal period with seizures, encephalopathy, and poor feeding. Metabolic acidosis, hyperammonemia, and hypoglycemia are indicators of a deficient metabolic enzyme.

Hyperbilirubinemia occurs in hemolytic disease and from inherited defects of conjugation. It is more common in infants of Asian or Hispanic descent. Neurons are particularly sensitive to high levels of bilirubin. Extracellular bilirubin is unconjugated and binds to phospholipids on the plasma membrane of cells, forming a complex with the cell membrane. Bilirubin then enters the cell and binds to mitochondria and the nucleus. Ligandin is an intracellular substance that binds to the bilirubin complex and removes its toxicity; neurons do not contain ligandin. Thus, neuronal cell death occurs. Therefore, acute bilirubin encephalopathy is associated pathologically with bilirubin staining of neurons, or "kernicterus." A later finding is neuronal necrosis. Premature infants are more susceptible to kernicterus at a lower level of total bilirubin compared to term infants.

Infants who survive kernicterus have severe neurological sequelae, including movement disorders such as chorea, ballismus, dystonia, and tremor. Also seen are gaze abnormalities, hearing loss, and cognitive deficits.

Seizures

Seizures occurring within 48 hours after birth are most likely from hypoxic-ischemic encephalopathy, intracranial hemorrhage, or hypoglycemia. Seizures occurring later are usually symptomatic seizures in the setting of infection, metabolic disturbance, pyridoxine deficiency, or inborn error of metabolism. Several types of seizures occur in the neonate and include tonic, clonic, myoclonic, and fragmentary. Fragmentary (or subtle) seizures may be challenging to manage since they are frequently associated with electroclinical dissociation. Neonates may have focal or generalized seizures; however, because the neonatal brain is not yet myelinated, generalized seizures consist of spread of focal activity, not the type of generalized convulsion that is seen in older age groups.

Other etiologies to consider include fifth-day fits, in which the seizures begin on the fifth day of life, are multifocal clonic activity, and disappear by 20 days of life. Familial neonatal seizures are recognized by the autosomal dominant family history of neonatal seizures.

Treatment of neonatal seizures consists of lorazepam in the acute setting and phenobarbital and/or fosphenytoin load for status epilepticus and for daily maintenance therapy.

Neurotoxin exposure

Neurotoxins that can affect the fetus include environmental toxins, prescription medications, and recreational drugs. Once substances consumed by the mother cross the placental barrier, levels in the fetus can be higher than in the mother. Toxins that affect the central nervous system (CNS), in particular, tend to be lipophilic and low in molecular weight and thus are able to penetrate into the fetal CNS. Environmental toxins such as heavy metals disrupt neuronal cell migration and formation of synapses, which in turn disrupts neurotransmitter function. Lead, a common heavy metal in the environment, particularly impairs formation of neurocircuitry by disrupting dopamine, glutamate, and acetylcholine. Mercury, found in fish, impairs glial formation and creates a state of higher vulnerability in which the brain is more susceptible to damage from other toxins. Organophosphates kill neurons, impair cell migration, and reduce synaptic number. In addition to disruption of brain formation and maturation, infants exposed to maternal drug use during pregnancy often exhibit neonatal abstinence syndrome (NAS), or withdrawal symptoms. These infants are often born prematurely with intrauterine growth restriction.

Alcohol interferes with many systems in addition to the brain, including the cardiovascular, gastrointestinal, and musculoskeletal systems. Severe cases of alcohol exposure can lead to fetal alcohol syndrome (FAS); however, most infants exposed to alcohol *in utero* do not manifest the typical dysmorphic features of FAS and may go unrecognized as having been exposed to alcohol. Withdrawal symptoms include irritability and seizures. *In utero* alcohol exposure kills neurons and stalls their migration, which leads to behavior problems. Tobacco use during pregnancy is associated with preterm birth and intrauterine growth restriction (IUGR), and postnatal withdrawal can occur with tremors and irritability in the infant. Nicotine impairs acetylcholine function, leading to cognitive impairments. Cocaine and amphetamines have been shown to interfere with monoamine function and change the maturation of cells that regulate focus and emotion.

NAS is most commonly seen with opiate exposure; however, women who use opiates during pregnancy are often using other drugs as well. Based on the metabolism and half-life of the drugs used, the time frame of presentation of withdrawal symptoms varies and can occur within 1 day to 3 weeks. Benzodiazepine and barbiturate withdrawal symptoms are similar to opiate withdrawal symptoms, but due to the longer half-life of these medications withdrawal symptoms may present as late as 2 weeks of age. Signs of withdrawal include rigidity, tremors, irritability, sneezing, yawning, and feeding problems, and these manifestations can be scored using a neonatal abstinence scoring system. Administering medications such as morphine, methadone, phenobarbital, lorazepam, or clonidine for treatment of NAS has been shown to lessen the incidence of withdrawal-related seizures, irritability, feeding problems, and tremors. These medications are administered using a stepwise weaning schedule, and, in combination with a low-stimulation environment, most neonates can be safely weaned off these medications within several weeks. However, once neonates have completed a weaning program, they often still manifest neurological abnormalities such as exaggerated startle reflex, restlessness, tremors, and developmental delays, with poor executive functioning in the school-age years.

Further reading

Bada HS, Das A, Bauer CR, *et al.* Low birth weight and preterm births: Etiologic fraction attributable to prenatal drug exposure. *J Perinatol* 2005;25(10):631–637.

Ellenberg JH, Nelson KB. Cluster of perinatal events identifying infants at high risk for death or disability. *J Pediatr* 1988;113(3):546–552.

Hudak ML, Tan RC. Neonatal drug withdrawal. *Pediatrics* 2012;129(2):e540–e560.

Shankaran S, Laptook AR, Ehrenkranz RA, *et al.* Whole-body hypothermia for neonates with hypoxic-ischemic encephalopathy. *N Engl J Med* 2005;353:1574–1584.

Sheth RD, Hobbs GR, Mullett M. Neonatal seizures: Incidence, onset, and etiology by gestational age. *J Perinatol* 1999;19(1):40–43.

162 Neurodevelopmental disorders

Adam L. Numis and Raman Sankar

Mattel Children's Hospital UCLA, David Geffen School of Medicine at UCLA, Los Angeles, CA, USA

Brain development is an intricate process beginning in the third week of gestation. Defects in neural development and maturation arise from varied genetic, infectious, immunological, and traumatic etiologies. This chapter provides a framework for the evaluation and management of neurodevelopmental disorders, and details several conditions with a genetic basis for which clinical criteria alone can be used for diagnosis.

Developmental delay and intellectual disability

Global developmental delay (GDD) refers to failure to meet expected milestones in two or more domains of development, including gross/fine motor, speech/language, cognition, social/personal, and activities of daily living in children under 6 years of age. Intellectual disability (ID) is characterized by deficits in intellectual and adaptive functioning that continue to be observed after 5 years of age and are diagnosed before 18 years of age, typically corresponding to an intelligence quotient from 65–75. While many children with GDD will meet criteria for ID, the two diagnoses are distinct, with clinical severity more reliably assessed in ID. GDD and ID are estimated to affect 1–3% of the population. Advances in laboratory, genetic, and radiological testing have expanded the ability to determine etiologies in GDD/ID. Specific diagnoses now allow for improvements in prognosis and, in certain scenarios, allow for tailored treatment regimens.

Clinical evaluation

Developmental surveillance in early childhood identifies those children who may benefit from further neurological and genetic evaluation for GDD/ID. Primary screening can include a focused history or use of screening tools such as the Denver Developmental Screening Test. Secondary neurodevelopmental evaluation by a neurologist or developmental pediatrician should include a detailed history focusing on behavioral, developmental, and educational milestones, prenatal and perinatal events, and a three-generation family pedigree. Physical examination should include a comprehensive multisystem evaluation, including measurement of growth parameters, evaluation of dysmorphic features, and attention to ophthalmological, dermatological, and neurological findings. Individuals often benefit from detailed neuropsychological testing to ascertain areas of relative strength and weakness. On detailed evaluation, approximately 85% of individuals with ID are diagnosed as mild, 10% as moderate, and 5% as severe.

Diagnostic approach

Children meeting criteria for GDD or ID may have historical and examination findings consistent with a particular diagnosis. For example, Trisomy 21 may be suspected based on clinical criteria alone. Children without distinctive syndrome features require further workup to evaluate for an underlying etiology. A study 15 years ago demonstrated a yield of only 4% for comprehensive diagnostic workup in children with developmental language disorder, while the yield was as high as 59% in children with isolated motor delay. The passage of time has dramatically improved the diagnostic yield in many non-focal cases of GDD/ID/ASD (autism spectrum disorder) due to advances in the availability of comparative genomic hybridization (CGH) array. Nevertheless, neuroimaging remains an important tool in the evaluation of GDD/ID, as brain computed tomography (CT) may contribute to the etiological diagnosis in 39% of cases and magnetic resonance imaging (MRI) in up to 66% of cases. Metabolic testing for inborn errors of metabolism may be warranted in children with particular clinical features, although yield is considered to be low in individuals who had previously undergone extensive newborn screening, likely less than 1%. Testing for inborn errors of metabolism may be enriched in populations with genetic homogeneity. Thus, metabolic testing, as well as additional biochemical testing (i.e., lead and thyroid function testing), should be considered on an individual basis.

First-line genetic evaluation in GDD/ID includes testing for Fragile X with assessment of CGG trinucleotide repeat number in the *FMR1* gene. This provides an etiological diagnosis in at least 2% of males and females with mild or moderate GDD/ID; sequencing of specific X-linked ID genes, including *ARX*, *JARID1C*, and *SLC6A8*, can increase the yield and provide diagnosis for an additional 8–10% of cases. Additional first-line genetic testing may also include genome-wide testing, referring collectively to karyotype analysis, sub-telomeric fluorescence *in situ* hydrization (FISH) testing, CGH array, gene sequencing panels, and whole-exome sequencing (WES). There is broad agreement now that the CGH array should replace traditional karyotyping, as it offers dramatically improved sensitivity as well as cost reduction. CGH and oligonucleotide arrays detect specific copy number changes with varying genome resolution, often ranging from 30000 base pairs to 1 million base pairs. Microarray studies provide an etiological diagnosis in approximately 8% of individuals with GDD/ID. The utility of WES may further increase the ability to determine an underlying diagnosis, although its availability remains limited by cost. An investigation of 250 individuals with a neurological diagnosis and negative

International Neurology, Second edition. Edited by Robert P. Lisak, Daniel D. Truong, William M. Carroll and Roongroj Bhidayasiri
© 2016 John Wiley & Sons, Ltd. Published 2016 by John Wiley & Sons, Ltd.

microarray testing demonstrated that WES provided a specific diagnosis in up to 33% of individuals. Further studies examining the yield of WES in GDD/ID are thus warranted.

Management

Medical management of individuals with GDD/ID is often symptomatic, with interventions focused on associated conditions such as visual and hearing impairment, epilepsy, behavioral disorders, constipation, and psychiatric comorbidities. ASD is a common comorbidity, with up to 28% of non-syndromic children with ID carrying dual diagnoses. Although few etiologies of GDD/ID have disease-modifying therapies, a specific diagnosis may lead to a tailored medication and behavioral therapy regimen with potential for clinical trial enrollment. The management of individuals with GDD/ID will also include psychological, physical, and educational support. These treatments focus on strengthening functional domains and optimizing transitions to adolescence and adulthood. Achievement of goals often requires a multidisciplinary team, including physical, occupational, behavioral, and speech/language therapists.

Selected genetic neurodevelopmental disorders

Tuberous sclerosis complex

Tuberous sclerosis complex (TSC) is a multisystem autosomal dominant disorder arising from mutations in either the *TSC1* or the *TSC2* gene. TSC has an incidence of 1 in 5800 live births, with 80% of cases arising from *de novo* mutations. The TSC1 (hamartin) and TSC2 (tuberin) gene products form a protein complex that regulates the mammalian target of rapamycin (mTOR) pathway. Dysfunction in either protein results in a lack of pathway suppression, with subsequent dysregulated cell growth and metabolism, ultimately leading to tumor formation.

Neurological features

The clinical manifestations of TSC are varied between individuals, even among familial cases. Symptoms are related to development of benign tumors in the brain, eyes, heart, kidney, lung, liver, and skin. Neurological involvement is felt to be secondary to the development of cortical tubers, white-matter changes, and formation of subependymal giant cell astrocytomas (SEGA). ID is diagnosed in approximately 50% of individuals with TSC, with 30% meeting the criteria for severe ID. Additionally, ASD is diagnosed in approximately 40% of individuals. Together, the constellation of ID, ASD, aggression, psychiatric disorders, and neuropsychological deficits is termed TSC-associated neuropsychiatric disorders (TAND). Further, epilepsy is diagnosed in up to 90% of individuals and often begins within the first year of life. Infantile spasms are the most common seizure type at diagnosis, occurring in 36–69% of individuals.

Diagnostic approach

TSC can be diagnosed based on clinical criteria (Table 162.1). Definitive diagnosis requires at least two major features *or* one major feature with two or more minor features. Possible diagnosis requires either one major feature *or* two or more minor features. Alternatively, definitive diagnosis can be based on identification of a pathogenic mutation in non-lesional tissue (i.e., serum) in the *TSC1* or *TSC2* gene.

Table 162.1 Clinical criteria for diagnosis of tuberous sclerosis complex.

Major features	Minor features
Hypomelanotic macules (≥3, at least 5 mm in diameter)	Dental enamel pits (≥4)
Angiofibromas (≥3) or fibrous cephalic plaque	Intraoral fibromas (≥2)
Ungual fibromas (≥2)	Retinal achromatic patch
Shagreen patch	Multiple renal cysts
Multiple retinal hamartomas	Non-renal hamartomas
Cortical dysplasias (cortical tubers and/or cerebral white-matter radial migration lines)	"Confetti" skin lesions (1–2 mm hypomelanotic macules)
Subependymal nodules	
Subependymal giant cell astrocytoma	
Cardiac rhabdomyoma	
Lymphangioleiomyomatosis	
Angiomyolipomas (≥2)	

Management

Individuals with TSC require treatment by a multidisciplinary specialty team. Surveillance guidelines are published through the 2012 International TSC Consensus Conference. From a neurological perspective, MRI is recommended at clinical diagnosis to assess for the presence of cortical dysplasias, subependymal nodules, and SEGAs. Follow-up MRI is planned every 1–3 years in asymptomatic individuals less than 25 years of age to evaluate for the emergence and/or growth of SEGAs. Routine electroencephalography (EEG) is recommended at diagnosis; if abnormal, a 24-hour EEG is suggested to evaluate for the presence of subclinical seizures. Given the prevalence of infantile spasms in this population, parental education on seizure semiology is likewise recommended.

Medical management in TSC remains symptomatic. Infantile spasms in TSC are treated with vigabatrin as the first-line medication given its demonstrated efficacy; steroid treatment, including prednisolone and adrenocorticotropin hormone (ACTH), should be reserved as a second-line therapy. There are no specific guidelines on the management of other seizure types in TSC, as no specific anticonvulsant therapy has been demonstrated to be superior. Epilepsy surgery and vagus nerve stimulators should be considered early on for individuals with medically refractory epilepsy, as seizure control in infancy and early childhood may improve neurodevelopmental outcome in this population. The management of SEGAs includes surgical resection, mTOR inhibitor therapy with everolimus, and when indicated cerebrospinal fluid shunt. The decision between medical versus surgical management should be made case by case based on tumor size, burden, and extraneurological manifestations.

The management of TAND may include treatment, with psychiatrists, social workers, and education support services. Clinical trials evaluating medical management of TAND with mTOR inhibition is currently underway. Likewise, treatment of medically refractory epilepsy with everolimus is being investigated. Further research is required to assess the impact of early mTOR inhibition on the natural history of TSC.

Neurofibromatosis type 1

Neurofibromatosis type 1 (NF1) is a neurocutaneous disorder with an incidence of 1 in 2500 to 1 in 3000 live births. NF1 is inherited in an autosomal dominant manner, with 50% of cases arising from *de novo* mutations in the *NF1* gene. *NF1* encodes the tumor suppressor gene neurofibromin, a GTPase-activating protein that converts the Ras proto-oncogene, involved in cellular signal transduction, to its inactive form. As Ras is upstream of several cell signaling cascades, including the mTOR and AKT (protein kinase B) pathways, dysfunction in neurofibromin can lead to subsequent cell proliferation and tumor formation.

Neurological features

NF1 affects multiple organ systems, with manifestations arising in the skin, bones, cardiovascular and gastrointestinal systems, eyes, peripheral nerves, and brain. Neurologically, ID is diagnosed in up to 4–8% of individuals, although moderate to severe cognitive impairments in one or more domains occur in up to 60% of individuals. Psychiatric comorbidities include anxiety, depression, attention deficit hyperactivity disorder, and ASD. Neurofibromas, or benign peripheral nerve sheath tumors, are found in over 99% of individuals with NF1. These lesions usually develop in adolescence and can be cutaneous, subcutaneous, or plexiform in character. The latter result in significant morbidity due to their growth along the length of a nerve or nerve branches, with concomitant pain, hemorrhage, or transformation to malignant peripheral nerve sheath tumors (MPNST). Other neurological manifestations in NF1 include optic pathway gliomas, often low-grade astrocytomas, which occur in 15% of individuals. Epilepsy is diagnosed in 4–13% of individuals with NF1, with onset from infancy through adulthood. Cerebrovascular disease, including arteriopathy and aneurysm formation, occurs in 3–6% of patients.

Diagnostic approach

NF1 can be diagnosed based on clinical criteria (Table 162.2). Definitive diagnosis requires the presence of at least two criteria. Genetic testing is available, and can be utilized to screen for family members of affected individuals or to confirm diagnosis in potential cases.

Table 162.2 Clinical criteria for diagnosis of neurofibromatosis type 1 (NF1) and classic/typical Rett syndrome (RTT).

NF1	RTT
Café-au-lait macules (≥6, at least 5 mm in diameter prepubertal and ≥15 mm postpubertal)	A period of regression followed by recovery or stabilization
Neurofibromas (≥2) or one plexiform neurofibroma	Partial or complete loss of acquired purposeful hand skills
Axillary or inguinal freckling	Partial or complete loss of acquired spoken language
Optic glioma	Gait abnormalities (dyspraxia or absence of gait)
Lisch nodules (Iris hamartomas, ≥2)	Stereotypic hand movements
First-degree relative with NF1	*Without:*
Distinctive bony lesion (i.e., sphenoid dysplasia or long bone cortical thickening)	– Abnormal psychomotor development in the first year of life *or* – Brain injury secondary to other cause

Management

The treatment of NF1 remains symptomatic. Cutaneous neurofibromas often require no treatment unless cosmetically disfiguring. However, plexiform neurofibromas may require surgical debulking due to persistent pain. Evaluation for the transformation of subcutaneous and plexiform neurofibromas to MPNST with MRI is indicated in patients with a rapid increase in tumor size, change in texture, persistent or nocturnal pain, or a new or unexplained neurological deficit. Treatment of MPNST requires surgical resection and adjunct radiotherapy. Given the relationship of the neurofibromin protein product within the mTOR pathway, clinical trials are underway to evaluate the efficacy of mTOR inhibition in the management of plexiform neurofibromas and MPNST.

Neuroimaging for evaluation of optic pathway glioma is recommended in patients with ophthalmological findings or complaints, including decreased visual acuity, visual field deficits, afferent pupillary defect, and optic disk swelling. Screening MRI is indicated in children for whom visual assessment cannot be performed. The presence of optic pathway glioma warrants close follow-up, although treatment is often not required. Therapy includes chemotherapy and/or surgery with debulking. As individuals with NF1 are at risk for additional gliomas along the neuraxis, symptoms and examination guide further neuroimaging. MRI may also reveal nonenhancing T2 hyperintensities throughout the cerebrum, which do not need further follow-up and may represent areas of dysplastic glial proliferation.

The treatment of seizures in NF1 is guided by seizure semiology, with no specific anticonvulsant therapy demonstrating superiority. Cognitive deficits and ID have been effectively treated with lovastatin in mouse models of NF1, although clinical trials are ongoing.

Rett syndrome

Rett syndrome (RTT) is a progressive X-linked neurodevelopmental disorder primarily affecting females, with an incidence of 1 in 10000 to 1 in 22000. RTT is classified into typical and atypical forms. Typical RTT is nearly exclusively caused by *de novo* mutations in the methyl-CpG binding protein 2 (*MECP2*) gene. Among the atypical forms, the early-seizure variant is frequently associated with mutations in the cyclin-dependent kinase-like 5 (*CDKL5*) gene, and the congenital variant is frequently associated with mutations in the foxhead box G1 (*FOXG1*) gene. The mechanism by which RTT-associated gene mutations result in neurological dysfunction is not well characterized and research in animal models is ongoing.

Neurological features

Typical RTT is characterized by normal development through the first 6 months of life. However, head growth often decelerates shortly after birth, before symptom onset. The stagnation of gross motor development, loss of fine motor and language abilities, and concomitant emergence of stereotypic hand movements takes place between 12 and 18 months. Thereafter, there is frequently a recovery of non-verbal communication with insidious regression of gross motor milestones. ID is present in all patients by this plateau phase. Gait apraxia and ataxia become prominent, with subsequent quadriparesis. Additional motor manifestations commonly include bruxism, drooling, and dystonia. Neuropsychiatric manifestations include self-injurious behaviors, uncontrolled screaming, and sleep disturbances, with many patients having prolonged periods of wakefulness or sleep. Epilepsy is diagnosed in approximately 60% of individuals, with seizure onset after 2 years of age in typical RTT. Epilepsy severity and seizure semiology are quite varied, although there is often an overall improvement in seizure burden over time. As individuals with RTT grow, the autonomic nervous system may demonstrate progressive dysfunction, with additional organ involvement in the cardiac, gastrointestinal, respiratory, and skeletal systems.

Atypical RTT variants share many, but not all features of typical RTT. The congenital variant is characterized by abnormal development from birth, earlier onset of neurological regression, and particular tongue stereotypies. The early-seizure variant is characterized by epilepsy onset before 5 months of life, prior to the developmental regression, and with more stereotyped seizure semiology including hypermotor, tonic, and infantile spasms; this variant shares fewer of the features associated with typical RTT.

Diagnostic approach

Typical RTT can be diagnosed based on clinical criteria (Table 162.2). Genetic testing confirms mutation in the *MECP2* gene in 95–97% of individuals who meet the clinical diagnostic criteria. Atypical RTT requires at least 2 of the 4 main criteria of typical RTT, with the addition of 5 out of 11 supportive criteria outlined by the 2010 RettSearch Consortium. Atypical variants of RTT may be associated with changes in the *CDKL5* and *FOXG1* genes; debate continues as to whether these RTT-like phenotypes represent a spectrum of RTT or disparate disease entities.

Management

Medical management is symptomatic in RTT, without known disease-modifying therapies. No specific anticonvulsant therapy has demonstrated superiority in the management of epilepsy in RTT. Lamotrigine, levetiracetam, carbamazepine, and valproic acid demonstrate modest success in case series, with smaller studies demonstrating the utility of the ketogenic diet and vagal nerve stimulator. Given nutritional deficiencies, decreased bone mineral density, and propensity for fractures, enzyme-inducing therapies should be minimized or avoided. The behavioral manifestations of RTT, including sleep disturbances, may require additional medical management, with several therapies showing modest efficacy. Several novel agents are being investigated in clinical trials in the treatment of RT in attempts to slow or halt regression.

Conclusion

Neurodevelopmental disorders arise from varied etiologies, although they often share similar features of impaired cognition and altered behavior. Differences in historical features and exam findings, as well as additional diagnostic testing, may lead to specific diagnoses allowing for improved prognosis, tailored treatment regimens, and perhaps evaluation of disease-modifying therapies.

One of the most exciting promises for the future will be the emergence of targeted molecular therapies that may supplement the neurocognitive and behavioral therapies on which we presently rely in the treatment of neurodevelopmental disorders. Extensive research using *Drosophila* and mouse models of these disorders has brought us increasing understanding of the molecular cascades and has even identified convergence among some (i.e., the interplay between Ras and mTOR pathways). Thus, there is promise that rapamycin analogues may improve learning in TSC, HMG-CoA reductase inhibitors (statins) may lower the RAS signaling in NF1, metabotropic glutamate receptor antagonists may have a potential therapeutic role in Fragile X, and the use of R-baclofen may improve behavior in certain forms of ASD. These examples of active translational approaches will herald a new era in the management of children diagnosed with GDD/ID/ASD.

Further reading

Ebrahimi-Fakhari D, Sahin M. Autism and the synapse: Emerging mechanisms and mechanism-based therapies. *Curr Opin Neurol* 2015;28:91–102.

Ferner R, Gutmann D. Neurofibromatosis type 1 (NF1): Diagnosis and management. *Handb Clin Neurol* 2013;115:939–955.

Ferner R, Huson S, Thomas N, et al. Guidelines for the diagnosis and management of individuals with neurofibromatosis 1. *J Med Genet* 2007;44:81–88.

Flore L, Milunsky J. Updates in the genetic evaluation of the child with global developmental delay or intellectual disability. *Semin Pediatr Neurol* 2012;19:173–180.

Krueger D, Northrup H, Roberds S, et al. Tuberous sclerosis complex surveillance and management: Recommendations of the 2012 International Tuberous Sclerosis Complex Consensus Conference. *Pediatr Neurol* 2013;49:255–265.

Michelson D, Shevell M, Sherr E, et al. Evidence report: Genetic and metabolic testing on children with global developmental delay. *Neurology* 2011;77:1629–1635.

Neul J, Kaufmann W, Glaze D, et al. Rett syndrome: Revised diagnostic criteria and nomenclature. *Ann Neurol* 2010;68:944–950.

Northrup H, Krueger D, Roberds S, et al. Tuberous sclerosis complex diagnostic criteria update: Recommendations of the 2012 International Tuberous Sclerosis Complex Consensus Conference. *Pediatr Neurol* 2013;39:243–254.

Shevell M, Ashwal S, Donley D, et al. Practice parameter: Evaluation of the child with developmental delay. *Neurology* 2003;60:367–380.

Yang Y, Muzny D, Reid J, et al. Clinical whole-exome sequencing for the diagnosis of Mendelian disorders. *N Engl J Med* 2013;369:1502–1511.

163 Floppy infant syndrome

Jong-Hee Chae[1] and Anna Cho[2]

[1] Department of Pediatrics, Seoul National University College of Medicine, Division of Pediatric Neurology, Seoul National University Children's Hospital, Seoul Korea

[2] Department of Pediatrics, Ewha Womans University School of Medicine, Seoul, Korea

Floppy infant syndrome is a disease in which infants present with generalized hypotonia at birth or early infancy. There are many possible etiologies, from many conditions involving the central nervous system to various kinds of neuromuscular disorders, which makes a specific diagnosis difficult. The expanding knowledge of genetic disorders has made non-invasive genetic testing available for specific diagnoses. In addition, the use of newly developed genetic technology such as next-generation sequencing and array chips as a diagnostic tool is increasing in clinical practice. However, a systemic approach to clinical diagnosis remains essential for the initial assessment of patients and in the interpretation of technical sequencing results. This chapter reviews the many possible etiologies of floppy infant syndrome, and proposes a systematic approach for the evaluation of this disorder.

Clinical features and evaluation

Floppy infants usually demonstrate a characteristic "frog-leg posture," excessive joint mobility, and profound weakness. These babies may also have limp and drooping limbs when they are held by the trunk, and a prominent head lag when traction is delivered. Muscle stretch reflexes are diminished or absent in floppy infants with neuromuscular disorders, whereas in those with central causes, these reflexes are usually present or even exaggerated.

Floppiness can have a variety of causes, which can affect the brain and any part of the motor units. It can be clinically useful to classify the syndromes into central and peripheral disorders (Table 163.1). Clinical features suggestive of central hypotonia include a history of hypoxic ischemic encephalopathy, impaired cognition in addition to motor delay, normal or brisk tendon reflex, dysmorphism implying a specific syndrome, and seizures. For appropriate and cost-effective investigations, it is essential to document the prenatal and perinatal history of infants in detail and to carry out careful physical and neurological examinations. Any history of gestational drug or teratogen exposure, breech presentation, reduced fetal movements, presence of polyhydramnios, or maternal diseases such as diabetes, myotonic dystrophies, myasthenia gravis, or epilepsies should be assessed. In addition, any family history of neuromuscular diseases and details of perinatal birth events such as birth trauma, birth asphyxia, or low APGAR scores should be included.

The presence of associated malformation of other organs and facial dysmorphic features, as in Down syndrome or Prader–Willi syndrome, can provide important clues for diagnosis. More than two-thirds of floppy infants have central nervous system (CNS) disorders as the primary cause. Seizures, impairment of consciousness, apnea, and delayed intellectual and language milestones suggest CNS disorders. Among those patients with central hypotonia, axial weakness is characteristic and prominent in early life. Hyperreflexia is noted over time. Usually, these findings can allow clinicians to make a diagnosis readily, without unnecessary electrophysiological studies or the need for muscle biopsies.

The presence of profound weakness with diminished or absent deep tendon reflexes suggests peripheral causes of this syndrome. Such children often show low-pitched weak crying, poor sucking power, and decreased spontaneous movements. A high-arched palate and typical myopathic face are often noted in infants with neuromuscular diseases. In addition, they are usually quite alert with bright eyes, unlike infants with central disorders. However, sometimes it is hard to make a clear distinction, because infants with lower motor neuron disorders may have suffered from perinatal asphyxia caused by abnormal uterine presentation or severe respiratory muscle weakness immediately after birth. Moreover, some disorders such as metachromatic leukodystrophy and Pelizaeus–Merzbacher disease have pathologies that affect both the central and peripheral nervous systems.

Laboratory investigations

The next step in the differential diagnosis is a cost-effective use of laboratory investigations. For infants with causes suggestive of central disorders, cytogenetic study (chromosome analysis or array comparative genomic hybridization/chromosomal microarray) and a neuroimaging study (ultrasonography, computed tomography [CT], or magnetic resonance imaging [MRI]) are recommended. Screening for inborn errors of metabolism should also be included for infants with multisystem involvements and hypotonia. The laboratory tests for metabolic disorders include ammonia levels, which can be elevated in urea cycle defects, organic acidemias, or fatty acid oxidation disorders. High lactate levels in blood and, more specifically, in CSF imply mitochondrial disorders or carbohydrate metabolism disorders. Quantitative analysis of amino acids in urine and blood, urine organic acid, tandem mass spectrometry for acylcarnitine profiles, very long chain fatty acid levels, and serum uric acid levels are investigated for detecting abnormal metabolites or biochemical markers for various metabolic disorders. Newborn screening programs for early detection of many treatable metabolic

International Neurology, Second edition. Edited by Robert P. Lisak, Daniel D. Truong, William M. Carroll and Roongroj Bhidayasiri
© 2016 John Wiley & Sons, Ltd. Published 2016 by John Wiley & Sons, Ltd.

Table 163.1 Possible causes of floppy infant syndrome.

Group	Diseases	Related genes
Central disorders		
Chromosomal abnormalities	Down syndrome	47, XY/XX, +21
	Turner syndrome	45, X
	Prader–Willi syndrome (PWS)	15q11–13
	Angelman's syndrome	15q11–13
Inborn errors of metabolism	Aminoacidopathy	
	Hyperammonemia	
	Hypoglycemia	
	Gangliosidosis	GM1, GM2
	Niemann–Pick disease	SMPD1
	Lowe's syndrome	OCRL1
Acute cerebral insult	Cerebrovascular accident (e.g., hemorrhage, thrombosis, embolism)	
	Hypoxic-ischemic encephalopathy	
	Cerebral infection	
Congenital malformation of brain development	Lissencephaly	17p13.3
Toxicity	Hyperbilirubinemia	
	Hypermagnesemia	
	Sedative drugs (e.g., phenobarbital)	
Spinal cord disorders	Syringomyelia	
	Spinal hypoxia	
Peripheral disorders		
Motor neuron	Spinal muscular atrophy (SMA)	SMN
	Poliomyelitis	
Peripheral nerve	Charcot–Marie–Tooth disease	PMP22
	Dejerine–Sottas disease	MPZ, PMP22, EGR2
	Familial dysautonomia	IKBKAP
Neuromuscular junction	Congenital myasthenic syndrome	DOK7, AGRN, RAPSN, CHAT
	Neonatal myasthenia gravis	
	Infantile botulism	
Muscle	Congenital myopathies (e.g., myotubular myopathy or nemaline myopathy)	ACTA1, NEB, RYR1, MTM1
	Congenital muscular dystrophies	LMNA, COL6A, FKTN
	Congenital myotonic dystrophies	DM1
	Glycogen storage disease (e.g., Pompe disease)	GAA
	Hypothyroidism	
	Polymyositis	

disorders are designed and performed around the world, and increasing number of disorders such as lysosome disorders are being added to the list of disorders for evaluation.

Classic laboratory tests including the evaluation of muscle enzymes, electromyography (EMG), nerve conduction studies (NCS), and muscle biopsies with enzyme histochemistry, immunohistochemistry, and electron microscopy are usually helpful for the diagnosis of peripheral neuromuscular disorders. In general, EMG is useful to differentiate between denervation and myopathy. However, in early infancy (within a few weeks of birth) or in infants with mild weakness, EMG and muscle pathology are sometimes not concordant. Thus, even if the electrophysiological studies and

muscle enzymes prove normal, muscle biopsies should be considered, especially in the diagnosis of suspected congenital myopathies and muscular dystrophies, because morphological diagnosis by muscle pathology plays a crucial role in the diagnosis and classification of these diseases.

Approach for genetic diagnosis

In floppy infant syndrome, genetic diagnosis is challenging in clinical practice, because one gene can cause a wide variety of clinical and/or pathological features and similar clinical features can be caused by mutations in different genes. Accurate genetic diagnosis is essential for appropriate management, carrier detection, prenatal diagnosis, and genetic counseling.

As mentioned earlier, the diagnostic approach to the investigation of floppy infant syndrome has significantly changed, thanks to the advancement of DNA-based diagnostic tests. The GeneTests website (https://www.genetests.org/) provides updated information about available genetic tests in various inherited disorders. An updated list of monogenic muscle diseases due to a primary defect residing in the nuclear genome is available in the GeneTable of Neuromuscular Disorders (http://www.musclegenetable.fr/).

Since next-generation sequencing (NGS) was introduced, it has been acknowledged that the increasing use of targeted sub-exomic sequencing as a diagnostic tool is likely to reduce the need for classic conventional diagnostic tests such as muscle biopsy as a first-line investigation. However, a careful phenotype analysis including pathological and clinical evaluation remains essential in the interpretation of sequencing results.

Special considerations for cost-effective genetic analysis

The neuromuscular causes in floppy infant syndrome include congenital myopathies, congenital muscular dystrophies, congenital myotonic dystrophy, spinal muscular atrophy, and congenital myasthenic syndromes. Considerations of the clinical and epidemiological characteristics of each disease group are necessary for cost-effective genetic testing.

The congenital myopathies are still classified into classic myopathies such as nemaline myopathy, central core disease, centronuclear or myotubular myopathy, and other myopathies such as congenital fiber type disproportion, multicore disease, and cytoplasmic body myopathy. Among them, severe neonatal hypotonia without any antigravity movements implies nemaline myopathy (*ACTA1* or *NEB* related), X-linked myotubular myopathy (*MTM1* related), or severe forms of core myopathies (*RYR1* related).

Congenital muscular dystrophies (CMD) are a group of clinically and genetically heterogeneous disorders, which usually present with severe weakness at birth as well as early joint contractures with mildly increased creatine kinase level and dystrophic features in muscle pathology. They are typically classified into two categories; classic CMD (CMD without mental retardation or nonsyndromic CMD) and CMD with mental retardation (syndromic CMD). Classic CMDs are divided into two groups depending on the presence of merosin (Laminin α2): a merosin-deficient form and a merosin-positive form. The most striking feature of merosin-deficient CMD, caused by mutations in *LAMA2*, is leukodystrophy with normal cognition. In the merosin-positive groups, Ullrich CMD, caused by mutations in the *COL6A1*, *COL6A2*, and *COL6A3* genes, shows a wide spectrum of severity in muscle weakness and associated features of rigid spine or severe distal joint laxity. With the growing numbers of clinical reports, lamin A/C-related CMD (*LMNA*) should be also included as a differential diagnosis for merosin-positive CMD. It is clinically characterized by a "drop head" phenotype with prominent neck flexor involvement. The other form, syndromic CMD, which includes Fukuyama type, Walker–Warburg syndrome, and muscle–eye brain diseases, has variable involvement of eye abnormalities and brain structural anomalies with mental retardation. The relative frequency of individual types of CMD varies in different populations. The merosin-deficient form of CMD is prominent in Western countries but rare in the Asian population.

In Japan, the most commonly diagnosed CMD subtype is Fukuyama CMD caused by a founder mutation in the *fukutin* gene, while *fukutin* mutations are very rare in other populations. In many countries where both merosin-deficient CMD and Fukuyama CMD are rare, Ullrich CMD has been reported to be the most common type. In CMDs, immunohistochemical examinations with muscle biopsies are particularly important for the classification, and brain MRI is useful to support clinical and pathological subtyping and further genetic research.

In several neuromuscular disorders such as spinal muscular atrophy and congenital myotonic dystrophy, rapid genetic tests are available (*SMN* and *DM1*, respectively). Spinal muscular atrophy (SMA) is an autosomal recessive disorder involving the anterior horn cells, almost 95% of which are attributed to mutations of the *SMN1* gene, located on chromosome 5q13. The presence of tongue fasciculation with striking proximal weakness suggests spinal muscular atrophy. If the child shows tented lips with facial weakness, severe respiratory muscle weakness with diaphragmatic eventuation, and foot deformities such as talipes, this strongly suggests congenital myotonic dystrophy. Therefore, an examination of the mother's face, particularly for evidence of eyelid closure weakness and grip myotonia, is important. These clinical situations will often confirm the clinical suspicion of a genetic disorder, and confirmation using DNA analysis and genotyping can then proceed without invasive diagnostic investigations such as muscle biopsies.

Although a neuromuscular junction disorder is not a common cause of floppy infant syndrome, it must be ruled out as a cause in the clinical setting. In mothers with myasthenia gravis, acetylcholine (ACh) receptor antibodies cross the placenta to the baby. This blockade of neuromuscular transmission (transient myasthenic syndrome) results in floppiness, which typically resolves in about 6 weeks. Congenital myasthenic syndromes (CMS) are genetic defects of neuromuscular transmission, including ion channels, acetylcholine receptors, or the recycling mechanism for ACh. These syndromes often present with easy fatigability of ocular, bulbar, and limb muscles and with a family history in those developing symptoms in later infancy. The variable causative genes for CMS identified to date are *CHAT, COLQ, LAMB2, AGRN, CHRNA1, CHRNB1, CHRND, CHRNE, CHRNG, RAPSN, SCN4A, MuSK, DOK7, PLEC1, GFPT1, DPAGT1, ALG2,* and *ALG14*. CMS are rare but underdiagnosed. Because of the early onset and prominent muscle involvement, scoliosis, possible contractures, and myopathic EMG pattern, patients are frequently misdiagnosed as having congenital myopathies, especially those with *DOK7* mutations. Different CMS subtypes may vary in onset and clinical course as well as in comorbidity and life expectancy based on the causative genes. However, accurate diagnosis is extremely important to start an early appropriate therapy to prevent life-threatening events and to improve the clinical course.

Therapeutic approach

The treatment strategy for floppy infant syndrome is mostly symptomatic and supportive, depending on the underlying disorders. Treatment includes physical therapy based on patient age, extent of hypotonia, and overall health. A significant number of infants require respiratory support. Timely assessment of needs for invasive or non-invasive ventilation and effective care by pulmonary specialists are important for these children. In many infants, sucking power is weak and adequate nutritional supports such as special nipples or nasogastric tubes are needed.

Specific treatments are available for a few conditions, including hypothyroidism (thyroxine), Pompe disease (myozyme), and congenital myasthenic syndromes (cholinesterase inhibitors or beta 2-adrenergic receptor agonists). As effective treatments can change the natural course of the syndrome in affected patients, early diagnosis and treatment are more critical in these diseases. Various clinical trials of antisense oligonucleotide therapies are still ongoing for the treatment of spinal muscular atrophy.

Conclusion

Floppy infant syndrome has highly variable etiologies, including both central and peripheral nervous system disorders. The evaluation of a hypotonic infant has to be comprehensive and requires a multidisciplinary approach. Although there are still some limitations and challenges using next-generation sequencing in clinical practice, it will be strongly anticipated to improve diagnosis, genetic counseling, and patient management.

Further reading

Bonnemann CG, Wang CH, Quijano-Roy S, et al. Diagnostic approach to the congenital muscular dystrophies. *Neuromuscular Disord* 2014;24(4):289–311.

North KN, Wang CH, Clarke N, et al. Approach to the diagnosis of congenital myopathies. *Neuromuscular Disord* 2014;24(2):97–116.

Prasad AN, Prasad C. Genetic evaluation of the floppy infant. *Semin Fetal Neonatal Med* 2011;16(2):99–108.

Swaiman KF. *Pediatric Neurology: Principles and Practice*, 5th ed. Philadelphia, PA: Elsevier/Saunders; 2012.

Volpe JJ. *Neurology of the Newborn*, 5th ed. Philadelphia, PA: Saunders/Elsevier; 2008.

164 Storage disorders

Jeffrey J. Ekstrand[1], Jason T. Lerner[2], and Raman Sankar[2]
[1] University of Utah School of Medicine, Primary Children's Hospital, Salt Lake City, UT, USA
[2] David Geffen School of Medicine at UCLA, Mattel Children's Hospital at UCLA, Los Angeles, CA, USA

Storage disorders consist of a clinically diverse group of individually relatively rare disorders that collectively constitute a significant medical burden to society. In most cases they result from a genetic mutation that causes an enzymatic defect in the catabolic process of large macromolecules. Historically, each subclassification of the various storage disorders was named based on the type of macromolecule being degraded. For example, the glycogenoses are a group of storage disorders that have a defect in the catabolic pathway of glycogen. However, there are also examples (e.g., the leukodystrophies) where the disease classification name is based on criteria established before there was a complete understanding of the underlying biochemistry. Most of the storage disorders can be characterized as lysosomal diseases, because many of the macromolecules are catabolized in this structure. The molecular defect is not always a primary degradative enzyme. Instead, a wide variety of protein functions, including but not limited to trafficking of macromolecules to specific organelles, transmembrane protein receptor targets, and chaperone molecules, can have an impact on the catabolic process.

Over the last decade, further progress has been made in identifying the impaired protein function and the genetic mutations responsible for these disorders. As such, improved screening and confirmatory genetic testing are now feasible. Unfortunately, for the majority of cases, the therapeutic options are still limited to mostly symptomatic treatment and supportive care. Definitive "cures" with gene therapy, hematopoietic bone marrow and stem cell transplantation, or enzymatic replacement therapy are still in their early and incompletely realized stage. However, despite the formidable challenges remaining with these strategies, particularly in treating neurological complications, there is still much optimism that progress will continue to be made.

The geographic regional differences observed for some of these disorders almost certainly result from the different distribution of ethnic populations with particular genetic endowments. This chapter will be limited to describing such differences when relevant, along with descriptions of the clinical characteristics, current diagnostic tools, and treatments, if available, of the more commonly observed conditions. The text is not meant to be exhaustive, nor is it intended to describe the often very complicated biochemical molecular genetics. For these features, the reader is referred to the Further reading and the Online Mendelian Inheritance in Man (OMIM) website.

Lipidoses

The lipidoses are storage diseases that are characterized by a defect in the metabolism of lipids, including lipoproteins or glycolipids. This defect results in the accumulation in cells of incompletely metabolized lipid intermediate products in a variety of tissues, including the brain, peripheral nervous system, liver, and bone marrow. There are a number of subcategories of lipid storage disorders that are named based on the starting complex macromolecule being metabolized, although each has a lipid component. These are neuronal ceroid lipofuscinosis, gangliosidosis, sphingomyelinosis, cerebrosidosis, and mucolipidosis. Other lipidoses that are not classified under this nomenclature include Fabry disease, abetalipoproteinemia, and Tangier disease. Finally, although Krabbe disease and metachromatic leukodystrophy are lipid storage diseases, they are discussed separately with the other leukodystrophies.

Neuronal ceroid lipofuscinosis

The neuronal ceroid lipofuscinoses (NCLs) are a group of neurodegenerative disorders that are characterized by the accumulation of autofluorescent lipopigment material within neuronal lysosomes. This results in a heterogenous clinical picture, although motor and mental deterioration with visual dysfunction is commonly seen. Historically, the NCLs were separated into four subclassifications based on age of presentation and electron microscopic appearance of the inclusions. More recently at least ten genetically distinct forms have been described. The childhood NCLs are inherited in an autosomal recessive fashion, while the adult disorder can be either recessive or dominant.

The infantile form (Santavuori–Haltia disease or CLN1) usually presents between 6 and 24 months of age with rapid mental deterioration, microcephaly, failure to thrive, and myoclonus. Visual impairment occurs with a brownish pigmentation of the macula, hypopigmentation of the fundi, and optic atrophy. Retinal blindness is evident by 2 years of age, and the electroretinogram (ERG) is unrecordable by 4 years. Ultrastructural examination of neuronal and other tissue demonstrates granular osmiophilic deposits. The defect is in a gene that codes for the lysosomal enzyme, palmityl-protein thioesterase 1 (*PPT1*), mapped to chromosome 1p32. This defect has also been occasionally seen in later-onset disease. Although observed worldwide, this disorder is particularly prevalent in Finland, with an incidence of 1 in 13000 and an estimated carrier rate of 1 in 70 (approximately 1 in 500 in the general population). This disease

International Neurology, Second edition. Edited by Robert P. Lisak, Daniel D. Truong, William M. Carroll and Roongroj Bhidayasiri
© 2016 John Wiley & Sons, Ltd. Published 2016 by John Wiley & Sons, Ltd.

progresses rapidly, with death usually occurring in early childhood. In addition to the classic infantile form, a severe congenital form (CLN10) has been described, which is caused by mutations in the lysosomal aspartic protease cathepsin D gene (*CTSD*). This congenital form presents with microcephaly, seizures, absent neonatal reflexes, and respiratory failure. Infants usually die within days.

The primary late infantile form (also called Jansky–Bielschowsky disease or CLN2) is considerably less common and it usually presents between 2 and 4 years of age with cognitive decline, ataxia, and either myoclonic or generalized seizures. As described later, considerable genetic variation has been found, and no specific genetic defect is uniquely responsible for this phenotypic presentation. Progressive visual decline usually follows. The ERG is abnormal at presentation and becomes undetectable in a short period of time. The visual evoked potential (VEP) shows abnormally large potentials early in the course of the disease and gradually disappears as the disease advances. Typically development is normal for the first 2 years of life, although in retrospect some mild clumsiness can be recalled after the diagnosis becomes apparent. The gene defect is in *TPP1*, which codes for a lysosomal enzyme, tripeptidyl-peptidase 1, mapped to chromosome 11p15.5. Ultrastructure examination shows a characteristic pattern of curved stacks of lamellae called curvilinear bodies. The disease has been observed worldwide, with an incidence of 0.46 per 100000 live births. There is also a variant of this more common late infantile form (Finnish-variant late infantile NCL or CLN5) that is prevalent in Finland, with an incidence of 1 in 21000 (estimated carrier rate of 1 in 115 in Finland). The gene defect encodes a soluble lysosomal protein of unknown function that maps to chromosome 13q21.1-q32. Other variants of this form have been even less well characterized and include CLN8 in Finland, CLN7 in Turkey, and CLN6 in multiple geographic areas (Costa Rica, South America, Portugal, and the United Kingdom). Death usually occurs by the end of the first decade.

The juvenile form (Batten disease, Spielmeyer–Vogt disease, CLN3) usually presents between 5 and 8 years of age with progressive visual loss, seizures, and ataxia. Although it has been described worldwide, the incidence is enriched in Finland, at 1 in 21000. The underlying gene defect is a transmembrane lysosomal protein of unknown function that maps to chromosome 16p12.1. Ultrastructure examination shows a "fingerprint" lamellae pattern distinct from the curvilinear bodies seen in CLN2. There is also a less well-characterized juvenile form (CLN9) for which the genetic/molecular basis is unknown. Death occurs in the late teens or early twenties.

The adult form (also called Kufs disease or CLN4) usually presents before age 30 years and is characterized by a more slowly progressive course. Visual dysfunction is not a frequent feature. The responsible mutation is in the *DNAJC5* gene, which codes for a cysteine string protein. It is the only autosomal dominant CLN. The adult form may also be occasionally inherited recessively due to a mutation in the late infantile CLN6 gene with a later presentation.

When the clinical suspicion for an NCL is present, the definitive diagnosis can be achieved by gene testing where available, an enzymatic assay, or morphological electron microscopy examination of sweat gland tissue showing the distinctive ultrastructure characteristics. The parents of an affected child are obligate heterozygotes (carriers of one mutant allele), and are generally completely asymptomatic. Carrier testing by DNA analysis is possible. In some regions where particular variant forms are more common, genetic mutation screening or sequencing may be available. Treatment is symptomatic and prognosis is poor.

Gangliosidoses

The gangliosidoses are a group of disorders characterized by the impaired breakdown of specific plasma membrane lipid macromolecules, primarily found in the gray matter of neuronal tissue ganglion cells. These macromolecules are composed of sphingosine, fatty acids, hexose, hexosamine, and neuraminic acid (see Figure 164.1 for the structure of sphingosine and its relationship with fatty acids and sugar molecules). The three most important gangliosidoses are Tay–Sachs disease, Sandhoff disease (both part of the GM2 gangliosidoses), and generalized GM1 gangliosidosis. All three are autosomal recessive with no sex predilection.

Tay–Sachs disease is the most common of the gangliosidoses and results from an enzyme defect in the alpha subunit of beta-hexosaminidase A. This defect is 100 times more common in Ashkenazi Jewish populations than in non-Jewish groups. The incidence is approximately 1 per 112000–360000 newborns in the general population, as opposed to 1 per 2500–3600 in Ashkenazi Jewish populations prior to the implementation of successful genetic screening programs. There also appears to be an increased frequency of this disease (comparable to that in the Ashkenazi Jewish population) in the Cordoba region of Argentina, French Canadians of the eastern St. Lawrence river valley, and isolated population groups of Cajuns in Louisiana. Although less than is observed in Ashkenazi Jewish populations, there is an increased frequency in Sephardic Jewish groups in both Morocco and Iraq. Children with Tay–Sachs disease develop normally for the first few months of life. Clinical symptoms usually begin between 3 and 10 months of age with developmental arrest or regression, hyperacusis (resulting in an exaggerated startle reflex), and generalized hypotonia. Examination of the fundus will invariably reveal the macular cherry-red spot that is due to the sparing of the red choroid of the fovea, surrounded by white, lipid-laden ganglion cells. The disease progresses with hearing loss, blindness, severe spasticity, seizures, and macrocephaly. Diagnosis is made initially on clinical grounds and confirmed with an assay for hexosaminidase A from peripheral blood leukocytes or cultured fibroblasts. This assay is also used as a carrier screening tool in very high-risk ethnic groups. Gene mutation analysis is also available, with two specific mutations (*TATC1238* and *IVS12*) accounting for 96% of the disease among the Ashkenazi Jewish population. There is no effective treatment for this disorder. Antiepileptic and antispasticity medications are used for symptomatic treatment. Death usually occurs by age 4 years.

Sandhoff disease results from an enzyme defect in the beta subunit of both beta-hexosaminidase A and beta-hexosaminidase B. The incidence is approximately 1 per 310000 newborns worldwide, and there is no increased frequency of this disease among Ashkenazi Jewish populations. An increased incidence of this disease has been observed in Creoles of northern Argentina, Metis Indians of northern Saskatchewan, individuals of Lebanese heritage, and a very high carrier rate in a small Maronite community in Cyprus. Sandhoff disease shares the same clinical symptoms and progression as Tay–Sachs disease. Additional symptoms include organomegaly, skeletal abnormalities, doll-like facies, and cardiac murmur. As with Tay–Sachs disease, there is no effective treatment for this disorder. Death usually occurs by age 4 years.

The generalized GM1 gangliosidoses result from an enzyme defect in beta-galactosidase. They are rare disorders occurring worldwide, with an unusually high incidence (1 in 3700 births) in the population of Malta. There are three forms based on the age of presentation. The early infantile GM1 presents prior to 1 year of age, often at birth. Symptoms include hypotonia, neurological degeneration,

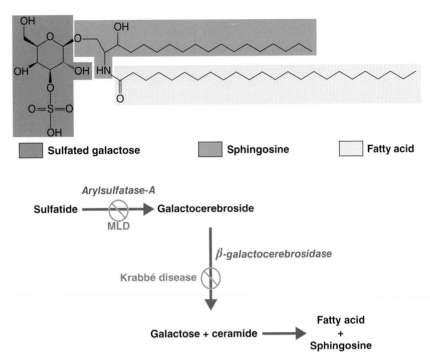

Figure 164.1 Sulfatides are sulfated galactosylceramides and are an important component of myelin. Deficiency of arylsulfatase A impairs removal of the sulfate moiety to generate galactocerebroside, which results in sulfatide accumulation and metachromatic leukodystrophy (MLD). A defect in breaking down galactocerebroside by removing the sugar moiety and releasing ceramide is responsible for Krabbe disease. Ceramide is formed by fatty acids connected by an amide bond to sphingosine.

seizures, hepatosplenomegaly, coarsening of facial features, dermal melanocytosis, skeletal abnormalities, and hyperacusis. In approximately half of cases a cherry-red spot is seen on fundal exam. The disease is rapidly progressive and death usually occurs by age 3 years. Late infantile GM1 presents between the ages of 1 and 3 years. Symptoms include ataxia, pronounced hyperacusis, seizures, slowly deteriorating mental function, and difficulties with speech. GM1 occurs between the ages of 3 and 30 years. Symptoms include progressive intellectual deterioration, ataxia, spasticity, and progressive athetosis or dystonia. Bony abnormalities, organomegaly, and cherry-red spots are not usually present in these two late-occurring forms. Diagnosis is usually made by showing lack of beta-galactosidase activity from peripheral blood leukocytes, cultured fibroblasts, or conjunctival biopsy. Gene mutation analysis is also available, with at least 102 separate defects in the beta-galactosidase gene identified to date. Treatment is symptomatic.

Sphingomyelinoses

The sphingomyelinoses are disorders associated with the accumulation of sphingomyelin, a macromolecule composed of sphingosine, fatty acid, phosphoric acid, and choline that is found abundantly in the spleen and is a major constituent of myelin. In this section the various types of Niemann–Pick diseases will be discussed. At least six types of Niemann–Pick disease have been described (types A–F), although the four most important types (types A–D) can be grouped into two broad biochemical pathological processes described further in what follows. Types E and F are not well-characterized adult forms that have minimal to no neurological symptoms and will not be discussed further. All are autosomal recessive with no clear sex predilection.

Niemann–Pick types A and B result from a defect in the lysosomal enzyme sphingomyelinase, which is responsible for the initial cleaving of sphingomyelin into phosphatidylcholine and ceramide (ceramide is fatty acid + sphingosine, shown in Figure 164.1). Type A is found in all ethnic groups, with an estimated incidence of 1 in 264000 live births. The rate is higher (1 in 40000) in Ashkenazi Jewish populations. Type B is also pan-ethnic, with the highest incidence occurring in individuals of Turkish, Arabic, and North African descent, but does not have a higher incidence among Ashkenazi Jewish populations. Niemann–Pick type A disease begins during infancy and presents with hepatosplenomegaly, growth retardation, hypotonia, macular cherry-red spot, and progressive neurodegeneration. The disease rapidly progresses with loss of motor development, increasing spasticity, and sometimes seizures. Death usually occurs by age 3 years. Niemann–Pick type B disease presents with hepatosplenomegaly, growth retardation, and problems with increased lung infections. There are few to no neurological problems and individuals usually survive into adulthood. The different clinical courses between these two diseases are believed to be due to the relative residual activity of sphingomyelinase present with each enzymatic defect.

Niemann–Pick diseases types C and D result from a disruption of cholesterol transport from endosomes to the plasma membrane. Both diseases show accumulations of intracellular cholesterol and sphingomyelin. Type C is further subdivided into C1 and C2 categories based on genotype. The C1 subtype represents 95% of cases of Niemann–Pick type C disease. Type D has now been shown to be an allelic variant of type C1 that was initially described in patients of Nova Scotia Acadian ancestry. The incidence of this disorder (combined C1, C2, and D) is estimated to be 1 in 150000 births.

The disease occurs in a much higher frequency in people of French Acadian descent in Nova Scotia and Cajuns in Louisiana, with an estimate of 1% (heterozygote carrier frequency between 10% and 26%). The clinical features can be quite heterogeneous, with the initial presentation ranging from infancy to adulthood; however, the more common course is relatively normal development in the first two years of life, followed by mild organomegaly, progressive neurological decline, ataxia, weakness, and vertical gaze palsy. Death often occurs by age 20.

Niemann–Pick types A and B can be diagnosed by demonstrating deficient sphingomyelinase activity in leukocytes and skin fibroblasts. Types C and D are diagnosed by showing increased amounts of unesterified cholesterol in fibroblasts. Another method is to demonstrate sea-blue histiocytes in the bone marrow. Gene mutation tests are also available where studies have reported mutations prevalent to specific regional/ethnic groups including three mutations (*R496L*, *L302P*, and *fsP330*), accounting for approximately 95% of type A disease in Ashkenazi Jewish populations, and a different mutation (*R608del*) in type B cases in North Africa. There is no established treatment other than symptomatic treatment for this disorder, although both enzyme replacement therapy and hematopoietic stem cell transplantation are under consideration for Niemann–Pick type B.

Cerebrosidoses

The cerebrosidoses are disorders of degradation of cerebrosides, which are glycosphingolipids that consist of a ceramide with a single sugar residue at the 1-hydroxyl moiety (see Figure 154.1 for this arrangement). The sugar residue can be either glucose (glucocerebrosides) or galactose (galactocerebrosides). The primary cerebrosidosis that will be discussed in this section is Gaucher disease, which results from an enzyme defect in the breakdown of glucocerebrosides. The disorder resulting from the defect for galactocerebrosides (Krabbe disease) will be discussed with the other leukodystrophies.

Gaucher disease is the most prevalent lipid storage disorder. The primary defect results from a deficiency in the lysosomal enzyme glucocerebrosidase. There are three specific clinical subtypes based on the presence of neuronal symptoms and rate of progression. All are autosomal recessive with no sex predilection. Type 1, the non-neuronopathic form, is the most common, with an estimated incidence of 1 in 40000. It is even more common in Ashkenazi Jewish populations, with a disease frequency of 1 per 855. It often presents in childhood with progressive hepatosplenomegaly, pancytopenia, and skeletal problems. There are no neurological manifestations initially, although a possible increased risk for Parkinson's disease in adulthood has been proposed. Type II Gaucher disease is an acute neuronopathic form with initial presentation in infancy. It has an estimated incidence of 1 in 100000 births. Patients are usually normal at birth, but develop hepatosplenomegaly, developmental regression, eye movement disorders, spasticity, and seizures. Death occurs by age 2 years. Type III Gaucher disease is the subacute neuronopathic form. It has a general estimated incidence of 1 in 100000 births, although it is observed with greater frequency in Swedish patients from the Norrbotten region with an incidence of 1 in 50000 births. It is characterized by more slowly progressive and milder symptoms compared to the type II form. Symptoms can begin in early childhood or adulthood and include hepatosplenomegaly, intellectual deterioration, ataxia, spasticity, skeletal abnormalities, horizontal supranuclear gaze palsy, anemia, and respiratory problems. Death often occurs by age 30 years.

Presumptive diagnosis can be made by detection of Gaucher cells in bone marrow aspirates in the correct clinical context. Definitive diagnosis can be made with an assay of glucocerebrosidase in leukocytes and fibroblast cultures. Complementary gene mutation analysis may also be available. Five gene defects have been reported to account for 96% of disease among Ashkenazi Jewish populations, but only 40–60% among non-Jewish populations.

There has been some progress in the treatment for this condition using enzyme replacement therapy and substrate reduction therapy to treat the systemic effects. However, because these therapies for the most part are limited by the problem of transport across the blood–brain barrier, their effect on established neurological symptoms is more marginal. Bone marrow transplantation has been shown to be effective when an appropriate HLA-compatible donor is available.

Mucolipidoses

The mucolipidoses are composed of four distinct clinical conditions (designated types I–IV) that result from the accumulation of lipid and carbohydrate molecules due to specific lysosomal enzyme defects. All are autosomal recessive with no sex predilection. Mucolipidosis type I, also referred to as sialidosis type II, results from an enzymatic defect in neuraminidase, which is involved in the initial cleavage of the sialic acid residue in glycoproteins. The incidence has been estimated at 1 in 2175000 individuals, and there has not been any documentation of regional or ethnic predilections. Symptoms present within the first year of life and include progressive mental retardation, myoclonus, ataxia, seizures, hypotonia, course facial features, macular cherry-red spot, corneal opacifications, macroglossia, hepatosplenomegaly, and skeletal malformations. Diagnosis is made by demonstrating deficient alpha-N-acetyl neuraminidase activity measured in leukocytes and fibroblasts. Gene mutation analysis may also be available. Treatment is symptomatic, and most infants die before the age of 1 year.

Mucolipidosis type II, also referred to as inclusion cell (I-cell) disease or mucolipidosis II alpha/beta, results from a defect in UDP-N-acetylglucosamine:N-acetylglucosaminyl-1-phosphotransferase, an enzyme that contributes to the marking of enzymes so that they are correctly targeted to lysosomes. In the absence of this step, lysosomal enzymes are incorrectly routed into the extracellular space. This disorder is rare, with an estimated incidence of 1 in 640000 births, although it may be higher in Saguenay-Lac-St. Jean, a French Canadian isolate. Symptoms present at birth and include hypotonia, coarse facial features, gingival hyperplasia, skeletal abnormalities, and progressive mental deterioration and microcephaly occurring over time. This condition is diagnosed by the presence of inclusion bodies in bone marrow cells and cultured fibroblasts. Death occurs in childhood. Treatments are limited for this disorder, although bone marrow transplantation has shown some promise.

Mucolipidosis type III, also called pseudo-Hurler polydystrophy or mucolipidosis III alpha/beta, is a milder form of type II possibly due to partially retained enzymatic activity with the defect. Symptoms do not occur until after age 2 years and include short stature, coarse facial features, skeletal abnormalities, and corneal clouding. Patients are generally of normal intelligence or have mild mental retardation. Prolonged survival into late adulthood can be observed.

Mucolipidosis type IV is due to a defect in mucolipin 1, a transmembrane protein that is involved in endosomal transport within the cell. Its relative incidence worldwide is unknown, although

Ashkenazi Jewish populations are believed to have a higher frequency, with 80% of patients with both mild and severe symptoms coming from this group. Symptoms include developmental delay, corneal clouding, hypotonia, achlorhydria with abnormal stomach pH, and hypoplastic corpus callosum. Diagnosis was previously made by demonstrating lysosomal inclusions by electron microscopy from conjunctival or skin biopsy studies. Gene mutation analysis is also available, where two specific mutations account for approximately 95% of the disease in Ashkenazi Jewish populations.

Fabry disease

Fabry disease results from an enzyme defect in alpha galactosidase A, which is necessary for the degradation of glycosphingolipids. As a result, globotriaosylceramide accumulates in blood vessels and other organ tissues. The disease has an X-linked recessive inheritance pattern, although heterozygous female carriers can sometimes also be affected, likely because of X-inactivation patterns during development. It is more common than many of the other lipid storage disorders, with an incidence of 1 in 40000. Symptoms present in early childhood or adolescence with anhidrosis, angiokeratomas, and burning pain of extremities, especially with warm weather, fever, or exercise. Ocular corneal whirling, vortex keratopathy, and high-frequency hearing loss may occur. Patients also have a 20-fold increased risk compared to the general population for small vessel transient ischemic event or stroke. Renal and cardiac complications are other systemic manifestations. The diagnosis in males is confirmed by observing a deficiency of alpha galactosidase A in serum leukocytes or cultured skin fibroblasts. Female patients must be diagnosed by mutation testing. Treatment has been relatively successful with enzyme replacement therapy.

Mucopolysaccharidosis

This group of lysosomal disorders result from a defect in the catabolism of mucopolysaccharides. There are now six major classifications (types I–IV and VI–VII), some with subtypes based on genetic enzyme defect. Mucopolysaccharides, also now more commonly referred to as glycosaminoglycans, are large polymers composed of a core protein with carbohydrate branches. Different polymers are important constituents found in bone, cartilage, connective tissue, skin, and cornea. Not surprisingly, in many cases these organ structures are affected to various degrees in each of the subtypes of the disorders.

Mucopolysaccharidosis type I (Hurler syndrome-type IH, Scheie syndrome-type IS, and Hurler–Scheie syndrome-type IH/S)

Mucopolysaccharidosis type I results from an enzymatic defect in alpha-L-iduronidase, which is essential for the metabolism of two glycosaminoglycans, heparan sulfate and dermatan sulfate. The disease is divided into three subtypes based on severity of clinical symptoms. All are autosomal recessive with no ethnic, regional, or sex predilection.

The most severe form is Hurler syndrome (mucopolysaccharidosis type IH). It has an estimated incidence of 1 in 144000 births. Affected children initially appear normal, although they may have frequent ear infections and an increased incidence of inguinal or abdominal hernia. Clinical symptoms usually present by 1 year with developmental delay, dysostosis multiplex, hepatosplenomegaly, cardiomegaly, corneal opacifications, and retinal degeneration. The typical child is small with a large head and coarse facial features. The bony deformities result in short stature (usually less than 4 feet in height), wide barrel chest, kyphosis, and short fingers prone to contractures. The face is dysmorphic with wide eyes, a depressed nasal bridge, large lips, and frontal bossing. Diagnosis can often be suspected based on these clinical characteristics, but can be confirmed either by demonstrating increased mucopolysaccharides output in urine or assaying for alpha-L-iduronidase in lymphocytes or cultured fibroblasts. Untreated, the disease progresses, and death often occurs by age 10 years from respiratory complications or congestive heart failure. Current treatment options have been improved by the use of bone marrow transplantation in children less than 2 years of age if the mental regression has not become severe. Enzymatic replacement therapy has also been used.

Scheie syndrome (mucopolysaccharidosis type IS) represents the least severe clinical manifestation in the continuum of alpha-L-iduronidase deficiency. It has an estimated incidence of 1 in 500000 births. Symptoms commonly occur after age 5 years and are often so mild that the diagnosis is not considered until adulthood. Affected individuals have stiff joints, clouding of the cornea, and a predisposition for aortic regurgitation and carpal tunnel syndrome. Intellectual deterioration and bony abnormalities are not present and individuals live to late adulthood.

Some individuals have a clinical course and symptoms intermediate between the severity of Hurler and Scheie syndromes. These cases are referred to as mucopolysaccharidosis type IH/S, with an estimated incidence of 1 in 115000 births. Symptoms present between the ages of 3 and 8 years with short stature, corneal clouding, joint stiffness, bony abnormalities, and hepatosplenomegaly. Although these features are shared with Hurler syndrome, symptoms tend to be milder and progress slower. There is also little to no intellectual deterioration and survival into adulthood is typical.

Mucopolysaccharidosis type II (Hunter syndrome)

Mucopolysaccharidosis type II, also referred to as Hunter syndrome, results from an enzyme defect in iduronate sulfatase. Like alpha-L-iduronidase in nucopolysaccharidosis type I, this enzyme is important in the metabolism of dermatan sulfate and heparan sulfate. Mucopolysaccharidosis type II is the only X-linked mucopolysaccharidosis. It has an estimated incidence of between 1 in 110000–165000 male births; however, there may be a slightly higher incidence in Jewish populations in Israel. Because of its X-linked recessive inheritance, it is almost exclusively found in males, although females may present with the disease due to inactivation of the paternal allele. The disorder is divided into two subgroups (types IIA and IIB) based on the severity of the disease and the presence of mental retardation. The most severe form, type IIA, usually presents between the ages of 2 and 4 years with mental deterioration, coarse facial features, skeletal deformities, short stature, joint stiffness, hepatosplenomegaly, seizures, hearing loss, and respiratory complications. Although retinal degeneration is present, corneal clouding (as seen in mucopolysaccharidosis type I) is usually not observed. Death from respiratory complications or cardiovascular failure usually occurs by age 15 years. The milder form, type IIB, presents with more mild facial features in early childhood. Short stature, skeletal abnormalities, hepatosplenomegaly, hearing loss, retinal degeneration, cardiomegaly, and respiratory complications are usually seen, but are less severe and more slowly progressive than in type IIA. Intellectual deterioration is not observed, and although premature death can occur due to respiratory and cardiac dysfunction, many individuals live into the fifth decade. Diagnosis is made by demonstrating deficient enzyme activity in serum, lymphocytes, or fibroblasts. Unlike mucopolysaccharidosis Type I, bone marrow transplantation does not prevent mental retardation.

Mucopolysaccharidosis type III (Sanfilippo syndrome)

Mucopolysaccharidosis type III, also referred to as Sanfilippo syndrome, results from a dysfunction in the catabolism of heparan sulfate. The disorder is divided into four subtypes (IIIA–D) based on distinct enzymatic gene defects. However, they are virtually indistinguishable clinically, except for possibly a slightly more severe course for type IIIA. Type IIIA results from a defect in heparan-N-sulfatase. Type IIIB results from a defect in N-acetyl-alpha-D-glucosaminidase. Type IIIC results from a defect in acetyl CoA alpha-glucosaminide acetyltransferase. Type IIID results from a defect in N-acetylglucosamine-6-sulfate sulfatase. All are autosomal recessive with no ethnic, regional, or sex predilection. All subtypes combined have an estimated incidence of 1 in 58000 births, making them the most common mucopolysaccharidoses. Symptoms usually present between the ages of 2 and 5 years with developmental delay and/or regression, coarse facial features, and mild hepatosplenomegaly. Growth retardation and corneal clouding are not typically observed. As the mental deterioration progresses, aggressive behavior and sleep disturbances become prominent features in many cases. Diagnosis can be made in suspected clinical cases by demonstrating urinary excretion of heparan sulfate, although definitive confirmation by enzymatic assay from serum, skin fibroblasts, or lymphocytes is often needed. Death usually occurs before age 20 years, and bone marrow transplantation does not appear to offer any benefit.

Mucopolysaccharidosis type IV (Morquio syndrome)

Mucopolysaccharidosis type IV, or Morquio syndrome, results from a defect in the metabolism of keratin sulfate and chondroitin-6-sulfate. There are two subtypes that are distinguished based on the specific enzymatic defect. Type IVA results from a defect in N-acetyl-galactosamine-6-sulfate sulfatase. Type IVB results from a deficiency of beta-galactosidase and, despite a very different clinical presentation, is an allelic variant with GM1 gangliosidosis (see later). Type IVA was previously believed to represent a more severe form, but with genetic analysis there now appears to be more overlap between the two subtypes. Both forms are autosomal recessive, with an estimated incidence of 1 in 200000 births, although the incidence may be higher in Northern Ireland. Symptoms usually present between the ages of 1 and 3 years with corneal clouding, skeletal dysplasia, short stature, joint stiffness, and predisposition for spinal odontoid hypoplasia. Neurological complications do not occur except secondarily to spinal compression from the skeletal abnormalities. Intelligence is not affected. The diagnosis is made by the presence of keratin sulfate in urine or enzymatic assay from leukocytes or fibroblasts. In the most severe cases, individuals generally do not live past the third or fourth decade.

Mucopolysaccharidosis type VI (Maroteaux–Lamy syndrome)

This disorder results from an enzymatic deficit in arylsulfatase B, an enzyme that is important for the catabolism of dermatan sulfate and chondroitin-4-sulfate. It is an autosomal recessive disorder with no ethnic, regional, or sex predilection. Its estimated incidence is 1 in 320000 births. Clinical presentation varies widely, but the most

severe form is similar to Hurler syndrome, except that intellectual function is preserved. It is diagnosed by demonstrating dermatan sulfate without heparan sulfate in the urine or by enzymatic assay. Treatment includes enzymatic replacement therapy.

Mucopolysaccharidosis type VII (Sly syndrome)

Mucopolysaccharidosis type VII, also known as Sly syndrome, results from a enzymatic defect in beta-glucuronidase, which is involved in the metabolism of heparan sulfate and dermatan sulfate. It is an autosomal recessive disorder with an estimated incidence of 1 in 250000 births. Clinical presentation varies widely, with the most severe form causing *hydrops fetalis* at birth. Other patients are less affected, with mild to no mental retardation, hepatosplenomegaly, and skeletal and facial abnormalities. Most children with mucopolysaccharidosis type VII live into the teenage or young adult years. Diagnosis is made with enzymatic assay from serum, leukocytes, or fibroblasts.

Glycogenoses

The glycogenoses refer to a group of disorders that result from a defect in the metabolism of glycogen. At least nine diseases have been enzymatically characterized. The three most prominent (types I, II, and V) are discussed here. All show an autosomal recessive inheritance pattern.

Glycogen storage disease type I (von Gierke's disease)

This disorder is also referred to as von Gierke's disease and it results from an enzymatic deficiency in glucose-6-phosphatase. The incidence of the disorder has been estimated at 1 in 100000–200000 births, without regional or ethnic predilections. Clinical symptoms usually present by age 2 years and include hypoglycemia, lactic acidosis, hepatomegaly, hyperlipidemia, growth failure, and joint problems. Neurological complications include seizures and chronic brain damage, usually provoked by episodes of hypoglycemia. Definitive diagnosis is made with liver biopsy. Treatment involves preventing hypoglycemia by providing a frequent source of carbohydrate.

Glycogen storage disease type II (Pompe disease)

Pompe disease results from a defect in acid alpha-glucosidase. It is the only glycogen storage disease that is a true lysosomal disease. It has an estimated incidence of 1 in 40000 births, although the highest frequency occurs in the African American population (1 per 14000 for the infantile category). Other regional areas with less well-characterized common mutations have been documented in Taiwan, southern China, and the Netherlands. The pathological process is due to progressive accumulation of glycogen in skeletal muscle, heart, liver, and central nervous system. Three subtypes have been described based on age of presentation. The infantile form presents in the first months of life with feeding problems, poor weight gain, muscle weakness, and hypotonia. Development is initially normal for the first few months, but slowly declines as the disease progresses. The heart is grossly enlarged due to the excess accumulation of glycogen (restrictive cardiomyopathy) and most infants die from cardiac or respiratory problems by 2 years of age. Glycogen accumulation results in progressive macroglossia, which can interfere with swallowing. In the juvenile form, symptoms appear in early to late childhood. Both this form and the adult form are characterized by progressive weakness of respiratory and other skeletal muscles. While the heart may be affected, it is generally not enlarged. Intelligence is also not affected. Diagnosis is made by muscle biopsy. The current treatment is with enzyme replacement therapy. In 2006, the drug alglucosidase alfa (Myozyme) received US Food and Drug Administration approval for the treatment of Pompe disease.

Glycogen storage disease type V (McArdle disease)

This disorder, also termed McArdle disease, is due to a deficiency in myophosphorylase. It has an estimated incidence of 1 in 100000 births. Although it is an autosomal recessive disorder, more male cases have been documented. No studies have documented any regional or ethnic preference. The disease primarily presents in the second or third decade of life, although an infantile form has been described. Symptoms include intermittent muscle pain, cramping, myoglobinuria, and weakness, often relieved by rest. Differential diagnoses include Tarui disease (phosphofructokinase deficiency, glycogen storage disease type VII) and the myopathic form of carnitine palmitoyltransferase II deficiency. Muscle biopsy shows increased glycogen and deficiency in muscle phosphorylase activity. The diagnosis can also be made by nuclear magnetic resonance (MR) spectroscopy.

Leukodystrophies

The leukodystrophies are a group of inheritable disorders that primarily affect the white matter of the central nervous system. Defects causing delayed myelination, dysmyelination, or demyelination have all been observed. The inheritance patterns, specific genes involved, and common imaging findings are detailed in Table 164.1.

Pelizaeus–Merzbacher disease

Pelizaeus–Merzbacher disease is an X-linked recessive disorder of dysmyelination. The defect is in proteolipid protein (*PLP1*), which results in myelin not forming properly. The incidence has not been well described, but has been estimated at 1 in 500000 births. It is found worldwide without any regional or ethnic predisposition. Symptoms present in infancy, usually before age 3 months, with a distinctive rotatory nystagmus. Hypotonia, poor head control, and delayed motor and cognitive development are also seen. Eventually, spasticity, optic atrophy, and mental retardation occur. Diagnosis is made based on X-linked inheritance in the right clinical setting

with abnormalities of white matter on MR imaging. The diagnosis can be confirmed with fluorescent *in situ* hybridization using a Planar Langmuir probe. There is no effective treatment for this condition.

Cockayne syndrome

Cockayne syndrome is an autosomal recessive demyelinating leukodystrophy that results from a defect involved in transcription-regulated DNA repair. There are at least two variants (types I and II) based on genotype. The disorder is rare, with an estimated incidence of less than 1 in 250000 births with no specific regional or ethnic predilection. It is a progressive disorder characterized by abnormal facial features of large ears and sunken eyes, premature aging, failure of growth starting by age 2 years, progressive intellectual deterioration, pigmentary retinal degeneration, and hypersensitivity of skin to sunlight. There is no effective treatment other than symptomatic care. Death usually occurs in adolescence, although survival into adulthood is possible.

Alexander disease

Alexander disease results from a defect in glial fibrillary acidic protein (GFAP). The infantile form accounts for 80% of cases, although juvenile and adult forms can be present. The disease is very rare, with fewer than 300 cases reported, but no studies have suggested a regional or ethnic predilection. Most cases are sporadic, although an autosomal dominant inheritance pattern can also be seen, especially in the adult form. In the infantile form, symptoms usually present by 6 months with macrocephaly (see Canavan disease in the next section), seizures, spasticity, and psychomotor and cognitive decline. MR imaging shows extensive cerebral white-matter signal changes with a frontal predominance. Histopathological examination shows a distinctive pattern of Rosenthal fibers. Diagnosis is made by a combination of neuroimaging and gene analysis in the correct clinical context. There is no effective treatment for this disorder and death usually occurs by the first decade.

Canavan disease

Canavan disease is an autosomal recessive leukodystrophy that results from a defect in the enzyme aspartoacylase, which hydrolyzes N-acetylaspartic acid to L-aspartic acid. The disorder is present worldwide, but is more common in Ashkenazi Jewish populations,

Table 164.1 Genetic and imaging characteristics of the leukodystrophies.

Disorder	Inheritance pattern	Genes	Imaging
Pelizaeus–Merzbacher disease	X-linked recessive	PLP1	Tigroid pattern = patchy distribution of dysmyelination with preserved patches of myelination
Cockayne syndrome	Autosomal recessive	ERCC3	Hypomyelination, calcifications (putamen > cortex and dentate), brain atrophy
Alexander disease	Autosomal dominant	GFAP	Frontal lobe early in the course and progresses posteriorly
Canavan disease	Autosomal recessive	ASPA	Diffuse high signal intensity (T2) throughout the white matter with subcortical U fibers preferentially affected and progressive atrophy
Krabbe disease (globoid cell leukodystrophy)	Autosomal recessive	GALC	Symmetric deep white-matter signal abnormalities in cortex and cerebellum, subcortical U fibers spared initially, progressive atrophy
Metachromatic leukodystrophy	Autosomal recessive	ARSA	Diffuse high signal intensity of periventricular white matter with sparing of subcortical U fibers, tigroid and "leopard-skin" pattern of demyelination suggests sparing of perivascular white matter
X-linked adrenoleukodystrophy	X-linked recessive	ABCD1	Demyelination begins in the posterior brain (peritrigonal white matter and across the corpus callosum splenium) and spreads anteriorly over time

where carrier rates as high as 1 in 40 have been observed. There may also be a higher incidence in families from Saudi Arabia, although this is less well documented. Symptoms present usually by 3–6 months with macrocephaly (see Alexander disease in the previous section), hypotonia, optic atrophy, and psychomotor and mental retardation. Children are characteristically quiet and apathetic (in contrast to the irritability seen in patients with Krabbe disease). Over time, seizures and progressive spasticity occur. Diagnosis is confirmed by demonstrating increased N-acetylaspartic acid in plasma, urine, or brain (by MR spectroscopy). There is no effective treatment. Death usually occurs by age 4 years, although some children survive into the second and third decades.

Krabbe disease (globoid cell leukodystrophy)

This is an autosomal recessive leukodystrophy resulting from a defect in degrading galactocerebrosides (see Figure 164.1; note the etiological relationship to metachromatic leukodystrophy). It can also be categorized as a cerebrosidosis, but is included here because of its specific pattern of white-matter pathology. The specific enzymatic defect is galactosylceramidase (galactocerebroside beta-galactosidase). The disorder has an estimated worldwide incidence of 1 in 100000 births, although in an isolated Druze community in Israel a much higher incidence of 6 in 1000 births has been reported. The incidence may also be slightly higher in Sweden, with a reported incidence of 1.8 in 100000 births. The most common presentation occurs in infancy, although juvenile and adult forms also occur. The infantile form is characterized by an onset before 6 months of age with irritability, decreased psychomotor and cognitive development, seizures, muscle weakness, spasticity, deafness, and optic atrophy. Diagnosis is made by typical white-matter changes on neuroimaging (deep white-matter signal abnormalities in cerebrum and cerebellum: increase in T2, decrease in T1) and showing near absence of beta-galactosidase activity in leukocyte or skin fibroblasts. Peripheral nerve involvement in the infantile form seems to be very early and is demonstrable by electrodiagnostics. Histopathological analysis also shows distinctive globoid cells near blood vessels of altered white matter. Untreated, the prognosis for the infantile form is poor, with death usually occurring before age 2 years. The prognosis has improved somewhat with early bone marrow transplantation and umbilical cord transplantation, although the best outcomes have occurred in the more mild juvenile and adult forms.

Metachromic leukodystrophy

Metachromic leukodystrophy results from a defect in the enzyme arylsulfatase A, which is required to hydrolyze sulfatides to cerebrosides. The disorder has an estimated worldwide incidence of 1 in 40000 births, making it one of the more common leukodystrophies. Higher incidences have also been reported in the western region of the Navajo nation, with an incidence of 1 in 2520 births, and it is also less well described in isolated Arab groups in Israel. The most common form occurs in infancy, although juvenile and adult forms also have been characterized. In the late infantile form symptoms present prior to 18 months of age with psychomotor retardation, developmental delay, muscle wasting, progressive loss of vision, and seizures. Death usually occurs by age 5 years. Diagnosis is confirmed by demonstrating reduced arylsulfatase A activity in leukocytes. Peripheral nerve involvement is common, and the nomenclature for this disease reflects the early observation of metachromasia (failure to stain "true" with a given stain, brown coloration with cresyl violet

in this case) in peripheral nerve biopsy specimens. There have been some promising results in delaying the progression of this disorder with bone marrow transplantation.

Adrenal leukodystrophy

Adrenal leukodystrophy is an X-linked peroxisomal disorder resulting in a defect in catabolism of very long chain fatty acids (VLCFA). The gene responsible is that for the D1 subtype of the ATP-binding cassette (*ABCD1*), which encodes a protein, ALDP, which is a member of the ATP-binding cassette transport system family. This protein is involved in the transport of fatty acids into peroxisomes. Because of the defect, fatty acid chains with 24–30 carbon atoms cannot undergo beta-oxidation and accumulate in a variety of tissues. This disease is the most common sudanophilic leukodystrophy, with an incidence of 1 in 20000 individuals. There is no regional or ethnic predilection. Three forms have been described based on age and severity of neurological symptoms. The most common form occurs between the ages of 5 and 10 years and presents with behavioral changes (either withdrawal or increased aggression), developmental regression, ataxia, seizures, adrenal insufficiency, and degeneration of visual and auditory systems. It is rapidly progressive and if untreated usually results in death or vegetative state by an early age. The second form, termed adrenomyeloneuropathy (AMN), has its onset in the third or fourth decade and is characterized with slowly progressive paraparesis. The third form is Addison's disease and usually presents in adulthood as isolated adrenal insufficiency without neurological symptoms. Diagnosis is made by measuring high levels of VLCFA in serum and cultured fibroblasts. In classic X-linked ALD, the MRI shows pathognomonic increased T2 signal bilaterally in the occipital white matter. The disease is treated mainly with bone marrow transplantation. Dietary modification with Lorenzo's oil lowers VLCFA in serum, but neurological deterioration is not significantly modified. At present a gene therapy trial involving a lentiviral vector is under way.

Refsum disease

Refsum disease (hereditary motor sensory neuropathy IV) results from a defect in phytanoyl-coenzyme A hydroxylase, which is involved in degrading phytanic acid. It is a rare disorder with only 60 published cases worldwide, but no specific regional or ethnic predilections have been reported. It typically presents in children age 2–7 years with peripheral neuropathy, increased night blindness due to retinal degeneration, anosmia, cerebellar degeneration, ichthyosis, skeletal abnormalities, and cardiac arrhythmias. Diagnosis is made by demonstrating a high level of phytanic acid in serum. Treatment involves dietary restriction of all foods with high levels of phytanic acid, including beef, lamb, and fatty fish.

Other lipidoses

There are two specific lipidoses that are often considered separately from the lysosomal lipid storage diseases. Rather than resulting from an enzymatic defect in a specific lysosomal degradative enzyme, these disorders result from a more fundamental error in lipid metabolic processing.

Abetalipoproteinemia

Abetalipoproteinemia, also termed Bassen Kornzweig syndrome, is a rare autosomal recessive disorder initially reported primarily in Ashkenazi Jewish populations that results in the complete lack of serum beta-lipoproteins. This is due to a decreased function in a microsomal triglyceride transfer protein (MTTP) that mediates the transfer of lipid molecules in the endoplasmic reticulum to nascent lipoprotein particles, including chylomicrons, very low-density lipoproteins, and low-density lipoproteins. As a consequence, absorption of fat and fat-soluble vitamins is deficient. The incidence of this condition has not been well established, although the carrier rate in one Ashkenazi Jewish population is 1 in 131 individuals. Symptoms present in the first year of life with failure to thrive, abdominal distention, diarrhea, and steatorrhea. Peripheral blood smears will show acanthocytosis. Confirmatory genetic testing is available, with over 30 mutations in the *MTTP* gene previously described. Neurological symptoms usually present between the ages of 2 and 17 years. Initially patients present with ataxia, proprioceptive loss, muscle weakness, and retinal degeneration resulting in night blindness. Imaging will show progressive combined posterior column degeneration. Approximately one-third of patients will develop mental retardation. The neurological symptoms are primarily due to the resultant vitamin E deficiency. Treatment involves supplementing vitamin E (100 mg/kg/day given orally) to prevent the development or progression of neurological or retinal deficits.

Tangier disease

Tangier disease is a rare autosomal recessive disorder characterized by a deficiency in high-density lipoprotein. Only 50 cases have been identified worldwide. The name is derived from the island off the coast of Virginia where the first two patients were discovered, although the disorder has now been observed in other countries as well. The defect responsible for this disease is the ATP-binding cassette transporter 1 (*ABCA1*), which is responsible for transporting cholesterol and phospholipids from inside the cell into the bloodstream. The most distinct symptom is the enlargement of the tonsils, which appear orange or yellow. Other symptoms include hepatosplenomegaly, early atherosclerosis, corneal clouding, retinitis pigmentosa, and relapsing asymmetric peripheral neuropathy.

Further reading

Bennett MJ, Rakheja D. The neuronal ceroid-lipofuscinoses. *Dev Disabil Res Rev* 2013;17(3):254–225.

Boustany RM. Lysosomal storage diseases – the horizon expands. *Nat Rev Neurol* 2013;9(10):583–598.

Kolter T, Sandhoff K. Sphingolipid metabolism diseases. *Biochim Biophys Acta* 2006;1758(12):2057–2079.

Lyon G, Fattal-Valevski A, Kolodny EH. Leukodystrophies: Clinical and genetic aspects. *Top Magn Reson Imaging* 2006;17(4):219–242.

Meikle PJ, Hopwood JJ, Clague AE, Carey WF. Prevalence of lysosomal storage disorders. *JAMA* 1999;281(3):249–254.

Menkes JH, Sarnat HB, Maria BL (eds.). *Child Neurology*, 7th ed. Philadelphia, PA: Lippincott, Williams and Wilkins; 2006.

Muenzer J. The mucopolysaccharidoses: A heterogeneous group of disorders with variable pediatric presentations. *J Pediatr* 2004;144(5 Suppl):S27–S34.

Online Mendelian Inheritance in Man (OMIM) Database, http://www.ncbi.nlm.nih.gov/sites/entrez?db=omim (accessed November 2015).

Poorthuis BJ, Wevers RA, Kleijer WJ, et al. The frequency of lysosomal storage diseases in The Netherlands. *Hum Genet* 1999;105(1–2):151–156.

Swaiman KF, Ashwal S, Ferriero DM, Schor NF (eds.). *Swaiman's Pediatric Neurology: Principles and Practice*, 5th ed. Edinburgh: Elsevier Saunders; 2012.

165 Fatty acid oxidation disorders

Thomas Wieser

Neurology and Pain Medicine, Fachkrankenhaus Jerichow, Jerichow, Germany

Disorders of fatty acid oxidation belong to the most prevalent group of monogenic conditions worldwide. Inherited defects in 17 proteins directly affecting either carnitine-dependent transport of long chain fatty acids or the process of β-oxidation itself have so far been described. These include glutaric aciduria type 2, primary carnitine deficiency, and deficiencies of carnitine palmitoyltransferase (CPT1a, CPT2), carnitine acylcarnitine translocase (CACT), (very) long chain acyl-CoA dehydrogenase ([V]LCAD), mitochondrial trifunctional protein (MTP), medium chain acyl-coenzyme A dehydrogenase (MCAD), medium and short chain hydroxyacyl-CoA dehydrogenase (M/SCHAD), short chain acyl-coenzyme A dehydrogenase (SCAD), and 2,4-dienoyl CoA reductase. Fatty acid oxidation disorders (FAOD) have three modes of clinical presentation. There is the hepatic presentation in the neonatal period or during early infancy, often triggered by catabolic states. With later onset, the presentation may consist predominantly of cardiac symptoms with hypertrophic cardiomyopathy and arrhythmias. Finally, there are milder adult-onset forms characterized predominantly by muscular symptoms. FAOD should also be considered in sudden unexplained infant death, as well as in cardiac conduction defect or ventricular tachycardia not otherwise explained.

Physiology

Carbohydrates and fatty acids comprise the major sources of energy in the mammalian organism. Glucose, the main carbohydrate fuel, is stored as glycogen in liver and muscle. Fatty acids are stored as triglycerides and in other lipids. In general, there is a hierarchy of usage for these substrates, with glucose as the primary fuel for short-term demands, its constant level maintained by glycogenolysis. Depletion of liver glycogen stores, as occurs during prolonged fasting, triggers a systemic switch to lipolysis and consequently oxidation of fatty acids, which predominantly occurs as β-oxidation in mitochondria.

This hierarchy of energy substrate use constitutes the connection between any disturbances of carbohydrate and fatty acid metabolism. If the use of carbohydrates is restricted, whether by a disorder of glucose metabolism, the inability to maintain glucose supply from glycogen breakdown, or a failure to create glycogen stores, the dependence on fatty acid oxidation is increased. Conversely, disturbances in the oxidation or restrictions in the availability of fatty acids, as in decreased lipolysis, or disturbances in their transport into cells and across the mitochondrial membrane to the site of β-oxidation, will immediately increase the dependence on

carbohydrate supply, which is both short term and quickly exhausted (e.g., during fasting).

Striated muscle and brain both have specific features of energy substrate usage that make them specifically, yet distinctly, vulnerable to any disturbance of energy metabolism. This is the essential use of fatty acids in long-term exercise in muscle and the unique dependence on glucose and ketone bodies in the brain, the latter formed as an end product of β-oxidation, which can neither be stored nor produced in the brain itself. The brain requires a stable blood level of both low molecular substrates. This can only be maintained when liver metabolism is intact. If, *secondary* to a disturbance in the liver due to a fatty acid oxidation defect, a shortage of these substrates occurs, the brain is readily affected and so-called hepatocerebral crises will occur. The clinical symptomatology is characterized by severe metabolic derangement with hypoketotic hypoglycemia, hyperammonemia, lethargy or reduced consciousness, seizures, and, potentially, cerebral edema.

A completely different situation is found in skeletal muscle and heart. Muscle cells possess the complete enzymatic apparatus required to form and break down both glycogen and triglycerides and, therefore, can utilize the entire range of fuels. While glycolysis and glycogenolysis are able to stave off acute peaks of energy demand, the main energy supply is through oxidation of fatty acids, especially during long-term exercise and fasting. With this unique feature of energy production, muscle and heart are *primarily* and predominantly affected whenever fatty acid oxidation is disturbed. Clinically, chronic muscle weakness, myopathy, and hypotonia develop as a result of chronic disruption of muscular function. Leaving patients with MCAD and CPT1a aside, cardiac involvement is found in 63%, particularly in long chain FAOD.

Muscle symptoms can be permanent and progressive, as in primary carnitine deficiency, where there is a defect of delivery of fatty acids at the site of β-oxidation and, consequently, triglyceride storage in the cytosol. On the other hand, patients with CPT2 deficiency are generally without symptoms and have normal muscle strength, but are prone to painful episodes of rhabdomyolysis and weakness, typically provoked by prolonged exercise or fasting.

Epidemiology and genetics

The spectrum of FAOD differs widely between ethnic groups, and newborn screening (NBS) has increased the rate of inborn errors identified worldwide. Calculations from reports from Australia, Germany, and the United States give a combined incidence of all

International Neurology, Second edition. Edited by Robert P. Lisak, Daniel D. Truong, William M. Carroll and Roongroj Bhidayasiri
© 2016 John Wiley & Sons, Ltd. Published 2016 by John Wiley & Sons, Ltd.

FAOD of approximately 1 in 9300. An unusually high prevalence was found in the Iberian population with a prevalence of 1 in 7960, mostly presenting as MCAD deficiency. There was a Gypsy origin for 90% of patients, revealing significant differences in the prevalence of FAOD even among different European populations.

The worldwide prevalence of MCAD ranges from 1 in 5000 to 1 in 20000, with the highest incidence seen in Northern Germany (about 1 in 5000) and the lowest in Far East populations (Japan and Taiwan).

The first inherited defects identified were CPT2 in 1973, PCD in 1975, and MCAD in 1976.

MCAD deficiency is the most common defect of the mitochondrial β-oxidation of fatty acids in humans. Since its inclusion in NBS programs, the spectrum of observed MCAD genotypes has changed dramatically. While reports from 2010 state that approximately 50% of individuals are homozygous for the common mutation p.Lys304Glu and approximately 40% are heterozygous for p.Lys304Glu (besides one of more than 90 rarer alleles), new data show that about 60% of MCAD patients are homozygous for the c.985 A>G (p.Lys329Glu) mutation.

For MCAD as well as other FAOD, the distinction between "normal" and "disease" is blurred into a spectrum of enzyme deficiency states caused by different mutations and possible epigenetic factors affecting intracellular protein processing and finally enzyme activity.

Screening for PCD has revealed a prevalence of 1 in 40000 births in the Akita prefecture in Japan and 1 in 120000 in Australia. The prevalence in the genetically homogenous population of the Faroe Islands is the highest reported in the world with 1 in 300. The frequency in the United States and Europe has not been defined, but from NBS data and reported cases the prevalence in the United States can be estimated as 1 in 50000.

PCD is caused by mutations in the *SLC22A5* gene on chromosome 5q31.1 encoding the sodium-dependent carnitine transporter OCTN2. More than 100 pathogenic variants have been reported in the Human Gene Mutation Database to date. The detection rate of mutant alleles is about 70% by direct sequencing.

CPT2 deficiency, which like all other disorders of fatty acid oxidation is inherited in an autosomal recessive mode, has been described in about 150 patients to date. Mutations are found in the *CPT2* gene on chromosome 1p32, with a "common" mutation (S113L) found in approximately 60% of mutant alleles. There is a fairly consistent genotype–phenotype correlation where missense mutations are associated with the muscle form and therefore called "mild mutations"; truncating mutations are frequently associated with the lethal neonatal forms and are therefore considered "severe" mutations. As expected, there are exceptions to the genotype–phenotype correlation.

Clinical features and pathophysiology

Clinical features and pathophysiology are closely interrelated in FAOD. How a specific disturbance in a metabolic pathway results in a certain phenotype will be outlined in the following section.

Acyl-CoA dehydrogenase deficiencies

The first step of mitochondrial β-oxidation is the dehydrogenation of acyl-CoA to enoyl-CoA. This step is catalyzed by different acyl-CoA dehydrogenases with distinct but somewhat overlapping substrate specificities (short chain, medium chain, and very long chain as well as branched chain fatty acids). The long chain activity is not mitochondrial and does not seem to play a role as a genetic defect.

Defects of this first step frequently result in abnormal lipid accumulation in muscle and carnitine deficiency, because acyl-CoA esters accumulated intra-mitochondrially are buffered as carnitine esters, which can permeate the mitochondrial membrane and are then excreted by the kidneys. Lipid accumulation in muscle as seen, for example, in MCAD deficiency is shown in Figure 165.1. Typically, when medium or very long chain activities are affected, there is also an increased bypass to ω-oxidation. The resulting dicarboxylic acids are diagnostic when detected in urine analysis or as carnitine esters in blood.

Clinical symptomatology varies based on the age of onset. Manifestation in childhood usually presents with multiorgan involvement affecting the liver, heart, kidneys, and central nervous system, with muscular symptoms playing only a minor role. In manifestations during adolescence or early adulthood, the symptoms are almost exclusively muscular. It is important to bear in mind that there is significant clinical heterogeneity seen in these disorders, even within families.

Children with MCAD deficiency seem normal at birth and manifestations occur between a few hours and 24 months of life; late manifestation in adulthood also occurs. One has to keep in mind that symptoms may appear before the results of newborn screening are available. A previously healthy child develops hypoketotic hypoglycemia, vomiting, lethargy, seizures, and encephalopathy, often precipitated by increased metabolic demand (e.g., due to infection, stress, or fasting). The risk of death in the first 72 hours is approximately 5%. Before extended NBS programs were implemented, 15–20% of affected children died during their first metabolic crisis; death is now a rare event. Once the defect is identified, prognosis is usually good. However, unexplained infant death is reported to occur in about 20% of families who have a child diagnosed with MCAD deficiency.

Carnitine deficiency

Long chain fatty acids are transported across the mitochondrial membrane with the help of the so-called carnitine shuttle. Carnitine, which is actively transported into the muscle cells using the

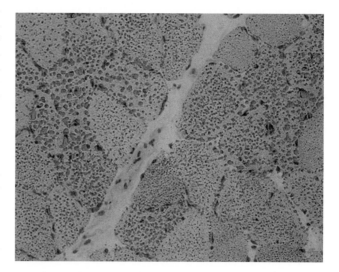

Figure 165.1 Pathological lipid storage in muscle. Intermyofibrillar accumulation of fatty acids as seen in lipid storage diseases, mitochondrial myopathies, and fatty acid oxidation disorders (Oil Red O staining). For color details, please refer to the color plates section.

sodium-dependent carnitine transporter (OCTN2), is esterified with long chain acyl residues and transferred from acyl coenzyme A esters by CPT1, translocated as acyl carnitines across the inner mitochondrial membrane by carnitine-acylcarnitine translocase (CAC), and then transferred back to coenzyme A by CPT2 to enter the β-oxidation cycle. The normal functioning of this shuttle is dependent on sufficient free carnitine in the cells derived both from the diet (meat and dairy products) and from biosynthesis in the liver, with 90% of body carnitine found in muscle.

Carnitine transporter defects due to mutations in the OCTN2 carnitine transporter gene SLC22A5 result in renal wasting of carnitine, low plasma carnitine levels (free carnitine <5 μM), and intracellular carnitine deficiency.

The systemic PCD phenotype encompasses a broad clinical spectrum ranging from metabolic decompensation in infancy, cardiomyopathy in childhood, fatigability in adulthood, to complete absence of symptoms.

In symptomatic patients, metabolic crises occur characterized by reduced consciousness, tonic–clonic seizures, hepatomegaly, hypoglycemia, acidosis, and liver failure. Age of onset varies between the eighth month of life and early adulthood. Early recognition and treatment with high doses of oral carnitine can be life saving. The average age of myopathic presentation is between 2 and 4 years, indicating that the myopathic manifestations of PCD may develop over a longer period of time compared to metabolic symptoms. Myopathic manifestations include dilated cardiomyopathy, hypotonia, skeletal muscle weakness, and elevated serum creatine kinase. Since newborn screening programs were introduced, some 80 patients have been identified who are "asymptomatic." Detailed examination in one study revealed symptoms in about 40%, with fatigue being the most prominent accompanied in half of patients by cardiac arrhythmias. There seems to be a fairly consistent genotype–phenotype correlation. The frequency of nonsense mutations is significantly increased in symptomatic patients as compared to asymptomatic persons.

Carnitine palmitoyltransferase deficiency

The carnitine palmitoyltransferase (CPT) system mediates the transport of long chain fatty acids into the mitochondrial matrix. This system includes two different enzymes, CPT1, located in the outer mitochondrial membrane, and CPT2, located in the inner membrane. These enzymes catalyze the exchange of acyl groups between acyl-coenzyme A (CoA) and acylcarnitine. Only a few cases have been described with CPT1 deficiency, presenting with severe episodes of hypoketotic hypoglycemia, usually occurring after fasting or illness, with onset in infancy or early childhood. Consistent epidemiological data for CPT2 are not available; however, more than 150 cases have been described to date. Three distinct clinical presentations occur. The first is the "lethal neonatal" form, manifesting within days after birth as liver failure with hypoketotic hypoglycemia, cardiomyopathy, cardiac arrhythmias, and seizures; it is often accompanied by malformations, including facial and neuronal migration defects, among others. Onset during the first year of life is characteristic of the "severe hepatocardiomuscular" form; liver failure, cardiomyopathy, seizures, hypoketotic hypoglycemia, abdominal pain, and peripheral myopathy are the main clinical features. Probably the most common presentation is the "adult onset muscular" form, with age of onset between the first and sixth decades of life. It is characterized by recurrent attacks of myalgia accompanied by myoglobinuria precipitated by prolonged exercise, especially after fasting. It may also be triggered by cold exposure or stress. Muscle weakness during attacks is possible. Characteristically, there are no signs of myopathy between attacks and patients are healthy and completely normal in neurological examination.

Both infantile and adult cases have been shown to be associated with a decreased amount of steady-state CPT2 protein. The lethal neonatal as well as the severe infantile forms are characterized by reduced CPT2 enzyme activity in multiple organs, reduced serum concentrations of total and free carnitine, and increased serum concentrations of long chain acyl carnitines and lipids. In the adult-onset type, reduced enzyme activity is also found. However, using the "isotope forward assay," enzyme activity is normal. Patients can be distinguished from controls based on significantly greater inhibition of enzyme activity by malonyl-CoA, a natural regulator of this pathway. This finding has led to the hypothesis that in the adult-onset muscular type of CPT2 deficiency, impaired regulation, rather than abnormal catalytic activity, is the underlying mechanism.

Investigations

Tandem mass spectrometry (MS/MS) permits efficient identification of FAOD. With implementation in NBS programs, an increasing number of conditions of uncertain clinical significance have been detected. Most FAOD have a spectrum of clinical presentations, which make confirmatory diagnostic procedures necessary and have still to be agreed. Findings suggestive of a defect in mitochondrial β-oxidation can be obtained not only in plasma or serum, but also in dried blood spots. C8/C2 ratio and C8 are the most accurate biomarkers of MCAD deficiency, while in PCD low levels of free carnitine (C0) are characteristic. In CPT2 elevation of C12–C18 acylcarnitines, notably of C16 and C18:1, is seen. Ultimately, measurement of the respective enzyme activities reveals the enzymatic defect. Mutation analysis in index patients may be performed to facilitate early or prenatal diagnosis.

Treatment and management

In contrast to other metabolic diseases like glycogenoses or defects of the respiratory chain, effective treatment is possible for fatty acid oxidation disorders. Therapeutic strategies include dietary recommendations as well as medication. Due to limited experience, published recommendations have to be treated with caution and close clinical monitoring and individualized treatment approaches are warranted. Close collaboration between metabolic centers and primary care providers is necessary. Specific information should be given to the families with regard to the potential danger of acute illness and the need for prompt medical attention, and social support for the family should be provided when needed.

Routine management should include echocardiography, sonography, and neurophysiology. Laboratory tests should include blood sugar, pH, liver enzymes, urea, aldolase, lactate dehydrogenase, and creatine kinase, as well as plasma acylcarnitines, plasma fatty acid (free or total), urine organic acids, and urine acylglycines.

Regarding diet, low-fat, high-carbohydrate diets are recommended (70% carbohydrates, less than 20% fat), preferably with multiple small meals and avoidance of fasting. Catabolic states that may easily aggravate to severe crisis should be avoided at any rate; timely application of intravenous glucose is important in any situation where supply of carbohydrate fuels might be impaired, such as infections, diarrhea, or fasting. A high rate of glucose intake not only normalizes the plasma glucose level but also efficiently suppresses lipolysis, diminishing the production of toxic long chain acylcarnitines in the case of a long chain fatty acid oxidation defect, and probably the production of other toxic metabolites such as octanoate in the case of medium chain or short chain defects. Long-term exercise should be avoided.

For MCAD deficiency, medical management strategies include avoidance of medium chain triglycerides, frequent feeding to shorten periods of fasting, and prompt medical attention during conditions of increased metabolic demand. When enzyme activity exceeds 10%, even prolonged fasting might be tolerated under normal conditions, as has been shown.

In PCD, metabolic decompensation and skeletal and cardiac muscle functions improve with 100–400 mg/kg/day oral levocarnitine (L-carnitine) if it is started before irreversible organ damage occurs. Hypoglycemic episodes are treated with intravenous dextrose infusion. Cardiomyopathy requires management by specialists in cardiology. Echocardiogram and electrocardiogram should be performed annually during childhood and continue less frequently into adulthood. Plasma carnitine concentration should be closely monitored until levels reach the normal range, and can then be reduced to measures three times a year during infancy and early childhood, twice a year in older children, and annually in adults. It is sufficient to look at serum creatine kinase concentration and liver transaminases only during acute illnesses.

For CPT II, it is recommended to avoid known triggers and reduce the amount of long chain dietary fat while covering the need for essential fatty acids. A large fraction of calories should be provided as carbohydrates to reduce body fat utilization and prevent hypoglycemia. Approximately one-third of the calories should be given as medium even chain triglycerides (MCT). Metabolism of the 8–10 carbon fatty acids in MCT oil, for example, is independent of CPT I, carnitine/acylcarnitine translocase, CPT II, very long chain acyl-CoA dehydrogenase (VLCAD), trifunctional protein, and long chain hydroxy-acyl-CoA dehydrogenase deficiency (LCHAD) enzyme activities.

Prenatal diagnosis

Prenatal diagnosis of fatty acid disorders can be offered to all parents with an increased familial risk. All enzymes of mitochondrial fatty acid oxidation are expressed in chorionic villi biopsies as well as cultured chorionic villous fibroblasts and amniocytes.

When the molecular defect of the index patient is known, direct analysis of the genetic mutation can be performed.

Conclusion

Generally, a careful history has to be taken with a special focus on metabolic derangements like episodes of rhabdomyolysis, myoglobinuria, hypoglycemia, encephalopathy or Rye-like symptoms, and muscular or cardiac symptoms. Family history regarding myopathy, encephalopathy, or sudden infant death is also of prime importance. As outlined, symptomatology is often not specific, but should lead immediately to further diagnostic procedures. Once the defect is identified, specific recommendations for management are available.

Further reading

Houten SM, Wanders RJA. A general introduction to the biochemistry of mitochondrial fatty acid ß-oxidation. *J Inherit Metab Dis* 2010;33:469–477.

Lund AM, Skovby F, Vestergaard H, Christensen M, Christensen E. Clinical and biochemical monitoring of patients with fatty acid oxidation disorders. *J Inherit Metab Dis* 2010;33:495–500.

Matter D, Rinaldo D. Medium chain ccyl coenzyme A dehydrogenase deficiency. In *Genereviews at GeneTests: Medical Genetics Information Resource* 2000 (updated 2012); Copyright University of Washington, Seattle 1997–2006. http://www.genetests.org (accessed November 2015).

Olpin SE. Pathophysiology of fatty acid oxidation disorders and resultant phenotypic variability. *J Inherit Metab Dis* 2013;36:645–658.

Wieser T. CPT II deficiency. In *Genereviews at GeneTests: Medical Genetics Information Resource* 2000 (updated 2014); Copyright University of Washington, Seattle 1997–2006. http://www.genetests.org (accessed November 2015).

166 Disorders of amino acid, organic acid, and ammonia metabolism

Stephen Cederbaum

Department of Psychiatry, Pediatrics, and Human Genetics, University of California, Los Angeles (UCLA), Los Angeles, CA, USA

Inborn errors of amino acid and organic acid metabolism are a subgroup of genetic disorders that involve the transformation of metabolites in the body. Amino acid and organic acid pathways involve small molecules that generally are ingested in the diet or are the result of tissue breakdown during the catabolism that accompanies a variety of acute intercurrent illnesses. These disorders are generally inherited in an autosomal recessive manner, although some are sex linked. Like all genetic diseases, their severity is dependent on the degree of enzyme deficiency caused by the specific mutation, and the input of other genetic and environmental influences that are difficult to identify and quantify.

The age at diagnosis of these disorders is getting earlier every year. Newborn screening with tandem mass spectrometry, widely used in the Western world for a decade or more, is becoming more prevalent worldwide. Depending on the structure of the screening program, diagnoses may be made, or at least suggested, at a week of life or sooner. The impact on those disorders that have an acute early onset is limited, but for those with a more indolent presentation, such as phenylketonuria, or those due to mutations causing only partial enzyme deficiencies, it may be profound. An unfortunate byproduct of the newborn screening programs is the ascertainment of patients with mutations so mild that clinical disease would not have occurred and for whom needless medical intervention is a burden.

A second evolving technology is having a profound effect on our understanding of these biochemical disorders and may have an even greater effect in the developing world. The technology is rapid, massive parallel DNA sequencing, often called next-generation sequencing. It can replace laborious, less accurate enzymatic analysis, which has often involved the shipping of fragile biological samples great distances with narrow windows of specimen viability and safety. DNA sequencing can be the reference confirmatory modality for abnormal biomarker levels, but cannot always be used to indicate the severity of the disorder. Mutation analysis can be accomplished from DNA extracted from dried blood spots, and when desired can be used for prenatal diagnosis in future pregnancies. The cost is less than $1,000 per sample and is falling all the time.

Neonatal disorders

Maple syrup urine disease

Maple syrup urine disease (MSUD), sometimes referred to as maple syrup disease, is caused by a genetic deficiency in branched chain keto acid decarboxylase, an enzyme complex that is responsible for the decarboxylation of the keto acids of the three branched chain amino acids, leucine, isoleucine, and valine. Its name derives from the odor given off by a byproduct of isoleucine accumulation that has the sweet smell that to North Americans resembles that of maple syrup. The odor may be particularly apparent on the skin and in the earwax. The three branched chain amino acids accumulate in the body with leucine predominating. The symptoms appear to correlate most closely with the level of leucine, although the precise pathogenic mechanism is not known.

Epidemiology

The disorder is infrequent (1 per 180,000 newborns) in a randomly mating population, but has a higher prevalence in some inbred groups such as the Old Order Amish and their Mennonite brethren who migrated from Switzerland and Germany to the United States in the eighteenth century.

Clinical features

In the most severe form due to complete or nearly complete enzymatic deficiency, onset occurs in the neonatal period and symptoms progress rapidly. The infants appear normal at birth, but then begin to deteriorate neurologically and become flaccid, alternating with hypertonicity and eventually with opisthotonic posturing. The cry becomes high pitched and the patients become unresponsive and are dependent completely on intravenous or enteral tube feeding. Seizures and lethargy can be accompanied by a severely abnormal electroencephalogram (EEG) with spikes, polyspikes, and triphasic waves; severe slowing and even bouts of a burst-suppression pattern may be seen. Magnetic resonance imaging (MRI) shows a specific and recognizable pattern of cerebral edema that regresses completely with effective treatment. It is in these more severely affected patients where the odor of maple syrup is most likely to occur.

With greater residual enzyme activity, onset may be delayed for weeks or months and the severity of the neurological illness may be diminished. The most mildly affected patients may go undiagnosed and be asymptomatic for years, or suffer from such mild episodes of intoxication that they are likely to be ascribed to some non-genetic cause. Despite this, severe catabolism can cause a sufficient accumulation of leucine so that the brain edema that results can be fatal. It is noteworthy that specialists in inborn errors are not infrequently confronted with healthy infants who have an odor resembling maple syrup. Their plasma amino acid levels are normal and the

International Neurology, Second edition. Edited by Robert P. Lisak, Daniel D. Truong, William M. Carroll and Roongroj Bhidayasiri
© 2016 John Wiley & Sons, Ltd. Published 2016 by John Wiley & Sons, Ltd.

condition appears to be due to some element in their environment, as least one of which is the herb fenugreek.

Diagnosis

If not picked up in the new, expanded newborn screening by tandem mass spectrometry (MS/MS), the diagnosis is relatively easy to make. Plasma amino acid determination reveals high levels of leucine, isoleucine, and valine, the former sometimes rising as high as 3,000-4,000 μM (versus normal value <300 μM in all laboratories). An isomer of isoleucine, alloisoleucine, is present in virtually all patients and is pathognomonic for the disorder. Organic acid analysis of urine reveals the keto acids of these three amino acids as the proximate product behind the site of the block. Ketones are detected in the urine during routine urinalysis.

Treatment

Acute episodes occurring in the immediate postnatal period or periodically thereafter are medical emergencies. It is essential that plasma levels of leucine be reduced rapidly and effectively. This is accomplished in two ways, used separately or together. The first and usually quite reliable method in older patients or those less severely affected is to feed an amino acid mixture lacking the branched chain amino acid precursors of the deficient enzyme step. This should be undertaken in collaboration with a metabolic disease specialist to prevent catabolism and exacerbation of the episode. This regimen promotes protein synthesis and utilizes the accumulated branched chain amino acids to complete the amino acid pool. In newborns, "normalization" of leucine levels may occur in 24–36 hours. It may be slower in older children. Because isoleucine and valine levels fall more rapidly than leucine, the more proximate toxin in this disorder, both isoleucine and valine must be supplemented within 36–48 hours to prevent levels from falling below normal and acting as a stimulus to protein catabolism.

The second approach to lowering the amino acid levels is dialysis, which effectively removes the excess branched chain amino acids (as well as the others present in normal amounts) from the body fluid space. This must be used in conjunction with proper nutritional support or body protein catabolism will occur and the salutary effect will be lost.

Treatment of intercurrent catabolic episodes or of those patients presenting later in life is simpler. These events can often be managed with fluid and electrolyte support and administration of non-branched chain amino acids. As with the treatment of all inborn errors, attention to adequate caloric intake, prevention of constipation, and special intervention during intercurrent illness are required. More recently, improved outcomes with liver transplantation have made this a viable option as a more definitive therapy for MSUD. With transplantation, patients are able to eat a normal diet and do not have acute episodes of metabolic decompensation.

Urea cycle disorders

The urea cycle is an eight-step cycle consisting of six enzymes operating sequentially and two transporters, all of which are essential for the conversion of ammonia generated from either endogenous or exogenous amino acids to urea. The six enzymes are N-acetylglutamate synthase, carbamoylphosphate synthase I, ornithine transcarbamylase (OTC), argininosuccinate synthase, argininosuccinate lyase, and arginase. The two transporters are both in the mitochondrial membrane, one transporting ornithine and the second transporting aspartate into the mitochondrion. The complete absence of

any of the first five enzymes in the cycle results in severe neonatal hyperammonemia, rapid neurological deterioration, coma, and then death. Like other inborn errors of metabolism, urea cycle disorders cannot be distinguished from a variety of other acute conditions of the neonatal period, such as sepsis or perinatal hypoxia. An elevated plasma ammonia level accompanied by relatively normal electrolyte balance is highly suggestive of such a disorder.

Epidemiology

Seven of the eight disorders of the urea cycle are inherited in an autosomal recessive manner, whereas ornithine transcarbamylase deficiency (OTCD) is inherited in a sex-linked co-dominant manner. A moderately large minority of female carriers of OTCD (30–40%) have protein intolerance or worse, and some may die or suffer permanent brain damage from hyperammonemia, particularly during parturition. With the possible exception of deficiency of the aspartate transporter (citrin deficiency), which may be more prominent in people of Japanese ethnicity, none of the disorders has any particular ethnic or geographic predilection. In the recessive disorders both sexes are affected with equal severity.

Clinical features

Newborn patients present as a catastrophic encephalopathy, with lethargy, poor feeding, a weak cry and suck, hypotonia, coma, and death, if successful treatment is not instituted. Older patients may present with slurred speech, ataxia, tremors, and confusion. This can progress to lethargy, obtundation, coma, and death. Those with partial deficiencies may exhibit learning disabilities, hyperactivity, and psychiatric disorders. Sometimes a history of protein aversion may be elicited (see Table 166.1).

Pathophysiology and treatment

Severe neonatal hyperammonemia constitutes a medical emergency and must be addressed immediately. The levels of ammonia and glutamine (with which it is in approximate equilibrium) must be reduced as rapidly as possible and prior to any determination of the precise site of the block. The most effective means of carrying this out is hemodialysis, which is more effective than peritoneal dialysis and certainly more effective than exchange transfusion, which has little utility or efficacy. The most immediate response to severe

Table 166.1 Neurological manifestations of urea cycle disorders. Source: Gropman 2007. Adapted with permission of Springer.

Classic proximal urea cycle defects	Partial enzyme deficiencies
Anorexia	Protein aversion
Vomiting	Hyperactive behavior
Cognitive and motor deficits	Self-injurious behavior
Lethargy	Stroke-like episodes
Ataxia	Psychiatric symptoms
Asterixis	
Brain edema	
Cytotoxic and vasogenic edema	
Hypothermia	
Seizures	
Coma	

hyperammonemia should be dialysis. In some larger centers, intravenous sodium benzoate combined with sodium phenylacetate is available and may be used to divert the ammonia from the urea cycle, to be excreted as benzoylglycine and/or phenylacetylglutamine. The resynthesis of glycine and glutamine in the body will then utilize one or two molecules of ammonia destined for the urea cycle to this synthetic reaction. Nutritional support with the guidance of a metabolic specialist can prevent the development of a catabolic state during treatment.

Dialysis is a very effective method for reducing plasma ammonia and glutamine and the failure to do so, if it is being carried out effectively, is usually due to the ongoing catabolism in the body and the production of ammonia. When ammonia comes down to a level of 200 μM, it then becomes imperative to add an essential amino acid mixture to the high calories being provided intravenously by glucose and lipids in order to inhibit endogenous catabolism and allow the body to begin to recover in a relatively normal manner, and to reestablish a balance in protein synthesis and breakdown.

Hyperammonemia is the cause of the brain damage, possibly acting through glutamine, with which it is in equilibrium. The most obvious and visible effect of ammonia intoxication is cerebral edema, although a number of other pathological mechanisms may be operating simultaneously. The degree of neurological damage correlates best with the length of time the patient spends in a coma, and to a much lesser degree with the level of ammonia. Few patients escape severe neonatal hyperammonemia without permanent neurological injury. At this stage, specific therapy for each disorder generally does not occur, although the severity of argininosuccinic aciduria may be mitigated by high arginine infusion (600 mg/kg/day in an infant). Deficiency in arginine biosynthesis is characteristic of seven of the eight urea cycle disorders and a lesser amount of arginine is used empirically in acute hyperammonemia of unknown etiology.

Chronic treatment consists of adequate calories and fluids, a diet low in natural protein and supplemented with an essential amino acid formula and sodium phenylbutyrate. In developing countries phenylbutyrate may prove to be too expensive or otherwise unavailable, but sodium benzoate, which is readily available and inexpensive, may be a suitable, albeit less effective substitute.

Liver transplantation is a definitive treatment for the hyperammonemia associated with the more acute-onset hyperammonemias and the outcome in the large majority of patients is favorable; the prior brain damage will, of course, be irreversible.

Newborn screening is particularly useful in detecting milder cases of argininosuccinate synthetase and lyase and arginase deficiencies, but so far has proven less reliable in detecting disorders whose enzyme deficiencies occur earlier in the cycle.

Propionic and methylmalonic acidemia

These two disorders involve sequential steps in the disposition of the carbon skeletons of four amino acids, threonine, methionine, isoleucine, and valine. Defects in either propionyl-CoA carboxylase or methylmalonyl-CoA mutase cause the propionic acid or methylmalonic acid to accumulate behind the site of the block. Because propionic acid is a precursor of methylmalonic acid, it accumulates as well in methylmalonic acidemia. These metabolites are toxic to the brain, heart, and bone marrow and can cause severe illness and death in their most severe form. Methylmalonyl-CoA mutase requires an activated form of vitamin B_{12} as a cofactor. This B_{12} gets to the site of action only after having undergone a series of meta-

bolic steps. Inherited defects in any of these steps may also cause homocytinemia. The most common of these defects is referred to as cobalamin C deficiency and is characterized by elevated body fluid levels of both methylmalonic acid and homocysteine. Remethylation of homocysteine to methionine also requires an activated form of vitamin B_{12} and shares many metabolic steps with the activated form, which serves as a cofactor for the mutase reaction.

Epidemiology
Like any autosomal recessive disorder, forms of propionic and methylmalonic acidemia may be found in increased frequency in population isolates and/or in populations that practice cousin marriage as a social custom. No large ethnic or gender predilection has been described for either condition.

Clinical features
The largest number of patients with both disorders have severe enzyme deficiencies present in the newborn period. Initial symptoms include decreased suck, poor feeding, irritability, lethargy, hypotonia, and seizures, which progress to stupor and coma. In the past when these conditions were poorly recognized, death ensued in most instances. Other manifestations include bone marrow depression, acidosis, hyperammonemia, hypotonia, and cardiac failure. The signs and symptoms may mimic neonatal sepsis and the neonatologist should be alert to the possibility of conditions like this, particularly in suspected cases of sepsis that are atypical in some manifestation(s).

In those countries and jurisdictions in which newborn screening uses tandem mass spectrometry (MS/MS), the majority of patients with these disorders will be ascertained by an elevation in C3 carnitine esters on the dried blood spot. In these jurisdictions, the level of suspicion in patients who have had a successful newborn screen will be altered and the position of these disorders on the list of diagnostic possibilities will be lowered.

Laboratory abnormalities found in these disorders include metabolic acidosis with an increase anion gap, elevated blood lactate, ketonuria, hyperammonemia, and bone marrow depression. Ketonuria in a newborn is exceedingly rare and is a telltale sign of a disorder of organic acid metabolism.

Pathophysiology
The pathophysiology of these conditions is not known with certainty. The resemblance between propionyl-CoA and acetyl-CoA is great, and propionyl-CoA is thought to compete with acetyl-CoA for the active site of enzymes using the latter substrate, particularly the biosynthesis of acetylglutamate and activation of the urea cycle.

Treatment
In the initial phases of diagnosis, the two disorders may be indistinguishable until the results of newborn screening or diagnostic urinary organic acid analysis becomes available. The treatment will, therefore, be generic, seeking to reduce the level of accumulated toxic metabolite and simultaneously diminishing the production of the offending compound. The most effective way of lowering the levels of either of these readily excreted organic acids, which could accumulate rapidly in the period of catabolism following birth, is by dialysis. The most effective means of dialysis is hemodialysis, but when this is not available peritoneal dialysis is an acceptable alternative. Exchange transfusion is largely ineffective. Treatment should include vitamin B_{12}, 1000 mg intramuscularly daily, until

it is demonstrated that the patient does not have a vitamin B_{12}-responsive form of methylmalonic acidemia. Intravenous carnitine 300 mg/kg is a frequently recommended adjunct to therapy. The usual supportive measures of maintenance of electrolyte balance and hydration are important in these patients and in general follow nursery protocol.

Infants rescued from the most acute manifestations of these disorders often will have suffered irreversible neurological damage and may over a period of years show mental retardation, growth delay, and a variety of neurological disabilities. Remarkably, some patients who have suffered grievously in the newborn period do remarkably well developmentally and may go on to live normal or near normal lives. Most patients will, after rescue, continue to make developmental progress and may achieve varying degrees of independence in aspects of daily life. These patients are prone, particularly in infancy and early childhood, to episodes of metabolic deterioration usually caused by intercurrent infection. The cause of these less frequent episodes in later life may not be apparent. Both propionic and methylmalonic acids are anorexogenic, probably due to chemically induced pyloric stenosis. As a consequence, most patients require some or virtually all of their enteral feedings through a gastrostomy tube, at least in infancy and for the first decade of life.

The jury is still out on the efficacy of liver transplantation in the treatment of patients who are particularly refractory to metabolic stabilization. The number of episodes of metabolic deterioration is reduced or eliminated in virtually all transplanted patients, but neurological disease is not reversed and in some patients may continue to progress to the basal ganglia strokes characteristic of methylmalonic acidemia in particular. Adequate calories, a diet limited in the precursors of these organic acids, prevention of constipation, carnitine supplementation, and metronidazole (to decrease the production of propionic acid by gut bacteria) are mainstays of long-term therapy.

In all disorders of metabolism, partial enzyme defects due to less severe mutations in the gene may result in attenuated disease. This more mild disease may manifest as chronic low-level intoxication resulting in little to moderate brain damage, may cause later-onset severe metabolic deterioration in response to catabolic stress, or may not manifest until later in life in response to such events as pregnancy and partutrition. The physician should always be alert to the possibility that a metabolic disorder lies behind undiagnosed cases of developmental delay or recurring episodes of acute encephalopathy. Cobalamin C deficiency is the most common form of methylmalonic acidemia observed in some screening programs and it is distinguished by its more indolent onset and response to injections of hydroxyl-vitamin B_{12}.

Progressive diseases of infancy and childhood

In contrast to the disorders already described, a number of metabolic disorders are characterized by the absence of acute manifestations in the newborn period, but rather by progressive or more insidious developmental delay or neurological disability. This section will describe these disorders.

Phenylketonuria

The most common of these metabolic disorders in countries for which accurate statistics are available is phenylketonuria (PKU), a disorder caused by deficiency of the enzyme phenylalanine hydroxylase. When deficiency of this enzyme is complete or nearly so, plasma phenylalanine levels rise to levels of 1200 μM or more when the patient is ingesting breast milk or an otherwise normal diet. This causes no obvious immediate symptoms, but the intoxicating effect is insidious. Depending on the individual patient and the astuteness of the parent and/or the physician, manifestations become apparent between 6 months and 1 year of age, by which time some degree of irreversible neurological damage has occurred.

Lesser degrees of enzyme deficiency lead to lower levels of plasma phenylalanine accumulation and correspondingly lower levels of jeopardy for short- or longer-term neurological damage. Although normally newborn phenylalanine levels in blood fall rapidly to adult levels of 100 μM or less, individual patients may tolerate levels up to 600 μM or slightly more without apparent neurological damage. There is some suspicion, however, that these individuals may be prone to a higher incidence of learning disability or attention deficit disorder.

Phenylketonuria was the flagship disorder for which newborn screening was developed by Robert Guthrie. When properly carried out, nearly all cases of PKU can be detected by an elevation in blood phenylalanine and/or by an elevated phenylalanine/tyrosine ratio after 24 hours of age, and preemptive therapy can be instituted. Evidence suggests that virtually all of these individuals will be protected from overt neurological damage and mental retardation and may be allowed to achieve success in professions requiring higher cognitive function, such as academics, medicine, law, and others. Evidence also suggests that the brain is continuously vulnerable to high phenylalanine levels and that the therapy that will be described here will have to be lifelong.

The advent of newborn screening and effective therapy for PKU is one of the great success stories in the field of metabolic disorders. It has taken a disorder in which the incidence of mental retardation was virtually 100% and has reduced it to the background level found in the population. However, it has raised the specter of maternal PKU. In this disorder, normal women with PKU and high phenylalanine levels are at risk of having children who become intoxicated *in utero* and who suffer a variety of adverse effects including microcephaly, mental retardation (virtually universally), and, in 15% of cases, congenital heart defects. The imperative for females to stay on the diet is therefore increased.

Epidemiology

The incidence of PKU varies greatly between countries and ethnic groups. Aside from genetic isolates such as a group of Gypsies (Travelers) in Great Britain, the frequency varies between about 1 in 4,000 births in Ireland and Turkey, to 1 in 100,000 in Japan, to virtually undetectable levels in Finland and among Ashkenazi Jews.

Clinical features

Untreated PKU has become a virtual historical oddity in those places where newborn screening is routine. Even many metabolic specialists are unfamiliar with the clinical features of mental retardation, a withdrawn autistic-like demeanor, spasticity, a "mousey" odor, and pigment dilution in hair and skin. There is a recent report in an Asian population that describes West syndrome in 10.9% of PKU patients who were not treated in the first 6 months of life and in 15% of those in whom treatment was delayed until 1 year. The

MRIs showed delayed myelination and increased T2 signal in the periventricular regions. With treatment, the average IQ is near normal, but some patients, even when well treated, have an increased incidence of attention deficit disorder and academic difficulties.

Treatment

This therapy usually consists almost exclusively of dietary restrictions. The diet is simple, effective, and onerous. The maintenance of the diet requires continuous discipline on the part of the family and, as the patient grows older and assumes greater responsibility for his or her own care, on the part of that individual as well. All high-protein foods must be eliminated, since the average individual, particularly in countries that ingest a relatively higher-protein diet, may consume about three times as much phenylalanine as is required by the body for growth and maintenance. The natural food component of the diet, therefore, consists of fruits and vegetables with low protein content, as well as special foods such as breads, pastas, and rice from which protein has been removed. This diet, if ingested without supplementation of the other amino acids handled normally by the body, would cause malnutrition. The missing nutrients are made up of special amino acid formulas from which phenylalanine has either been removed or to which it has not been added. The main difficulty for many patients lies in the tedium of a diet that does not have a lot of variation, but to which, with imagination, spices and sauces can be added to make the foods far more palatable.

More recently, it has been discovered that a fraction of patients with phenylalanine hydroxylase deficiency may respond with increased enzyme activity to the addition of tetrahydrobiopterin (BH_4), the natural cofactor in the phenylalanine hydroxylase reaction (see later). This increases phenylalanine hydroxylase activity and boosts the degree of tolerance to phenylalanine in these patients. About 10% of patients with severe phenylalanine hydroxylase deficiency may be responsive in whole or in part to this treatment; approximately half with more moderate phenylalanine elevations on a natural diet may be responsive, and the majority of those with phenylalanine levels under 600 μM on a normal diet will respond. Tetrahydrobiopterin is an expensive product available in Europe and the United States, and in some other countries as well. All patients detected with elevated phenylalanine in the newborn period in more affluent countries will undergo a trial of BH_4 prior to the institution of the diet, and those who are responsive will, in those venues that can afford it, be maintained on this therapy while receiving no special diet or one that is far less stringent.

Recently there has been increased awareness that dietary supplements with high levels of large neutral amino acids may compete with phenylalanine for their shared intestinal transporter. This competition has been shown in limited studies to lower plasma phenylalanine levels by as much as 30%. This treatment may be particularly relevant in patients who are unable or unwilling to adhere to a low phenylalanine diet, who may respond partially to BH_4, and for whom the cost–benefit ratio of this treatment may be unfavorable. The need for an adult to take as many as 45 pills a day may be a deterrent to this therapy.

Tetrahydrobiopterin-deficient hyperphenylalaninemia

As already noted, the phenylalanine hydroxylase reaction requires a cofactor, BH_4, to carry out a complex oxidation reaction for which it is responsible. BH_4 is synthesized in the body from guanidine triphosphate (GTP) in a multistep process. In the course of the phenylalanine hydroxylase reaction, BH_4 is oxidized to BH_2 and must be regenerated by yet another enzyme, dihydropteridine reductase. A genetic deficiency in any of the enzymes in the biosynthesis of the pteridine or of the regeneration of BH_4 will lead to hyperphenylalaninemia that on the basis of phenylalanine levels alone cannot be distinguished from phenylalanine hydroxylase deficiency. Unfortunately, BH_4 functions as a cofactor in the hydroxylation of tyrosine to L-DOPA and of tryptophan to 5-hydroxytryptophan. These are both essential neurotransmitter precursors whose deficiency leads to an early-onset and relatively severe neurological condition that does not respond to the normalization of phenylalanine levels by diet.

Epidemiology

A number of conditions leading to BH_4 deficiency are inherited in an autosomal recessive manner. No unambiguous ethnic or geographic predilection for these conditions is known. In contrast to the West, in which BH_4 constitutes no more than 1% of the hyperphenylalaninemic population ascertained by newborn screening, the rate is closer to 10% in Japan. This is caused not by an increased frequency of these disorders, but rather by the lower frequency of phenylalanine hydroxylase deficiency.

Diagnosis

Symptoms most frequently occur in patients with hyperphenylalaninemia who respond appropriately with lowered phenylalanine levels in blood, but who continue to deteriorate neurologically. Symptoms include progressive neurological deterioration, variability in muscle tone, temperature instability, seizures, and abnormal movements.

Fortunately, this condition is generally ascertained in the newborn period by elevation of plasma phenylalanine, and it is now routine to do urinary pterin studies and measure dihydropteridine reductase in red blood cells and institute appropriate therapy rapidly. Early treatment vastly improves the outlook for these patients and allows them to be normal in many instances. Other disorders of neurotransmitter metabolism more distal to the hydroxylation reactions are not ascertained through elevation in plasma phenylalanine and are diagnosed when the index of suspicion is high by analyzing neurotransmitter metabolites in cerebral spinal fluid. The BH_4 deficiency syndromes are collectively referred to as biopterin-dependent hyperphenylalanemias.

Treatment

Treatment consists of BH_4 supplementation and the addition of L-DOPA (with carbidopa) and 5-OH-tryptophan to the regimen. The latter two drugs are widely available and are relatively inexpensive.

Homocystinuria (homocystinemia)

Classic homocystinuria was first described in 1968, simultaneously in retarded infants and in adults seen in an ophthalmology clinic. The latter are individuals who, for reasons unknown, escaped the retardation that often occurs in homocystinuria due to cystathionine β-synthase deficiency and who only later manifest a characteristic feature of the disorder, lens dislocation. Subsequently, those affected in an intermediate manner manifesting retardation at variable ages were found as well. The cardinal biochemical features are greatly elevated methionine in the blood and greatly elevated homocysteine in the blood and the urine to levels 10 times normal.

Methionine is a critical amino acid in the body and plays a role not only in protein synthesis but also as a major methyl group donor in methylation reactions, including the synthesis of neurotransmitters. The product of these methylation reactions is homocysteine, which may have two fates in the body. During periods of low or no methionine intake, a fraction of homocysteine that may be high as 50% is remethylated to methionine to allow physiological methylation reactions to continue. The other variable fraction is metabolized by cystathionine β-synthase, ultimately ending up as cysteine, another important but non-essential amino acid, with the excess as part of the carbon pool and as sulfate. Thus, lower levels of cysteine are a characteristic feature of homocystinuria.

Disorders of remethylation of homocysteine to methionine have been mentioned previously in the discussion of methylmalonic acidemia. While many, if not most, members of this family of disorders are ascertained by the elevated levels of plasma and urine levels of methylmalonic acid, those that involve homocysteine accumulation alone must be found through increased levels of this metabolite, or sometimes by low methionine levels.

Epidemiology

Cystathionine β-synthase deficiency is far less common than PKU and less is known about its population frequency in various countries. Therefore, no general ethnic predilection is known. It is the least frequent of any of the disorders discussed in this section.

The vascular features, at least, are thought to be largely caused by the elevations in homocysteine levels. The symptoms of cystathionine β-synthase deficiency alone will be discussed, as they are more distinctive than those of the remethylation defects, which share with it only the homocysteine-related predilection for precocious arterial and venous thrombosis. The cardinal clinical manifestations of "classic" homocystinuria are a thin and marfanoid-like habitus, mental retardation in a significant fraction of affected patients, a predisposition to arterial and venous thrombosis, and an elevated risk of stroke, osteopenia, and dislocation of the ocular lenses. It is easily ascertained by the presence of hypermethioninemia, although accurate measurement of levels of homocysteine requires an independent study in which the sulfhydryl bonds between homocysteine and the plasma proteins are broken. It cannot be reliably diagnosed by MS/MS-based newborn screening.

Treatment

When homocystinuria is diagnosed in infancy, the treatment is a rigid low-methionine diet with supplementation by a dietary product from which this amino acid is excluded. This diet is more rigorous and onerous than those for many other metabolic disorders and long-term compliance is difficult. However, outcome in early-treated patients may be quite good. Instituting this rigorous diet in adulthood is extremely problematic and compliance is typically poor. Because of the tendency toward precocious thrombosis, the use of aspirin and other antiplatelet aggregation medications is indicated. Prophylaxis for venous thrombosis is rarely specifically undertaken. In addition, betaine is useful in providing an alternative pathway from homocysteine back to methionine, and may work in an adjunctive fashion to lower the toxic levels of homocysteine. High levels of methionine are far less likely to be intoxicating or to cause symptoms. The remethylation defects also respond to treatment with betaine, vitamin B$_{12}$, and antiplatelet adhesion therapy. Folate supplementation is used in all of the hyperhomocysteinemias.

Disorders of lysine and tryptophan metabolism: Glutaric acidemia type I

Although a number of disorders in the breakdown of lysine are known, glutaric acidemia alone appears to have severe clinical consequences. This disorder, due to a deficiency of glutaryl-CoA dehydrogenase, may present in the newborn period, but more commonly presents with acute and devastating symptoms at a later stage in infancy and in association with intercurrent infection or, less frequently, another type of catabolic event. This should be distinguished from the misnamed glutaric acidemia type II, more properly called multiple acyl-CoA dehydrogenase deficiency (MADD). Biochemically, glutaric acidemia type I is characterized by the accumulation of glutarate and glutarylcarnitine in the blood and glutarate and 3-hydroxyglutarate in the urine. Unfortunately, some patients may have very low plasma and urine levels of these metabolites outside of the times when they are in metabolic crisis. Most, but not all, affected infants are picked up on newborn screening by MS/MS technology, and preemptive therapy is an important factor in eliminating or reducing the pathological consequences of this disorder. Newborn screening by MS/MS has, however, led to the diagnosis of a number of patients who never experience a metabolic crisis and no apparent intellectual or neurological deficit.

Epidemiology

Like maple syrup urine disease, glutaric acidemia type I appears in high frequency in the Old Order Amish community. It is also more frequent in the Ojibway Indian tribe of Canadian Indians. No other ethnic or national predilection is known.

Pathophysiology

Much effort has been invested into understanding the pathophysiology of this condition, but despite the availability of a reasonably faithful knockout mouse model, it remains to be elucidated. Genotype–phenotype correlation is poor, and the plasma and urine levels of glutarate do not seem to be an accurate gauge of the severity of clinical symptoms.

Clinical features

The majority of symptomatic patients present with macrocephaly, hypotonia, and a basal ganglia–type injury resulting in dystonia and athetosis. In some, spasticity eventually develops. The patients may be more devastated neurologically than they are cognitively, although many affected individuals are mentally retarded as well. Seizures may occur although they are not a defining part of the phenotype. In contrast to many other inborn errors of metabolism, there may be a characteristic MRI picture suggesting corticovenous lakes as a prominent feature and perhaps as a contributor to the macrocephaly that occurs. Macrocephaly may occur in asymptomatic patients.

Treatment

Therapy consists of a semisynthetic low-lysine diet and great care in the prevention of acute episodes of deterioration. Families are urged to come to the emergency room very quickly on the onset of infection, evidence that fluid and food intake is diminishing, or that the level of alertness is decreased. Supportive intravenous therapy with 10% glucose and insulin may prevent the development of acute neurological deterioration. A distinctive feature of this disorder in contrast to many others is the relative immunity to further neurological damage after emergence from infancy, and almost invariably after the age of 5 or 6 years. Carnitine and riboflavin supplementation is frequently used, but has never been subjected to rigorous study.

Biotinidase deficiency

Biotin is an essential vitamin whose requirement is mitigated by its reuse in the body. In normal metabolism, biotin is bound covalently to lysine groups on a number of enzymes with carboxylate carbon skeletons; these include propionyl-CoA carboxylase, methylcrotonyl-CoA carboxylase, pyruvate carboxylase, and acetyl-CoA carboxylase. When these enzymes are degraded, the biotinilated lysine or biocytin releases free biotin to be reutilized in a reaction catalyzed by biotinidase. In the absence of biotinidase, the biocytin is lost in the urine and the body becomes biotin deficient.

Pathophysiology

Patients with biotinidase deficiency excrete variable amounts of the precursors of each of the impaired enzymatic reactions and these were thought to be toxic. More recently, a far broader role for biotin in the regulation of gene expression has been found, so that the breadth of metabolic derangements that might be involved in the disease pathogenesis has grown.

Clinical features

Biotinidase deficiency rarely presents with symptoms in the neonatal period. The symptoms usually begin in the first few months of life and consist of skin rashes, alopecia, visual difficulties, hearing difficulties leading to deafness, and ultimately a neurological syndrome with developmental delay and retardation. In one series, 55% of the symptomatic children had seizures. In 38% of the enzyme-deficient patients, seizures were the presenting symptom. Patients may lose the ability to walk and become mute.

Biotinidase is easy to measure and is now a part of many newborn screening programs. Generally, individuals with biotinidase activity 10% or more of normal are usually free of symptoms; lower levels of activity occurring about 1 in 100,000 in many Western populations are generally required for the development of overt symptoms. In addition to the deficiency of biotinidase in plasma, the enzymatic defects that occur in consequence of deficiency of the normal cofactor lead to an abnormal acylcarnitine profile in plasma and urinary organic acid abnormalities in which metabolites of propionyl-CoA carboxylase, methylcrotonyl-CoA carboxylase, and pyruvate carboxylase accumulate. Unfortunately, the accumulation of these metabolites is variable and occurs after infancy, and there is not a reliable means of ascertaining this disorder by MS/MS technology.

Treatment

Biotinidase deficiency is readily treated with complete protection from neurological damage by administering 10–20 mg per day of biotin. The adequacy of therapy may be monitored using urinary organic acid analysis and more recently acylcarnitine analysis. Biotin therapy results in rapid control of medically refractory seizures in these patients and is accompanied by improvement in the EEG.

Further reading

Blau N, Duran M, Gibson KM, et al. (eds.). *Physicians Guide to the Diagnosis, Treatment and Followup of Metabolic Disease*, 2nd ed. New York: Springer-Verlag; 2014.
Gropman AL, Summar M, Leonard JV. Neurological implications of urea cycle disorders. *J Inher Metab Dis* 2007;30:865–869.
OMIM (Online Mendelian Inheritance in Man). http://www.ncbi.nlm.nih.gov/sites/entrez?db=omim (accessed November 2015).
Saudubray J-M, van den Berghe G, Walter JH (eds.). Inborn Metabolic Diseases: Diagnosis and Treatment, 5th ed. New York: Springer-Verlag; 2012.
Valle D (ed.). *The Online Metabolic and Molecular Bases of Inherited Disease*. New York: McGraw-Hill Medical. http://OMMBID.MHMedical.com/book.aspx?bookid=971 (accessed November 2015).

167 Pediatric neurotransmitter diseases

Stephen R. Deputy

Department of Neurology, Louisiana State University School of Medicine, Louisiana State University Health Sciences Center, New Orleans, LA, USA

The pediatric neurotransmitter disorders represent a challenging group of rare neurometabolic disorders classified on the basis of alterations in neurotransmitter metabolic pathways. The disorders are currently classified into disturbances of monoamines (dopamine, serotonin, and norepinephrine) and gamma-aminobutyric acid (GABA) metabolism. One of the challenging aspects of these disorders is their varied clinical presentation, ranging from mental retardation to epilepsy to movement disorders. Another challenging aspect is their diagnosis, which often relies on measuring neurotransmitter metabolites in the cerebrospinal fluid (CSF), as analysis of amino acids in the plasma and organic acids in the urine are uninformative. Disorders of monoamine metabolism include guanosine triphosphate (GTP) cyclohydrolase I deficiency, tyrosine hydroxylase deficiency, aromatic L-amino acid decarboxylase deficiency, and sepiapterin reductase (SR) deficiency. Disorders that fall under the spectrum of GABA metabolism include succinic semialdehyde dehydrogenase deficiency, pyridoxine-dependent epilepsy, and GABA-transaminase deficiency.

Pathophysiology

The normal synthesis and metabolism of the monoamine neurotransmitters serotonin, dopamine, and norepinephrine and their analyzable metabolites are shown in Figure 167.1. Figure 167.2 shows the synthesis and metabolic pathways of GABA. Figure 167.3 shows the metabolism of pyridoxine to its active metabolite pyridoxal-5-phosphate.

Monoamine neurotransmitter disorders

DOPA-responsive dystonias

The DOPA-responsive dystonias all share the biochemical feature of impaired synthesis of dopamine and the clinical feature of improved symptoms in response to treatment with oral L-DOPA. To date, there have been three identified disorders that fall into this category: GTP-cyclohydrolase I deficiency, tyrosine hydroxylase deficiency, and sepiapterin reductase deficiency. Figure 167.4 gives

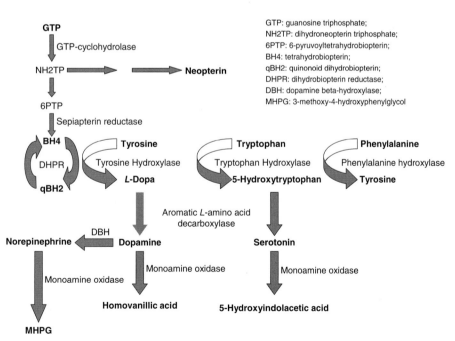

GTP: guanosine triphosphate;
NH2TP: dihydroneopterin triphosphate;
6PTP: 6-pyruvoyltetrahydrobiopterin;
BH4: tetrahydrobiopterin;
qBH2: quinonoid dihydrobiopterin;
DHPR: dihydrobiopterin reductase;
DBH: dopamine beta-hydroxylase;
MHPG: 3-methoxy-4-hydroxyphenylglycol

Figure 167.1 Monoamine metabolism.

International Neurology, Second edition. Edited by Robert P. Lisak, Daniel D. Truong, William M. Carroll and Roongroj Bhidayasiri

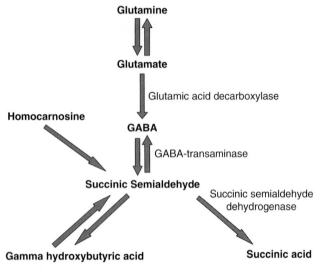

Figure 167.2 GABA metabolism.

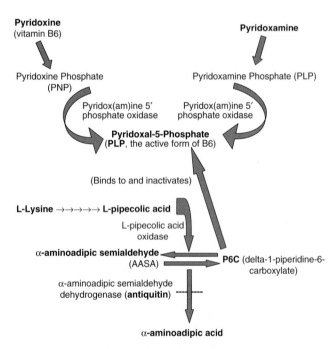

Figure 167.3 Pyridoxal-5-phosphate and cerebral lysine metabolism.

CSF Metabolite	CGH-I Deficiency	TH Deficiency	SPR Deficiency
Biopterin	↓	Normal	Normal to Mildly ↑
Neopterin	↓	Normal	↑
HVA	Normal to mildly ↓	↓	↓↓
5-HIAA	Normal to mildly ↓	Normal	↓↓
MHPG	Normal to mildly ↓	↓	↓

Figure 167.4 Comparison of DOPA-responsive disorders.

GTP-cyclohydrolase I catalyzes the first step of tetrahydrobiopterin synthesis from GTP. Tetrahydrobiopterin is an essential cofactor for tyrosine hydroxylase, tryptophan hydroxylase, and phenylalanine hydroxylase (see Figure 167.1). These enzymes are responsible for the synthesis of dopamine (phenylalanine hydroxylase and tyrosine hydroxylase) as well as for serotonin (tryptophan hydroxylase). Reduced enzymatic activity of GTP-cyclohydrolase I also results in reduced formation of neopterin.

Clinical symptoms usually begin with monomelic postural dystonia (often pes equinovarus) beginning at early school age, which then gradually progresses to affect all extremities over the next 10–15 years. There is a marked diurnal fluctuation of the dystonia severity at the onset of the disease that diminishes over time. GTP-cyclohydrolase I deficiency is often mistaken for cerebral palsy, which is not progressive and does not show diurnal fluctuation of symptoms. On physical examination, deep tendon reflexes are exaggerated with flexor plantar responses. Linear growth is often impaired, whereas cognitive function is usually spared. Clinically, there is a marked, sustained improvement of all neurological deficits in response to low doses of orally administered L-DOPA. Prolonged use of L-DOPA does not tend to produce dyskinesias, as it often does with Parkinson's disease. Neuroimaging studies are generally normal.

The pathophysiology of GTP-cyclohydrolase I deficiency results from reduced levels of dopamine within the striatum without destruction of the dopamine nerve terminals. Tyrosine hydroxylase activity is also markedly reduced within the striatum.

The diagnosis of GTP-cyclohydrolase I deficiency is strongly suggested by reduced levels of tetrahydrobiopterin, neopterin, homovanillic acid, and 5-hydroxyindolacetic acid in the CSF. The disease can also be genetically confirmed in 60% of patients who exhibit mutations of the *GCH1* gene. An initial trial of low dose L-DOPA may be undertaken in those patients with clinical features of GTP-cyclohydrolase I deficiency. This intervention usually results in significant and sustained improvement of the dystonia. As such, this may be a more affordable approach to making the diagnosis compared to gene sequencing or CSF analysis of neurotransmitter metabolites.

Tyrosine hydroxylase deficiency

Tyrosine hydroxylase (TH) catalyzes the hydroxylation of tyrosine to L-DOPA. This reaction requires reduced tetrahydrobiopterin, which serves as a cofactor (see Figure 167.1). TH is the rate-limiting step in the biosynthesis of the catecholamines dopamine and norepinephrine (and ultimately epinephrine). TH deficiency is a rare, autosomal recessive disorder caused by pathological biallelic

a quick reference to the biochemical differences found among these disorders within the CSF.

GTP-cyclohydrolase I deficiency (GCH-1 deficiency, Segawa disease)

This autosomal dominant form of DOPA-responsive dystonia was first described by Masaya Segawa in 1971 as a hereditary progressive basal ganglia disease with marked diurnal fluctuation. GTP-cyclohydrolase I deficiency is caused by mutations of the *GCH1* gene located on 14q22.1–q22.2. There is a female:male ratio of 3:1 due to less complete penetrance in males than in females. The worldwide incidence is estimated to be at least 1:1000000, as the disorder may often go undiagnosed.

mutations of the TH gene, which has been mapped to chromosome 11p15.5.

Children with autosomal recessive TH deficiency may present with progressive hypokinesia and rigidity with overriding dystonia within the first year of life. These patients generally respond fairly well to oral L-DOPA therapy. An earlier, more complex presentation of TH deficiency consists of infantile encephalopathy with bradykinesia, hypotonia, myoclonus, ptosis, and oculogyric crises. Life-threatening paroxysmal episodes of lethargy, sweating, body temperature instability, and drooling are common. Only the motor manifestations of the early-onset form of TH deficiency are partially responsive to treatment with L-DOPA; the encephalopathy and autonomic crises are not.

A diagnosis of TH deficiency may be suggested by elevated serum prolactin levels due to reduced dopamine production and subsequent diminished aminergic inhibition of prolactin secretion. Diagnosis of TH deficiency is confirmed by the findings of low or undetectable levels of homovanillic acid and 3-methoxy-4-hydroxyphenylglycol (MHPG) in the CSF. These are the end products of dopamine and norepinephrine metabolism, respectively. In addition, normal levels of biopterin and 5-hydroxy-indolacetic acid are found in the CSF, reflecting normal synthesis of tetrahydrobiopterin and serotonin that are not affected by deficient tyrosine hydroxylase activity (see Figure 167.1).

Sepiapterin reductase deficiency

Only 12 known cases of sepiapterin reductase (SR) deficiency have been reported in the literature. All have shown dystonia with spasticity and psychomotor retardation. SR is responsible for the conversion of 6-pyruvoyl-tetrahydrobiopterin (6PTP) to tetrahydrobiopterin (BH4). As previously mentioned, reduced biopterin in the form of BH4 serves as an essential cofactor for tyrosine, tryptophan, and phenylalanine hydroxylase enzymes. Hence, diagnosis of SR deficiency rests on the presence of elevated biopterin and neopterin in the presence of reduced levels of 5-hydroxyindolacetic acid and homovanillic acid in the CSF (see Figure 167.1). This disorder is felt to be transmitted in an autosomal recessive pattern and the SR gene has been mapped to chromosome 2p14–p12. Treatment has been attempted with L-DOPA and 5-hydroxytryptophan, with variable success.

Other monoamine neurotransmitter disorders

Aromatic *L*-amino acid decarboxylase deficiency

Aromatic *L*-amino acid decarboxylase deficiency (AADC), which requires pyridoxine (vitamin B$_6$) as a cofactor, is responsible for decarboxylating L-DOPA and 5-hydroxytryptophan into dopamine and serotonin, respectively (see Figure 167.1). AADC deficiency results in a combined catecholamine and serotonin deficiency. The rare disorder is transmitted in an autosomal recessive pattern and is caused by mutations within the dopa decarboxylase (aromatic *L*-amino acid decarboxylase) (*DDC*) gene mapped to chromosome 7p12.2.

Children with AADC deficiency share a characteristic movement disorder that is present by 6 months of age and consists of intermittent oculogyric crises with limb dystonia and athetosis. Ocular convergence spasm, myoclonic jerks, orofacial dystonia, limb tremor, blepharospasm, and breath-holding spells have been frequently reported. Autonomic dysfunction, including paroxysmal sweating, impaired gastric motility with reflux, hypothermia, sudden cardiorespiratory arrest, and abnormal sympathetic modulation of heart rate and systolic blood pressure have been reported.

All children reported have variable degrees of mental retardation and several have epilepsy. Treatment with dopamine receptor agonists and monoamine oxidase inhibitors has been reported to reduce the frequency of paroxysmal spells and to improve voluntary movements, although many patients suffer from dyskinesias. While all patients are treated with supplemental pyridoxine, no obvious direct benefit has been reported.

Diagnosis is based on the findings of low levels of homovanillic acid and 5-hydroxyindolacetic acid, elevated levels of L-DOPA, 5-hydroxytryptophan, and 3-*O*-methyldopa levels, and normal pterin levels in the CSF. Many patients have also been noted to have markedly increased urinary secretion of L-DOPA, 5-hydroxtryptophan, and 3-methoxytyrosine.

GABA neurotransmitter disorders

Succinic semialdehyde dehydrogenase deficiency (SSADH deficiency, 4-hydroxybutyric aciduria)

Succinic semialdehyde dehydrogenase (SSADH) is necessary for the degradation of GABA (see Figure 167.2). In SSADH deficiency, GABA is preferentially metabolized to gamma-hydroxybutyric acid (GHB), which accumulates and becomes the primary neurotoxic metabolite in this disorder. This disorder is transmitted in an autosomal recessive manner and the gene for SSADH, *ALDH5A1*, has been mapped to chromosome 6p22.

Presenting clinical features may vary, although the most consistent clinical findings are those of developmental delay and hypotonia. Ataxia is frequent and generally improves slightly over time. Many patients also suffer from agitation, insomnia, hyperactivity, hallucinations, aggression, and self-injurious behavior. Absence and convulsive seizures have been reported in about half of patients, despite elevated GABA levels. Magnetic resonance imaging (MRI) has revealed in some patients an increased T2 signal within the globus pallidus and subcortical white matter bilaterally, and MR spectroscopy has shown elevated peaks of GABA and GABA metabolites when they have been specifically evaluated.

Diagnosis is based on the presence of elevated levels of 4-hydroxybutyric acid on urinary organic acid analysis. Other GABA metabolites, such as 3,4-dihydroxybutyric acid, 3-oxo-4-hydroxybutyric acid, and glycolic acid, may also be identified. Unlike other disorders of organic acid and fatty acid metabolism, metabolic acidosis and hypoglycemia are not features of SSADH deficiency. CSF analysis has shown significant elevations of GHB and free GABA. SSADH deficiency is confirmed either through analysis of the SSADH enzymatic activity of leukocytes or through sequencing of the *ALDH5A1* gene.

Treatment has been attempted with vigabatrin, an irreversible inhibitor of GABA transaminase, which should theoretically inhibit the formation of succinic semialdehyde and therefore GHB. The treatment response has been limited at best, however. Symptomatic treatment of epilepsy with lamotrigine or carbamazepine has been shown anecdotally to be more effective. There is a theoretical contraindication to valproate use, as it may inhibit residual SSADH activity.

Pyridoxine-dependent epilepsy

Most children with pyridoxine-dependent epilepsy (PDE) present in the neonatal period with frequent seizures and an epileptic encephalopathy that are unresponsive to traditional anticonvulsant medications. It is an autosomal recessive disorder with a point prevalence that ranges from 1:20000 in Germany (where pyridoxine challenges in neonatal seizures are quite common) to 1:687000 in the United Kingdom and Ireland for definite and probable cases. The diagnosis of definitive PDE is suggested by the complete cessation of seizures within 7 days of pyridoxine administration, the recurrence of seizures following withdrawal of pyridoxine, and the subsequent remission of seizures when pyridoxine is readministered. While most children present in the newborn period, convincing cases with epilepsy onset as late as 7 years of age have been reported. While the full spectrum of clinical symptomatology has not been fully elucidated, some children with PDE appear to be cognitively normal, whereas others have been reported to have autism or mental retardation. Seizure types vary from infantile spasms to recurrent partial motor seizures, generalized convulsive seizures, and/or myoclonus.

Diagnosis of PDE is suggested by normalization of the interictal electroencephalogram (EEG) and cessation of seizures following intravenous injection of 50–100 mg of pyridoxine. If there is not an immediate clinical and electrical response to this dose, additional dosages of 100 mg of pyridoxine given every 10–15 minutes may be administered up to a total 500 mg to determine whether a response exists. Pyridoxine, through its active metabolite, PLP, is an essential cofactor for glutamic acid decarboxylase and is necessary for the conversion of glutamic acid into GABA (see Figure 167.3). Patients with PDE who are treated with intravenous pyridoxine may become hypotonic and apneic due to the sudden increase in CSF GABA concentrations, and artificial respiration may be required. There are, however, reported cases of PDE who do not immediately respond to intravenous pyridoxine, but who do gradually but completely respond to ongoing oral pyridoxine administration at dosages of 30/mg/kg/day.

Most patients with PDE have been found to have point mutations in the *antiquitin* gene (*ALDH7A1*) on chromosome 5q31. This gene encodes the enzyme alpha-aminoadipic semialdehyde dehydrogenase, which is part of the cerebral lysine degradation pathway (see Figure 167.3). Dysfunction of this enzyme leads to accumulations of alpha-aminoadipic semialdehyde (AASA) as well as delta-1-piperidine-6-carboxylate (P6C) and *L*-pipecolic acid in serum, urine, and CSF. P6C inactivates pyridoxal-5-phosphate, which is the active form of pyridoxine. Several children with PDE have been found to have significant elevations of pipecolic acid in the serum prior to administration of pyridoxine treatment and milder elevations that have persisted once treatment was begun. Likewise, significant elevations of serum and urine AASA have been reported in PDE even after treatment.

Once a diagnosis of PDE is confirmed (either through pyridoxine treatment criteria or by documenting elevated levels of serum pipecolic acid or AASA), ongoing maintenance therapy with oral pyridoxine at dosages ranging from 50–200 mg/day or more should be instituted. The dosage should be titrated upward until all seizures stop. Titrating the dosage until there is normalization of CSF glutamate levels has also been suggested.

Two other forms of vitamin-responsive neonatal epileptic encephalopathies are folinic acid–responsive seizures and pyridoxal phosphate-dependent seizures.

With folinic acid–responsive seizures, patients respond to supplemental treatment with 2.5 mg folinic acid twice a day. High-performance liquid chromatography (HPLC) of CSF neurotransmitter metabolites has revealed a pattern of two unidentifiable chemicals not seen in other patients. Of even more clinical interest is that in some cases of folinic acid–responsive seizures, patients were shown to have elevations of AASA and pipecolic acid in the CSF as well as mutations in the *ALDH7A1* gene, suggesting that these patients are identical to PDE patients, with the exception of the two unidentified chemicals on the HPLC CSF analysis. Other patients who have shown variable degrees of clinical and electrographic response to pyridoxine have responded well to the combination of folinic acid and pyridoxine.

Pyridoxal phosphate–dependent seizures do not respond to pyridoxine administration, but rather to pyridoxal-5-phosphate (PLP) administration. The disorder is believed to be caused by deficient pyridoxamine phosphate oxidase, which converts both pyridoxine phosphate and pyridoxamine phosphate to PLP, the active form of pyridoxine (see Figure 167.3). This disorder has been linked to mutations in the *PNPO* gene, which encodes the enzyme pyridoxamine 5'-phosphate oxidase and is inherited in an autosomal recessive fashion. Diagnosis of pyridoxal phosphate-dependent seizures can be evaluated by a challenge of pyridoxal phosphate (not pyridoxine) at 50 mg/kg intravenously, followed by 12.5 mg/kg by mouth every 6 hours to look for a significant reduction or elimination of seizures. Some authors have even suggested starting neonates or older children with unexplained refractory epilepsy or infantile spasms on pyridoxal phosphate and bypassing the pyridoxine challenge, since PLP is the active form of pyridoxine that is inactivated in pyridoxine-dependent epilepsy and produced in reduced amounts in pyridoxal phosphate-dependent seizures (see Figure 167.3).

GABA transaminase deficiency

GABA transaminase (GT) deficiency is an extremely rare disorder of GABA catabolism that has been reported in only two families. The affected children had early-onset generalized convulsions that were unresponsive to treatment, along with lethargy, hypotonia, feeding difficulties, and hyperreflexia. EEGs have shown a burst-suppression pattern in all affected patients. CSF analysis revealed elevated levels of GABA and homocarnosine (see Figure 167.2). The disease has been fatal by 2 years of age in all three affected patients.

Conclusion

Pediatric neurotransmitter diseases are a heterogeneous group of disorders affecting the synthesis or metabolism of GABA or the monoamine neurotransmitters. Several of these disorders, such as the dopa-responsive dystonias and pyridoxine-dependent epilepsy, can be diagnosed and treated with a combination diagnostic and therapeutic trial of neurotransmitter precursors or cofactors. More sophisticated diagnostic genetic testing or neurotransmitter metabolite analysis can be used to confirm the diagnosis in affected patients.

Further reading

Charlesworth G, Bhatia K, Wood N. The genetics of dystonia: New twists in an old tale. *Brain* 2013;136:2017–2037.

De Vivo D, Johnston MJ. Supplement: Pediatric neurotransmitter diseases. *Ann Neurol* 2003;54(6):S1–S109.

Gospe, SM. Neonatal vitamin-responsive epileptic encephalopathies. *Chang Gung Med J* 2010;33(1):1–12.

Plecko B, Paul K, Paschke E, *et al*. Biochemical and molecular characterization of 18 patients with pyridoxine-dependent epilepsy and mutations of the antiquitin (ALDH7A1) gene. *Hum Mutat* 2007;28(1):19–26.

Wang HS, Chou ML, Hung PC, *et al*. Pyridoxal phosphate is better than pyridoxine for controlling idiopathic intractable epilepsy. *Arch Dis Child* 2005;90:512–515.

168 Mitochondrial encephalomyopathies

Stacey K. H. Tay[1], Caterina Garone[2], and Salvatore DiMauro[3]

[1] Department of Paediatrics, Yong Loo Lin School of Medicine, National University of Singapore, Singapore
[2] Medical Research Council Mitochondrial Biology Unit, Cambridge, UK
[3] Department of Neurology, Columbia University Medical Center, New York, USA

Mitochondrial diseases are a heterogeneous group of disorders characterized by impaired mitochondrial function. Because of the ubiquitous distribution of mitochondria in tissues, clinical phenotypes involve multiple organ systems and often encompass a bewildering variety of symptoms. Mitochondrial function is especially important in tissues with high-energy requirements such as brain and skeletal muscle, so it is not unusual for symptoms to predominantly affect those tissues. Given the functional complexity of the nervous system, the neurological manifestations of mitochondrial diseases are diverse and include seizures, cognitive regression or dementia, ataxia, myoclonus, strokes, migraine, myopathy, and peripheral neuropathy. However, some patients may have isolated organ involvement, most frequently isolated myopathy, whereas others have multisystemic disorders that may progressively involve more organ systems with age. Because many respiratory chain disorders involve both the brain and skeletal muscle, they are also known as "mitochondrial encephalomyopathies" and they are the subject of this chapter.

Given the complexity of phenotypes, it is not surprising that mitochondrial diseases are often at the top of the differential diagnosis of "difficult-to-diagnose patients." Nonetheless, there are important clinical clues that can orient clinicians toward the correct diagnosis. This chapter aims to give an overview of current knowledge and recent advances on the genetics of mitochondrial diseases affecting both central and peripheral nervous systems.

Mitochondrial genetics

Genomic organization

Mitochondria are relics of bacterial intruders that developed a symbiotic relationship with proto-eukaryotic cells over a billion years ago. A positive consequence of this "invasion" is that mitochondria have conferred on these cells the ability to meet cellular energy requirements by using oxygen as a substrate. This unusual relationship also resulted in mitochondria retaining their original circular DNA (mtDNA), which encodes only 13 of the approximately 90 proteins of the respiratory chain (Figure 168.1). Thus, the mitochondria are "slaves" of the nuclear genome, because most proteins of the respiratory chain are themselves components of individual complexes, while many other proteins assemble individual

complexes. Other proteins encoded by nuclear DNA (nDNA) are in charge of controlling mtDNA translation; others are needed to put together the phospholipids of the inner mitochondrial membrane (IMM), to direct mitochondrial dynamics (motility, fission, and fusion), and many are needed for mtDNA maintenance (replication and integrity of mtDNA). Together, the 13 mtDNA-encoded and the more than 75 nDNA-encoded proteins of the respiratory chain are assembled into five enzyme complexes embedded in the inner mitochondrial membrane (IMM), where electron transfer and proton translocation generate adenosine triphosphate (ATP) through the action of a magnificent "turbine" complex V (ATP synthase).

The human mitochondrial genome is a double-stranded circle of 16569 base pairs and contains only 37 genes, of which 13 encode essential polypeptides and the rest form the ribosomal machinery necessary for protein translation: two ribosomal RNAs (12S and 16S rRNA) and 22 transfer RNAs (tRNAs). As already mentioned, the thirteen polypeptides are subunits of the respiratory chain: seven subunits of complex 1 (ND1, 2, 3, 4, 4L, 5, and 6), one subunit of complex III (cytochrome b), three subunits of complex IV, or cytochrome c oxidase (*COXI*, *COXII*, and *COXIII*), and two subunits of ATP synthase (ATPase 6 and ATPase 8). To date, about 200 pathogenic point mutations of mtDNA have been described, and the number of nuclear gene mutations is expected to be much more numerous and is rapidly escalating.

Replication, transcription, and translation of mtDNA

Some features of mtDNA replication are reminiscent of bacterial DNA replication. Replication of mtDNA is controlled by a combination of RNA and DNA polymerases that synthesize the daughter strands simultaneously in a bidirectional fashion. The mitochondrial replisome is thought to consist of several proteins: polymerase γ (POLG), Twinkle (with 5′ to 3′ helicase activity), and a mitochondrial single-stranded binding protein. Replication ends with the formation of a pair of circles, each containing a double helix of one "parent" strand and one "daughter" strand. This pair of catenated circles is then separated by topoisomerase II.

The mode of mtDNA replication has been under debate. According to the original "Clayton model," replication was thought to occur by strand displacement, in which the origin of replication is in the heavy G and T nucleotide-rich strand (O_H). A short stretch of

International Neurology, Second edition. Edited by Robert P. Lisak, Daniel D. Truong, William M. Carroll and Roongroj Bhidayasiri
© 2016 John Wiley & Sons, Ltd. Published 2016 by John Wiley & Sons, Ltd.

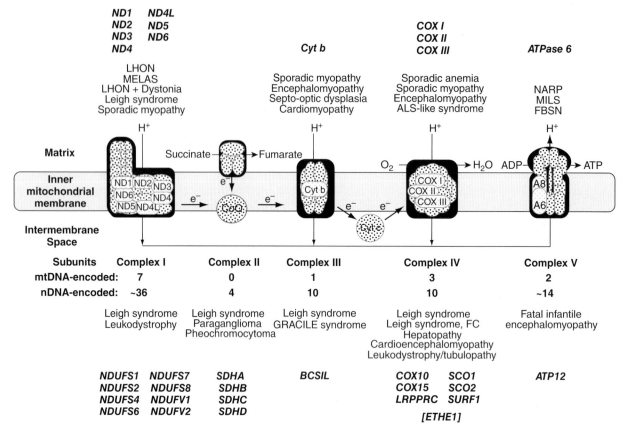

Figure 168.1 Schematic view of the mitochondrial respiratory chain, showing subunits encoded by nuclear DNA (nDNA) in blue and subunits encoded by mitochondrial DNA (mtDNA) in red. As electrons (e^-) flow down the electron-transport chain, protons (H^+) are pumped from the matrix to the intermembrane space through complexes I, III, and IV, then back into the matrix through complex V (ATP synthetase). Coenzyme Q (CoQ) and cytochrome c (Cyt c) are electron carriers. The genes responsible for mitochondrial disorders are listed above or below the clinical entities.

RNA is needed to prime DNA synthesis from O_H and binds to the lighter C and A nucleotide-rich L strand, displacing a portion of H strand in the O_H region (the so-called displacement loop or "D-loop"). As replication progresses and reaches the "8 o'clock" position of the circle, synthesis of the light strand begins at the origin of light strand replication (O_L) and proceeds in the opposite direction. The alternative "Holt model" is a modification of the classic bacterial "theta" replication, named after the shape of the DNA generated by the bidirectional replication from a single origin. Recent two-dimensional gel electrophoresis studies support this latter model, in which the mechanism of leading and lagging strands of DNA replication is coordinated.

MtDNA transcription is also reminiscent of the bacterial system in that the mtDNA genes are transcribed in two giant 16 kb polycistronic precursor transcripts, cleaved precisely from precursor RNAs, and processed to produce individual tRNA and mRNA molecules.

Translation of the mitochondrial mRNAs takes place on mitochondrial ribosomes and involves the mtDNA-encoded 12 S and 16 S rRNAs as well as imported ribosomal proteins. The mtDNA genetic code differs from the "universal code" of nDNA at 4 of the 64 triplet positions: AUA specifies methionine instead of isoleucine; UGA specifies tryptophan instead of stop codon; and AFA and AGG encode stop codons instead of arginine.

Mitochondrial DNA inheritance and transmission

Human mtDNA is maternally inherited. A woman transmits her mtDNA to all her children regardless of gender, but only her daughters will pass their mitochondria on to their children. Paternal mitochondria are known to enter the ovum at fertilization, but are destroyed selectively through an unknown mechanism. It has been reported that a patient with mitochondrial myopathy and a two base pair (bp) pathogenic deletion in the *ND1* gene had inherited most of his muscle mtDNA (but not the mutation) from his father. However, this appears to be a rare exception and maternal inheritance of mtDNA is still the rule. Current genetic counseling still considers that fathers with mtDNA mutations do not risk transmitting the defect to their children.

A mutation in mtDNA can affect all genomes (which is known as homoplasmy) or only some genomes. The latter results in the coexistence of two mtDNA populations, which is known as heteroplasmy. Neutral mutations (polymorphisms) are usually homoplasmic, whereas most–but not all–pathogenic mutations are heteroplasmic. Both homoplasmic and heteroplasmic mtDNA mutations are transmitted to all maternal offspring. Genetic counseling, however, becomes complicated for disorders due to homoplasmic mtDNA mutations, because nuclear genetic factors are important in regulating the expression of the disease. In Leber's hereditary optic neuropathy (LHON), for example, 50% of males and only 10%

of females develop impaired vision, implying the involvement of a genetic modifier. Environmental factors are also important in the expression of diseases associated with homoplasmic mtDNA mutations. For example, the 12 S rRNA A1555G mutation causes sensorineural hearing loss only following exposure to aminoglycoside antibiotics.

Heteroplasmic mtDNA mutations may be transmitted to the offspring in different proportions because of the genetic bottleneck, during which there is a random shift of mutation load from the primordial germ cell to primary oocytes, and also at implantation, when the cells of the inner cell mass multiply to populate the embryo. The "bottleneck hypothesis" states that the number of mtDNAs transmitted from mother to child is quite small, so that–even if the germ line is heteroplasmic–purification to homoplasmy can progress within a few generations. Heteroplasmic patients have inherited pathogenic mutations that have slipped through the mitochondrial bottleneck between mother and child. Therefore, the mutation load may vary widely and unpredictably between individuals in the same family. On the other hand, certain pathogenic homoplasmic mutations may be seen rarely, because they may result in oocyte failure or embryonic lethality.

Heteroplasmy and threshold effect

Each mitochondrion contains 2–10 copies of mtDNA, and each cell contains hundreds of mitochondria, depending on oxidative demands. In conditions of heteroplasmy, mutant mtDNAs coexist with wild-type genomes, and the clinical features of the corresponding mitochondrial disease depend on several factors. First, the clinical features depend on the proportion of pathogenic mtDNA mutation. If and when this proportion exceeds the tissue "threshold," clinically evident mitochondrial dysfunction will result. The threshold for disease is lower in tissues that are highly dependent on oxidative metabolism, such as brain, heart, skeletal muscle, retina, renal tubules, and endocrine glands, explaining why patients with the same heteroplasmic mutation may have variable tissue involvement and variable overall clinical severity. The T8993G mutation illustrates this concept nicely. Patients with a mutation load of about 70–90% present with a syndrome characterized by neuropathy, ataxia, and retinitis pigmentosa (NARP), while those with a mutation load >90% present with maternally inherited Leigh syndrome (MILS), a more severe form of infantile encephalomyopathy.

Second, the distribution of the mutation may vary in different tissues, which affects clinical expression. In patients with large-scale single mitochondrial deletions, infants may present with Pearson syndrome, a severe sideroblastic anemia, where most deleted mtDNA is in bone marrow stem cells. If these children survive the original hematological dysfunction, they usually develop a multisystemic mitochondrial disorder, Kearns–Sayre syndrome (KSS), in which deleted mtDNA is present in multiple tissues, resulting in the typical KSS phenotype of external ophthalmoplegia, ptosis, cardiac conduction block, and pigmentary retinopathy.

Although mtDNA mutations are mostly heteroplasmic and neutral polymorphisms are homoplasmic, there are exceptions to this truism. A good example is that of the LHON-related mutations (G11778 A mutation in the *ND4 L* gene, G3460 A mutation in *ND1*, and T14484 C mutation in *ND6*), which are homoplasmic. Another example is that of a severe but reversible form of infantile COX-deficient mitochondrial myopathy for which homoplasmic mutations were found (T14674 C in the *tRNA^{Glu}* gene in 17 patients of various ethnic origins and T14674G in 8 Japanese patients). The pathogenicity of this mutation has been proven, but does not explain the reversibility of the condition; a developmentally-regulated nuclear modifying factor has been postulated. The plot thickened when eight new patients from six families harbored mutations in the *TRMU* gene, which modifies a wobble uridine base in glutamine tRNA. Skeletal muscle from reversible infantile respiratory chain deficiency (RIRCD or reversible COX deficiency) in the initial symptomatic phase showed significantly decreased 2-thiouridylation due to defective TRMU activity and exacerbating the effect of the *tRNA^{Glu}* mutation by triggering a mitochondrial translation defect. Thus, the original homoplasmic *tRNA^{Glu}* mutation–postulated to be related to mitochondrial genetics–explains how the mtRNA translation defect can further explain the reversible clinical benefits, and the tissue-specific and time-related COX reversibility.

Several factors may influence the expression of homoplasmic mtDNA mutations, including the mtDNA haplotype, nDNA background, and epigenetic factors. Epigenetic factors have been shown to play a role in homoplasmic patients with LHON due to increased penetrance by the European mtDNA haplogroup J and, in affected males, due to a protective effect of estrogens in women.

Segregation

The random redistribution of organelles at the time of cell division can change the proportion of mutant mtDNAs received by daughter cells; if and when the pathogenic threshold in a previously unaffected tissue is surpassed, the phenotype can also change. This explains the age-related, and even tissue-related, variability of clinical features frequently observed in mtDNA-related disorders.

The numbers of organelles and their mtDNA content may also vary among cells and tissues as well as during development and aging. Certain conditions that increase the oxidative demands of a tissue, including acclimatization to high altitude or endurance training, may also increase its mitochondrial content. Conversely, aging may result in progressive accumulation of mitochondrial mutations, leading to a progressive decline in mitochondrial function.

Genetic and functional classification

Disorders of mtDNA

Disorders of mtDNA can be classified according to the type of genetic defect as large-scale rearrangements, such as mitochondrial deletions or duplications, or point mutations (Table 168.1). A functional classification divides mutations that affect mitochondrial protein synthesis and those that affect protein-coding genes. In the following sections, we describe eight of the most common mtDNA syndromes.

Kearns–Sayre syndrome

Kearns–Sayre syndrome (KSS) is a multisystem disorder characterized by a triad of progressive external ophthalmoplegia, pigmentary retinopathy, and onset before 20 years of age, as well as at least one of the following features: conductive cardiac block; cerebrospinal fluid (CSF) protein >100 mg/dL; and cerebellar ataxia. Other supportive findings include short stature, hearing loss, dementia, limb weakness, dysphagia, and various endocrinopathies. Large-scale deletions of mitochondrial DNA have been found in over 90% of KSS patients, and large-scale duplications in some.

Table 168.1 Classification of mtDNA disorders according to the underlying genetic defect.

Functional defect	Genetic defect	Disorder	Inheritance
Mutation in protein synthesis genes	Large-scale rearrangements MtDNA deletions	Kearns–Sayre syndrome (KSS)	Usually sporadic
		Progressive external ophthalmoplegia (PEO)	
		Pearson syndrome (congenital pancytopenia with sideroblastic anemia, and intestinal malabsorption)	
	Point mutations (tRNA genes)	Mitochondrial encephalomyopathy, lactic acidosis, and stroke-like episodes (MELAS)	Usually maternally inherited
		Myoclonic epilepsy with ragged red fibers (MERRF)	
Mutations in protein-coding genes	Point mutations (protein-coding genes)	Leber's hereditary optic neuropathy (LHON)	
		Neuropathy, ataxia, retinitis pigmentosa (NARP) syndrome	
		Maternally inherited Leigh syndrome (MILS)	

ALS = amyotrophic lateral sclerosis; FBSN = familial bilateral striatal necrosis; GRACILE = growth retardation, aminoaciduria, iron overload, lactic acidosis, early death; LS = Leigh syndrome; LHON = Leber's hereditary optic neuropathy; MELAS = mitochondrial encephalomyopathy, lactic acidosis, and stroke-like episodes; MILS = maternally inherited Leigh syndrome; NARP = neuropathy, ataxia, retinitis pigmentosa

Although KSS is multisystemic, a muscle biopsy is ideal to confirm the presence of mtDNA deletions, which are often undetectable in blood. Deletions vary in size and location within the mitochondrial genome, but there is a deletion hotspot between nucleotides 8469 and 13147. This 4.9-kb "common deletion" accounts for one-third of cases of KSS.

Blood creatine kinase (CK) may be modestly elevated, but lactate and pyruvate levels are often significantly increased. CSF protein is greatly elevated, usually >100 mg/dL. Magnetic resonance (MR) brain imaging often shows cerebral and cerebellar atrophy and, more commonly, abnormal T2-weighted signal in the subcortical white matter. Electrocardiography (ECG) characteristically shows cardiac conduction defects and should be performed at regular intervals, because timely placement of a pacemaker is often life-saving. Ophthalmological evaluation shows pigmentary retinopathy and electroretinography (ERG) may show retinal degeneration. Sensorineural hearing loss should be assessed with brainstem auditory evoked responses. Muscle biopsy usually demonstrates "ragged red fibers" (RRF) due to subsarcolemmal aggregates of abnormal mitochondria on the modified Gomori trichrome stain. Using COX histochemistry, most RRF (and many non-RRF) are COX deficient.

This condition is progressive, but several measures can improve quality of life. Patients with cardiac conduction block should have a pacemaker inserted to prevent complete heart block. Management of ptosis with eyelid "crutches," blepharoplasty, or frontalis muscle–eyelid sling placement improves vision and cosmesis. Aerobic exercise may improve strength and prevent deconditioning. Dysphagia may be treated with cricopharyngeal myotomy or gastrostomy feeding.

Progressive external ophthalmoplegia

Progressive external ophthalmoplegia (PEO) is one of the most common clinical manifestations of mitochondrial myopathy. It may appear in isolation or in association with other features suggestive of a specific mitochondrial syndrome such as KSS or mitochondrial neurogastrointestinal encephalopathy (MNGIE) disease. PEO may be sporadic, maternally inherited (mtDNA disorder), or Mendelian in inheritance (nDNA disorder). Sporadic PEO is most frequently

due to a single large-scale mtDNA rearrangement, similar to that in KSS, but PEO affects the muscles alone and is characterized by progressive bilateral ptosis, ophthalmoplegia, exercise intolerance, and muscle weakness.

Diagnosis has to be made by muscle biopsy because the mtDNA deletions are not found in blood. Electroretinography and visual-evoked potential testing are usually normal.

Pearson syndrome

Pearson syndrome (PS) is the most severe of the conditions caused by large-scale mtDNA rearrangements. This infantile disorder includes sideroblastic anemia, exocrine pancreatic dysfunction with malabsorption, chronic diarrhea, failure to thrive, lactic acidemia, and various endocrine abnormalities. PS is almost universally fatal, and the few patients who survive the initial severe sideroblastic anemia tragically develop the multisystemic symptoms of KSS later on in life.

Mitochondrial encephalopathy, lactic acidosis, and stroke-like episodes

Mitochondrial encephalopathy, lactic acidosis, and stroke-like episodes (MELAS) is a relatively common multisystem mitochondrial disorder characterized by (1) stroke-like episodes before 40 years of age; (2) encephalopathy, with seizures and/or psychomotor retardation/regression; (3) myopathy with ragged red fibers; and (4) lactic acidosis.

The stroke-like episodes are often occipital in location, resulting in cortical blindness, do not correspond to vascular territories, and involve predominantly the cortex and adjacent white matter, with deeper white matter spared. These stroke-like episodes may not be due to acute ischemia, but rather a combination of metabolic dysfunction with decreased oxidative phosphorylation and altered cerebrovascular autoregulation. Other neurological features of MELAS include ataxia, myoclonus, episodic encephalopathy, optic nerve atrophy, sensorineural hearing loss, retinopathy, ophthalmoplegia, and migraine-like headaches. Psychiatric disturbance such as depression or schizophrenia may also be present. Non-neurological features include cardiac dysfunction with cardiomyopathy, arrhythmias, or conductive heart block, endocrine dysfunction with diabetes mellitus, short stature, gastrointestinal dysfunction with dysmotility, and renal dysfunction with nephropathy.

The age at onset varies and the disease sometimes starts in infancy or early childhood with developmental delay, seizures, learning disability, failure to thrive, and exercise intolerance. However, in many patients a stroke-like episode is the first presentation, which may occur in childhood, adolescence, or, less frequently, later in life.

Point mutations in mtDNA almost always underlie MELAS. This syndrome illustrates one of the key concepts of mitochondrial genetics; namely, genotypic diversity. The most common mutation is A3243G in the $tRNA^{Leu(UUR)}$ gene, which is seen in about 80% of patients, but many mutations have been described in other tRNA genes, including $tRNA^{Leu}$, $tRNA^{Val}$, $tRNA^{Phe}$, and $tRNA^{Glu}$, as well as mutations in protein-coding genes such as complex I (*ND1*, *ND4*, *ND5*, *ND6*) and complex IV (*COXIII*) genes. Interestingly, mutations in *ND1* (G3376A) and *ND5* (G13513A, A13045C, and A13084T) often cause overlapping phenotypes of MELAS, LHON, and Leigh syndrome.

Lactic acidosis is one hallmark of the syndrome and increased lactic acid levels in the CSF and in the brain parenchyma can be appreciated by magnetic resonance spectroscopy (MRS). Neuroimaging findings on MRS include (1) stroke-like lesions with increased signal in T2-weighted or fluid attenuation inversion recovery (FLAIR) images; (2) increased signal on diffusion-weighted images (DWI), with normal or increased apparent diffusion coefficient (ADC) values suggestive of vasogenic edema; (3) relatively normal angiograms; (4) basal ganglia calcifications; (5) variable cerebral atrophy; and (6) increased lactate in the ventricular CSF and in the brain parenchyma. Positron emission tomography (PET) studies may reveal reduced cerebral oxygen metabolism. Single photon emission computed tomography (SPECT) often shows decreased tracer accumulation in acute and subacute lesions, possibly due to focal loss of metabolically active cells.

Blood screening for the common mtDNA mutations is usually diagnostic. However, in oligosymptomatic or asymptomatic relatives of MELAS patients, the mutation is often undetectable in blood, although it is readily detectable in easily accessible urinary sediment. Muscle biopsy shows scattered ragged red fibers, which are positive for COX activity, and blood vessels with increased succinate dehydrogenase (SDH) and COX staining. Biochemical analysis of the respiratory chain enzymes suggests partial defects in the activities of complexes containing mtDNA-encoded subunits (I, III, and IV), contrasting with normal activities of the nDNA-encoded complex II (succinate dehydrogenase) and citrate synthase.

Treatment of MELAS includes "cocktails" of vitamins and dietary supplements, symptomatic management of seizures and other medical complications (e.g., diabetes mellitus), and avoidance of metabolic stressors. Patients with severe neurosensory hearing loss may need cochlear implants. L-arginine, a nitric oxide precursor that may favor vascular dilatation, has been shown to improve outcomes in stroke-like episodes when used acutely within the first 3 hours after onset of the event, and to decrease the frequency and severity of stroke-like episodes when administered between episodes.

Myoclonic epilepsy and ragged red fibers

Myoclonic epilepsy and ragged red fibers (MERRF) is a multisystem mitochondrial disorder dominated by myoclonus, which is often the first symptom, followed by generalized epilepsy, ataxia, weakness, and dementia. Onset is usually in childhood, although onset in adulthood has been described. Other common findings include sensorineural hearing loss, short stature, optic atrophy, and cardiomyopathy with Wolff–Parkinson–White syndrome. Occasionally, pigmentary retinopathy and multiple lipomatosis may be observed.

Neuropathological studies have demonstrated degeneration of the cerebellum, brainstem, and spinal cord, which may explain the prominent ataxia in some patients. In addition, there is significant cortical hyperexcitability, resulting in cortical reflex myoclonus.

The mitochondrial $tRNA^{Lys}$ gene is a hotspot for mutations causing MERRF (A8344G, T8356C, G8361A, G8363A), although MERRF-like syndromes have also been associated with point mutations in $tRNA^{Phe}$, $tRNA^{Ser(UCN)}$, $tRNA^{His}$, and $tRNA^{Leu\ (UUR)}$. The most common mutation (80% of cases) is the A8344G point mutation. In the absence of the common mutations, however, muscle biopsy is useful, because the presence of COX-negative RRF confirms the suspicion of a mitochondrial disorder. It should also be noted that several $tRNA^{Lys}$ mutations (A8344G, T8356C, G8363A) cause symptoms overlapping with MELAS and Leigh syndrome.

Treatment is supportive, and there are no comparative studies of the relative efficacy of different anticonvulsants. Myoclonus has been reported to improve in several patients with the use of levetiracetam.

Leber's hereditary optic neuropathy syndrome

Leber's hereditary optic neuropathy syndrome (LHON) is an mtDNA disorder causing subacute visual loss, predominantly in young men. There is a rapid and painless loss of central vision, which affects both eyes simultaneously in 50% of cases and within 6 months in the remainder of patients. During the acute phase, there is loss of central and color vision. Fundoscopic evaluation reveals peripapillary telangiectasia, microangiopathy, and disc pseudoedema (from swelling of the nerve fiber layer around the disc). This is followed by the atrophic phase, when there is progressive optic atrophy and decline in visual acuity.

In 95% of cases, LHON is caused by homoplasmic mutations in one of three ND genes, G11778A (*ND4*), G3460A (*ND1*), and T14484C (*ND6*). Only 50% of men and 10% of women harboring LHON mutations actually develop the symptoms of LHON, stressing the role of mitochondrial or nuclear modifier genes. Several patients with mutations in *ND5* have shown overlap with MELAS symptoms, while patients with mutations in *ND4* or *ND6* may show, in addition to LHON, basal ganglia degeneration and symptoms of dystonia and spasticity. The clinical course may also vary depending on the mutation: more patients with the T14484C mutation show recovery compared with those with the G11778A mutation (71% vs. 4%).

Neuropathy, ataxia, retinitis pigmentosa syndrome

Neuropathy, ataxia, retinitis pigmentosa (NARP) syndrome is a maternally inherited mitochondrial disorder of young adulthood defined by the presence of sensory neuropathy, ataxia, and retinitis pigmentosa. This is caused by either a T8993G or a T8993C mutation in the mitochondrial ATP synthase subunit 6 gene (*ATPase6*). The diagnosis of NARP is suggested by peripheral neuropathy, which may be sensory or sensorimotor axonal, ataxia with cerebellar atrophy, and retinitis pigmentosa, plus seizures and dementia. The retinopathy usually has a "salt and pepper" appearance, although a more severe appearance with classical bone spicules may also be seen. Optic atrophy may appear later in the course of the disease. Muscle biopsy does not show RRF.

Patients with NARP typically have mutation loads ranging between 70% and 90%. Patients with higher mutation loads (>90%) are affected by maternally inherited Leigh syndrome (MILS); see the next section.

Maternally-inherited Leigh Syndrome

Maternally-inherited Leigh Syndrome (MILS) is characterized by progressive psychomotor degeneration, features of brainstem and basal ganglia abnormalities, and raised lactate in both blood and CSF. Both neuroimaging and pathology show the hallmarks of Leigh syndrome (LS), including symmetric necrosis of the basal ganglia, thalamus, and brainstem. About 40% of patients with MILS also have retinitis pigmentosa; this should be a clue to clinicians regarding the underlying molecular defect, because retinitis pigmentosa is rarely, if ever, seen in other forms of LS. Adult-onset MILS has been described in association with $tRNA^{Val}$ mutations, and MILS with spinocerebellar ataxia with $tRNA^{Lys}$ mutations.

Important new causes of MILS have been identified, including mutations in *ND5* and *ND3*, which can also cause MELAS or MELAS/LHON overlap syndromes. Mutations in *ND3* are more characteristically associated with MILS.

Disorders of nDNA

The nuclear genome encodes hundreds of mitochondrial proteins that are essential for various mitochondrial functions besides maintenance and replication of mtDNA (i.e., intergenomic signaling). Mitochondrial diseases may therefore result from a plethora of abnormalities, affecting mitochondrial motility, fission, or fusion (i.e., mitochondrial dynamics), protein importation, and phospholipid membrane composition, with or without direct involvement of the respiratory chain (Table 168.2).

Clinical syndromes due to nDNA mutations tend to be more stereotyped than those due to mtDNA mutations, as they are not subject to the variable mutation load and differential tissue distribution of mutant mtDNA. Several common syndromes are discussed here.

Leigh syndrome

Leigh syndrome (LS) is a condition of subacute necrotizing encephalomyelopathy with typical pathological findings of symmetric foci of spongiform degeneration in the basal ganglia, thalami, brainstem, dentate nuclei, and optic nerves. Most patients with LS present in infancy with psychomotor regression, although later onset in childhood or even adolescence is possible. Other features include hypotonia, visual impairment, progressive external ophthalmoplegia, hearing impairment, nystagmus, ataxia, and seizures. Respiratory insufficiency is fairly common and is an important cause of mortality.

Clinical diagnostic criteria include (1) progressive neurological disease with motor and intellectual developmental delay; (2) signs and symptoms of brainstem and/or basal ganglia disease; (3) raised lactate concentration in blood and/or CSF; and (4) one or more of the following: (a) characteristic features of Leigh syndrome on neuroimaging, which include symmetrically increased signal in the basal ganglia and brainstem on T2-weighted or FLAIR images; (b) typical neuropathological changes including multiple symmetric foci of degeneration and necrosis with capillary proliferation, demyelination and gliosis in the basal ganglia, brainstem, thalamus, cerebellum, and spinal cord; and (c) typical neuropathology or neuroimaging findings in a similarly affected sibling.

Leigh syndrome is genetically heterogeneous because it may be caused by mtDNA mutations (MILS) or nDNA mutations. LS is caused by nDNA mutations in genes encoding for subunits of the pyruvate dehydrogenase complex (PDHC), genes encoding respiratory chain components of complex I (*NDUFS2*, *NDUFS4*, *NDUFS8*, *NDUFV1*, *NDUFS1*, *NDUFS7*) or complex II (*SDHA*), or genes encoding proteins needed for the assembly or maintenance of respiratory chain function (*SURF1*, *COX10*, *COX15*, *SCO1*, *SCO2*, *LRPPRC*). Underlying all these diverse genetic defects, however, is the unifying problem of impaired adenosine triphosphate (ATP) synthesis.

Specific defects of the pyruvate dehydrogenase and mitochondrial respiratory chain can guide the molecular genetic workup in patients. When the criteria of Leigh syndrome are not completely fulfilled, additional signs such as liver or kidney involvement together with the biochemical defect may suggest a mitochondrial depletion syndrome (e.g., *SUCLA2* or *SUCLG1* mutations in hepatoencephalopathy) or coenzyme Q_{10} (CoQ_{10}) deficiency (e.g., *PDSS2* mutations in renal insufficiency).

Autosomal dominant or recessive progressive external ophthalmoplegia

As described earlier in this chapter, PEO is a mitochondrial myopathy with ptosis, paralysis of the extraocular muscles, and proximal limb weakness. It may be isolated or associated with other clinical features of mitochondrial syndromes. Autosomal dominant (adPEO) and autosomal recessive (arPEO) PEO are associated with multiple mtDNA deletions. These myopathies begin in adolescence or in early adulthood, and are usually slowly progressive. The genes responsible for adPEO include *POLG* (polymerase gamma being the only mtDNA polymerase), *ANT1* (muscle-specific isoform of mitochondrial adenine nucleotide translocator), and *PEO1* (Twinkle, a helicase involved in mtDNA replication). *POLG*, *TK2*, and *RRM2B* mutations have been described in arPEO. *POLG* mutations appear to be associated with more severe and complex clinical manifestations, including sensory ataxia, dysphagia, dysphonia, and less frequently parkinsonism, cerebellar ataxia, chorea, gastrointestinal dysmotility, and psychiatric disturbances. In contrast to adPEO, arPEO tends to begin in childhood or adolescence, and may be part of multisystem disorders like MNGIE or autosomal recessive cardiomyopathy and ophthalmoplegia (ARCO).

Mitochondrial neurogastrointestinal encephalomyopathy

Mitochondrial neurogastrointestinal encephalomyopathy (MNGIE) is an autosomal recessive disorder associated with mtDNA depletion, multiple deletions, and site-specific point mutations, and is caused by mutations in the thymidine phosphorylase (*TYMP*) gene that regulates the mitochondrial nucleotide pools. This condition is characterized by PEO, severe gastrointestinal dysmotility, and cachexia, peripheral neuropathy, and leukoencephalopathy. The peripheral neuropathy is demyelinating in half of patients and axonal in the other half. The leukoencephalopathy seen on magnetic resonance imaging (MRI) is usually asymptomatic. Allogeneic hematopoietic stem cell transplantation (AHSCT) has been performed, with normalization of biochemical features and subjective improvement in several patients, although AHSCT remains risky in patients in poor medical condition.

Table 168.2 Classification of nDNA disorders according to the underlying biochemical and genetic defects.

Functional defect	Biochemical/ genetic defect	Defective gene	Disorder	Inheritance
Mutation in structural components of the respiratory chain: "direct hits"	Complex I	NDUFS2, NDUFS4, NDUFS8, NDUFV1, NDUFS1, NDUFS7	Leigh syndrome	AR
		NDUFS2, NDUFV2	Cardioencephalomyopathy	AR
	Complex II	Flavoprotein subunit of SDH and assembly factor	Leigh syndrome	AR
		SDHB, SDHC, SDHD	Hereditary paraganglioma or pheochromocytoma	AD
	Complex II	UQCRB	Hypoglycemia, lactic acidosis	AR
Mutations in ancillary proteins of respiratory chain: "indirect hits"	Complex I	B17.2L	Early-onset progressive encephalopathy	AR
		ACAD9	Cardioencephalomyopathy or myopathy	AR
	Complex III	BCS1L	Encephalopathy, tubulopathy, hepatopathy	AR
	Complex IV	SURF1	Leigh syndrome	AR
		SCO2, COX14, COX15, COA5, FAM36A, TACO1	Infantile cardioencephalomyopathy	AR
		SCO1	Infantile hepatoencephalopathy	AR
		COX10	Infantile nephroencephalopathy	AR
		LRPPRC	French Canadian Leigh syndrome	AR
	Complex V deficiency	ATPAF2	Early-onset encephalopathy, lactic acidosis	AR
	Defect of mitochondrial protein import	Tim 8/9 (DDP)	Deafness-dystonia (Mohr–Tranebjaerg syndrome)	XLR
		HSP60 (HSPD1)	Spastic paraplegia 13; hypomyelinating leukodystrophy	AD AR
Defects of mtDNA maintenance	Multiple mtDNA deletions	DNA2	Encephalomyopathy	AR
		POLG	adPEO, arPEO, Alpers syndrome, SANDO syndrome	AR/AD
		ANT1, Twinkle helicase (C10ORF2)	adPEO	AD
	mtDNA depletion	TK2	Infantile myopathy	AR
		dGK	Infantile hepatopathy and encephalopathy	AR
		FBXL4	Infantile encephalopathy	
	mtDNA depletion/deletions	TK2	Adult myopathy	AR
		MGME1	Encephalomyopathy	AR
		TYMP	Mitochondrial neurogastrointestinal encephalopathy	AR
Defects of mtDNA translation	Ribosomal protein assembly	MRPS16	Fatal neonatal lactic acidosis	AR
		MRPS22	Fatal neonatal lactic acidosis	AR
		RMND1	Fatal neonatal lactic acidosis	AR
	Translation elongation	EFG1	Severe hepatoencephalopathy and lactic acidosis	AR
		EFTu	Severe infantile leukodystrophy and polymicrogyria	AR
	tRNA synthetase	DARS2	Leukoencephalopathy, brainstem and spinal cord involvement, lactic acidosis	AR
		EARS2	Leukodystrophy	AR
		YARS2	Mitochondrial myopathy, lactic acidosis and sideroblastic anemia	AR
		AARS2	Ovario-leukodystrophy	AR
		RARS2	Pontocerebellar hypoplasia	AR
	Translation activators	TACO1	Late-onset Leigh syndrome with COX deficiency	AR
		LRPPRC	French Canadian Leigh syndrome	
	tRNA base modifiers	TRMU	Reversible hepatopathy	AR
		PUS1	Myopathy, lactic acidosis, sideroblastic anemia	AR
		TRNT1	Sideroblastic anemia with immunodeficiency, fevers, and developmental delay	AR

(continued)

(contiuned)

Functional defect	Biochemical/ genetic defect	Defective gene	Disorder	Inheritance
		GTPBP3	Hypertrophic cardiomyopathy, lactic acidosis, and encephalopathy	AR
		TRIT1	Encephalopathy and myoclonic epilepsy	AR
		MTFMT	Leigh syndrome	AR
Defects of mitochondrial membrane function	Cardiolipin defect	Tafazzin (G4.5)	Barth syndrome	XLR
	CoQ$_{10}$deficiency	COQ2, PDSS2, COQ6	Infantile encephalomyopathy with nephropathy	AR
		ADCK3	Ataxia	AR
		COQ4	Myopathy	AR
	Phosphotidyl-choline defect	CHKB	Encephalomyopathy with giant displaced mitochondria	AR
	Phosphatidic acid deficiency	AGK	Senger syndrome	AR
	Accumulation of phosphatidic acid and lysophospho-lipids	LPIN1	LPIN1 myopathy	AR
	Altered phospholipid modeling	SERAC1	MEGDEL syndrome	AR
Defects of mitochondrial dynamics	Impaired motility	OPA1	Dominant optic atrophy	AD
		KIF5A	Hereditary spastic paraplegia	AD
		DYNC1H1	Charcot–Marie–Tooth disease type 2 O; lower extremity dominant spinal muscular atrophy	AD
	Mitochondrial fusion/fission	Mitofusin (MFN2)	Charcot–Marie–Tooth disease type 2 A	AD
		GDAP1	Charcot–Marie–Tooth disease type 4 A	AR
		DNM2	Centronuclear myopathy; Charcot–Marie–Tooth disease type 2M	AD
		DNM1 L (DRP1)	Fatal infantile microcephaly and lactic acidosis	AR
		MFF	Fatal infantile microcephaly and lactic acidosis	AR
Defects of iron homeostasis	Iron storage	Frataxin (FRDA)	Friedreich's ataxia	AR
	Iron transport	ABC7	X-linked sideroblastic anemia with ataxia	XL
Defects of mitochondrial metabolism	PDH E1α subunit	PDHA1	X-linked Leigh syndrome	XL
	Ethylmalonic acid metabolism	ETHE1	Encephalopathy, ethylmalonic aciduria	AR
Others	Chaperone function	SPG7	Spastic paraplegia	AR

AD = autosomal dominant; adPEO = autosomal dominant progressive external ophthalmoplegia; AR = autosomal regressive; arPEO = autosomal recessive progressive external ophthalmoplegia; COX = cytochrome c oxidase; MEDGEL = methylglutaconic aciduria, deafness, encephalopathy and Leigh-like disease; SANDO = sensory ataxia, neuropathy, dysarthria and ophthalmoplegia; XLR = X-linked recessive

Hepatocerebral syndromes

Mitochondrial liver disease can present acutely in a child with no history of hepatic dysfunction with neonatal liver failure due to genetic defects in mtDNA synthesis (*DGUOK, POLG, MPV17, TWINKLE*), mtDNA translation (*FARS2, TRMU, TSFM, EFG1, EF-Tu, MRPS16*), mitochondrial respiratory chain defects (*BSC1 L, SCO1*), Krebs cycle defect (*SUCLA2, SUCLG1*), or carnitine cycle/fatty acid oxidation defects (*HADHA/LCHAD*, tri-functional protein deficiency, or *CPTI* and *CPTII* deficiency (*SLC25A20*). Correct diagnosis and identification of central nervous system (CNS) involvement are important when liver transplant is considered.

Ataxia syndromes

Patients with syndromic mitochondrial disease may present with sensory or cerebellar ataxia. Sensory ataxia is often due to *POLG*

defect with three different clinical forms: (1) myoclonic epilepsy, myopathy, sensory ataxia (MEMSA); (2) ataxia neuropathy spectrum (ANS); or (3) sensory ataxic neuropathy, dysarthria, and ophthalmoparesis (SANDO). Cerebellar ataxia is most often caused by coenzyme Q$_{10}$ (CoQ$_{10}$) deficiency. CoQ$_{10}$ is an important quinone that transfers electrons from complexes I and II to complex III of the respiratory chain, and its deficiency has been associated with myopathy, ataxia, or infantile encephalomyopathy and nephropathy. Primary CoQ$_{10}$ deficiency is associated with molecular genetic defects in genes involved in CoQ$_{10}$ biosynthesis (*PDSS21, PDSS2, CoQ2, CoQ4, CoQ6, ADCK3*). Mutations in *ADCK3* are the most common causes of primary CoQ$_{10}$ deficiency.

Secondary forms of CoQ$_{10}$ deficiency have been associated with mutations in the aprataxin gene (*APTX*) in patients with ataxia and oculomotor apraxia. CoQ$_{10}$ deficiency is also associated with lipid storage myopathy and mutations in the gene encoding the enzyme electron transport flavoprotein dehydrogenase (*ETFDH*). *ETFDH* normally discharges electrons from the beta-oxidation pathway to CoQ_{10} in the respiratory chain. It is important to keep in mind that for all of these conditions, oral supplementation with CoQ_{10} is beneficial and should be instituted as early as possible.

Encephalomyopathy syndromes

Mitochondrial encephalomyopathies due to nDNA-encoded genes are mostly due to defects in protein regulation of mtDNA synthesis. The pathogenic mechanisms may include defects in deoxynucleotide pool balance (*TK2*, *RRM2B*), in polymerase that synthesizes mtDNA (*POLG*), or in genes encoding proteins that regulate or initiate mtDNA synthesis (*MGME1* and *DNA2*). These may present as a spectrum: (1) severe infantile myopathy with or without renal dysfunction (*TK2* or *RRM2B*); (2) childhood-onset myopathy mimicking spinal muscle atrophy with severe mtDNA depletion (*TK2* mutation); (3) juvenile-onset myopathy, ptosis, and progressive external ophthalmoplegia with multiple mtDNA deletions with low-level mtDNA depletion (*TK2*); or (4) adult-onset ptosis and progressive external ophthalmoplegia and multiple deletions of mtDNA (*TK2* or *RRM2B*). Other variants include mutations in the *DNA2* gene, presenting with late onset and slowly progressive limb-girdle muscle weakness, ptosis, and ophthalmoparesis, and in the *C20orf72* (or *MGME1*) gene, presenting with PEO with emaciation and respiratory failure.

Mitochondrial leukodystrophies

White-matter lesions in the infratentorial or supratentorial regions are readily recognized in mitochondrial leukoencephalopathies. There is an emerging group of leukodystrophies in which chronic and progressive white-matter involvement is the main presentation, and is caused by a defect in mitochondrial proteins.

Leukoencephalopathy with brainstem and spinal cord involvement and lactate elevation (LBSL) is a rare autosomal recessive disease characterized by juvenile onset of slowly progressive ataxia, spasticity, dorsal column dysfunction, and a highly distinctive MRI pattern, consisting of signal abnormalities in the periventricular cerebral white matter and specific brainstem and spinal cord tracts, with high lactate peak on MRS. In 2007, Scheper and colleagues identified the molecular genetic defect in the gene *DARS2* that encodes mitochondrial aspartyl-tRNA synthetase, defining LBSL as a disorder of mitochondrial translational defects.

Defects in other mitochondrial translation proteins, *EARS2* and *AARS2*, have been described in two different leukodystrophies. Defective *EARS2* protein has been associated with an MRI pattern of extensive symmetric cerebral white-matter abnormalities sparing the periventricular rim, and symmetric signal abnormalities of the thalami, midbrain, pons, medulla oblongata, and cerebellar white matter, and high lactate on MRS. *EARS2*-related leukodystrophy may present with a severe clinical course such as neonatal hypotonia, spasticity, dystonia, visual impairment, and seizures, and elevated lactate. In mild disease, patients have normal development or mild developmental delay followed by clinical regression with spasticity, seizures, and extreme irritability. Unexpectedly, clinical, biochemical, and MRI pattern improvement may occur in some from the second year onward.

Progressive leukoencephalopathy with ovarian failure (ovarioleukodystrophy) is an autosomal recessive disorder characterized by ataxia, spasticity, cognitive decline, and premature ovarian failure in young adulthood. Progressive signal abnormalities in the deep white matter are seen on MRI. Mutations have been previously found in the *eIF2B* gene, but recently also in the *AARS2* (mitochondrial alanyl-tRNA synthetase) gene. Patients with *AARS2* gene mutations had tract-like signal abnormalities involving the corpus callosum and descending connections, predominantly involving the frontal and parietal periventricular and deep white matter, sparing a segment of white matter in between.

Even though the most common defects are in tRNA synthetase proteins, mitochondrial leukodystrophies are not restricted to mitochondrial translational defects, as demonstrated by a recent report of *APOPT1* (Apoptogenic-1) gene mutations associated with severe COX deficiency and a distinctive brain MRI pattern characterized by posterior-predominant cavitating leukodystrophy.

Neurodegenerative disorders

There is little question that mitochondrial dysfunction has a role in apoptosis and in the pathogenesis of neurodegeneration. Late-onset neurodegenerative disorders, including Parkinson's disease (PD), Huntington's disease (HD), Alzheimer's disease (AD), and amyotrophic lateral sclerosis (ALS), have been associated with oxidative stress. Nonetheless, the relative contributions of mitochondrial and various environmental factors to the aging process remain to be clearly defined.

Epidemiology

Epidemiological evidence suggests that mutations in mtDNA are not uncommon, although these numbers may be underestimated. The prevalence of the common MELAS A3243G mutation is estimated at 16.3/100000 in north Finland. LHON has a minimum prevalence of 11.82/100000 in northeastern England. In northeastern England, the cumulative frequency of mtDNA mutations in adult and child populations has been estimated to be 9.2 to 16.5/100000. In western Sweden, the prevalence of mitochondrial diseases in preschool children has been estimated to be 1 in 11000. Based on conservative estimates from epidemiological studies in northern England, northern Finland, western Sweden, and Australia, the prevalence of mitochondrial DNA mutations in adults and children is approximately 11.5 per 100000 (about 1 in 8500), underlining the fact that collectively these are not rare diseases. Large-scale epidemiological data from different ethnic or racial groups are lacking.

Neurological manifestations

The range of neurological manifestations of mitochondrial disorders is vast. CNS manifestations may include fluctuating encephalopathy, cognitive decline, loss of motor skills, psychiatric disturbance, migraine-like headaches, stroke-like episodes, seizures, dystonia, myoclonus, spasticity, ataxia, dysarthria, dysphagia, hypotonia, and visual problems. Peripheral nervous system manifestations include myopathy or neuropathy (demyelinating or axonal neuropathy).

Some patients may have a constellation of symptoms or signs typical enough to allow recognition of specific mtDNA syndromes (Table 168.3). Certain disorders affect a single organ, such as aminoglycoside-induced deafness or pure myopathies, while others involve multiple organ systems but often with predominant neurological or neuromuscular features.

Abnormalities of the CNS may also be secondary to mitochondrial dysfunction in other organs. Endocrine dysfunctions may

Table 168.3 Clinical features of mitochondrial diseases associated with mtDNA mutations.

Tissue	Symptom/sign	Δ-mtDNA		tRNA		ATPase	
		KSS	Pearson	MERRF	MELAS	NARP	MILS
CNS	Seizures	–	–	+	+	–	+
	Ataxia	+	–	+	+	+	±
	Myoclonus	–	–	+	±	–	–
	Psychomotor retardation	–	–	–	–	–	+
	Psychomotor regression	+	–	±	+	–	–
	Hemiparesis/hemianopia	–	–	–	+	–	–
	Cortical blindness	–	–	–	+	–	–
	Migraine-like headaches	–	–	–	+	–	–
	Dystonia	–	–	–	+	–	+
PNS	Peripheral neuropathy	±	–	±	±	+	–
Muscle	Weakness	+	–	+	+	+	+
	Ophthalmoplegia	+	±	–	–	–	–
	Ptosis	+	–	–	–	–	–
Eye	Pigmentary retinopathy	+	–	–	–	+	±
	Optic atrophy	–	–	–	–	±	±
	Cataracts	–	–	–	–	–	–
Blood	Sideroblastic anemia	±	+	–	–	–	–
Endocrine	Diabetes mellitus	±	–	–	±	–	–
	Short stature	+	–	+	+	–	–
	Hypoparathyroidism	±	–	–	–	–	–
Heart	Conduction block	+	–	–	±	–	–
	Cardiomyopathy	±	–	–	±	–	±
GI	Exocrine pancreatic dysfunction	±	+	–	–	–	–
	Intestinal pseudoobstruction	–	–	–	–	–	–
ENT	Sensorineural hearing loss	–	–	+	+	±	–
Kidney	Fanconi's syndrome	±	±	–	±	–	–
Laboratory	Lactic acidosis	+	+	+	+	–	±
	Muscle biopsy: RRF	+	±	+	+	–	–
Inheritance	Maternal	–	–	+	+	+	+
	Sporadic	+	+	–	–	–	–

CNS = central nervous system; ENT = ear, nose, and throat; GI = gastrointestinal; KSS = Kearns–Sayre syndrome; MELAS = mitochondrial encephalopathy, lactic acidosis, and stroke-like episodes; MERRF = myoclonic epilepsy and ragged red fibers; MILS = maternally inherited Leigh syndrome; NARP = neuropathy, ataxia, and retinitis pigmentosa; PNS = peripheral nervous system; RRF = ragged red fibers

cause Hashimoto's or diabetic encephalopathy, and liver and/or kidney failure may cause hepatic or uremic encephalopathy. It should also be remembered that specific drugs may worsen or unmask symptoms of mitochondrial disorders. For example, valproic acid may cause hepatic failure in patients with Alpers syndrome, and statin drugs may cause rhabdomyolysis in patients with MELAS.

Diagnosis

Because of the bewildering range of clinical phenotypes, the diagnosis of mitochondrial diseases is fraught with difficulty even for the most experienced neurologist. In general, mitochondrial disorders should be suspected in the differential diagnosis of any multisystem disorder. Specific red flags should be looked for in the history and on clinical examination, and a judicious range of investigations chosen to document mitochondrial dysfunction.

History

A careful and detailed history of the patient's symptoms is essential to obtain an accurate diagnosis. Red flags in the history include exercise intolerance, migraine headaches, diabetes mellitus, short stature, hearing loss, neuropathy, hypertrophic cardiomyopathy, and, in children, unexplained developmental delay or failure to thrive. Family history is also important in distinguishing maternal from Mendelian forms of inheritance. Careful screening of red flags in the extended pedigree is also necessary. Consanguinity may suggest an autosomal recessive nDNA disorder.

A history of mid-trimester or late pregnancy loss or infant death (often with a dubious label of "sepsis") should also be noted. While mitochondrial disorders may manifest at any age, it is useful to remember that in general, nuclear DNA abnormalities tend to appear in infancy and childhood, while mtDNA abnormalities often – but not always – present in late childhood or adult life.

Exposure to drugs such as aminoglycosides, valproic acid, and other drugs known to compromise mitochondrial function should also be carefully recorded.

Physical examination

A careful physical examination may yield clues to the diagnosis. Failure to thrive in a child, or short stature in an adolescent or adult, may be significant. Ptosis and external ophthalmoplegia are telltale signs of KSS or PEO after excluding myasthenia gravis. Multiple lipomatosis is a typical feature of MERRF. Fundoscopic examination may show a pigmentary retinopathy (often with "salt and pepper" appearance) in KSS, NARP, MILS, and, less commonly, MELAS and MERRF. Peripheral neuropathy is typical of NARP, but may also be present in MELAS and MERRF, and among the Mendelian conditions is very common in adPEO or arPEO with *POLG* mutations and in patients with MNGIE.

Systematic examination of other organ systems is equally important, as it may reveal other pointers to the underlying mitochondrial syndrome.

Investigations

An extensive evaluation is necessary in patients with a complex neurological picture or with a single neurological symptom with organ involvement. The strategy for evaluation is greatly simplified when the clinical picture is typical of a specific mitochondrial syndrome (such as KSS, MELAS, or MERRF), because studies of blood mtDNA can be targeted to the appropriate mutations, starting with the most common. Should the clinical picture be non-specific but still suggestive of a mitochondrial condition, simpler laboratory tests such as lactate levels and metabolic testing should be performed first.

Basic laboratory tests

Laboratory evaluation should include full blood count, renal and liver function tests, and lactate and pyruvate levels. Lactate and pyruvate are often elevated at rest in mitochondrial diseases and may increase further with exercise. A higher carbohydrate intake is also associated with increased lactate levels. In general, the lactate/pyruvate ratio of patients with mitochondrial disease should be >30:1. However, lactate may not be raised in conditions like NARP, and often repeated lactate levels are necessary to confirm the lactic acidosis. Creatine kinase (CK) is usually mildly elevated in mitochondrial disorders, but may be markedly raised in the myopathic form of mtDNA depletion. Should there be a suggestive history, other investigations may be considered, such as fasting blood glucose for diabetes mellitus or hormonal tests for thyroid, parathyroid, and pituitary function.

Metabolic workup should include plasma amino acids, urinary organic acids, and plasma acylcarnitine levels. Increased plasma alanine can suggest a mitochondrial dysfunction. Increased excretion of methylmalonic acid may suggest *SUCLG1* or *SUCLA2* defects in patients with Leigh-like syndrome and mtDNA depletion.

CSF studies may be useful to demonstrate cerebral lactic acidosis. CSF protein may be raised in MELAS and KSS (especially KSS, where protein is often more than 100 mg/dL), and oligoclonal bands may also be present. Lactate may be raised following stroke-like events or generalized seizures.

Electrocardiogram (ECG) may reveal conductive heart block in KSS or MELAS, and pre-excitation in MELAS and MERRF. 2D-echocardiography may confirm hypertrophic cardiomyopathy in some patients.

Neuroimaging

Computed tomography (CT) scans of the brain in patients with mitochondrial disorders may show non-specific findings, such as white matter and basal ganglia hypodensity, calcification of the cortex and basal ganglia, atrophy of the pons and cerebellum, or hypotrophy of the corpus callosum. MRI of the brain is extremely useful to demonstrate certain characteristic patterns in specific syndromes. For example, the diagnosis of LS is dependent on bilateral symmetric signal hyperintensity of the basal ganglia and brainstem. Acute stroke-like events in MELAS are demonstrated on MRI as lesions with increased signal on T2-weighted and FLAIR images, with no conformation to large vessel territories, and affecting the cortex and adjacent white matter. These lesions also show increased diffusion-weighted signal with normal or increased ADC values, typical of vasogenic edema rather than cytotoxic edema. Other common findings on MRI include diffuse signal abnormalities of the central white matter (KSS, MERRF, MNGIE, PEO), basal ganglia calcifications (KSS, MELAS), supratentorial cortical atrophy (PEO, MNGIE), and cerebellar atrophy (KSS); see Table 168.4.

MRS is useful to reveal CNS lactate accumulation. In fact, MRS may reveal abnormal lactate peaks in oligosymptomatic carriers of the A3243G mutation. Lactate peaks may even precede stroke-like lesions in MELAS patients. This modality has also proven to be useful in carriers of the A3243G mutation who subsequently went on to have manifestations of disease. ^{1}H-MRS imaging has shown significantly raised N-acetyl-L-aspartate (NAA), total choline, total creatine, and lactate levels in carriers who subsequently developed MELAS compared with carriers who did not.

Neurophysiological studies

Electroencephalography (EEG) may show focal or diffuse slowing, and various focal and generalized epileptiform discharges. Visual

Table 168.4 Combinations of MRI abnormalities seen in various mitochondrial disease syndromes.

Mitochondrial syndrome	Basal ganglia signal abnormalities or calcification	Cerebellar signal abnormalities or atrophy	Brainstem signal abnormalities or atrophy	Leucoencephalopathy	Cortical atrophy	Stroke-like episodes
MELAS	±	±	−	−	±	±
MERRF	±	−	−	±	±	−
KSS	±	±	±	±	±	±
MNGIE	±	±	±	+	−	−
LS	±	±	±	±	−	−

KSS = Kearns–Sayre syndrome; LS = Leigh syndrome; MELAS = mitochondrial encephalopathy, lactic acidosis, and stroke-like episodes; MERRF = myoclonic epilepsy and ragged red fibers; MNGIE = mitochondrial neurogastrointestinal encephalopathy evoked potentials (VEP) may show prolonged P100 latencies, especially in patients with LHON and retinopathy, but sometimes also in the absence of clear morphological changes. Brainstem auditory evoked responses (BAER) are used to demonstrate sensorineural hearing loss, which may be present even in asymptomatic individuals.

Exercise physiology

Formal exercise testing with near-infrared spectroscopy and measurement of oxygen consumption is available in specialized centers. These tests assess the respiratory chain function non-invasively, revealing abnormal results in patients with mitochondrial disorders. While useful, these tests may not be applicable to young children because of the need for their active cooperation.

Muscle biopsy

Muscle biopsy is performed with two main objectives: histochemistry (with modified Gomori trichrome, SDH, and COX staining) and enzyme biochemical assays to assess the various complexes of the respiratory chain (Table 168.5). Ultrastructural studies may show mitochondrial proliferation, enlarged mitochondria with disorganized cristae, or abnormal mitochondrial inclusions. The RRF seen with the modified Gomori trichrome staining have abnormal subsarcolemmal and, less prominently, intermyofibrillar collections of mitochondria. SDH, NADH-TR (nicotinamide dehydrogenase-tetrazolium reductase), and COX stains can also demonstrate excessive mitochondrial proliferation, and may identify isolated enzyme defects. Disorders of protein synthesis usually have COX-negative RRF, with the exception of MELAS, where there may be relative preservation of COX staining. Certain conditions like LHON and NARP usually do not have abnormal histology or any respiratory chain enzyme defects.

Biochemical assays of respiratory chain function may be performed either in isolated mitochondrial fractions or in whole tissue homogenates. The following assays are usually performed: (1) NADH-cytochrome c reductase (complexes I + III); (2) NADH-CoQ reductase (complex I); (3) NADH dehydrogenase (complex I); (4) succinate-cytochrome c reductase (complexes II + III); (5) reduced CoQ-cytochrome c reductase (complex III); (6) cytochrome c oxidase (complex IV); (7) succinate dehydrogenase (complex II); and (8) citrate synthase, a matrix enzyme of the Krebs cycle. Citrate synthase, which is encoded by nDNA, is a good marker of mitochondrial abundance, and we refer the activities of respiratory chain enzymes to those of citrate synthase to correct for increased (or more rarely decreased) numbers of mitochondria. Conditions with multiple deletions or depletion of mtDNA usually have multiple partial defects of the respiratory chain enzymes, although in some cases these defects may not be apparent. Isolated defects of complex I, II, or IV activity suggest mutations in mtDNA genes encoding subunits of that complex, or in nDNA genes encoding subunits or assembly proteins of the same complex. Enzyme assays should always be interpreted in the light of the clinical presentation and caution should be used in assessing data in very young and very old patients. When a defect in mtDNA translation is suspected, one-dimensional or two-dimensional (2D) Blue Native PAGE (polyacrylamide gel electrophoresis) for mitochondrial proteins extract from muscle homogenate or any affected tissue available should be performed to identify the defect.

Molecular genetic testing

The choice of the appropriate DNA test is a complex decision that requires review of the clinical features, histology, and biochemical results. If a mitochondrial syndrome such as MELAS, MERRF, NARP, MILS, or NARP is evident, the appropriate mutations can be screened in blood. Other easily accessible tissues may also be used, such as urinary sediment, buccal mucosa, hair follicles, or cultured skin fibroblasts. If there is a history suggestive of PEO or KSS,

Table 168.5 Summary of clinical syndromes, genetic and pathological classification, as well as associated lactic acidosis, type of ragged red fibers (with cytochrome c oxidase COX staining), and patterns of respiratory chain complex deficiencies in the muscle.

Genetic defect	Functional defect	Clinical features	LA	RRF	Muscle biochemistry
mtDNA mutations	Defects of protein synthesis	KSS; PS; CPEO; MELAS; MERRF	+	COX−	I+ III+ IV
	Protein-coding gene mutations	LHON; NARP/MILS/ MELAS overlaps	− +/−	− +/−	I; V
		Myopathy	+	COX+	I; III
Inter-genomic signaling defects (nDNA)	Multiple mtDNA deletions	adPEO; arPEO; ARCO; MNGIE; SANDO	+	COX−	I+ III+ IV
	mtDNA depletion	Hepatocerebral; myopathic; Alpers	+	COX−	I+ III+ IV
	Defects of mtDNA translation	Hepatocerebral; generalized; MLASA	+	COX−	I+ III+ IV
Other nDNA mutations	RC subunits	LS	+	−	I; II
	Assembly proteins	LS; LSFC; EE; GRACILE	+	−	I; III; IV; V
	Fusion/fission/motility	AD-optic atrophy; CMT; HSP	+/−	−	?
	Lipid milieu	Barth syndrome	−	+	IV

adPEO = autosomal dominant progressive external ophthalmoplegia; ARCO = autosomal recessive cardiopathy and ophthalmoplegia; arPEO = autosomal recessive progressive external ophthalmoplegia; CMT = Charcot–Marie–Tooth disease; CPEO = chronic progressive external ophthalmoplegia; EE = ethylmalonic encephalopathy; HSP = hereditary spastic paraplegia; GRACILE = growth retardation, aminoaciduria, iron overload, lactic acidosis, early death; KSS = Kearns–Sayre syndrome; LA = lactic acidosis; LHON = Leber's hereditary optic neuropathy; LS = Leigh syndrome; LSFC = Leigh syndrome, French Canadian type; MELAS = mitochondrial encephalopathy, lactic acidosis, and stroke-like episodes; MERRF = myoclonic epilepsy and ragged red fibers; MILS = maternally-inherited Leigh syndrome; MLASA = mitochondrial myopathy and sideroblastic anemia; MNGIE = mitochondrial neurogastrointestinal encephalopathy; NARP = neuropathy, ataxia, and retinitis pigmentosa; PS = Pearson syndrome; RRF = ragged red fibers; SANDO = sensory ataxia, neuropathy, dysarthria and ophthalmoplegia

Southern blot to detect single or multiple mtDNA deletions should be performed. In pure sporadic myopathy, muscle is the tissue of choice, as the mutant mtDNA is not found in other tissues.

Leigh syndrome is a particularly difficult condition to define because of its striking biochemical and genetic heterogeneity. Certain clinical features may be useful; for example, retinitis pigmentosa is almost pathognomonic for MILS. X-linked transmission suggests mutations in the PDHC E1α subunit. A history suggestive of autosomal recessive inheritance should trigger biochemical analysis of muscles to look for a specific complex deficiency for which the specific genes can then be screened (Table 168.2).

With the advent of high-throughput next-generation sequencing such as targeted or whole-exome sequencing, sequential sequencing of mitochondrial genes may soon be a strategy of the past. Recent targeted exomic studies (sequencing of the whole mitochondrial genome and about 1500 known mitochondrial genes) resulted in increased identification of molecular defects by approximately 20%. As these technologies become more affordable over time, it is likely that next-generation sequencing will be the cornerstone of mitochondrial genetic diagnosis.

Mitochondrial disease scales

Mitochondrial disease scales are important in natural history studies of this diverse group of diseases and are also critical in evaluation of outcomes in therapy. These scales remain the mainstay of periodic assessments, as there is no single effective biomarker for mitochondrial disorders. At present, several age-appropriate disease scales exist, including the Newcastle Mitochondrial Disease Adult Scale (NMDAS) and the Newcastle Paediatric Mitochondrial Disease Scale (NPMDS), which can be used to rate quantitatively the degree of disease involvement in different organ systems of affected patients, as well as the patients' quality of life.

Therapy

Therapy for mitochondrial diseases is woefully inadequate. To date, treatments have been palliative or have involved the use of vitamins, cofactors, and antioxidants with the aim of mitigating, postponing, or circumventing the potential damage to the respiratory chain. Because of the clinical diversity of mitochondrial disorders and their unpredictable clinical course, rigorous, controlled therapeutic trials are difficult to perform, and therefore most interventions are not evidence-based. Commonly used laboratory measures such as lactate levels, neurophysiological responses, MRS, or strength testing may not adequately reflect the efficacy of treatment. Class 1 evidence is therefore unlikely to be obtained in evaluating treatments of mitochondrial disorders.

Symptomatic therapy

Treatment of specific symptoms is important in patients with mitochondrial encephalomyopathies. Seizures usually respond to anticonvulsants, although valproic acid should be used with caution because it inhibits carnitine uptake, which could worsen myopathy or trigger fulminant hepatic failure in patients with Alpers syndrome. PEO can be treated with surgery for ptosis and sensorineural hearing loss with cochlear implants. Episodes of recurrent myoglobinuria should be treated aggressively with fluid hydration and urine alkalinization.

Exercise training may benefit patients not only by improving their oxidative capacity, but also potentially by inducing regeneration of muscle fibers that have lower amounts of mutant mtDNA than mature muscle fibers.

In general, most anesthetic and surgical procedures are well tolerated by patients with mitochondrial disorders. Problems with anesthesia are usually related to preexisting clinical conditions such as seizures, respiratory compromise, and cardiac arrhythmias. Careful preoperative assessment is necessary and patients with myopathy should avoid the use of inhalational agents and depolarizing muscle relaxants that may trigger malignant hyperthermia.

Dietary measures such as the ketogenic diet may be useful in selected conditions, such as PDHC deficiency, and potentially even in KSS, where ketogenic treatment has been shown to decrease deleted mtDNA in cell cultures.

Pharmacological therapy

The strategy for pharmacological treatment of mitochondrial disorders is to minimize the metabolic derangements resulting from respiratory chain dysfunction by removing toxic metabolites, to improve respiratory chain function by introducing electron chain acceptors, vitamins, and cofactors essential to respiratory chain function, and to decrease oxidative stress by giving oxygen radical scavengers.

Removal of noxious metabolites

Dichloroacetic acid (DCA) is a pyruvate dehydrogenase kinase inhibitor, which keeps PDH in the active form and favors lactic acid oxidation, thereby decreasing lactic acidosis. While it is useful for treatment of acute lactic acidosis, the side effects of chronic therapy, specifically peripheral neuropathy, suggest that DCA should not be used over extended periods of time.

Administration of electron acceptors

Primary CoQ_{10} deficiency can be treated with high-dose CoQ_{10} supplementation (300–1500 mg/day) in severe infantile encephalopathic and myopathic primary CoQ_{10} deficiency. Patients with the ataxic form tend to respond less well, probably due to inadequate drug bioavailability in the cerebellum or irreversible cerebellar damage.

Administration of vitamins and cofactors

Various cocktails of vitamins (riboflavin, thiamine, folic acid) and cofactors (CoQ_{10}, L-carnitine, creatine, and lipoic acid) have been used based on anecdotal reports. Some of these compounds may be decreased in patients (e.g., carnitine deficiency secondary to partial impairment of β-oxidation), warranting supplementation, while others are considered to be neuroprotective because they supposedly favor ATP production and counteract free radical generation and apoptosis. Anecdotal evidence also supports the use of folinic acid because of an abnormal CSF:serum folate ratio.

Alteration of nitric oxide (NO) homeostasis is thought to underlie endothelial dysfunction in MELAS patients, resulting in stroke-like episodes. Intravenous administration of L-arginine (0.5 g/kg) during the acute phase and interictal oral administration (0.15–0.3 g/kg/day) diminished the frequency and severity of stroke-like episodes in open-label trials.

Administration of oxygen radical scavengers

In order to decrease free radical damage in energy-challenged cells, several oxygen radical scavengers have been used, such as vitamin E, CoQ_{10}, idebenone, glutathione, and dihydrolipoate. Recent trials of EPI-743, a para-benzoquinone analogue with potent cellular protective activity against oxidative stress, has shown promising results in several open-label studies in patients with mitochondrial disorders and Leigh syndrome, with improvements in the oxidative state of the brain on SPECT scans.

Gene therapy

Gene therapy for mtDNA disorders is not available, mainly because no investigator has been able to transfect DNA into mitochondria in a heritable fashion. Currently, one of the most promising strategies is to force a shift in heteroplasmy, reducing the ratio of mutant to wild-type genomes. This can be achieved by inhibiting replication of mutant genomes with peptide nucleic acids, importing RNAs into the mitochondria, importing polypeptides into the mitochondria, selecting for respiratory function, inducing muscle regeneration, and inducing mitochondrial fusion. Most of these approaches have shown promising results *in vitro*, but none is readily applicable to patients.

Gene therapy for nDNA disorders is similar to that for other Mendelian disorders. Proof-of-principle studies have been performed by inserting transgene ANT1 protein into the mitochondrial inner membrane of transgenic *Ant1* mutant mice, ameliorating their muscle pathology. The efficacy and safety of this approach have also been demonstrated in *MPV117*, *ETHE1*, and thymidine phosphorylase/uridine phosphorylase mouse models.

Cytoplasmic transfer

As many mtDNA diseases are devastating and life threatening and prenatal diagnosis is of limited use, there are few reproductive options for carrier women. Cytoplasmic transfer is an approach where the nuclear genome is transferred between the oocyte from a carrier to an enucleated oocyte from a normal donor. In this process, the embryo will have the nDNA of the biological parents, but the mtDNA of a normal woman. Nuclear genome transfer has been shown to be a promising technique, as it did not reduce the developmental efficiency to the blastocyst stage and genomic integrity was maintained by transferring incompletely assembled spindle-chromosomal complexes in one study. Although mtDNA was transferred together with the nuclear genome, this was an extremely low amount (less than 1%). Therapeutic application of this technique is pending approval in the United States and it has been approved in the United Kingdom.

Nucleoside and nucleotide treatment

Mitochondrial nucleotide pool unbalance represents the pathogenic pathway for a group of mtDNA depletion syndromes in which key enzymes in the salvage pathway of deoxypurine and deoxypyrimidine are defective. *In vivo* and *in vitro* studies have recently demonstrated the efficacy and safety of oral supplementation with the specific reduced dNTPs to rescue the mtDNA depletion and consequently mitochondrial dysfunction. This represents an example of disease-modifying treatment that has potential for human use.

Mitochondrial biogenesis modulators

Mitochondrial disorders have common dysfunction in the oxidative phosphorylation (OXPHOS) system, with ATP depletion and overproduction of reactive oxygen species (ROS), resulting in activation of compensatory mechanisms in the expression of antioxidant enzymes, mitochondrial biogenesis, overexpression of respiratory chain subunits, or metabolic shift to glycolysis. New therapeutic approaches have been developed specifically targeting mitochondrial biogenesis, including bezafibrate targeting the PGC-1alpha axis, AICAR modulating the AMPK pathway, or NAD+ and its precursor, vitamin B3, regulating the sirtuin proteins. Clinical trials for safety and efficacy are still necessary.

Conclusion

The nervous system is one of the most frequently affected organs in mitochondrial diseases and therefore should be extensively investigated if mitochondrial disease is suspected. While therapy for mitochondrial disorders continues to be woefully inadequate at present, rapidly increasing knowledge of different molecular defects and their pathogenic mechanisms may allow individualized treatments in future.

Further reading

Barragan-Campos HM, Vallee JN, Lo D, *et al.* Brain magnetic resonance imaging findings in patients with mitochondrial cytopathies. *Arch Neurol* 2005;62:737–742.

DiMauro S. Mitochondrial encephalomyopathies – fifty years on: *The Robert Wartenberg Lecture. Neurology* 2013;81:281–291.

DiMauro S, Quinzii CM, Hirano M. Mutations in coenzyme Q10 biosynthetic genes. *J Clin Invest* 2007;117:587–589.

Maresca A, la Morgia C, Caporali L, Valentino ML, Carelli V. The optic nerve: A "mito-window" on mitochondrial neurodegeneration. *Mol Cell Neurosci* 2013;55:62–76.

Molleston JP, Sokol RJ, Karnsakul W, *et al.* Evaluation of the child with suspected mitochondrial liver disease. *J Pediatr Gastroenterol Nutr* 2013;57:269–276.

Paull D, Emmanuele V, Weiss KA, *et al.* Nuclear genome transfer in human oocytes eliminates mitochondrial DNA variants. *Nature* 2013;493:632–637.

Pearce S, Nezich CL, Spinazzola A. Mitochondrial diseases: Translation matters. *Mol Cell Neurosci* 2013;55:1–12.

Pfeffer G, Horvath R, Klopstock T, *et al.* New treatments for mitochondrial disease–no time to drop our standards. *Nat Rev Neurol* 2013;9:474–481.

Schaefer AM, Taylor RW, Turnbull DM, Chinnery PF. The epidemiology of mitochondrial disorders - past, present and future. *Biochim Biophys Acta* 2004;1659:115–120.

Viscomi C, Bottani E, Zeviani M. Emerging concepts in the therapy of mitochondrial disease. *Biochim Biophys Acta* 2015;1847:544–557.

169 Disorders resulting from transporter defects

Anna Czlonkowska[1], David Gloss[2], and Tomasz Litwin[3]

[1] Institute of Psychiatry and Neurology and Warsaw Medical University, Warsaw, Poland
[2] Geisinger Health System, Danville, PA, USA
[3] Institute of Psychiatry and Neurology, Warsaw, Poland

Transporter defects are a group of mostly rare diseases that span many areas of neurology. This chapter describes some of the best-understood and most well-known transporter defects (Wilson's disease, Menkes disease, and carnitine *O*-palmitoyltransferase 2 deficiency), as well as four very rare disorders–namely, other copper transporter AP1S1 (MEDNIK syndrome), manganese transporter deficiency (HMDPC), glucose transporter 1 (GLUT1) deficiency syndrome, and hereditary folate malabsorption (HFM)–to demonstrate the range of transporter defects with neurological manifestations.

Disorders of copper transporters

Copper is an essential trace metal taken in through food and present in nearly every cell in the body. It is found in the highest concentrations in the liver and brain, but levels are also relatively high in the other organs. It is used by the body as a cofactor for a variety of enzymes (cytochrome *c* oxidase, dopamine beta hydroxylase, superoxidase dismutase) that are required for normal neurological development and function. Copper is also a potential source of free radicals and oxidative stress, and excess copper can lead to neurodegeneration. Copper metabolism is regulated by a complex system that allows it to be utilized where needed while also protecting the brain and other organs from the toxic effects of the metal. Dysfunction in transporters involved in copper metabolism can therefore lead to significant damage to many organ systems.

There are two main disorders of copper metabolism related to transporters: Wilson's disease of ATP7B and Menkes disease of ATP7A. While the proteins encoded by these genes are identical in function, the unique signs and symptoms of these diseases occur as a result of localization of the proteins in different tissues. There is also another protein involved in copper transport, AP1S1. AP1S1 dysfunction can lead to copper disturbances and a syndrome consisting of biochemical signs of both of the main copper metabolic disorders.

Wilson's disease

Wilson first described this disease in 1912 in the United Kingdom. It is autosomal recessive disease, the exact frequency of which is not known. Older European and North American studies have shown a prevalence of 1 in 30000 live births, but more recent data indicate that frequency may be higher, at 1 in 7000 in Europe and 1 in 3000 in East Asia. The frequency is much higher in isolated populations. It seems likely that a large number of patients remain undiagnosed and/or that penetrance of the gene is reduced in these populations.

Clinical features

Wilson's disease can first present at a range of ages, with typical cases presenting at ages 6–35 years, but later diagnosis is now more common. Three main forms of the disease are distinguished: (1) hepatic (hepatic symptoms without neurological signs); (2) neurological (due to common behavioral or psychiatric symptoms; this form is also named neuropsychiatric); and (3) presymptomatic (when disease is diagnosed based on family screening before development of clinical signs). Typically, if the initial presentation occurs before the age of 10 years, Wilson's disease manifests with hepatic symptoms only. If the presentation is later, neurological symptoms more often present, but that is not always the case. Wilson's disease is usually fatal if not recognized. Diagnosis in advanced stages of the disease worsens prognosis.

In more than 50% of patients with Wilson's disease, the presenting feature is hepatic dysfunction. It can be only a mild increase in transaminase or acute hepatitis, or it can manifest as chronic active hepatitis and as cirrhosis. Acute liver failure, often with hemolytic anemia, accounts for about 10% of referrals for emergency liver transplantation. Cirrhosis may develop in a cryptogenic way, and is detected in most cases that present clinically with neurological signs. Liver injury may lead to hepatic encephalopathy, in which pyramidal signs, asterixis, and disturbances of consciousness are often observed. These features are not characteristic of the neurological form of the disease. However, in some cases it is difficult to distinguish neurological and behavioral signs caused by hepatic encephalopathy from those caused by the neurological form.

The neurological symptoms of Wilson's disease are also quite variable. Three main phenotypes are recognized: parkinsonian, dystonic, and ataxic. However, most patients have signs from more than one system, making it difficult to distinguish clearly between these phenotypes. Initial signs may be very mild and worsen without treatment, leading to severe disability. Different types of tremor can be observed: intentional, positional, and resting. Tremors are often asymmetric at the beginning. The characteristic

International Neurology, Second edition. Edited by Robert P. Lisak, Daniel D. Truong, William M. Carroll and Roongroj Bhidayasiri
© 2016 John Wiley & Sons, Ltd. Published 2016 by John Wiley & Sons, Ltd.

"wing-beating tremor" is observed in later stages of the disease. Dystonia can be focal initially, followed later by segmental or generalized dystonia with painful contractures. Hypomimia (masked facies), facial grimacing with jaw opening and lip retraction, and drooling are often present. As the disease progresses, risus sardonicus is very characteristic. Dysarthria of various types is usually observed during the early stage of the disease and, in severe forms of dystonia, can progress to permanent aphonia. Gait is affected relatively later in the disease course, and can become parkinsonian, ataxic, or dystonic.

Most patients have mild behavioral features, but severe irritability and aggression may occur. Severe psychiatric syndromes such as depression, mania, and hallucinations are also observed. Behavioral and psychiatric symptoms may precede the first neurological symptoms by many years or may occur in the context of hepatic injury. Decline in school performance is often observed in children.

About 95% of patients with neurological impairment, half with only liver disease, and some in the presymptomatic stage have a brownish-yellow discoloration of the limbus due to copper deposition in Descemet's membrane in the cornea, called a Kayser–Fleischer ring. Sunflower cataract is rarely observed. Hematological abnormalities (low platelets, leukopenia, anemia), renal, cardiac, or musculoskeletal involvement may also occur.

Pathophysiology

Wilson's disease arises from a defect in the *ATP7B* gene on chromosome 13q14.3–q21.1. The Wilson's disease protein (ATP7B) is a copper-transporting P-type ATPase. It is possibly responsible for transport of copper across the trans-Golgi network and into transport vesicles. This protein directs the incorporation of copper into apo-ceruloplasmin and lysosomes. The copper in the vesicular compartment is excreted into bile. Impaired synthesis of ceruloplasmin and copper excretion from hepatocytes leads to cell overload, necrosis, and release of free copper into the blood, which further accumulates in other tissues. A high amount of copper is also excreted through the kidney in urine. There are more than 500 identified mutations of *ATP7B*, the most common of which in Europe is H1069Q, which may occur in about 50% of patients with Wilson's disease and has a tendency to be associated with a later and neurological presentation. In different world regions various predominances of mutations are observed due to the founder effect.

Diagnosis

Due to the variable clinical signs, diagnosis may be difficult. The disease should be suspected in persons with liver disorder of unknown origin and patients with atypical extrapyramidal/cerebral signs for common neurological diseases (e.g., Parkinson's disease, essential tremor, cerebellar atrophy).

A careful medical history is important, with red flags noted in patients with liver disease and later neurological or psychiatric symptoms, as well as hepatic or neurological diseases in the family. Standard laboratory tests may show liver and often hematological abnormalities. More specific tests for abnormal copper metabolism are ceruloplasmin concentration in blood, 24-hour copper excretion with urine, and total copper in blood. Ceruloplasmin usually is decreased below 50% of the lower laboratory range, but in the hepatic form can be in the normal range. Copper excretion in the urine is usually markedly increased (above 40 μg/24 hr), but in early stages of the disease may be borderline. Total blood copper is decreased (due to low ceruloplasmin), but this test has the lowest

diagnostic value. Due to different methods used across laboratories, results must be compared with laboratory norms.

DNA analysis to identify mutations is now more commonly available. It is regarded as the gold standard diagnostic test. Due to a high number of mutations, as a first step patients should be tested for mutations that predominant in their particular region, and later, if that is negative, by full gene sequencing. Lack of detection of two mutations does not exclude the disease. Slit-lamp examination to look for Kayser–Fleischer rings is recommended during the initial evaluation, but the rings are not always present in the hepatic form of the disease. Kayser–Fleischer rings, while sensitive, are not highly specific, since they can also be found in patients with chronic cholestatic diseases as well as in disorders with a high serum copper level (e.g., neoplasms) and during estrogen intake. Other components of the diagnostic evaluation can include hepatic copper concentrations on liver biopsy (copper concentration is usually above 250 μg/g dry tissue), radiolabeled copper testing, and brain imaging. Magnetic resonance brain imaging in the neurological form usually shows pathology in basal ganglia, thalamus (Figure 169.1), and, in more advanced stages, also in the brainstem. Changes can be asymmetric at the beginning. In many cases with atypical extrapyramidal signs, imaging directs the diagnosis.

There is a scoring system that is used by many neurologists to establish a diagnosis (Table 169.1, recommended by the European Association for the Study of the Liver). The scoring system includes mutation analysis as one of the criteria; this may not be feasible or accessible in developing countries. However, even without the ability to perform mutation analysis, the scoring system can be useful in diagnosis. Siblings of patients should be screened for Wilson's disease. Recent studies on disease gene frequency indicate that it is reasonable to screen children of the proband, as their risk of disease is 4%.

Treatment

The goal of pharmacological treatment is to remove copper overload in tissues and stop further accumulation of copper. There are two main groups of drugs: chelators (d-penicillamine, trientine), which bind copper in blood and tissues and facilitate its excretion

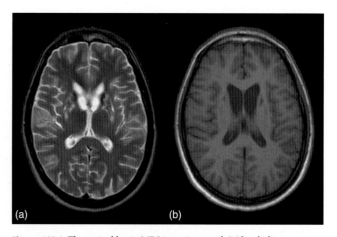

Figure 169.1 The typical brain MRI in patients with Wilson's disease–symmetrically increased signal intensity in T2 weighted sequences in both putamen and globus pallidus (a), with hypointensive signal in T1 sequences (b).

Table 169.1 Scoring system for diagnosis of Wilson's disease. Source: European Association for the Study of the Liver 2012. Reproduced with permission of Elsevier under the Creative Commons License.

Clinical signs and symptoms and other tests used in diagnosis	Evaluation (in points)		
Kayser–Fleisher rings	0 = absent	2 = present	
Neurological symptoms	0 = absent	1 = mild	2 = severe
Serum ceruloplasmin*	0 if normal (>0.2 g/L)	1 if 0.1–0.2 g/L	2 if <0.1 g/L
Coombs negative hemolytic anemia	0 = absent	1 = present	
Liver copper (in absence of cholestasis)	-1 if (normal <50 µg/g)	1 if 50–250 µg/g or 1 if rhodanine positive granules if unable to perform quantitative liver copper	2 if >5x upper limit of normal (ULN) (>250 µg/g)
Urinary copper (in absence of acute hepatitis)	0 = normal	1 if 1–2x ULN	2 if >2x ULN 2 if normal but >5x after D-penicillamine
Mutation analysis	0 if no mutation found	1 if on one chromosome	4 if on both chromosomes

≥4 diagnosis established, 3 diagnosis possible, 0–2 diagnosis very unlikely

in urine; and zinc salts, which inhibit intestinal copper absorption. Both treatment approaches are effective and in the great majority of cases can stop disease progression, in others leading to clinical improvement. In presymptomatic cases, early therapy may delay symptom onset. Therapeutic effects depend on the stage of the disease. Severe neurological impairment is usually non-reversible. Treatment must be maintained for the whole life and drug compliance is crucial for good long-term prognosis. The choice of therapy depends on drug availability, price, and physician experience. There is no direct evidence that chelating agents are better than zinc salts. They both may be used as initial and maintenance therapy.

D-penicillamine is usually given in the initial dose 1000–1500 mg/day in 3 divided doses, one hour before each meal. It is important to start therapy with small doses, 100 mg per day, increasing the dose every few days and reaching the full dose by 1 month. Rapid introduction of the drug may lead to severe, even permanent, neurological deterioration. The long-term dose can be 1000 mg, but basic laboratory tests and copper excretion in urine should be monitored. Adverse effects of D-penicillamine include leukopenia, skin rash, proteinuria, and autoimmune diseases, but in the great majority of cases the drug is well tolerated and patients stay on it for decades.

Trientine has not been studied as extensively, but, based on preliminary data, it appears to work as well as D-penicillamine, with probably fewer side effects. It was originally introduced as an alternative to D-penicillamine. The initial daily dose is 900–2700 mg, and the maintenance dose is 900–1500 mg. Therapy also should be started with small doses.

Zinc salts (sulphate, acetate, gluconate) are given in daily doses of 150–180 mg of zinc (in children, between 50 mg and 75 mg), 30 min before or after meals, divided into 3 doses. The most common adverse effect is gastritis. Taking the drug after meals causes fewer adverse effects.

No symptomatic drugs improve neurological recovery. Any drugs that modulate dopaminergic transmission, especially neuroleptics, should be avoided, as they may cause severe and rapid neurological deterioration. Symptomatic therapy in liver disease should be administered according to hepatologists' recommendations (diuretics, vitamin K, lactulose, etc.).

Treated patients should undergo periodic clinical examination. Liver function tests and other basic laboratory tests should be performed. Copper metabolism should also be studied. It may help to monitor drug compliance and overtreatment. High urinary 24-hour copper excretion after a few years of treatment indicates non-compliance. Generally, patients taking chelators should have urinary copper levels lower than before the initiation of therapy, but higher than the upper limit of normal. Patients treated with zinc should have values below the normal range. Low values of total copper indicate copper deficiency, which may cause leukopenia and myelopathy.

Liver transplantation is recommended only in cases of acute, severe liver failure or decompensated liver cirrhosis. Transplantation should not be done for improvement of neurological signs. Patients awaiting transplant should receive anti-copper treatment.

Menkes disease

Clinical features

Menkes disease was first described by John Menkes in 1962. It is an X-linked recessive disorder of copper metabolism that is detectable during the prenatal period. A multisystem disease, it is progressively degenerative and fatal. Onset of symptoms occurs within 1–2 months after birth and the disorder has a relentless course, ending in death between the ages of 1 and 3 years. Clinically, it is characterized by scant, white, silver, or gray, stubby, kinky hair (the disease is also known as kinky hair disease); skin pallor; growth retardation; hypothermia with acute illness; long bone metaphyseal demineralization; tortuosity of cerebral vessels; and diffuse cerebral atrophy with subdural fluid collection. Seizures often complicate the picture. Other symptoms include bone spurs and pudgy rosy cheeks. The incidence of Menkes disease is estimated to be 1 in 100000. Since it is X-linked recessive, it is a rare disease in females. In the few female cases that have been reported, expression of the disease is variable.

Several variants of the disorder have been reported, but due to the paucity of cases it is difficult to determine whether these cases are truly related. There are Japanese cases that do not show the characteristic kinky hair. There is an occipital horn syndrome (OHS) with occipital exostoses that do not develop until age 3 or 4 years with skin laxity, dysarthria, and chronic diarrhea. Late-onset and asymptomatic cases have also been described. Finally, ATP7A-related distal motor neuropathy with ATP7A dysfunction can occur. This genotype differs from classic Menkes disease and OHS, with symptoms manifesting between 5 and 50 years of age with atrophy and weakness of distal muscles, deep tendon reflex loss, and pes cavus foot deformity. However, biochemical disturbances in serum copper and copper metabolism are not seen in these cases.

Pathophysiology

Menkes disease results from a defect of the *ATP7A* gene on chromosome Xq13.3. *ATP7A* is present in the brain, intestines, kidneys, and other organs, but not in the liver. This gene codes for an ATPase that is integral to transmembrane copper transport and mediates the transport of copper across the intestinal mucosa, the blood–brain barrier, and the blood–cerebrospinal fluid barrier. The ATP7A protein transports copper and is located on the trans-Golgi network. When this transport system fails, copper cannot reach cells that require copper for the structure and function of enzymes involved in various bodily processes. When intracellular copper levels become too high, the protein translocates to the cell membrane to excrete the copper. As a result of defective intestinal copper transport, there is deficient transport of dietary copper in the intestine, but accumulations in the duodenum, kidney, pancreas, placenta, and skeletal muscle. Patients with Menkes disease have abnormally low levels of copper in the brain and blood.

There is a diverse group of genetic mutations in *ATP7A* that cause Menkes disease, some of which result in complete loss of transporter function. Variation among the types of mutations on the *ATP7A* gene may underlie the variety of clinical manifestations. A large deletion or a frame-shift mutation is thought to cause infantile-onset Menkes disease, while mutations causing either reduced levels of ATP7A or reduced function of ATP7A are believed to cause the occipital horn syndrome.

The symptoms of Menkes disease can be explained by the effect of the gene mutation on the essential enzymes that need copper to function. The loss of hair and skin pigment may be explained by dysfunction of the copper-containing enzyme tyrosinase, which catalyzes the production of melanin from tyrosine by oxidation. Arterial defects are due to abnormalities in an extracellular copper enzyme, lysyl oxidase, which is involved in cross-linking collagens and elastin. Kinky hair is related to monoamine oxidase dysfunction. Hypothermia may be explained by cytochrome *c* oxidase dysfunction, and the long bone demineralization may be due to peptidylglycine monooxygenase dysfunction (which leads to decrease of different endocrine factors, e.g., kalcytonine) as well as ascorbate oxidase dysfunction.

Diagnosis

Diagnosis is generally clinical, and is suspected when infants have typical neurological and hair changes, with confirmation by high placental copper levels, low serum copper and ceruloplasmin levels (after 6 weeks of age), or abnormal catecholamines. Because copper is an essential cofactor for dopamine β-hydroxylase, the ratio of urinary excretion of the dopamine metabolite homovanillic acid (HVA) is increased over that of the norepinephrine metabolite vanillylmandelic acid (VMA). The latter two can be tested at birth. More recently, some neurologists have used a skin cell fibroblast culture and molecular genetic testing with multiplex ligation-dependent probe amplification (MLPA).

Treatment

The treatment for Menkes disease is subcutaneous administration of copper chloride and *L*-histidine in an attempt to restore normal copper levels to the body. Although some children do not respond, those who do respond will have normal blood and cerebrospinal levels of copper within 6 weeks, accompanied by a regression of symptoms other than connective tissue manifestations. Unfortunately, the neurological symptoms may or may not respond. It is thought that copper administration may work only for those children with some functioning ATP7A.

MEDNIK syndrome

Clinical features

MEDNIK syndrome is a rare, autosomal recessive disorder. The mental retardation, enteropathy, deafness, neuropathy, ichthyosis, and keratodermia. The other clinical symptoms include dysmorphic features (resembling Down syndrome facial appearance, low-set ears, growth retardation, and others), osteoporosis, hair pathology similar to Menkes disease, and erythrodermia, as well as liver disease (hepatomegaly with signs of intrahepatic cholestasis). The phenotypic presentation of the disease mostly combines the symptoms of both Wilson's and Menkes diseases.

Pathophysiology

The disease is caused by mutations in the *AP1S1* gene on the 7q22.1 chromosome, encoding a small subunit of the adaptor protein (AP1). This protein mediates intracellular signals, also affecting copper metabolism by perturbing copper ATPases, leading to decreased levels of serum ceruloplasmin and total copper and increased hepatic copper storage and urinary copper excretion, as in Wilson's disease.

Diagnosis

Diagnosis is based on clinical presentation as well as copper metabolism abnormalities including decreased serum ceruloplasmin and total copper and increased serum non-ceruloplasmin-bound copper and daily copper urinary excretion. It is confirmed by genetic analysis (homozygous mutation in the *AP1S1* gene on the 7q22.1 chromosome).

Treatment

Treatment with zinc salts (only zinc acetate is used) is effective, with significant improvement in clinical symptoms and copper metabolism; however, due to the limited number of MEDNIK cases, the treatment experience is very limited.

Manganese transporter deficiency

Clinical features

Manganese transporter deficiency disease was first described as an autosomal recessive disorder in 2012. The clinical symptoms of the disease include features of liver disease and movement disorders. Consequently, the disease is also known as HMDPC (hypermanganesemia with dystonia, polycythemia, and cirrhosis). As in Wilson's disease, the severity of liver disease varies widely, from asymptomatic increases in liver enzyme, through liver cirrhosis to liver failure.

The neurological symptoms of the disease, in most cases, begin during the first decade of life (2–14 years) with predominant dystonia (usually generalized); other symptoms such as spastic paraparesis or motor neuropathy rarely occur. In the two adulthood-onset cases described to date (45- and 47-year-old patients), asymmetric parkinsonism with early postural instability was reported. Due to brain manganese accumulation, HMDPC patients present a specific abnormality on brain magnetic resonance imaging (MRI), with symmetric hyperintense signal in T1 sequences from bilateral globus pallidus. The other symptoms of the disease include hypermanganesemia, polycythemia with iron storage depletion (decrease level of ferritin), and high total iron binding capacity (TIBC).

Pathophysiology

The disease is caused by a mutation in the manganese transporter *SLC30A10* (Solute Carrier Family 30, Member 10) gene, located on chromosome 1q41, which causes manganese accumulation in the brain (mainly in the basal ganglia and cerebellum) and the liver. Currently, more than 10 mutations have been reported.

Diagnosis

The diagnosis of HMDPC is based on (1) clinical symptoms (i.e., the coexistence of liver disease and movement disorders); (2) polycythemia, which is required for a diagnosis; (3) the tissue affected (e.g., liver) and serum hypermanganesemia (normal Mn2+ serum range <320nmol/L; in HMDPC patients described so far, the manganese serum levels were between 1145 and 6370 nmol/L); and (4) low serum ferritin and increased TIBC5 confirmed by genetic testing.

Treatment

The treatment of HMDPC consists of (1) manganese chelation treatment with repeated infusions of Na2Ca-EDTA, which increases manganese urinary excretion; and (2) oral iron supplementation, which decreases manganese absorption from the digestive tract. Due to the actions of chelators on the metabolism of different metals, regular monitoring of serum zinc, copper, iron, and manganese should be performed to verify treatment safety. The proposed treatment is effective and leads to clinical improvement in most cases.

Carnitine O-palmitoyltransferase 2 deficiency

Carnitine O-palmitoyltransferase 2 (CPT 2) deficiency is the most common metabolic disorder of skeletal muscle. It has an autosomal recessive pattern of inheritance.

Clinical features

There are three different manifestations of this disorder. The neonatal form is universally fatal, with non-ketotic hypoglycemic encephalopathy, respiratory failure, seizures, and arrhythmia leading to cardiac arrest. These neonates often display dysmorphic features. This is the least common form and symptom onset has been noted within hours of birth in some cases, but typically within the first 4 days of life.

The second presentation, the so-called severe infantile hepatocardiomuscular form, typically presents between 6 months and 2 years of age, with most cases presenting in infants under 1 year. This form affects multiple organ systems. Episodes may be brought on by infection, fasting, or fever. This form is primarily characterized by loss of consciousness and seizures due to hypoketotic hypoglycemia. Acute liver failure, hepatomegaly, and cardiomyopathy with severe arrhythmia may also occur. Individuals with this presentation are at risk for liver failure, coma, and sudden death.

The best-known form typically presents in the teen to young adult years, with muscle pain and swelling after either fasting or sustained exercise. During exacerbation of the disease rhabdomyolysis and myoglobinuria occur, sometimes leading to kidney failure. There is increased risk of malignant hyperthermia in patients with this deficiency. Importantly, most patients affected with this presentation have no signs or symptoms of the disease between episodes. There are significant differences in the penetrance of the disease even among members of the same family. There is some evidence that peripheral neuropathy and migraines may develop.

Pathophysiology

Carnitine is ingested largely through dietary meats and dairy products. Carnitine O-palmitoyltransferase 2 is present on the inner membrane of mitochondria and it is involved in the transport of hydrophobic fatty acids. While not a transporter per se, it is a necessary part of a three-enzyme group–carnitine O-palmitoyltransferase 2, acetyl-CoA synthase, and carnitine/acylcarnitine translocase–which allows fatty acids to be transferred into mitochondria to undergo oxidation and energy production.

The *CPT2* gene encodes the CPT 2 enzyme; the gene locus has been identified as 1p32. To date, 60 mutations in the coding process have been identified–in a protein 658 amino acids long–that are known to cause disease, the majority of which cause critical amino acid deletions or substitutions.

Diagnosis

Diagnosis is accomplished by measuring creatine phosphokinase (CPK) and urinary myoglobin after exercise. Muscle histology is typically normal during attacks. Muscle biopsy with carnitine O-palmitoyltransferase 2 measurement confirms the diagnosis. Tandem mass spectrometry is a rapid and non-invasive method for measuring CPT 2 deficiency. Other methods used in diagnosis include enzymatic studies in fibroblasts and/or lymphocytes and other laboratory testing. Metabolic acidosis and hyperammonemia may be observed in neonates and infants. Adults often have myoglobin, creatine kinase, and transaminase levels up to 400 times the upper limit of normal during an attack.

Treatment

Treatment is largely supportive, consisting of exercise restriction and dietary guidelines. A diet with carbohydrate loading can be protective; restriction of lipid intake is also recommended. Patients should be cautioned not to fast. Prolonged exercise should be avoided. A small amount of data suggests that prolonged exercise may be safe with intravenous glucose during exercise, but this is not practical. Carnitine supplementation combined with replacement of long chain with medium chain triglycerides may be beneficial. In adult-onset patients, triheptanoin, a medium chain fatty acid, has been shown to be effective.

GLUT1 deficiency syndrome

GLUT1 (facilitated glucose transporter-1) deficiency (GLUT1 DS) was first described by De Vivo in 1991, and is sometimes called De Vivo disease. It is caused by a genetic defect in glucose transport into the brain. Most often the disease is transmitted as an autosomal dominant disorder (90% of individuals present with *de novo* mutation), but there are also rare reports presenting an autosomal recessive inheritance.

Clinical features

The clinical manifestations of the disease occur in one of two forms:

- Classic GLUT1 DS phenotype (which occurs in almost 90% of patients)–with predominant epileptic seizures, also with delayed neurological development (epileptic encephalopathy), acquired microcephaly, dysarthria, and a wide spectrum of movement disorders (dystonia, ataxia, chorea). Characteristic of this form is the onset of epileptic seizures between the ages of 1 month and 6 months as the first manifestation of the disease. The initial infantile epileptic episodes include apneic episodes, cyanosis, focal seizures, paroxysmal eye movements, complex absence, and tonic seizures, as well as rarely myoclonic astatic epilepsy (MAE). Over time the seizures become generalized tonic, myoclonic, absence, atonic, or unclassified.
- Non-epileptic GLUT1 DS form (10% of patients affected)–without seizures, but with paroxysmal dyskinesias such as choreoathetosis, dystonia, intermittent ataxia, or alternating hemiplegia.

The other neurological symptoms that generally occur intermittently in both forms of GLUT1 DS include sleep disturbances, lethargy, headaches, migraine, a wide spectrum of movement disorders (e.g., chorea, dystonic tremor, cerebellar action tremor, writer's cramp, parkinsonism, myoclonus), and dyspraxia.

There are also newer deficiency syndromes that have recently been described. GLUT1 deficiency syndrome 2, also known as paroxysmal exercise-induced dyskinesia (PED), is much less severe than the type 1 syndrome. It is associated with a combination of dystonia, ballism, and choreoathetotic movements after prolonged exercise and only in the exercised limbs. It is sometimes associated with seizures. Further, previously known dystonia 9 (DYT9) syndrome–paroxysmal choreoathetosis with spasticity–and dystonia 18 (DYT18) syndrome–paroxysmal exercise-induced dyskinesia and epilepsy–are currently recognized also as part of GLUT1 DS spectrum disease.

Pathophysiology

The gene locus is 1p31–35, where it encodes the *SLC2A1* gene. GLUT1 is present in all tissues at low levels. Its highest concentration is in the erythrocytes and cerebral capillary endothelial cells, such as those associated with the blood–brain barrier. Such localization of transporter causes normal serum glucose, low or normal cerebrospinal fluid lactate, and otherwise unexplained hypoglycorrhachia, with typical values being approximately one-third of the serum values. This lack of metabolic energy substrate affects brain development.

Diagnosis

Diagnosis has not been standardized. It can be accomplished through appropriate cerebrospinal fluid (CSF) studies, performed after a 4-hour fast. Most patients with GLUT1 deficiency will have CSF glucose <40 mg/dL, a CSF glucose:blood glucose ratio of 0.33–037, and a CSF lactate value of 0.5–1.4 mmol/L. The GLUT1 deficiency type 2 is characterized by CSF glucose <65 mg/dL, and a CSF glucose:blood glucose ratio of <0.6 (which is near normal). Most reported cases do not have brain abnormalities on MRI, but there is one reported case of delayed myelination.

Treatment

Treatment is the ketogenic diet. Acetoacetate and β-hydroxybutyrate are products of fatty acid metabolism that can be transported across the blood–brain barrier. The brain is well adapted to utilize ketone bodies as fuel. The ketogenic diet has been shown to treat the seizures associated with this condition. Seizure medications have been ineffective. Some medications, including diazepam, valproate, and phenobarbital, may actually exacerbate the condition due to their negative effect on GLUT1 transport. Others, such as phenytoin and carbamazepine, do not seem to worsen the condition, but also do not provide benefit. The ketogenic diet may also improve associated motor symptoms and, to some extent, developmental delay.

In 2014, the US Food and Drug Administration granted orphan drug status to triheptanoin for the treatment of GLUT1 deficiency syndrome. Triheptanoin is a synthetic triglyceride that is metabolized to heptanoate that crosses the blood–brain barrier and is converted to glucose. Heptanoate can be further metabolized to ketones in the liver, can cross the blood–brain barrier, and can regenerate new glucose in the brain. Triheptanoin is currently in Phase 2 clinical trial testing in the United States and Europe in patients who have breakthrough seizures in spite of following the ketogenic diet.

Hereditary folate malabsorption

Clinical features

The clinical symptoms of hereditary folate malabsorption (HFM) occur in early childhood, and have been reported as early as the age of 2 months. The age at symptom onset depends on the folate stores accumulated *in utero*. The clinical symptoms of folate deficiency can be divided into (1) systemic folate deficiency symptoms; and (2) neurological folate deficiency symptoms. The systemic HFM symptoms include megaloblastic anemia (even severe, needing transfusions before HFM diagnosis), less frequently thrombocytopenia and leukopenia, immunodeficiency (humoral and cellular), leading often to severe and reversible infections (prior to folate supplementation) and mimicking severe combined immune deficiency (SCID) symptoms, and diarrhea (as a malabsorption symptom). Neurological HFM symptoms include developmental delay and motor impairment (e.g., ataxia, athetosis, and other movement disorders), peripheral neuropathy, and seizures. In brain CT or MRI basal ganglia calcifications are observed. It is unknown why some patients do not present with neurological symptoms, because all affected patients presented with low folate concentrations in CSF. Most of the reported cases have parental consanguinity. Many children with this disorder may die in the first few months of life without the disorder being recognized.

Pathophysiology

HFM was first described in 1965. It is now known to be caused by homozygous or heterozygous mutations in the *SLC46A1* gene located on chromosome 17q11.2, and encoding the proton-coupled folate transporter (PCFT) protein. This defect leads to impaired intestinal folate absorption, resulting in systemic folate deficiency and impaired transport of folate into the central nervous system (CNS), and ultimately CNS folate deficiency.

Diagnosis

Diagnosis is made by the clinical constellation of megaloblastic anemia with leukopenia, thrombocytopenia, low concentrations of serum immunoglobulin IgG, IgM, and IgA, and low serum and erythrocyte folate concentrations in early infancy. The diagnosis is confirmed by (1) impaired absorption of an oral folate load–baseline serum folate concentration in HFM is very low and after an oral load of 5-formyltetrahydrofolate (5-formylTHF), measurement over more than 4 hours demonstrates no increase or very little increase in serum folate; and (2) a low level of CSF folate (0–1.5 nM in HFM patients) with positive intramuscular administration of 5 mg 5-formylTHF and increased CSF folate concentrations after 1–2 hours, with a decrease to baseline level during a maximum of 24 hours. Finally, recently available molecular genetic testing for mutations in the *SLC46A1* gene can additionally confirm the HFM diagnosis.

Treatment

Folate substitution with 5-formylTHF (oral or parenteral), or with active isomer 6(S)5-formylTHF (parenteral) or (6 S) methylTHF (oral), usually leads to complete reversal of the systemic symptoms of HFM. Correcting neurological deficits due to folate deficiency is more difficult, but it is possible over a longer time period. Systematic assessment by a pediatric neurologist is needed to verify the improvement of motor and cognitive functions, sometimes correlated with CSF folate concentrations of affected patients. Seizures respond variably to folate supplementation and may be controlled with a combination of folate, cyanocobalamin, and methionine. It is important to note that folic acid should not be used for HFM treatment, because exogenous folate could block folate receptors, leading to further worsening of HFM symptoms.

Conclusion

Transporter disorders due to different pathophysiology and underlying problems are a very heterogeneous group of rare genetic neurodegenerative disorders, usually presenting with a wide spectrum of movement disorders and/or epilepsy. Due to advances in metabolic and genetic testing, many of these syndromes can be identified early and successfully treated pharmacologically or with diet (as in GLUT1 DS). The correct and early diagnosis is key for treatment success. Disorders due to transported defects should be included in the differential diagnosis of movement disorders and epilepsy.

Further reading

Dusek P, Litwin T, Czlonkowska A. Wilson disease and other neurodegenerations with metal accumulations. *Neurol Clin* 2015;33:175–204.

European Association for the Study of the Liver. Clinical practice guidelines: Wilson's disease. *J Hepatol* 2012;56:671–685.

Jebnoun S, Kacem S, Mokrani C, *et al*. A family study of congenital malabsorption of folate. *J Inherit Metab Dis* 2001;24:749–750.

Klepper J, Voit T. Facilitated glucose transporter protein type 1 (GLUT1) deficiency syndrome: Impaired glucose transport into the brain–a review. *Eur J Pediatr* 2002;161:295–304.

Vladutiu GD, Bennett MJ, Fisher NM, *et al*. Phenotypic variability among first-degree relatives with carnitine palmitoyltransferase II deficiency. *Muscle Nerve* 2002;26:492–498.

170   The porphyrias

Frank J. E. Vajda

Department of Medicine and Neuroscience, University of Melbourne, Melbourne, VIC, Australia

Porphyria comprises a group of largely inherited inborn errors of metabolism that result from a deficiency of enzymes involved in the production of heme molecules along a complex pathway. Figure 170.1 shows the biochemical pathway for heme synthesis. These enzyme deficiencies are the preferred basis of classification. Porphyrias are overproduction syndromes, with potentially toxic metabolites causing clinical disease. Porphyrias have been classified into hepatic and erythropoietic, based on the site of the metabolic defect, but they also may be classified into acute types of porphyric attacks that differ clinically with the production of chronic skin disorders.

There are seven types of porphyria, of which three, acute intermittent porphyria (AIP), variegate porphyria (VP), and hereditary coproporphyria (HC), commonly give rise clinically to neuropsychiatric syndromes. AIP does not give rise to skin manifestations, but HC and VP can do so. Two erythropoietic porphyrias manifest as skin disorders, as does porphyria cutanea tarda (PCT). The

Glycine + Succinyl coenzyme A

⇓   (Aminolevulinic synthetase)
Aminolelulinic acid

⇓   (Aminolevulinic dehydratase)
Porphobilinogen

⇓   (Hydroxymethylbilane synthetase)
Hydroxymethylbylane

⇓   (Uroporphyrinogen synthetase)
Uroporphyrinogen III

⇓   (Uroporphyrinogen decarboxylase)
Coproporphyrinogen III

⇓   (Coproporphyrinogen oxidase)
Protoporphyrinogen IX

⇓   (Protooporphyrinogen oxidase)
Protoporphyrin IX

⇓   (Ferrochelatase)
Heme

Figure 170.1 Biochemical pathway for heme synthesis.

condition of aminolevulinic dehydratase (ALD) deficiency or plumboporphyria is exceedingly rare. The prevalence of hepatic porphyrias varies between 1 in 10000–20000 to 1 in 125000 of the population. Table 170.1 shows different types of porphyria with regard to specific metabolic errors and modes of genetic transmission.

An X-linked dominant protoporphyria (XLDPP) was first reported in 2008. It has a phenotype similar to erythropoietic protoporphyria, but is distinguished by higher concentrations of erythrocyte protoporphyrin and a higher incidence of liver disease.

Porphyria may be potentially serious or even life threatening, yet it tends to be underdiagnosed. The diagnosis is corroborated by clinical and genetic identification of family history. In the presence of otherwise unexplained neurological symptoms, biochemical and genetic testing must be performed rapidly on relatives to identify asymptomatic carriers. Treatment depends on the specific disorder and also varies by individual, particularly with regard to identifying precipitating factors that must be avoided as part of the treatment approach.

Ascertainment of porphyria is often incidental. Neurological complications tend to precede the definitive biochemical diagnosis. The clinical picture is frequently complex and heterogeneous. Neurological complications are common, but the clinical picture may be transient, often initially disregarded. Although different enzymatic defects account for each of the acute porphyrias, there is no clear difference in the spectrum of neuropsychiatric features associated with an acute attack.

Pathogenesis of neurological dysfunction

Neurological dysfunction may underlie not only nervous system–related symptoms but also non-neurological manifestations. Histopathology may reveal edema, irregularity of myelin sheaths, axonal vacuolization, and degeneration of autonomic nerves. Evidence from electrophysiological data shows muscle denervation and slow nerve conduction.

A possible protective effect of melatonin has been proposed, based on its reduced urinary excretion in non-epileptic AIP patients compared to matched controls. A possible direct epileptogenic effect of δ-aminolevulinic acid (ALA) was postulated after ALA was shown to interfere with γ-aminobutyric acid (GABA) and, possibly, glutamate activity.

ALA neurotoxicity has been demonstrated in chick embryo neuronal and glial cells. Some cases of acute toxic neuropathy (e.g., lead poisoning) are associated with increased ALA urinary excretion, but a clear causative effect has not been established. Another

International Neurology, Second edition. Edited by Robert P. Lisak, Daniel D. Truong, William M. Carroll and Roongroj Bhidayasiri
© 2016 John Wiley & Sons, Ltd. Published 2016 by John Wiley & Sons, Ltd.

Table 170.1 Classification of porphyric syndromes, inheritance, and enzyme defects.

Clinical condition	Enzyme deficiency	Chromosome location	Inheritance
Congenital erythropoietic porphyria (CEP)	Uroporphyirinogen III synthetase	10q25.2→q26.3	Autosomal recessive
Erythropoietic protoporphyria	Ferrochelatase	18q21.3	Autosomal dominant
ALA dehydratase deficiency porphyria	ALA dehydratase	9q34	Autosomal recessive
Acute intermittent porphyria (AIP)	Hydroxymethylbilane synthetase	11q23.3	Autosomal dominant
Hereditary coproporphyria	Coproporphyrinogen oxidase	3q12	Autosomal dominant
Variegate porphyria	Protoporphyrinogen oxidase	1q23	Autosomal dominant
Porphyria cutanea tarda (PCT)	Uroporphyrinogen decarboxylase	1p34	Variable
Hepatoerythropoietic porphyria	Uroporphyrinogen decarboxylase	1p34	Autosomal recessive

ALA = δ-aminolevulinic acid

observation is the potential auto-oxidation of ALA in the presence of iron or other heavy metals, potentially inducing the formation of free radicals, causing oxidative stress on mitochondria and increased Ca^{++} uptake in cortical neurons. Eight patients affected by end-stage protoporphyric liver disease showed neurological clinical features similar to those observed in the acute attacks.

Epidemiology

The overall prevalence and incidence of porphyrias are geographically variable. The hepatic form appears to be far more common than the erythropoietic form. The acute syndromes have a higher prevalence in Scandinavia and the United Kingdom. AIP has been estimated to have a prevalence of 1 in 10000 in Sweden. PCT has a prevalence of 1 in 25000 in the British population. In contrast, a prevalence of 1 in 125000 has been reported in Argentina, whereas in the same country VP has a prevalence of 1 in 600000.

An update on the molecular diagnosis of porphyrias was produced in Italy, together with a flow chart to facilitate the identification of mutations in heme biosynthetic genes. The molecular analysis permitted identification of the molecular defects underlying the disease in 66 probands with different porphyrias (acute intermittent porphyria, variegate porphyria, porphyria cutanea tarda, and erythropoietic protoporphyria). No Italian patients with defects in the coproporphyrinogen oxidase gene, responsible for HC, have been detected. The rarity of AIP in Africans has been emphasized by various authors. An increasing number of cases have been recently reported in Nigeria. Most of them have initially been misdiagnosed and only later found to be AIP. Doctors working among African populations should be alerted about this disease. A simple Watson–Schwartz test for porphobilinogens will save many patients from unnecessary hazards of treatment.

Information about morbidity associated with acute porphyrias is mostly derived from the clinical experience of specialty porphyria centers.

The Norwegian Porphyria Registry (NAPOS) includes 70% of Norwegians registered as having porphyria. The prevalence of PCT in Norway is approximately 10 in 100000 and that of AIP approximately 4 in 100000. Diagnostic delay varies from 1–17 years depending on the type of porphyria.

Genetic heterogeneity is also a prominent feature of some porphyrias. The mutation R116W, which has a high prevalence in Dutch and Swedish population, was found on three different haplotypes in three Norwegian families and five Swedish families.

Congenital porphyrias are rare. Only 15% of carriers of mutations develop clinical syndromes and more than 30% of patients have no family history. However, in China, out of a total of 145 cases, 75.2% were erythropoietic purpura (EPP; 109 cases), but only 28 cases (19.3%) were PCT. This prevalence differs from that in other parts of the world. Early diagnosis of EPP using the fluorescence microscopic test for determination of red blood cell (RBC) protoporphyrin is important. The complication of hepatobiliary aspects in PCT and EPP was noted. Liver disease seems to be an important precipitating factor in China.

A study measuring levels of ALA, porphobilinogen (PBG), and total urine porphyrin (TUP) excreted in urine was conducted in 20 patients with AIP following an attack of acute porphyria and showed elevated urinary metabolites for periods of 3 months to 23 years after their last documented acute attack. Urinary concentrations of all metabolites remain elevated for many years. This study highlights the difficulties of using urinary analysis for diagnosing recurrent attacks, and also raises important questions about the pathophysiology of the condition.

Clinical features

Erythropoietic porphyrias

Erythropoietic porphyrias (EP), including X-linked sideroblastic anemia, congenital erythropoietic porphyria (CEP), and erythropoietic protoporphyria, are rare. There are just 50 documented cases of CEP in the literature. The clinical picture is characterized by hemolytic anemia, severe photosensitivity, and epidermal bullae, the latter caused by accumulation of porphyrins in the skin derived from bone marrow erythrocytes, with consequent phosphosensitization. Chronic liver failure is occasionally observed, due to protoporphyrin accumulation. Although there have been isolated reports of sensorimotor neuropathy in EPP, neurological manifestations do not generally occur in the erythropoietic porphyrias.

Hepatic porphyrias

Hepatic porphyrias are characterized by systemic involvement including gastrointestinal symptoms, cardiovascular symptoms, diffuse erythematous reaction and subsequent vesicles, and, rarely, chronic liver failure. Sideroblastic anemia is the most common hematological complication. Several commonly used medications may induce or aggravate porphyric attacks. Infections, pregnancy, and menstrual irregularities are also considered potential triggering factors.

Neurological sequelae can affect both central and peripheral nervous systems. Peripheral neuropathy is most common, affecting predominantly motor nerves, with a rapid onset of symmetric weakness affecting all limbs. Cranial nerve involvement, sensory disturbances, consistent pain, and an asymmetric pattern of weakness occur, spreading to trunk and legs, and rarely progressing to paresis. Tachycardia and hypotension may be present in the acute phase.

When acute hepatic porphyria is triggered by pregnancy, it usually presents with gastrointestinal symptoms and personality changes. In its rare neurological manifestation it can lead to untreatable convulsions.

Neurological manifestations

Epilepsy is not infrequent in porphyric patients. The etiology of seizures is multifactorial, attributable to hyponatremia consequent to vomiting or diarrhea, brain structural pathology, or supposed neurotoxic and epileptogenic effects of some porphyrins. Psychiatric and cognitive disturbances have also been documented, including mood disturbances, anxiety, depression, psychosis, restlessness, insomnia, schizophrenic symptoms, impulsive behavior, persecutory delusions, and catatonia. Acute attacks consisting of neuropsychiatric manifestations without abdominal pain are rare, but there are reports of isolated neuropathy, encephalopathy, and psychosis as the sole manifestations of an attack.

Both transient and permanent structural brain damage has been reported in patients with porphyria. Evidence of cortical and subcortical structural damage has been shown by radiology (or imaging) and pathology techniques. Ischemic brain damage was also reported in a patient showing transient cortical blindness. Bi-occipital lesions were noted on magnetic resonance imaging (MRI) in two patients with AIP. A hemiparesis and abnormal brain MRI study was noted in a patient with hepatoerythropoietic porphyria. Transient MRI T2 hyperintense lesions have also been reported, as well as multiple, reversible cortical lesions, predominantly posteriorly.

Seizures are not uncommon during exacerbations of porphyric attacks, occurring in 2.2% of patients with known AIP and 5.1% of those with manifest AIP. About 30% of teenagers and 10–20% of adults with acute porphyria also suffer from seizures. Seizures may precede the presentation of porphyria by many years. Complex partial seizures are most common; absence, myoclonic, and tonic–clonic seizures and EEG abnormalities have also been recorded. Precipitating factors include a variety of almost 200 drugs, which include antiepileptic drugs, sulfonamides, methyldopa, tetracycline, antihistamines, amphetamines, cocaine, and excessive quantities of alcohol. Infections may also be precipitants. In women, pregnancy and premenstrual seizures are considered potential triggering factors for a relapse. Treatment with sex hormones may also precipitate an acute attack of porphyria.

The differential diagnoses to be considered are polyneuropathy, especially acute polyneuritis, Guillain–Barré syndrome, epilepsy, psychiatric illness including cognitive and affective disorders, and unusual causes of neurological syndromes due to vasculitis, systemic lupus erythematosus, and polyarteritis nodosa.

Extra-neurological manifestations

Extra-neurological manifestations include acute attacks of abdominal pain, nausea, constipation, vomiting, or gastrointestinal upset. Tachycardia and postural hypotension may be present due to autonomic disturbances. Cutaneous manifestations are associated with PCT, but are also present in VP and HC; these manifestations are attributed to accumulation of porphyrins in the skin and include a burning sensation after exposure to sunlight, diffuse erythema and tense fluid-filled vesicles, fragile skin, pigmentation, and hypertrichosis, which may also present diagnostic challenges.

Differential diagnosis

Porphyrias are called "the little imitators." The differential diagnoses involve neurological disturbances ranging from polyneuropathy, autonomic disturbances, seizures, and a wide range of psychiatric disorders referred to earlier. The cutaneous manifestations form a differential diagnosis for photosensitization, bullae, dermatitis, vesicles, and pigmentation.

Porphyric attacks caused by antiepileptic medications

Many antiepileptic drugs (AEDs) can induce the isoenzyme of cytochrome P450 and have been reported to worsen or induce attacks of AIP and PCT, accelerating catabolism by uroporphyrinogen decarboxylase and hydroxymethylbilane synthetase, and altering the feedback mechanism on heme biosynthesis.

A worsening of acute porphyric attacks has been reported in patients treated with phenytoin, carbamazepine, phenobarbital, sodium valproate, and lamotrigine. Topiramate and tiagabine increase liver porphobilinogen content, and the latter has been demonstrated to be potentially porphyrogenic in chicken embryos. Seizures have been successfully treated with gabapentin and oxcarbazepine in patients with acute porphyria, not associated with exacerbation of acute attacks. However, oxcarbazepine can induce hyponatremia, which may induce or complicate porphyric attacks. Levetiracetam was reported to be safe in AIP, HC, and PCT. Propofol has been used safely in refractory status epilepticus.

Treatment

Porphyrinogenic agents should be stopped. Various pharmacological and hormonal agents promote overproduction of the porphyrins and their precursors, mainly by inducing the hepatic cytochrome P450 enzyme system. Commonly implicated drugs are alcohol, AEDs, sulfonamide antibiotics, rifampicin, estrogen, and progesterone.

Fluctuations in the menstrual cycle can trigger acute episodes. In patients with recurrent premenstrual attacks, treatment with luteinizing hormone-releasing hormone analogues may be beneficial. The oral contraceptive pill should only be used with caution. Patients should avoid fasting or low-calorie diets and infections should be treated promptly, as these situations upregulate the heme synthetic pathway.

Management should focus on supportive therapy and reduction of the activity of the heme synthetic pathway. Paracetamol or opiates (excluding tramadol) are safe to use in an acute attack. Beta blockers can be used for hypertension and tachycardia. Chlorpromazine is recommended for sedation. A high-carbohydrate diet should be followed.

The mainstay of treatment of a severe attack is the end product of the heme synthetic pathway, heme. Two commercial preparations are hematin and heme arginate. They replenish the depleted heme pool of porphyrin precursors. An intravenous infusion of 3–4 mg/kg daily for 4 days may be given. These preparations effectively reduce plasma concentration and urinary excretion of porphyrin precursors. Levels may rebound on cessation of the infusion.

Liver transplantation has been performed successfully in patients with AIP and VP, with subsequent normalization of biochemical abnormalities and prevention of further attacks. Progress in laboratory research into gene therapy for AIP may potentially lead to a therapeutic option.

Conclusion

Prompt diagnosis and treatment of porphyria have to date been suboptimal because of under-recognition of clinical features, importance of family history, poor availability of biochemical tests, and false negative test results during asymptomatic periods. The clinical picture is often transient and the diagnosis may be missed if porphyria is not considered at the time of the acute symptoms. From the neurologist's viewpoint there is a challenge in trying to identify and characterize the psychiatric abnormalities. Better epidemiological data and understanding of the comorbidities of porphyrias are needed.

Metabolic imbalances that can induce seizures during porphyric attacks have been identified. It is important to perform serum and urinary porphyrin measurements during the attack, as their specificity is very high in hepatic porphyrias. Sensitivity of the analysis does not allow a reliable exclusion in asymptomatic AIP patients.

The possible neurotoxicity of ALA seems to be contradicted by some *in vivo* experiments. An alternative toxic role of protoporphyrin, porphobilinogen, or other porphyrins or a neural metabolic failure due to heme deficiency has not been confirmed. Animal models do not explain completely the clinical effects observed.

Some patients appear reluctant to accept the diagnosis of porphyria because of the psychiatric implications. A register for porphyric patients, focusing on family history and results of genetic testing, is gaining acceptance.

A list of over 200 drugs that have been reported to be unsafe in patients with porphyria is available at http://www.uq.edu.au/porphyria. Key references are also provided by Michael Moore of the University of Queensland at http://www.drugs-porphyria.org.

Acknowledgments

We thank the Porphyria Association of Australia and our colleagues at St. Vincent's Hospital, Monash University, and Melbourne University. Formatting assistance provided by Simon Raoul Vajda.

Further reading

Albers JW, Fink JK. Porphyric neuropathy. *Muscle Nerve* 2004;30(4):410–422.

Crimlisk HL. The little imitator – porphyria: A neuropsychiatric disorder. *J Neurol Neurosurg Psychiatry* 1997;62:319–328.

Desnick RJ. The porphyrias. In: Braunwald E, Fauci AS, Kasper DL, *et al.* (eds.). *Harrison's Principles of Internal Medicine*, 15th ed. New York: McGeaw Hill; 2001: 2261–2267.

Kauppinen R. Porphyrias. *Lancet* 2005;365(9455):241–252.

Simon N, Herkes G. The neurologic manifestations of the acute porphyrias. *J Clin Neurosci* 2011;18(9):1147–1153.

Solinas C, Vajda F. Epilepsy and porphyria: New perspectives. *J Clin Neurosci* 2004;11:356–361.

171 Traumatic brain injury

Christopher C. Giza

UCLA Brain Injury Research Center, David Geffen School of Medicine and Mattel Children's Hospital, Los Angeles, CA, USA

Traumatic brain injury (TBI) refers to any biomechanically induced acquired brain injury. It is the most common cause of death and disability in young persons in many countries, often resulting in chronic neurological, cognitive, and behavioral impairments. The World Health Organization (WHO) estimates that TBI will surpass many diseases as the major cause of death and disability by 2020. TBI occurs in a spectrum from mild to severe, typically classified based on clinical signs as determined by the Glasgow Coma Score (GCS; Table 171.1). TBI encompasses a range of pathophysiological injuries, from simple concussions to intracranial hematomas to profound cerebral edema with ischemic secondary damage.

Epidemiology

TBI occurs in a trimodal age distribution, with peaks in infancy, adolescence/young adulthood, and senescence. There is a male:female predominance of 2–3:1. Specific mechanisms of injury are quite variable in terms of the biomechanical forces imparted to the brain and the severity of the injury.

The mildest injuries (concussions) typically involve lower forces and may be associated with only transient neurological signs and symptoms. These represent the majority (70–80%) of all TBI. Recurrent mild concussions are most commonly seen in sports-related settings, although the specific sport may differ based on geographic location. Football is by far the biggest contributor to mild TBI in the United States, while in many other countries soccer, rugby, and, to some extent, boxing are more common causes. In Asia, the various forms of contact martial arts constitute other contributors to mild TBI.

It is estimated that 60% of TBI worldwide is caused by road traffic accidents (RTAs), 20–30% due to falls, 10% to violence, and another 10% due to a combination of work and sports injuries. Mechanisms underlying moderate and severe TBI vary by age and geography.

Agewise, infants and toddlers are more commonly injured by inflicted TBI (child abuse) and falls. Teenagers and young adults are more often affected by RTAs. Worldwide, in 2002, RTAs resulted in 1.2 million deaths and between 20 million and 50 million people becoming disabled. The specific mechanisms of RTAs causing TBI vary considerably by geographic location. In developed countries, the most common types of RTA causing TBI involve automobile-to-automobile crashes, and rates are declining. In developing countries, RTAs involving pedestrians or motorized scooters are

Table 171.1 The Glasgow Coma Scale.

Eye opening (E)	
• Spontaneous	4
• To speech (to shout)	3
• To pain	2
• None	1
Motor response (M)	
• Obeys commands	6
• Localizes pain	5
• Withdraws	4
• Abnormal flexion	3
• Extensor response	2
• None	1
Verbal response (V)	
• Oriented	5
• Confused conversation	4
• Inappropriate words	3
• Incomprehensible sounds	2
• None	1
Verbal response, modified for infants	
• Babbles, coos appropriately	5
• Cries, but consolable	4
• Cries inconsolably	3
• Grunts or moans to pain	2
• None	1

more common and have generally been on the rise. In Thailand and Malaysia, 55–70% of RTA deaths involve motorized cycles. In India, Indonesia, and Sri Lanka, motorized cycles are involved in 40% of RTA deaths and pedestrians in another 40%. In more developed countries such as the United States and Australia, motorized four-wheeled vehicles constitute 70–80% of RTA-related deaths. These numbers suggest the need for marked differences in the approach to treatment and prevention.

While RTAs occur all over the world, other mechanisms of TBI also vary by location. India has the highest rate of TBI due to falls. Violence is associated with higher rates of TBI in sub-Saharan Africa and Latin America, while war-related TBI is estimated to be highest in sub-Saharan Africa and in the Middle Eastern crescent.

Pathophysiology

The underlying pathophysiology of TBI varies by injury severity, but the basic neurobiological processes include acute, biome-

International Neurology, Second edition. Edited by Robert P. Lisak, Daniel D. Truong, William M. Carroll and Roongroj Bhidayasiri
© 2016 John Wiley & Sons, Ltd. Published 2016 by John Wiley & Sons, Ltd.

chanical strain on neuronal membranes, causing indiscriminate ionic flux and glutamate release in both animal models and human patients. Acute energy demands compromise neuronal function and, if severe, result in cell death. Subsequently, cerebral glucose metabolism is reduced for 7–10 days in experimental animals and days to months in humans. The duration of metabolic depression appears to be related to injury severity.

Other cellular processes involved in the response to TBI include inflammatory processes, neurotransmitter dysfunction, delayed cell death, gliosis/scarring, and axonal injury. Impairment of neurotransmission may be especially relevant during the recovery period, particularly in children and adolescents whose brains are still undergoing development. Axonal injury is also an important mechanism that may have unique consequences in terms of neural connectivity during the state of coma and in recovery.

Based on understanding of pathophysiology, the most clinically relevant intervention consists in the detection, avoidance, and treatment of secondary insults. This refers to deleterious physiological events that are distinct from the primary injury itself, such as hypotension/ischemia, hypoxia, seizure, and hyperthermia. The presence of a secondary insult is the single most important treatable factor in improving TBI outcome. The ability to address these remediable conditions varies greatly depending on geographic location and medical resources. Both pre-hospital care and adequate hospital intensive care are crucial to monitor and treat these important problems. In developed nations, reductions in mortality following severe TBI (as seen in the 1970 and 1980 s) can be directly traced to the development of pre-hospital emergency medical services (EMS) and to improved monitoring and treatment of complications in the hospital in specialized intensive care units (now, neuro-intensive care units). The establishment and optimal operation of these systems are still a major obstacle in many developing nations and regions experiencing armed conflict.

Clinical features

The hallmarks of TBI are neurological dysfunction and impairment of mental status, but the range of clinical features varies greatly depending on injury severity. Here it is best to discuss mild TBI/concussion separately from moderate–severe TBI.

Mild traumatic brain injury/concussion

Concussion has been defined as any transient disturbance of neurological function imparted by injury due to biomechanical forces. This type of injury can occur with any TBI mechanism, but is generally associated with short falls and sports-related head injuries. The most common clinical hallmarks of concussion include memory impairment, headaches, confusion, nausea, dizziness, and visual disturbances. Loss of consciousness may occur, but is not necessary for a diagnosis of concussion. On average, these symptoms recover relatively rapidly, with adolescents taking longer (14–28 days) than young adults (7–10 days). However, symptoms may become persistent for months or even years in a minority (5–10%) of individuals.

Mild TBI is historically defined as TBI with a GCS of 13–15. Concussion may be thought of as a subset of mild TBI with neurological symptoms in the absence of demonstrable structural brain injury. Repeated concussion (described further subsequently) results in more prolonged symptoms (including headaches, dizziness, and cognitive problems) and may be associated with late neurodegeneration.

Moderate to severe traumatic brain injury

More severe TBI incorporates a broad range of distinct injury processes and pathology. Moderate TBI is defined by an initial GCS of 9–12, while severe is defined by a GCS of 3–8. The underlying mechanisms here are assault (including inflicted TBI or child abuse), high falls, gunshot wounds, and RTAs. These head injuries are divided into closed head injuries and penetrating injuries. Penetrating injuries will be associated with skull fracture and the primary destruction of brain parenchyma, as well as intracranial hemorrhage and often foreign bodies. Gunshot wounds tend to be more common in urban areas, but, worldwide, can be attributed to warfare. In developing countries, significant penetrating injuries are likely to result in death, as operative interventions and methods to prevent subsequent infection may not be readily available. Closed head injuries are far more common, and may include nondisplaced skull fractures, intracranial hemorrhage (epidural, subarachnoid, and subdural), and parenchymal brain damage such as contusions and diffuse axonal injury.

Blast injuries may represent a unique type of TBI due to proximity to an explosive device, as might occur during terrorism or warfare. Mechanisms of blast TBI include the primary blast overpressure wave, being struck by objects propelled by the explosion, being flung against an object/ground by the blast wind, or associated injuries due to heat or toxic exposures.

The clinical signs of moderate–severe TBI include altered mental status/coma, amnesia, focal neurological deficits, and seizures. Physical examination may reveal scalp hematomas or lacerations, palpable skull step-offs (indicating fractures), hemotympanum or otorrhea (associated with basilar skull fractures), and raccoon eyes or rhinorrhea (associated with orbitofrontal skull fractures).

Moderate–severe TBI results in many persistent neurological sequelae that may fall to neurologists for ongoing management. Sequelae of severe TBI include post-traumatic epilepsy, spasticity, headaches, and occasionally hydrocephalus. Furthermore, TBI can result in varying degrees of behavioral or cognitive deficits, particularly personality change, impulsivity, poor attention, and memory impairment. For pediatric patients with moderate–severe TBI, careful longitudinal follow-up is warranted, as late neurobehavioral problems may emerge and become more evident as ongoing development proceeds.

Investigations

Most mild TBI/concussion will not require additional diagnostic testing, as concussion is a clinical diagnosis, made primarily on the basis of history, initial signs/symptoms, and neurological examination. The routine use of skull X-rays to evaluate mild TBI has not been supported in the literature; however, if there is clinical suspicion of a skull fracture at a facility where head computed tomography (CT) is not available, skull X-ray has some clinical utility. In these circumstances, the presence of a skull fracture on X-ray strongly suggests the need for transport to a facility with head CT capability, as the risk of intracranial pathology is increased 21- to 80-fold.

Diagnostic evaluation of moderate–severe TBI is best accomplished by a non-contrast head CT. This method can quickly and definitively diagnose conditions requiring neurosurgical intervention, such as space-occupying lesions (epidural and subdural hematomas, and contusions; Figure 171.1 a, b, and c, respectively), and delayed complications of TBI (hydrocephalus and cerebral infarction). Magnetic resonance imaging (MRI) is not

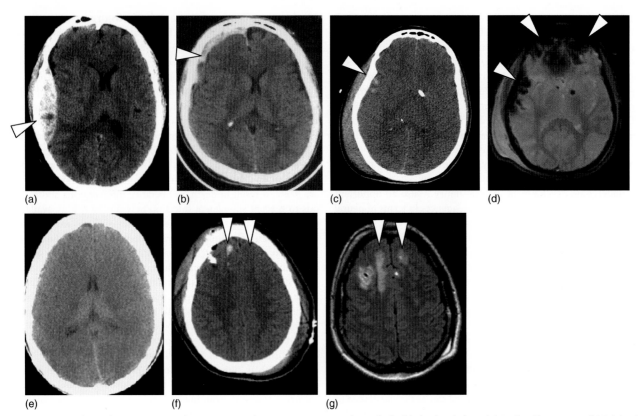

Figure 171.1 Radiographic appearances of acute traumatic brain injury. Arrows indicate the highlighted pathology. (a) Epidural hematoma. (b) Subdural hematoma. (c) Cerebral contusion on computed tomography (CT). (d) Multiple cerebral contusions evident on magnetic resonance imaging (MRI) done the same day as the CT scan in (c). (e) Diffuse cerebral edema. (f) Diffuse axonal injury on CT. (g) More extensive diffuse axonal injury evident on MRI done the same day as the CT in (f).

indicated acutely, but may be valuable subacutely for patients with persistent coma by identifying the extent of lesions not optimally seen on CT (Figure 171.1 c vs. d for contusions, f vs. g for diffuse axonal injury).

Treatment

Mild traumatic brain injury/concussion

The foundation of management of mild TBI is careful clinical assessment and observation. Determination of risk factors (high-force impact, very young or old age, prolonged or continuing alteration in mental status, loss of consciousness, seizure, repeated vomiting, focal neurological signs, or intoxication of patient) is important to triage these patients properly. In the vast majority of cases, a normal or improving neurological exam in the early post-injury hours and an absence of clinical risk factors will permit management solely with observation, forgoing the need for neuroimaging. As already indicated, however, there are circumstances where skull X-ray or non-contrast head CT would be prudent.

There is an increasing focus on management and return to contact risk after mild TBI/concussion, particularly in the setting of sports and military service. Multiple guidelines recommend immediately removing a concussed individual from contact risk, using a multimodal assessment to help diagnose concussion (symptoms, cognition, balance, reaction time), serial monitoring of neurocognitive function in the hours and days after injury, and gradual

return to activity and, eventually, to contact risk. There is a 3- to 6-fold increased risk of repeat concussion after an initial concussion, particularly if an individual returns to contact risk prior to full recovery. Furthermore, there is growing evidence that repeated mild TBI/concussion may predispose to more chronic sequelae (post-concussion syndrome) or even initiate premature neurodegenerative changes, such as Alzheimer's disease, Parkinson's disease, or chronic traumatic encephalopathy.

Moderate to severe traumatic brain injury

More severe brain injuries warrant more aggressive intervention – beginning outside of the hospital. Evidence-based guidelines for the management of severe TBI have been published and recently revised. Pre-hospital management of TBI varies worldwide based on the availability of EMS, but basic care can still have a significant impact on the outcome by interventions to reduce secondary injuries. This includes immediate assessment of airway, breathing, and circulation as well as instituting proper resuscitative efforts. Maintenance of an adequate airway may be achieved using oral or nasopharyngeal airways and proper head position. Careful assessment and immobilization for concomitant cervical spine injury should be undertaken. Supplemental oxygen can be administered as soon as it is available, and intravenous (IV) access should be established for fluid resuscitation to address hypotension and shock, as well as to provide a means of rapid drug delivery.

The mainstay of management for moderate–severe TBI centers on identification and treatment of elevated intracranial pressure (ICP) and maintenance of adequate cerebral perfusion pressure (CP = mean arterial pressure – ICP). In the initial assessment, elevated ICP and/or impending cerebral herniation may be detected based on clinical signs (declining mental status, unilateral dilated pupil, hemi-motor signs, or posturing) or neuroimaging. Increased ICP can occur due to a space-occupying lesion (such as a hematoma; Figure 171.1 a, b) or cerebral edema (as occurs adjacent to a contusion or diffusely; Figure 171.1 c, e). Surgical intervention is warranted in cases of a significant mass lesion. For severe TBI, ICP monitoring in an intensive care unit may be the standard of care in locations where such resources are available, with clinical signs being utilized where monitoring resources are limited. ICP may be measured via a surface transducer or by a ventriculostomy. The latter is preferred because it allows both measurement of ICP and therapeutic drainage of cerebrospinal fluid (CSF). Medical interventions are important in the management of elevated ICP. It is recommended that these interventions occur in a stepwise fashion, from less aggressive to an increasing intensity of therapy.

The first steps include slight elevation of the head of the bed (15–30°) and maintenance of the head in a neutral position to facilitate jugular venous drainage. Next are sedation and analgesia, followed by neuromuscular blockade. The resulting reduction of intrathoracic pressures can help in lowering ICP, particularly in intubated patients who may struggle against positive pressure breathing. Hyperosmolar agents may be administered intravenously – mannitol (0.25–1 g/kg IV every 3–6 hrs) is the agent of choice. Hypertonic saline (3%) may also be used. Finally, controlled ventilation or mild hyperventilation (pCO_2 = 30–35) can be used, but care should be taken not to overventilate, which may result in vasoconstriction of cerebral vasculature and secondary ischemic injury. In a setting of clinical herniation, airway control and hyperventilation are usually the most rapid means of reducing ICP in the absence of a ventriculostomy. IV hyperosmolar agents should follow closely. This process takes slightly longer; however, it results in more sustained ICP reductions and is less likely to lead to ischemia.

Second-tier therapies are reserved for refractory elevations of ICP in the absence of a surgical lesion and include metabolic suppressive therapy, severe hyperventilation, and decompressive craniectomy. Pharmacological suppression of cerebral activity is typically accomplished with barbiturate coma and continuous electroencephalogram (EEG) monitoring. More aggressive hyperventilation (pCO_2 <30) can be safely implemented if monitoring for cerebral ischemia is available via jugular venous O_2 saturation or newer tissue oxygenation monitors. Systemic hypothermia has not proven effective for TBI.

The third set of therapies is considered supportive and includes avoidance of hyperthermia, prophylaxis against early post-traumatic seizures, deep vein thrombosis (DVT) prophylaxis, and caloric supplementation. The use of corticosteroids is *not* recommended.

Chronic management of sequelae

In most cases of mild TBI/concussion, symptoms will resolve within days to weeks. As already mentioned, a small subset will develop chronic postconcussion syndrome. In these cases, further evaluation should be undertaken to identify and treat comorbid conditions. Persistent headaches may be due to migraine, evolution to chronic daily headache, cervicogenic causes, occipital neuralgia, hydrocephalus, CSF leak, and medication overuse headache. Chronic headaches are often best addressed by preventive

pharmacotherapies such as tricyclics (amitriptyline, nortriptyline), anticonvulsants (gabapentin, topiramate), anti-inflammatories, and herbal treatments (Butterbur). Discrete acute migraine attacks can be treated with abortive medications. Maintaining a simple headache diary may allow more effective titration of medications. Cervicogenic headaches and occipital neuralgia may respond to physical therapy, neck stretching and strengthening, anti-inflammatories, or local injections. Care should be taken in any patient with chronic headaches to avoid medication overuse or rebound headache. Anxiety and mood disturbances are frequent in patients suffering chronic problems. Once the underlying diagnosis has been made, proper long-term treatment may be initiated.

Moderate–severe TBI almost always results in significant long-term sequelae of some sort. Chronic headaches may be managed as described earlier for milder injuries. Post-traumatic epilepsy is most frequently localization-related, and thus treatment may be targeted to either focal epilepsy medications (carbamazepine, oxcarbazepine, etc.) or broad-spectrum medications (levetiracetam, lamotrigine, topiramate, etc.). In intractable cases, more aggressive interventions include vagal nerve stimulation or even, in selected cases, epilepsy surgery. Motor disturbances including spasticity may be addressed by antispasticity medications (baclofen, tizandine, dantrolene), bracing, and physical/occupational therapy. Sometimes a local injection or orthopedic release of contractures is needed. Cognitive-behavioral sequelae are ubiquitous after more severe injuries; often the initial step is to obtain formal neuropsychological testing to quantitate their strengths and weaknesses more objectively, followed by cognitive therapy or off-label use of nootropic medications or stimulants. In some of the most severely injured patients, autonomic disturbances may respond to beta blockers, sedatives, gabapentin, baclofen, and bromocriptine. Patients in a persistent vegetative or minimally conscious state may benefit from amantadine, which has been shown to be effective in a randomized placebo-controlled trial.

General supportive care includes maintaining adequate hydration, providing good nutrition, and proper sleep hygiene. The long-term burden of TBI is poorly understood on a global level, although undoubtedly it has major social costs, including lost productivity, disability, unemployment, need for chronic care, and associated issues related to mental health, addiction, and law enforcement. Another global challenge is understanding the sequelae of TBI in children, which causes more death and disability than all other pediatric problems combined.

Further reading

Giza CC, Kutcher JS, Ashwal S, et al. Summary of evidence-based guideline update: Evaluation and management of concussion in sports. *Neurology* 2013;80(24):2250–2257. http://www.neurology.org/content/80/24/2250.full (accessed November 2015).

Guidelines for the Acute Medical Management of Severe Traumatic Brain Injury in Infants, Children and Adolescents. *Pediatr Crit Care Med* 2012;13(1):supplement.

Guidelines for the Management of Severe Traumatic Brain Injury. *J Neurotrauma* 2007;24(supplement 1).

Hyder AA, Wunderlich CA, Puvanachandra P, Gururaj G, Kobusingya OC. The impact of traumatic brain injuries: A global perspective. *NeuroRehabilitation* 2007;22:341–353.

McCrory P, Meeuwisse WH, Aubry M, et al. Consensus statement on concussion in sport: The 4th International Conference on Concussion in Sport held in Zurich, November 2012. *Br J Sports Med* 2013;47:250–258. http://bjsm.bmj.com/content/47/5/250.full (accessed November 2015).

World Health Organization. *World Report on Road Traffic Injury Prevention*. Geneva: WHO; 2004. http://www.who.int/violence_injury_prevention/publications/road_traffic/world_report/en/ (accessed November 2015).

Spinal injury

Enver I. Bogdanov and Aisylu T. Faizutdinova

Department of Neurology and Rehabilitation, Kazan State Medical University, Kazan, Russia

Spinal cord injury (SCI) is a potentially catastrophic event for individuals and for society. The causes and incidence of SCI, its consequences and complications often reflect the complex interaction and problems of the socioeconomic and health-related areas of society.

Approximately 20% of SCI patients do not survive to reach acute hospitalization. More than 48% of SCI patients die within 24 hours after injury. After acute hospitalization less than 30% of patients showed improvements in functional independence. The incidence of disabling pain in patients with SCI is 30–40%. Death from suicide is the one of the leading causes of death among SCI patients with paraplegia.

SCI results in different motor, sensory, and autonomic dysfunction below the level of injury. In all acute SCI the full extent of injury may not be apparent initially. Better functional recovery was observed in patients with lower neurological levels of the lesion. Persons with SCI may be required to have surgical or conservative orthopedic treatment, and also long-term continuous rehabilitation.

Epidemiology

Epidemiological data on SCI vary considerably from country to country (Figure 172.1). The reasons for these geographic differences are multifactorial.

SCI is most frequent in young adults and is often associated with vertebral fracture. The main causes of injuries in developed countries are road traffic and sporting accidents, whereas falling from a height is the most common cause in developing regions. In Bangladesh, SCI after falling while carrying a heavy load on the head is frequent. Injuries due to intentional violence are a relatively common cause of cord injury in particular areas, including parts of South America and Africa. Universally, there is a large predominance in males (the male:female ratio is 3–4:1).

Pathophysiology

The mechanisms of SCI can be broadly subclassified into five types – dislocation, lateral bending, axial loading, rotation, and hyperflexion/hyperextension – although severe injuries often result from a combination of more than one of these types. Intra- and extramedullary circulatory impairment occurs not only at the initial impact level, but also in the adjacent levels. The presence of constitutional or spondylotic narrowing of the spinal canal seems to predispose to lesions of the cord. In 50% of cases the cervical spine is affected, followed by the thoracic and lumbosacral spine, respectively.

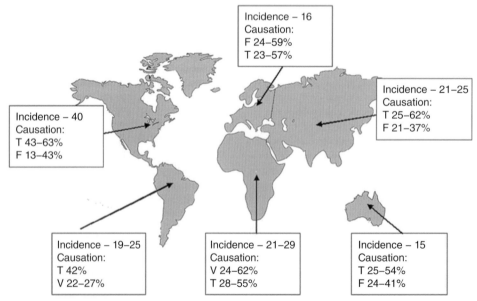

Figure 172.1 The incidence (per million) and causation (traffic accidents [T], falls [F], violence [V]) of spinal cord injuries on different continents.

International Neurology, Second edition. Edited by Robert P. Lisak, Daniel D. Truong, William M. Carroll and Roongroj Bhidayasiri

© 2016 John Wiley & Sons, Ltd. Published 2016 by John Wiley & Sons, Ltd.

Clinical features

Spinal shock is characterized by a state of areflexia below the level of the SCI. It is manifested by flaccidity in the legs, which gradually disappears and is replaced by increasing muscle tone. The duration of spinal shock varies from several hours to 1–2 weeks. Sparing of sensation in lower sacral segments may be the only predictive sign that some recovery may occur. The onset of some voluntary movement within 72 hours of SCI is a good prognostic sign. Flaccidity remains in lower motor neuron lesions associated with permanent cauda equina damage. Traumatic "cauda equina" syndrome consists of sensory disturbance, characteristically in the perineal region, as well as difficulty in walking due to weakness of the legs. Autonomic disturbances are less common and can include bowel and bladder dysfunction. In the setting of acute trauma, hypotension without tachycardia should raise concern for severe SCI. Acute SCI above Th6 may lead to the interruption of sympathetic control that results in neurogenic shock (hypotension, bradycardia, peripheral vasodilatation, and associated hypotermia). By 6–7 weeks, patients present an average of seven contractures.

Approximately 30% of blunt contusive human SCI results in a complete loss of continuity of central nervous system tissue that is clinically indistinguishable from spinal cord transection. The neurological completeness/incompleteness of an injury at any stage can be graded according to the American Spinal Injury Association (ASIA) from A to E, as follows: A = complete with no sensory or motor function preserved in S4–5; B = incomplete with sensory but no motor function preserved below the neurological level and extending through S4–5; C = incomplete with motor function preserved below the neurological level, the majority of key muscles present a grade <3; D = incomplete with motor function preserved below the neurological level, the majority of key muscles present a grade ≥3; E = normal motor and sensory function. The neurological level of injury refers to the most caudal intact segment with normal sensory and motor function.

Incomplete injuries may be classified into four types: anterior spinal syndrome; central cord syndrome (CCS); Brown–Séquard syndrome; and mixed types. The anterior cord syndrome typically results in some degree of paralysis, with a loss of pain and temperature sensation below the level of the lesion and relative sparing of touch, vibration, and proprioception. CCS typically occurs following trauma to the cervical spinal cord, and an elderly patient with preexisting cervical spondylosis is a classic presentation. An associated fracture of a cervical vertebra is uncommon. CCS is characterized by symmetrically incomplete quadriplegia, affecting the upper more than the lower limbs; sensory impairment is variable and urinary retention is common. The "burning hands syndrome" is a variant of CCS characterized by burning dysesthesia of the hands and associated weakness in the hands and arms. Most symptoms resolve quickly. Brown–Séquard syndrome consists of ipsilateral weakness and loss of proprioceptive sensation due to disruption of the corticospinal tracts and dorsal columns. Pain and temperature sensations are lost on the contralateral side due to the affected spinothalamic tract.

Approximately two-thirds of SCI patients may develop new symptoms several weeks or even years after injury. Pain is a common problem and has a major impact on patients with chronic SCI. Delayed post-traumatic pain commonly begins in the first 6–9 months post injury, but can start several years after. Several types of pain may occur, which can be divided into musculoskeletal pain, visceral pain, and above-level, at-level, and below-level neuropathic pains indicated by descriptions such as burning, shooting, electric shock-like, and hypersensitivity. Progressive post-traumatic myelomalacic myelopathy (PPMM) and syringomyelia are the well-known "late" post-traumatic complications of SCI. PPMM has been reported in 0.3–3.2% of patients with chronic spinal cord injury and can occur as soon as 2 months and up to 30 years following injury. PPMM is a possible precursor of syringomyelia. Clinically, PPMM and post-traumatic syringomyelia are neurologically indistinguishable; however, magnetic resonance imaging (MRI) can be used to differentiate the two entities. Syringomyelia occurs in 3–4% of cases; it can manifest as early as 8 weeks after injury or may be delayed in onset for several years. It is caused by cystic degeneration of the injured spinal cord at or near the site of the trauma. The clinical presentation in post-traumatic syringomyelia is non-specific. Most patients present with ascending sensory signs and motor deficit. The treatment consists of shunting the syrinx, with improvement of symptoms in the majority of patients. Spinal cord atrophy is a third type of lesion found in the chronic stage of spinal cord injury. It is usually observed many years after the traumatic event and occurs in approximately 15–20% of patients. Occasionally, it is difficult to differentiate atrophy from a subarachnoid cyst with cord compression and from "postsyrinx" syndrome.

Investigations

The trauma patient who is alert, oriented, and neither sedated nor distracted may or may not have neck pain or tenderness on clinical examination. The probability of structural injury in such patients is close to zero; it is increasingly recognized that imaging such patients is unnecessary.

A plain, three-view radiograph is usually performed for patients with neurological signs, although multislice computed tomography (CT) is usually recommended for initial evaluation of spinal trauma patients and clarification as to whether a fracture is present. MRI typically serves as a problem-solving technique when CT is unable adequately to assess the cause of neurological deficits, determine acuity of a fracture, or assess the presence of ligamentous injury. MRI can show transection, hemorrhage, contusion, or edema of the spinal cord. It can also demonstrate ligamentous injuries, muscular lesions, facet joint dislocations, and bone marrow edema. The presence of abnormalities on MRI in a patient with a complete cord syndrome is generally a bad prognostic sign. Absence of spinal cord edema is a strong predictor of full recovery in patients with acute central cervical cord injury involving only the upper extremities.

Clinical examination and imaging can be complemented by electrophysiological recordings to deduce the degree of involvement of different spinal pathways. Corticospinal, spinothalamic, dorsal column, and sympathetic pathway functions may be quantifiably measured by motor evoked potentials, laser evoked potentials, somatosensory evoked potentials, and sympathetic skin response techniques, respectively.

Spinal cord injury without radiographic abnormality (SCIWORA) refers to spinal injuries, typically located in the cervical region, in the absence of identifiable bony or ligamentous injury on plain radiographs or CT. With the increased availability of MRI, the diagnosis of "real" SCIWORA is less common. Among patients with SCIWORA, using MRI allows the identification of different patterns of SCI, including transection, contusive hemorrhage, traumatic edema, and concussion. Currently, the discussion of SCIWORA is of practical importance mainly for situations with limited diagnostic resources.

Probably the development of this form of SCI can contribute some premorbid factors and the mechanism of injury.

SCIWORA is well known in the pediatric population (with an incidence of 5–35%). Relative to adults, anatomic features in children (especially in infants and children up to 8 years) predispose to hypermobility of the spinal column in the absence of apparent bony injury. The mechanism underlying adult SCIWORA is the compression of the cord during sudden hyperflexion anteriorly with the posterior longitudinal ligament and mildly protruded discs, and posteriorly with the laminae and ligamentum flavum. SCIWORA should be suspected in patients subjected to blunt trauma who report early or transient symptoms of neurological deficit that range from transient paresthesiae to complete motor paralysis and sensory loss. SCIWORA should not be confused with symptoms of peripheral brachial plexus injuries (cervical "burners" or "stingers").

Conventional MRI and diffusion-weighted MRI (DWI) of the region of suspected injury, and flexion-extension radiographs in the acute setting and at late follow-up, are recommended for diagnosis and to allow a better prognostic evaluation of recovery from SCIWORA. Acute management priorities for SCIWORA consist of maintenance of external spinal immobilization for up to 12 weeks and avoidance of "high-risk" activities for up to 6 months.

Treatment

In general, trauma patients with SCI should be managed by immobilization to attain anatomic alignment. In the acute setting, initiation of intravenous methylprednisolone treatment as a bolus dose of 30 mg/kg over 15 minutes within 8 hours after SCI (the "time window"), followed by 5.4 mg/kg/hour for the ensuing 23 hours, is recommended. Subsequent treatments must be individualized and depend on the degree of neurological deficit, spinal level, and severity of deformity. Occasionally, spinal surgery is required (e.g., when there are bony fragments compressing the cord). For a compression fracture of the upper lumbar spine (typically occurring in older osteoporotic patients), the decision between bracing and surgery is based on the degree of spinal stability (classified according to the Denis three-column model), spinal stenosis, and neurological deficit. Bracing is a low-risk, cost-effective method to treat neurologically intact patients with traumatic thoracolumbar fractures without stenosis. Secondary medical complications for acute SCI such as respiratory failure, deep venous thrombosis, and urological complications should be appropriately corrected. Related to prolonged immobility, the leading causes of death among persons with SCI are pneumonia and septicemia. Spasticity, pain, autonomic dysreflexia, and contractures are common complications associated with chronic SCI, requiring pharmacological measures and physical therapy.

Further reading

Bogdanov EI, Heiss JD, Mendelevich EG. The post-syrinx syndrome: Stable central myelopathy and collapsed or absent syrinx. *J Neurol* 2006;253:707–713.

Hoffman JR, Mower WR, Wolfson AB, *et al.* Validity of a set of clinical criteria to rule out injury to the cervical spine in patients with blunt trauma. *N Engl J Med* 2000;343:94–99.

Kramer KM, Levine AM. Posttraumatic syringomyelia: A review of 21 cases. *Clin Orthop Relat Res* 1997;334:190–199.

Lee TT, Arias JM, Andrus HL, *et al.* Progressive posttraumatic myelomalacic myelopathy: Treatment with untethering and expansive duraplasty. *J Neurosurg* 1997;86:624–628.

Roselle C, Aarabi B, Dhall S, *et al.* Spinal cord injury without radiographic abnormality (SCIWORA). *Neurosurgery* 2013;72:227–233.

Singh A, Tetreault L, Kalsi-Ryan S, *et al.* Global prevalence and incidence of traumatic spinal cord injury. *Clin Epidemiol* 2014;6:309–331.

173 Whiplash injury

Anthony Ciabarra

Neurology Center of North Orange County, Fullerton, CA, USA

Whiplash-associated disorders (WAD) are a frequent cause of disability. Acceleration–deceleration forces applied to the neck, particularly with flexion-extension movements, commonly result in whiplash injury. Whiplash injury is most frequently caused by automobile accidents, but may also be caused by other mechanisms including falls, contact sports resulting in a blow to the head, and the violent shaking of a child. The term whiplash should be used to describe an injury mechanism. Whiplash injury results in a mechanical sprain or strain, often with tissue edema or contusion. The posture of the neck and direction of forces dictate the injury sustained. Acceleration strain of the spine may occur in the sagittal plane resulting in extension, flexion, or translational injury; in the frontal plane resulting in lateral inclination or translational injury; or in the axial plane resulting in rotational injury.

Epidemiology

Considerable variability exists in the frequency and prognosis of whiplash injuries sustained in different geographic regions. These differences may be partially attributable to societal differences, including such factors as traffic volume, expectations with regard to outcome, and legal and financial ramifications associated with the injury. Reported rates of WAD range from 10 to more than 1000 per 100000 worldwide. The rate of WAD has been reported as 70 per 100000 inhabitants in Quebec, 106 per 100000 in Australia, and 250 per 100000 in the Netherlands. Risk factors for whiplash injury include the speed of impact, being the driver or front-seat passenger, and rear-end collision or frontal collision rather than side collision. The speed limit necessary to produce whiplash injury is generally considered to be above 6–8 km/hour. Female gender has been reported in some studies to be a risk factor, but other studies have found no gender differences. Age, socioeconomic status, and level of educational attainment have not been consistently shown to influence the rate of whiplash injury.

WAD results in substantial socioeconomic costs in the industrialized world. Personal injury claims related to whiplash injury in the United Kingdom exceed €3 billion per year. Studies of the incidence and outcome of whiplash injuries in Saskatchewan following a change in the compensation system from a tort-based system with payments for pain and suffering to a no-fault system suggest that compensation based on pain may promote persistent illness and disability. In Singapore and Lithuania, where such compensation systems are absent, the prevalence of chronic symptoms is low.

Pathophysiology

The precise pathophysiology of WAD is controversial. An acute whiplash injury follows sudden hyperextension, hyperflexion, or rotation of the neck. In mild cases, tissue edema or contusion may be present consistent with a sprain injury. Injury to structures including zygoapophyseal joints, cervical discs, and ligaments are present to varying degrees in some patients. Zygoapophyseal joints are considered to be a significant source of neck pain, particularly in those who are chronically affected. More serious injuries may result from whiplash mechanisms including anterior subluxation, spinous process fractures, facet dislocation, cervical radiculopathy, and vertebral compression fractures. Augmented central pain processing mechanisms have also been suggested to play a role.

Clinical features

Quebec Task Force guidelines established grades of WAD in 1995 (Table 173.1) and this classification continues to be used throughout the world. The term whiplash is generally used to refer to grades 1–2. The diagnosis of cervical sprain and strain resulting from a whiplash injury is a clinical one. Whiplash injury can be associated with a variety of physical and psychosocial symptoms. Pain and stiffness in the neck and shoulders, with limitation in movement, are felt within 24 hours of the injury. Headache, particularly at the occiput, is frequently reported. Dizziness, vertigo, paresthesias, and weakness in the extremities are also reported.

Chronic whiplash syndrome (CWS) is defined by the presence of symptoms beyond 6 months after the underlying injury. CWS is often accompanied by a combination of symptoms including persistent headache, neck pain and stiffness, paresthesias, and often memory disturbance, fatigue, and anxiety. Observed behavior and

Table 173.1 Quebec Task Force classification of whiplash-associated disorders.

Classification grade	Criteria
0	No neck complaints or physical signs
1	Neck pain or stiffness in the absence of physical signs
2	Neck complaints and musculoskeletal signs including decreased range of motion and point tenderness
3	Neck complaints and neurological signs including decreased or absent reflexes, sensory loss, or weakness
4	Neck complaints and fracture or dislocation

International Neurology, Second edition. Edited by Robert P. Lisak, Daniel D. Truong, William M. Carroll and Roongroj Bhidayasiri
© 2016 John Wiley & Sons, Ltd. Published 2016 by John Wiley & Sons, Ltd.

the presence of non-physiological sensory loss must be carefully assessed. Prognostic indicators for the development of CWS include initial pain level, initial disability level, symptoms of post-traumatic stress, negative expectation of recovery, fear of neck movement, depressed mood, past history of neck pain, and cold hyperalgesias. Prognostic factors for CWS yielding inconsistent results in studies include age, gender, and compensation factors.

Considerable variability has been noted between clinical studies with regard to prognosis, which may be attributed to differences in patient selection or the definition of whiplash used. After 1 month symptoms improve in most patients and 75% are able to perform their regular duties. More than 88% of patients will return to normal daily activities by 1 year. In one study of 680 patients with WAD, 71% of patients had recovered within 6 months of injury, with a median time to recovery of 97 days. Those suffering from continued pain and inability to work after 1 year are likely to have persistent symptoms.

Investigations
Examining for signs of muscular spasm, point tenderness, and neurological deficits is critical. Cervical spine X-rays consisting of a standard series of three views should be obtained in patients 65 years or older with neck pain or midline tenderness. Younger patients should also undergo X-ray examination if evaluation of neck movement is considered unsafe or if there are risk factors for severe injury, such as paresthesias in the extremities, a high-speed collision >100 km/hour, a fall from greater than 1 meter, or a bicycle collision. Computed tomography (CT) scan evaluation of the cervical spine is indicated if plain films reveal a definite abnormality, are deemed inadequate, or clinical suspicion of more serious injury is present despite normal radiographs. Magnetic resonance imaging (MRI) is indicated in patients with neurological signs and is useful to delineate cervical disc injury, posterior longitudinal, and interspinous ligament injuries. CT myelogram may be employed if MRI is not available or not tolerated. Electrodiagnostic studies are indicated in patients with persistent radicular symptoms, numbness, or weakness.

Treatment
Randomized controlled trials of acute WAD support mobilization and return to normal activities as effective early interventions. Soft collars and rest do not reduce the duration of neck pain and may prolong recovery. A recent randomized controlled trial determined that a comprehensive exercise program in grades 1–2 acute WAD was no more effective than verbal and written advice provided by a physician and physiotherapist. Advice emphasized the importance of exercise and avoidance of immobility as well as the likely favorable prognosis. Missed work time was found to be reduced by high-dose methylprednisolone administered within 8 hours of injury in one study; however, it is uncertain whether the risks outweigh the benefits. Muscle relaxants alone or in combination with nonsteroidal anti-inflammatory medications were shown to provide little relief in a randomized controlled study in acute WAD. Multimodal programs including exercise and cognitive and behavioral therapies may be useful, but randomized trials are lacking. Cognitive and behavioral therapies administered by a neuropsychologist may include stress management, coping strategies, and realignment of perceptions and expectations. Evidence of the benefits of intra-articular steroid injections is conflicting. Botulism neurotoxin A (BoNTA) and traction have not been found to be beneficial. Evidence of the effectiveness of acupuncture in the treatment of WAD is limited. The efficacy of exercise therapy in CWS is uncertain. For those with pain after 6 months, percutaneous frequency neurotomy may be beneficial if a response to local anesthetic injections of facet joints is helpful.

Conclusion
Whiplash-associated disorders are encountered frequently in clinical practice and may result from a variety of mechanisms, with automobile accidents being the most common. Current evidence supports early mobilization, reassurance, and active intervention as the best treatment options in WAD grades I–III. Socioeconomic factors may play a role in extending disability in some patients. WAD carry a favorable prognosis for the majority of patients.

Further reading
Pearce JMS. Polemics of chronic whiplash injury. *Neurology* 1994;44:1993–1997.
Rodriquez AA, Barr KP, Burns SP. Whiplash: Pathophysiology, diagnosis, treatment, and prognosis. *Muscle Nerve* 2004;29(6):768–781.
Spitzer WO, Skovron ML, Salmi LR, *et al.* Scientific monograph of the Quebec Task Force on Whiplash-Associated Disorders: Redefining "whiplash" and its management. *Spine* 1995;20(8 Suppl):1 S—73 S.
Sterling M. Physiotherapy management of whiplash-associated disorders (WAD). *J Physiotherapy* 2014;60:5–12.

174 Decompression sickness

Leon D. Prockop[1], Andreas Koch[2], and Günther Deuschl[3]

[1] Department of Neurology, University of South Florida, Tampa, FL, USA
[2] German Naval Medical Institute, Christian-Albrechts-University Kiel, Kiel, Germany
[3] Department of Neurology, Christian-Albrechts-University Kiel, Kiel, Germany

In scuba diving, caisson work, flying, and simulated altitude ascents, changes in ambient pressure can cause pressure-related medical issues, such as barotrauma, arterial gas embolism (AGE), and decompression sickness (DCS). The relationship between pressure and volume is governed by Boyle's law, which states that the volume of a fixed mass of gas is inversely proportionate to the absolute pressure. The solubility of gases is ruled by Henry's law, which says that the solubility of a gas in a liquid is directly proportional to the partial pressure of the gas above the liquid. The term "barotrauma" encompasses disorders related to a mismatch between changes in pressure and its equalization in a gas-filled cavity, such as the middle ear, predominantly during pressure increase. Here, pain, hearing dysfunction, and vertigo or even bleeding can occur.

An inadequate rapid reduction in ambient pressure, on the other hand, may allow an excessive formation of bubbles from inert gases, especially nitrogen, normally dissolved in body tissues according to Henry's law, causing a decompression incident (DCI). Bubble formation is caused by the growth of gas nuclei in predominantly fatty tissues and musculature, and transported via the venous catchment to the right heart and the lungs. In cases of transpulmonary passage after massive bubble formation with pulmonary air embolism (known as "dysbaric chokes"), or cardiac shunting of gas bubbles, peripheral embolic decompression sickness (DCS) can occur. Even more dangerous is the accidental overexpansion of the lung during a rapid ascent, which can result in lung rupture and subsequent arterial gas embolism (AGE) due to the direct penetration of pulmonary gas into the systemic circulation. The resulting lesions involve the limbs, cardiopulmonary system, and central nervous system (CNS). Besides the embolic way, it is still under discussion whether extravascular autochthonous bubble formation directly inside the tissues, for instance in the spinal cord, may also contribute to DCS. In addition, the possible role of microparticles in the genesis of DCS needs to be elucidated.

In divers, DCS primarily affects the CNS and the spinal cord. Aviators may develop characteristic musculoskeletal or neurological DCS symptoms while at altitude, with resolution of symptoms frequently occurring on return to sea level. Other medical problems that may occur during diving and/or flying include nitrogen narcosis, hypoxia, CNS and pulmonary oxygen toxicity, hypercapnia, and hypocapnia.

Epidemiology

The incidence of neurological DCS in divers is rather low, about 2.3 cases per 10000 dives in divers without a patent foramen ovale (PFO), and 5.7 cases per 10000 dives in PFO-positive divers.

Pathophysiology

Although the spinal cord is the most common site of neurological lesions, encephalopathy is also well described. Electrophysiological studies, experimental models, and isolated postmortem examinations of patients have shown predominant involvement of the posterolateral and posterior columns in the watershed areas of the thoracic, upper lumbar, and lower cervical cord. Ischemic perivascular lesions are usually confined to the white matter, but subsequent petechial hemorrhage may occur and extend into the gray matter. Lesions result from bubbles occluding vessels or directly disrupting tissue. Coincident intra-arterial embolism may cause cerebral damage.

Clinical features

DCS manifestations include limb pain; itching and skin markings; non-specific constitutional symptoms such as headache, fatigue, malaise, nausea, vomiting, and anorexia; enlarged and tender lymph nodes; vertigo and deafness; and cardiovascular or pulmonary compromise. Neurological signs range from subtle and subjective to unconsciousness or tetraplegia. With cord damage, radicular symptoms are followed by leg paresthesia, paresis, and bladder and bowel dysfunction. When the brain is affected, neurological signs and symptoms include visual impairment, vertigo, hemiparesis, loss of consciousness, and seizures. Unless adequate therapy of the DCS is achieved promptly, the signs, including paralysis, may become permanent. Preventive medical clearance and proper scuba diving techniques are essential, and a DCS should be considered in case of any diving-related new onset of suspicious symptoms. Absolute neurological contraindications to scuba diving include a history of any of the following: a seizure occurring other than in childhood or febrile; transient ischemic attack or stroke; and prior DCS with residual deficit. Other neurological conditions of serious concern in preventive evaluation include complicated migraine, head injury, herniated nucleus pulposus,

---

International Neurology, Second edition. Edited by Robert P. Lisak, Daniel D. Truong, William M. Carroll and Roongroj Bhidayasiri
© 2016 John Wiley & Sons, Ltd. Published 2016 by John Wiley & Sons, Ltd.

multiple sclerosis, trigeminal neuralgia, and a history of cerebral gas embolism. There are also relative and absolute contraindications for diving in those presenting other body system diseases (such as intracardiac right-to-left shunt).

Treatment

Manifestations of DCS, including any neurological symptoms and signs, are a medical emergency. Current therapy consists of immediate 100% normobaric oxygenation via demand valve or face mask and fluids, oral or intravenous. Hyperbaric oxygenation in a pressure chamber should be administered as soon as possible. Results of treatment vary, but the sooner therapy is begun, the better the outcome. Although the use of drugs to improve outcomes is being investigated, no particular adjunctive pharmacotherapy has been proven effective. Some writers advise the use of steroids or lidocaine. MRI can document the extent of brain and spinal cord damage. For chamber locations and emergency information, US physicians should contact the Divers Alert Network at 919–684–9111, a 24-hour hotline. The website for the Diving Division Research Center in Derriford, United Kingdom, is

http://www.ddrc.org. For locations of hyperbaric chambers worldwide, consult http://scuba-doc.com/listchmbr.htm.

Further reading

Bove AA. Risk of decompression sickness with patent foramen ovale. *Undersea Hyperb Med* 1998;25(3):175–178.

Cianci P, Slade JB, Jr. Delayed treatment of decompression sickness with short, no-air-break tables: Review of 140 cases. *Aviat Space Environ Med* 2006;77(10):1003–1008.

Dutka AJ. Long term dffects on the central nervous system. In: BrubakkAO, NeumanTS (eds.). *Bennett and Elliott's Physiology and Medicine of Diving*, 6th ed. New York: W. B. Sanders; 2003.

Gronning M, Risberg J, Skeidsvoll H, *et al.* Electroencephalography and magnetic resonance imaging in neurological decompression sickness. *Undersea Hyperb Med* 2005;32(6):397–402.

MacDonald RD, O'Donnell C, Allan GM, *et al.* Interfacility transport of patients with decompression illness: Literature review and consensus statement. *Prehosp Emerg Care* 2006;10(4):482–487.

Naval Sea Systems Command. *U.S. Navy Diving Manual: Revision 6.* Washington, DC: US Government Printing Office. http://www.usu.edu/scuba/navy_manual6.pdf (accessed November 2015).

Yang M, Kosterin P, Salzberg BM, *et al.* Microparticles generated by decompression stress cause central nervous system injury manifested as neurohypophysial terminal action potential broadening. *J Appl Physiol* 2013;115(10):1481–1486.

175 Pain

Guillermo García-Ramos[1], Bernardo Cacho-Díaz[2], and Bruno Estañol-Vidal[1]

[1] Neurology and Neurophysiology Department, Instituto Nacional de Ciencias Médicas y Nutrición Salvador Zubiran, Mexico City, Mexico

[2] Neuroscience Unit, Instituto Nacional de Cancerología, Mexico City, Mexico

Global statistics show that approximately 1 in 5 adults (20%) suffers from pain, which may be acute, chronic, intermittent, or a combination, and 1 in 10 adults (10%) is newly diagnosed with chronic pain each year. The most frequent complaint in an emergency room or physician's office visit is pain. Pain is defined by the International Association for the Study of Pain (IASP) as "an unpleasant sensory and emotional experience associated with actual or potential tissue damage, or described in terms of such damage." Even in cases where pain does not have a clear etiology, it should be considered pathological and should always be treated.

Classification of pain

Pain is divided into nociceptive, neuropathic, or visceral types. Nociceptive pain results from the physiological activity of normal pain receptors with no primary dysfunction of the nervous system. Neuropathic pain results from dysfunction of the central or peripheral nervous system and involves two different kinds of pain, reflecting several different pathophysiological mechanisms. Visceral pain is the result of activation of sensory afferents from the internal organs, and it is often accompanied by accentuated motor and autonomic reflexes.

Pathophysiology of pain

Nociceptors

Pain is the consequence of stimulation of pain-sensitive structures (nociceptors) and is often, but not always, a sign of tissue damage. Nociceptors do not consist of a homogenous group of afferents; no single criterion can reliably define a nociceptor. Nociceptors can be subclassified by an array of anatomical, physiological, and biochemical criteria. One common criterion is the response profile of the afferent: afferents that respond to mechanical, thermal, and chemical stimuli are referred to as polymodal nociceptors; those that respond to mechanical and cold stimuli are referred to as C-MC (mechano-cold) nociceptors; and those that do not respond to mechanical stimuli are referred to as MIA (mechanically insensitive afferents) nociceptors.

Pain and temperature are sensations mediated at a primary afferent level by fibers of a smaller diameter than those mediating touch, vibration, and position sense. Cold sensation is transmitted by small myelinated (poorly myelinated) Aδ fibers, whereas warm sensation is transmitted by unmyelinated warm-specific C fibers. Pain is mediated by small myelinated Aδ nociceptors and unmyelinated C nociceptors. The skin subcutaneous tissues, muscles, and joints are sensitive to a variety of potentially harmful mechanical, thermal, and chemical stimuli. Although the ultrastructural characteristics of pain receptors are not well known, classically two types have been characterized, depending on their fiber characteristics: unmyelinated C and those associated with Aδ fibers. A third type of cutaneous nociceptor has been described, which is activated only during inflammation and modulates information through unmyelinated C fibers. In the absence of inflammation, these receptors usually do not respond even to a highly noxious stimulus. These receptors have also been named mechano-insensitive and heat-insensitive (MiHi) receptors. These receptors probably mediate hyperalgesia and itch in different populations.

Glabrous and hairy skin is richly innervated by nociceptors with unmyelinated C fibers. These are known as C-polymodal nociceptors (CPNs) because they respond to a variety of noxious stimuli (mechanical, thermal, and chemical). A single CPN innervates an area of skin approximately 1 cm square. CPNs respond to capsaicin and to temperatures below 15 °C.

Aδ nociceptors seem to be stimulated mainly through mechanical provocation; these display a smaller, usually punctiform receptive field and have higher mechanical and heat thresholds than CPNs. Excitation of cutaneous CPNs evokes a pure burning sensation. Aδ nociceptors evoke sharp pain that is projected to a punctiform area. CPNs are also involved in inflammation; excitation triggers the release of algogenic substances from nociceptive terminals in the skin, causing vasodilatation and thus local redness of the skin; this reaction spreads some centimeters around the site of stimulation through an axonal reflex that depends on a network of fine dermal afferent fibers, described as a nocifensor system.

Hyperalgesia occurring at the site of injury is defined as primary hyperalgesia and is a characteristic response to heat and mechanical stimuli. Secondary hyperalgesia is hyperalgesia that occurs at a wider area of undamaged surrounding skin. The first type of hyperalgesia is the consequence of sensitization of CPNs at the site of injury, whereas the latter is due to plastic changes in the central nervous system (CNS) and probably in the peripheral nervous system (PNS). MiHi receptors develop heat and mechanical sensitivity in areas of secondary hyperalgesia.

International Neurology, Second edition. Edited by Robert P. Lisak, Daniel D. Truong, William M. Carroll and Roongroj Bhidayasiri
© 2016 John Wiley & Sons, Ltd. Published 2016 by John Wiley & Sons, Ltd.

Steps in the pain pathway

Transduction

The first step is transduction. Transduction is recognized as the process by which noxious stimuli are converted to electrical signals by "pain" receptors – nociceptors – that do not have a specialized structure but rather are free nerve endings. Nociceptors do not respond to non-noxious stimuli and do not adapt; that is, continued stimulation results in continuous or repetitive firing of the nociceptor and, in some cases, continued stimulation actually results in a decrease in the threshold at which the nociceptor responds. Nociceptive afferent fibers come from pseudounipolar neurons, whose bodies reside at the dorsal root ganglia. The neurotransmitters produced by these cells are released at both terminals of the neuron, so that the neuron has both afferent and efferent neurotransmitter release. There is not only an afferent function of the primary afferent nociceptor, but also an efferent function, which reflects the release of excitatory transmitter from the peripheral terminals. This may result in the release of other mediators, which can produce further sensitization and/or activation of primary afferent fibers or nearby primary afferent nociceptors. This process is the "axon reflex," which leads to peripheral changes that are clinically recognized as indicators of pain (e.g., redness, swelling, and tenderness).

Transmission

Transmission is the second stage of processing noxious signals. Information from the periphery is relayed to the spinal cord, then to the thalamus, and finally to the cortex. Noxious information is relayed mainly via two types of primary afferent nociceptors. C fibers are nonmyelinated fibers that conduct impulses in the range of 0.5–2 m/s. Nociceptive C fibers transmit noxious information from a variety of sensory modalities, including mechanical, thermal, and chemical, and thus have been termed C polymodal nociceptors. These receptors transmit their information through the release of substance P and glutamate. Aδ fibers are thinly myelinated fibers that conduct impulses in the range of 2–20 m/s. All Aδ fibers respond to high-intensity mechanical stimulation and therefore are termed high-threshold mechanoreceptors. Some, but not all, receptors also respond to thermal stimuli and are thus named mechano-thermal receptors.

These fibers then synapse on a second-order neuron in the superficial layer of the spinal cord, whose axons are sent across the midline and form the ascending spinothalamic tract, where they reach a third-order neuron in the thalamus and then are transmitted to the sensory cortex.

The second-order neurons also have the capacity to change their response patterns in the circumstance of sustained discharge of afferent fibers (e.g., injury). Under these conditions, these neurons respond to lower thresholds and from inputs over a broader area in the periphery (i.e., they have expanded receptive fields); this phenomenon is termed central sensitization and contributes to hyperalgesia and allodynia.

Once the nociceptive afferents have terminated in the dorsal horn of the spinal cord, they transmit the signal from the periphery by releasing specific neurotransmitters. One of the most important pain neurotransmitters and the primary afferent is glutamate, which can interact with both NMDA and non-NMDA receptors. Another very important neurotransmitter is substance P, which interacts with the tachykinin receptor family (G protein-coupled receptor).

Nociceptive neurons are located mainly in lamina I of Rexed and they receive inputs mainly from primary nociceptive afferents. These neurons project to the contralateral spinothalamic tract (STT) and their activity is modulated by local interneurons. Wide dynamic range (WDR) neurons respond more vigorously to inputs from nociceptive afferents, but also discharge in response to non-noxious stimuli; they are mostly located in lamina V, but can be found in laminae I and II as well. They are thought to project to the contralateral STT. Second-order nociceptive neurons also project to higher regions through the spinoreticular, spinomesencephalic, and spinocervical tracts, and some project into the posterior columns. The spinomesencephalic and spinocervical tracts project to the reticular formation, the thalamus, and the periaqueductal gray (PAG) nuclei.

Third-order neurons are mainly localized in the ventral posterior lateral (VPL) nucleus. This nucleus receives input from neurons in laminae I and V and projects to the primary somatosensory cortex. The ventral posterior medial nucleus receives input from the second-order nociceptive neurons of the trigeminal nuclei. The intralaminar nuclei receive input from the deep dorsal horn laminae and the reticular formation of the brainstem; this thalamic region is probably concerned with arousal rather than with pain sensation itself. The facial sensations of pain and temperature are carried by cranial nerve V and ascend separately to the thalamus.

In the primary somatosensory cortex, two main types of neurons have been described. One group, which receives inputs from the VPL thalamus, displays a small, contralateral receptive field. The second group comprises neurons that have wide receptive fields, usually bilateral, and that probably receive inputs from the medial thalamic nuclei. The thalamocortical projections and the primary sensory cortex in the parietal lobe have a homuncular sensory pattern, in which projections for the face are closest to the sylvian fissure, those for the hand and arm are above, and those for the leg lie near the central sulcus.

Ascending modulation

The third process, modulation, involves changes in the nervous system's response to noxious stimuli and allows noxious signals received at the dorsal horn of the spinal cord to be selectively inhibited, so that the transmission of the signal to higher centers is modified. An endogenous pain modulation system that inhibits transmission of the pain signal consists of intermediate neurons (superficial layers of the spinal cord) and descending neural tracts. Opiates can act on the presynaptic terminal of the primary afferent nociceptors via the mu opioid receptor by indirectly blocking voltage-gated calcium channels as well as opening potassium channels. This leads to hyperpolarization of the cell and inhibition of pain neurotransmitter release from these fibers, which produces analgesia. Opioids have a second site of action at the spinal cord, on the postsynaptic neuron. When activated by an opioid, potassium channels are indirectly opened and lead to hyperpolarization of these neurons. Activation of the cortical descending neural system is thought to involve the supraspinal release of β-endorphins and enkephalins. These peptides represent two families of endogenous peptides that are associated with pain relief, especially under conditions of stress.

Descending modulation

Activation of descending modulation systems by endorphins occurs through opioid receptors. These systems are activated in and around the PAG mesencephalic (midbrain) region. These neurons project to sites in the medullary reticular formation and the locus ceruleus (primary areas for production of serotonin and norepinephrine, respectively). These descending fibers then project to the dorsal horn of the spinal cord along a tract called the dorsolateal funiculus to synapse with either the incoming primary afferent neuron, second-order neuron, or interneurons. These descending pain modulatory neurons either (1) release neurotransmitters in the spinal cord, especially serotonin (5-HT) and norepinephrine (NE), both of which directly inhibit release of pain transmitters from the incoming nociceptive afferent signal or inhibit the second-order pain transmission cell; or (2) activate small opioid-containing interneurons in the spinal dorsal horn to release opioid peptides.

Neuropathic pain

Perception of pain is frequently triggered by a noxious stimulus, but it also can be elicited by lesions in the peripheral or central nervous system such as in diabetic neuropathy or stroke. It is important to realize that pain can occur without nociception. Pain due to nerve injury does not respond to analgesics such as morphine as efficiently as pain caused by tissue damage, indicating the complex relation between injury and pain. Another relevant issue is that the intensity of chronic pain frequently bears little or no relation to the extent of tissue injury or of other quantifiable pathology.

Visceral pain

There are two common principles that apply to all visceral pain. The first is that the neurological mechanisms of visceral pain differ from those involved in somatic pain, and therefore findings in somatic pain research cannot necessarily be extrapolated to visceral pain. The second principle is that the psychophysics (perception and psychological processing) of visceral pain also differs from that of somatic pain.

Visceral pain has five important characteristics: (1) it is not evoked from all viscera – organs such as liver, kidney, most solid viscera, and lung parenchyma are not sensitive to pain; (2) it is not always linked to visceral injury – cutting the intestine causes no pain and is an example of visceral injury with no subsequent pain, whereas stretching the bladder is painful and is an example of pain with no injury; (3) it is diffuse and poorly localized; (4) it is referred to other locations; and (5) it is accompanied by motor and autonomic reflexes, such as the nausea, vomiting, and lower back muscle tension in renal colic.

These features of visceral pain are due to functional properties of the peripheral receptors of the nerves that innervate certain visceral organs, and to the fact that many viscera are innervated by receptors that do not evoke conscious perception of pain and thus are not sensory receptors in the strict sense. Visceral pain tends to be diffuse because of the organization of visceral nociceptive pathways in the central nervous system, particularly the absence of a separate visceral sensory pathway and the low proportion of visceral afferent nerve fibers compared with those of somatic origin.

There are two distinct classes of nociceptive sensory receptors that innervate internal organs. The first class of receptors have a high threshold to natural stimuli (mostly mechanical); high-threshold receptors have been identified in the heart, veins, lungs and airways, esophagus, biliary system, small intestine, colon, ureter, urinary bladder, and uterus. The second class of receptors

are intensity-encoding receptors that have a low threshold to natural stimuli (mostly mechanical) and an encoding function that spans the range of stimulation intensity from innocuous to noxious. These receptors are intensity encoding in that they encode stimulus intensity in the magnitude of their discharges; they have been identified in the heart, esophagus, colon, urinary bladder, and testes.

Silent receptors, a third nociceptive receptor family that play a role in visceral pain, have been increasingly studied. These are normally unresponsive to discrete stimuli and become activated only in the presence of inflammation. This class of sensory receptors contributes to the signaling of chronic visceral pain, to long-term alterations of spinal reflexes, and to abnormal autonomic regulation of internal organs. They comprise no more than 40–45% of total afferent visceral innervation of the colon and bladder.

High-threshold receptors and intensity-coding receptors contribute to the peripheral encoding of noxious events in the viscera. Brief acute visceral pain could be triggered initially by the activation of high-threshold afferents. More extended forms of visceral stimulation result in the sensitization of high-threshold receptors and bring into play previously unresponsive silent nociceptors. Once sensitized, these nociceptors will begin to respond to the innocuous stimuli that normally occur in internal organs. As a consequence, the central nervous system receives an increased afferent barrage from peripheral nociceptors that is initially due to the acute injury, but is also influenced by the physiological activity of the internal organ and persists until the process of peripheral sensitization subsides completely. In this way, the pain is intensified and its duration extended by a central mechanism brought into action by the peripheral barrage.

Damage and inflammation of the viscus also affect its normal pattern of motility and secretion, which produces dramatic changes in the environment that surrounds the nociceptor endings. The altered activity of the viscus further increases the excitation of sensitized nociceptors and may even be sufficient to excite more distant nociceptors not affected by the initial insult. Therefore, afferent discharges due to viscus activity after an injury or inflammation may be greater in magnitude and duration than the discharges produced by acute injury, and visceral pain may persist even after the initial injury is on its way to resolution.

Fine-caliber unmyelinated primary afferents that innervate somatic and visceral tissues have two distinct biochemical classes: the first class contains neurons that express peptide neurotransmitters, such as substance P and calcitonin gene-related peptide (CGRP); the other class does not express these substances. These two classes can also be distinguished by various enzymes, such as fluoride-resistant acid phosphatase (non-peptide group), and receptors such as the nerve-growth-factor receptor tyrosine kinase A. They also differ with regard to trophic requirements.

The peptide-containing afferents of the somatic system terminate in the outermost layers of the posterior horn, lamina I, outer lamina II, and lamina V, whereas the non-peptide groups terminate in inner lamina II. In contrast to the somatic fine afferent fibers, most visceral afferent fibers seem to belong to the peptide class that expresses peptide neurotransmitters and does not express carbohydrate group characteristics of the non-peptide class. As with somatic peptide-containing afferents, visceral afferents also terminate on spinal cord laminae I and V. Peptides seem to have more importance in the transmission of information from the viscera; substance P may have a specific role in visceral hyperalgesia.

Several pathways have been found to be responsible for transmission of visceral pain: traditional crossed anterolateral pathways, mainly the spinothalamic and spinoreticular tracts, were believed to be the only pathways, but the dorsal column pathway, the spinal(trigeminal)–parabrachio–amygdaloid pathway, and the spinal–hypothalamic pathway have also been demonstrated to transmit pain.

Currently available information underscores the complexity of visceral pain integration in the brain. For example, there are descriptions of responses to visceral sensory signals in neurons in the visual cortex that emphasize the convergent nature of most sensory messages, but do not deny the primary role of the visual cortex in visual perception. Microstimulation of the thalamus can evoke visceral pain experiences such as angina or labor pain. This observation highlights the integrative role of the thalamus in processing memories of pain and the existence of long-lived neural mechanisms capable of storing painful experiences. Enteric representation in healthy volunteers who received acute noxious stimulation of the rectum evoked brain activity in the anterior cingulate cortex, a region associated with the perception of the affective emotional qualities of the pain experience; the precise components of the cingulate cortex activated by visceral stimulus differ from those normally activated by somatic stimulation.

The so-called functional abdominal pain syndromes, which include irritable bowel syndrome, functional dyspepsia, and other conditions, may be the result of sensitization of the peripheral nociceptors or of alterations of central processing that lead to increased activation of visceral nociceptive pathways.

Neuralgias and neuropathic pain syndromes

Peripheral nerve injury usually results in numbness and sensory deficit in the territory of the involved nerve. Occasionally tingling or pins-and-needles sensations (paresthesias) are reported. Pain as a manifestation of nerve injury is difficult to predict; for instance, up to 50% of diabetics develop neuropathy during the course of their disease, but only 10% of those patients will complain of pain.

Three cardinal features of neuropathic pain are usually present to variable degrees: (1) continuous pain, commonly described as burning, an icy feeling, or intense tightness; (2) paroxysmal pain, described as lancinations, jabbing, or shooting; or (3) allodynia, defined as an aberrant sensation of pain response to what is normally an innocuous stimulus (e.g., a light touch).

The are two primary mechanisms of ongoing pain after nerve injury. The first is nerve injury–induced changes in transduction. Inappropriate activation of transducers may arise from several sources, including (1) emergence of mechanical or thermal transducers (or both) at or near the cut ends of damaged axons or within the ganglia; (2) de novo expression of transducers in neurons that do not normally express them; (3) decreases in inhibitory transducers (i.e., opioid receptors) and/or increases in excitatory transducers (i.e., P2×3); (4) changes in the expression of receptors, the release of endogenous ligands, or both; (5) changes in the coupling between transducers and signaling pathways; and (6) emergence of aberrant sources of nociceptor activation. The second mechanism is nerve injury–induced changes in membrane stability, which may arise from changes in the distribution, expression, and biophysical properties of ion channels.

There are a number of physical signs of neuropathic pain, including hyperalgesia, characterized by an intensely painful response to modest irritation such as a pinprick; hyperpathia, an abnormally prolonged sensation of a stimulus, usually painful, after the stimulus has stopped; and dysesthesia, or the disagreeably abnormal sensations evoked when an area of abnormal sensation is touched. In addition, neuropathic pain may include abnormally sensitive area disturbances after the initial nerve injury, and accumulation of sodium channels at the site of neuroma formation at the axon and at the dorsal root ganglia. All these sites are foci of ectopic impulses. In addition to firing spontaneously, these sites may produce prolonged discharges causing nearby fibers and inactive fibers to respond excessively, thereby generating a broader than normal location of pain distribution.

Classification of painful neuropathies is based on the localization or distribution of affected nerves. In symmetric polyneuropathies, distal areas are usually affected, and hyporeflexia and trophic changes are seen. Symmetric polyneuropathies result from conditions that have a diffuse effect on the PNS, such as diabetes mellitus, alcohol abuse, renal failure, toxicity, paraneoplastic syndromes, and chronic inflammatory demyelinating polyneuropathy (CIDP). In focal neuropathies the affected areas follow a specific nerve territory as in entrapment neuropathies (e.g., carpal tunnel syndrome), tumor infiltration, trigeminal neuralgia, postherpetic neuralgia, and post-traumatic neuralgia. Multifocal mononeuropathies are characterized by a patchy pattern of distribution due to simultaneous or sequential damage to non-contiguous nerves. This type of neuropathy can be found in patients with diabetes mellitus, vasculitis, and brachial or lumbar plexitis. Finally, small fiber neuropathy, one of the most painful neuropathies, presents with allodynia and changes in proprioception or vibration along with regional autonomic dysfunction (e.g., abnormal sweating, temperature changes, erythema). Examples include amyloid neuropathy, diabetes mellitus, Fabry disease, and Tangier disease.

Motor deficits tend to dominate the clinical picture in acute and chronic inflammatory demyelinating neuropathies, multifocal motor neuropathy with conduction block, hereditary neuropathies, and neuropathies associated with myeloma, porphyria, lead or organophosphate intoxications, and hypoglycemia. Predominant sensory involvement may be a feature seen in neuropathies associated with diabetes, carcinoma, Sjögren's syndrome, dysproteinemia, human immunodeficiency virus (HIV), vitamin B_{12} deficiency, cisplatinum, or pyridoxine use, among others.

Entrapment neuropathies

Entrapment neuropathies are a group of focal neuropathies caused by mechanical compression or distortion of a nerve in an anatomic tunnel or fibrous canal, or less frequently by nearby structures such as bone, ligament, or connective tissue.

Compression, constriction, angulation, or stretching are the physical mechanisms that harm the nerve at certain vulnerable areas. The mechanism of harm is induced by morphological changes that lead the nerve into demyelination, remyelination, axonal, or, in severe cases, wallerian degeneration. There can also be endoneural inflammation, collagen proliferation, and thickening of perineural structures. All of these changes induce a self-perpetuating cycle of compression–ischemia–edema. The characteristic feature of entrapment neuropathy is either conduction delay or conduction block across the site of entrapment.

Complex regional pain syndromes

At present, postinjury pain syndromes have been divided into complex regional pain syndrome type I (CRPS I), also referred to as reflex sympathetic dystrophy (RSD), and complex regional pain syndrome type II (CRPS II or causalgia). CRPS I develops without evidence of nerve injury, whereas in CPRS II a nerve lesion is usually present. The sympathetic nervous system has been implicated in the pathogenesis of both types of CRPS. Causalgia means burning pain. It is defined by the IASP as "burning pain, allodynia, and hyperpathia, usually in the hand or foot after partial injury of a nerve or one of its major branches." RSD is defined by the IASP as a "continuous pain in a portion of an extremity after trauma which may include fracture, but does not involve a major nerve, associated with sympathetic hyperactivity." CRPS usually involves the distal extremity adjacent to a traumatized area and the main feature is pain described as burning, continuous, exacerbated by movement, cutaneous stimulation, or stress, with onset usually weeks after injury.

The CRPS Severity Score can assist in monitoring the disease and is made up from (1) symptoms (allodynia or hyperpathia; temperature, skin color, sweating, edema asymmetry; trophic or motor changes; active range of motion); and (2) signs (hyperpathia, allodynia, temperature, darkening of skin color, sweating, edema, trophism, motor changes, and range of motion). Therapeutic modalities include glucocorticoids, bisphosphonates, topical dimethyl sulfate, and/or pain medications with physical therapy. Sympathetic block or sympathectomy should be performed if long-term results are not achieved with repeated blocks.

Central pain syndromes

In lesions of the CNS, deafferentation of secondary neurons in the posterior horns or of sensory ganglion cells that terminate on them may cause the deafferentated cells to become continuously active and, if stimulated, to reproduce pain. In the patient with spinal cord transection, there may be intolerable pain below the level of the lesion that can be exacerbated or provoked by movement, fatigue, or emotion, and projected to areas disconnected from suprasegmental structures. In lesions of the pons and medulla, loss of descending inhibitory systems seems a likely explanation. This may also explain the pain of the Déjerine–Roussy thalamic syndrome (painful anesthesia).

Pain due to systemic disorders

Patients with different diseases complain of pain that is usually poorly defined and difficult to explore. Examples of diseases accompanied by pain include cancer, multiple sclerosis, diabetes, and fibromyalgia.

Pain in patients with cancer

Pain is one of the most common and dreaded symptoms associated with cancer. It occurs in one-quarter to one-half of patients with newly diagnosed malignancies. Overall, 75% of patients with cancer experience pain severe enough to require treatment with opioids. Pain in 90% of patients with cancer results from the tumor or its evaluation or therapy. In 70% of patients, pain develops from tumor invading or compressing soft tissue, bone, or neural structures. It has been suggested that 85% of patients with cancer pain can be well palliated using oral opioids. Addiction is extremely rare in patients with cancer who are taking opioids.

Pain due to undiagnosed medical disease

The source of pain is usually peripheral and caused by a lesion that irritates and destroys nerve endings. Carcinomatosis is the most frequent example. Osseous metastases, peritoneal implants, invasion of retroperitoneal tissues or the hilum of the lung, and involvement of the nerves of the brachial or lumbosacral plexuses can be extremely painful. It is sometimes necessary to repeat all diagnostic procedures months after a negative investigation in order to reach an accurate diagnosis. Treatment is directed to relieving pain and, if possible, stopping the progression of primary disease.

Psychiatric patients usually have pain as the predominant symptom. Examples of psychiatric diseases associated with pain are depression, malingering, and hysteria. A psychiatric evaluation is very helpful in diagnosing and treating patients who complain of chronic pain. The diagnosis of a psychiatric condition causing pain should always be done after excluding other causes.

Approach to the patient with pain

Whether or not a stimulus becomes painful depends on many factors aside from physical disorders, including characteristics of the host such as genetics, gender, endogenous pain control, anxiety, depression, coping behavior, cognition, disease history, socialization, lifestyle, traumas, expectations, and roles.

Although pain is not always associated with tissue damage, a complete past and present history, physical examination, and special examinations must be done to exclude damage to the corresponding tissue before labeling pain as idiopathic. It is of the utmost importance to identify factors that initiate and maintain pain. We recommend that the term psychological pain or conversive pain should be withheld, because pain most often includes a psychological component regardless of etiology.

Suffering is a state of severe distress associated with events that threaten the intactness of the person and occurs when one's physical or psychological integrity is vulnerable. It is a negative response induced by pain and also by fear, anxiety, stress, loss of loved objects, and other psychological states. Not all pain causes suffering, and not all suffering expressed as pain, or coexisting with pain, stems from pain. It must be recognized that patients are dynamic psychological and social entities. Thus, suffering is the consequence of perceived, impending destruction of the person or of some essential part of the person, and entails a disparity between what one expects of oneself and what one does or is. For a given painful condition, vulnerability to suffering depends partially on who one is and what one does in society.

Pain is essentially subjective and the measurement of quality and severity is based on verbal concepts. Several subjective measures of pain based on verbal descriptions have been developed, including unidimensional scales such as verbal rating and/or visual analogue scales, and multidimensional scales such as the McGill Pain Questionnaire, Wisconsin Brief Pain Inventory, Memorial Pain Assessment Card, and the Hopkins Pain Rating Instrument.

Treatment

The goal of therapy is to control pain and to rehabilitate patients so that they can function as well as possible. A major goal of pain management is to provide pain relief that is clinically meaningful, sustained, and associated with minimum and reversible adverse effects.

Most of the time, treating patients in pain involves a multidisciplinary approach, in which each member of the treatment team should play a significant role. In patients with chronic pain, physicians, psychologists, nurses, physical and occupational therapists, vocational counselors, pharmacists, and perhaps others should work together to provide comprehensive and coordinated care with the most important member of the therapeutic team: the patient.

In managing patients with pain, it is important to keep in mind that an injury usually unleashes the production of cytokines and chemokines (tumor necrosis factor alpha, growth factors, interleukin-1beta, interleukin-8), surface antigens, adenosine triphosphate, cannabinoids, and neuropeptides that, in turn, induce the release of excitatory chemicals including glutamate, bradykinin, cyclo-oxygenase 2, and nitric oxide, ultimately leading to sensitization of the central nervous system.

A treatment algorithm for chronic pain is presented in Figure 175.1. Once the physician has established the working diagnosis and has identified that medication is necessary, the usual approach is to start with a non-opioid analgesic such as a non-steroidal anti-inflammatory drug (NSAID) or acetaminophen for mild to moderate pain. If this is inadequate and if there is an element of sleep loss, the next step may be to add an antidepressant with analgesic qualities. If there is a component of neuropathic pain, then one of the anticonvulsant analgesic agents is appropriate (i.e., gabapentin or pregabalin). If these steps are inadequate, then an opioid analgesic may be added.

Key strategies in treating patients with acute pain – defined as the normal, predicted physiological response to an adverse chemical, thermal, or mechanical stimulus, associated with surgery, trauma, or acute illness – include (1) assess options for pain control with each patient and provide instruction in simple, cognitive-behavioral techniques; (2) assess pain routinely, just like monitoring vital signs; (3) treat pain as early as possible; (4) use non-drug and drug interventions together; (5) select treatment according to the clinical setting and promptly modify it according to the patient's response; and (6) provide continuity of pain control after discharge. One should identify and treat as soon as possible any causative lesion, and always recall that multiple neural and biochemical mechanisms may be operative and multiple modalities and treatment may be required. Multidisciplinary treatment is a better approach.

Depending on their mechanism and diagnostic tests, we can divide the pharmacological treatments as seen in Table 175.1. As already mentioned, it is important in patients suffering with neuropathic pain to distinguish peripheral neuropathic pain as stimulus-evoked pain or stimulus-independent pain (spontaneous).

Opioids

There is a growing body of evidence that controlled-release opioid analgesics have a role to play in a subset of patients with chronic pain, including neuropathic pain. Table 175.2 summarizes the principles of practice for the use of opioid analgesics in chronic non-cancer pain.

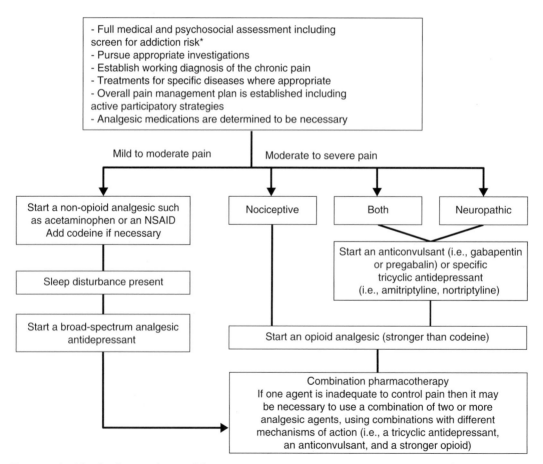

Figure 175.1 Treatment algorithm for pharmacotherapy of chronic non-cancer pain.

NSAID = non-steroidal anti-inflammatory drug

Table 175.1 Mechanism, clinical features, molecular target(s), and drugs proposed for treatment of patients with pain.

Mechanism	Diagnostic feature(s)	Molecular targets	Drugs proposed
General sodium channels: redistribution or altered expression	Spontaneous pain, paresthesia	Sodium channels sensitive to tetrodotoxin	Local anesthetics, antiepileptics, antiarrhythmics, tricyclic antidepressants
Specific sodium channels	Spontaneous pain	Sodium channels resistant to tetrodotoxin	Selective blockers
Central sensitization	Hyperalgesia (in response to touch, cold, pinprick)	NMDA receptor (glutamate, glycine), neurokinin 1 receptor (bradykinin), neuronal nitric oxide synthase, protein kinase	NMDA antagonist (ketamine, dextromethorphan, memantine), glycine site antagonists, neurokinin 1 receptor antagonists, neuronal nitric oxide synthase inhibitors, protein kinase inhibitors
Peripheral sensitization	Hyperalgesia in response to pressure	Vanilloid receptor	Capsaicin, cannabinoids
	Hyperalgesia in response to thermal stimuli	Neurokinin 1 receptor	Neurokinin 1 receptor antagonist
	Neurogenic inflammation	Nerve growth factor	Nerve growth factor antagonist
Sympathetic activity	Spontaneous pain	Adrenergic receptors (alpha adrenergic), nerve growth factor, or trKA	Phentolamine, guanethidine, clonidine, nerve growth factor antagonists
Reduced inhibition	Hyperalgesia	Opioid receptors, GABA transaminase, neurokinin 1, adenosine, purine, kainite, cholecystokinin, acetylcholine (nicotinic)	Morphine, gabapentin

GABA = gamma-aminobutyric acid; NMDA = N-methyl-d-aspartate; trKA = tyrosine receptor kinase A

Table 175.2 Principles of practice for the use of opioid analgesics in chronic non-cancer pain.

Evaluate the patient	Detailed history and physical Assessment of impact of pain on significant others Review previous investigations and assessments and perform additional investigations, if necessary, to complete diagnostic workup Assess comorbidity
Establish diagnosis	Identify nociceptive versus neuropathic mechanisms underlying the pain
Assess psychological aspects	Identify comorbid psychiatric diagnoses; note that pain leads to psychological suffering and address this aspect in treatment
Assess risk of addiction	Identify patients who may need a more detailed assessment Ask: has your use of alcohol or other drugs ever caused a problem for you or those close to you?

Office screening tools

SISAP+	CAGE-AID++
1. If you drink, how many drinks do you have in a typical day? 2. How many drinks do you have in a typical week? 3. Have you used marijuana or hashish in the past year? 4. Have you ever smoked cigarettes? 5. What is your age?	In the past have you ever: 1. Felt that you wanted or needed to CUT down on your drinking or drug abuse? 2. Been ANNOYED by other's complaining about your drinking or drug abuse? 3. Felt GUILTY about the consequences of your drinking or drug abuse? 4. Had a drink or drug in the morning (EYE-OPENER) to decrease hangover or withdrawal symptoms?

Patients with a history of addiction will require more careful prescribing and closer follow-up

Indications for trial of opioid therapy	Patients with moderate to severe pain that is nociceptive, neuropathic, or both. Patients with mild to moderate pain that has failed to respond to other treatments (modality based or pharmacological)
Establish an overall management plan	Treatment with chronic opioids should take place with an overall pain management plan that includes consideration of all appropriate therapies for that individual patient
Identify reasonable goals of treatment	Improved pain control is a reasonable and appropriate goal. It is also useful to develop functional goals; however, failure to attain all functional goals should not necessarily be construed as therapeutic failure
Obtain full informed consent	Review: risks and benefits of opioid therapy including possible side effects, small risk of addiction in low-risk patients, tolerance, physical dependence, and withdrawal risk if suddenly discontinued; risk of additive side effects with other potentially sedating agents; conditions under which opioids will be prescribed. Written consent is preferred.
Use time-contingent dosing	The goal is to try to keep breakthrough doses to a minimum once stabilization is accomplished
Consult appropriate pain, addiction, or psychological specialists when necessary	This will also depend on availability of the appropriate specialists
Periodic review ("5 As")	Assess: Analgesia, Activities, Adverse effects, Abuse behaviors, Adequate documentation
Manage adverse effects of opioids/lack of efficacy	Institute treatment of side effects; if there is a decrease in function or intolerable side effects, gradual reduction of opioid may be indicated
Document, document, document	Document evaluation process, rationale for opioid therapy in context of overall management plan, follow-up, and compliance with federal regulations

+ When applying the Screening Instrument for Substance Abuse Potential (SISAP) tool, use caution in the following patients: men who exceed 4 drinks/day or 16 drinks/week; women who exceed 3 drinks/day or 12 drinks/week; recreational use of marihuana or hashish for euphoriant effects; a patient younger than 40 years of age who smokes.
++ One positive answer to any of the CAGE-AID questions would suggest caution; two or more positive responses should strongly suggest assessment by an addiction specialist before embarking on chronic opioid therapy.

Table 175.3 Selected guideline recommendations related to mitigating the risk of opioid therapy during long-term use for chronic non-cancer pain.

Recommendation	Comment
Dose that warrants scrutiny, mg of morphine equivalents per day	Most patients successfully treated with lower doses; higher doses associated with adverse effects and overuse (doses >90–200 mg of morphine or equivalent)
Medications and formulations	Methadone: risks for QTc prolongation and bioaccumulation; only experienced providers should prescribe methadone Fentanyl patch: limit to opioid-tolerant patients; variable absorption, exercise, and heat increase risk of overdose Immediate-release fentanyl: limit to opioid-tolerant patients; safety unknown for chronic non-cancer patients Codeine: ability to convert to morphine varies greatly
Initiation and titration of dose	Start low-dose, short-acting opioid, visit 2–3 days
Switching between opioids	Dose reduction: equianalgesic dosing tables omit variability, decrease dose by 25–50% Switching to methadone: conversion ratios vary with dose
Drug–drug interactions	Sedative hypnotics: risk for sedation, cognitive impairment, motor vehicle accidents, and overdose; especially for benzodiazepines Pharmacokinetic interactions: other medications affect the metabolism of opioids
Drug–disease interaction	Preexisting substance abuse disorders increase risk of overdose or misuse Mood, personality, and cognitive disorders increase risk of overdose and misuse Sleep and obstructive pulmonary disorders are exacerbated Chronic kidney disease: consider hydromorphone; may increase methadone, descrease oxymorphone; may accumulate active metabolites of morphine
Screening tools for assessing risk for misuse (in addition to patient history)	Recommended
Written treatment agreements (in addition to informed consent)	Strongly recommended
Urine drug testing	Recommended at least at baseline and randomly thereafter

Although the guidelines for opioid use involve varied development methods and clinical emphases, a consensus has emerged across them on several issues, such as the recommendations related to mitigating the risk of opioid therapy described in Table 175.3. They generally agree about the need for caution in prescribing doses greater than 90–200 mg of morphine equivalents per day, having knowledgeable clinicians manage methadone, recognizing risks associated with fentanyl patches, titrating with caution, and reducing doses by at least 25–50% when switching from one opioid to another. They also agree that opioid risk assessment tools, written treatment agreements, and urine drug testing can be helpful when opioids are prescribed for long-term use.

Respiratory depression is kept to a minimum when appropriate regular doses of opioid are given to patients with chronic pain. Appropriate titration keeps serious adverse effects minimal. Some of the common opioids include morphine, diamorphine, meperidine, methadone, hydromorphone, oxycodone, fentanyl, and buprenorphine (mixed agonist/antagonist). It is probable that not all types of pain respond equally well to all opioids.

Fast onset of effect is not a critical factor if the patient is receiving continual analgesics for chronic pain, but may be relevant in patients taking the drug on an as-needed basis. When prescribing opioids one should keep in mind that drug doses should be decreased substantially if creatinine clearance is less than 30 mL/min per 1.73 m^2.

Adverse effects include nausea, dizziness, somnolence, and constipation. The first two commonly abate. Tolerance is the need for a higher dose (or increased plasma concentration) to achieve the same pharmacological effect. There is scant information about the therapeutic window for opiates, so close follow-up is important when increasing doses.

Chronic cancer pain and non-cancer pain are not always relieved by opioids. Opioid-insensitive pain can be defined as pain that does not respond to progressively increasing opioid dose. The most common causes are nerve compression and nerve destruction. A useful clinical rule is that when pain is localized in a numb area, opioids may not be as effective. The usual pharmacological solutions for neuropathic pain include oral antidepressants, anticonvulsants, and local anesthetics in the form of spinal infusions of local anesthetics and opioid mixtures used for treating non-relieved patients. In some patients losing effectiveness of pain relief with opioids, the addition of clonidine may provide additional benefit.

As a guide in prescribing opioids for chronic non-malignant pain, one should take the following steps: (1) contract with the patient–only one prescriber, amount to be dispensed, no additional prescriptions, consequences of breaking contract; (2) monitor the patient–titration of doses, use of short-acting opioids, use of injectable opioids at home, prescription of more than one opioid, assessment at intervals of 6–9 weeks; (3) educate the patient to avoid alcohol and drug problems; (4) focus on improved function (quality of life) not pain relief, use of long-acting opioids, make prescriptions tamper proof.

Further reading

Birklein F, O'Neill D, Schlereth T. Complex regional pain syndrome. *Neurology* 2015;84:89–96.

Cervero F, Laird JMA. Visceral pain. *Lancet* 1999;353:2145–2148.

Gilron I, Jensen TS, Dickenson AH. Combination pharmacotherapy for management of chronic pain: From bench to bedside. *Lancet Neurol* 2013;12:1084–1095.

Gold MS, Gebhart GF. Nociceptor sensitization in pain pathogenesis. *Nat Med* 2010;16(11):1248–1257.

Holdcroft A, Power I. Management of pain. *BMJ* 2003;326:635–639.

Lynch ME, Watson CPN. The pharmacotherapy of chronic pain: A review. *Pain Res Manage* 2006;11(1):11–38.

Merkskey H, Bogduk N. *Classification of Chronic Pain.* Seattle: International Association for the Study of Pain Press; 1994.

Moayedi M, Davis KD. Theories of pain: From specificity to gate control. *J Neurophysiol* 2013;109:5–12.

Nuckols TK, Anderson L, Popescu I, *et al.* Opioid prescribing: A systematic review and critical appraisal of guidelines for chronic pain. *Ann Intern Med* 2014;160:38–47.

Van den Beuken-van Everdingen MH, de Rijke JM, Kessels AG, *et al.* Prevalence of pain in patients with cancer: A systematic review of the past 40 years. *Ann Oncol* 2007;18:1437–1449.

Vanderah TW. Pathophysiology of pain. *Med Clin N Am* 2007;91:1–12.

176   Headache

Stephen D. Silberstein

Department of Neurology, Jefferson Medical College, Thomas Jefferson University, and Jefferson Headache Center,
Thomas Jefferson University Hospital, Philadelphia, PA, USA

The International Classification of Headache Disorders (ICHD-2) divides headaches into primary and secondary disorders. A primary headache disorder is one in which headache itself is the illness and no other etiology is diagnosed. Headache attributed to an identifiable structural or metabolic abnormality constitutes a secondary headache disorder. Migraine, tension-type headache, and cluster headache are examples of primary headache disorders, while low-pressure headache and idiopathic intracranial hypertension are examples of secondary headache disorders. Migraine and tension-type headache can be episodic (headaches fewer than 15 days a month) or chronic (headaches 15 or more days a month).

Migraine headache

Epidemiology

In the United States, 18% of women, 6% of men, and 4% of children have migraine. The disorder usually begins in the first three decades of life, and prevalence peaks in the fifth decade.

Chronic daily headache (CDH) refers to a group of disorders characterized by very frequent headaches (15 or more days a month). The major primary disorders defined by ICHD-2 are chronic migraine (CM), hemicrania continua (HC), chronic tension-type headache (CTTH), and new daily persistent headache (NDPH). Patients who have daily headaches that persist for months often have chronic migraine, and have a past history of episodic migraine that typically began in their teens or 20 s. Most of these patients are women, 90% of whom have a history of migraine without aura. The headaches grow more frequent, and the associated symptoms of photophobia, phonophobia, and nausea become less severe and less frequent than during typical migraine. Patients often develop a pattern of daily, or nearly daily, headaches that phenomenologically resemble CTTH, with mild to moderate pain but with photophobia, phonophobia, or gastrointestinal features. Other features of migraine, including unilaterality and aggravation by menstruation and other trigger factors, may persist. Attacks of full-blown migraine superimposed on a background of less severe headaches often occur. Many patients with transformed migraine overuse symptomatic medication. Stopping the overused medication frequently results in distinct headache improvement. Depression is experienced by 80% of patients with transformed migraine, but it frequently lifts when the pattern of medication overuse and daily headache is interrupted.

Pathophysiology

Migraine aura is probably due to cortical spreading depression (CSD), a slowly spreading wave (at a rate of 2–3 mm/min) of neuronal and glial depolarization that lasts about 1 minute. CSD develops within brain areas, such as the cerebral cortex, cerebellum, or hippocampus, after electrical or chemical stimulation. CSD is associated with a marked decrease in neuronal membrane resistance, a massive increase in extracellular K^+ and neurotransmitters, and an increase in intracellular Na^+ and Ca^{++}. It is believed that patients with migraine have a reduced threshold for CSD. How CSD is triggered in the human cortex during a migraine attack is uncertain.

Headache probably results from activation of meningeal and blood vessel nociceptors combined with a change in central pain modulation. Trigeminal sensory neurons contain substance P, calcitonin gene-related peptide, and neurokinin A. Stimulation results in the release of substance P and calcitonin gene-related peptide from sensory C fiber terminals and neurogenic inflammation. The neuropeptides interact with the blood vessel wall, producing dilation, plasma protein extravasation, and platelet activation. Neurogenic inflammation sensitizes nerve fibers (peripheral sensitization), which then respond to previously innocuous stimuli, such as blood vessel pulsations, causing, in part, the pain of migraine. Central sensitization (CS) of trigeminal nucleus caudalis neurons can also occur. CS may play a key role in maintaining the headache. The migraine aura can trigger headache, as CSD activates trigeminovascular afferents. How does a headache begin in the absence of aura? CSD may occur in silent areas of the cortex or the cerebellum. In addition, direct activation of the trigeminal nerve can occur.

Migraine may be the result of a change in pain and sensory input processing. The aura is triggered in the hypersensitive cortex (CSD). Headache is generated by central pain facilitation and neurogenic inflammation. CS can occur, in part mediated by supraspinal facilitation. Decreased antinociceptive system activity and increased peripheral input may be present.

Clinical features

The migraine attack can be divided into four phases: (1) the prodrome, which occurs hours or days before the headache; (2) the aura, which immediately precedes the headache; (3) the headache itself; and (4) the postdrome. Migraine with aura may occur with or without the headache, but migraine without aura requires the headache for its diagnosis.

International Neurology, Second edition. Edited by Robert P. Lisak, Daniel D. Truong, William M. Carroll and Roongroj Bhidayasiri
© 2016 John Wiley & Sons, Ltd. Published 2016 by John Wiley & Sons, Ltd.

The migraine aura is a complex of focal neurological symptoms (positive or negative phenomena) that precedes or accompanies an attack. Most aura symptoms develop over 5–20 minutes and usually last less than 60 minutes. The aura can be characterized by visual, sensory, or motor phenomena and may also involve language or brainstem disturbances.

The typical migraine headache is unilateral, throbbing, moderate to marked in severity, and aggravated by physical activity. The pain may be bilateral at the onset or start on one side and become generalized. The pain usually lasts between 4 and 72 hours in adults and 2 and 48 hours in children. The average migraineur experiences from one to three headaches a month.

The pain of migraine is accompanied by other features. Anorexia is common, nausea occurs in almost 90% of patients, and vomiting occurs in about one-third of patients. Many patients have photophobia, phonophobia, and osmophobia, and seek a dark, quiet room. Following the headache, during the postdrome phase, the patient may feel tired, "washed out," irritable, and listless, and may have impaired concentration, scalp tenderness, or mood changes. A variety of migraine clinical subtypes have been described. Attacks of migraine lasting longer than 72 hours define *status migrainosus*.

Differential diagnosis

Similar headaches may occur as a result of abnormalities of the brain, including tumors, infections, and vascular malformations. Idiopathic intracranial hypertension (IIH), low-pressure headache, and intracranial neoplasms may also mimic migraine, as may hypoxia, hypoglycemia, dialysis, pheochromocytoma, and various chemicals and medications. Sinusitis or glaucoma may occasionally resemble migraine. Other primary headache disorders, such as TTH, cluster headache, and hypnic headache, should be considered.

Investigations

Patients who have normal neurological examinations and benign recurrent headaches that fit ICHD-2 criteria do not require brain imaging. Patients who have an abnormal neurological examination, an atypical history, or a sudden, unexplained change in the frequency or major characteristics of their headaches should be imaged.

Treatment

The two strategies of migraine treatment are (1) acute treatment, to terminate attacks; and (2) preventive treatment, to prevent future attacks. Acute treatment can be specific or non-specific. Non-specific medications–analgesics, antiemetics, anxiolytics, non-steroidal anti-inflammatory drugs (NSAIDs), steroids, neuroleptics, and opioids–are used to control the pain and associated symptoms of migraine or other pain disorders, while specific medications (ergots and triptans) control the migraine attack but are not useful for other pain disorders. Analgesics are used for mild to moderate headaches. Triptans or dihydroergotamine (DHE) are first-line drugs for severe attacks and for less severe attacks that do not adequately respond to analgesics. The sooner acute treatment is begun, the more effective it will be. Early intervention prevents escalation and may increase efficacy. Triptans can prevent the development of cutaneous allodynia (CA), and CA predicts triptans' effectiveness.

The goals of preventive treatment are to reduce the frequency, duration, or severity of attacks, improve responsiveness to acute attack treatment, improve function, and reduce disability. Preventive drug treatments include antidepressants, beta blockers, calcium channel blockers, NSAIDs, serotonin antagonists, and anticonvulsants.

Preventive treatment is used because of (1) recurring migraine that significantly interferes with the patient's daily routine despite acute treatment; (2) frequent headaches (>4 attacks/month); (3) contraindication to, failure with, overuse of, or intolerance to acute therapies; (4) frequent, very long, or uncomfortable auras; (5) patient preference; or (6) certain migraine conditions, including hemiplegic migraine, basilar migraine, migraine with prolonged aura, or migrainous infarction.

Preventive medication should be chosen based on documented efficacy, side effect profiles, ease of use, and comorbid conditions. Medications can be divided into five major categories: (1) drugs that have been proven effective (some beta blockers, amitriptyline, topiramate, divalproex, and methysergide); (2) drugs that are probably effective (gabapentin, fluoxetine, venlafaxine, cyproheptadine, MIG-99 [feverfew], coenzyme Q_{10}, and vitamin B_2); (3) drugs that are possibly effective (verapamil); (4) drugs for which evidence is inadequate or conflicting; and (5) drugs that are probably ineffective.

Medication should be started at a low dose and increased slowly until headache severity or frequency decreases, the maximum recommended dose is reached, or adverse effects develop. When the headaches have been controlled, attempts can be made to taper and discontinue therapy. Patients should be monitored for acute medication overuse, which may result in chronic refractory headaches and withdrawal symptoms when the medication is discontinued. Some studies support the use of topiramate, tizanidine, and gabapentin for CM. Amitriptyline is perhaps the most commonly used medication, but evidence only exists for CTTH, not for CM.

Tension-type headache

Epidemiology

Tension-type headache (TTH) is very common, with a lifetime prevalence of 69% in men and 88% in women. TTH can begin at any age, but onset during adolescence or young adulthood is most common.

Pathophysiology

TTH is not the result of sustained contraction of the pericranial muscles. The muscle ache of a TTH attack may be due to increased neuronal sensitivity and pain facilitation due to chronic or intermittent dysfunction of the monoaminergic or serotonergic function in the hypothalamus, brainstem, and spinal cord.

Clinical features

Episodic TTHs can be either infrequent (<1 day/month or 12 days/year) or frequent (>1 but <15 days/month or >12 but <180 days/year). The ICHD-2 requires at least 10 previous headaches, each lasting 30 minutes to 7 days (median 12 hours), with at least two of the following characteristics: a pressing/tightening (non-pulsating) quality; mild to moderate intensity; bilateral location; and no aggravation with physical activity. In addition, the patient should not have nausea or vomiting or a combination of photophobia and phonophobia. Episodic TTH occurs fewer than 15 days a month, whereas CTTH occurs 15 or more days a month. The pain is a dull, achy, non-pulsatile feeling of tightness, pressure, or constriction (vise-like or hatband-like), and it is usually mild to moderate, in contrast to the moderate to severe pain of migraine. Most patients have bilateral pain.

Differential diagnosis

Migraine is the headache disorder that is most confused with TTH. Both can be bilateral, non-throbbing, and associated with anorexia. Migraine is more severe, often unilateral, and frequently associated with nausea. IIH, brain tumor headache, chronic sphenoid sinusitis, and cervical, ocular, and temporomandibular disorders need to be considered. What we call episodic TTH may be two distinct disorders. The first disorder may be attacks of mild migraine. The second may be a pure TTH that is not associated with other features of migraine (nausea, photophobia, or sensitivity to movement) or with attacks of severe migraine.

Investigations

Most patients with a long history of unchanged episodic TTHs do not require extensive evaluation if they have normal neurological examinations and are otherwise healthy. A metabolic screen, complete blood count, electrolytes, and kidney and thyroid function studies are also appropriate prior to treatment.

Treatment

TTH patients usually self-medicate with over-the-counter analgesics. If these medications are not effective, prescription NSAIDs or combination analgesic preparations can be used. Narcotics and combination analgesics that contain sedatives should be limited, because overuse may cause dependence.

Preventive therapy should be administered when a patient has frequent headaches that produce disability or may lead to symptomatic medication overuse. Medications used for TTH prevention include antidepressants, beta blockers, and anticonvulsants. Antidepressants are the medication of first choice. An adequate trial period of at least 1–2 months must be allowed. Biofeedback therapy may improve the therapeutic benefit derived from antidepressants.

Episodic TTH usually improves with time. Some patients may, however, progress to CTTH, especially when analgesic overuse occurs.

Cluster headache

Epidemiology

Cluster headache prevalence (0.01–1.5%) is lower than that of migraine or TTH. Prevalence is higher in men than in women and in African American patients compared with Caucasian patients. The most common form of cluster headache is episodic cluster. Cluster headache can begin at any age, but it generally begins in the late 20 s.

Pathophysiology

Cluster events are probably related to alterations in the circadian pacemaker, which may be due to hypothalamic dysfunction. Neurogenic inflammation, carotid body chemoreceptor dysfunction, central parasympathetic and sympathetic tone imbalance, and increased responsiveness to histamine have been proposed as the cause of cluster pain.

Clinical features

Patients with cluster headache have multiple episodes of short-lived (30–90 minutes) but severe, unilateral, orbital, supraorbital, or temporal pain. At least one of the following associated symptoms must occur: conjunctival injection, lacrimation, nasal congestion, rhinorrhea, facial sweating, miosis, ptosis, or eyelid edema. Episodic cluster consists of headache periods of 1 week to 1 year, with remission periods lasting at least 1 month, whereas chronic cluster headache has either no remission periods or remissions that last less than 1 month.

The pain of a cluster attack rapidly increases (within 15 minutes) to excruciating levels. The attacks often occur at the same time each day and frequently awaken patients from sleep. The pain is deep, constant, boring, piercing, or burning in nature, located in, behind, or around the eye. It may radiate to the forehead, temples, jaws, nostrils, ears, neck, or shoulder. During an attack, patients often feel agitated or restless. Most patients have one or two cluster periods a year that last 2–3 months, with one or two attacks a day.

Differential diagnosis

This includes chronic paroxysmal hemicrania, migraine, trigeminal neuralgia, temporal arteritis, pheochromocytoma, Raeder's paratrigeminal syndrome, Tolosa–Hunt syndrome, sinusitis, and glaucoma.

Investigations

In most cases, a careful history is all that is needed to make the diagnosis. Magnetic resonance imaging (MRI) of the head is justified only in atypical cases or cases with an abnormal neurological examination (except when the abnormality is a Horner's syndrome).

Treatment

Patients should avoid alcohol and nitroglycerin. Effective acute treatments include oxygen, sumatriptan, DHE, and (perhaps) topical local anesthetics. Preventive therapy includes ergotamine, calcium channel blockers, lithium, corticosteroids, divalproex, topiramate, melatonin, and capsaicin. If medical therapy fails completely, occipital, sphenopalatine ganglia, or vagal nerve stimulation may be beneficial. Since cluster headache is a chronic headache disorder that may last for the patient's life, the prognosis is guarded.

Idiopathic intracranial hypertension

Epidemiology

IIH with papilledema occurs with a frequency of about 1 case per 100000 per year in the general population and 19.3 cases per 100000 per year in obese women aged 20–44 years. The patient with IIH is commonly a young, obese woman with chronic daily headaches, normal laboratory studies, an empty sella, and a normal neurological examination (except for papilledema).

Pathophysiology

IIH is a disorder of increased intracranial pressure of unknown cause. Some authors suggest that most patients with IIH have partial venous sinus stenosis. One explanation is that increased cerebrospinal fluid (CSF) pressure, through external compression, could account for narrowing of the venous sinuses.

Clinical features

Headache, commonly bifrontotemporal, occurs in most, but not all, patients. The headache can be unilateral. Transient visual obscuration (visual clouding in one or both eyes lasting seconds) occurs with all forms of increased intracranial pressure with papilledema. Pulsatile tinnitus, diplopia, and visual loss can occur. Friedman and

Jacobson have proposed diagnostic criteria: symptoms only those of generalized intracranial hypertension or papilledema; signs only those of generalized intracranial hypertension or papilledema; documented elevated intracranial pressure; normal CSF composition; MRI/MRV (magnetic resonance venography) with no hydrocephalus, mass, or structural or vascular lesion (except for empty sella); not attributable to another cause.

Differential diagnosis

IIH may be either truly *idiopathic*, with no clear identifiable cause, or *symptomatic*, a result of venous sinus occlusion, radical neck dissection, hypoparathyroidism, vitamin A intoxication, systemic lupus erythematosus, renal disease, or drug side effects (nalidixic acid, danocrine, steroid withdrawal).

Investigations

The diagnosis of IIH is based on lumbar puncture following neuroimaging (paying attention to empty sella and sinus thrombosis). If CSF biochemical and cytological analyses are unremarkable and intracranial pressure is elevated to greater than 200 mm H_2O (in non-obese subjects), IIH is the likely diagnosis.

Treatment

Obese patients should be encouraged to lose weight. If patients are asymptomatic and do not have visual loss, treatment is not indicated. In these cases, careful ophthalmologic follow-up is necessary. If headache is associated with visual loss or papilledema, aggressive treatment should be instituted.

The headache of IIH frequently responds to the same treatments as used for migraine and TTH. If rigorous headache therapy is unsuccessful, or if there is visual loss, then a 4–6-week trial of furosemide or a potent carbonic anhydrase inhibitor (acetazolamide) should be given. Some physicians use topiramate because it is also a carbonic anhydrase inhibitor. High-dose steroids may be effective, but headache commonly recurs when they are withdrawn. Lumbar puncture typically relieves the headache that occurs with IIH and papilledema. Surgical treatment of IIH has been directed toward preventing visual loss secondary to papilledema, and many patients experience headache improvement with optic nerve sheath fenestration.

Most patients with IIH and papilledema can be managed successfully. The prognosis for headache control of IIH without papilledema is more guarded, although there appears to be no risk of visual deterioration.

Low-pressure headache

Epidemiology

The incidence of spontaneous or secondary intracranial hypotension is unknown. Postlumbar puncture headache is more common in women, who are affected twice as often as men, and in younger patients. An atraumatic needle reduces the risk of postlumbar puncture headache.

Pathophysiology

The most common cause of low-pressure headache is a lumbar puncture. Spontaneous intracranial hypotension is often due to occult dural tears. Mokri believes that the disorder is primarily that of

hypovolemia; hypotension is usually, but not always, present. Low CSF volume leads to brain sagging, with compression of the pituitary–hypothalamic axis and further reduction in CSF production. Occult CSF leakage may also be a major cause of low CSF volume. A history of minor trauma is often elicited.

Clinical features

The headache may be frontal, occipital, or diffuse. It is accentuated by the erect position and relieved with recumbency. The pain is severe, dull, or throbbing in nature and is usually not relieved with analgesics. It is aggravated by head-shaking, coughing, straining, sneezing, and jugular compression. The longer the patient is upright, the longer it takes the headache to subside with recumbency. Physical examination is usually normal; however, mild neck stiffness and a slow pulse rate (so-called vagus pulse) may be present. Spinal fluid pressure usually ranges from 0–65 mm. The CSF composition is usually normal, but there may be a slight protein elevation and a few red blood cells in the fluid. Reversible Arnold–Chiari-type malformation has been reported in association with a low CSF pressure headache.

Investigations

Diffuse pachymeningeal enhancement is the most commonly seen abnormality on head MRI. Descent of the brain is common and is manifested by descent of the cerebellar tonsils, decrease in the size of the prepontine cistern, inferior displacement of the optic chiasm, effacement of perichiasmatic cisterns, and crowding of the posterior fossa. Subdural fluid collections are usually but not always bilateral. Decrease in ventricle size is best noted by comparing a head MRI obtained after recovery with an MRI taken during the symptomatic phase. Other abnormalities include pituitary enlargement, engorged venous sinuses, and elongation of the brainstem in the anteroposterior plane.

Treatment

Intravenous or oral caffeine therapy is effective. If the patient continues to be symptomatic, a blood patch should be used, even if the site of the leak is unknown. If treatment is unsuccessful, one should reevaluate the patient with radioisotope cisternography, using nasal pledgets if a cribriform plate leak is possible, or myelography to identify CSF leaks, which can be caused by very small dural tears or nerve avulsions. MRI of the spine may also identify cryptogenic leaks. If the headache of intracranial hypotension recurs, a repeat blood patch can be performed or a continuous intrathecal saline infusion attempted. A cervical or upper thoracic blood patch has been reported to be effective when lumbar blood patches fail.

Most patients with intracranial hypotension can be cured once the diagnosis is made. Occasionally, none of the treatments provides relief for a patient with a refractory CSF leak or a refractory low-pressure headache without apparent cause.

Other headache syndromes

Cough and exercise headache

Benign cough headache is a bilateral, throbbing headache of sudden onset, lasting less than 1 minute and precipitated by coughing in the absence of any intracranial disorder. Benign exertional headache lasts from 5 minutes to 24 hours and is produced by physical exercise without any associated systemic or intracranial disorder. Benign exertional headache starts at a younger age than benign cough headache (mean age of onset is 55 years).

MRI must be performed to rule out posterior fossa abnormalities, which can cause these headache syndromes. Symptomatic cough headache is more likely to be associated with a Chiari malformation and to begin at an earlier age than benign cough headache. Symptomatic exertional headaches begin later in life and last longer than benign exertional headaches. Patients with benign cough headache often respond dramatically to indomethacin.

Benign thunderclap headache

Thunderclap headache is a sudden-onset headache that reaches maximum intensity in less than 30 seconds. It usually lasts up to several hours, with a less severe headache that lasts weeks. Attacks may be precipitated by exercise or sexual intercourse. They may be accompanied by nausea and vomiting, a variant of which has been called "crash migraine." Thunderclap headache may be accompanied by diffuse focal vasospasm in very large arteries at the circle of Willis and second- and third-order segments. If focal symptoms or stroke accompany the vasospasm, Call–Fleming syndrome is present. The differential diagnosis of thunderclap headache includes acute hypertensive crisis, carotid artery dissection, cerebral venous sinus thrombosis, benign (idiopathic) thunderclap headache, pituitary apoplexy, spontaneous intracranial hypotension, spontaneous retroclival hematoma, subarachnoid hemorrhage, and unruptured intracranial aneurysm.

Diagnostic evaluation includes early computed tomography (CT), lumbar puncture, MRI with MRA (magnetic resonance angiography) or CTA (computed tomography with angiography), and venography.

Further reading

Headache Classification Committee. The International Classification of Headache Disorders, 2nd edition. *Cephalalgia* 2004;24:1–160.

Lay CL, Campbell JK, Mokri B. Low cerebrospinal fluid pressure headache. In GoadsbyPJ, SilbersteinSD (eds.). *Headache*. Boston, MA: Butterworth-Heinemann; 1997:355–368.

Manzoni GC, Prusinski A. Cluster headache: Introduction. In: Olese nJ, Tfelt-Hansen P, Welch KMA (eds.). *The Headaches*. Philadelphia, PA: Lippincott, Williams & Wilkins; 2000:675–678.

Matchar DB, Young WB, Rosenberg JA, *et al.* Evidence-based guidelines for migraine headache in the primary care setting: Pharmacological management of acute attacks. *Neurology* 2000;55:754. http://tools.aan.com/professionals/practice/pdfs/gl0090.pdf (accessed November 2015).

Mokri B. Headache associated with abnormalities in intracranial structure or function: Low cerebrospinal fluid pressure headache. In: Silberstein SD, Lipton RB, Dalessio DJ (eds.). *Wolff's Headache and Other Head Pain*. New York: Oxford University Press; 2001:417–433.

Silberstein SD. Chronic daily headache and tension-type headache. *Neurology* 1993;43:1644–1649.

Silberstein SD. Pharmacological management of cluster headache. *CNS Drugs* 1994;2:199–207.

Silberstein SD. Migraine. *Lancet* 2004;363:381–391.

Silberstein SD. Transformed and chronic migraine. In: Goadsby PJ, Silberstein SD, Dodick DW (eds.). *Chronic Daily Headache for Clinicians*. Hamilton: B. C. Decker; 2005:21–56.

Silberstein SD, Goadsby PJ. Migraine: Preventive treatment. *Cephalalgia* 2002;22: 491–512.

Silberstein SD, McKinstry RC, III. The death of idiopathic intracranial hypertension? *Neurology* 2003;60:1406–1407.

177 Facial and neck pain

Kammant Phanthumchinda

Department of Medicine, Chulalongkorn University, Bangkok, Thailand

In general, patients presenting with facial and/or neck pain need specific treatments for the underlying causes. Some of these patients, however, do not demonstrate any recognizable structural abnormalities, causing a great deal of confusion regarding the true etiology, appropriate investigation, and management. A thorough history and physical examination are essential in providing clues to the selection of appropriate diagnostic tests. The International Classification of Headache Disorders, 3rd edition (ICHD-3, beta version) has defined and proposed diagnostic criteria for facial pain, cranial neuralgia, and cervicogenic headache as a standard tool for the evaluation of these syndromes. This chapter briefly summarizes the challenging syndromes of facial and neck pain encountered in clinical practice.

Facial pain

Clinicians can usually diagnose common facial and orofacial pain associated with a clearly defined pathological process (e.g., dental pain, sinus headache). The most commonly undiagnosed pain conditions in this anatomic region include cranial neuralgia and myofascial pain. The etiology and pathophysiological mechanisms of these pain syndromes are poorly understood.

Trigeminal neuralgia

Epidemiology
The incidence of trigeminal neuralgia is 4.3/100000(year. This disorder affects women more commonly than men and the incidence increases with age.

Pathophysiology
Although the exact mechanism underlying trigeminal neuralgia is unclear, a theory of central and peripheral hypersensitivity of the trigeminal nerve has been proposed. Hypersensitivity may occur as a result of focal demyelination of the trigeminal nerve or a central demyelinating process occurring at the nerve root entry zone. The demyelination may cause epiphatic action potentials and set up a centrally mediated disinhibition of neuralgic pain.

Clinical features
Trigeminal neuralgia is characterized by short-lived episodes of neuralgic pain affecting one or more divisions of the trigeminal nerve. Patients may describe these episodes of excruciating pain as superficial, jabbing, stabbing, sharp, shooting, burning, searing, or an electric shock sensation. The pain is usually sudden and paroxysmal, lasting from a fraction of a second to minutes. The episodes are typically separated by pain-free intervals lasting several seconds, and stimulation of the trigger area will cause no pain during these periods (referred to as refractory periods). However, the pain often comes in clusters at very short intervals and aching between paroxysms may occur. The attacks are usually stereotyped in the individual patient and the number of attacks varies. The episodes may occur spontaneously, but they can be triggered by a variety of non-noxious stimuli, including eating, talking, smiling, brushing the teeth, or touching a small area of nasolabial fold and/or chin (trigger area). The patient with classical trigeminal neuralgia may not tolerate any touch or exposure of these areas, which can differentiate this neuralgia from other facial pain conditions for which patients may rub or massage their face to relieve pain. Remissions may occur that last for months. However, the syndrome is usually recurrent and chronic.

Causes of trigeminal neuralgia include classic trigeminal neuralgia and secondary or symptomatic trigeminal neuralgia. In classic trigeminal neuralgia, the facial pain is typically unilateral and follows the distribution of maxillary and mandibular divisions of the trigeminal nerve. Physical examination regularly reveals no cranial neuropathy.

Classic trigeminal neuralgia is usually associated with neurovascular compression of the trigeminal nerve in the prepontine cistern at the level of the nerve entry zone. Secondary trigeminal neuralgia is caused by other pathological processes affecting the trigeminal nerve or trigeminal pathway, such as tumor, multiple sclerosis, vascular anomalies, aneurysm, inflammation, and infection. Atypical presentations include onset under 50 years of age, bilateral symptomatology, focal neurological deficits, lack of triggered pain, poor response to carbamazepine, and presence of active systemic diseases. In these cases, causes other than a vascular compression should be investigated.

Differential diagnosis of orofacial pain with neuralgic-like symptoms includes orofacial pain of dental origin and trigeminal autonomic cephalalgia. Dental evaluation for pulpitis, an infected tooth, or cracked tooth syndrome should be performed. In trigeminal autonomic cephalalgia, especially chronic paroxysmal hemicranias (CPH), short-lasting unilateral neuralgiform headache with conjunctival

International Neurology, Second edition. Edited by Robert P. Lisak, Daniel D. Truong, William M. Carroll and Roongroj Bhidayasiri
© 2016 John Wiley & Sons, Ltd. Published 2016 by John Wiley & Sons, Ltd.

injection and tearing (SUNCT), and short-lasting unilateral neuralgiform headache attacks with cranial autonomic symptoms (SUNA), the location of pain is in the orbitofrontal area and is usually associated with pronounced autonomic features that are uncommon in classic trigeminal neuralgia. However, mild to moderate cranial autonomic syndrome may occur in classic trigeminal neuralgia. In addition, patients with CPH experience a dramatic response to indomethacin, which is frequently used as a therapeutic diagnosis. SUNCT has prominent features of lacrimation and conjunctival injection as its diagnostic clues. In SUNA, the location of maximal pain may be prominent in the distribution of maxillary and mandibular divisions of the trigeminal nerve, and nasal symptoms are common. Based on the evidence of the overlap of clinical profiles, neuroimaging findings as well as therapeutic response to medical and surgical treatments, SUNCT, SUNA, and trigeminal neuralgia may be variants or a continuum of the same malady.

Investigations

Magnetic resonance imaging (MRI) is the investigation of choice for the evaluation of trigeminal neuralgia. The technique can identify various pathological processes that involve the trigeminal nerve and related pain pathway. However, MRI may be insensitive for assessing the vascular compression loop. In patients with associated systemic diseases or other neurological diseases, appropriate diagnostic tests should be applied accordingly.

Treatment

Secondary or symptomatic trigeminal neuralgia should be treated according to its underlying cause. Medical treatment to initiate a remission period for a classic trigeminal neuralgia should be started with carbarmazepine or oxcarbamazepine. If patients experience side effects and do not benefit from carbamazepine or oxcarbamazepine, alternative agents, including lamotrigine, baclofen, diphenylhydantoin, gabapentin, pregabalin, or other anticonvulsants, should be considered. Tricyclic antidepressants may be helpful in some cases. If the pain subsides for months, a reduction of the medication may be attempted and the therapy may be restarted if the pain recurs. Botulinum toxin type A can be used as a therapeutic option for refractory classic trigeminal neuralgia. When patients become intractable to medical management, surgical interventions may be considered. Common indications for surgical intervention include intolerability of medication side effects and patient's expectation of "cure." Microvascular decompression, which is a non-destructive intervention, is the most effective and safe procedure, with a high rate of long-term remission. The other destructive strategies include gamma-knife radiosurgery, radiofrequency rhizotomy, balloon microcompression, and percutaneous retrogasserian glycerol rhizotomy.

Glossopharyngeal–vagoglossopharyngeal neuralgia

Epidemiology

Glossopharyngeal–vagoglossopharyngeal neuralgia is far less prevalent than trigeminal neuralgia. The incidence is 0.7/100000(year. The disorder affects women more often than men and the age of onset is usually over 50 years.

Pathophysiology

The mechanisms are proposed to be similar to trigeminal neuralgia.

Clinical features

Neuralgic pain in glossopharyngeal neuralgia affects the area supplied by somatosensory branches of the glossopharyngeal and the vagus nerves. The painful areas include tonsils, base of tongue, throat, larynx, neck, angle of jaw, and external auditory meatus, in any combination. The attacks consist of abrupt, severe stabbing, shooting, knife-like, electric-shock sensations, and scratching episodes similar to trigeminal neuralgia. The pattern of attack is always paroxysmal. There is often sensation between paroxysms in the form of hard or sharp sticking or foreign body sensation or a dull, deep, continuous pain at the affected sites. Rare associated symptoms during the attack include vigorous coughing, hoarseness of voice, syncope from sick sinus syndrome, severe bradycardia, asystole, and severe hypotension. Seizures may result from cerebral hypoperfusion due to hypotension.

The trigger phenomena are stimulation in the pharyngeal area such as swallowing (especially cold liquids and food with a sharp sensation of taste and smell), talking, coughing, chewing, yawning, and clearing the throat. Other tactile triggers in the external auditory meatus, lateral aspect of the neck, and pre- and postauricular area, as well as rapid head movement and ipsilateral arm elevation, can precipitate the neuralgia.

Glossopharyngeal neuralgia usually has a relapsing and remitting course. It may be side-switching or bilateral (unilateral preceding, non-synchronously, or simultaneously affected), with nocturnal attacks, which is different from trigeminal neuralgia. Ipsilateral glossopharyngeal and trigeminal neuralgia may occur in the same patient. Physical examination is usually normal, but the ear on the affected side may be painful. Symptomatic or secondary glossopharyngeal neuralgia is far less common than trigeminal neuralgia and the underlying pathological processes include neoplasms, infections, elongated ossified styloid process (Eagle's syndrome), and multiple sclerosis. Vascular compression from ectatic blood vessels has recently been reported as a frequent cause of glossopharyngeal neuralgia.

Investigations

MRI is the neuroimaging procedure of choice for identification of the lesions causing secondary glossopharyngeal neuralgia. It can also demonstrate compressed and distorted ninth and tenth cranial nerves at the nerve entry zone by tortuous vertebrobasilar vessels. Skull radiography can depict elongated ossified styloid process in Eagle's syndrome.

Treatment

Anticonvulsants, including carbamazepine, oxcarbamazepine, diphenylhydantoin, lamotrigine, and gabapentin, are the treatment of choice. Baclofen is also effective. When medical therapy fails, microvascular decompression as well as vagus and glossopharyngeal nerve rhizotomies are advocated. The other interventions are gamma knife radiosurgery, radiofrequency rhizotomy, and balloon microcompression.

Neck pain and headache

Headache caused by disorders of the cervical spine occurs only in cases with well-defined structural lesions in the craniovertebral junction and/or upper cervical spines (e.g., developmental anomalies or acquired lesions such as tumor, trauma, infection, and inflammatory processes). Controversy exists as to the contribution of degenerative spine and/or trivial spinal disorders to the development of various primary headache disorders such as cervicogenic headache, migraine, and occipital neuralgia. ICHD-3 has provided diagnostic criteria for cervicogenic headache and other headache attributed to disorder of the neck. Three conditions with conflicts and contradictions are discussed.

Occipital neuralgia

Epidemiology
The incidence of occipital neuralgia is 3.2/100000(year.

Pathophysiology
The pathophysiology is unclear. However, microtrauma as well as entrapment and irritation of the nerve from myofascial spasm have been proposed, and the lesion causing neuralgia may be proximal to the occipital nerve.

Clinical features
Neuralgic pain in occipital neuralgia is distributed in the areas supplied by the greater and lesser occipital nerves. The pain is usually sharp, lancinating, and electric shock-like in character. The episodes of pain are paroxysmal and may be unilateral or bilateral. The attacks of pain can be triggered at the emergence of the involved nerve. Neurological examination is usually normal, but patients may experience dysesthesia or allodynia in the affected area. Limitation of motion and tenderness over the nerve trunk as it crosses the superior nuchal line may be observed. In general, occipital neuralgia is not a common cause of headache, and other disorders should be carefully considered. Unlike the C2 root, which is more vulnerable to trauma, nerve entrapment, meningioma, inflammatory processes, and venous anomalies, the occipital nerves are not usually prone to these lesions. Pain from occipital neuralgia should be differentiated from referred pain from C2–C3 joint and craniovertebral junction anomalies, including upper cervical spine and posterior fossa lesions. The referred pain is usually continuous without neuralgic character or impairment of sensation.

Investigations
MRI is used to exclude other causes of referred pain that can mimic occipital neuralgia. Response to anesthetic agents or nerve block of the related structures may be helpful for clarification of the precise origin of occipital pain.

Treatment
Effective treatments for occipital neuralgia are still inconclusive. Physical therapy and medications, for instance carbamazepine, gabapentin, pregabalin, baclofen, and tricyclic antidepressants, are helpful. In severe intractable cases, neuromodulation with pulsed radiofrequency or occipital nerve stimulation is an option.

Carotidynia

Epidemiology
The syndrome of carotidynia is usually associated with many disorders, such as benign or idiopathic carotidynia, migraine-related entity, dissection of cerebral vessel, and giant cell arteritis. The epidemiological data therefore vary according to the underlying diseases.

Pathophysiology
Stimulation of the carotid artery wall, especially at its bifurcation, will cause pain at the jaw, throat, cheek, gum, nose, eye, and teeth via sensory branches of the vagus nerve. The syndrome may be caused by various pathological processes. In migraine-related carotidynia, the pain may be induced by vascular hypersensitivity.

Clinical features
The pain, characterized by unilateral neck and/or facial pain, may radiate to the ear, eye, nose, gum, cheek, jaw, or scalp. The character of the pain as well as its associated physical findings are heavily related to the underlying diseases. The pain may be continuous and dull, with the possibility of throbbing or pounding episodes. Stabbing, burning, sharp, ice-pick-like jabs, or neuralgic features may be observed. The pain is usually aggravated by head and neck movements, swallowing, coughing, sneezing, yawning, and chewing. The maximal tenderness is at the carotid bifurcation occurring along its entire length. Moreover, swelling of the overlying soft tissue may occasionally be detected.

Important clues to the causes of carotidynia are related to the natural history of pain and its associated conditions. In benign or idiopathic carotidynia, which is an acute monophasic disease with or without an associated viral infection, the clinical course is less than 2 weeks and the proposed etiology could be reactive vasculitis or viral infection. In cases with subacute course associated with neurological signs (e.g., Horner's syndrome), it may be associated with the dissection of the carotid artery, ruptured atherosclerotic plaque, or giant cell arteritis. In cases with recurrent or daily attacks that last hours and are associated with a throbbing headache that responds to ergotamine or triptan, migraine may be the possible diagnosis.

Investigations
Investigation should be focused on the non-invasive diagnostic tests that are appropriate for carotid lesions (e.g., MRI angiography, carotid ultrasound). Vascular imaging can detect dissection, ruptured atherosclerotic plaque, and inflammation of the carotid artery and perivascular tissue. Erythrocyte sedimentation rate (ESR), temporal artery biopsy, and a therapeutic trial with prednisolone may be appropriate for elderly individuals who are suspected of having giant cell arteritis. In cases with monophasic illness, the evaluation should include systemic inflammatory processes and viral infection.

Treatment
Carotidynia is a pain syndrome in which treatment depends on the underlying causes. In benign or idiopathic carotidynia, non-steroidal anti-inflammatory drugs (NSAIDs) are usually effective. Corticosteroid should be considered in cases with a protracted course.

Cervicogenic headache

Epidemiology
The epidemiological data of cervicogenic headache are still inconclusive due to the heterogeneity of the diagnostic criteria and the controversial concept of the syndrome itself.

Pathophysiology
Identifiable diseases or pathological processes causing dysfunction of structure in the neck can generate and cause referred pain to the head via the trigeminocervical nucleus caudalis, spinal tract of

the trigeminal nerve, upper cervical spinal nerves, and ophthalmic division of the trigeminal nerve. In cases with poorly defined lesions, the possible source of cervicogenic headache may lie in the structures such as synovial joints, cervical muscles, intervertebral discs, dura of the upper cervical cord, and posterior fossa, as well as vertebral and carotid arteries.

Clinical features

Sjaatad's cervicogenic headache is a syndrome or "reaction pattern" of dysfunction or disease in the neck. The syndrome is still controversial and the etiology, affected tissue sites, and mechanisms remain unclear. The main cardinal features of the headache include episodic, unilateral, side-locked neck/occipital pain associated with specific neck movement and/or posture. The headache is chronic and frequently relapses. The pain may spread forward bilaterally and evolve into persistent headache. The pain may be triggered by neck movement or sustained awkward neck positioning and is frequently associated with ipsilateral shoulder and arm discomfort. Physical examination reveals a specific affected site in the upper cervical (occipito-atlas axis) region as the cervical site of the pain (e.g., limitation of movement of the head or neck, flexion–extension, head tilt, or reproduction of the symptom from cervical maneuver). Apart from the cardinal features, some patients may have other associated migrainous symptoms such as photophobia, phonophobia, nausea, dizziness, ipsilateral blurred vision, or autonomic disturbance such as conjunctival injection, lacrimation, or periocular edema. However, the clinical profiles must not fulfill the International Headache Society criteria for other primary headaches, such as migraine, tension-type headache, or trigeminal autonomic headache, and symptoms should not exhibit a dramatic response to ergotamine, triptans, or indomethacin.

Investigations

Computed tomography (CT) scan and MRI are the diagnostic tests of choice for viewing the upper cervical segment, particularly the craniovertebral junction and surrounding soft tissue. Neuroimaging findings will establish the specific causes of cervicogenic headache when there are overt, structurally visible lesions and the lesions are clinically correlated with the headache syndrome. When the neuroimaging fails to reveal a relevant pathology or disease, diagnostic local anesthetic block should then be considered.

Treatment and management

Correction of the causative disorder is a mainstay of treatment. Treatment of Sjaatad's cervicogenic headache or cervicogenic headache with poorly defined lesions is controversial and management tends to focus on physical therapy. Therapeutic evidence on nerve blocks, facet joint injections, epidural steroid injections, botulinum toxin type A injections, oral medications, and surgical interventions is limited.

Further reading

Antonaci F, Sjaastad O. Cervicogenic headache: A real headache. *Curr Neurol Neurosci Rep* 2011;11(2):149–155.

Blumenfeld A, Nikolskaya G. Glossopharyngeal neuralgia. *Curr Pain Headache Rep* 2013;17(7):343.

Dougherty C. Occipital neuralgia. *Curr Pain Headache Rep* 2014;18(5):411.

Fernández-de-las-Peñas C, Cuadrado ML. Therapeutic options for cervicogenic headache. *Expert Rev Neurother* 2014;14(1):39–49.

Gadient PM, Smith JH. The neuralgias: Diagnosis and management. *Curr Neurol Neurosci Rep* 2014;14(7):459.

Headache Classification Committee of the International Headache Society (IHS). The International Classification of Headache Disorders, 3rd edition (beta version). *Cephalalgia* 2013;33(9):629–808.

Lambru G, Matharu MS. SUNCT, SUNA and trigeminal neuralgia: Different disorders or variants of the same disorder? *Curr Opin Neurol* 2014;27(3):325–331.

Reddy GD, Viswanathan A. Trigeminal and glossopharyngeal neuralgia. *Neurol Clin* 2014;32(2):539–552.

Shephard MK, Macgregor EA, Zakrzewska JM. Orofacial pain: A guide for the headache physician. *Headache* 2014;54(1):22–39.

Stanbro M, Gray BH, Kellicut DC. Carotidynia: Revisiting an unfamiliar entity. *Ann Vasc Surg* 2011;25(8):1144–1153.

178   Chronic fatigue syndrome

Jasem Yousef Al-Hashel

Department of Neurology, Ibn Sina Hospital, Safat, Kuwait

The terms chronic fatigue syndrome and myalgic encephalomyelitis (ME/CFS) describe a complex physical illness. It is characterized by debilitating fatigue, postexertional malaise, pain, cognitive problems, sleep dysfunction, and an array of other immune, neurological, and autonomic symptoms. It follows a relapsing and remitting course.

The term myalgic encephalomyelitis (ME) was introduced in 1956 to describe a well-documented cluster outbreak of a fatiguing illness in London (United Kingdom). The name chronic fatigue syndrome (CFS) was proposed following the investigation of a cluster outbreak of a similar fatiguing illness in Nevada (United States) in 1984. CFS replaced the preliminary name, chronic Epstein–Barr virus syndrome, because clinical studies were unable to confirm Epstein–Barr virus as the putative cause. The name ME is more commonly used in Europe and Canada, while CFS is more often used in the United States and Australia. The US National Institutes of Health (NIH) use the combined term myalgic encephalomyelitis/chronic fatigue syndrome (ME/CFS) to describe the condition.

Several studies have shown that the term "chronic fatigue syndrome" affects patients' perceptions of their illness as well as the reactions of others, including medical personnel, family members, and colleagues. This label can trivialize the seriousness of the condition and promote misunderstanding of the illness.

The term "myalgic encephalomyelitis" is not appropriate because there is a lack of evidence for encephalomyelitis (brain inflammation) in patients with this disease, and myalgia (muscle pain) is not a core symptom of the disease.

The US Institute of Medicine (IOM) committee recommends the name *systemic exertion intolerance disease* (SEID) for this disorder. This new name captures a central characteristic of this condition: the fact that exertion of any sort (physical, cognitive, or emotional) can adversely affect patients in many organ systems and in many aspects of their lives.

Epidemiology

ME/CFS affects 836,000–2.5 million Americans. Its true prevalence is unknown. Women are affected more often than men. Most patients currently diagnosed are Caucasian. The average age of diagnosis is between 30 and 40 years, although ME/CFS has been reported in patients younger than 10 years and older than 70 years.

Etiology

Researchers have suggested that an inciting event triggers an immune response and promotes immune and/or neuroendocrine dysregulation, which perpetuates the body's response and symptom experience that become ME/CFS. Viral etiologies have been predominantly studied; however, no specific virus or other infectious agent has been identified. ME/CFS may be inherited or familial.

Pathophysiology

ME/CFS is a multisystem disorder. This includes immune and neuroendocrine abnormalities; brain dysfunction and neurocognitive defects; cardiovascular and autonomic disturbances; abnormalities in energy production, including mitochondrial dysfunction; and changes in the expression of certain genes. Brain imaging studies with single photon emission computed tomography (SPECT), positron emission tomography (PET), and magnetic resonance imaging (MRI) have found abnormalities in both white and gray matter.

Diagnosis

Because there is no specific test to diagnose ME/CFS, the diagnosis is made through clinical and laboratory examinations, mainly to exclude other conditions. A detailed patient history and thorough physical and mental examination will help in making the diagnosis. A series of laboratory tests will help identify or rule out other possible causes of symptoms. A diagnosis of ME/CFS-like illness could be made if a patient has been fatigued for 6 months or more, but does not meet the criteria for ME/CFS.

Although many healthcare providers are aware of ME/CFS, they may misunderstand the disease or lack knowledge of how to diagnose it; this may delay the diagnosis and the management of patients' symptoms. Therefore, the US Department of Health and Human Services (HHS), the NIH, the Agency for Healthcare Research and Quality, the Centers for Disease Control and Prevention, the Food and Drug Administration (FDA), and the Social Security Administration asked the IOM to convene an expert committee to examine the evidence base for ME/CFS. The committee proposed new diagnostic criteria that will facilitate timely diagnosis and care and enhance understanding among healthcare providers and the public.

Proposed diagnostic criteria for ME/CFS

Diagnosis requires that the patient have the following three symptoms: (1) a substantial reduction or impairment in the ability to engage in pre-illness levels of occupational, educational, social, or personal activities, which persists for more than 6 months and is accompanied by fatigue, which is often profound, of new or definite onset (not lifelong), is not the result of ongoing excessive exertion,

International Neurology, Second edition. Edited by Robert P. Lisak, Daniel D. Truong, William M. Carroll and Roongroj Bhidayasiri.
© 2016 John Wiley & Sons, Ltd. Published 2016 by John Wiley & Sons, Ltd.

Table 178.1 Differential diagnosis of myalgic encephalomyelitis/chronic fatigue syndrome.

Psychiatric	**Hematological**	**Autoimmune**
Bipolar disorder	Anemias	Polymyalgia rheumatica
Generalized anxiety disorder	Hemochromatosis	Rheumatoid arthritis
Major depressive disorder	Leukemia or lymphoma	Systemic lupus erythematosus
Post-traumatic stress disorder	Myelodysplastic syndromes	**Cardiovascular**
Respiratory	**Infections**	Cardiomyopathy
Asthma or allergies	Acute mononucleosis (Coxsackie)	Claudication
Sarcoidosis	Brucellosis	Heart valve disease
Sleep disorders	Hepatitis B or C	Pulmonary hypertension
Central sleep apnea	Human immunodeficiency virus (HIV)	**Endocrine/metabolic**
Obstructive sleep apnea	Leptospirosis	Addison's disease
Narcolepsy	Lyme disease	Hyper- and hypothyroidism
Periodic leg movements	Post-polio syndrome	Hyper- and hypocalcaemia
Miscellaneous	Q fever	Menopause
Alcohol or drug abuse	Toxoplasmosis	Vitamin B_{12} or D deficiency
Gulf war syndrome	Tuberculosis	**Gastrointestinal**
Lead, mercury, or other heavy	**Neuromuscular**	Celiac disease
metal poisoning	Multiple sclerosis	Inflammatory bowel diseases
Organophosphate pesticide	Myasthenia gravis	**Malignancy**
poisoning	Myopathies and neuropathies	Primary and secondary cancers
	Parkinson's disease	

and is not substantially alleviated by rest; (2) postexertional malaise; and (3) unrefreshing sleep. At least one of the two following manifestations is also required: (1) cognitive impairment; or (2) orthostatic intolerance. (See Table 178.1 for differential diagnoses.)

Some explanation of the terms used in the definition will help. Post-exertional malaise is a prolonged exacerbation of a patient's baseline symptoms after physical/cognitive/orthostatic exertion or stress. Unrefreshing sleep can be defined as feeling unrefreshed after sleeping for many hours. Cognitive impairments are problems with thinking exacerbated by exertion, effort, or stress. With orthostatic intolerance, symptoms worsen on assuming and maintaining an upright posture and are improved, although not necessarily abolished, by lying back down or elevating the feet.

Treatment

There is no cure for ME/CFS. Although there are therapies available to manage the symptoms, their efficacy is not yet known. The goal of treatment is to reduce symptoms and improve quality of life based on a collaborative therapeutic relationship. Although not all patients will improve, the potential for improvement, which ranges from modest to substantial, should be clearly communicated. Tricyclic antidepressants, cognitive behavioral therapy (CBT), and exercises are some of the treatment options. Alternative therapies such as herbal medications, massage, and acupuncture are very attractive to some patients, but their efficacy has not been tested in clinical trials.

Further reading

Carruthers BM, van de Sande MI, De Meirleir KL, *et al.* Myalgic encephalomyelitis: International consensus criteria. *J Intern Med* 2011;270(4):327–338.

Friedberg F, Bateman L, Bested AC, *et al. ME/CFS: A Primer for Clinical Practitioners.* Chicago, IL: International Association for Chronic Fatigue Syndrome/Myalgic Encephalomyelitis; 2012.

Institute of Medicine. *Beyond Myalgic Encephalomyelitis/Chronic Fatigue Syndrome: Redefining an Illness.* Washington, DC: National Academies Press; 2015.

Light AR, Bateman L, Jo D, *et al.* Gene expression alterations at baseline and following moderate exercise in patients with chronic fatigue syndrome and fibromyalgia syndrome. *J Intern Med* 2012;271(1):64–81.

Yoshiuchi K, Farkas J, Natelson BH. Patients with chronic fatigue syndrome have reduced absolute cortical blood flow. *Clin Physiol Funct Imaging* 2006;26(2):83–86.

179 Fibromyalgia

Saeed Bohlega and Hussam Abou Al-Shaar

Division of Neurology, Department of Neurosciences, King Faisal Specialist Hospital and Research Centre, and College of Medicine, Alfaisal University, Riyadh, Saudi Arabia

Fibromyalgia (FM) is a chronic heterogeneous condition characterized by widespread musculoskeletal pain and tenderness. It is one of the most frequent causes of non-articular rheumatism. It involves the muscles and soft tissue rather than joints. FM is one phenotype of a central sensitivity syndrome that encompasses a spectrum of clinical syndromes, including some not involving muscles or soft tissues. Therefore, it is not uncommon for FM patients to experience various symptoms such as non-restorative sleep disturbances, migraine headaches, irritable bowel, fatigue, diffuse pain, and cognitive dysfunction.

Epidemiology

FM is highly prevalent in rheumatology clinics, pain centers, general medicine, and family practice clinics. Its prevalence increases steadily with age. Patients usually present after their third decade of life. The global mean prevalence of FM is estimated to be 2.7%, ranging from 0.4% in Greece to 9.3% in Tunisia. Women are more commonly affected than men, with a mean global prevalence of 4.2% in women and 1.4% in men. The female-to-male ratio is 3:1. An incidence rate of 6.88 new cases per 1000 person-years for males and 11.28 new cases per 1000 person-years for females was reported in some studies. FM is more prevalent among people with a low educational level and socioeconomic status.

FM appears to coexist sometimes with other rheumatological disorders such as rheumatoid arthritis, osteoarthritis, and systemic lupus erythematosus. Head trauma and sleep apnea may increase the risk in men, while hypothyroidism and hyperprolactinemia are reported to increase the risk in women.

Pathogenesis

FM does not have a distinct cause or pathology; several mechanisms have been postulated to underline the diffuse lowering of nociceptive threshold. The presence of other centrally associated phenomena such as sleep disturbances and blunted stimulus response, as well as the diffuse nature of pain, suggest that a central mechanism may be involved.

Several other mechanisms have been postulated, including alteration of the brain concentration of regulatory neurotransmitters such as serotonin, endorphin, and substance P, trauma, psychological conditions, neuroendocrine and autonomic nervous system changes, infections, genetic familial factors, abnormal blood supply to muscles, and low level of insulin-like growth factor (IGF-1). The interplay between these factors leads to chronic central nervous system hyperexcitement, with the resultant central sensitization and intense widespread pain.

No microscopic, ultrastructural, biochemical, or metabolic abnormalities have been consistently demonstrated in muscle biopsy specimens from patients with FM. However, patients with fibromyalgia classically display "alpha-delta intrusion" on electroencephalography, which may explain the increased fatigue and pain in such patients.

Diagnosis

The American College of Rheumatology (ACR) first established classification criteria for the diagnosis of fibromyalgia in 1990, based on the presence of widespread pain for more than 3 months and at least 11 of 18 tender points. The same group introduced new preliminary diagnostic criteria in 2010, which did not require tender point examination. In 2011, the ACR group published a modification of the 2010 ACR criteria, which allowed individual self-reporting through a survey questionnaire in order to aid epidemiological and clinical studies (Table 179.1).

These criteria have a sensitivity of 96.6% and a specificity of 91.8%. The authors recently published the summed Widespread Pain Index and Symptom Severity Score, called the Polysymptomatic Distress Scale.

Clinical features

Approximately 50% of patients complain of pain that is "all over"; the pain is frequently associated with marked stiffness, especially postexertional, and sometimes lasts all day. Additional sources of pain are headache, sore throat, and eye or pelvic pain. Other notable features are often debilitating fatigue, joint swelling, disturbed sleep pattern, paresthesia of hands and feet, anxiety, panic attacks, and depression.

The presence of tender points according to the 1990 ACR-specified anatomic sites may aid in establishing the diagnosis. The tender points are widely distinctive and symmetric, but generally do not produce referred pain. However, it is important to note that 25% of patients diagnosed as having FM do not have 11 tender points.

Other physical findings include skin fold tenderness, reactive hyperemia, myofascial trigger points, and decreased pain threshold.

International Neurology, Second edition. Edited by Robert P. Lisak, Daniel D. Truong, William M. Carroll and Roongroj Bhidayasiri
© 2016 John Wiley & Sons, Ltd. Published 2016 by John Wiley & Sons, Ltd.

Table 179.1 Modified 2010 American College of Rheumatology (ACR) criteria for fibromyalgia. Source: Adapted from Wolfe 2010.

Criteria

A patient satisfies modified ACR 2010 fibromyalgia diagnostic criteria if the following three conditions are met:

(1) Widespread Pain Index ≥7 and Symptom Severity Score ≥5 or Widespread Pain Index between 3 and 6 and Symptom Severity Score ≥9.

(2) Symptoms have been present at a similar level for at least 3 months.

(3) The patient does not have a disorder that would otherwise sufficiently explain the pain.

Ascertainment

(1) Widespread Pain Index (WPI): Note the number of areas in which the patient has had pain over the last week. The score will be between 0 and 19.

Shoulder girdle, left	Hip (buttock, trochanter), left	Jaw, left	Upper back
Shoulder girdle, right	Hip (buttock, trochanter), right	Jaw, right	Lower back
Upper arm, Left	Upper leg, left	Chest	Neck
Upper arm, right	Upper leg, right	Abdomen	
Lower arm, left	Lower leg, left		
Lower arm, right	Lower leg, right		

(2) Symptom Severity Score: fatigue; waking unrefreshed; cognitive symptoms.
For each of these three symptoms, indicate the level of severity over the past week using the following scale: 0 = No problem; 1 = Slight or mild problems: generally mild or intermittent; 2 = Moderate: considerable problems, often present and/or at a moderate level; 3 = Severe: pervasive, continuous, life-disturbing problems.

The Symptom Severity Score is the sum of the severity of the three symptoms (fatigue, waking unrefreshed, and cognitive symptoms) plus the sum of the number of the following symptoms occurring during the previous 6 months: headaches, pain or cramps in lower abdomen, and depression (0–3). The final score is between 0 and 12.

Differential diagnosis

The differential diagnosis is broad and diverse (Table 179.2). Some of these conditions may also coexist with FM. Therefore, physicians should be aware of these conditions in order not to misdiagnose patients with FM.

Management

The reality of patients' symptoms must be acknowledged by the physician; the benign, non-deforming, and non-life-threatening nature of FM and the absence of infection should be emphasized.

A combination of pharmacological and non-pharmacological treatment is the basis for management of patients with fibromyalgia. There is a wide range of pharmacological agents available. However, the complexity of FM and the presence of multiple symptoms make the assessment of effective treatments with clinical trials very challenging.

Antidepressants, primarily tricyclics such as amitriptyline, clomipramine, and doxepin, are widely used and researched because they promote sleep and help depression, but they have a relatively narrow therapeutic index and their anticholinergic side effects (e.g., dry mouth, weight gain, and occasional daytime sedation) are limiting factors.

Selective serotonin reuptake inhibitors (SSRIs) have better tolerability than tricyclics and play an important role in improvement of mood and fatigue. However, they do not appear to be effective in relieving FM pain. The combination of fluoxetine and amitriptyline was shown to be more effective than either agent alone or placebo.

Serotonin-norepinephrine reuptake inhibitors (SNRIs), such as venlafaxine, milnacipran, and duloxetine, are effective in treating pain, fatigue, and sleep disturbances, with fewer side effects than tricyclics.

Many studies have shown that tramadol, a weak μ-opioid receptor agonist, is effective in the treatment of FM pain.

Table 179.2 Differential diagnosis of fibromyalgia.

Condition	Key features
Myofascial pain	Pressure on some axial or fascial points will evoke a transient twitch of the taut muscle band, with restricted range of motion. Pain can be alleviated by local injection into these tender points or by passively stretching the involved muscles.
Seronegative spondyloarthropathies	Subtle inflammatory findings, diffuse body and back pain, morning stiffness, and disturbed sleep.
Polymyalgia rheumatica	Usually seen in the elderly with pain and stiffness of the shoulder girdle and other associated symptoms, including general stiffness, weight loss, fatigue, and jaw and lingual claudication. Elevation of erythrocyte sedimentation rate (ESR) and a prompt response to low-dose glucocorticoid treatment.
Hypothyroidism	Substantial fatigue, myalgia, and malaise. Serum creatine kinase (CK) levels may be elevated.
Polymyositis	Proximal muscle weakness and elevation of serum CK levels.
Statin-related myopathy	Muscle weakness or pain or a combination of both. Serum CK levels are often elevated.
Inflammatory diseases (e.g., rheumatoid arthritis, systemic lupus erythematosus, Sjögren's syndrome)	Synovitis, multisystem abnormalities, sicca symptoms, or other systemic manifestations.
Vitamin D deficiency	Proximal muscle weakness and low vitamin D levels

Other opioids are generally not recommended because of concern about addictive potential. Muscle relaxants, sedatives, analgesics, and hypnotics have been shown to have positive results in open-label trials. Pregabalin and gabapentin, which have been approved by the US Food and Drug Administration for the management of fibromyalgia, inhibit the release of neurotransmitters associated with pain pathways like substance P. In addition, they are well tolerated and reduce many of the symptoms associated with FM.

It is important always to follow the "start low and go slow" dosing strategy in order to improve patient compliance, reduce complications, and optimize outcomes.

Aerobic exercises, stress-reduction techniques, and cognitive-behavioral therapy are among the main non-pharmacological modalities utilized in the management of such patients.

Other modalities that have been used with some reports of efficacy but with little scientific evidence include acupuncture, chiropractic therapy, balneotherapy, massage, passive and active manipulation of skeletal muscles, deep heat, ultrasound, and transcutaneous electrical nerve stimulation (TENS). Physical therapy is an important part of a patient's overall treatment and response should be used to measure progress.

Finally, the patient's psychological state and the impact of this painful condition should be addressed. Psychotherapy and relaxation therapies such as biofeedback, stress reduction, and behavioral modification will give patients significant help and satisfaction.

Further reading

Hawkins RA. Fibromyalgia: A clinical update. *J Am Osteopath Assoc* 2013;113(9): 680–689.

Jay GW, Barkin RL. Fibromyalgia. *Dis Mon* 2015;61(3):66–111.

Queiroz LP. Worldwide epidemiology of fibromyalgia. *Curr Pain Headache Rep* 2013;17(8):356.

Wolfe F, Clauw DJ, Fitzcharles MA, *et al.* The American College of Rheumatology preliminary diagnostic criteria for fibromyalgia and measurement of symptom severity. *Arthritis Care Res* 2010;62(5):600–610.

Wolfe F, Clauw DJ, Fitzcharles MA, *et al.* Fibromyalgia criteria and severity scales for clinical and epidemiological studies: A modification of the ACR preliminary diagnostic criteria for fibromyalgia. *J Rheumatol* 2011;38(6):1113–1122.

Index

Illustrations are comprehensively referred to from the text. Therefore, significant items in illustrations (figures and tables) have only been given a page reference in the absence of their concomitant mention in the text referring to that illustration. 'vs' indicated a differential diagnosis.

International Neurology, Second edition. Edited by Robert P. Lisak, Daniel D. Truong, William M. Carroll and Roongroj Bhidayasiri
© 2016 John Wiley & Sons, Ltd. Published 2016 by John Wiley & Sons, Ltd.